NMS
Medicine
5th edition

NMS Medicine

5th Edition

Editor

Allen R. Myers, MD
Professor of Medicine
Section of Rheumatology
Department of Medicine
Temple University School of Medicine
Philadelphia, Pennsylvania

LIPPINCOTT WILLIAMS & WILKINS
A **Wolters Kluwer** Company
Philadelphia • Baltimore • New York • London
Buenos Aires • Hong Kong • Sydney • Tokyo

Editor: Donna Balado
Managing Editor: Emilie Linkins
Marketing Manager: Scott Lavine
Production Editor: Caroline Define
Designer: Doug Smock
Compositor: Circle Graphics
Printer: Data Reproductions Corp.

351 West Camden Street
Baltimore, Maryland 21201-2436 USA

530 Walnut Street
Philadelphia, Pennsylvania 19106

Printed in the United States of America

Library of Congress Cataloging-in-Publication Data

Medicine / [edited by] Allen R. Myers.—5th ed.
p. ; cm.—(The National medical series for independent study)
Includes index.
ISBN 0-7817-5468-2
1. Internal medicine—Outlines, syllabi, etc. 2. Internal medicine—Examinations, questions, etc. I. Myers, Allen R. II. Series
[DNLM: 1. Internal Medicine—Examination Questions. 2. Internal Medicine—Outlines.
WB 18.2 M489 2004]
RC59.M44 2004
616—dc22

2004048302

To purchase additional copies of this book, call our customer service department at **(800) 638-3030** or fax orders to **(301) 824-7390.** For other book services, including chapter reprints and large quantity sales, ask for the Special Sales department.

For all other calls originating outside of the United States, please call **(301) 714-2324.**

***Visit Lippincott Williams & Wilkins on the Internet:* http://www.lww.com.** Lippincott Williams & Wilkins customer service representatives are available from 8:30 am to 6:00 pm, EST, Monday through Friday, for telephone access.

04 05 06 07 08
1 2 3 4 5 6 7 8 9 10

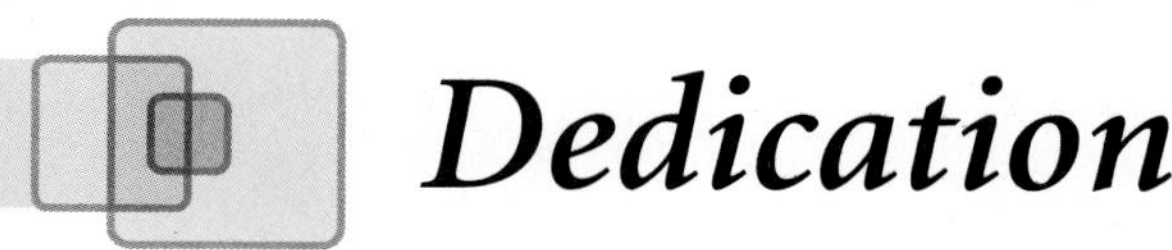

Dedication

To Rosina and Ellis Myers, for having the foresight to point me in the right direction, one of lasting interest and continuing pleasure.

To Ellen, for journeying with me and being a superb partner.

To David, Rob and Scott, for their inspiration and understanding.

To Alexandra, Haley, Camryn, and Spencer, for bringing incredible joy into my life.

To Doris and Nathan Patz, for their strong encouragement to pursue my goals.

To my teachers, for stimulating my interest, sharing their knowledge, and being excellent role models.

To the legions of hardworking and inquisitive medical students and residents who constantly seek knowledge in their quest for clinical excellence.

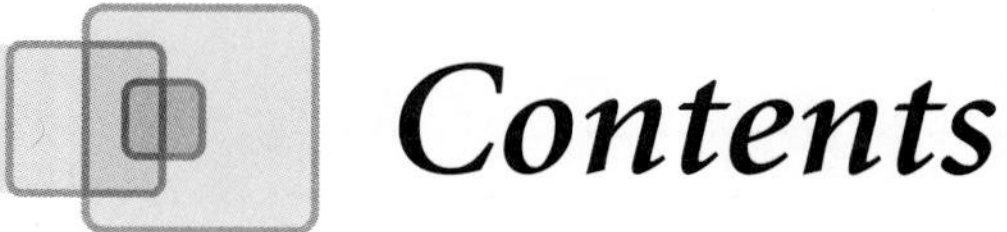

Contents

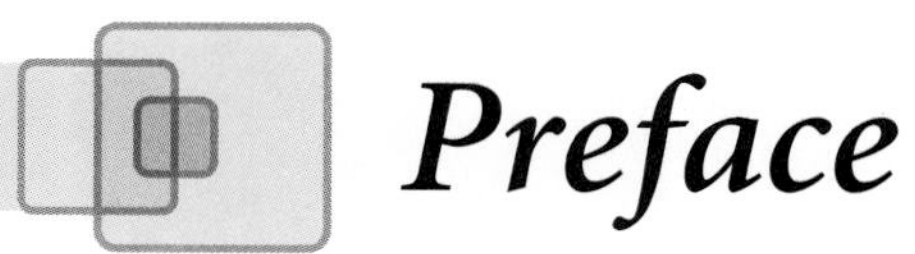

Preface

The easiest and surest way of acquiring facts is to learn them in groups, in systems, and systematized knowledge is science. You can very often carry two facts fastened together more easily than one by itself. . . .
—Oliver Wendell Holmes, "Scholastic and Bedside Teaching" from *Medical Essays*

In the natural method of teaching, the student begins with the patient, continues with the patient, and ends his studies with the patient, using books and lectures as tools, as means to an end.
—William Osler, 1901

Internal medicine is a vast and complicated field that is based upon strong scientific and clinical foundations. While certain pedagogical learning is unavoidable, an understanding of basic sciences, particularly pathophysiology, allows some meaning to be made of seemingly unrelated facts.

Any effort to provide a comprehensive review of internal medicine is destined to fall short of its goal. Despite this limitation, the authors have provided a framework for a working knowledge of internal medicine. It is not all-inclusive but nonetheless provides the essentials of the subject in an easily read and well-organized format. By necessity, NMS *Medicine* must be used as a companion to more extensive texts and monographs, but it can be considered a starting point. Internal medicine cannot be fully learned in a year or two, or in a lifetime, but its essence can be appreciated by students and house officers.

Medicine has been written primarily for students and residents. However, the authors believe it also can be used by all others who deal with patients who have medical illnesses.

This fifth edition has been extensively updated. The study questions with explanations have been carefully revised and, as an aid to learning and preparing for the new computer-based USMLE Step 2, are provided in both print and electronic format. The section on problem-solving exercises has been expanded in order to help the student develop clinical reasoning skills. A chapter on Dermatologic Disorders has been added with a companion CD-ROM containing images of the major dermatologic lesions. The CD will also include some materials from other chapters as well as the Comprehensive Examination. A chapter on dermatologic disorders (Chapter 12) has been added. The companion CD-ROM contains color images of the major dermatologic lesions as well as of hematologic diseases (Chapter 3) and infectious diseases (Chapter 8) along with study questions and the comprehensive examination. The result of our efforts is a "user-friendly" review of internal medicine that enhances the educational process.

Allen R. Myers

Acknowledgments

The editor and contributing authors are grateful to Lippincott Williams & Wilkins for their support of this endeavor. Particular thanks go to Emilie Linkins for her patience, dedication, and extraordinary hard work and to Neil Marquardt, senior acquisitions editor.

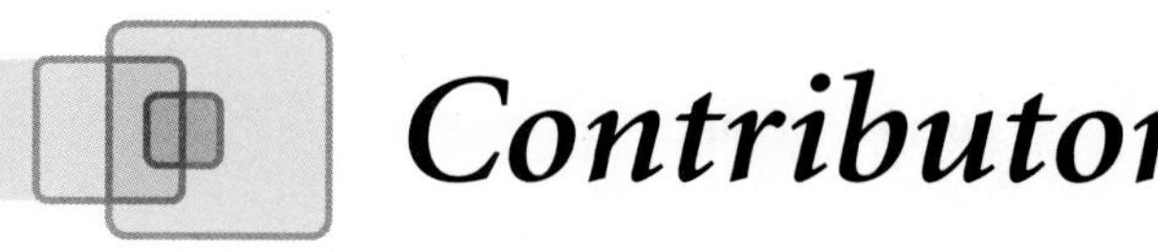

Contributors

E. Victor Adlin, MD
Associate Professor of Medicine Emeritus
Endocrinology and Metabolism Section
Department of Medicine
Temple University School of Medicine
Attending Physician
Temple University Hospital
Philadelphia, Pennsylvania

Jack M. Becker, MD
Associate Professor of Pediatrics
Drexel University College of Medicine
Chief, Section of Allergy
Saint Christopher's Hospital for Children
Philadelphia, Pennsylvania

Hossein Borghaei, DO, MS
Assistant Member
Department of Medical Oncology
Fox Chase Cancer Center
Philadelphia, Pennsylvania

Blase A. Carabello, MD
Professor of Medicine
Baylor College of Medicine
Chief, Department of Medicine
Houston Veterans Affairs Medical Center
Houston, Texas

Gerard J. Criner, MD
Professor of Medicine
Director, Pulmonary and Critical Care Medicine
Temple University School of Medicine
Philadelphia, Pennsylvania

Anthony J. DiMarino, Jr., MD
William Rorer Professor of Medicine
Thomas Jefferson Medical College
Chief, Division of Gastroenterology
Thomas Jefferson University Hospital
Philadelphia, Pennsylvania

Thomas Fekete, MD
Professor of Medicine
Infectious Diseases Section
Department of Medicine
Temple University School of Medicine
Attending Physician
Temple University Hospital
Philadelphia, Pennsylvania

Stanley Goldfarb, MD
Associate Dean for Clinical Education
University of Pennsylvania School of Medicine
Philadelphia, Pennsylvania

Donald P. Goldsmith, MD
Professor of Pediatrics
Drexel University College of Medicine
Chief, Section of Rheumatology
St. Christopher's Hospital for Children
Philadelphia, Pennsylvania

S. Christine Kovacs, MD, MPH
Division of Rheumatology
Lahey Clinic
Burlington, Massachusetts

Stuart R. Lessin, MD
Senior Member and Director of Dermatology
Fox Chase Cancer Center
Professor of Medicine (Dermatology)
Chief, Division of Dermatology
Department of Medicine
Temple University School of Medicine
Philadelphia, Pennsylvania

Allen R. Myers, MD
Professor of Medicine
Section of Rheumatology
Department of Medicine
Temple University School of Medicine
Philadelphia, Pennsylvania

Ronald N. Rubin, MD
Professor of Medicine
Section of Hematology
Department of Medicine
Temple University School of Medicine
Chief, Clinical Hematology
Temple University Hospital
Philadelphia, Pennsylvania

Barney J. Stern, MD
Professor of Neurology
Department of Neurology
University of Maryland School of Medicine
Baltimore, Maryland

Louis M. Weiner, MD
Professor of Medicine
Temple University School of Medicine
Chairman, Department of Medical Oncology
Senior Member, Division of Medical Science
Fox Chase Cancer Center
Philadelphia, Pennsylvania

Fuad N. Ziyadeh, MD
Professor of Medicine
Division of Renal, Electrolyte, and Hypertension
Department of Medicine
University of Pennsylvania School of Medicine
Attending Physician
Hospital of the University of Pennsylvania
Veterans Affairs Medical Center
Philadelphia, Pennsylvania

chapter **1**

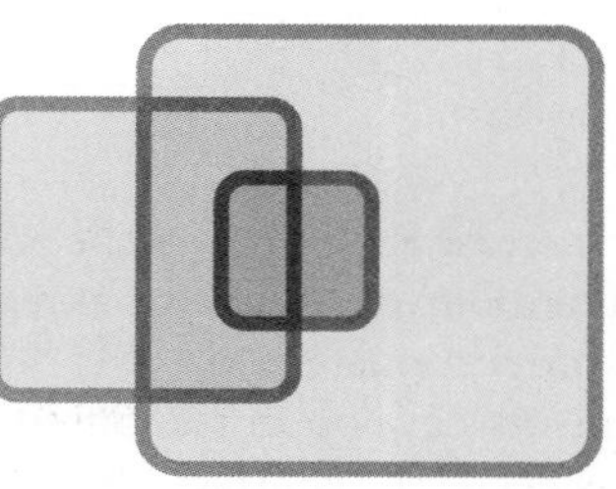

Cardiovascular Diseases

BLASE A. CARABELLO

I CONGESTIVE HEART FAILURE (CHF)

A Definition CHF is the inability of the heart, working at normal or elevated filling pressure, to pump enough blood to meet the oxygen requirements of the body tissues. CHF should never be considered a diagnosis. Rather, it is a syndrome resulting from many diseases that interfere with cardiac function. In acting as a muscular pump, the heart does only two things: it contracts (systole) and it relaxes (diastole). Therefore, heart failure can result from only two broad abnormalities—systolic dysfunction and diastolic dysfunction.

B Etiology

1. **Systolic dysfunction.** Systole is governed by three cardiac properties, **contractility**—the ability of myocardium to generate force, **afterload**—the force against which the heart must contract, and preload—the sarcomere stretch before contraction.
   a. **Decreased contractility.** Most cases of CHF occur when an insult to the myocardium reduces its ability to generate force, thus reducing its contractility.
      (1) **Myocardial infarction (MI).** In MI, a portion of the myocardium undergoes necrosis and can no longer generate force, resulting in weakening of the ventricle. If extensive areas of the myocardium are infarcted, CHF results.
      (2) **Valvular heart disease** results in stenosis or regurgitation of the cardiac valves, which places a **pressure** or **volume overload,** respectively, on the ventricles. Initially, compensatory mechanisms [see I B 1 c] accommodate these overloads and maintain normal cardiac output at acceptable filling pressures. However, eventually these mechanisms fail, and heart failure ensues.
      (3) **Hypertension.** Many patients who develop CHF have had systemic hypertension at some time in the clinical course of their illness. **Persistent severe hypertension** is associated with a **contractile deficit** that leads to CHF. Today, hypertension is more likely to cause diastolic rather than systolic dysfunction, however (I B 2 b).
      (4) **Cardiomyopathies** are diseases that directly injure the myocardium.
         (a) **Toxic.** Substances directly toxic to the myocardium (e.g., ethanol, catecholamines) may damage its force-generating ability. Prolonged exposure to these agents may lead to the development of CHF.
         (b) **Idiopathic.** When the contractile function of the myocardium fails in the absence of a known etiology, a viral cause often is implied but frequently cannot be proven.
         (c) **Infiltrative.** Infiltration of the myocardium by a variety of substances (e.g., amyloid) may reduce contractility.
   b. **Increased afterload.** Increasing the afterload makes it harder for the ventricular muscle fibers to shorten, reducing cardiac output. Afterload can be quantified by calculating the systolic force on the myocardium using the Laplace equation for stress:

$$Stress = (pressure \times radius)/(2 \times thickness)$$

Thus, disease states that increase either the systolic pressure (hypertension, aortic stenosis) or chamber radius (dilated cardiomyopathy, valvular regurgitation) increase afterload unless the wall thickness increases proportionately.

c. **Compensatory mechanisms** develop in response to the ventricular pressure and volume overload that accompany decreased contractility.

(1) The **Frank-Starling mechanism** is activated when reduced ventricular emptying results in more volume retained in the ventricles at the end of systole, which leads to a greater volume at the end of diastole. Increased end-diastolic volume increases sarcomere stretch (preload), which increases the number of systolic actin–myosin cross-bridges that develop. The greater number of cross-bridges increases the strength of contraction.

(2) **Cardiac hypertrophy** provides additional muscle mass to bear the burden of various overloads.

(3) **Adrenergic stimulation** by endogenous catecholamines increases the inotropic state.

2. **Diastolic dysfunction.** Diastole is governed by **active** and **passive** properties. Active relaxation occurs early in diastole as calcium is pumped out of the myocardium, resulting in the near cessation of actin–myosin cross-bridge interaction. Passive filling occurs as the mitral valve opens, allowing the blood stored in the atria to fill the ventricles.

a. **Abnormalities in active relaxation.** Active relaxation is impaired when there is delay in calcium reuptake at the beginning of diastole. Myocardial ischemia and ventricular hypertrophy are two common causes of impaired active relaxation.

b. **Abnormalities of passive filling.** Passive relaxation is impaired when the myocardium is stiffer than normal. Stiffness is defined as a change in pressure (ΔP) per unit change in volume (ΔV), or $\Delta P/\Delta V$. When stiffness is increased, any change in volume requires or causes a greater increase in pressure. Thus, to fill the heart to an adequate volume, high filling pressure occurs, which in turn leads to pulmonary and systemic congestion. Increased passive stiffness of the ventricles occurs when concentric hypertrophy causes the chamber wall to be thicker than normal as might occur in hypertension or when the myocardium is infiltrated by abnormal substances such as amyloid.

C Descriptive terminology

1. **High-output failure** is characterized by cardiac output that may be several times higher than normal but still is not adequate to maintain tissue perfusion needs or, if adequate, is maintained with a higher-than-normal filling pressure. A classic example of high-output failure is **chronic severe anemia,** which causes reduced oxygen-carrying capacity. In chronic severe anemia, the following occurs:

a. Compensation is provided by increased forward cardiac output, which is facilitated by cardiac enlargement, decreased total peripheral resistance, and increased venous return to the heart. This causes a volume overload of ventricles.

b. Eventually, the demands on the heart lead to cardiac failure; cardiac output, although high, still is not adequate to meet the circulatory demands placed on the heart by the anemia. Some other causes of high-output failure include arteriovenous fistula, beriberi, and thyrotoxicosis.

2. **Left-sided failure** indicates that the left ventricle is the failing chamber. A disease that primarily affects the left ventricle (e.g., MI) may reduce its contractile force, while the right ventricle continues to pump normally. Thus, left ventricular failure can occur without right ventricular failure.

3. **Right-sided failure** indicates that the right ventricle has failed, either as a result of left ventricular failure or in isolation from the left ventricle.

a. The **most common cause** of right ventricular failure is **left ventricular failure.** When left ventricular failure occurs, the filling pressure in the left ventricle becomes elevated, increasing the workload of the right ventricle (the chamber responsible for filling the left ventricle). Thus overtaxed, the right ventricle eventually fails also.

b. The right ventricle also may fail in isolation from the left ventricle. In the presence of **chronic obstructive pulmonary disease (COPD),** increased pulmonary vascular resistance develops as a result of architectural changes in the lungs. The higher pulmonary vascular resistance produces a pressure overload on the right ventricle, which leads to increased right ventricular work and eventual failure. Pulmonary embolism and primary pulmonary hypertension are some other causes of right-sided failure.

D Clinical features

1. **Symptoms**
   a. **Dyspnea** is the most frequently encountered symptom of CHF.
      (1) The feeling of breathlessness is caused by **vascular congestion,** which reduces pulmonary oxygenation. In addition, the vascular congestion diminishes lung compliance, increasing the work of breathing, thus adding to the feeling of breathlessness.
      (2) Dyspnea also results from **reduced cardiac output to the periphery,** which triggers the symptom through neurohumoral mechanisms. In the early stages of CHF, dyspnea occurs only with exertion. As heart failure progresses, the amount of exertion required to produce dyspnea becomes progressively less until dyspnea may occur at rest.
   b. **Orthopnea** refers to dyspnea that occurs in the recumbent position and is relieved by elevation of the head. Orthopnea results from volume pooling in the central vasculature during recumbency, which leads to increased cardiac volume and, in turn, to increased left ventricular filling pressure, pulmonary congestion, and the feeling of dyspnea. The physician may gauge the degree of orthopnea by noting the number of pillows the patient uses to sleep. However, it should be recognized that many patients sleep on more than one pillow out of habit, not because of breathlessness. **Nocturnal cough,** which has the same pathophysiology as orthopnea, may occur together with, or instead of, nocturnal dyspnea.
   c. **Paroxysmal nocturnal dyspnea** is the occurrence of sudden dyspnea that awakens the patient from sleep. Like orthopnea, it occurs during recumbency as a result of pooling in the central vasculature, which increases left ventricular filling pressure. Paroxysmal nocturnal dyspnea may occur in the orthopneic patient who inadvertently slips off the pillows used to elevate the upper body. Usually, the patient awakens from sleep and feels the need to sit upright or to go to an open window for increased ventilation. The symptom usually subsides after the patient has been in the upright position for 5–20 minutes.
   d. **Nocturia** develops in CHF as a result of increased renal blood flow when the patient is recumbent and asleep.
      (1) **During the day,** when the skeletal muscles are active, limited cardiac output is shifted away from the kidney toward the skeletal musculature. The kidney interprets this reduction in blood flow as **hypovolemia** and becomes sodium avid via activation of the **renin–angiotensin system.**
      (2) **At night,** when the patient is at rest, cardiac output is shifted toward the kidney, and diuresis ensues.
   e. **Edema.** There are many causes of peripheral edema, several of which are noncardiac. **Cardiac edema** occurs when the systemic hydrostatic venous pressure is greater than the systemic oncotic venous pressure. Thus, cardiac edema is a sign of **right-sided failure;** it occurs because of the increased systemic venous pressure that results from right ventricular dysfunction.
   f. **Anorexia** may occur as a late manifestation of CHF. The exact mechanism leading to anorexia is unknown, but the occurrence of anorexia seems to correlate with hepatic congestion and right-sided failure.
2. **Physical signs**
   a. **Tachycardia.** Increased heart rate occurs in heart failure due to increased release of catecholamines as a compensatory mechanism for maintaining cardiac output in the presence of decreased stroke volume. Catecholamines increase both the force and the rate of cardiac

contraction. However, note that in chronic heart failure adrenergic down-regulation occurs, so heart rates over 100 bpm in the absence of arrhythmia are distinctly unusual. Therefore, when tachycardia does exist in the patient with chronic CHF, arrhythmia should be ruled out.

b. **Pulmonary rales.** The increased left ventricular filling pressure associated with CHF is referred to the left atrium and pulmonary veins. The increased hydrostatic pressure produces transudation of fluid into the alveoli. As air circulates through the alveoli, cracking sounds (rales) are produced. Note that there are multiple causes of pulmonary rales; the mere presence of rales does not necessarily indicate CHF.

c. **Cardiac enlargement.** As the failing heart relies more and more on the Frank-Starling mechanism, it dilates and may develop eccentric hypertrophy. In the presence of cardiac enlargement, the point of maximal impulse (PMI) of the left ventricle is shifted downward and to the left. This shift is detected during a physical examination. Although much of the cardiac examination should be performed with the patient in the left lateral decubitus position, this position may artifactually shift the PMI. Thus, the PMI should be established with the patient lying supine.

d. **Fourth heart sound (S_4).** Patients in sinus rhythm and heart failure often have an S_4 (atrial gallop). The S_4 is produced as left atrial systole propels volume into the left ventricle just before ventricular systole. In CHF, the left ventricle is noncompliant and the S_4 probably results from the reverberation of the blood ejected from the left atrium into the left ventricle. In elderly patients, however, an S_4 may indicate reduced compliance of a stiff left ventricle as a result of aging rather than heart failure. The S_4 also may be heard over the right ventricle in right ventricular failure.

e. **Third heart sound (S_3).** An S_3 **(ventricular gallop),** which occurs early in diastole, probably is the single most **reliable sign of left heart failure** revealed during physical examination. The S_3 occurs during rapid filling of the left ventricle. Increased left atrial pressure (which propels the blood forward with increased force) and noncompliance of the left ventricle are two important factors in the production of this extra sound. Although an S_3 is a reliable sign of heart failure in individuals over the age of 40 years a similar sound is a normal finding in young, healthy athletes.

f. **Neck vein distention.** The neck veins can be considered manometers attached to the right atrium and, as such, reflect right atrial pressure.

   (1) When the right ventricle fails, it relies increasingly on the Frank-Starling mechanism for compensation. This results in increased right ventricular volume and pressure, which is referred back to the right atrium.

   (2) To estimate central venous pressure in cm H_2O, the patient's back is elevated or lowered so the point demarcating the distended from the nondistended portion of the neck vein can be discerned clearly. The vertical height is measured from this point to the manubrium. The average depth of the right atrium inside the chest cavity (5 cm) is added to the height of the neck vein. This sum approximates the right atrial pressure.

g. **Hepatic enlargement.** Elevated central venous pressure can lead to hepatic congestion, in turn causing hepatomegaly. On occasion, rapid hepatic enlargement may also cause liver tenderness.

h. **Edema.** Lower extremity and presacral edema occur in right-sided failure as increased venous pressure results in transudation of fluid into these areas. For edema to be attributable to CHF, distended neck veins indicative of elevated right-sided filling pressure also should be present.

i. **Ascites.** Transudation of fluid into the **peritoneal space** also may occur as a result of increased systemic venous pressure. When ascites is caused by CHF, the neck veins typically are elevated, and the liver is distended from passive congestion.

E Diagnosis

1. **Etiologic approach.** Because CHF is a syndrome that results from a disease, the management of CHF must focus on the cause of the heart failure, not simply on relieving the symptoms. Although a careful history and physical examination are the most important tools available in

arriving at a diagnosis, in many cases a diagnosis may not be reached. In these instances, the following studies often are helpful:

a. The **electrocardiogram (ECG)** frequently is nonspecific. However, the presence of Q waves helps confirm that MI has been the cause of the CHF.

b. The **chest radiograph** is useful in demonstrating cardiac chamber enlargement and in documenting congestion in the lungs. It provides objective evidence that heart failure is present.

c. The **echocardiogram** is essential in identifying chamber enlargement and in quantifying left ventricular function and valvular function. The most commonly used descriptor of ventricular function is the **ejection fraction,** which is the percentage of the end-diastolic volume expelled during systole. For example, if a patient's end-diastolic volume is 150 mL and the stroke volume is 100 mL, then 67% (100/150) of the diastolic contents was ejected.

   (1) The end-diastolic and stroke volumes can be estimated from the echocardiogram.

   (2) Ejection fractions between 55% and 76% are normal.

d. **Doppler interrogation** measures the direction and velocity of blood flow through the cardiac chambers and great vessels. This technique is useful for detecting blood flow moving in an abnormal direction, which is characteristic of valvular regurgitation and intracardiac shunts. In addition, Doppler interrogation can detect and quantify valvular stenoses by measuring how much velocity is necessary to maintain constant blood flow through a stenotic valve.

e. **Radionuclide ventriculography** is used to measure right and left ventricular ejection fraction. It is an excellent noninvasive procedure to use when quantifying precisely the degree of systolic cardiac dysfunction is necessary.

f. During **cardiac catheterization,** intracardiac pressures, chamber size, valvular stenosis, valvular regurgitation, and coronary anatomy can be evaluated. Cardiac catheterization remains the gold standard for assessing coronary anatomy. However, assessment of valve and chamber function has largely been supplanted by echocardiography because, unlike the noninvasive tests mentioned earlier, catheterization has a small but finite risk, and echocardiography has become extremely accurate. Therefore, cardiac catheterization is performed in patients with CHF when the additional information the procedure provides is necessary for proper patient management. For example, cardiac catheterization may be necessary to help determine whether valve replacement will correct heart failure in a patient with valvular heart disease when the noninvasive data conflict with the clinical impression of the diagnosis.

2. **Symptomatic approach.** In cases in which the definitive cause is not thought to be important in the management of CHF (e.g., a patient with terminal cancer), some objective evidence of cardiac dysfunction is still advisable before therapy. Frequently, a patient with dyspnea on exertion and orthopnea is treated for CHF, but the symptoms have another cause. The chest radiograph and echocardiogram are useful adjuncts to the physical examination in providing objective evidence of cardiac dysfunction before therapy and also for gauging the effects of treatment.

F Therapy

1. **Etiologic therapy.** It is important, when possible, to direct treatment at the etiologic agent of the CHF. For example, if aortic stenosis is the cause, aortic valve replacement is the most effective therapy.

2. **Symptomatic therapy.** If the etiologic agent cannot be found, if the patient's condition does not permit direct intervention, or if the patient refuses to consider corrective surgery even if indicated, the physician must resort to therapy aimed at relieving the symptoms of heart failure.

   a. **Systolic dysfunction**

      (1) **Increasing the contractile state.** Contractile dysfunction is the most common mechanism that produces heart failure; therefore, increasing the contractile state may result in symptomatic improvement.

         (a) **Cardiac glycosides** (e.g., **digoxin**) increase the contractile state by impeding the Na^+-K^+-ATPase–controlled intracellular pump. This results in the net influx of calcium into the myocardium, which increases contractile strength. The efficacy of cardiac glycosides in the chronic treatment of CHF has been the subject of controversy. However, it now seems clear that digitalis can reduce symptoms and the need for hospitalization. Digitalis does not affect mortality.

(b) **β-Adrenergic agonists** (e.g., **catecholamines**) increase contractile function by increasing the production of cyclic adenosine monophosphate (cAMP), which results in greater myocardial calcium release. In end-stage heart failure, intravenous infusion of dobutamine for several days may help restore and maintain pump performance even after the infusion is discontinued. The mechanism by which the positive effect persists after the therapy is stopped is not well understood.

(c) **Phosphodiesterase inhibitors** increase contractile function by inhibiting the breakdown of cAMP. The most commonly used cardiac-specific phosphodiesterase inhibitor is **milrinone.** These agents act to enhance the inotropic state and reduce afterload by causing vasodilation. Currently, they are administered by intravenous infusion and are for short-term use only.

(2) **Reducing afterload.** Agents that cause arteriolar dilation reduce impedance of the outflow of blood from the left ventricle. By diminishing resistance to ejection, these agents cause cardiac output to rise because the left ventricle can eject more completely against a lower afterload. The net effect is increased cardiac output without a serious fall in blood pressure, leading to symptomatic improvement.

(a) **Several vasodilators** are used in the treatment of CHF to reduce afterload, including **angiotensin-converting enzyme** (ACE) **inhibitors** (e.g., **captopril, enalapril, lisinopril), nitrates,** and **hydralazine.**

(3) **Reducing preload and left ventricular filling pressure.** The increased preload resulting from volume retention in the ventricles is a compensatory mechanism that helps increase forward cardiac output by use of the Frank-Starling mechanism; however, an excessive increase in preload is associated with an increase in left ventricular and right ventricular filling pressures, which is responsible for symptoms of pulmonary and systemic congestion. Judicious reduction in filling pressures without excessive reduction in preload is indicated in the therapy of CHF.

(a) **Diuretics** reduce renal tubular absorption of sodium and water and increase the clearance of these substances from the body. The result is a reduction in central volume and in cardiac filling pressure.

(b) **Vasodilators,** which increase the capacity of the systemic venous system, transfer central volume to the periphery, thus reducing central preload and filling pressure. The nitrates and ACE inhibitors are effective as preload-reducing vasodilators.

(4) **The neurohumoral hypothesis of heart failure: systems blockade.** Heart failure leads to the persistent activation of many neurohumoral systems and hormones, including the renin-angiotensin-aldosterone system, the adrenergic nervous system, inflammatory cytokines, endothelin, vasopressin, and many more. Although once thought of as compensatory, persistent overactivation of these agents is cardiotoxic, in turn leading to a progressive decline in cardiac function. Thus, blockade of these systems should be beneficial in treating CHF.

(a) **Renin-angiotensin system blockade.** The combination of an ACE inhibitor and diuretics has been shown to reduce mortality associated with CHF and to extend life by 6 months to 1 year. Because many vasodilators have failed to improve survival despite reducing afterload, properties of ACE inhibitors other than vasodilation are thought to be operative. Blocking the overactivity of the renin-angiotensin system is probably beneficial. In patients who develop coughing due to ACE inhibitors, **angiotensin receptor blockers** (losartan, candesartan, etc.) may be substituted. Additional blockade of the renin-angiotensin system, using **spironolactone** to block the final product of this system, aldosterone, adds additional benefit. Indeed, the observation that blockade of the renin-angiotensin system enhanced prognosis led to the neurohumoral hypothesis.

(b) **Use of β-blocking agents.** Because stimulation of the β-receptor increases the force of cardiac contraction, β-agonists have been used in the therapy of CHF [see I F 2 a (2) (b)]. Paradoxically, cautious use of β-receptor antagonists has also been effective in reversing the same syndrome. The mechanism of action for this class of agents in the treatment of heart failure probably stems from protection of the heart from the toxic effects of prolonged exposure to the high levels of circulating catecholamines.

(5) **Cardiac resynchronization.** Many patients with advanced heart failure develop electrical conduction disturbances, including left bundle branch block, which delays the impulse signaling contraction from getting to the left ventricle. This delay discoordinates contraction, in turn causing a further reduction in cardiac output. Recent studies have shown that inserting a pacemaker to resynchronize contraction improves both hemodynamics and symptoms.

(6) **Physical conditioning.** An important adjunct to the medical treatment of CHF, physical conditioning permits the peripheral tissues to use cardiac output more efficiently. Thus, the patient experiences an increase in tolerance to physical activity without an increase in cardiac output.

(7) **Cardiac transplantation** may offer an improved quality of life to selected patients in whom control of CHF is not possible and prognosis is poor. The increasingly effective use of the immunosuppressive agents cyclosporine and tacrolimus injection (Prograf) have greatly increased the success of this therapy. Currently, approximately 75% of patients undergoing cardiac transplantation achieve a 5-year survival rate. The paucity of cardiac donors is the primary factor limiting the use of this therapy. Left ventricular assist devices (LVADs) may provide a bridge to transplantation.

b. Pulmonary edema. Pulmonary edema is the most extreme example of CHF, in which profound transudation of fluid into the pulmonary alveoli occurs because of a high left ventricular filling pressure. The result is impaired oxygenation and, if untreated, death. The goal of therapy is to improve oxygenation, to reduce left ventricular filling pressure, and to increase forward cardiac output.

(1) **Oxygen.** A mainstay in the treatment of acute pulmonary edema, oxygen should be administered by facemask, because patients in pulmonary edema are so dyspneic that they breathe primarily through their mouths.

(2) **Diuretics. Furosemide** probably is the single most commonly used medication in the treatment of acute pulmonary edema. This rapid-acting loop diuretic promotes an immediate diuresis in most cases.

(3) **Morphine sulfate.** This opioid reduces patient anxiety, which may help relieve the arterial vasoconstriction often present in acute pulmonary edema. This, in turn, helps increase forward cardiac output. Morphine also is a venodilator; therefore, it reduces central volume and left ventricular filling pressure.

(4) **Other vasodilators. Nitroglycerine** (administered sublingually or intravenously) or **nitroprusside** (administered intravenously) often is effective in treating pulmonary edema when other therapies fail. Recently nesiritide, an analog of B-type naturetic hormone that causes veno and arteriolar vasodilation, has been approved for the acute intravenous therapy of CHF. These drugs reduce central volume by venodilation and also increase cardiac output secondary to arteriolar vasodilation. However, the potent vasodilating ability of these drugs requires that blood pressure be monitored constantly during administration to avoid hypotension.

(5) **Intubation and positive-pressure ventilation.** If the patient's oxygenation does not improve rapidly with the above therapies, intubation may be necessary to provide mechanical ventilation and improve oxygenation.

(6) **Invasive hemodynamic monitoring.** Most cases of pulmonary edema resolve quickly, making invasive hemodynamic unnecessary. However, in cases of recalcitrant pulmonary edema with severe cardiac compromise, exact knowledge of intracardiac filling pressure may be useful in guiding therapy. Hemodynamic monitoring (via Swan-Ganz catheterization) provides this information so that optimal filling pressure and cardiac output may be obtained.

c. **Diastolic heart failure**

(1) **Physiology** (Figure 1–1). Increased wall stiffness results in a higher filling pressure for any specific filling volume (curve B). The ultimate goal is to return the patient's ventricle to the normal state (curve A), but this cannot be accomplished acutely. For example, if hypertension has led to ventricular hypertrophy, which in turn has increased ventricular stiffness, treatment of the hypertension may result in regression of hypertrophy but only over months or years. In the meantime, the therapies available treat the symptoms but do not actually improve the pressure–volume relationship of the ventricle.

(2) **Diuretics.** Diuretics are the mainstay of therapy. By reducing ventricular volume, they lower ventricular pressure and reduce the symptoms of congestion. However, reduced ventricular volume also lowers stroke volume and cardiac output. Therefore, diuretics must be used with caution.

(3) **Introduction of bradycardia.** Slowing the heart rate increases the time available for ventricular filling. β-Blockers and rate-responsive calcium channel blockers (verapamil and diltiazem) are used to cause relative bradycardia.

(4) **Relief of ischemia.** In patients with coronary disease, ischemia impairs the active relaxation phase of diastole by impairing calcium reuptake by the sarcoplasmic reticulum. Thus, standard therapy for angina is also effective in improving diastolic function [see III A 5 a (4)].

(5) **Maintenance of sinus rhythm.** The normal atrial "kick" afforded by atrial contraction improves the efficiency of ventricular filling that is lost in atrial fibrillation. Thus, every effort should be made to maintain sinus rhythm (see II).

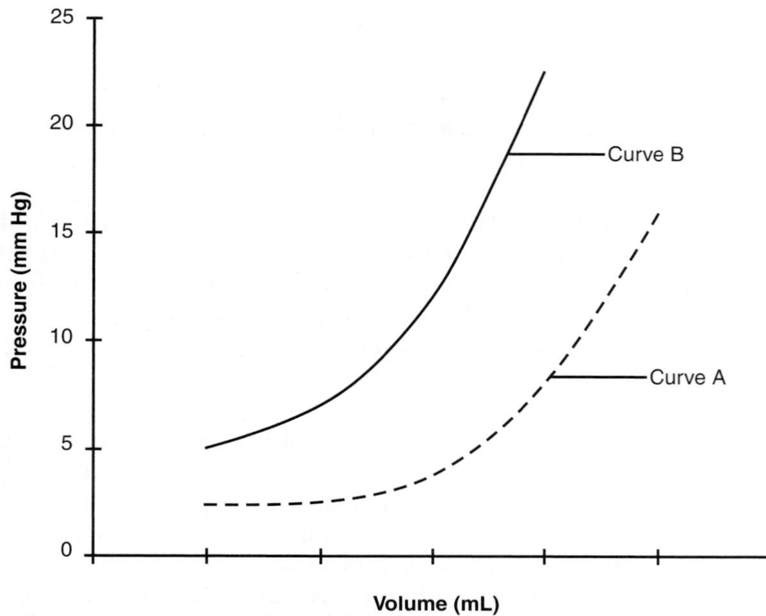

FIGURE 1–1 The diastolic left ventricular pressure–volume relationships for a normal subject (*curve A*) and a patient with diastolic dysfunction (*curve B*). In curve B, the filling pressure is higher at any filling volume.

II CARDIAC ARRHYTHMIAS

A Introduction Bradyarrhythmias result from inadequate sinus nodal impulse production or from blocked impulse propagation and usually are not cause for concern unless syncope or presyncope develops. Sustained atrial tachyarrhythmias usually permit adequate cardiac output and are less dangerous than sustained ventricular arrhythmias, which often cause collapse or death.

B Atrial tachyarrhythmias The atrial tachyarrhythmias can be classified into two subcategories, those that produce a regular cardiac rhythm and those that produce an irregular cardiac rhythm. In general, atrial tachyarrhythmias do not interfere with inter- or intraventricular conduction of the cardiac impulse, and therefore the QRS complex (which is generated from the ventricles) remains narrow in form. Occasionally, however, atrial arrhythmias cause aberrant ventricular conduction with a wide QRS complex, which may mimic arrhythmias of ventricular origin.

1. **Regular atrial tachycardias**
   a. **Sinus tachycardia.** Sinus tachycardia represents a physiologic or pathophysiologic increase in the sinus rate (> 100 bpm) and is usually secondary to some other disease process. In general, the physician should treat the condition that is causing the sinus tachycardia, not the tachycardia itself. However, in some patients, such as those suffering from coronary artery disease, sinus tachycardia must be controlled to prevent myocardial ischemia. In this instance, β-blocking agents or calcium antagonists (either verapamil or diltiazem) may be effective in controlling heart rate.
   b. **Paroxysmal atrial tachycardia.** As the name implies, this arrhythmia is of sudden onset. This condition, which often exists in patients with otherwise normal hearts, is characterized by a heart rate of 150–250 bpm.
      (1) **ECG identification.** As demonstrated in the rhythm strip shown in Figure 1–2, the P waves are often not visible because they are buried in the QRS complex or the T wave.
      (2) **Therapy**
         (a) Therapies should be administered in a **quiet setting,** and patients should be made as comfortable as possible to reduce sympathetic discharge. As in the therapy of all arrhythmias, countershock may be necessary if patients are hemodynamically unstable or if the arrhythmia has caused worsening of angina or CHF.

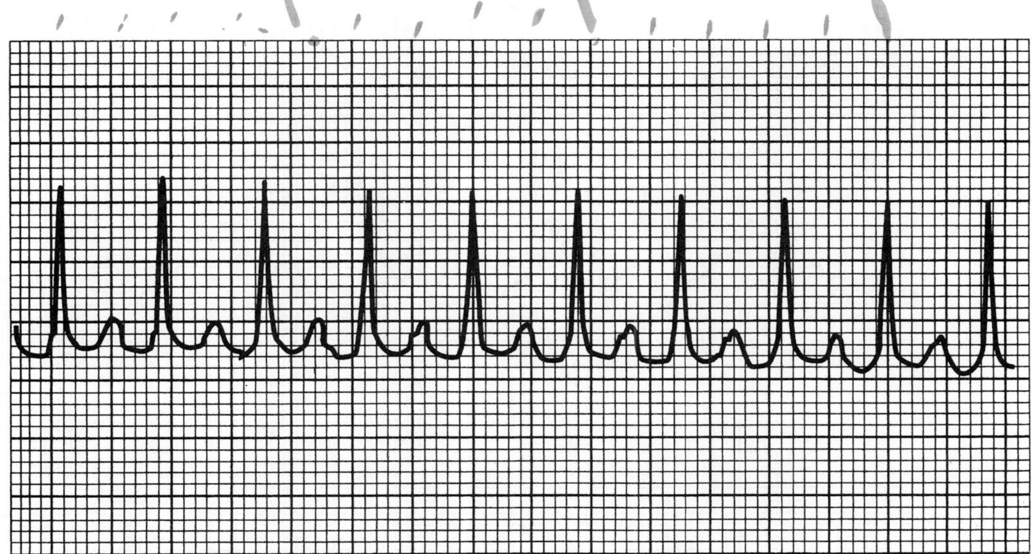

FIGURE 1–2 This rhythm strip demonstrates an episode of paroxysmal atrial tachycardia. The QRS complexes are narrow, and the heart rate is 165 bpm. The P waves are hidden in the T waves.

(b) Because **most episodes** of paroxysmal atrial tachycardia are **secondary to electrical reentry around the atrioventricular (AV) node,** therapies that increase vagal tone usually succeed in halting the arrhythmia.

(i) **Mechanical maneuvers** such as **carotid sinus massage,** the **Valsalva maneuver,** and **head immersion in cold water** are often effective in terminating the arrhythmia. These are especially important because they can be self-administered by the patient prior to seeking medical assistance.

(ii) **Medical therapy** includes the intravenous administration of **verapamil, esmolol, digoxin,** or **adenosine.**

c. **Atrial flutter with constant conduction** usually occurs in patients with antecedent heart disease, including coronary artery disease, pericarditis, valvular heart disease, and cardiomyopathy. Atrial flutter is characterized by an atrial rate of 220–400 bpm and is usually conducted to the ventricle with block so that the ventricular rate is a fraction of the atrial rate.

(1) **ECG identification.** As shown in Figure 1–3, this arrhythmia produces a classic sawtooth pattern on the ECG. In this example, there is 2:1 AV block with an atrial rate of 220 bpm and a ventricular rate of 110 bpm.

(2) **Therapy**

(a) Although intravenous administration of **digoxin, esmolol,** or **verapamil** may be effective in converting the arrhythmia to normal sinus rhythm, conversion is less likely than in paroxysmal atrial tachycardia. Usually these medications control the ventricular response, which, in turn, helps maintain hemodynamic stability. Once the ventricular rate has slowed as a result of increased AV block (3:1 or 4:1 conduction), **ibutilide** or another antiarrhythmic agent can be administered to restore sinus rhythm.

(b) If medical therapy does not convert the patient to normal sinus rhythm, atrial flutter will usually self-convert over time, either to atrial fibrillation or to normal sinus rhythm.

(c) As in all arrhythmias, **direct current (DC) cardioversion** is necessary if the arrhythmia has already produced hemodynamic instability.

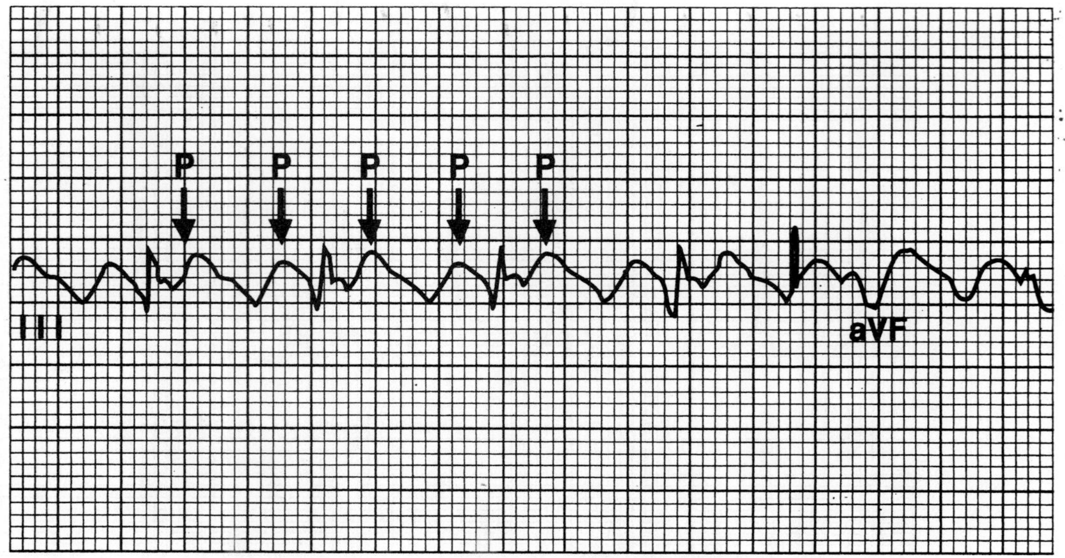

FIGURE 1–3 An episode of atrial flutter with 2:1 atrioventricular (AV) block is demonstrated. Note the frequency of the P waves, which represent the depolarization of the atria.

2. **Irregular atrial tachycardias**
   a. **Atrial fibrillation.** Atrial fibrillation is an **irregularly irregular** arrhythmia in which there is no ordered contraction of the atria but, rather, multiple discoordinate wave fronts of depolarization that send a large number of irregular impulses to depolarize the AV node. The irregular impulses produce an irregular ventricular response, the rate of which depends on the number of impulses that are conducted through the AV node. Selected causes of atrial fibrillation include stress, fever, excessive alcohol intake, volume depletion, pericarditis, coronary artery disease, MI, pulmonary embolism, mitral valve disease, thyrotoxicosis, and idiopathic (lone) atrial fibrillation.
      (1) **ECG identification.** An example of atrial fibrillation is shown in Figure 1–4.
      (2) **Therapy**
         (a) If patients with atrial fibrillation are hemodynamically unstable or demonstrate an increase in angina pectoris or worsening of CHF, immediate DC synchronous cardioversion is indicated.
         (b) If patients are hemodynamically stable, the physician should first focus on controlling the ventricular response to the atrial fibrillation while simultaneously treating the cause of the arrhythmia. The ventricular response may be controlled by the intravenous administration of digoxin, verapamil, diltiazem, or esmolol.
         (c) Once the ventricular response has been controlled, cardioversion to sinus rhythm may be spontaneous. Alternatively, it may be induced by administration of ibutilide, sotolol, or quinidine; or by DC synchronous cardioversion.
         (d) If the atrial fibrillation has been present for more than 2 days prior to cardioversion, the risk of intra-atrial thrombus, and therefore, embolization, increases.
            (i) Many authorities advocate anticoagulation therapy for 10 days or longer prior to either pharmacologic or electrical cardioversion.
            (ii) An alternative strategy undergoing intensive investigation is the use of transesophageal echocardiography to image the left atrium and its appendage. If no thrombus is present, anticoagulation with heparin is begun, and cardioversion is performed 24–48 hours later. Oral anticoagulation is then continued for up to 4 weeks. Postcardioversion anticoagulation is advantageous because atrial mechanical activity often lags behind restoration of normal electrical activity, potentiating thrombus formation. Postcardioversion anticoagulation is required whether or not precardioversion anticoagulation is used.
   b. **Multifocal atrial tachycardia.** In this arrhythmia, there is synchronous atrial contraction, but the contraction arises from many sites in the atria, not from the sinus node. In the majority of cases of multifocal atrial tachycardia, patients have severe antecedent pulmonary disease.
      (1) **ECG identification.** The multiple sites of origin of the atrial contraction produce many different P-wave configurations and different R-R intervals. At least three different P-wave morphologies are required to make this diagnosis.

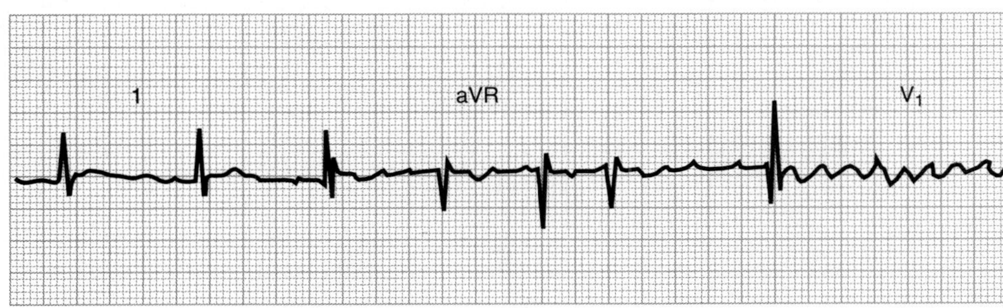

FIGURE 1–4 The irregularly irregular pattern of atrial fibrillation is demonstrated on this strip. Note the coarse fibrillatory waves in lead V_1. Although these could be confused with flutter waves, they are too irregular to be atrial flutter.

(2) **Therapy.** Treatment is directed primarily at improving oxygenation, ventilation, and airway mechanics. If these measures fail, **verapamil** may be useful in controlling the heart rate.

c. **Atrial flutter with irregular conduction.** If atrial flutter is conducted with varying block, the rhythm is irregular. This arrhythmia is treated identically to atrial flutter with constant block [see II B 1 c (2) (a)–(c)].

C Bradyarrhythmias

Bradyarrhythmias occur when sinus node impulse generation is slowed or when normal sinus node impulses cannot be conducted to the ventricles because of AV nodal block or ventricular conducting system disease. In general, bradyarrhythmias are a cause for concern only when patients have become symptomatic with presyncope or syncope from the reduced cardiac output that the low heart rate produces [see IX C 1 a (1)–(2)].

1. **Sinus bradycardia**
   a. Sinus bradycardia may be a physiologic and normal response to cardiovascular conditioning, as in trained athletes. In such cases, the arrhythmia is obviously a normal finding and requires no therapy. However, extreme sinus bradycardia (< 35 bpm) as a result of sinus node dysfunction may cause symptoms.
   b. **Therapy. Atropine** may be useful in temporarily increasing the sinus rate. The definitive therapy for symptomatic bradycardia is **pacemaker implantation.**
2. **Sinus pause.** This bradyarrhythmia is caused by the failure of the sinus node to generate an impulse on time. Such pauses may last for several seconds and induce syncope. Definitive therapy requires pacemaker implantation.
3. **AV block.** In AV block, some of the impulses generated from the sinus node are not conducted to the ventricles.
   a. **Types of AV block**
      (1) **Mobitz type I (Wenckebach) block.** There is a progressive prolongation in the P-R interval until a generated P wave is not conducted. This type of block usually occurs at the level of the AV node and is demonstrated in Figure 1–5. It rarely produces symptoms.

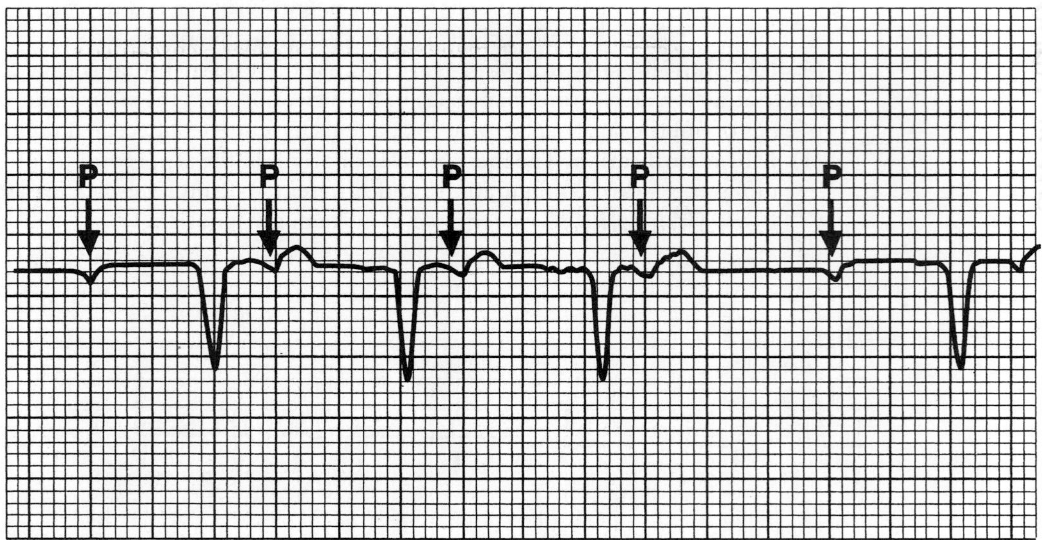

FIGURE 1–5 Electrocardiogram (ECG) rhythm strip produced by Mobitz type I second-degree atrioventricular (AV) nodal block. There is progressive prolongation of the P-R interval until finally a P wave is not conducted. In this example, there are four P waves for every three QRS complexes, resulting in a 4:3 Wenckebach block.

(2) **Mobitz type II block.** There is no prolongation of the P-R interval before the dropped beat. Often conduction in a 2:1 ratio is of long enough duration to cause symptomatic bradycardia. This type of block can occur at the AV node or in the His-Purkinje system.

(3) **Complete heart block.** No impulses are conducted (Figure 1–6), and the ventricular rate becomes dependent on spontaneous ventricular depolarizations. Severe symptomatic bradycardia characterized by a heart rate of 25–40 bpm is the rule.

b. **Therapy. Atropine** and **isoproterenol** are often effective in temporarily increasing the ventricular response. If this therapy fails, transcutaneous pacing temporarily increases heart rate. However, most forms of symptomatic AV block require the implantation of either a temporary (in the case of inferior MI) or a permanent **cardiac pacemaker.**

D Ventricular tachyarrhythmias

1. **Types of ventricular arrhythmias**

a. **Premature ventricular contraction (PVC).** In this arrhythmia, heart beats arise directly from the ventricles, bypassing the specialized cardiac His-Purkinje conduction system.

(1) **ECG identification**

(a) Because the His-Purkinje system is bypassed, the **QRS configuration** is typically **widened and bizarre** in appearance.

(b) PVCs usually do not affect atrial depolarization, which proceeds normally and in dissociation with the PVC. Thus, the next sinus beat occurs at the same time it would have occurred if no PVC had been present. Accordingly, a **full compensatory pause** usually follows a PVC (Figure 1–7). The normally occurring P wave is usually buried in the PVC–QRS complex.

(2) **Therapy.** Most isolated PVCs are benign and should not be treated.

b. **Ventricular tachycardia** is a regular rhythm that occurs paroxysmally and exceeds 120 bpm. **AV dissociation,** which causes the ventricular arrhythmia to proceed independently of the normal atrial rhythm, is the hallmark of the arrhythmia. During ventricular tachycardia, cardiac relaxation is impaired. This factor, together with loss of AV synchrony (i.e., loss of the atrial "kick") and loss of the electrical coordination of the contraction by the His-Purkinje system, usually leads to severely reduced cardiac output, producing hypotension. **Sustained ventricular tachycardia is usually a life-threatening arrhythmia that degenerates into ventricular fibrillation and death if untreated.**

(1) **Physical examination.** In many cases of ventricular tachycardia, severe decompensation precludes performance of a detailed physical examination.

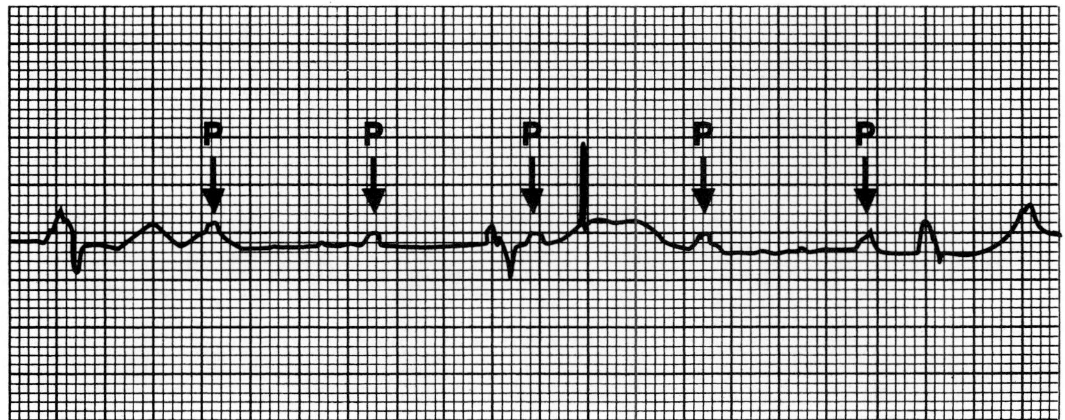

FIGURE 1–6 Complete heart block. In this strip, the P waves are regular, and the atrial rate is 85. However, no relationship between the P waves and QRS complexes is present, indicating the presence of complete heart block.

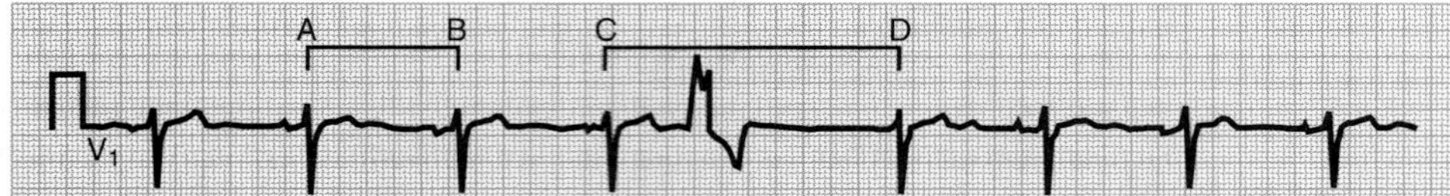

FIGURE 1–7 Premature ventricular contraction (PVC). The QRS is widened and bizarre in appearance and is followed by a compensatory pause—the R-R-interval. *C–D* is exactly twice the R-R interval *A–B*.

(a) If patients are relatively stable, physical diagnosis reveals AV dissociation, manifested by the appearance of **cannon a waves** in the neck veins. These waves occur intermittently when right atrial contraction occurs during ventricular contraction. Because the atrial blood cannot go forward against the closed tricuspid valve, backward flow produces a large bulge in the neck veins.

(b) **Variability in intensity of the S_1,** caused by variable positioning of atrial and ventricular contraction, can be auscultated.

(2) **ECG identification** (Figure 1–8)

(a) The **QRS complex is widened and bizarre in appearance** because the arrhythmia does not use the specialized conducting system of the heart. Because the ventricles

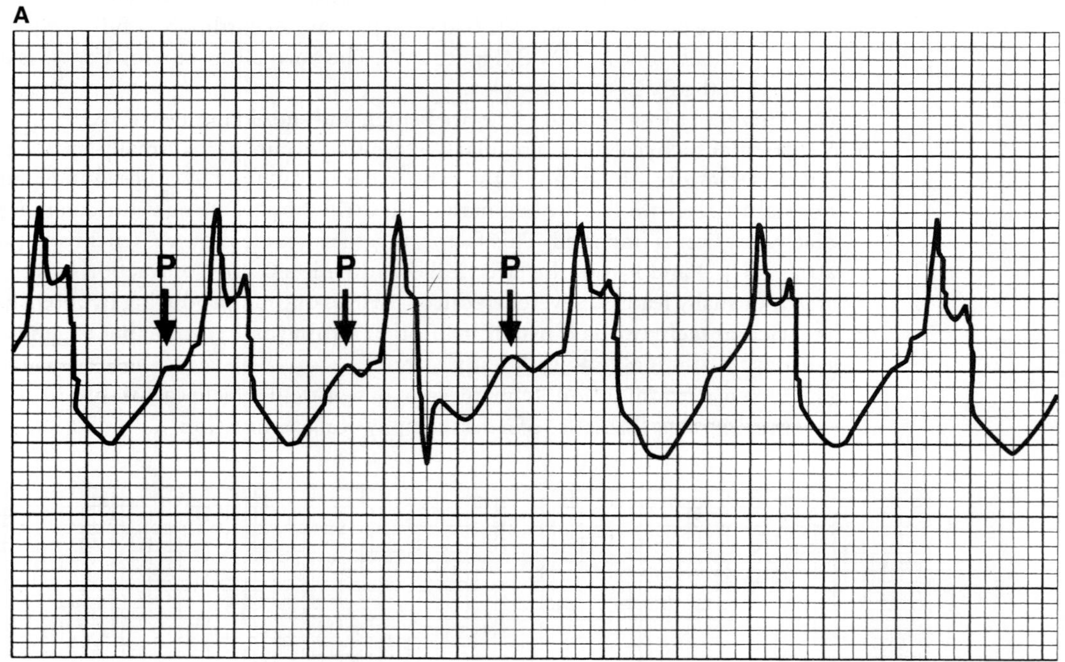

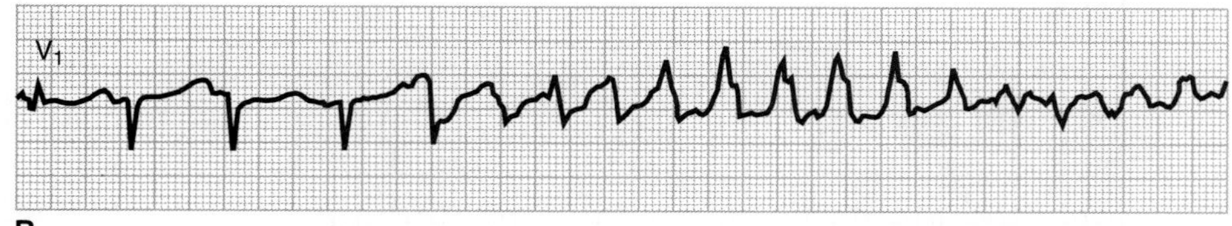

FIGURE 1–8 (*A*) Monomorphic ventricular tachycardia. There is a widened bizarre QRS complex, which has an inconsistent relationship to the preceding P wave. (*B*) Polymorphic ventricular tachycardia in a patient with a prolonged Q-T interval (torsades de pointes).

are operating independently of the atria, there is **no constant relationship between the P wave and the QRS complex.**

(b) The QRS complex may be **monomorphic** (i.e., of one shape), as shown in Figure 1–8A, or it may be **polymorphic,** as shown in Figure 1–8B. When the axis of a polymorphic arrhythmia appears to revolve about a central point and is associated with a prolonged Q-T interval, the arrhythmia is termed **torsades de pointes.**

(3) **Therapy.** Because of the unstable and life-threatening nature of this arrhythmia, **DC cardioversion** is urgently required in most cases. While preparations are being made for DC cardioversion, intravenous administration of **amiodarone, lidocaine, bretylium,** or **procainamide** may be useful in returning the rhythm to normal.

c. **Ventricular fibrillation** is characterized by a lack of ordered contraction of the ventricles; therefore, there is no cardiac output. Thus, **ventricular fibrillation is synonymous with death unless conversion to an effective rhythm can be accomplished.** The physician should begin cardiac resuscitation, including mechanical ventilation, cardiac compression, and drug and electrical therapy, immediately on recognizing the presence of ventricular fibrillation.

2. **Prevention and treatment of ventricular arrhythmias.** Table 1–1 lists the current classification and some of the side effects of drugs currently available for long-term prevention of ventricular

TABLE 1–1 Antiarrhythmic Agents

Class	Major Electrophysiologic Properties	Specific Agents	Major Side Effects
Sodium channel blockers	Ia Inhibit rapid inward current Prolong repolarization	Quinidine	Proarrhythmia Diarrhea
		Procainamide	Proarrhythmia Lupus-like syndrome
		Disopyramide	Proarrhythmia Congestive heart failure Anticholinergic effects
	Ib Inhibit rapid inward current	Lidocaine	CNS effects Proarrhythmia CNS effects
	Accelerate repolarization	Tocainide	Neutropenia
		Mexiletine	CNS effects
		Phenytoin	CNS effects
	Ic Inhibit rapid inward current Little effect on repolarization	Flecainide	Congestive heart failure Proarrhythmia
Beta-blockers	II Reduce ischemia	Propranolol	Bradycardia Bronchospasm Congestive heart failure
	Reduce sympathetic arrhythmogenicity	Acebutolol	Congestive heart failure
Potassium channel blockers	III Prolong action potential duration	Amiodarone	Pulmonary fibrosis Hypo- and hyperthyroidism
		Bretylium	Orthostatic hypotension
		Sotalol	Proarrhythmia
		Ibutilide	Proarrhythmia
Calcium channel blockers	IV Depress slow inward current	Verapamil (atrial arrhythmias)	Bradycardia

CNS = central nervous system.

arrhythmias. Such therapy is used when ventricular fibrillation occurs in the absence of an MI (because of a high likelihood of recurrent arrhythmia) or with the occurrence of symptomatic or sustained ventricular tachycardia. Today, insertion of an implantable cardiac defibrillator accompanies anti-arrhythmic agents in most cases of life-threatening arrhythmias.

III ISCHEMIC HEART DISEASE

A Atherosclerotic coronary artery disease (ASCAD)

1. **Definition.** ASCAD is the focal narrowing of the coronary arteries as a result of intimal proliferation of smooth muscle cells and the deposition of lipids. The basic lesion is called a **plaque,** the chief components of which are diagrammed in Figure 1–9. These include:
   a. **Intimal smooth muscle cells,** which proliferate, probably as a result of endothelial damage
   b. **Lipids** (cholesterol esters and crystals), which are deposited at the center of the plaque and also accumulate within smooth muscle cells
   c. A **fibrous cap** made of connective tissue
2. **Incidence and risk factors.** Currently in the United States, the overall incidence of death as a result of ASCAD is 0.5 in 1000 and decreasing. However, ASCAD differs in frequency in subpopulations with the following risk factors:
   a. **Age.** The incidence of ASCAD increases progressively with age. The risk of death is 1.5 in 1000 individuals at age 50.
   b. **Gender.** ASCAD is more prevalent in men than in women. This difference is most marked in premenopausal women compared with men of similar age. By the time men reach the age of 50 years, they are affected five times more often than women of the same age, and the difference declines as age increases.
   c. **Serum cholesterol.** The incidence of ASCAD increases with increasing total serum cholesterol levels, as shown in Figure 1–10.
      (1) Total serum cholesterol is carried in the blood by **low-density lipoprotein (LDL), very low-density lipoprotein (VLDL),** and **high-density lipoprotein (HDL).**
         (a) The higher the percentage of total cholesterol carried by LDL in relation to HDL, the higher the risk of ASCAD. Patients with LDL-to-HDL ratios of greater than 4:1 are par-

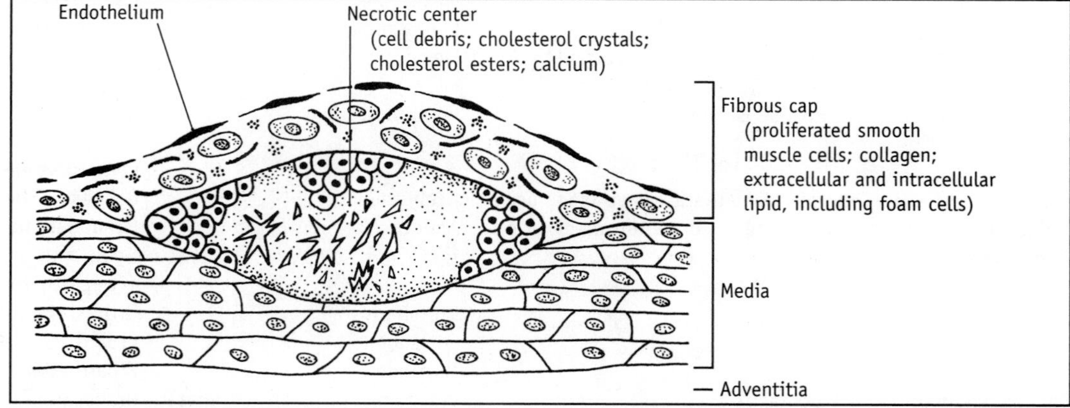

FIGURE 1–9 Diagrammatic representation of an atherosclerotic plaque, showing its composition. The *fibrous cap* of the plaque is linked to clinical events because of its tendency to fracture and ulcerate. The *necrotic core* of the plaque has clinical consequence as a result of its size, consistency, and thromboplastic components. (Adapted from Braunwald E: *Heart Disease,* 2nd edition. Philadelphia, WB Saunders, 1984, p 1186.)

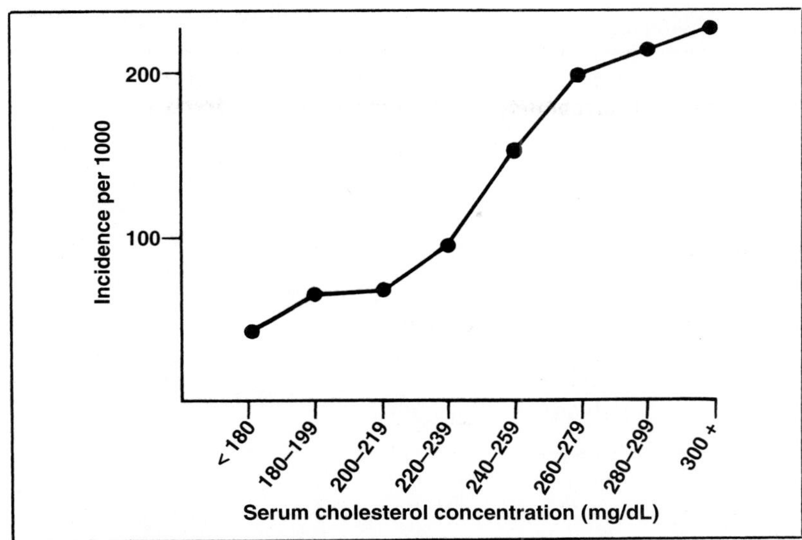

FIGURE 1–10 Graph showing the effect of increasing serum cholesterol concentration on the incidence of atherosclerotic coronary artery disease in men age 30–49 years. (Adapted from Cohn PF: *Diagnosis and Therapy of Coronary Artery Disease.* Boston, Little, Brown, 1979, p 27.)

ticularly prone to ASCAD. Conversely, high levels of HDL seem to be protective. One theory is that HDL may allow for elution of cholesterol out of the coronary vessel.

(b) It is desirable for the total cholesterol level to be less than 200 mg/dL.

(i) The LDL cholesterol level should be less than 130 mg/dL; in patients with known coronary disease, it should be less than 100 mg/dL.

(ii) The HDL cholesterol level should exceed 40 mg/dL.

(2) Several types of hyperlipidemia exist, and many are associated with an increased incidence of coronary artery disease. Table 1–2 presents an overview of the hyperlipidemias.

d. Smoking. Compared with nonsmokers, cigarette smokers are 60% more likely to develop ASCAD when other risk factors are controlled for statistically. Smoking increases carbon monoxide levels in the blood, which may, in turn, damage the coronary endothelium. Smoking also increases platelet adhesiveness and thus the likelihood of thrombotic coronary occlusion.

e. Hypertension. The higher either the systolic or diastolic blood pressure, the more likely the development of ASCAD. This likelihood is apparent in both men and women and becomes more pronounced with advancing age.

f. Diabetes mellitus is associated with a 50% increase in the incidence of ASCAD in men and a 100% increase in women, explained in part by the increased platelet adhesiveness and increased serum cholesterol levels associated with diabetes. In general, however, there is a poor correlation between the severity of the diabetes and the severity of ASCAD.

g. Family history. A familial predisposition to coronary artery disease exists in part due to inheritance of the above risk factors (except smoking). However, family history is the only risk factor in about one third of individuals with ASCAD.

h. Oral contraceptives are associated with an increased incidence of MI, a clinical consequence of ASCAD. The incidence of MI rises from 0.01% to 0.04% in nonsmoking women between the ages of 30 and 40 who use oral contraceptives and, more dramatically, from 0.06% to 0.25% in similar women who also smoke.

i. Obesity. Recently, obesity has been recognized as an independent risk factor for ASCAD.

TABLE 1–2 The Hyperlipidemias

Type of Hyperlipidemia	Lipid Abnormality	Lipoprotein Abnormality	Clinical Manifestations	Therapy
I Lipoprotein lipase deficiency	↑ Triglycerides	↑ Chylomicrons	Pancreatitis Eruptive xanthomas Lipemia retinalis	Fat-free diet
IIa LDL receptor deficiency	↑ Cholesterol	↑ LDL	Coronary disease Tendon xanthomas Xanthelasma	Restricted diet Bile acid–binding resins Nicotinic acid HMG-CoA reductase inhibitors
IIb	↑ Cholesterol ↑ Triglycerides	↑ LDL ↑ VLDL	Coronary disease	Restricted diet Bile acid–binding resins Nicotinic acid Gemfibrozil HMG-CoA reductase inhibitors
III Dysbetalipoproteinemia	↑ Triglycerides ↑ Cholesterol	↑ VLDL Remnants	Palmar fatty streaks Tuberous xanthomas Coronary disease Peripheral vascular disease Hypothyroidism	Gemfibrozil
IV	↑ Triglycerides	↑ VLDL	Eruptive xanthomas Pancreatitis Diabetes ± Coronary artery disease	Restricted diet Gemfibrozil
V	↑ Triglycerides	↑ VLDL ↑ Chylomicrons	Eruptive xanthomas Pancreatitis Diabetes ± Coronary artery disease	Restricted diet Gemfibrozil

HMG-CoA = β-hydroxy-β-methylglutaryl coenzyme A; LDL = low-density lipoproteins; VLDL = very-low-density lipoproteins.

j. **Other risk factors.** Gout, "type A" personality, premature arcus corneae, hyperhomocysteinemia, hypertriglyceridemia, and a diagonal ear lobe crease are other conditions associated with an increased risk of ASCAD.

3. **Pathogenesis.** The previously mentioned risk factors do not constitute a known mechanism for ASCAD. The major theory of atherogenesis is the **response to injury theory.**
   a. This theory states that some injurious stimulus (e.g., hypertension or hypercholesterolemia) causes endothelial damage, resulting in the release of various growth factors. These growth factors cause smooth cell proliferation and migration of macrophages into the vessel wall. At the same time, the now injured endothelium becomes more permeable, admitting lipid and cholesterol into the intima.
   b. These changes result in plaque formation, which may eventually compromise the vessel lumen enough to impede blood flow. If the plaque is disrupted, platelets are activated, leading to thrombus formation and worsening obstruction.

4. Pathophysiology (leading to ischemia)

a. Supply–demand relationship. As wall stress and heart rate increase (e.g., with exercise), myocardial oxygen consumption rises. Autoregulated increases in coronary blood flow normally meet this increased demand. However, if demand exceeds supply, ischemia results. The product of heart rate and left ventricular systolic pressure or wall stress roughly approximate the oxygen needs of the myocardium (see I B 1 b).

(1) **Increased demand.** In patients with ASCAD, stenosis of the coronary artery prevents the increase in coronary blood flow needed to compensate for an increased demand, resulting in an oxygen demand that exceeds the oxygen supply. **Myocardial ischemia** is the result of this imbalance.

(2) **Reduced supply.** The atherosclerotic stenosis was once viewed as a fixed obstruction to coronary blood flow. In fact, the diseased area of the coronary artery often remains dynamic, and the effective lumen of the artery undergoes constant change. Changes are produced by vasoconstriction of the coronary artery, by production and degradation of local thrombi at the site of stenosis, and by progressive enlargement of the atherosclerotic plaque. Acute changes in lumen diameter may reduce the supply of coronary blood flow and, thus, produce ischemia without an increase in demand.

b. Myocardial infarction (MI). The necrosis of myocardial tissue occurs as a result of prolonged ischemia. The rapidity and extent of the infarction process are determined by the extent of reduction of blood flow to the area. In some cases, **collateral flow** may supply enough blood flow to prevent infarction despite a total coronary occlusion.

(1) Although the cause of **transmural (ST segment elevation myocardial infarction [STEMI]) infarction** has been debated for much of the last century, it is now clear that most transmural MIs are associated with early occlusion of a coronary artery by a **thrombus.**

(a) Usually, the thrombus is located adjacent to an atherosclerotic coronary stenosis. Dissolution or rupture of the fibrous cap over the atherosclerotic plaque precedes thrombosis. Activation of inflammatory cytokines may lead to matrix metalloproteinase activation, which is partially responsible for dissolution of the fibrous cap.

(b) Aggressive lysis of the thrombus with agents such as **streptokinase** and **tissue plasminogen activator (t-PA)** or balloon angioplasty reestablishes coronary blood flow, relieves pain, reestablishes contractile function of the segment of myocardium supplied by the thrombosed artery, and reduces myocardial damage [see III A 5 b (5) (b)]. These observations indicate that the thrombus is not merely a coincident event in MI; rather, it is central to the pathogenesis of the infarction.

(2) The pathogenesis of **nontransmural (non–STEMI) infarction** is less clear, but the presence of total coronary occlusion is significantly less common, occurring in less than 50% of cases.

5. Clinical consequences

a. Angina pectoris is chest pain or pressure produced by myocardial ischemia.

(1) **Characteristic features**

(a) **Relation to exertion.** The single most important feature of angina pectoris is its precipitation by exertion. Exertion increases myocardial oxygen demand beyond the supply capabilities of diseased coronary arteries, producing ischemia. Other factors that increase myocardial oxygen demand (e.g., emotional upset, eating a meal, or the peripheral vasoconstriction caused by walking in cold weather) also may precipitate angina. In some patients, angina occurs predominantly at rest. When rest pain occurs, it probably is produced by a reduction in coronary blood flow or by spontaneous increases in blood pressure, heart rate, or both.

(b) **Quality of pain.** Although many patients perceive angina as **chest pain,** others report a feeling of **pressure** in the chest area or complain of a **burning** sensation. In some patients, **exertional dyspnea** may represent an anginal equivalent.

(c) **Radiation of pain.** Radiation of anginal pain to the left arm is well known. Pain also may radiate to the right arm, jaw, teeth, or throat. Occasionally, these radiation sites may be the only sites of pain, and the chest is free of discomfort; or the chest discomfort, when present, may not radiate at all.

(d) **Progression of ischemia and duration of symptoms.** Whatever the anginal symptom quality for a given patient, repeated episodes of ischemia usually reproduce that same quality. The symptom complex usually begins at a low intensity, increases over 2–3 minutes, and lasts a total of less than 15 minutes. Episodes longer than 30 minutes suggest that MI may have occurred. **Sudden onset of severe chest pain does not suggest ischemic pain.**

(2) **Types of ischemic episodes**

(a) **Chronic stable angina** is angina that recurs under similar circumstances and with a similar frequency over time.

(b) **Silent ischemia** refers to the usual occurrence of four to five episodes of asymptomatic ischemia for every episode of symptomatic ischemia that the patient suffers. These episodes, which can be detected by ECG monitoring, are less severe in nature and shorter in duration than the episodes that the patient perceives as angina. In some patients, especially those with diabetes mellitus, documentable ischemia occurs without any patient perception of ischemic symptoms.

(c) **Unstable angina** is a term applied to angina when a change in status occurs (e.g., new-onset angina; angina of increasing severity, duration, or frequency; or angina occurring at rest for the first time). It is the progressive nature of unstable angina that is ominous, and the physician and the patient should be aware that close observation and intensive therapy are required. Unstable angina represents a more serious clinical situation than chronic stable angina because unstable angina may be an immediate precursor of MI.

(i) **Rest angina.** Angina at rest is particularly worrisome because it implies that decreased supply, rather than increased demand, is causing the angina. This concept in turn suggests that arterial occlusion and possible infarction may be imminent.

(ii) **New-onset angina.** In cases of new-onset angina, it is difficult to generalize about clinical outcome. New-onset angina that progresses in frequency, severity, or duration over 1 or 2 months is worrisome. Conversely, some cases of new-onset angina may simply be the first episode in what becomes a chronic stable anginal pattern.

(d) **Variant (Prinzmetal's) angina**

(i) The **hallmark** of variant angina is the appearance of transient **S-T segment elevation** on the ECG during the angina attack. The S-T segment elevation represents **transmural ischemia** produced by a sudden reduction in coronary blood flow.

(ii) The reduction in flow results from **transient coronary spasm,** which may or may not be associated with a fixed atherosclerotic lesion. The spasm produces total but transient coronary occlusion. The cause of the spasm and its release are unknown.

(iii) Variant angina usually occurs at rest (often at night), and episodes frequently are complicated by complex ventricular arrhythmias.

(e) **Acute coronary syndromes.** Because the definitions of unstable angina, rest angina, and non-ST segment elevation MI are often blurred but require the same therapy, this group of ischemic events are often referred to as acute coronary syndromes rather than by a more specific term.

(3) Diagnosis. When a patient exhibits chest pain characteristic of angina, the diagnosis can be suspected strongly on the basis of patient history alone. The suspicion that coronary disease is present is heightened by the presence of one or more coronary risk factors. However, the following procedures are useful in confirming the diagnosis.

(a) Physical examination. Patients experiencing an episode of angina are usually uncomfortable and anxious. Blood pressure and pulse rate are increased in most cases. Palpation of the precordium may reveal a **dyskinetic impulse** over the apex of the left ventricle. A new S_4 may appear, and **transient mitral regurgitation** as a result of ischemically produced papillary muscle dysfunction may produce a **holosystolic murmur.**

(b) Resting electrocardiography. The ECG taken in the absence of pain in patients with angina pectoris with no history of MI is normal in 50% of cases. However, in many cases, efforts to obtain an ECG while the patient is experiencing chest pain are more rewarding.

(i) The presence of **new horizontal** or **downsloping S-T segments** on the ECG is highly suggestive of myocardial ischemia. **New T-wave inversion** also may occur, but this finding alone without S-T segment depression is less specific.

(ii) In the presence of variant angina, an acute current of injury indicated by transient S-T segment elevation is diagnostic. The S-T segment elevation normalizes as the pain wanes and no Q waves appear.

(c) Stress electrocardiography. Recording the ECG during exercise substantially increases the sensitivity and specificity of electrocardiography. In addition, a formal exercise test permits quantification of the patient's exercise tolerance and observation of the effects of exercise on the patient's symptoms, heart rate, and blood pressure.

(i) The appearance of horizontal or downsloping S-T segment depression of 1 mm or more during exercise has a sensitivity of approximately 70% and a specificity of 90% for the detection of coronary disease.

(ii) The S-T criteria for positivity are less accurate in women than in men. The presence of **bundle branch block** or **left ventricular hypertrophy** or the use of **digitalis** by the patient **all reduce the accuracy of this test.**

(d) Stress scintigraphy, when used in combination with the stress ECG, has yielded increased sensitivity (80%) and specificity (92%) over the standard stress ECG alone. Therefore, it is a particularly useful diagnostic tool when the standard stress ECG is expected to be of low yield (e.g., in women and in patients with bundle branch block) and in patients in whom a previous stress ECG has produced equivocal results.

(i) Method. When the radioactive isotope **thallium 201** (^{201}TI) or the technetium-based isonitrile **sestamibi** is injected into the peripheral venous blood, a portion of the substance is taken up by the myocardium. The myocardial distribution of the substance is affected by blood flow and ischemia, with areas of less blood flow and ischemia taking up less ^{201}TI or sestamibi than areas of normal blood flow. Normally, blood flow and, thus, the isotope, are distributed equally throughout the myocardium. With exercise, blood flow increases, but in patients with coronary artery disease, those parts of the myocardium supplied by diseased coronary arteries and areas of MI take up less ^{201}TI or sestamibi than normal areas, as shown in the scintigram in Figure 1–11. In patients unable to exercise, infusion of dobutamine (to increase oxygen demand) or dipyridamole (to cause coronary vasodilatation) are used to alter coronary flow in place of exercise.

(ii) Enhancements. Thallium and sestamibi imaging can be further enhanced using **single-photon emission computed tomography (SPECT).** This technique

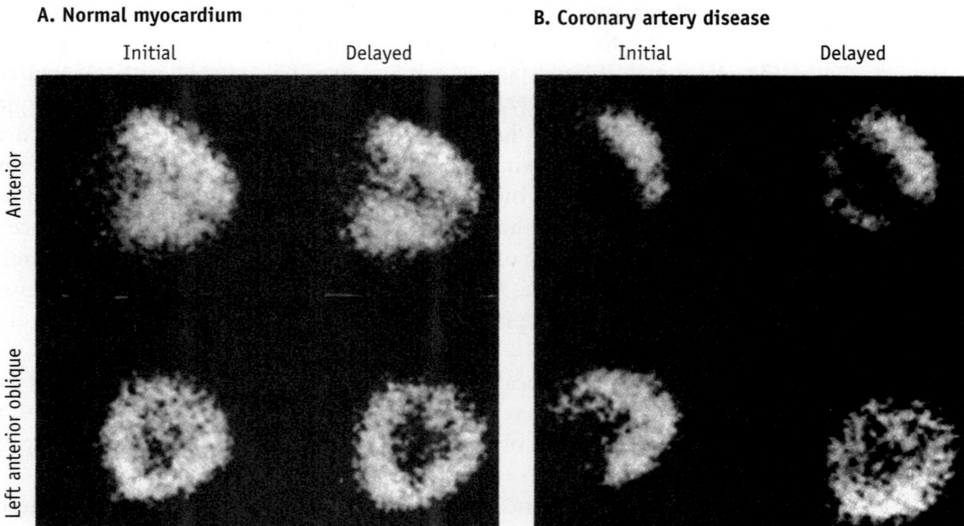

FIGURE 1–11 Stress scintigraphy in a normal patient (*A*) and in a patient with coronary artery disease (*B*). (*A*) Normal thallium study shows initial (i.e., immediately after exercise) and delayed thallium 201 (^{201}TI) images in the anterior and left anterior oblique views. ^{201}TI is taken up and released homogeneously throughout the myocardium, indicating equal coronary blood flow to all portions of the left ventricle. (*B*) A large defect (*black area from 5 o'clock to 11 o'clock*) is seen in the initial scintiscan in the anterior view. This area corresponds to the inferoapical area of the left ventricle. A defect also is seen in the left anterior oblique view (*black area from 6 o'clock to 9 o'clock*), which corresponds to the inferior portion of the left ventricular septum. Areas of decreased perfusion eventually demonstrate ^{201}TI uptake, as seen in the delayed scintiscan. This study is consistent with exercise-induced hypoperfusion of the inferolateral and septal areas of the left ventricle and with obstructive disease of the right coronary artery. (Reprinted with permission from Johnson R, et al: *The Practice of Cardiology*. Boston, Little, Brown, 1980, p 1046.)

uses a rotating gamma camera to acquire data at 32 to 64 stops in a 180- or 360-degree arc around the patient. A computer reconstructs the data into a two-dimensional image and assigns different colors to different levels of ^{201}TI uptake. The sensitivity for detecting coronary disease with SPECT imaging is as high as 90%.

(e) **Stress radionuclide ventriculography**

(i) **Method.** Pyrophosphate, injected peripherally, binds the radionuclide **technetium** to red blood cells (RBCs). Radionuclide-tagged RBCs in the blood pool of the left ventricle can be used to produce a scintigraphic image of the left ventricle. By gating the fluctuations in tagged RBC count that occur within the ventricles over a number of cardiac cycles, a radionuclide ventriculogram can be produced.

(ii) **Interpretation.** Coronary disease produces regional dysfunction by ischemia or infarction of those areas of the left ventricle not receiving an adequate blood supply. Exercise-induced ischemia produces transient regional dysfunction, which can be detected by radionuclide angiography. For example, in a patient with disease in the left anterior descending coronary artery, the anterior left ventricular wall may move normally at rest but become dyskinetic with exercise as a result of ischemia.

(iii) **Sensitivity.** This test is sensitive (90%) for the detection of coronary artery disease but is not as specific because heart disease other than coronary artery disease may produce exercise-induced regional dysfunction.

(f) **Stress echocardiography.** This technique is based on the same principles of ischemia as stress radionuclide ventriculography, but an echocardiograph, rather than a radioactive blood pool, is used to produce the images of wall motion abnormalities.

(g) **Cardiac catheterization with coronary arteriography** allows for direct visualization of the coronary arteries by selective injection of radiographic contrast material. This procedure is the **most sensitive and specific test commonly used for coronary artery disease.**

(i) **Risk.** Unlike the previously mentioned tests, cardiac catheterization is an invasive procedure that carries a small but finite risk. The overall risk of mortality during coronary arteriography is approximately 0.2%.

(ii) **Applications.** Cardiac catheterization should be reserved for cases in which the diagnosis is uncertain after noninvasive testing or when more information is needed to help determine whether medical or surgical therapy is most appropriate for the patient's coronary disease. If surgery is contemplated, the arteriograms obtained at catheterization guide the surgeon's placement of the bypass grafts.

(h) **Intravascular ultrasound** using an echo transducer attached to a coronary catheter is an ultrasensitive technique currently under investigation for the diagnosis of ASCAD. However, this procedure carries a risk that probably exceeds that of arteriography.

(4) **Therapy.** Treatment of angina pectoris is directed either at reducing myocardial oxygen demand to compensate for impaired flow through diseased coronary arteries or at increasing myocardial oxygen supply (i.e., blood flow).

(a) **Nitrates.** This class of drugs produces venodilation and, to a lesser extent, arteriolar vasodilatation.

(i) Venodilation and arteriolar vasodilatation decrease blood pressure and reduce cardiac size, thereby reducing left ventricular wall stress and myocardial oxygen demand.

(ii) Direct coronary arterial vasodilation also may increase coronary blood flow, because even diseased portions of the coronary artery have been shown to dilate.

(iii) Sublingual, oral, dermal, and intravenous nitrate preparations are available and effective.

(b) **β-Adrenergic blocking agents.** β-Adrenergic receptor stimulation results in an increase in heart rate and in the force of myocardial contraction. Both events increase myocardial oxygen demand. β-Adrenergic blocking agents counteract these effects and **limit myocardial oxygen demand.**

(i) Recent evidence suggests that β-blockers also may diminish platelet activation, which could be important in stabilizing the coronary plaque and in preventing reduction in coronary blood flow.

(ii) Currently, the **five β-blockers approved for use in treating angina are propranolol, metoprolol, atenolol, nadolol,** and **timolol.**

(iii) These drugs may precipitate CHF in some patients with severe systolic dysfunction. In addition, β-blockers may precipitate bronchospasm in asthmatics and in patients with obstructive lung disease. They also may cause severe bradycardia in patients with sinoatrial (SA) node or AV node disease and can aggravate peripheral vascular disease.

(c) **Calcium antagonists.** Calcium regulates the contraction of smooth muscle, which is present in the walls of the coronary and peripheral arteries.

(i) Calcium antagonists are particularly **effective in preventing the coronary spasm that causes variant angina.** They are also useful in treating cases of typical angina, in which they **act as coronary and peripheral arterial vasodilators.** Diltiazem and verapamil also reduce heart rate.

(ii) **Nifedipine, verapamil, diltiazem, amlodipine,** and **nicardipine** are the calcium antagonists currently approved for the treatment of both typical and variant angina.

(iii) All calcium blockers may cause hypotension. Verapamil and, more rarely, diltiazem may precipitate CHF or severe bradycardia.

(d) **Percutaneous transluminal angioplasty (PCTA).** Removing or reducing the obstructive coronary atherosclerotic lesion can alleviate the angina.

(i) During angioplasty, a small balloon is inserted into a femoral or brachial artery and guided to the obstruction of the affected coronary artery. The balloon is inflated, dilating the stenosis and reducing the obstruction.

(ii) The initial success rate of PCTA approaches 90%, although there is a 33% restenosis rate after 6 months, making it necessary to repeat the procedure in some patients. The mortality rate is 1%, and 5% of the patients undergoing PCTA require immediate surgery as a result of PCTA-related occlusions. Placement of small wire **stents** reduces the rate of restenosis and now accompanies the majority of angioplasties. Today stents are coated with sirolimus or paclitaxel, which reduces the restenosis rate to approximately 5%. Coadministration of abciximab, a IIb–IIIa platelet receptor antibody, or eptifibatide, a IIb–IIIa receptor antagonist, also enhances short- and long-term patency.

(e) **Atherectomy.** In some patients in whom PCTA is ineffective, atherectomy can be performed. **Rotational atherectomy** involves the use of a high-speed drill to remove the plaque.

(f) **Coronary artery bypass surgery.** Surgery offers a high incidence of symptomatic improvement (85%) at a 2%–5% operative risk and, thus, is indicated for patients whose lifestyles are seriously compromised by angina despite medical therapy. In addition, coronary bypass surgery increases longevity in most patients with severe disease of the main left coronary artery and some anatomic distributions of left anterior descending and triple-vessel coronary disease (see III A 6).

(g) **Therapy for acute coronary syndromes (ACS).** ACS are ominous because they indicate sudden decrease in blood supply, suggesting plaque instability. Bed rest, aspirin, intravenous heparin, and nitroglycerin are the mainstays of initial therapy. In most centers, low-molecular-weight heparins such as enoxaparin have replaced unfractionated heparin because low-molecular-weight heparins do not require PTT monitoring and are associated with fewer bleeding complications. Addition of eptifibatide or tirofiban further reduces the risk of MI. Cardiac catheterization is then performed to gauge the potential for revascularization.

b. **Myocardial infarction (MI)** occurs when the myocardium is deprived of its blood supply (and therefore, oxygen) for a significant amount of time. **Transmural (STEMI) MI** results from the obstruction of the coronary arteries by **thrombi** or **coronary spasm.** Spasm is especially common in cocaine abusers. The cause of nontransmural (**subendocardial**) infarction remains uncertain.

(1) **Pathogenesis.** An abrupt change in the atherosclerotic plaque seems to be one of the events precipitating an MI. Plaque rupture and its roughened surface attracts platelets that trigger thrombus formation, leading to total occlusion of the vessel. Antecedent endothelial dysfunction enhances potential for both vasospasm and thrombus formation.

(2) **Symptoms.** The patient usually experiences **severe, oppressive chest pain** or **pressure** that persists for more than 30 minutes and is unrelieved by nitroglycerin. The pain radiates in a pattern similar to that of angina pectoris.

(a) Frequently, **nausea, vomiting, diaphoresis,** and **shortness of breath** accompany the pain.

(b) The pain usually occurs when the patient is **at rest** or involved in minimal activity. However, recent studies show that MI can be triggered by discrete events (e.g., **shov-**

eling snow), and an unusually large number of infarctions occur **between 6 A.M. and 10 A.M., when catecholamine levels increase on awakening.**

(3) **Diagnosis**

(a) **Physical examination.** The patient experiencing MI is in obvious pain, is quite apprehensive, and often appears ashen. If the infarction is extensive, hypotension and tachycardia may be present. There also may be signs of CHF (e.g., elevation of the neck veins, pulmonary rales, and a cardiac gallop rhythm). The new murmur of mitral regurgitation may be present.

(b) **Electrocardiography.** The ECG is diagnostic in approximately 85% of cases. The remaining 15% of patients may experience MI without manifesting clearcut evidence on the ECG.

(i) When **transmural MI** is present, an injury current usually is demonstrated by S-T segment elevation in those leads reflecting the area of the MI. As the S-T segments fall, Q waves appear, and the T waves become inverted.

(ii) In the presence of **subendocardial infarction,** the electrocardiographic diagnosis is less certain, and S-T segment depression may be the only finding.

(iii) Because the presence or absence of Q waves on the ECG does not correlate well with transmural versus subendocardial infarction at autopsy, the current practice is to classify MIs as either **Q wave or non–Q wave,** as opposed to transmural or subendocardial.

(c) **Cardiac enzyme studies**

(i) As myocardial necrosis occurs, the myocardium releases **creatine kinase (CK), aspartate aminotransferase [AST (SGOT)],** and **lactic acid dehydrogenase (LDH),** thereby increasing serum concentrations of these enzymes.

(ii) CK elevation appears 6 hours after infarction, AST elevation appears 12 hours after infarction, and LDH elevation appears 24 hours after infarction.

(iii) Although these enzymes may be elevated in other disease states, isoenzyme studies can determine with a high probability whether the enzymes are cardiac in origin. The amount of the **MB isoenzyme** (i.e., the CK isoenzyme found primarily in the myocardium) increases in the presence of MI. In addition, **LDH_1** isoenzyme levels are elevated so that they exceed LDH_2 isoenzyme levels.

(iv) **Myocardial proteins.** Because the enzymes noted above still lack perfect sensitivity and specificity, the release of cardiac-specific **troponin I** is now also routinely monitored to enhance the diagnosis of MI and high-risk unstable angina.

(4) **Complications.** An MI can occur with little clinical consequence; indeed, many are silent. The complications of MI, however, produce clinically significant events.

(a) **Arrhythmias.** A patient having an acute MI is subject to acute, **lethal ventricular arrhythmias** (i.e., ventricular tachycardia or ventricular fibrillation), as well as **less serious atrial arrhythmias** (e.g., atrial fibrillation, atrial flutter).

(i) Lethal arrhythmias often occur without warning, often within 24 hours of the infarction. Although many patients experience frequent PVCs as a harbinger of lethal ventricular arrhythmias, other patients have sudden arrhythmias without lesser, premonitory rhythm disturbances.

(ii) The need for detection of cardiac arrhythmias fostered the concept of the **coronary care unit.** By closely monitoring the patient with MI, it is possible to detect and prevent severe cardiac arrhythmias before they become fatal.

(b) **Acute conduction system abnormalities.** The specialized conducting system of the heart is itself myocardium, which may become ischemic or infarcted during an MI. This may lead to bradyarrhythmias, heart block, or both.

(i) **Inferior MI** usually occurs when the right coronary artery is diseased. Because this artery supplies the SA node in 55% of patients and the AV node in 85% of patients, it is not surprising that **sinus bradycardia** and varying degrees of **AV**

nodal block occur during inferior MIs. Heart block occurring during inferior infarction is almost always transient.

(ii) On the other hand, **anterior MI** usually occurs from occlusion of the anterior descending coronary artery, which supplies the interventricular septum. Because the bundle branches course through the septum, acute **right** or **left bundle branch block** may occur during anterior MIs. **Complete heart block** also may occur due to dysfunction of both bundle branches or the bundle of His.

(c) **Pump failure**

(i) When 30% of the myocardium is infarcted from one or more MIs, **CHF** is likely to ensue.

(ii) If more than 40% of the myocardium becomes infarcted, **cardiogenic shock** is likely to develop. In true cardiogenic shock, there is not enough myocardium to generate enough cardiac output to sustain bodily function. One definition of cardiogenic shock is a systolic blood pressure of less than 90 mm Hg together with a urinary output of less than 20 mL/hr in the presence of adequate left ventricular filling pressure. When cardiogenic shock occurs, the mortality rate is 50%–75%.

(d) **Mitral regurgitation.** The **papillary muscles,** which are projections of the myocardium, tether the mitral valve. Dysfunction or infarction of the papillary muscles together with ventricular dilatation may lead to systolic prolapsing of the mitral valve into the left atrium, causing varying degrees of mitral regurgitation. If the mitral regurgitation is severe, the cardiac output is decreased profoundly because a large part of the left ventricular stroke volume is ejected backward. At the same time, there is a precipitous rise in the left ventricular filling pressure that is transmitted to the lungs, resulting in pulmonary edema.

(e) **Ventricular septal defect.** The left ventricular septum may become infarcted in either anterior or inferior MI, leading to rupture of the septum. Thus, a free communication between left and right ventricles (an acute ventricular septal defect) is formed. This defect diverts a significant percentage of the left ventricular stroke volume into the right ventricle, compromising forward cardiac output. Rupture of the septum occurs in approximately 2% of patients, usually 2–5 days after infarction.

(f) **Cardiac rupture.** MI of the free wall may lead to eventual perforation of the heart. This complication, which results in overwhelming **cardiac tamponade,** is nearly always fatal.

(g) **Left ventricular aneurysm.** The infarcted zone of the myocardium may evaginate and heal with fibrous connective tissue, forming a "fifth chamber" attached to the left ventricle. This useless chamber saps a portion of the left ventricular stroke volume. Left ventricular aneurysms may produce cardiac failure and angina, and they also may be the source of severe left ventricular arrhythmias and systemic emboli.

(5) **Therapy.** When a patient enters the hospital with an MI, an intravenous cannula is placed percutaneously for use in administering medications. Intramuscular injections should be avoided because they may confuse interpretation of the cardiac enzymes. Oxygen is traditionally delivered via a nasal cannula. An aspirin is administered immediately.

(a) **Pain relief**

(i) **Nitroglycerin.** Because approximately 4% of all acute MIs are thought to be caused by **coronary spasm** (as opposed to thrombotic occlusive disease), sublingual nitroglycerin should be administered in case the patient is suffering from coronary spasm.

(ii) **Morphine sulfate.** If nitroglycerin is not effective in relieving pain, enough morphine sulfate should be given intravenously to relieve pain and anxiety.

(b) **Thrombolysis**

(i) The use of **thrombolytic agents** (e.g., streptokinase, t-PA, urokinase, anistreplase) to dissolve the occlusive thrombus and promote reperfusion of the infarct-related artery significantly reduces the mortality from MI when administered within 6 hours of the onset of chest pain. Substantial evidence exists that if reperfusion can be accomplished within 3 hours of the onset of chest pain, a significant amount of myocardium can be salvaged, leading to lower acute mortality and, often, better left ventricular function. Concomitant administration of aspirin enhances the effectiveness of streptokinase, whereas coadministration of heparin, and perhaps aspirin, enhances the effectiveness of t-PA. The antiplatelet agent clopedrogrel is also effective.

(ii) In centers that are expert in coronary intervention, **direct PCTA** of the occluded vessel is preferred over thrombolytic agents.

(c) **Antiarrhythmic therapy.** If serious ventricular arrhythmias occur, amiodarone or lidocaine is infused. Additional drugs may be necessary to control arrhythmias if lidocaine is ineffective. **Bretylium tosylate, procainamide, and intravenous β-blockers** may be useful in controlling acute recalcitrant arrhythmias. These agents are given intravenously with caution.

(d) **Correction of serious conduction disturbances.** As noted, high-degree AV nodal block may occur during acute MI, producing significant bradycardia and hypotension. Therapies for restoring heart rate include:

(i) **Atropine** (1 mg intravenously) may restore conduction and increase heart rate, especially in inferior infarctions. If this fails, an infusion of a positive chronotropic agent such as **isoproterenol** (or use of a **transcutaneous electronic pacemaker**) increases heart rate. These therapies are directed at maintaining heart rate until **temporary transvenous pacemaking** can be performed.

(ii) In cases of severe left ventricular dysfunction, atrial systole must be preserved to maintain cardiac output, and **AV sequential pacemaking** is the preferred treatment.

(iii) The occurrence of new **bundle branch block**—particularly the combination of right bundle branch block and left anterior hemiblock—may be an indication for **temporary prophylactic pacemaking** because these disturbances may presage the occurrence of complete heart block; however, this tactic is controversial and obviated by the availability of transcutaneous pacing.

(e) **Treatment of heart failure**

(i) Mild CHF in patients with MI can be treated with **diuretics.**

(ii) The use of **digitalis** during acute MI is safe but of limited efficacy.

(iii) In more advanced cases of CHF, **vasodilators** may be useful in reducing cardiac afterload, allowing increased cardiac output.

(f) **Treatment of cardiogenic shock.** Shock in the presence of MI usually is attributable to inadequate left ventricular filling, severe muscle damage, or a mechanical complication of the MI. When shock ensues, an **echocardiogram** is performed to assess ventricular function, and a **Swan-Ganz catheter** should be placed to measure left ventricular filling pressure.

(i) If the pulmonary capillary wedge pressure is less than 18 mm Hg, **volume is infused to maximize left ventricular filling** and cardiac output. In addition, if a new cardiac murmur is detected, the echocardiogram and the Swan-Ganz catheter are useful in making the diagnosis of acute mitral regurgitation or acute ventricular septal defect.

(ii) Alternatively, if cardiogenic shock is caused by severe muscle damage, **pressor agents** (e.g., dobutamine, dopamine) and **intra-aortic balloon pumping** may be used to stabilize the patient until coronary arteriography and reestablishment of coronary blood flow by **PCTA** are carried out. However, the prognosis for such patients remains very poor despite therapy.

(g) **Treatment of mitral regurgitation and acute ventricular septal defect**

(i) **Arteriolar vasodilator therapy** to lower systemic vascular resistance is the mainstay of medical therapy for these complications. Reduction of systemic vascular resistance preferentially increases forward cardiac output and reduces nonproductive cardiac output, either into the left atrium (in the case of mitral regurgitation) or through the ventricular septal defect.

(ii) **Intra-aortic balloon pumping,** which also increases forward cardiac output and reduces nonproductive cardiac output, is useful in stabilizing patients with mitral regurgitation or acute ventricular septal defect, especially in hypotensive patients, where the use of vasodilators is contraindicated.

(iii) **Surgical correction of mechanical complications** often is required.

(h) **Adjunctive therapy**

(i) **β-Blockers** administered hours to days after MI reduce early mortality by reducing ventricular arrhythmias and the risk of reinfarction. Generally, however, these agents are avoided in patients with severe CHF, antecedent cardiac bradyarrhythmias, or bronchospasm. They are currently underutilized despite proven efficacy.

(ii) **ACE inhibitors.** Changes in the infarct zone and forces placed on the noninfarcted portion of the ventricle lead to ventricular dilation, which reduces ventricular efficiency. **Captopril** (and probably all ACE inhibitors) reduces the extent of remodeling and the incidence of late mortality.

(iii) **Anticoagulants.** In anterior infarction, especially an infarct involving the apex of the heart, there is a high risk of developing a mural thrombus, which can become a systemic embolus. Echocardiography should be performed during the first few days following anterior infarction. If a thrombus is detected, anticoagulation with heparin followed by oral administration of warfarin is indicated.

(iv) **Aspirin.** Administration of aspirin following acute MI reduces subsequent mortality. The dose is controversial, but 81 mg per day is recommended.

(v) **Diltiazem.** Postinfarction administration of diltiazem in patients with non-Q wave infarcts reduces mortality.

(vi) **Prevention.** In patients who have survived an MI, it is important to prevent subsequent infarctions. Administration of aspirin, ACE inhibitors, and β-blockers can reduce the risk of reinfarction [see III A 5 b (5) (h)]. In addition, modification of major risk factors (e.g., hypercholesterolemia, hypertension, and smoking) reduces the risk of a second MI.

c. **Sudden death** in patients with coronary artery disease is common; in fact, approximately one-third of patients with coronary disease experience sudden death without antecedent angina or MI.

(1) **Precipitating causes.** It is believed that most patients die of **acute ventricular arrhythmias** precipitated by ischemia. Although sudden death may be the result of an MI secondary to coronary artery disease, most patients who die suddenly and are resuscitated do not have an acute MI documented. It is likely that in these patients, ischemia produces heterogeneous depolarization of the ventricle, which leads to ventricular tachycardia and ventricular fibrillation.

(2) **Acute therapy**

(a) **Cardiopulmonary resuscitation** (i.e., mouth-to-mouth resuscitation and external chest compression) must be initiated in the euthermic patient within 4 minutes of the cessation of effective ventricular contraction to preserve neurologic and myocardial function. The mechanism by which closed chest compression causes circulation of blood is controversial. It may actually compress the heart, or the valves in the systemic veins may allow chest compression to produce a pressure gradient between the relatively low pressure in the extrathoracic veins and the relatively high pressure in the intrathoracic cavity, thereby creating forward cardiac flow.

(b) Electrical defibrillation and **drug support** should be provided as soon as possible.

(3) Preventive therapy. It is estimated that cardiac resuscitation of patients experiencing out-of-hospital cardiac arrest is fully successful in only 10%–20% of cases. The goal of preventive therapy, then, is to identify high-risk patients and prevent sudden death from occurring. Patients with the following conditions are recognized as being at high risk for an episode of sudden death.

(a) Previous sudden death. Patients who have experienced one episode of sudden death and have been successfully resuscitated have a 30%–50% chance of a second episode if the first episode occurred in the absence of an MI.

(i) In such patients, intensive diagnostic workup is indicated and should include **invasive electrophysiologic testing** and **intensive antiarrhythmic therapy** (see Table 1–1).

(ii) If medical antiarrhythmic therapy fails to control the arrhythmia, **surgical or catheter ablation of the arrhythmogenic area** of the myocardium may be effective.

(iii) An alternative to medical therapy is insertion of an **implantable defibrillator.** Electrode patches connect this device (usually implanted in the abdominal wall) with the heart. When a lethal arrhythmia is detected by the defibrillator, it automatically discharges a defibrillating electrical shock to the myocardium, thereby restoring effective cardiac contraction.

(b) Sustained ventricular tachycardia. The risk of sudden death is several times greater in patients with ventricular tachycardia on ECG than in patients without such abnormalities. Treatment of affected individuals is similar to therapy for sudden death.

(c) Prolonged Q-T intervals. Patients who demonstrate prolonged Q-T intervals on ECG are also at risk for sudden death. Prolonged Q-T syndromes may be congenital or acquired.

6. Prognosis. The prognosis of patients with coronary artery disease is determined primarily by three variables: age, the extent of coronary disease in terms of the **number of vessels affected** by the disease, and the **extent of left ventricular damage** present as a result of previous MIs.

a. Patients with uncorrected **main left coronary artery disease** have approximately a 20% mortality rate in the first year after its discovery.

b. Patients with **single-vessel coronary artery disease** have approximately a 2% annual mortality rate, those with **double-vessel disease** have approximately a 3%–4% annual mortality rate, and those with **triple-vessel disease** have approximately a 5%–8% annual mortality rate. Proximal anterior descending disease also increases risk.

c. The presence of significant **left ventricular dysfunction** (as identified by an ejection fraction of less than 40%) approximately doubles the yearly mortality rate at each level of extent of coronary disease.

d. Revascularization improves the prognosis for patients with main left coronary disease, for those with triple-vessel disease associated with left ventricular dysfunction, and for those with proximal left anterior descending disease.

B Nonatherosclerotic coronary artery disease Although the majority of cardiac ischemic events are caused by atherosclerotic coronary disease, nonatherosclerotic disease also may produce clinical ischemia.

1. **Coronary embolism** occurs in infective endocarditis, from mural thrombus formation following MI, and in the presence of atrial fibrillation. Coronary embolism frequently produces MI.
2. **Collagen vascular disease.** The collagen vascular diseases that affect medium-sized arteries, including the coronary arteries, are: **polyarteritis nodosa, Wegener's granulomatosis, systemic lupus erythematosus** (SLE), and, occasionally, **rheumatoid arthritis.**
3. **Radiation therapy.** Tumor irradiation, in which the field of radiation includes the heart, damages the coronary arteries and leads to nonatherosclerotic coronary artery disease.
4. **Transplantation.** The development of coronary disease following cardiac transplantation is a major factor in limiting the success of this therapy. Post-transplantation coronary disease tends to be distal in location and diffuse in nature. It is probably partially attributable to chronic rejection of the organ and is not closely related to the presence of the standard risk factors for coronary disease.

IV VALVULAR HEART DISEASE

A Aortic stenosis

1. Etiology
   a. **Congenital aortic stenosis** usually is detected in pediatric patients but occasionally becomes apparent in early adulthood.
   b. **Senile calcific aortic stenosis** occurs when scarring and calcification of a tricuspid aortic valve lead to orifice narrowing in the sixth, seventh, and eighth decades of life. While once considered a "degenerative" idiopathic disease, it is now clear that the pathology leading up to severe aortic stenosis has much in **common with coronary artery disease.** The initial valve lesion resembles the plaque of CAD, and both diseases hold the same risk factors in common. Indeed, early evidence suggests that the rate of progression of aortic stenosis can be slowed by administration of HMG Co-A reductase inhibitors (statins)
   c. **Bicuspid aortic valve** is a common congenital cardiac abnormality. The flow characteristics of the bicuspid valve are more turbulent than those of the normal valve, leading to valve injury, calcification, and stenosis in the fourth and fifth decades of life. The disease affecting these valves also appears similar to that of CAD.
   d. **Rheumatic aortic stenosis** never occurs alone and always is associated with mitral valve disease.
2. **Pathophysiology.** Aortic valve stenosis produces a pressure overload on the left ventricle due to the greater pressure that must be generated to force blood past the stenotic valve.
   a. As shown in Figure 1–12, obstruction to outflow causes the systolic pressure inside the left ventricle to be greater than in the aorta, producing a pressure gradient across the aortic valve.

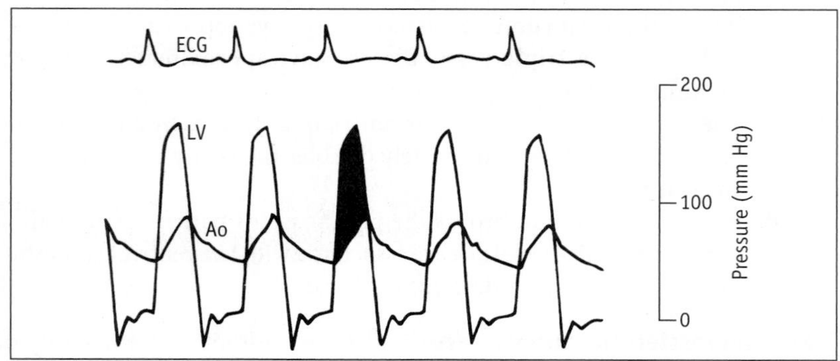

FIGURE 1–12 Diagram showing simultaneous recording of the electrocardiogram (*ECG*), left ventricular pressure tracing (*LV*), and aortic pressure tracing (*Ao*) in a patient with aortic stenosis. A large pressure gradient (*black area*) is evident. (Reprinted with permission from Grossman W: *Cardiac Catheterization and Angiography,* 2nd edition. Philadelphia, Lea & Febiger, 1980, p 128.)

The pressure overload produced by the disease leads to the development of concentric left ventricular hypertrophy.

b. Hypertrophy is a compensatory mechanism that reduces wall stress (afterload) on the left ventricle during systole. Thus, increased thickness of the ventricular wall as a result of concentric hypertrophy helps offset the increased pressure, which, in turn, reduces wall stress (the force each unit of myocardium must generate in order to shorten) (see I B 1 b).

3. Clinical features

a. Symptoms. Asymptomatic patients with aortic stenosis are at little risk for sudden death. However, this risk increases dramatically when symptoms develop.

(1) **Angina** occurs in 35%–50% of patients with aortic stenosis.

(a) Fifty percent of patients who develop this symptom die within 5 years of its onset unless aortic valve replacement is performed.

(b) Although the exact mechanism of angina is unknown, current data suggest that coronary blood flow reserve is impaired in the severely hypertrophied left ventricle. Impairment of the coronary blood flow reserve limits oxygen delivery to the myocardium and produces angina during exercise.

(2) **Syncope** occurs during exercise when total peripheral resistance falls due to local autoregulatory mechanisms [see IX B, C 1 b (2) (b)]. When aortic stenosis is present, cardiac output across the stenotic aortic valve cannot increase during exercise. Because total peripheral resistance falls, blood pressure must also fall, and syncope occurs.

(a) **Other causes** of syncope in aortic stenosis include a reflex vasodepressor response to high intraventricular pressure, **atrial** or **ventricular arrhythmias,** and **heart block** as a result of conduction system calcification.

(b) After syncope occurs in patients with aortic stenosis, expected survival is 2–3 years without valve replacement.

(3) **Heart failure.** Fifty percent of patients who develop heart failure die within 1–2 years of presentation if the stenosis is not corrected. Heart failure occurs because the afterload placed on the myocardium becomes excessive and also because both contractile dysfunction and diastolic muscle dysfunction occur when the myocardium is exposed to a prolonged, severe pressure overload.

b. Physical signs

(1) **Delayed carotid upstroke.** In the presence of aortic stenosis, the carotid upstroke typically is delayed in timing and reduced in volume. This finding is the most reliable physical sign in gauging the severity of the disease.

(2) **Systolic ejection murmur.** A harsh, late-peaking systolic ejection murmur is heard in the aortic area and is transmitted to the carotid arteries. The murmur also may be reflected to the mitral area, producing the false impression that mitral regurgitation also is present **(Gallavardin's phenomenon).**

(3) **Soft, single S_2.** Because the aortic valve is stenotic, its motion is severely impaired. The reduction in motion of the valve causes the **aortic component (A_2)** of the S_2 to be absent. Thus, the only component of the S_2 that is heard is the **pulmonic component (P_2),** which is normally soft.

(4) **S_4.** An S_4 usually is heard as a result of the reduced left ventricular compliance that occurs in left ventricular hypertrophy.

(5) **Sustained, forceful apex beat.** The point of maximal cardiac impulse usually is not displaced unless heart failure has occurred; however, the impulse is sustained and forceful throughout systole.

4. Laboratory diagnosis

a. Electrocardiography. The ECG usually shows evidence of left ventricular hypertrophy.

b. Echocardiography can rule out significant aortic stenosis if valve motion is shown to be normal, but the standard echocardiogram generally cannot prove that severe aortic stenosis definitely is present. However, Doppler examination of the aortic outflow tract during echocardiography can accurately measure the pressure gradient across the aortic valve, more precisely defining the severity of the pressure overload produced by the stenotic valve.

c. **Cardiac catheterization.** Diagnosis and evaluation of the severity of aortic stenosis may be confirmed by cardiac catheterization, during which the pressure gradient across the valve is measured and the degree of stenosis is calculated.

5. **Therapy**
   a. **Palliative therapy**
      (1) **Medical therapy** has no definitive role in the treatment of aortic stenosis, but **digitalis** and **diuretics** may temporarily improve heart failure until mechanical relief of the obstruction is performed.
      (2) Insertion and inflation of a large balloon in the aortic valve orifice (**balloon valvuloplasty**) also may produce a moderate improvement in the amount of obstruction and in the symptoms, but relief using this technique is usually only temporary. It does not reduce the mortality expected if the disease is left untreated.
   b. **Curative therapy** requires **aortic valve replacement,** which may be performed using a preserved human homograft valve, a bioprosthetic heterograft valve, a mechanical valve, or a pulmonary autograft.
      (1) **Homograft valves.** The hemodynamic flow pattern is excellent, and patients with homograft valves do not require anticoagulation therapy. Availability of these valves is limited, because most suitable donors are also acceptable for whole heart donation in cardiac transplantation.
      (2) **Heterograft valves.** Patients with heterograft valves do not require anticoagulation therapy, but the durability of the valve is limited, and deterioration after 10 years is common.
      (3) **Mechanical valves.** Patients with mechanical valves do require anticoagulation therapy. However, these valves are more durable than bioprostheses.
      (4) **Autograft (Ross procedure).** In this procedure, the patient's normal pulmonary valve is transplanted into the aortic position, where it has excellent durability and longevity. A homograft is then inserted into the pulmonary position, where low pressure enhances homograft longevity. In practiced hands, the results of this procedure are excellent.

B Mitral stenosis

1. **Etiology.** Almost all cases of mitral stenosis in adults are **secondary to rheumatic heart disease.** Most cases occur in women.
2. **Pathophysiology**
   a. Mitral valve stenosis impedes left ventricular filling, thereby increasing left atrial pressure as a pressure gradient develops across the mitral valve. Elevated left atrial pressure is referred to the lungs, where it produces **pulmonary congestion.** As the stenosis becomes more severe, it may significantly reduce forward cardiac output.
   b. Because the right ventricle is responsible for filling the left ventricle, the burden of propelling blood across the stenotic mitral valve is borne by the right ventricle. The overload on the right ventricle may be increased further when secondary pulmonary vasoconstriction occurs. Thus, the right ventricle must generate enough force both to overcome the resistance offered by the stenotic valve and to propel blood through constricted pulmonary arteries. Consequently, pulmonary arterial pressure may increase to three to five times normal, eventually resulting in **right ventricular failure.**
3. **Clinical features**
   a. **Symptoms**
      (1) **Left-sided failure. Dyspnea on exertion, orthopnea,** and **paroxysmal nocturnal dyspnea** occur as a result of reduced left ventricular output and increased left atrial pressure.

In mitral stenosis, the symptoms of left ventricular failure usually are not attributable to left ventricular dysfunction but, rather, to the mitral stenosis itself.

(2) **Right-sided failure.** When pulmonary hypertension occurs, the right ventricle may fail, producing **edema, ascites, anorexia,** and **fatigue.**

(3) **Hemoptysis.** The high left atrial pressure produced in mitral stenosis may lead to rupture of small bronchial veins, producing hemoptysis.

(4) **Systemic embolism.** Stagnation of blood in the enlarged left atrium and left atrial appendage occurs in mitral stenosis, particularly if atrial fibrillation is present. Under these circumstances, a thrombus may form in the left atrium and can become a source of systemic embolism.

(5) **Hoarseness** may occur in mitral stenosis as the enlarged left atrium impinges on the left recurrent laryngeal nerve (Ortner's syndrome).

b. **Physical signs**

(1) **Atrial fibrillation.** Frequently, an irregularly irregular cardiac rhythm indicative of atrial fibrillation is present.

(2) **Pulmonary rales.** Bilateral pulmonary rales occur secondary to elevated left atrial and pulmonary venous pressures.

(3) **Increased intensity of the S_1.** The S_1 usually increases in intensity because the transmitral gradient limits spontaneous diastolic mitral valve closure. Thus, the mitral valve remains open until ventricular systole closes it forcibly, resulting in an increase in S_1 intensity. Late in the course of the disease, the valve may become so stenotic that it no longer opens or closes, reducing the intensity of S_1.

(4) **Increased intensity of the P_2** component of the S_2. The P_2 component of the S_2 is usually increased in intensity if pulmonary hypertension has developed.

(5) **Opening snap.** An **opening snap is heard following the S_2** as the stenotic valve is forced open in diastole by the high left atrial filling pressure. The higher the pressure, the sooner the mitral valve opens. Thus, a short interval (< 0.10 second in duration) indicates relatively high left atrial pressure and severe stenosis.

(6) **Diastolic rumble.** The murmur of mitral stenosis is a low-pitched apical rumble, which begins after the opening snap. If the patient is in sinus rhythm, atrial systole produces a presystolic accentuation of this murmur.

(7) **Sternal lift.** Enlargement of the right ventricle as a result of pulmonary hypertension produces a systolic lift of the sternum.

(8) **Other symptoms. Neck vein distention, edema, hepatic enlargement,** and **ascites** may be present if right ventricular failure occurs.

4. **Laboratory diagnosis**

a. **Electrocardiography.** The ECG may show atrial fibrillation as well as signs of left atrial enlargement and right ventricular hypertrophy.

b. **Chest radiography**

(1) Straightening of the left heart border and a double density along the right heart border (formed by the right and left atria) occur as a result of left atrial enlargement.

(2) Signs of pulmonary venous hypertension, including an increase in pulmonary vascular markings and **Kerley's lines,** are likely to be present.

(3) When **pulmonary hypertension** leads to right ventricular enlargement, the lateral view shows a **loss of the retrosternal airspace.**

c. **Echocardiography** usually provides excellent images of the mitral valve.

(1) The echocardiogram shows reduction in the excursion of the valve leaflets and thickening of the valve. Two-dimensional echocardiography can be used to visualize and measure the residual mitral valve orifice. Invariably, left atrial enlargement is present.

(2) Doppler examination of the mitral valve may also help to quantify the severity of the stenosis.

5. **Therapy**
   a. **Medical therapy** is reserved for patients with mild-to-moderate symptoms of left-sided failure.
      (1) **Diuretics.** The mainstay of treatment, these agents are used to **control pulmonary congestion** and to **limit dyspnea and orthopnea.**
      (2) **Digitalis.** Because left ventricular muscle function usually is normal in mitral stenosis, the use of digitalis is of little benefit to patients in sinus rhythm. In patients in **atrial fibrillation,** however, digitalis is used to slow ventricular rate. A rapid ventricular rate in mitral stenosis shortens diastole, thereby reducing left ventricular filling, which, in turn, further increases left atrial pressure and reduces cardiac output. **β-Blockers** and **diltiazem** or **verapamil** may be added to digoxin if further heart rate control is necessary.
      (3) **Anticoagulants.** Patients with mitral stenosis and coexistent atrial fibrillation have a **high incidence of systemic embolism.** In such patients, anticoagulation therapy (e.g., with **warfarin**) usually is indicated.
   b. **Balloon valvuloplasty.** Unlike balloon valvuloplasty for aortic stenosis, balloon valvuloplasty for mitral stenosis can offer effective long-term improvement. The best candidates for balloon mitral valvuloplasty are those in sinus rhythm with relatively mild mitral regurgitation and mild-to-moderate thickening of the mitral valve leaflets.
      (1) Valvuloplasty for mitral stenosis produces a commissurotomy similar to that produced at open heart surgery. During balloon mitral valvuloplasty, transseptal catheterization of the interatrial septum is performed, allowing passage of the balloon catheter from right atrium to left atrium. From the left atrium, the balloon catheter is advanced to the mitral valve and inflated.
      (2) Although long-term follow-up data are still being gathered, it is likely that this technique will be as effective as surgery in reducing symptoms and prolonging life.
   c. **Surgical therapy** is effective in relieving the symptoms of mitral stenosis and in prolonging life in symptomatic patients. Surgery should be performed prior to the development of pulmonary hypertension, which increases surgical risk. However, if pulmonary hypertension is present and surgery is successful, pulmonary hypertension usually regresses postoperatively.
      (1) **Mitral commissurotomy.** In young patients without significant valvular calcification or mitral regurgitation, commissurotomy allows relief of the stenosis without valve replacement.
      (2) **Mitral valve replacement.** If commissurotomy cannot be performed, valve replacement relieves the stenosis and the symptoms.

C Aortic regurgitation

1. **Etiology**
   a. **Idiopathic aortic root dilatation.** Aortic root dilatation, a common cause of aortic regurgitation, occurs more frequently in patients with hypertension but correlates best with increasing age. It is also seen more frequently in patients with bicuspid aortic valves.
   b. **Rheumatic heart disease.** Aortic insufficiency usually is present to some degree in most cases of rheumatic heart disease. Mitral stenosis usually predominates, but occasionally aortic insufficiency is the most severe manifestation of rheumatic heart disease.
   c. **Infective endocarditis.** Infection of the aortic valve may lead to **perforation or partial destruction of one or more aortic leaflets,** producing aortic insufficiency.
   d. **Marfan syndrome** may produce aortic insufficiency in two ways.
      (1) **Proximal root dilatation.** The extreme expansion of the proximal aortic root seen in Marfan syndrome may produce aortic insufficiency.
      (2) **Aortic root dissection.** The advanced cystic medial necrosis present in Marfan syndrome may lead to an intimal tear and dissection of the aorta. If the dissection involves the proximal aortic root, the supporting structures of the aortic valve are disrupted, and the valve is rendered incompetent.

e. **Aortic dissection.** Any cause of aortic dissection other than Marfan syndrome may lead to aortic insufficiency.

f. **Syphilis** may produce **aortitis,** which may extend to the aortic valve and produce aortic incompetence.

g. **Collagen vascular disease.** Systemic lupus erythematosus (SLE) and ankylosing spondylitis may cause aortic insufficiency.

2. **Pathophysiology**

a. A portion of the left ventricular stroke volume ejected during systole regurgitates into the left ventricle during diastole. If no compensation occurs, left ventricular forward output decreases. However, chronic regurgitation of blood into the left ventricle stimulates sarcomere replication in series, producing eccentric cardiac hypertrophy and an increase in end-diastolic volume. Because the stroke volume equals the end-diastolic volume minus the end-systolic volume, the total stroke volume increases, helping to compensate for the volume that is regurgitated. The increase in total stroke volume leads to an increase in pulse pressure and increased systolic pressure. The additional development of concentric hypertrophy compensates this second type of overload. **The additional volume and pressure that the left ventricle must generate eventually lead to left ventricular dysfunction and CHF.**

b. An additional pathophysiologic consequence of aortic insufficiency is a **reduction in systemic diastolic blood pressure.**

3. **Clinical features**

a. **Symptoms**

(1) **Left ventricular failure**

(a) **Chronic aortic insufficiency** may cause left ventricular dysfunction, leading to symptoms of **dyspnea, orthopnea,** and **paroxysmal nocturnal dyspnea.**

(b) In **acute aortic insufficiency,** normal muscle function may coexist with heart failure. In this circumstance, reduced forward output and elevated left ventricular filling pressure occur prior to **compensatory left ventricular enlargement.**

(2) **Syncope.** Reduction in diastolic systemic arterial pressure produces a reduction in mean arterial pressure. If the mean arterial pressure is reduced significantly, cerebral perfusion is compromised, and syncope may occur.

(3) **Angina** occurs less commonly in aortic insufficiency than in aortic stenosis. The cause of angina in aortic insufficiency is **reduced coronary blood flow.** Coronary blood flow occurs primarily in diastole and is driven by the aortic diastolic blood pressure. This driving pressure is reduced in aortic insufficiency, in turn reducing coronary blood flow.

b. **Physical signs**

(1) **Left ventricular impulse.** The PMI is **hyperdynamic** and is **displaced downward and to the left** as a result of left ventricular enlargement.

(2) **Diastolic murmur.** The murmur of aortic insufficiency is a **high-pitched, diastolic blowing murmur** heard along the left sternal border. Often the murmur is heard best when the patient is sitting up and leaning forward.

(3) **Austin Flint murmur.** A **low-pitched diastolic rumble** similar to that heard in mitral stenosis may be present in patients with aortic insufficiency. The Austin Flint murmur **usually indicates moderate-to-severe insufficiency.** The murmur is believed to be caused by reverberation of the regurgitant flow against the mitral valve, although the exact mechanism is unclear.

(4) **Total stroke volume** and consequently, **pulse pressure, increases** in chronic aortic insufficiency, because of the following relationship:

$$\text{Pulse pressure} = \frac{\text{stroke volume}}{\text{aortic elasticity}}$$

The increased stroke volume and pulse pressure lead to many physical signs, some of which are listed below. These signs are usually absent in *acute* aortic insufficiency because compensatory increases in end-diastolic volume and stroke volume have not yet occurred. In fact, the clinical picture of acute severe aortic insufficiency is remarkably bland. The apical impulse is not enlarged. S_1 is soft because increased left ventricular end diastolic pressure closes the mitral valve before systole. This finding marks a poor prognosis for patients treated without valve replacement. When acute aortic insufficiency is suspected, blood cultures and echocardiography are essential in making the diagnosis. Transthoracic echocardiography usually is performed first, and, if unrevealing, is followed by more sensitive transesophageal echocardiography.

(a) **Corrigan's pulse.** The carotid pulse has a rapid rise and full upstroke with a rapid fall in diastole.

(b) **Hill's sign** refers to a disproportionate increase of systolic blood pressure (i.e., > 30 mm Hg) when measured in the leg, as compared with the systolic blood pressure measured in the arm. This sign suggests severe aortic insufficiency.

(c) **Pistol-shot femoral pulses.** Auscultation over the femoral arteries reveals a pulse that sounds like a pistol shot.

(d) **Duroziez's sign.** A stethoscope is placed over the femoral artery with enough pressure to produce a systolic bruit. The concomitant occurrence of a diastolic bruit constitutes Duroziez's sign.

(e) **de Musset's sign** refers to a bobbing movement of the head caused by the increased stroke volume and pulse pressure.

(f) **Quincke's pulse** is systolic blushing and diastolic blanching of the nail bed when gentle pressure is placed on the nail.

4. **Diagnosis**
   a. **Electrocardiography.** The ECG usually shows left ventricular hypertrophy. In endocarditis, a prolonged P-R interval may indicate abscess formation involving the conduction system.
   b. **Chest radiography.** Unless the aortic insufficiency is mild or acute, **cardiac enlargement** is usually present, and often, the proximal aorta is dilated. The absence of cardiac enlargement is evidence against the diagnosis of severe chronic aortic insufficiency.
   c. **Echocardiography.** Evidence of an enlarged left ventricular cavity is usually present in aortic insufficiency. Frequently, diastolic vibration of the mitral valve, produced by the regurgitant flow striking the valve, is present. Doppler examination of the aortic outflow tract reveals abnormal diastolic flow from the aorta to the left ventricle.
   d. **Cardiac catheterization.** Aortography is performed during cardiac catheterization. Contrast material is injected into the aorta, and the amount that regurgitates into the left ventricle is analyzed qualitatively. The regurgitant volume also can be calculated.

5. **Therapy.** If aortic insufficiency is severe, eventual **aortic valve replacement** is necessary.
   a. Timing of surgery is difficult, however, because the lesion may be tolerated for several years. Careful follow-up is required to detect early signs of decompensation; at this time, valve replacement is advisable. In most cases, valve replacement should be performed before the left ventricular echocardiographic end-systolic dimension exceeds 55 mm and the ejection fraction falls below 55%.
   b. If surgery is not possible, therapy with **digitalis, diuretics,** and **vasodilators may afford symptomatic relief.**

D Mitral regurgitation

1. **Etiology**
   a. **Mitral valve prolapse and click-murmur syndrome** are terms that describe a common group of diseases in which the mitral valve or chordae are redundant, permitting systolic prolapse of the mitral valve into the left atrium with resultant mitral regurgitation.

(1) This syndrome usually is benign, but in some cases it may be associated with significant mitral regurgitation. Additional complications include atypical chest pain, cardiac arrhythmias, and an increased risk of embolic stroke. Most clinically important sequelae occur in those patients whose mitral valves are clearly thickened and echocardiographically abnormal.

(2) A midsystolic click and a late systolic murmur typically are heard on physical examination.

b. Coronary artery disease may lead to ischemia or infarction of the papillary muscles to which the mitral valve is tethered, thereby producing mitral incompetence.

c. Rheumatic heart disease. Scarring and retraction of the mitral leaflets as a result of rheumatic heart disease causes mitral regurgitation.

d. Ruptured chordae tendineae. Spontaneous rupture of the chordae tendineae may occur in otherwise healthy individuals. Chordal rupture permits prolapse of a portion of a mitral valve leaflet into the left atrium, rendering the valve incompetent.

e. Infective endocarditis. Infection of the mitral valve may cause its destruction with subsequent regurgitation.

2. Pathophysiology. Mitral regurgitation permits a portion of the left ventricular stroke volume to be pumped backward into the left atrium instead of forward into the aorta, resulting in **increased left atrial pressure and decreased forward cardiac output.** Preload is increased by the volume overload, and afterload is initially decreased as the left ventricle empties a portion of its contents into the relatively (i.e., compared with the aorta) low-pressure left atrium. This augments ejection performance and helps compensate for the regurgitation.

a. Initially, compliance of the left atrium is low, and the regurgitant volume produces high left atrial pressure with resultant congestive symptoms.

b. With time, the left atrial compliance and volume increase, allowing accommodation of the regurgitant volume at more physiologic filling pressures.

c. The development of left ventricular eccentric cardiac hypertrophy restores forward stroke volume.

d. After a prolonged period of compensation, left ventricular muscle dysfunction eventually occurs, resulting in a fall in ejection fraction from supranormal to normal or even subnormal values.

3. Clinical features

a. Symptoms. Characteristics include those of left ventricular failure (i.e., **dyspnea, orthopnea,** and **paroxysmal nocturnal dyspnea**).

(1) If mitral regurgitation is severe and chronic, **pulmonary hypertension** and **symptoms of right-sided failure** also may occur.

(2) Patients in atrial fibrillation may experience **symptoms of systemic embolization.** The risk of embolization appears to be less in patients with mitral regurgitation than in those with mitral stenosis, although this is debatable.

b. Physical signs

(1) **Left ventricular impulse.** As with aortic regurgitation, the PMI is hyperdynamic and displaced downward and to the left.

(2) **Murmur.** The murmur of mitral regurgitation is a holosystolic apical murmur that radiates to the axilla and frequently is **accompanied by a thrill.** It does not vary in intensity with variation in R-R interval.

(3) An S_3 usually is heard in mitral regurgitation and may occur even in the absence of overt heart failure. The S_3 is caused by the rapid filling of the left ventricle by the large volume of blood accumulated in the left atrium during systole.

4. Diagnosis

a. Electrocardiography. The ECG shows signs of left ventricular hypertrophy and left atrial enlargement.

b. Chest radiography shows cardiac enlargement. Vascular congestion indicates heart failure.

c. **Echocardiography**
   (1) In cases of a **ruptured chorda** or **mitral valve prolapse,** the mitral valve can be seen extending into the left atrium during systole.
   (2) When the mitral valve has been damaged by **endocarditis,** vegetations on the mitral leaflets frequently are demonstrated. Transesophageal echocardiography is better than transthoracic echocardiography for detecting vegetations.
   (3) Regardless of the cause of the mitral regurgitation, **left atrial** and **left ventricular enlargement occur** if the condition is both chronic and severe.
   (4) Doppler examination reveals abnormal systolic flow from the left ventricle into the left atrium.

d. **Cardiac catheterization.** Right-heart catheterization yields a **pulmonary capillary wedge tracing** that often displays a **large v wave** representative of the systolic volume overload on the left atrium. **Left ventriculography** demonstrates systolic regurgitation of contrast material into the left atrium.

5. **Therapy**
   a. **Medical treatment.** The goal of medical therapy is to relieve symptoms by increasing forward cardiac output and reducing pulmonary venous hypertension.
      (1) **Digitalis.** When atrial fibrillation occurs, digitalis is useful in controlling heart rate. In chronic mitral regurgitation with muscle dysfunction, this agent may be useful in increasing the inotropic state. In cases of acute mitral regurgitation when no inotropic deficit exists, it is not indicated.
      (2) **Diuretics** are used to reduce central volume overload, which in turn reduces pulmonary venous hypertension and congestion.
      (3) **Vasodilators.** Arteriolar vasodilators are **particularly useful** in managing acute mitral regurgitation. These agents **reduce resistance to aortic outflow,** thereby preferentially increasing forward output while reducing the amount of regurgitation. Vasodilators also **reduce left ventricular size,** which helps to reestablish mitral competence.
      (4) **Anticoagulants.** Patients with mitral regurgitation and atrial fibrillation are at some risk for systemic embolism; thus, anticoagulants usually are indicated.
   b. **Surgical treatment.** Mitral valve replacement or repair is indicated for chronic mitral regurgitation, even if symptoms are mild, if there is evidence of ventricular dysfunction.
      (1) **Valve replacement** must be performed prior to the onset of significant muscle dysfunction, which limits the success of operative intervention. To help ensure preservation of ventricular function, surgery should occur before the ejection fraction falls below 60% or the end-systolic dimension exceeds 45 mm.
      (2) **Valve repair** offers several advantages over replacement, including eliminating the introduction of a prosthesis and decreasing the need for anticoagulation therapy. Furthermore, repairing rather than replacing, the valve helps preserve left ventricular function because the mitral valve apparatus, which plays an important role in ventricular contraction is preserved.

E Tricuspid regurgitation

1. **Etiology**
   a. **Infective endocarditis.** In drug abusers who inject drugs under septic conditions, infective endocarditis is a common cause of tricuspid regurgitation.
   b. **Right ventricular failure.** Sustained pressure or volume overload on the right ventricle leads to right ventricular dilatation and improper alignment of the papillary muscles, which produces tricuspid regurgitation.
   c. **Rheumatic heart disease.** In rheumatic heart disease, tricuspid regurgitation may occur, secondary to right ventricular pressure overload from left-sided valvular lesions. Tricuspid regurgitation also may occur as a result of primary rheumatic involvement of the tricuspid valve.

2. **Pathophysiology.** During systole, the dysfunctioning tricuspid valve allows blood to flow backward into the right atrium, leading to systemic venous congestion and venous hypertension.
3. **Clinical features**
   a. **Symptoms.** Right-sided failure (i.e., **edema, ascites**) occurs. In severe and acute cases, **hepatic congestion** may be extensive enough to produce **right upper quadrant pain.** Passive hepatic congestion also may lead to hepatocellular damage and **jaundice.**
   b. **Physical signs**
      (1) **Right ventricular lift.** The enlarged right ventricle may be palpated as a systolic lift of the sternum.
      (2) **Murmur.** A holosystolic murmur that increases with inspiration is heard along the left sternal border.
      (3) **Jugular venous pulsation.** A large **v wave** is seen in jugular veins during systole.
      (4) **Pulsatile liver.** Systolic expansion of the liver frequently is present.
4. **Diagnosis**
   a. **Chest radiography** shows right ventricular enlargement as an obliteration of the retrosternal airspace on the lateral view.
   b. **Echocardiography** demonstrates enlargement of the right atrium and right ventricle. Doppler examination is highly effective in demonstrating tricuspid regurgitation.
5. **Therapy.** Left-sided failure frequently is the cause of right-sided failure and tricuspid regurgitation. Effective treatment of left-sided failure reduces right ventricular pressure overload, which may decrease right ventricular size, thus restoring valvular competence. If tricuspid regurgitation is caused by organic valvular disease, surgical repair or replacement of the tricuspid valve may be necessary.

V CARDIOMYOPATHIES

A Dilated (congestive) cardiomyopathy

1. **Definition.** Dilated cardiomyopathy is defined as a diminution in the contractile function of the left, right, or both ventricles in the absence of pressure overload, volume overload, or coronary artery disease. The loss of cardiac muscle function results in CHF.
2. **Etiology.** The cause of most cases of dilated cardiomyopathy is unknown. Viral infection has been implicated in the pathogenesis of this disease, but proof of cause generally is lacking. The following other conditions have been linked to cardiomyopathy.
   a. **Prolonged ethanol abuse** is the most common reversible cause of cardiomyopathy.
   b. **Doxorubicin therapy.** High doses of doxorubicin, a commonly used antitumor drug, may result in irreversible dilated cardiomyopathy.
   c. **Exposure to mercury, lead,** or **high-dose catecholamines** may cause myocardial damage and dilated cardiomyopathy.
   d. **Endocrinopathies,** including **thyrotoxicosis, hypothyroidism,** and **acromegaly,** have been reported to cause dilated cardiomyopathy. In thyrotoxicosis and in hypothyroidism, the myopathy usually is reversed when the endocrinopathy is corrected.
   e. **Metabolic disorders** (e.g., **hypophosphatemia, hypocalcemia, thiamin deficiency**) may produce reversible cardiomyopathy.
   f. **Hemoglobinopathies** (e.g., **sickle cell anemia, thalassemia**) are associated with myocardial dysfunction.
   g. **Genetic abnormalities.** In some families, the development of dilated cardiomyopathy is linked to specific genetic abnormalities.
   h. **Prolonged tachycardia** (persisting for weeks or months) may result from uncontrolled atrial arrhythmias, causing a dilated cardiomyopathy that may be reversed within weeks, after heart rate is controlled.

3. **Clinical features**
   a. **Symptoms** of dilated cardiomyopathy are those of both left- and right-sided CHF as described in I D 1.
      (1) Generally, the symptoms of left-sided failure (i.e., **orthopnea, paroxysmal nocturnal dyspnea,** and **dyspnea on exertion**) precede those of right-sided failure.
      (2) **Chest pain** may occur in the absence of obstructive coronary disease. The cause of the chest pain may be the excessive oxygen demands of an enlarged, thin-walled ventricle with high wall stress.
   b. **Physical signs** in dilated cardiomyopathy are those of CHF. A gallop rhythm is usually present. The murmur of mitral regurgitation also may be present. Mitral regurgitation occurs as a result of ventricular dilatation and improper alignment of the papillary muscles.
4. **Diagnosis**
   a. **Electrocardiography** reveals frequent left ventricular hypertrophy and nonspecific S-T–and T-wave abnormalities. Left bundle branch block is common.
   b. **Chest radiography** shows an enlarged heart, and there is evidence of pulmonary vascular congestion.
   c. **Echocardiography** reveals dilated and poorly contracting left and right ventricles. In addition, secondary left and right atrial enlargement usually is seen.
   d. **Gated blood pool scanning** in dilated cardiomyopathy reveals reduction of the ejection fraction of both ventricles. There usually is global dysfunction, but regional contractile abnormalities also may exist.
   e. **Cardiac catheterization** usually is not necessary to make the diagnosis of dilated cardiomyopathy. However, because surgical correction of ischemic heart disease can occasionally improve left ventricular function, ischemic heart disease should be excluded prior to making the diagnosis of cardiomyopathy. In such cases, cardiac catheterization may be indicated.
5. **Therapy**
   a. **Removal of an offending agent.** The most hopeful situation is one in which incessant tachycardia or a known toxin has caused ventricular dysfunction. Heart rate control or removal of the toxin from the patient's environment may lead to significant improvement in ventricular function.
   b. **Supportive therapy.** When dilated cardiomyopathy is idiopathic, the symptoms of CHF can be improved by such measures as **salt restriction** and **administration of cardiac glycosides, diuretics, vasodilators,** and **neurohumoral blockers.** Evidence shows that the addition of ACE inhibitors to a standard regimen of diuretics increases longevity. Gradual introduction of β-blockers also prolongs life.
   c. **Cardiac transplantation.** Cardiac transplantation may offer an improved quality of life to selected patients when control of CHF is not possible and prognosis is poor.

B Hypertrophic obstructive cardiomyopathy

1. **Definition.** Hypertrophic obstructive cardiomyopathy, which previously was referred to as **idiopathic hypertrophic subaortic stenosis** or **asymmetric septal hypertrophy,** is a disorder in which the interventricular septum hypertrophies excessively. The hypertrophied septum and the anterior leaflet of the mitral valve produce left ventricular outflow obstruction.
2. **Etiology.** Most cases are inherited through an autosomal dominant mode of transmission, but sporadic cases also occur. Specific abnormalities in the genes coding for cardiac myosin and other cardiac proteins have been identified.
3. **Pathophysiology**
   a. **Methods of obstruction** include the following:
      (1) As shown in Figure 1–13, the hypertrophied septum encroaches on the left ventricular outflow tract and comes into close approximation with the anterior leaflet of the mitral valve.

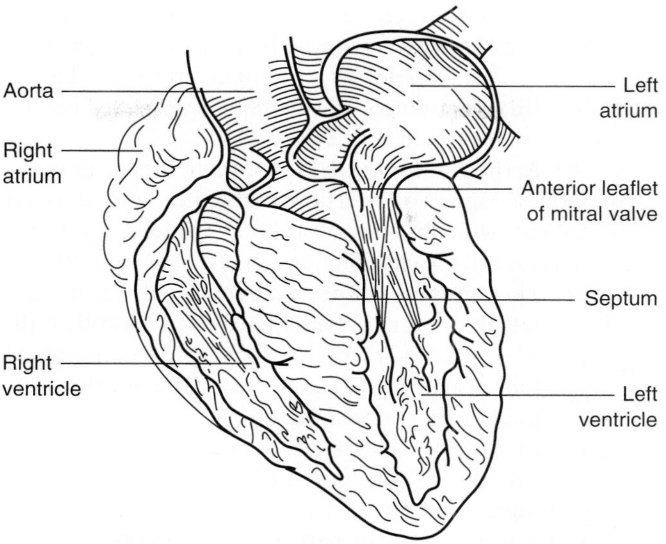

FIGURE 1–13 Cardiac cross-section cut from the apex to the base in a patient with hypertrophic obstructive cardiomyopathy. The upper portion of the septum is thickened and comes into close proximity with the anterior leaflet of the mitral valve. (Adapted from Johnson R, et al: *The Practice of Cardiology*. Boston, Little, Brown, 1980, p 648.)

(2) During systole, a low-pressure zone may develop as blood flow accelerates through the narrowed area between the septum and the anterior leaflet, generating a **Bernoulli effect.** Thus, the anterior leaflet of the mitral valve is drawn into the septum (systolic anterior motion), leading to outflow obstruction.

(3) The septum itself shortens very little during systole because of its catenoid shape. Because the septum does not shorten, it cannot thicken. Therefore, it is the anterior leaflet of the mitral valve that plays the active role in creating the obstruction.

b. The **degree of outflow obstruction** varies from patient to patient and from time to time in the same patient.

(1) Physiologic conditions that enlarge the left ventricle (e.g., increases in preload and afterload) separate the septum and anterior leaflet of the mitral valve and reduce the obstruction.

(2) Physiologic conditions that make the ventricle smaller or that increase the velocity of blood flow (e.g., dehydration, positive inotropic drugs) increase the degree of obstruction.

c. The obstruction to outflow may cause secondary cardiac hypertrophy of the nonseptal portions of the ventricle, but septal thickness generally remains greater than that of the free wall of the ventricle.

4. Clinical features

a. Symptoms

(1) **Angina.** Patients with obstructive cardiomyopathy frequently complain of chest pain.

(**a**) The pain usually has **atypical features;** that is, the pain may occur at rest and is not always related to exercise.

(**b**) The pathophysiology of angina in hypertrophic obstructive cardiomyopathy is unclear, but coronary blood flow is subnormal, potentially causing ischemia.

(2) **Syncope**

(**a**) Syncope usually occurs after exercise in patients with obstructive cardiomyopathy as a result of reduced left ventricular size and the consequent increased obstruction to outflow.

(i) After exercise, **afterload is reduced** because of peripheral vasodilatation.

(ii) **Preload is reduced** because of the decreased activity of the contractions of the leg muscles, which help to return blood to the heart.

(iii) The **inotropic state remains elevated** because of the increased catecholamine level after exercise.

(b) **Arrhythmias,** which are common in this disorder, also may precipitate syncope.

(3) **CHF.** Dyspnea on exertion, orthopnea, and paroxysmal nocturnal dyspnea occur in patients with obstructive cardiomyopathy. Systolic function usually is normal or supranormal and the ejection fraction often exceeds 80%.

(a) The symptoms of heart failure usually are not caused by systolic malfunction, but rather, occur as a result of increased diastolic stiffness.

(b) The thickened myocardium requires an increased filling pressure for adequate diastolic distention. The increased filling pressure is reflected to the lungs and produces pulmonary congestive symptoms.

(c) In the later stages of the disease, however, systolic dysfunction also may occur, contributing to the symptoms of CHF.

b. Physical signs

(1) **Carotid upstroke.** In patients with the obstructive form of the disease, the carotid upstrokes have a **spike and dome character** (Figure 1–14). This configuration indicates early systolic outflow followed by a period of obstruction, during which flow falls. The dome portion of the curve reflects the period near the end of systole when obstruction diminishes and aortic outflow again commences.

(2) **Murmur.** The murmur is a systolic ejection murmur, heard along the left sternal border. Unlike the murmur in valvular aortic stenosis, it does not usually radiate to the neck.

(a) **Increasing the intensity of the murmur**

(i) Maneuvers that diminish left ventricular size (e.g., the **Valsalva maneuver**) cause an increase in both the obstruction to outflow and the intensity of the cardiac murmur. Thus, the Valsalva maneuver, which diminishes the murmur in valvular aortic stenosis by diminishing flow, increases the murmur in obstructive cardiomyopathy by increasing obstruction.

(ii) Having the patient stand or inhale amyl nitrite also diminishes left ventricular size and therefore increases the intensity of the murmur.

(b) **Diminishing the intensity of the murmur. Squatting,** which increases myocardial afterload and venous return to the heart, increases cardiac size and, therefore, diminishes the murmur.

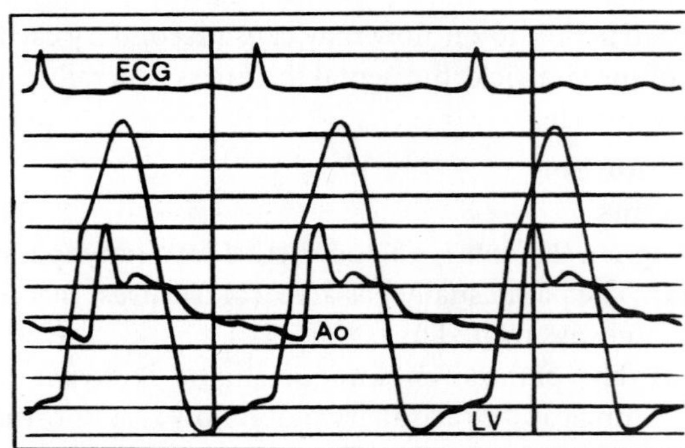

FIGURE 1–14 Diagram showing simultaneous recording of the electrocardiogram (*ECG*), left ventricular pressure tracing (*LV*), and aortic pressure tracing (*Ao*) in a patient with hypertrophic obstructive cardiomyopathy. A large pressure gradient exists between the left ventricle and aorta. The aortic pressure tracing (similar to the carotid pulse) demonstrates a spike and dome configuration. (Reprinted with permission from Cohn PF, Wynne J: *Diagnostic Methods in Clinical Cardiology*. Boston, Little, Brown, 1982, p 147.)

5. Diagnosis

a. **Electrocardiography** almost always is abnormal. The ECG usually shows evidence of left ventricular hypertrophy, nonspecific S-T–and T-wave abnormalities, and left atrial enlargement.

b. **Echocardiography** establishes the diagnosis in most patients.

(1) In patients with **asymmetric septal hypertrophy without obstruction,** increased septal thickness results in a **septum-to-free wall thickness ratio of 1.3:1** or greater.

(2) **Findings in the obstructive form** of the disease include **systolic anterior motion of the mitral valve, systolic fluttering of the aortic valve leaflets,** and **early closure of the aortic valve,** corresponding to the spike and dome seen in the carotid pulse.

c. **Cardiac catheterization** is performed in patients with obstructive cardiomyopathy to quantify the degree of obstruction prior to surgery and to assess coronary anatomy.

6. Therapy. Unlike aortic stenosis, in which relief of valvular obstruction relieves symptoms and prolongs life, there is no conclusive evidence that surgical relief of obstruction in obstructive cardiomyopathy prolongs life. Therefore, medical therapy is used first in an attempt to improve symptoms.

a. **Medical therapy**

(1) **β-Adrenergic blocking agents** (e.g., **propranolol**) are effective in relieving symptoms in this disease.

(a) β-blockade **slows the heart rate,** which increases left ventricular filling and size, diminishing obstruction.

(b) β-blockade also reduces the vigor of left ventricular contraction and, thus, **decreases the velocity of blood flow,** which also reduces the degree of obstruction.

(2) **Calcium channel blocking agents.** Although currently not approved for treatment of obstructive myopathy, rate-reducing calcium channel blockers have been shown to **diminish the left ventricular outflow gradient. Verapamil** is the calcium channel blocker most widely used in the treatment of this disease. Caution must be exercised in patients with CHF, because verapamil may worsen failure and precipitate acute pulmonary edema.

(3) **Digitalis** is **contraindicated in the hyperdynamic phase** of the disease when obstruction is present and the left ventricular cavity is small, because digitalis increases the vigor of left ventricular contraction and thus increases the outflow obstruction. In the end stages of the disease **when ventricular dilatation has occurred,** standard therapy for CHF (i.e., **digitalis** and **diuretics**) **may be beneficial.**

b. **Surgical therapy**

(1) **Myomectomy.** Surgical reduction of the thickness of the left ventricular septum relieves the outflow gradient and symptoms in those patients who have not responded to medical therapy.

(2) **Mitral valve replacement.** Because it is the anterior leaflet of the mitral valve that produces the obstruction, mitral valve replacement is also effective in relieving obstruction.

(3) **Pacemaker implantation.** Recent studies have shown that implantation of an AV sequential pacemaker can reduce outflow obstruction, probably by altering the sequence of septal contraction in relation to the rest of the ventricle. However, recent trials have not demonstrated long-term efficacy of this therapy.

(4) **Intentional septal infarction** (experimental). Transcatheter instillation of ethanol into the septal artery is performed to infarct the septum and reduce obstruction. This procedure shows promise.

c. **Antiarrhythmic therapy.** Most patients with hypertrophic myopathy die suddenly. Patients with a family history of sudden death or a personal history of syncope or ventricular tachycardia are at high risk and should undergo electrophysiologic testing. Many patients receive implantable defibrillators.

C Restrictive cardiomyopathy

1. **Definition.** The restrictive cardiomyopathies are a group of diseases in which the composition of the myocardium has changed so that it becomes stiffer. The **increased stiffness of the myocardium** restricts left ventricular filling, reducing stroke output and increasing left ventricular filling pressure.
2. **Etiology. Infiltrative diseases** of the myocardium, which produce restrictive cardiomyopathy, include **amyloidosis, hemochromatosis, idiopathic eosinophilia, carcinoid syndrome, sarcoidosis,** and **endomyocardial fibroelastosis.**
3. **Pathophysiology.** Systolic function usually is normal in the early stages of the disease, but the altered properties of the myocardium increase diastolic stiffness. Thus, the left ventricular pressure is above normal at any diastolic left ventricular volume. Increased filling pressure produces pulmonary congestion. As the infiltrative process progresses, systolic function also is compromised.
4. **Clinical features**
   a. **Symptoms of both left-sided and right-sided CHF** usually are present; the symptoms of right-sided failure are usually more prominent.
   b. **Physical signs** include those present in left-sided and right-sided CHF.
5. **Diagnosis**
   a. **Electrocardiography.** The ECG frequently shows low QRS voltages and nonspecific S-T– and T-wave abnormalities. Conduction abnormalities are common.
   b. **Radiographs.** Signs of pulmonary vascular congestion may coexist with normal heart size, because even when left ventricular systolic function fails in the later stages of the disease, the restriction to cardiac filling prevents cardiac dilatation.
   c. **Echocardiography**
      (1) The echocardiogram demonstrates thickening of the left and right ventricles. The combination of increased left ventricular thickness on the echocardiogram and decreased left ventricular voltage on the ECG is highly suggestive of restrictive cardiomyopathy.
      (2) Left and right ventricular chamber sizes usually are normal, whereas the left and right atria are increased in size.
      (3) In amyloidosis, the myocardium may appear brighter than normal.
   d. **Cardiac catheterization.** Often it is difficult to distinguish restrictive cardiomyopathy from constrictive pericarditis.
      (1) A **dip** and **plateau** in the left and right ventricular filling pressures may be seen in both diseases.
      (2) In restrictive cardiomyopathy, **left and right atrial pressures and left and right ventricular filling pressures** usually are **not identical,** as they are in constrictive pericarditis.
      (3) **Endomyocardial biopsy** during cardiac catheterization may help establish the diagnosis.
6. **Therapy.** Treatment for this group of diseases is limited.
   a. In cases with a **reversible etiology** (e.g., hemochromatosis), **direct therapy** such as iron chelation may result in improvement.
   b. When the cause of the disease cannot be treated, **symptomatic therapy with diuretics** to reduce the symptoms of congestion is indicated. **Vasodilators** must be used with caution because a reduction in preload causes a reduction in both left ventricular filling and cardiac output.

VI PERICARDIAL DISEASE

A Acute pericarditis

1. **Etiology**
   a. **Myocardial infarction (MI).** Pericarditis may occur in the first 24 hours following transmural MI, because the inflamed surface of the infarcted area of myocardium produces **pericardial irri-**

tation. A second type of pericarditis, called **Dressler's syndrome,** also may be seen from 1 week to several months after MI and may occur as the result of an autoimmune reaction to the damaged heart muscle. Pericarditis following infarction has become rare in the thrombolytic era.

b. **Viral infection.** Many cases of acute pericarditis have no known etiology. However, because **pericarditis frequently follows upper respiratory tract viral infections,** a viral etiology has been implicated.

c. **Collagen vascular disease.** Acute pericarditis may be a clinical manifestation of SLE, or, less commonly, scleroderma.

d. **Infectious pericarditis.** Tuberculosis, streptococcal infection, staphylococcal infection, and the sequelae of infective endocarditis all may produce pericarditis.

e. **Drugs.** Commonly used drugs that may cause acute pericarditis include **procainamide, hydralazine,** and **isoniazid.**

f. **Malignancy.** Pericarditis may occur secondary to metastatic involvement of the pericardium. **Pulmonary and breast carcinomas** are the most **common primary sites.**

g. **Uremia.** Pericarditis is common in untreated or undertreated severe chronic renal failure.

h. **Postpericardiotomy syndrome.** During open heart surgery, the pericardium is incised. Usually, the pericarditis that arises from this injury is short-lived; however, it may be protracted and severe in some patients.

i. **Radiation.** Radiation therapy delivered to the chest for thoracic malignancies may cause pericarditis.

2. **Clinical features**

a. **Symptoms.** The most common symptom in pericarditis is **inspiratory chest pain.**

(1) The pain is located in the left side and often is lessened when the patient sits up and leans forward.

(2) Occasionally, the pain may be similar to that of myocardial ischemia and may radiate to the neck and arm.

b. **Physical signs.** The **classic sign** of acute pericarditis is the **pericardial friction rub,** which is a scratchy, leathery sound heard during both systole and diastole. Atrial contraction may add a third component to the rub.

3. **Diagnosis**

a. **Physical examination.** The presence of a **pericardial friction rub** confirms the diagnosis of pericarditis.

b. **Electrocardiography.** Epicardial inflammation produces a diffuse current of injury with S-T segment elevation throughout the ECG. There is no reciprocal S-T segment depression, as is seen in acute MI. **Depression of the P-R segment is unique to pericarditis.**

c. **Echocardiography.** The echocardiogram frequently demonstrates a pericardial effusion, which helps confirm the diagnosis.

4. **Therapy**

a. **Specific therapy** should be directed toward the cause of the pericarditis, if the cause is known.

b. **Nonsteroidal anti-inflammatory drugs** (**NSAIDs**) such as **aspirin, indomethacin,** and **ibuprofen** usually are effective in reducing the inflammation and relieving the chest pain.

c. **Colchicine.** Intractable cases of pericarditis, as may occur with Dressler's syndrome and postpericardiotomy syndrome, may require glucocorticoid therapy for relief of symptoms. Recently, colchicine has replaced steroids at many centers.

B Pericardial effusion

1. **Pathophysiology.** The inflammation caused by acute pericarditis often produces exudation of fluid into the pericardial space. When fluid accumulates slowly, the pericardium expands to accommodate it, but when fluid accumulates rapidly, it compresses the heart, thus inhibiting cardiac filling. This latter condition is known as **cardiac tamponade** (see VI C).

2. **Clinical features**
   a. **Symptoms.** The mere presence of a pericardial effusion does not cause symptoms. However, symptoms of acute pericarditis may coexist with a pericardial effusion.
   b. **Physical signs.** As the effusion accumulates, it acts as a cushion around the heart.
      (1) The precordium becomes quiet, palpation of the PMI becomes difficult, and the heart tones become distant and soft.
      (2) Although the accumulation of fluid between the layers of pericardium may diminish a pericardial friction rub, a friction rub still may exist in the presence of a large effusion.

3. **Diagnosis**
   a. **Electrocardiography.** The ECG demonstrates low voltage; electrical alternans often is present.
   b. **Chest radiography.** Cardiac enlargement occurs as the effusion develops. Typically, the cardiac silhouette has a **"water bottle" appearance.** The presence of an extremely enlarged heart without signs of vascular congestion suggests the diagnosis of pericardial effusion.
   c. **Echocardiography.** An echocardiogram demonstrating an **echo-free space between the two layers of the pericardium** is diagnostic of a pericardial effusion.
   d. **Pericardiocentesis.** The presence of a pericardial effusion may be confirmed by the aspiration of fluid from the pericardial sac. Examination of the fluid helps establish the cause of the effusion.
      (1) The fluid should be sent for a cell count and differential, bacterial and fungal cultures, stains and cultures for *Mycobacterium tuberculosis,* protein content, and LDH content.
      (2) An additional aliquot of fluid should be centrifuged and examined for tumor cells.
      (3) Bloody effusions are characteristic of certain etiologies (e.g., neoplasia, tuberculosis). However, bloody effusions can also occur if the needle is passed too far and ventricular blood is aspirated by mistake. It is possible to distinguish the two because ventricular blood clots, whereas a bloody effusion does not.
   e. **Therapy.** Treatment for a pericardial effusion is the same as that for acute pericarditis, but also involves aspiration.

C Cardiac tamponade

1. **Definition and pathophysiology.** Cardiac tamponade is a **life-threatening condition** in which a pericardial effusion has developed so rapidly or has become so large that it compresses the heart.
   a. The heart cannot fill adequately, and because the heart can pump out only what it takes in, impaired filling causes a profound reduction in cardiac output.
   b. The external pressure produced by the fluid on the four chambers of the heart is dispersed equally. Because external pressure usually rises to a greater level than the normal cardiac filling pressures, intrapericardial pressure, left and right atrial pressures, and left and right ventricular pressures all become equal in diastole.

2. **Clinical features**
   a. **Symptoms.** Most patients with cardiac tamponade complain of **dyspnea, fatigue,** and **orthopnea.**
   b. **Physical signs**
      (1) **Pulsus paradoxus.** This finding, the normal fall in systolic blood pressure that occurs during inspiration, is exaggerated in tamponade. A pulsus paradoxus of more than 10 mm Hg occurs in 95% of patients with cardiac tamponade. The presence of pulsus paradoxus implies that stroke volume is falling during inspiration, probably as a result of the following mechanisms:
         (a) **Septal shift.** During inspiration, right ventricular filling is augmented by negative intrathoracic pressure, which increases venous return. This causes transient enlargement of the right ventricle and pushes the ventricular septum into the left ventricle, thus reducing the size and output of the left ventricle.

(b) **Tensing of the pericardium.** Inspiration produces downward traction on the pericardium, further compressing the cardiac structures and reducing left ventricular output.

(c) **Right ventricular enlargement.** The enhanced right ventricular filling during inspiration also distends the right ventricle, causing it to take up more room in the pericardial space. This further limits left ventricular filling.

(d) **Negative intrathoracic pressure.** During inspiration, the negative pressure inside the chest subtracts pressure from the extrathoracic vasculature, further reducing blood pressure.

(e) **Expansion of the pulmonary vascular bed.** The pulmonary vascular bed expands during inspiration, increasing its capacity and, thus, reduces left atrial filling.

(2) **Neck vein distention.** The intrapericardial pressure and right atrial pressure is reflected by extreme elevation of the jugular venous pressure. However, Kussmaul's sign (i.e., increased neck vein distention with inspiration) usually is absent in this condition.

(3) **Narrowed pulse pressure.** Reduction in left ventricular stroke volume leads to a reduction in systolic pressure; the tachycardia that usually occurs as a compensatory mechanism diminishes diastolic runoff and maintains diastolic pressure. Thus, pulse pressure is narrowed; however, less severe cases of cardiac tamponade may coexist with a normal pulse pressure.

(4) **Shock.** The carotid upstroke is diminished in volume, the systolic blood pressure is reduced, and the periphery is cold and clammy because of the vasoconstriction present in reduced cardiac output states.

3. **Diagnosis.** Elevated neck veins and pulsus paradoxus in a patient exhibiting symptoms of compromised cardiac output strongly suggest the diagnosis.
   a. A chest radiograph that shows an enlarged heart, together with an echocardiogram that confirms the presence of a pericardial effusion, increases the likelihood of tamponade if the cardinal clinical signs and symptoms are present.
   b. Cardiac catheterization, which would confirm that left and right atrial pressures are equal, further strengthens the diagnosis.

4. **Therapy.** The only effective therapy for cardiac tamponade is removal of fluid from the pericardial sac. Thus, **emergency pericardiocentesis** is indicated. The use of **pressor agents** and volume **expansion** is of limited benefit until pericardiocentesis can be performed.

D Constrictive pericarditis

1. **Definition.** Constrictive pericarditis is the diffuse thickening of the pericardium in reaction to prior inflammation, which results in reduced distensibility of the cardiac chambers. Cardiac output is limited, and filling pressures are increased to match the external constrictive force placed on the heart by the pericardium.

2. **Etiology.** Most conditions that cause acute pericarditis may lead to chronic constrictive pericarditis.

3. **Clinical features**
   a. **Symptoms.** The clinical picture typically is dominated by **symptoms of right-sided failure** rather than left-sided failure.
      (1) Most patients with constrictive pericarditis complain of **dyspnea on exertion** as a result of limited cardiac output. Although approximately 50% of patients complain of **orthopnea,** paroxysmal nocturnal dyspnea is rare.
      (2) Symptoms related to systemic venous hypertension frequently are reported and include **ascites, edema,** and **jaundice.**
   b. **Physical signs**
      (1) **Jugular venous distention.** The jugular veins are distended, indicating systemic venous hypertension. Neck vein distention increases with inspiration **(Kussmaul's sign).**

(2) **Heart sounds.** The heart sounds are distant. Early in diastole, a pericardial knock may be heard, which falls in the same cadence as an S_3 but is higher pitched.

(3) **Other signs of systemic venous hypertension. Ascites, edema, hepatic tenderness,** and **hepatomegaly** are frequently present. It is not uncommon for constriction to masquerade as end-stage liver disease.

4. **Diagnosis**
   a. **Electrocardiography.** The ECG shows low voltage in the limb leads. **Atrial arrhythmias** are common.
   b. **Chest radiography** reveals **pericardial calcification** in 50% of patients. This finding is seen as a **radiopaque ring around the heart** in the lateral view. The heart usually is normal in size, although cardiomegaly occasionally is noted.
   c. **Echocardiography.** Although pericardial thickening often can be detected, reliable diagnosis of constrictive pericarditis by echocardiography is difficult. However, Doppler interrogation of the mitral valve usually demonstrates an abnormal decrease in flow during inspiration.
   d. **Magnetic resonance imaging (MRI)** gated to the cardiac cycle is an imaging technique capable of measuring pericardial thickness.
   e. **Cardiac catheterization** reveals equal pressures in the four cardiac chambers during diastole; in addition, all pressures usually are elevated. A marked **Y descent** is present in the right atrial pressure tracing. Left and right ventricular pressure tracings demonstrate a characteristic **dip** and **plateau** or **"square root" sign.**

5. **Therapy.** Surgical removal of the pericardium is curative. However, immediate relief of constrictive symptoms may not occur for up to 6 weeks after **pericardiectomy.**

VII CONGENITAL HEART DISEASE IN THE ADULT

A Atrial septal defect

1. **Classification**
   a. An **ostium secundum atrial septal defect** occurs in the **midportion** of the intra-atrial septum and is caused by failure of the septum secundum to form properly.
   b. An **ostium primum atrial septal defect** results from improper septation of the endocardial cushion portion of the septum. It invariably involves the **mitral valve,** which is cleft and often regurgitant.
   c. A **sinus venosus–type atrial septal defect** occurs **high in the atrial septum** and frequently is associated with anomalous drainage of one or more of the pulmonary veins into the right atrium.
   d. **Holt-Oram syndrome** is characterized by the presence of a **secundum defect** together with **bony abnormalities of the forearms and hands.** This syndrome is a **hereditary** disease that is transmitted in an autosomal dominant fashion.

2. **Pathophysiology**
   a. Left and right atrial pressures usually are equal in atrial septal defect; thus, no pressure gradient exists between the atria. However, the increased thickness of the left ventricle as compared with the right ventricle makes the left ventricle less compliant and, therefore, harder to fill. Blood flow takes the path of least resistance and thus is shunted from the left atrium to the right atrium. The net effect is to increase the volume work of the right ventricle.
   b. The increased volume pumped through the pulmonary vasculature may lead to architectural changes in the pulmonary vasculature and to the development of irreversible pulmonary hypertension—a serious but rare complication.

3. **Clinical features**
   a. **Symptoms.** Patients with atrial septal defect may have a **prolonged symptom-free period.** Eventually, symptoms develop and may include **palpitations** as a result of atrial arrhythmias,

fatigue, dyspnea on exertion, orthopnea, frequent respiratory tract infections, and **symptoms of right ventricular failure.**

b. **Physical signs**

(1) **Wide and fixed splitting of the S_2 is the classic finding** in atrial septal defect. The increased cardiac flow through the right ventricle delays pulmonic valve closure, widening the normal splitting of the S_2. Inspiration produces relatively little change in right-sided flow, so there is little respiratory variation in the splitting of the S_2.

(2) **Murmur.** Under low pressure, blood flow from the left to the right atrium occurs through a wide aperture and produces no turbulence or murmur. However, the increased pulmonary blood flow in atrial septal defect produces a **systolic ejection murmur,** which is **heard in the pulmonic area.** The increased flow also may produce a **diastolic rumble across the tricuspid valve** if the left-to-right shunt ratio is greater than 3:1.

(3) **Neck vein distention, ascites,** and **edema** are indicative of right ventricular failure.

4. **Diagnosis**

a. **Electrocardiography.** In ostium secundum defects, incomplete right bundle block and right axis deviation are common findings. Ostium primum defects usually involve the anterior fascicle of the left bundle, producing left anterior hemiblock and left axis deviation.

b. **Chest radiography**

(1) Increased pulmonary blood flow produces increased pulmonary vascular markings in the lungs, which is called **shunt vascularity.**

(2) Right ventricular enlargement may encroach on the retrosternal airspace, reducing it in the lateral view.

(3) Enlargement of the pulmonary artery segment in the posteroanterior view also may be seen.

c. **Echocardiography**

(1) The echocardiogram shows enlargement of the right ventricle, and the atrial septal defect itself may be seen in many cases.

(2) A **saline injection,** which carries with it micro bubbles of air, shows a **negative-contrast image at the site** of the defect.

(3) **Doppler examination** of the interatrial septum demonstrates the abnormal presence of left-to-right blood flow across the septum.

d. **Cardiac catheterization**

(1) During cardiac catheterization, the diagnosis can be confirmed by passage of the catheter across the atrial septal defect.

(2) Left and right atrial pressures usually are equal.

(3) Oxygen samples drawn from the superior vena cava and right atrium demonstrate a **step-up in oxygen concentration** in the right atrium, as highly oxygenated left atrial blood is shunted into the right atrium. Oxygen saturations can be used to quantitate the magnitude of the left-to-right shunt.

5. **Therapy**

a. **Surgical correction,** which has a low operative mortality rate, is indicated for shunts with a pulmonary-to-systemic flow ratio of greater than 2:1, even in asymptomatic patients. Shunts of this magnitude may lead to the development of pulmonary hypertension, usually become symptomatic, and worsen with age.

b. Alternatively, several catheter-based devices for defect closure are under investigation.

B Ventricular septal defect

1. **Pathophysiology.** In ventricular septal defect, the left ventricle actively propels the blood into the right ventricle, resulting in the taxation of both ventricles and in increased pulmonary blood flow. Pulmonary hypertension is more severe and more frequent in ventricular septal defect than in atrial septal defect.

2. **Clinical features.** Because most ventricular septal defects lead to symptoms and are corrected in childhood, significant congenital ventricular septal defect rarely is diagnosed for the first time in adulthood.
   a. **Symptoms** of ventricular septal defect are those of both **left-** and **right-sided CHF.**
   b. **Physical signs**
      (1) **Displacement of the PMI** to the left is indicative of left ventricular enlargement.
      (2) **Sternal lift** is indicative of right ventricular enlargement.
      (3) **Murmur.** A **harsh, holosystolic murmur** is heard along the left sternal border. The murmur often is accompanied by a **thrill** and radiates to the right of the sternum.
      (4) **Aortic regurgitation.** Ventricular septal defects may involve the right coronary cusp of the aortic valve, producing insufficient support for this valve leaflet and, hence, aortic regurgitation. Approximately 6% of patients with ventricular septal defect have signs of aortic insufficiency.
3. **Diagnosis**
   a. **Electrocardiography.** The ECG typically shows **biventricular hypertrophy.**
   b. **Chest radiography.** Cardiac enlargement is the rule. If the shunt is greater than 2:1 in magnitude, **shunt vascularity** usually is present.
   c. **Echocardiography.** The septal defect frequently can be demonstrated during two-dimensional echocardiography. Left and right ventricular enlargement is seen as well. Doppler examination reveals abnormal blood flow from the left ventricle to the right ventricle.
   d. **Cardiac catheterization**
      (1) A left ventriculogram obtained in the left anterior oblique position demonstrates flow of contrast from the left ventricle across the septum into the right ventricle.
      (2) During cardiac catheterization, an **oxygen step-up** occurs at the level of the right ventricle. Pulmonary hypertension, if present, can be quantified.
4. **Therapy.** Because patients with ventricular septal defects are prone to pulmonary vascular complications and bacterial endocarditis, ventricular septal defects with a magnitude of 2:1 or greater should be corrected surgically.

C Patent ductus arteriosus

1. **Pathophysiology.** In patent ductus arteriosus, blood flows from the aorta into the pulmonary artery after the takeoff of the left subclavian artery. Volume overload is imposed on the left ventricle, which must pump blood into both the systemic and pulmonary circulations, and in time may lead to left ventricular failure. The increased pulmonary blood flow created by this lesion may lead to the development of pulmonary hypertension, imposing a pressure overload on the right ventricle.
2. **Physical signs**
   a. **Murmur.** Throughout the cardiac cycle, the vascular resistance and pressure in the pulmonary circuit are lower than the resistance and pressure in the aorta. Therefore, blood is shunted from left to right in both systole and diastole, and a **continuous murmur** with systolic and diastolic components is heard.
   b. **Pulses.** The presence of a low-pressure, low-resistance pathway allows for increased aortic runoff in diastole, which produces **bounding, full pulses** similar to those found in aortic insufficiency.
3. **Diagnosis**
   a. **Chest radiography** reveals an enlarged cardiac silhouette with the presence of shunt vascularity. In adults, the patent ductus may become calcified, rendering it visible on the chest radiograph.
   b. **Echocardiography** may reveal the patent ductus. Doppler interrogation detects abnormal flow of blood from the aorta to the pulmonary artery.

c. **Cardiac catheterization**
   (1) During cardiac catheterization, the catheter usually can be passed from the pulmonary artery into the descending aorta, confirming the presence of a patent ductus arteriosus.
   (2) **Oximetry** can be used to quantify the magnitude of the left-to-right shunt.
   (3) **Aortography** demonstrates the flow of contrast from the aorta through the patent ductus into the pulmonary artery.

4. **Therapy.** Surgical closure of the patent ductus is indicated in adults with a shunt ratio of greater than 2:1. Catheter techniques for ductus closure are under investigation.

D **Coarctation of the aorta** This defect is a stenosis of the aorta, usually at the site of the ductus arteriosus.

1. **Pathophysiology.** Coarctation of the aorta often leads to hypertension.
   a. If the stenosis is severe, it limits aortic blood flow distal to the constriction. Distal tissues are perfused by an extensive collateral arterial circulation.
   b. Whereas renal blood flow and renal function usually are normal in the adult with coarctation of the aorta, the kidneys still are perfused at a subnormal blood pressure.
   c. Some investigators have found elevated renin levels and activation of the renin–angiotensin system in adults with coarctation, which helps explain the hypertension.

2. **Clinical features.** If the coarctation does not cause heart failure due to pressure overload in childhood, it may not be detected until it manifests as hypertension in the adult.
   a. **Symptoms.** Patients with coarctation may complain of **headache, claudication,** and **leg fatigue.**
   b. **Physical signs**
      (1) **Blood pressure** determined in the arms usually is elevated, whereas pulses and blood pressure in the legs usually are reduced, representing the gradient across the coarctation.
      (2) **Habitus.** The upper body usually is well developed, whereas the legs occasionally appear underdeveloped.
      (3) **Murmur.** Typically, a **midsystolic** murmur is heard over the back. If the stenosis is severe, a continuous murmur may be heard. Continuous murmurs also may be heard diffusely over the chest cavity as the result of increased flow through collateral vessels.

3. **Diagnosis**
   a. **Electrocardiography.** The ECG shows left ventricular hypertrophy.
   b. **Chest radiography. Cardiac enlargement** usually is seen. Dilatation of the aorta proximal and distal to the coarctation with indentation at the site of the coarctation may cause the aorta to assume a **figure "3" appearance.** Dilatation of chest wall arteries forming the collateral pathways produces **rib notching.**
   c. **Cardiac catheterization.** During cardiac catheterization, the gradient across the coarctation can be measured. Aortography also allows visual demonstration of the coarctation.

4. **Therapy. Surgical correction** of the coarctation is standard therapy. **Percutaneous balloon aortoplasty** appears effective in some cases and is under investigation as an alternative to surgery.

5. **Complications. Hypertension, infective endocarditis, dissection of the thoracic aorta,** and **rupture of cerebral (berry) aneurysms** frequently are seen. Hypertension may persist even after the coarctation is repaired.

E **Ebstein's anomaly of the tricuspid valve**

1. **Pathophysiology.** In Ebstein's anomaly, the tricuspid valve is situated abnormally low in the right ventricle. Part of the tricuspid valve is tethered directly to the right ventricle. Thus, a portion of the right ventricle actually lies above the AV groove and is "atrialized," reducing the size of the right ventricle and usually resulting in **tricuspid regurgitation.** A **coexistent atrial septal defect** occurs in approximately 75% of cases.

2. **Clinical features**
   a. **Symptoms.** Depending on the degree of tricuspid regurgitation and whether an atrial septal defect exists, a patient's status may **range from asymptomatic to cyanotic.**
      (1) Dyspnea on exertion, peripheral edema, and other **symptoms of right ventricular failure** frequently are encountered.
      (2) Palpitations also are common in this anomaly, which is associated with **Wolff-Parkinson-White (WPW) syndrome** in approximately 10% of patients. WPW syndrome is characterized by abnormal ventricular conduction as the result of a congenital short circuit of the conducting system. Tachyarrhythmias are common.
   b. **Physical signs**
      (1) **Tricuspid regurgitation.** A **large v wave** in the neck veins and a pulsatile liver reflect tricuspid regurgitation.
      (2) **Heart sounds.** Wide splitting of the S_1 and S_2 is heard. Because an S_3 and an S_4 often exist also, a quadruple or quintuple cadence is a common auscultatory finding.
      (3) **Murmur.** The **holosystolic murmur of tricuspid regurgitation** is heard along the sternal border and may be accompanied by a systolic thrill.
3. **Diagnosis**
   a. **Electrocardiography.** The ECG may show evidence of WPW syndrome (a short P-R interval and a slurred QRS upstroke). Other findings include giant P waves and right bundle branch block.
   b. **Echocardiography.** The echocardiogram in Ebstein's anomaly shows delayed closure of the tricuspid valve in relation to the mitral valve. The inferior and leftward displacement of the tricuspid valve usually can be demonstrated.
4. **Therapy.** Tricuspid valve replacement and closure of the atrial septal defect may be useful in patients who have developed early signs of right ventricular failure.

F Eisenmenger's syndrome

1. **Pathophysiology.** In Eisenmenger's syndrome, which can occur with any intracardiac shunt, the **left-to-right shunt is reversed** to produce a right-to-left shunt. Reversal occurs as a result of pulmonary vascular disease that leads to increased pulmonary vascular resistance. Increased pulmonary vascular resistance leads to decreased right-sided compliance and increased right-sided pressures, which produce right-to-left shunting.
2. **Clinical features**
   a. **Cyanosis** may be constant or noted only during exercise. **Differential cyanosis** may occur in the presence of a patent ductus arteriosus; the preductal tissues (including the upper trunk) are pink, and the postductal tissues are cyanotic.
   b. **Angina.** Patients with Eisenmenger's syndrome may suffer from exertional chest pain, which occurs even in the presence of normal coronary arteries. Reduced myocardial oxygenation and increased right ventricular wall stress may be factors causing the symptom.
   c. **Heart failure.** Dyspnea on exertion, ascites, and peripheral edema are common.
3. **Diagnosis**
   a. **Electrocardiography.** Right ventricular hypertrophy invariably is present.
   b. **Echocardiography. Saline injection** demonstrates right-to-left shunting of micro bubbles in the presence of either an atrial or a ventricular septal defect. **Doppler examination** also demonstrates the abnormal right-to-left blood flow at the site of the shunt.
   c. **Hemogram.** Patients with Eisenmenger's syndrome are **polycythemic.** Hemoglobin concentrations in excess of 20 g/dL are common.
   d. **Cardiac catheterization.** Right-sided pressures are extremely elevated. Oximetry is used to quantitate the right-to-left shunt. Administration of 100% oxygen via a rebreathing mask does not significantly correct the arterial desaturation.

4. **Therapy.** Surgical therapy generally is not successful.
   a. **Closure of the shunt site,** which acts as an escape valve for the right ventricle, increases right ventricular pressures and causes worsening of right ventricular failure.
   b. **Phlebotomy** may be necessary to avoid hyperviscosity by maintaining the hemoglobin level at less than 20 g/dL.

VIII VENOUS THROMBOSIS

A Deep venous thrombosis

1. **Definition.** Deep venous thrombosis occurs when a blood clot forms in the lower extremities or in the pelvic veins. The exact initiating events are unknown. The gravity of deep venous thrombosis stems from the tendency of the thrombi to become pulmonary emboli; this tendency is especially pronounced for clots located above the popliteal fossa.
2. **Predisposing factors**
   a. **Immobilization.** The muscles in the legs act as pumps to maintain venous return from the lower extremities. Inactivity of these muscles leads to **venous stasis,** with subsequent development of **thrombophlebitis.** Stasis is likely to occur during surgery, prolonged bed rest, and prolonged periods in one position.
   b. **Venous incompetence.** Venous valvular incompetence and the presence of varicose veins increase the incidence of thrombophlebitis.
   c. **CHF.** In CHF, cardiac output is reduced, as is venous return from the legs.
   d. **Injury.** Direct mechanical injury to the lower extremities may lead to blood clot formation and the development of thrombophlebitis.
   e. **Hypercoagulable states. Malignancy, estrogen use,** and **hyperviscosity syndrome** may produce a hypercoagulable state, increasing the risk of thrombophlebitis.
3. **Clinical features**
   a. **Symptoms.** The patient usually presents with **unilateral leg pain** and **swelling.**
   b. **Physical signs.** In general, the physical examination is unreliable. Tenderness on compression of the calf muscles, pain during dorsiflexion of the foot (**Homans' sign**), and an increase in the circumference of the affected leg by at least 1 cm suggest the presence of deep venous thrombosis.
4. **Diagnosis**
   a. **Noninvasive studies. Impedance plethysmography** and **Doppler ultrasonography** are useful tests for the detection of deep venous thrombosis.
   b. **Invasive studies. Contrast venography** currently is the most effective way to demonstrate the area of blood clot. This technique is associated with complications, including adverse reactions to the contrast agent and postvenography thrombophlebitis.
5. **Therapy. Anticoagulants** prevent additional clot formation and allow the body's autolytic system to lyse effectively and heal deep venous thrombosis. Anticoagulation therapy is usually maintained for 3–6 months.
   a. Anticoagulation with **intravenous heparin** is indicated in the acute treatment of deep venous thrombosis. Low–molecular-weight heparin (LMWH) appears to be as effective as unfractionated heparin. Although the low–molecular-weight form is more expensive, it does not require laboratory monitoring. In cases of heparin-induced thrombocytopenia, hirudin should be substituted for heparin.
   b. After adequate treatment with heparin, **oral anticoagulation with warfarin** is begun.
6. **Prophylaxis.** There is substantial medical evidence that the incidence of deep venous thrombosis for hospitalized patients can be reduced by the following methods.
   a. **Rapid mobilization.** Prolonged bed rest should be avoided when possible. The increasingly rapid mobilization of patients following MI has significantly reduced the incidence of thromboembolic complications following this disease.

b. **Increasing deep venous flow**

(1) **Antithromboembolic stockings** compress the superficial veins, thereby increasing deep venous flow and reducing stasis and the incidence of thromboembolism.

(2) **Foot exercises** and **avoidance of leg crossing** are further methods of preventing deep venous thrombosis.

c. **"Minidose" heparin.** Intermittent doses of subcutaneous heparin given at 8- to 12-hour intervals inhibit factors X and XI in the clotting cascade without producing overt anticoagulation. This treatment significantly reduces the incidence of deep venous thrombosis in both medical and surgical patients on bed rest.

B Superficial thrombophlebitis Unlike deep venous thrombosis, in which a thrombus may break off and become a pulmonary embolism, superficial thrombophlebitis has **little potential for embolic complications.** Patients with superficial thrombophlebitis may present with a painful tender cord that can be easily palpated in the lower extremities. In the absence of concomitant deep venous thrombosis, **anticoagulation is not indicated.** Superficial thrombophlebitis is **treated with elevation of the legs,** heat, and **administration of salicylates or other NSAIDs.**

IX CARDIOVASCULAR SYNCOPE

A Definition Syncope is a sudden loss of consciousness of brief duration.

B Pathophysiology Cardiovascular syncope occurs when the brain's metabolic needs cannot be met by the available blood supply. Adequate perfusion is dependent on an adequate systemic blood pressure: BP = CO × SVR (where BP = blood pressure, CO = cardiac output, and SVR = systemic vascular resistance). Therefore, a fall in cardiac output or a fall in systemic vascular resistance can precipitate a fall in blood pressure, leading to syncope. Because CO = SV × HR (where SV = stroke volume and HR = heart rate), either inadequate stroke volume or inadequate heart rate reduces cardiac output, potentially leading to hypotension and syncope.

C Etiology

1. **Reduced cardiac output**

a. **Bradycardia**

(1) **Heart block.** A block in the cardiac conduction pathway may prevent the SA nodal electrical signal for ventricular contraction from being transmitted, in turn causing bradycardia. Whether syncope occurs depends on whether an alternative, lower pacemaker (e.g., the AV junction) produces an escape rate that is sufficiently fast to maintain blood pressure.

(a) **Types of heart block**

(i) **Complete heart block,** which indicates that no SA nodal impulses are conducted to the ventricle

(ii) **Second-degree heart block,** which indicates that some SA nodal impulses are conducted while others are not

(b) **Causes of AV block** include MI, idiopathic degeneration of the conducting system, amyloidosis, sarcoidosis, and drugs that interfere with cardiac conduction (e.g., digitalis, calcium channel blockers, β-blockers).

(2) **Sick sinus syndrome** occurs when there is a deficit in impulse generation from the sinus node, which may lead to bradycardia and syncope.

(a) Profound sinus bradycardia, sinus arrest or exit block, and the tachycardia–bradycardia syndrome are the arrhythmias that constitute the sick sinus syndrome. The tachycardia–bradycardia syndrome is one of atrial instability where supraventricular tachycardia halts abruptly and is followed by severe bradycardia.

(b) Sick sinus syndrome may result from ischemic heart disease and idiopathic or inflammatory degeneration of the SA node.

b. **Impaired stroke volume.** The rhythmic filling and emptying of the left ventricle generates its stroke volume; therefore, conditions that either inhibit left ventricular filling or inhibit left ventricular emptying can severely reduce stroke volume, leading to hypotension and syncope.

(1) **Conditions that limit left ventricular filling**

(a) **Obstruction to inflow.** Any mechanical block in the cardiovascular system that inhibits filling of the left ventricle impairs its output. Such obstructions include mitral stenosis, left atrial myxoma, right atrial myxoma, pulmonary embolism, and pulmonic stenosis.

(b) **Tachycardia.** Both ventricular tachycardia and very rapid supraventricular tachycardia reduce the diastolic filling period of the left ventricle, limiting its filling and reducing its stroke volume. In ventricular tachycardia, the shortened diastolic filling period is compounded by incomplete ventricular relaxation, which further limits filling.

(c) **Impaired systemic venous return.** Failure of adequate systemic venous return to the right heart subsequently impairs its output to the left heart, impairing left ventricular stroke volume.

(i) Typically, impaired venous return occurs when the supine patient assumes the upright posture.

(ii) Normally, the tendency for gravity-induced venous pooling of blood in the legs is offset by venous vasoconstriction, which helps maintain venous return. However, in the face of dehydration, antihypertensive drugs, or autonomic dysfunction, impaired venous return may produce **orthostatic syncope.** Autonomic dysfunction may be idiopathic; familial; surgically induced; or result from diabetes, alcoholism, or pyridoxine deficiency.

(2) **Conditions that impair left ventricular emptying.** The left ventricle may be impaired from emptying either as a result of a severe, sudden depression in myocardial contractile function or as a result of outflow obstruction.

(a) **Decreased myocardial contractility.** The sudden and severe degree of contractile depression required to cause syncope is almost invariably caused by global ischemia produced by main left or triple-vessel coronary disease or acute MI.

(b) **Obstruction to outflow.** Obstruction of left ventricular outflow that produces syncope is caused by valvular aortic stenosis and hypertrophic obstructive cardiomyopathy.

2. **Reduced total peripheral resistance.** If cardiac output is maintained but total peripheral resistance falls, blood pressure also falls, potentially causing syncope.

a. An inappropriate fall in total peripheral resistance is usually operative in the **common fainting spell.** Increased blood flow to the skeletal muscles due to a fall in total peripheral resistance may divert flow from the brain and result in fainting. Venodilation and relative bradycardia may further compound the **"vasovagal faint"** by reducing venous return and cardiac output.

b. Reduced total peripheral resistance leading to syncope may also occur in drug-induced, familial, or idiopathic autonomic dysfunction.

D Diagnosis

A single fainting episode or episode of light-headedness occurs in more than 50% of the population at some point in a lifetime. It would be impossible to explore the cause of the event extensively in every affected patient. A good history and physical examination should be adequate to exclude potentially serious causes of a single episode of syncope. However, recurrent syncope requires a more extensive workup.

1. **History.** A thorough patient interview can reveal clues that may point to a specific etiology for the recurrent syncope.

a. A history of palpitations might indicate an arrhythmia.

b. The observation that syncope occurred upon assumption of an upright position suggests orthostatic hypotension.

c. A history of chest pain might indicate an ischemic event or pulmonary embolism.

d. A change in antihypertensive medication or a recent episode of dehydration are additional clues.

2. **Physical examination.** Those maneuvers that might reveal a reason for hypotension and possible syncope should be emphasized.

   a. **Blood pressure**

      (1) The blood pressure should be recorded in both arms in both the supine and the sitting or standing positions.

      (2) On assuming an upright posture, it is normal for systolic blood pressure to fall slightly while diastolic pressure increases. There is also usually a slight increase in heart rate.

         (a) A frank decline in systolic and diastolic pressure on assuming an upright posture may indicate volume depletion or sympathetic compensation that is inadequate to counteract the change in posture.

         (b) A fall in diastolic pressure of more than 10 mm Hg is significant and may suggest an orthostatic etiology of the syncope.

   b. **Heart rate and rhythm.** The pulse should be examined for an extended period of time in an effort to detect arrhythmia or bradycardia.

   c. **Valvular obstruction.** The murmurs and physical findings associated with mitral stenosis, aortic stenosis, pulmonic stenosis, or idiopathic hypertrophic subaortic stenosis should be recognized as indications of potentially correctable mechanisms for syncope.

   d. **Thromboembolism.** Thrombophlebitis in the lower limbs indicates a source of pulmonary emboli, which can cause syncope. Physical evidence that a pulmonary embolus is present includes wheezing, increased intensity of the pulmonary component of the S_2, and jugular venous distention.

3. **Electrocardiography.** If second- or third-degree AV block is detected, it demonstrates the likely cause of the syncope. Bundle branch block and arrhythmias, or both, on the standard ECG should raise suspicion that heart block or arrhythmia are syncopal etiologies.

4. **Holter monitoring.** If the patient interview, physical examination, and ECG point to an arrhythmia as the potential cause of the syncope, Holter monitoring may be performed.

   a. This tape recording, which documents each heart beat over a 24-hour period, increases the period of observation for the detection of arrhythmias and constitutes an exceptional piece of positive evidence in arriving at the diagnosis.

   b. Unfortunately, because most arrhythmias occur sporadically, most Holter monitor examinations are negative even when an arrhythmia is the source of the syncope. Newer monitoring devices can be activated at the time of symptoms but may have to be worn for weeks if symptoms are infrequent.

5. **Electrophysiologic testing.** If the initial workup demonstrates that heart disease is present but fails to demonstrate a specific cause of syncope, electrophysiologic stimulation may provoke the arrhythmia responsible for the syncope. Having established an arrhythmic cause, the proper therapy may then be instituted.

E Therapy

1. **Therapy of bradyarrhythmias.** When a bradyarrhythmia has been established as the cause of the syncope, drug-induced bradycardia should be ruled out as a cause by discontinuing potentially offending drugs. Subsequent insertion of a permanent pacemaker protects the patient from subsequent syncope.

2. **Therapy for tachyarrhythmias**

   a. **Drug therapy** for both ventricular and superventricular tachyarrhythmias that have caused an episode of syncope is clearly indicated [see II D 1 b (3)]. In general, such therapy should be guided by electrophysiologic testing.

b. **Antitachycardia pacemakers** or **implantable defibrillators** may be used to electrically correct arrhythmias if drug therapy fails.

3. **Therapy for autonomic dysfunction.** If autonomic dysfunction is the cause of orthostatic hypotension and syncope, little can be done directly to treat the underlying cause. Instead, therapies to protect the patient from possible hypotension should be instituted. These include high salt intake to ensure volume expansion, support stockings to prevent venous pooling, and atrial pacemaking if an inappropriate lack of tachycardia during hypotension is part of the underlying syndrome.

4. **Correction of mechanical obstructions to cardiac inflow or outflow.** Any fixed valvular lesion that has caused an episode of syncope should be corrected. If idiopathic hypertrophic subaortic stenosis is determined to be the cause of the syncope, standard therapy with propranolol or verapamil is indicated to reduce the amount of outflow obstruction. If medical therapy fails, myomectomy may be necessary.

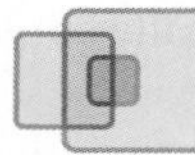

Study Questions

A 52-year-old man presents with fever, chills, and arthralgia. On physical examination: temperature is 102.2°F, pulse is 106 beats/min, blood pressure is 100/60 mm Hg, respiratory rate 22. S_1 is soft. There is a short II/VI diastolic blowing murmur at the left sternal border. There are no rashes or petechiae. The results of the rest of the examination are unremarkable.

1. What is the most likely diagnosis?

A Viral syndrome with flow murmur
B Acute systemic lupus erythematosus with aortic valve involvement
C Infective endocarditis of the aortic valve with probably mild insufficiency
D Infective endocarditis of the mitral valve
E Infective endocarditis of the aortic valve with probably severe insufficiency

2. Which of the following statements is true of the condition of the patient in #1?

A The cardiac physical examination is hyperdynamic.
B S_1 is soft because of aortic valve preclosure.
C Mitral valve preclosure indicates a poor prognosis without aortic valve replacement.
D The appearance of a diastolic murmur is usually benign.
E Hill's sign is a good predictor of severity.

3. The diagnostic test(s) that should be performed next is/are

A A chest x-ray
B Blood cultures
C Cardiac catheterization
D A radionuclide ventriculogram
E Exploratory thoracotomy

A 56-year-old man enters the emergency department complaining of dyspnea that began about 3 weeks ago and has progressed so that he now has difficulty walking across a room. He has begun sleeping on 3 pillows. On physical examination: temperature 99.0°, pulse 102 beats/min, BP 130/90 mm Hg, RR 24. There is jugular venous distension, and estimated central venous pressure is 10 cm H_2O. Other findings include bibasilar rales and an S_3 gallop.

4. What is the most likely diagnosis in this patient?

A Pulmonary embolism
B Congestive heart failure
C Emphysema
D Pneumonia
E Atrial septal defect

5. Which of the following tests is most appropriate to aid in establishing therapy for this patient?

A A chest X-ray
B An echocardiogram
C An electrocardiogram
D A heart catheterization
E A radionuclide ventriculogram

6. Which of the following is true about the treatment of the condition of the patient in #4?

A The cause of the condition should be treated whenever possible.
B Systolic versus diastolic dysfunction usually cannot be established.
C ACE inhibitors improve symptoms but do not prolong life.
D Diuretics are the court of last resort.
E β-blockers are dangerous and should be avoided.

On a routine office visit, a 45-year-old man complains that recently he has noted right-sided chest pain while mowing his lawn with a push lawn mower. The pain develops suddenly, lasts 2–3 minutes, and subsides when he rests. He denies smoking or a history of hypertension, diabetes, or hyperlipidemia. His physical examination is unremarkable. An ECG shows nonspecific T wave abnormalities.

7. This patient is most likely suffering from which of the following?

A Angina pectoris
B Hiatal hernia
C Pleuritis
D A nonspecific chest pain syndrome
E There is not enough information to arrive at a diagnosis

8. What should be the next step in establishing the diagnosis for this patient?

A Repeat the ECG
B Perform a cardiac catheterization
C Obtain cardiac enzymes and a troponin level
D Perform a stress ECG
E Perform a stress echocardiogram

9. If coronary disease is found in this patient, indications for revascularization will include which of the following?

A Occasional angina
B A severe lesion in the circumflex coronary artery
C Three-vessel disease with left ventricular dysfunction
D Disease in the distal left anterior descending
E Disease of the right and circumflex coronary arteries

A 56-year-old man with a history of hypertension is seen for the evaluation of chest pain that began an hour ago. The pain was centered in the left side of the chest and radiates to the left arm. It was associated with nausea and vomiting. His physical examination findings are:

BP 80/60, P 58, RR 16

Chest: clear

Heart: no gallops or murmurs

ECG: Acute anterior myocardial infarction and sinus bradycardia

10. What should be the next step in management of this patient?

A Insertion of a temporary pacemaker
B Administration of nitrates
C Fluid resuscitation
D Insertion of an intra-aortic balloon pump
E Administration of a β-blocker

11. After the patient in #10 is stabilized, he should:

- A Be transferred to the critical care unit
- B Undergo immediate percutaneous coronary angioplasty if available
- C Receive warfarin
- D Receive nifedipine
- E Receive intravenous lidocaine

12. On the second hospital day, the patient becomes diaphoretic and hypotensive. A III/VI holosystolic murmur is heard. Which of the following is likely?

- A He has developed pericardial tamponade.
- B There has been acute ventricular septal rupture.
- C He has an acute atrial septal defect.
- D He has developed mitral valve endocarditis.
- E The murmur was old but obscured by the reduced cardiac output from his MI.

13. Ultimately this patient's prognosis will be determined most by which of the following?

- A The amount of myocardial damage he has sustained.
- B His LDL cholesterol level
- C His HDL cholesterol level
- D The ratio of LDL to HDL cholesterol
- E Blood pressure control

A 25-year-old woman presents with chest pain that worsens when she inspires. Her physical examination findings are BP 120/70 mm Hg, pulse 76 beats/min, RR 14, Heart: 2-component friction rub.

14. Which of the following statements is true of the friction rub?

- A It is generated by movement of the parietal and visceral layers of the pericardium.
- B It is generated by the visceral layers of the pericardium and pleura.
- C It indicates the absence of an effusion.
- D It indicates that the cause of the pericarditis is a malignancy.
- E It often persists through effective therapy.

15. What would be the best first-line therapy for the patient in #14?

- A Acetaminophen
- B Aspirin
- C Ibuprofen
- D Prednisone
- E Colchicine

16. Several days later, the patient develops dyspnea and jugular venous distension. The likely diagnosis now is:

- A Right-sided heart failure
- B Myocardial infarction
- C Pulmonary embolism
- D Pericardial tamponade
- E Pneumonia

A 75-year-old man reports chest pain while climbing stairs. On physical examination, there is a II/VI systolic ejection murmur that radiates to the neck. The carotid upstrokes are delayed and diminished in volume.

17. The most likely diagnosis is:

- A Hypertrophic cardiomyopathy
- B Aortic stenosis
- C Mitral stenosis
- D Pulmonary stenosis
- E Vasovagal syncope

18. The best test to confirm the diagnosis is:

- A An ECG
- B An exercise stress test
- C An echocardiogram
- D A radionuclide ventriculogram
- E A chest X-ray

19. The recommended therapy is:

- A Immediate aortic valve replacement
- B An angiotensin-converting enzyme inhibitor
- C Nitroglycerine
- D A calcium channel blocker
- E A β-blocker

A murmur is detected on the routine examination of a 35-year-old woman. She is entirely asymptomatic and engages in aerobic exercise classes without difficulty. On physical examination, there is II/VI systolic ejection murmur heard best in the left second interspace. S_1 is normal. S_2 is widely split and does not vary with respiration.

20. The likely diagnosis is:

- A Pulmonary stenosis
- B Aortic stenosis
- C Ventricular septal defect
- D Atrial septal defect
- E A flow (innocent) murmur

21. Which of the following is true about the condition of this patient?

- A It likely developed in childhood.
- B It is associated with an increased risk of infective endocarditis.
- C It will have little consequence if left uncorrected.
- D It may lead to ventricular arrhythmias.
- E It may be associated with bony abnormalities of the forearm.

A 55-year-old man complains of increasing dyspnea on exertion, peripheral edema, and increasing abdominal girth. He denies orthopnea or paroxysmal nocturnal dyspnea. Physical examination findings are as follows:

BP 100/70, P 80. RR 18

Marked jugular venous distension

Lungs: clear

Heart: loud P_2, no murmurs

Extremities: Pitting edema

22. What is the predominant syndrome present in this patient?

A Left-sided heart failure
B Right-sided heart failure
C Biventricular failure
D Noncardiac edema
E Pure volume overload

23. Which of the following is a likely cause of this condition?

A Mitral stenosis
B Constrictive pericarditis
C Pulmonary embolism
D Ventricular septal defect
E Dilated cardiomyopathy

A 35-year-old white woman enters the emergency department complaining of episodic chest pain that usually lasts for 5–10 minutes. Sometimes it is related to exercise, but on other occasions, it occurs at rest. The pain does not radiate. The woman is a nonsmoker and has no history of hypertension. Two other family members have died of heart disease, one at 50 years of age and the other at 56 years of age. On physical examination, the patient is in no acute distress. Her blood pressure is 120/70 mm Hg and her pulse is 70. Examination of the precordium finds that the point of maximal impulse (PMI) is forceful. There is a II/VI systolic ejection murmur heard along the left sternal border that increases in intensity when the patient stands up. The electrocardiogram (ECG) shows nonspecific S–T segment and T-wave abnormalities.

24. Which of the following is the most likely diagnosis?

A Innocent flow murmur
B Aortic stenosis
C Hypertrophic obstructive cardiomyopathy
D Mitral stenosis
E Pulmonic stenosis

25. Which of the following tools would be best to use when diagnosing this patient?

A Chest radiograph
B Cardiac catheterization
C Thallium scanning
D Echocardiography
E Myocardial biopsy

26. Which of the following therapies is most appropriate for this patient?

A Immediate surgery
B A β-blocker
C Vasodilators
D Digoxin
E Furosemide

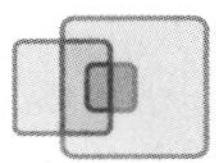

Answers and Explanations

1. **The answer is E** [IV C 3 b]. The diastolic murmur is typical of that of aortic insufficiency. The fever chills and arthralgia suggest infection, making infective endocarditis the most likely diagnosis. The soft S_1 suggests mitral valve preclosure, indicating severe disease. This syndrome could be seen in acute lupus, but this is less likely in a man without other evidence of the disease. Increased flow from any cause does not produce aortic insufficiency. A lesion on the mitral valve creates systolic, not diastolic, murmurs.

2. **The answer is C** [IV C 3 b]. Mitral valve preclosure, caused by high ventricular diastolic filling pressure, greater than left atrial pressure, indicates severe disease that is usually fatal without aortic valve replacement. In acute aortic insufficiency such as that seen in endocarditis, LV dilatation has not yet occurred, stroke volume is not increased very much, and thus the circulation is not hyperdynamic. Therefore Hill's sign is also absent. In general, diastolic murmurs are not benign and indicate valve pathology.

3. **The answer is B** [IV C 4]. Blood cultures to confirm a bloodstream infection and echocardiography to identify valve lesions and valve function are the mainstays of diagnosis in infective endocarditis. Although a chest X-ray might be useful, it is never diagnostic of endocarditis. Valve surgery would not be contemplated without the diagnosis of endocarditis being established first. Cardiac catheterization is rarely indicated in endocarditis today because echocardiography provides more information more safely. A radionuclide ventriculogram would give information about cardiac performance but would not confirm the diagnosis.

4. **The answer is B** [I D 1–2]. The gradual onset of dyspnea, the pulmonary rales, and the S_3 gallop are all typical of congestive heart failure. Although a pulmonary embolus could cause all of the findings in this patient, even a right-sided S_3, sudden onset is the norm in that condition. The other conditions all could cause dyspnea but would not cause gallop rhythm.

5. **The answer is B** [I E]. An echocardiogram will yield data about systolic and diastolic function, chamber size, and valvular abnormalities. All of the other tests are useful, but all except catheterization give less information than the echocardiogram. Cardiac catheterization has a higher risk and is only employed when the information gained outweighs that risk. Thus, in CHF, echocardiography provides the "biggest bang for the buck."

6. **The answer is A** [I F]. Congestive heart failure is a syndrome, and its cause should be sought and treated directly whenever possible. It is usually helpful to establish whether the root cause is systolic or diastolic dysfunction, a distinction made easily with echocardiography. Diuretics form the mainstay of therapy, but adding both ACE inhibitors and β-blockers prolongs life.

7. **The answer is E** [III A 5 a (1)]. His presentation with exertional pain is typical of angina, but the location, duration, and lack of risk factors are atypical. No diagnosis can be made based on this information.

8. **The answer is E** [III A 5 a (3)]. A stress echocardiogram will give information about cardiac function and the presence of coronary disease (90% sensitivity). Repeating the ECG is unlikely to give new information. The brevity of the pain makes it very unlikely that myocardial damage has occurred, and thus troponin is likely to be normal. The stress ECG will be of limited use because the resting ECG is already abnormal. Cardiac catheterization could be employed, but because of its invasive nature it is usually not the first step in arriving at a diagnosis.

9. **The answer is C** [III A 5 a (4)]. Revascularization increases the life span in main left coronary disease, in proximal left anterior descending (LAD) disease, and in three-vessel coronary disease when left ventric-

ular dysfunction already exists presumably because revascularization forestalls further damage to an already damaged myocardium. Longevity is not increased by revascularization in two-vessel disease not involving the LAD nor in distal LAD disease. Because there is a risk to all revascularization procedures, they would not be entertained for mild symptoms alone.

10. The answer is C [III A 5 b (5) (f)]. The patient is hypotensive, as he has no signs of volume overload or heart failure; thus, fluid resuscitation should be performed first. Although both β-blockers and nitrates are indicated in MI, their use here would only exacerbate the hypotension. A pacemaker might improve blood pressure but only if A-V sequential pacing, a sometimes complex procedure, were used. In fact, pacemakers are rarely used for mild sinus bradycardia. Intra-aortic balloon pumping would be used only if other measures failed to restore blood pressure.

11. The answer is B [III A 5 b (5) (b)]. If acute angioplasty is available, it should be performed immediately to restore coronary blood flow without transferring the patient to the CCU, because every minute counts in preserving myocardium. Dihydropyridine calcium channel blockers such as nifedipine are contraindicated in MI because they increase mortality. Lidocaine is no longer used prophylactically against cardiac arrhythmias because of possible cardiac standstill. Although heparin is an essential part of therapy, warfarin, which takes days to become effective, is not.

12. The answer is B [III A 5 b (4) (e)]. Hemodynamic decompensation and a new cardiac murmur after MI indicate either acute ventricular septal rupture or acute mitral valve dysfunction. Atrial septal defect is not a consequence of MI. There is no indication that the patient has developed endocarditis. If anything, the patient's output has been still further reduced, as indicated by his change in vital signs. There are no signs of tamponade, such as pulsus paradoxus or neck vein distension.

13. The answer is A [III A 6]. Prognosis is dependent most on the amount of muscle damage (and therefore the amount the ventricular dysfunction that develops), the patient's age, and the extent of coronary disease. Although improving the status of known coronary risk factors such as hyperlipidemia and hypertension reduces subsequent risk, the effect on prognosis is not as large as are muscle damage, age, and extent of disease.

14. The answer is A [VI A 2]. The rub is caused by movement of the inflamed parietal and visceral layers of the pericardium. A rub is indicative of pericarditis from any cause and does not imply malignancy. Rubs can still occur even when an effusion separates the two layers of the pericardium. Rubs usually disappear with effective therapy.

15. The answer is C [VI A 4]. Nonsteroidal anti-inflammatory agents (NSAIDS) such as ibuprofen form the first line of therapy. High-dose aspirin is effective but is more likely to cause GI side effects. Although acetaminophen might relieve the pain, it would not treat the inflammation. Prednisone and colchicine are reserved for NSAID failures.

16. The answer is D [VI B 2]. The onset of dyspnea and neck vein distension should immediately trigger concern for tamponade in a patient with known pericarditis. As fluid builds up in the pericardial sac, it compresses the heart, limits its output, and raises the pressure in all four cardiac chambers; hence the neck vein distension. Whereas MI, right-sided failure, pulmonary embolism, and pneumonia are all possible occurrences, there are no findings to confirm their presence in this otherwise healthy young woman.

17. The answer is B [VI A 3 a–b]. The murmur and delayed carotid upstrokes are typical of the fixed LV outflow obstruction of aortic stenosis. Pulmonary stenosis also can cause chest pain and a systolic ejection murmur but would not cause carotid delay. Hypertrophic cardiomyopathy causes a spike and dome of the carotid upstrokes, that is, a sharp upstroke followed by fall and a flatter secondary rise. The murmur of mitral stenosis is diastolic. Although the syncope could have been attributable to a vasovagal faint, this could only be a diagnosis of exclusion in the face of obvious aortic stenosis.

18. The answer is C [IV A 4]. Echocardiography with Doppler interrogation of the valve will show the aortic stenosis, quantify its severity, and assess LV function. The ECG and chest X-ray are nonspecific in this disease. Although useful in asymptomatic patients, stress testing is dangerous in symptomatic aortic stenosis. A radionuclide study would give information about LV function but not about lesion severity.

19. The answer is A [IV A 5 b]. The only accepted therapy for symptomatic aortic stenosis is aortic valve replacement. Nitrates can be used cautiously for angina until the valve is replaced but only as a temporizing measure. The other agents listed could cause hypotension and should not be used.

20. The answer is D [VII A 3 b]. The widely split S_2 that does not vary with respiration is pathognomonic of atrial septal defect. The murmur is caused by increased flow across the pulmonic valve, which is not stenotic. The murmur of a VSD is holosystolic. The murmur of aortic stenosis is associated with a soft single S_2 because the aortic valve neither opens nor closes well.

21. The answer is E [VII A 1 d]. Atrial septal defect associated with bony abnormalities of the hands and forearms is called Holt-Oram syndrome. ASD is a congenital abnormality and thus does not develop in childhood. If left untreated, it will lead to atrial arrhythmias and will significantly reduce life span, but it is not associated with an increased risk of endocarditis.

22. The answer is B [I D]. The syndrome is that of right-sided heart failure with elevated neck veins, ascites, and edema. There is no orthopnea or pulmonary rales to indicate concomitant left-sided CHF. Pure volume overload would not cause the loud P_2 indicative of pulmonary hypertension.

23. The answer is C [I D 3]. The most likely cause of pulmonary hypertension listed is pulmonary embolus. Mitral stenosis can cause the condition, but there are no physical signs to indicate its presence. Constrictive pericarditis also presents with predominantly right-sided findings but does not usually cause pulmonary hypertension. Dilated cardiomyopathy would present with findings of both left- and right-sided failure.

24. The answer is C [V B 4]. The most likely diagnosis is hypertrophic cardiomyopathy, as evidenced by the increased intensity of the systolic ejection murmur when the patient stands up. When a patient with hypertrophic cardiomyopathy stands up, blood pools in the legs, decreasing left ventricular size and bringing the anterior leaflet of the mitral valve in closer contact with the hypertrophied ventricular septum. This increases the obstruction and makes the murmur louder. Conversely, innocent flow murmurs and the murmurs associated with pulmonic and aortic stenosis decrease when the patient stands, because the temporary pooling of central volume in the legs decreases forward cardiac output, thereby decreasing turbulent flow in the valve. The murmur of mitral stenosis is a diastolic murmur, not a systolic murmur.

25. The answer is D [V B 56]. The echocardiogram is a highly effective diagnostic tool in hypertrophic cardiomyopathy, provided the patient can be visualized adequately. Asymmetric hypertrophy of the septum compared with the free cardiac wall confirms the diagnosis. If obstruction is present, there will also be systolic anterior motion of the mitral valve. There are no particular features of hypertrophic cardiomyopathy demonstrable on a chest radiograph. Thallium scintigraphy may show the hypertrophied septum, but this is not the optimum form of imaging. Cardiac catheterization can certainly confirm the diagnosis, but this invasive test needs to be performed in only a minority of patients when echocardiography cannot adequately visualize the patient's heart.

26. The answer is B [V B 6 a]. Symptoms of hypertrophic cardiomyopathy may be relieved with propranolol, a β-adrenergic blocking agent. By decreasing heart rate, propranolol allows increased left ventricular filling, thereby increasing separation of the anterior leaflet of the mitral valve and the septum and reducing the amount of obstruction. Unlike valvular aortic stenosis (where death may be imminent after the development of symptoms unless surgery is performed) in hypertrophic cardiomyopathy, there is no evidence that surgery prolongs life. Both digoxin (by increasing the force of that contraction) and furosemide (by decreasing left ventricular size) would worsen the obstruction and likely exacerbate the patient's symptoms.

chapter **2**

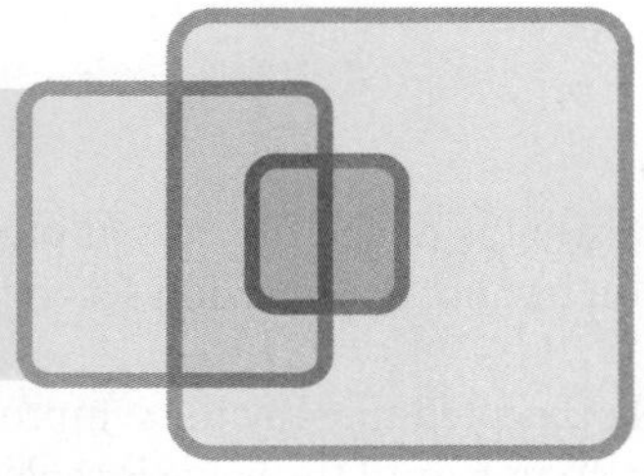

Pulmonary Diseases

GERARD J. CRINER

I PULMONARY FUNCTION STUDIES

A Introduction Tests of pulmonary function provide three basic kinds of information:

1. **Lung volumes** are the volumes of the various intrapulmonary compartments.
   a. **Static lung volumes** reflect the elastic properties of the lungs and chest wall.
   b. **Dynamic lung volumes** reflect the patency of the airways.
2. The **expiratory flow rate** is the maximal rate of airflow during forced expiration.
   a. The rate of airflow is influenced by lung volume and by effort (i.e., force of expiration). Airflow increases with increasing effort, especially at high lung volumes [>75% of the vital capacity (VC)].
   b. Other factors influencing flow rate include the elastic recoil of the lung, small peripheral airway resistance, and the cross-sectional area of larger central airways.
3. **Diffusing capacity (DL_{CO})** is the efficiency of gas transfer from alveoli to pulmonary capillary blood.

B Spirometry

1. **Definition.** Spirometry is a simple, easy test of pulmonary function. The spirometer device plots a tracing (the **spirogram**) of the lung volume against time (in seconds) while the patient takes as deep a breath as possible and then exhales all of the inspired air as rapidly and forcefully as possible.
2. **Uses.** Spirometry can aid in distinguishing obstructive from restrictive lung diseases (Table 2–1) as well as suggest the severity of functional impairment and its reversibility with treatment. It is useful both as a diagnostic aid and as a monitoring tool.

C Values obtainable from the spirogram Many spirogram measurements are stated as a percentage of **predicted values** that are determined from many normal individuals grouped on the basis of sex, age, and height. The range of normal is 80%–120% of the predicted value.

1. **Tidal volume (V_T)** is the volume of air in one breath during normal quiet breathing. The V_T (normal, 500–800 mL) varies according to effort and level of ventilation. The portion of the V_T that participates in gas exchange is the **alveolar volume (V_A);** the remainder, approximately 30% of the V_T, is "wasted" or **"dead space."**
2. **Vital capacity (VC)** is the maximal volume of air that can be expelled from the lungs after a maximal inspiration. Because VC decreases progressively with restrictive lung disease, it is useful, in conjunction with DL_{CO} (see I E 1), for monitoring the course and response to therapy in a patient with a restrictive lung disorder.
3. **Forced vital capacity (FVC)** is the same as VC, except that the inhalation is performed as rapidly and forcefully as possible. Forced expiration causes the airways to narrow, slowing the rate of expiration.

TABLE 2–1 Obstructive and Restrictive Lung Disorders

- **Primarily obstructive ventilatory defects** (disorders characterized by reduced flow rates)
  - Chronic obstructive pulmonary disease
    - Chronic bronchitis
    - Pulmonary emphysema
    - Asthma
    - Cystic fibrosis
- **Primarily restrictive ventilatory defects** (disorders characterized by reduced lung volumes)
  - Parenchymal disorders
    - Alveolar and interstitial processes (e.g., edema, fibrosis, infection)
    - Large space-occupying lesions
    - Atelectasis
    - Resection of pulmonary tissue
  - Chest wall disease
    - Obesity
    - Kyphoscoliosis
    - Ankylosing spondylitis
  - Pleural disease
    - Effusion
    - Pneumothorax
    - Fibrothorax
  - Neuromuscular diseases
    - Guillain-Barré syndrome
    - Spinal cord injury
    - Muscular dystrophies
    - Poliomyelitis

4. **Forced expiratory volume in 1 second (FEV_1)** is the volume of air forcefully expired during the first second after a deep breath, or the portion of the FVC exhaled in 1 second. The FEV_1 primarily reflects the status of large airways. It is often expressed as a percentage of the VC (normal $FEV_1 = 75\%$ VC).
5. **FEV_1/FVC** is the ratio of the FEV_1 to FVC, expressed as a percentage (normal, $\geq 70\%$).* The FEV_1/FVC is **effort dependent** (i.e., it increases with increasing expiratory effort). FEV_1/FVC is particularly useful in evaluating obstructive disorders but is also helpful in the evaluation of restrictive disorders. If only the FEV_1 is low ($FEV_1/FVC < 70\%$), obstruction is suggested; if both the FEV_1 and FVC are low ($FEV_1/FVC \geq 70\%$), restriction is suggested.
6. **$FEF_{25\%-75\%}$** is the forced expiratory flow rate over the middle half of the FVC (i.e., between 25% and 75%); it is also called the **maximal mid-expiratory flow rate (MMEFR** or **MMFR).** The $FEF_{25\%-75\%}$ primarily reflects the status of the small airways, and it is more sensitive than the FEV_1 for identifying early airway obstruction. The $FEF_{25\%-75\%}$ is **effort independent.**

D **Other lung volumes** (Figure 2–1) Obtaining the following values requires the use of spirometry and either helium dilution (which measures the volume of gas in the lungs) or, preferably, body plethysmography (which measures intrathoracic gas volume).

1. **Total lung capacity (TLC)** is the volume of air in the lungs after a maximal inspiratory effort.
2. **Functional residual capacity (FRC)** is the volume of air remaining in the lungs at the end of a normal expiration. The FRC reflects the resting position of the lungs and chest wall; it is the lung

*In this case, percentage is not a percentage of predicted normal.

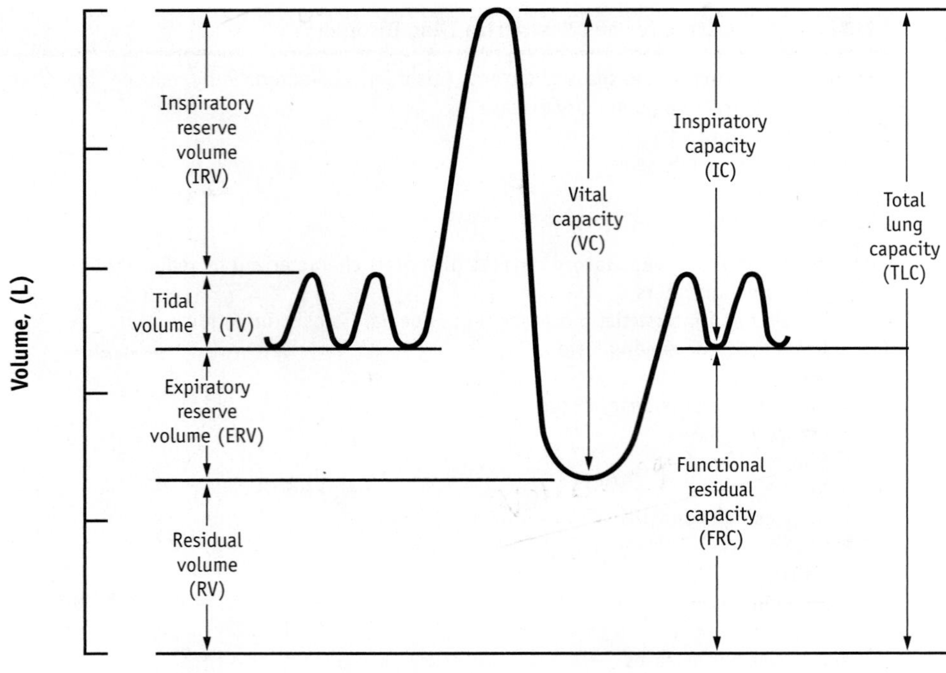

FIGURE 2–1 The subdivisions of lung volume as recorded by a spirometer. The record is generated on paper calibrated for volume in the vertical direction and time in the horizontal. The term *capacity* is applied to a subdivision composed of two or more volumes.

volume at which the inward recoil of the lungs is balanced by the outward recoil of the chest wall. The FRC has two components:

a. The **expiratory reserve volume (ERV)** is the amount of the FRC that can be expelled by a maximal expiratory effort.

b. The **residual volume (RV)** is the volume of air remaining in the lungs after a maximal expiratory effort (normal, 25%–30% of FRC).

3. **Lung volume relationships** are as follows:

a. TLC = VC + RV

b. RV = FRC − ERV

E Other tests of pulmonary function

1. **Diffusing capacity of carbon monoxide (DL_{CO}).** The DL_{CO} indicates the adequacy of the alveolar–capillary membrane.

a. The DL_{CO} is determined by measuring the amount of carbon monoxide (CO) transferred from the alveolar gas to the pulmonary capillary blood after the patient inhales a known amount of CO (0.1%); it is expressed in mL/min/mm Hg.

b. The DL_{CO} has a number of uses. It helps distinguish between asthma, chronic bronchitis, and emphysema, indicates the severity of emphysema, and provides a useful monitoring tool in sarcoidosis and interstitial lung disease.

c. The effects of various disorders on the DL_{CO} are shown in Table 2–2.

2. **Compliance curve.** The **elastic properties of the lung** can be assessed from the relationship between change in lung volume and change in transpulmonary pressure (the pressure in the alveoli minus the pressure within the pleural space; $Pa - P_{PL}$).

TABLE 2–2 Effect of Various Disorders on Diffusing Capacity (DL_{CO})

Disorders that decrease DL_{CO}
Emphysema
Interstitial fibrosis
Multiple pulmonary emboli
Pulmonary edema
Sarcoidosis
Pulmonary alveolar proteinosis
Pulmonary resection (due to reduced binding of CO by hemoglobin)
Anemia
Disorders that increase DL_{CO}
Pulmonary hemorrhage (due to uptake by intra-alveolar RBCs)
Intracardiac left-to-right shunt
Vascular congestion, but only prior to edema
Polycythemia vera (early)

CO = carbon monoxide; RBCs = red blood cells.

a. A given volume of air in the lung requires a certain amount of pressure to achieve that degree of inflation. This pressure is a combination of the elastic (inward) recoil of the lung and the elastic (outward) recoil of the chest wall.

(1) At the normal resting end-expiratory position of the lungs (i.e., at FRC), the elastic recoil of the lung is exactly balanced by the elastic recoil of the chest wall.

(2) At full inspiration (i.e., at TLC), the lungs reach their maximal elastic recoil.

(3) At full expiration (i.e., at RV), the chest wall reaches its maximal elastic recoil, unless age or airway disease causes the airways to close prematurely, trapping gas within the lungs.

b. Plotting the lung volume against a range of transpulmonary pressures gives the **compliance curve** for the lung. **Compliance (C)** is determined from the slope of the pressure–volume (P–V) curve over the tidal volume range: $C = V/P$ (normal, 200 mL/cm H_2O) (Figure 2–2).

c. Changes in lung elastic recoil inversely affect the compliance curve.

(1) Loss of lung elastic recoil (e.g., in emphysema) increases compliance, shifting the compliance curve to the left.

(2) Increased lung elastic recoil (e.g., in restrictive lung diseases such as idiopathic pulmonary fibrosis) decreases compliance, shifting the compliance curve downward and to the right.

3. Airway resistance (Raw). Measuring Raw primarily reflects the status of large airways, because 80%–90% of the resistance to airflow is in the large central airways.

a. Raw is usually determined from dynamic lung volumes and expiratory flow rates; when a more accurate measure is needed, body plethysmography is used.

b. Raw is increased in obstructive lung disease and decreased in restrictive lung disease.

F Patterns of pulmonary function impairment

1. Obstructive lung disorders

a. Flow rates. A **reduced FEV_1/FVC** (> 70%) is the time-honored indicator of obstructive airway disease. However, the FEV_1/FVC may be normal even with considerable peripheral airway obstruction. A reduced $FEF_{25\%-75\%}$ (60% or less of predicted value) may detect airway obstruction when the FEV_1/FVC is normal. However, the range of normal $FEF_{25\%-75\%}$ values is wide.

b. Lung volumes. Changes in lung volume may be seen in moderate-to-severe obstructive airway disease.

(1) Lung volume measurements are useful in identifying hyperinflation caused by premature airway closure.

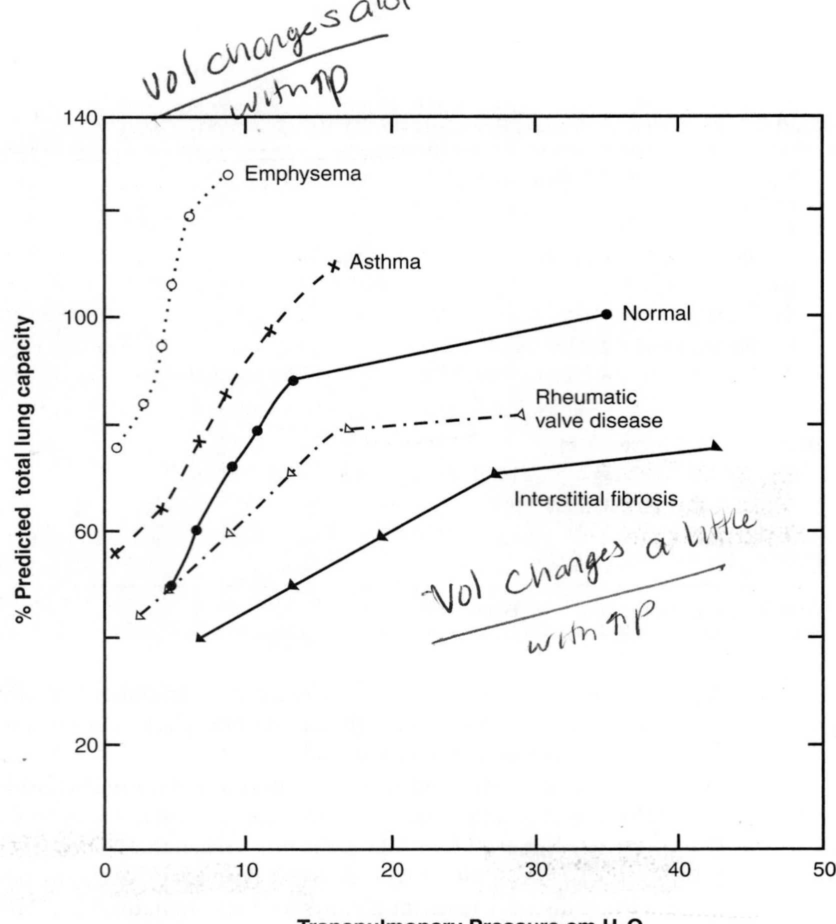

FIGURE 2–2 Pressure–volume curves of the lung. The curves for emphysema and asthma (during bronchospasm) are shifted upward and to the left, whereas those for rheumatic valve disease and interstitial fibrosis are flattened. (Reprinted with permission from Bates DV, Macklem PT, Christie RV: Respiratory Function in Disease, 2nd Ed. Philadelphia: WB Saunders, 1971:9.)

(a) During a forced expiration, if the terminal airways close before all the air is expelled, hyperinflation results, causing an increase in the FRC, RV, and RV/TLC.

(b) In small airway disorders, because of air trapping, the RV may increase while the FRC and FEV_1 remain normal.

(2) In emphysema, the alveolar wall destruction and loss of lung elastic recoil cause an increase in the TLC.

c. Compliance is increased in emphysema, because lung elastic recoil is reduced.

d. **Raw** is increased in obstructive lung disease.

2. **Restrictive lung disorders**

a. **Flow rates.** FEV_1/FVC and $FEF_{25\%-75\%}$ may be normal or increased because of increased traction on the intrathoracic airway walls.

b. **Lung volumes**

(1) A **reduction in VC and TLC** is the most useful indicator of a restrictive ventilatory defect.

(2) Lung stiffness in restrictive diseases increases the lung elastic recoil, thus lowering the FRC.

(3) Chest wall stiffness (e.g., in kyphoscoliosis) lowers lung volumes because it restricts lung expansion.

c. **Compliance** is reduced because lung elastic recoil is increased.

d. **Raw** is decreased because the elastic forces maintain wider airways at any lung volume.

G **Arterial blood gases** The partial pressures of oxygen (**Pa_{O_2}**) and carbon dioxide (**Pa_{CO_2}**) as well as the **pH** of arterial blood are important in assessing pulmonary function, because these data indicate the status of gas exchange between the lungs and the blood.

1. **Pa_{O_2}** and **Pa_{CO_2}**. The Pa_{O_2} and Pa_{CO_2} show the net effect of lung disease on gas exchange.
   - **a.** The Pa_{O_2} normally decreases with age as a result of the loss of lung elasticity (normal Pa_{O_2} is approximately 90 mm Hg at age 20 years and approximately 75 mm Hg by age 70 years). A lower than normal Pa_{O_2} indicates hypoxemia. However, tissue oxygenation is not significantly reduced until the Pa_{O_2} decreases to less than approximately 60 mm Hg.
   - **b.** The Pa_{CO_2} (normal, 35–45 mm Hg) reflects alveolar ventilation—**hypercapnia** (respiratory acidosis, a high Pa_{CO_2}) indicates **hypoventilation,** and **hypocapnia** (respiratory alkalosis, a low Pa_{CO_2}) indicates **hyperventilation.**
2. **pH**
   - **a.** Comparing the arterial pH (normal, 7.35–7.45) with the Pa_{CO_2} helps distinguish respiratory from metabolic abnormalities. For example, if the Pa_{CO_2} and pH are related **inversely** (one declining while the other increases), the acid–base imbalance is respiratory.
   - **b.** Clinically, however, results often are not straightforward, being complicated by the nature of the patient's disorders and any medications being taken.

H **Ventilation–perfusion ($\dot{V}/\dot{Q}$) mismatch** (inequality of pulmonary gas exchange)

1. **$\dot{V}/\dot{Q}$ relationships**
   - **a.** Ventilation and blood flow through the lung should match if there is to be adequate uptake of oxygen and adequate elimination of carbon dioxide (Figure 2–3).
   - **b.** The overall $\dot{V}/\dot{Q}$ of the lung is 0.8. Thus, there is a normal **"physiologic $\dot{V}/\dot{Q}$ mismatch,"** equivalent to a 2% **shunting** of pulmonary arterial (mixed venous) blood directly into the pulmonary venous circulation without gas exchange.
2. **Significance of $\dot{V}/\dot{Q}$ mismatch**

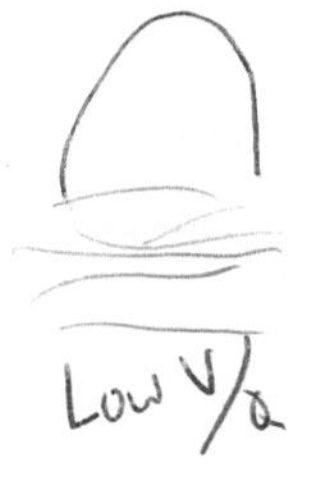

   - **a.** A **low $\dot{V}/\dot{Q}$** signifies inadequate ventilation of an adequately perfused area of the lung. The result is a lowered Pa_{O_2} or hypoxemia.
     - (1) Unless the alveoli are occluded or fluid filled, the hypoxemia can be corrected by administering oxygen, because the oxygen reaches the areas of alveolar hypoxia.
     - (2) If an area of the lung has **no alveolar ventilation,** it has no gas exchange at all (**$\dot{V}/\dot{Q} = 0$**) (Figure 2–4). The result is **right-to-left shunting** of blood; that is, true venous blood mixes with arterial blood. This form of hypoxemia is refractory to oxygen therapy because the oxygen cannot reach the alveolar–capillary membrane (Figure 2–5).
   - **b.** A **high $\dot{V}/\dot{Q}$** signifies adequate ventilation of a poorly perfused area of the lung. Oxygen exchange is inefficient because the available hemoglobin can only take up so much oxygen.
     - (1) If an area of the lung has **no blood flow** at all, it has no gas exchange at all ($\dot{V}/\dot{Q} = \infty$). All of the oxygen going to that area of alveolar dead space is wasted ventilation.
     - (2) Alveolar dead space results in carbon dioxide retention as well as hypoxia. The hypercapnia stimulates the respiratory center, thereby increasing the work of breathing but also increasing ventilation. Even though this may normalize the Pa_{CO_2}, it does not improve the lowered Pa_{O_2}.

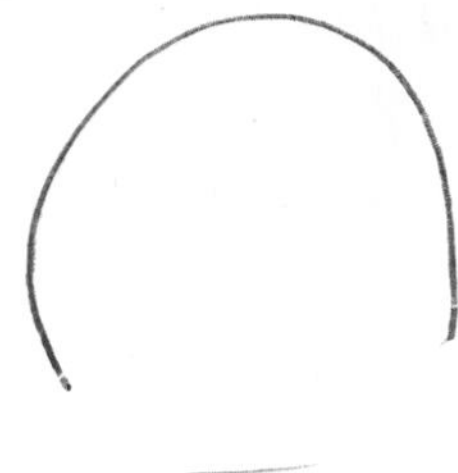

   - **c.** Typically, in patients with $\dot{V}/\dot{Q}$ abnormalities, the reduction in Pa_{O_2} is much more marked than the increase in Pa_{CO_2}. However, as lung disease progresses, ventilation cannot increase any further. The result is hypoxemia and hypercapnia (i.e., acute respiratory failure).
3. **Alveolar–arterial oxygen gradient** (**A-a D_{O_2}**) is the difference (i.e., gradient) between the **alveolar P_{O_2}** (**$P_{A_{O_2}}$**) and the **arterial P_{O_2}** (**Pa_{O_2}**). **A decrease in the A-a D_{O_2} reflects an increase in the $\dot{V}/\dot{Q}$**.
   - **a.** Calculating the A-a D_{O_2} may help distinguish hypoventilation from other causes of hypoxemia and indicate the severity of lung disease.

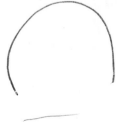

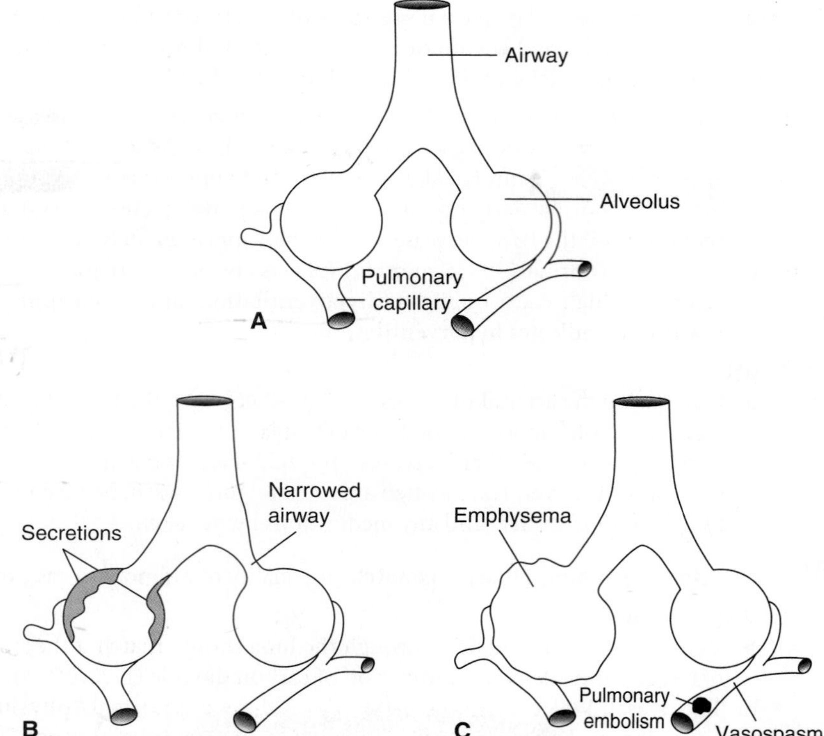

FIGURE 2–3 Examples of ventilation perfusion and the quality: a) normal idealized alveolar capillary exchange unit; b) examples of decreased ventilation–perfusion units, as a result of alveolar secretions or airway obstruction; c) examples of increased ventilation–perfusion units owing to the presence of emphysema or problems in the pulmonary vascular bed, such as pulmonary embolism or pulmonary vasospasm. (Reprinted with permission from Pulmonary Pathophysiology, Fence Creek Publishing, 1999 LLC Madison, Connecticut. Editors: Criner and D'Alonzo.)

(1) The PaO_2 is calculated from the simplified alveolar gas equation:

$$\boldsymbol{PaO_2} = FIO_2\,(P_B - PH_2O) - PaCO_2/R$$

where FIO_2 = the fraction (percentage) of oxygen in the inspired air (0.21 mm Hg for room air at sea level); P_B = atmospheric pressure (760 mm Hg); PH_2O = partial pressure

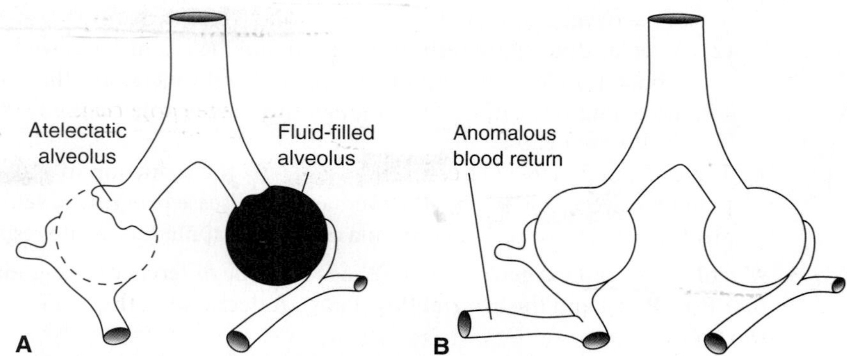

FIGURE 2–4 Examples of intrapulmonary shunt: a) collapse of fluid-filled alveolus; b) the effect of anomalous blood return of mixed blood bypassing the alveolus, and contributing to intrapulmonary shunt. (Reprinted with permission from Pulmonary Pathophysiology, Fence Creek Publishing, 1999 LLC Madison, Connecticut. Editors: Criner and D'Alonzo.)

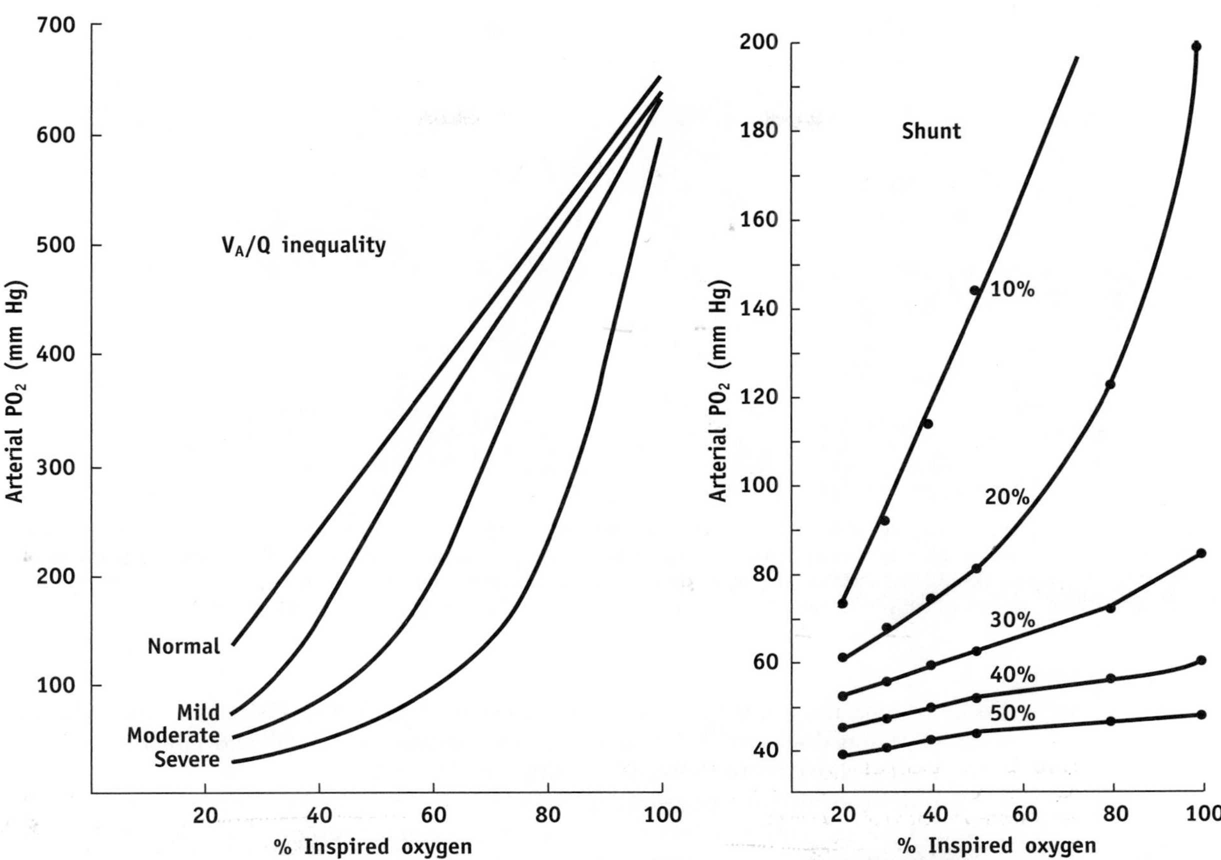

FIGURE 2–5 Response of ventilation–perfusion inequality of intrapulmonary shunt to supplemental oxygen: A) Even with the presence of severe V_A/Q inequity, high levels of supplemental oxygen have a profound impact on increasing arterial PO_2; b) By contrast, intrapulmonary shunts of 30% or greater are relatively refractory to supplemental oxygen, increasing arterial Pa_{O_2} with supplemental oxygen. Adapted from Dantzker MD, David R. Pulmonary Gas Exchange, in Bone R. Ed., Pulmonary and Critical Care Medicine. St. Louis: Mosby, 1997.

of water vapor (47 mm Hg—included in the formula because inspired air is saturated with water vapor); and R = respiratory exchange ratio (0.8).

(2) The Pa_{O_2} is determined directly from a blood sample.

(3) **The A-a D_{O_2} is therefore:**

$$A - a\,D_{O_2} = F_{IO_2}(P_B - P_{H_2O}) - \frac{Pa_{CO_2}}{R - Pa_{O_2}}$$

b. The Pa_{O_2} is normally 5–15 mm Hg lower than the Pa_{O_2} because of ***a normal degree of*** physiologic $\dot{V}/\dot{Q}$ mismatch; the difference increases with age. Thus, the A-a D_{O_2} is normally less than 15 mm Hg and increases with age.

II CHRONIC OBSTRUCTIVE PULMONARY DISEASE (COPD)

A Introduction

1. **Definition.** COPD is defined as a disease state characterized by the presence of airflow obstruction caused by chronic bronchitis or emphysema. The airflow obstruction is generally progressive, may be accompanied by airway reactivity, and may be partially reversible (Figure 2–6). COPD is a common disorder usually characterized by progressive obstruction to airflow and a

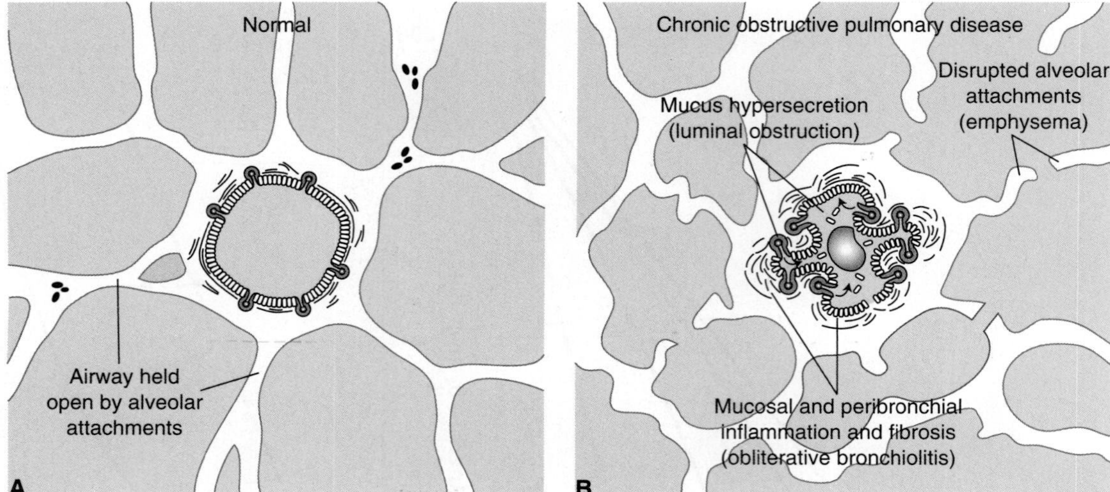

FIGURE 2–6 Examples of normal and COPD small airways. Normal peripheral airways have no evidence of inflammation or goblet cell hypertrophy and the airways are held open by alveolar attachments. By contrast, in chronic obstructive pulmonary disease, a loss of alveolar attachments, due to emphysema, contributes to small airway closure. In addition, mucous hypersecretion, and peribronchial inflammation and fibrosis contribute to obliterative bronchiolitis and luminal obstruction. Reprinted with permission from Barnes P. N Engl J Med 2000;3(43)269–280.

history of inhalation of irritants (e.g., tobacco smoke). COPD also is referred to as **chronic obstructive lung disease (COLD), chronic airway obstruction (CAO),** and, either individually or together, as chronic bronchitis and emphysema.

a. **Chronic bronchitis** may be defined in terms of clinical symptoms (i.e., excessive mucus secretion in the bronchial tree leading to productive cough for at least 3 months during each of 2 successive years).
b. **Emphysema** can be described in terms of morbid anatomy (i.e., destruction of alveolar walls and abnormal enlargement of air spaces distal to the terminal nonrespiratory bronchiole).
c. Many patients have, in varying degrees, a combination of these two entities. Therefore, the more general term COPD is appropriate.

2. The **social and economic consequences** of COPD are staggering. Screening studies of the general population suggest that 5% of individuals have significant airflow obstruction. Approximately 18 billion dollars are expended annually in health care dollars to treat COPD patients; another $9.9 billion are lost annually because of decreased work productivity.
3. The **death rate** attributable to COPD has doubled every 5 years in the past 2 decades. COPD is the fourth leading cause of death in the United States. Unlike many other diseases (coronary heart disease, stroke, and other cardiovascular diseases) for which there has been a 20%–60% decline in mortality rate over the past 20 years, the incidence of COPD has increased by 70% over the same period.

B **Etiology** The precise scientific etiology of COPD is unknown; however, the most important environmental etiologic agent is chronic inhalation of tobacco smoke (Figure 2–7). Premature birth, poor lung maturation, lower socioeconomic status, and airways hyperreactivity are believed to be additional important factors.

1. **Tobacco smoke.** Smoking in **pack-years** (the number of years a patient has smoked × the number of packs smoked per day) is directly related to ventilatory dysfunction and pathologic changes in the lung. Smoking stimulates inflammatory cytokines and depresses alveolar macrophages, reduces the functional integrity of pulmonary surfactant, retards mucus transport, enhances the

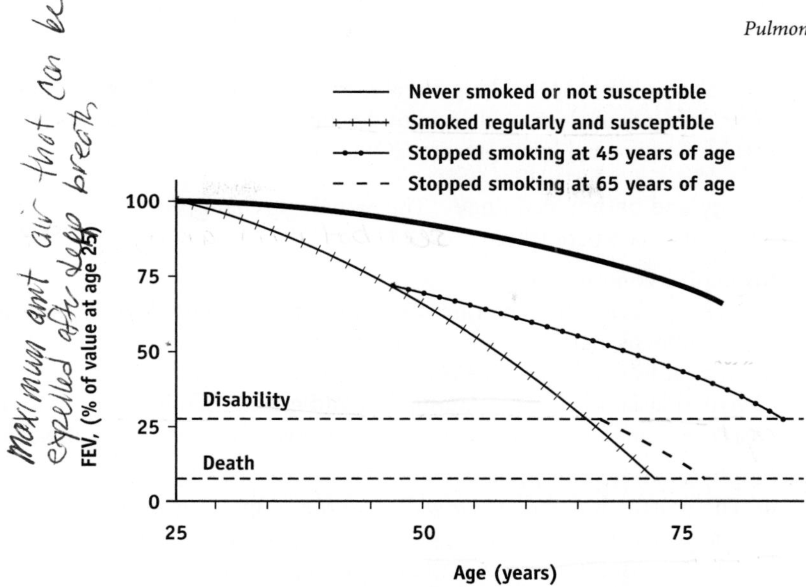

FIGURE 2–7 Age-related rate of decline in lung function in various patient groups. *FEV*$_1$ = forced expiratory volume in 1 second. (Modified with permission from Snider GL, Saling LJ, Renard SI: Chronic bronchitis and emphysema. In Murray JF, Nadel JA, eds. Textbook of Respiratory Medicine. Philadelphia: WB Saunders, 1994:1342.).

release of lysosomal enzymes, and produces numerous other effects believed to be involved in the pathogenesis of COPD.

2. **Other environmental factors**
   a. The extent that urban and industrial **air pollution** contributes to the pathogenesis of COPD is not entirely known. Studies comparing patients who live in areas of clean air with those who reside in highly polluted areas indicate a higher incidence of COPD in the latter group.
   b. The role of **infections** in the development and progression of COPD is receiving increasing attention. Evidence suggests that upper respiratory **viral infections** in childhood may predispose patients to COPD in adulthood, and viral infections are frequent precipitating factors in symptomatic exacerbations of COPD. **Bacterial infections** also have been reported to be involved in acute exacerbation of chronic bronchitis.
3. **α_1-Antitrypsin deficiency** is a well-recognized genetic factor that predisposes patients to emphysema. It accounts for approximately 2% of all cases of emphysema.
   a. Presumably, this deficiency increases the susceptibility of pulmonary tissue to autodigestion by naturally occurring proteases.
   b. Emphysema may develop early in life in individuals with homozygous deficiency. Cigarette smoking accelerates the process. In its pure form (see also Chapter 5 IX C 1), α_1-antitrypsin deficiency manifests as hepatic cirrhosis, absence of the α_1-globulin peak on serum protein electrophoresis, negligible amounts of serum α_1-antitrypsin, and advanced panlobular emphysema, predominantly in the base of the lungs.

C **Pathogenesis** Evidence suggests that COPD begins in the small airways (i.e., those <2 mm in diameter). Normally, these airways contribute only a small amount of the total resistance to airflow in the tracheobronchial tree. In COPD, however, the small airways are the sites of extensive disease and airflow limitation. Recent evidence suggests that inflammation is commonly found in histopathologic samples, involving the airway, alveolar tissue, and in some studies, the pulmonary vascular bed.

1. Histopathologic abnormalities of the small airways are common findings at autopsy in young smokers. This small-airway disease is presumed to progress over approximately 30 years to the characteristic clinical picture of disabling COPD.

2. If young smokers stop smoking, the abnormalities observed in tests of small airway function tend to resolve. It is unclear at what point during the course of the disease the changes become irreversible and inevitably progress to COPD.

D **Pathology and pathophysiology** The pathologic changes of COPD are seen in both the airways and the pulmonary parenchyma.

1. **Bronchitic component**
   a. In early disease, the small airways demonstrate mucus plugging, inflammation, peribronchiolar fibrosis, narrowing, and obliteration.
   b. In established disease, the bronchitic component includes varying degrees of mucus gland hyperplasia, mucosal inflammation and edema, bronchospasm, and impacted secretions. These elements contribute to airway narrowing and increased airway resistance.

2. **Emphysematous component**
   a. The destruction of alveolar walls and the supporting structure produces widely dilated air spaces. The loss of tissue support for the airways is believed to contribute to airway narrowing; the unsupported airways tend to collapse dynamically during expiration to low lung volumes. In addition, the loss of the alveolar capillary membrane reduces DL_{CO}.
   b. Anatomically, emphysema is classified as either **centrilobular** or **panlobular.**
      (1) **Centrilobular emphysema** often is associated with **chronic bronchitis** and **bronchial inflammation.** It is the most common type of emphysema encountered in clinical practice. The condition is rare in nonsmokers.
         (a) Centrilobular emphysema is believed to represent a destructive lesion of the respiratory bronchiole. It originates at the center of the lobule and is distinct from the periphery of the acinus with its septae and vessels.
         (b) Centrilobular emphysema is variable and patchy and has a predilection for upper lung zones. The greatly dilated respiratory bronchioles coalesce and may produce bullous cysts.
      (2) **Panlobular emphysema,** in contrast to centrilobular emphysema, has little association with chronic bronchitis and is seen commonly in patients with α_1-antitrypsin deficiency, or those with prior intravenous ritalin abuse. It is thought to evolve from dilated alveolar ducts at the periphery of the lobules to markedly enlarged air spaces.

E **Clinical features**

1. **Typical history.** COPD is an insidious, long-term process that typically develops as follows:
   a. In teenagers who smoke, mild but asymptomatic changes develop in the small airways.
   b. As adults, these smokers experience chronic cough and symptoms suggestive of an upper respiratory infection.
   c. By middle age, these smokers have significant bronchial disease characterized by progressive airway obstruction that produces dyspnea on exertion. This condition occurs in 25%–50% of smokers and frequently goes unrecognized with the patients' more sedentary lifestyle.
   d. When an unrelated health problem places the smokers' respiratory system under stress, the presence of COPD becomes evident. Pneumonia, surgery, and trauma are common precipitating events.

2. **Clinical syndromes**
   a. **Two classic types of COPD** exist and are given various names. Patients with "emphysematous," "dyspneic," or "type A" COPD are referred to as **pink puffers;** those with "bronchitic," "tussive," or "type B" COPD are referred to as **blue bloaters.**
      (1) **Pink puffers** have predominant emphysema and show symptoms at a relatively advanced age (often >60 years). There is progressive exertional dyspnea, weight loss, and little or no cough and expectoration.

(a) Pulmonary function testing indicates mild hypoxia, hypocapnia, decreased DL_{CO}, only a mild increase in Raw, and little improvement in airflow after treatment with bronchodilators.

(b) These patients usually undergo a slowly progressive downhill course.

(2) **Blue bloaters** have predominant chronic bronchitis and, at a relatively young age, experience chronic cough and expectoration, episodic dyspnea, and weight gain. Wheezing and rhonchi frequently are heard in the chest, and cor pulmonale often develops, accompanied by edema and cyanosis.

(a) Pulmonary function testing indicates severe hypoxia, hypercapnia, polycythemia, increased Raw, improved airflow after treatment with bronchodilators, and relatively preserved lung volumes and DL_{CO}.

(b) Pathologically, there is minimal emphysema but significant bronchiolitis, bronchitis, mucous gland hyperplasia, and right ventricular hypertrophy. This contrasts with pathologic findings in pink puffers.

b. Patients with emphysema have proportional and matched losses of ventilation and perfusion and, hence, are spared severe hypoxemia. In contrast, patients with chronic bronchitis have marked V/Q mismatch, resulting in severe hypoxemia. The hypoxia in chronic bronchitis is worsened by the hypercapnia, which may be the result of respiratory muscle dysfunction or an acquired or congenital reduction in central respiratory drive.

F Diagnosis

The diagnosis of COPD may be suspected based on the patient's history, symptoms, and physical signs, or it may become obvious through chest radiograph and clinical circumstances.

1. Spirometric screening may be used to diagnose COPD in middle-aged smokers.
2. On physical examination, the findings might include hyperinflation, poor diaphragmatic movement, the use of accessory muscles of respiration, and decreased breathing sounds and wheezing on auscultation.
3. The chest radiograph may show hyperinflation, a loss of vascularity, a flattened diaphragm, and a small heart. In addition, patients with chronic bronchitis often exhibit thickened bronchial walls and "dirty" lung fields.
4. Diagnosis should not rest solely on the basis of radiographic findings. Objective documentation of expiratory flow obstruction by pulmonary function testing is necessary for the diagnosis of COPD.

G Clinical course and prognosis

1. COPD tends to be a progressive disorder unless there is some form of intervention (i.e., cessation of smoking, removal of other irritants, or medical therapy). Once COPD is well advanced, specific medical treatment may not slow the progression of disease. However, cessation of smoking may alter the decline in pulmonary function in all but far-advanced disease.
2. The FEV_1 declines by approximately 50–75 mL/yr in typical patients with COPD, as compared with a normal decline of approximately half that rate.
3. Survival is statistically related to the degree of ventilatory function that exists when patients are first evaluated. For example, among patients with an initial FEV_1 of less than 0.75 L, the 5-year survival rate is 25%, whereas among those with an initial FEV_1 and 1 L, the 5-year survival rate is approximately 50%.

H Therapy

1. **Bronchodilation.** Overall, most patients with COPD show improvement in pulmonary function after sufficient bronchodilator therapy.

   a. COPD is not always an irreversible process. A patient may have airflow reactivity even when pulmonary function studies performed after bronchodilator therapy have indicated nonreversible airflow obstruction. It appears that 15%–20% of COPD patients in this category have reversible airflow obstruction.

b. The three major classes of bronchodilators are **β-adrenergic agonists, anticholinergics** (ipratropium bromide), and **xanthines** (theophylline-type agents). These agents may be used separately or in combination. The newer, selective β-adrenergic agonists offer advantages over the older agents in terms of a longer duration of bronchodilating action (β_2 effect) and reduced cardiac stimulation (β_1 effect). Some newer β agonists have acute as well as long-acting effects.

2. **Corticosteroid therapy.** The use of corticosteroids in the treatment of the bronchospasm associated with COPD is controversial. However, some patients clearly have an asthma-like component to their disease and ***may*** likely respond to steroid therapy to some extent. Delivery of inhaled corticosteroids by a metered-dose inhaler (MDI) is the preferred route of administration, although the role of these agents in COPD is not clearly defined.

3. **Sputum mobilization.** Traditional expectorants and mucolytic agents appear to have little beneficial effect in COPD patients. Bland hydrating aerosols and physical therapy may improve bronchial drainage transiently, but the long-term benefit is not known. Postural drainage usually is reserved for patients with bronchiectasis.

4. **Management of infection.** Patients presenting in exacerbation are more likely to be infected with *Haemophilus influenza, Moraxella catarrhalis,* or *Streptococcus pneumoniae.* In addition, patients with this disease should receive annual vaccination against influenza as well as a vaccine for pneumococcal infection.

5. **Pulmonary rehabilitation programs.** Participation in these programs may improve exercise performance, decrease dyspnea, and improve quality of life. Patients are instructed in exercise programs aimed at increasing exercise tolerance and respiratory muscle stamina. In addition, counseling and nutritional guidance are available.

6. **Surgery**

a. The **resection** of large localized bullae (e.g., bullectomy) may benefit patients with large bullae that occupy more than one third of a hemithorax, without evidence of diffuse underlying emphysema.

b. Single and double lung transplantations have been performed in patients with COPD, and they improve quality of life and exercise tolerance. However, bronchiolitis obliterans continues to be the major obstacle to long-term success; 5-year mortality still approaches 50%.

c. A new technique, lung volume reduction surgery (LVRS), has been shown to improve lung function, exercise performance, quality of life, and even survival in select patients with emphysema. Upper lobe predominant emphysema by CT scan appears to be the key prognostic factor in predicting success with LVRS. By decreasing lung volume in hyperinflated subjects, LVRS improves respiratory muscle function, chest wall mechanics, and increases lung recoil, thereby facilitating enhanced expiratory flow.

7. **Oxygen.** Oxygen is the only therapeutic modality other than LVRS that can improve survival. Its value, however, is only demonstrable in those patients with a PaO_2 of 55 mm Hg or less on room air at rest.

8. **α_1-Antitrypsin.** For those patients with a deficiency of α_1-antitrypsin, replacement therapy is available.

I Prevention Avoidance of smoking is by far the best means of disease prevention. In addition, patients should avoid chronic exposure to other bronchial irritants. Simple spirometric screening of high-risk patients can help detect early disease and prevent further deterioration.

J Complications of COPD include cor pulmonale, polycythemia, infection, respiratory failure, bronchogenic carcinoma, nocturnal hypoxia, general disability, and (for unknown reasons) a proclivity for peptic ulcer disease.

1. **Pneumonia** occurring in a COPD patient is of special concern because of its relative severity and its potential for precipitating respiratory failure.
2. **Respiratory failure** may be precipitated by many conditions, including heart failure, sedation, infection, acute bronchospasm, and trauma.
3. Although **bronchogenic carcinoma** is not strictly a complication of COPD, it occurs in COPD patients with high frequency, presumably because of the common denominator of tobacco smoking.
4. General disability, although expected by the degree of lung impairment in COPD patients, appears also to result from concomitant peripheral muscle weakness. Whole-body rehabilitation may be an important adjunct in most moderately to severely afflicted patients.

III ASTHMA

A Definition Asthma is a reversible airway obstruction that is characterized by hyperirritability and inflammation of the airways. Substances that have no effect when inhaled by normal individuals can cause bronchoconstriction in patients with asthma. Asthma per se does not cause emphysema or other chronic diseases, but it alone may be a significant cause of disability. A principal feature of asthma is its **extreme variability,** both from patient to patient and from time to time in the same patient. Another feature of asthma that is important to its pathophysiology and treatment is the presence of **airway inflammation.**

B Incidence and etiology

1. Asthma occurs in 3%–8% of the population. Etiologic or pathologic classification of the disease is difficult; however, asthma traditionally is divided into two forms.
   a. An **allergic form,** responsible for most cases of asthma in children, is immunologically mediated—it is caused by type I (immediate) hypersensitivity to inhaled antigens.
   b. An **intrinsic form,** which occurs in adults, shows no evidence of immediate hypersensitivity to specific antigens.
2. In patients in whom the evidence of immediate hypersensitivity to antigen is absent or equivocal, most attacks do not appear to be provoked by inhalation of antigens, and there is a poor correlation between the severity of symptoms and the levels of specific antigens circulating as airborne particles. These observations indicate that asthmatic bronchospasm may not necessarily require an immunologically mediated hypersensitivity reaction.

C Pathogenesis

1. **Biochemical mediators**
   a. The **mediators of immediate hypersensitivity** and their mechanisms of action are discussed in Chapter 7 II A.
   b. **Other biochemical mediators,** including serotonin, prostaglandins, thromboxanes, and endoperoxides, also cause tissue inflammation and may be particularly important in the pathogenesis of **nonallergic** asthma (Figure 2–8).
   c. The physiologic changes seen in asthma can be directly induced by mediators that diffuse locally to mucous glands, vessels, and smooth muscle. Clearly, however, the simple release of mediators is not sufficient to cause an asthmatic attack.
2. **Airway hyperirritability**
   a. The tracheobronchial tree of asthmatic individuals appears to have an exaggerated reactivity, sometimes called **nonspecific bronchial hyperreactivity,** to distinguish it from the bronchospasm provoked by immunologically specific antigens. The ubiquity of bronchial hyperreactivity has caused pathogenetic theories to shift in focus from the **nature of biochemical mediators** to the **responsiveness of the end organ.**

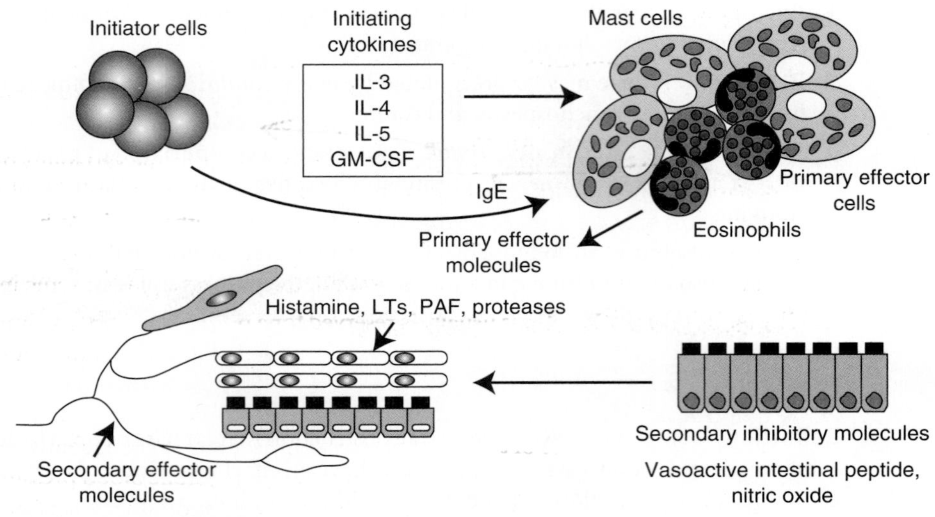

FIGURE 2–8 Pathogenesis of the potential events contributing to asthmatic airways obstruction. Reprinted by permission of Jeffrey Drazen, MD. www.uptodate.com.

b. The mechanism underlying bronchial hyperreactivity is unknown, but a number of factors have been suggested.

(1) **Muscle reactivity.** A change in the contractile mechanisms of airway smooth muscle may induce hyperreactivity.

(2) **Autonomic reactivity.** The abnormality may exist in the nerves that regulate the tone of the muscle, not in the muscle itself.

(a) The **parasympathetic system** appears to mediate the reflex bronchial constriction caused by inhalation of nonspecific irritants such as dust or sulfur dioxide.

(b) A deficiency in the **sympathetic nervous system** may be responsible for bronchial hyperreactivity.

(c) The **nonadrenergic inhibitor system,** a third system of autonomic innervation, may exist in the bronchial muscles as it does in the gut, where it seems to inhibit constriction of intestinal smooth muscle. Congenital absence of this system leads to Hirschsprung's disease (see Chapter 5 V C), in which the distal bowel is intensely constricted. A similar deficiency in the airway conceivably could cause recurrent constriction of bronchial smooth muscle.

(3) **Environmental factors.** Bronchial reactivity is temporarily increased by upper respiratory viral infections and by exposure to pollutants such as ozone, nitrogen dioxide (NO_2), and industrial fumes. By amplifying the response to the materials released from mast cells, this increased reactivity could be responsible for the exacerbations of asthma seen with viral infections, occupational exposures, and exposure to severe pollution.

D Pathophysiology

1. Pathophysiologically, asthma is characterized by constriction of airway smooth muscle, hypersecretion of mucus, edema and inflammatory cell infiltration of the airway mucosa, and thickening of the basement membrane underlying the airway epithelium.

2. These pathophysiologic changes are not uniformly distributed. Some airways may display a predominance of bronchospasm, others may be occluded by mucous plugging, and still others may appear unaffected.

E Clinical features

1. Classic **presentation** involves episodic bouts of coughing, dyspnea, chest tightness, and expiratory wheezing. Upper respiratory viral infection, exposure to allergens, emotional stress, and many nonspecific precipitating events may provoke asthmatic attacks.
2. The **symptoms** exhibit a wide spectrum of severity, reflecting the variability of the underlying airway obstruction. Some patients display only occasional attacks of exertional dyspnea and wheezing, which respond to inhaled bronchodilators alone. Other patients have chronic symptoms requiring continuous use of orally inhaled medications. Although this latter group of patients may have irreversible thickening of the airway walls, their illness still is episodic in occurrence.
3. The term **status asthmaticus** usually is reserved for a prolonged, severe asthmatic attack that does not respond to treatment and involves bronchospasm so severe that the patient is at risk for ventilatory failure.
   a. The clinical manifestations of severe asthma include fatigue, a pulse rate of more than 100 bpm, and cyanosis. The use of accessory muscles for respiration is frequently evident.
   b. An inspiratory decrease of more than 20 mm Hg in systolic blood pressure (i.e., **pulsus paradoxus**) indicates gross overinflation of the lung and wide swings in pleural pressure.

F Diagnosis

1. **Physical examination** typically shows tachycardia; tachypnea with prolonged expiration; overinflation of the chest with poor movement of the diaphragm; and diffuse, high-pitched expiratory wheezing.
2. **Sputum analysis.** Sputum may appear purulent because of an increased eosinophil content or an inflammatory response to a viral tracheobronchitis. Sputum smears may reveal **Curschmann's spirals** (i.e., mucus that forms a cast of the small airways) or **Charcot–Leyden crystals** (i.e., breakdown products of the eosinophils).
3. **Hematologic studies** indicate a modest leukocytosis and eosinophilia in both the allergic and intrinsic forms of the disease.
4. **Pulmonary function testing**
   a. The FVC is reduced; the FEV_1/FVC is reduced but may improve after inhalation of a bronchodilator. RV, TLC, and lung compliance usually are increased, and the DL_{CO} frequently is increased.

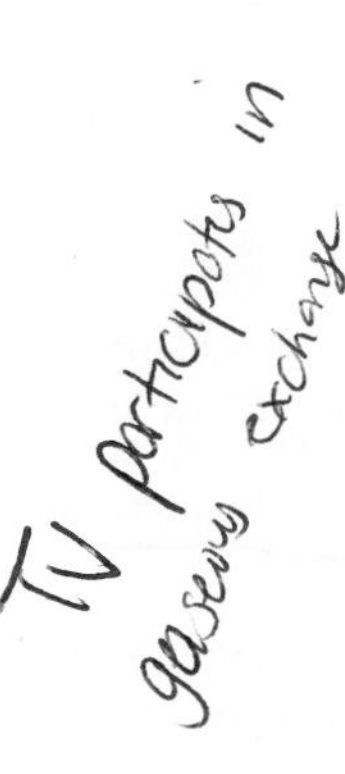

   b. After symptomatic recovery, TLC and lung compliance return to normal, but the maximal expiratory flow rate may remain reduced at low lung volumes, and an abnormal distribution of ventilation may persist, reflecting resistant obstruction of small airways.
5. **Chest radiography** usually shows nothing more than overinflation. Occasional findings include localized density caused by a large mucous plug and the ominous sign of pneumothorax or pneumomediastinum, reflecting the rupture of alveolar tissue caused by high intra-alveolar pressure.
6. **Arterial blood gas studies.** The Pa_{CO_2} usually is low (i.e., < 36 mm Hg). An increased Pa_{CO_2} or a normal Pa_{CO_2} (40 mm Hg) indicates severe obstruction. Arterial hypoxemia is common despite the increased ventilation and is due to underventilation of lung segments supplied by narrowed airways (i.e., there is a $\dot{V}/\dot{Q}$ mismatch).

G **Therapy** is based on an understanding of the underlying pathophysiologic mechanisms. Effective management of asthma relies on four integral components: objective measures of lung function, pharmacologic therapy, environmental measures to control allergens and irritants, and patient education.

1. **Goals of therapy.** The goals of therapy are to:
   a. Maintain near-normal pulmonary function
   b. Maintain normal activity levels

c. Prevent chronic and troublesome symptoms (e.g., cough, nocturnal symptoms)
d. Prevent recurrent exacerbations
e. Avoid adverse effects from asthma medications

2. **Principles of treatment.** Asthma is a **chronic condition with acute exacerbations.**
   a. **Prevention** of exacerbations is particularly important.
   b. **Early intervention** when treating acute exacerbations of asthma is important to reduce the likelihood of developing severe airway narrowing.
   c. **Control of airway inflammation** is a key factor in treating asthma, as suggested by evidence of the presence of airway inflammation in all subjects with asthma. Morphologic studies show that bronchial infiltration with inflammatory cells is most evident in mild-to-severe asthma. The increased levels of inflammatory mediators are associated with airway hyperresponsiveness.

3. **Pharmacologic therapy**
   a. **Anti-inflammatory agents** (e.g., **corticosteroids, cromolyn sodium, cromolyn-like compounds**), which interrupt the development of bronchial inflammation, have a prophylactic or preventive action. They also may modulate ongoing inflammatory reactions. These agents decrease the severity of acute asthma attacks as well as chronic asthma.
      (1) Administration may be oral or via an inhaler.
      (2) Oral or intravenous routes are recommended in acute attacks; aerosolized corticosteroids are for long-term use.
   b. **Bronchodilators** act principally to dilate the airways by relaxing bronchial smooth muscle. Agents include sympathomimetics, methylxanthines, and anticholinergics.
      (1) **Methylxanthines** (theophylline) and **sympathomimetics** (β_2-agonists) are used during acute attacks of asthma. Methylxanthines are given intravenously at a loading dose, followed by continuous infusion, and β_2-agonists are inhaled.
      (2) **Anticholinergic agents** (e.g., ipratropium) are used primarily as supplements to other bronchodilators during acute attacks.
   c. **Leukotriene modifiers** are a newer class of drugs that are useful in long-term control of a select group of asthmatics. They act by inhibiting different parts of the arachidonic cascade, which plays an important role in asthma and airway inflammation.
   d. Anti-IgE antibody therapy may be helpful in some asthmatics with elevated IgE serum levels.

IV BRONCHIECTASIS, CYSTIC FIBROSIS, AND LUNG ABSCESS

A Bronchiectasis

1. **Definition.** Bronchiectasis is a pathologic, irreversible dilatation of the bronchi caused by destruction of the bronchial wall, usually resulting from suppurative infection in an obstructed bronchus.
2. **Etiology and pathogenesis**
   a. The small bronchi of childhood are most susceptible to bronchial infection and to obstruction by impacted secretions, foreign bodies, or compressing lymph nodes. Seventy-five percent of patients can recall experiencing symptoms of bronchiectasis as early as the age of 5 years.
   b. The most common cause of bronchiectasis is bacterial pneumonia, which may be primary or may be a complication of measles, aspiration of gastric contents or particulate matter, or tumor.
   c. Predisposing conditions include congenital disorders (e.g., congenital cystic disease of the lung, bronchial stenosis, or compression of bronchi by anomalous arteries to the lung); immune deficiencies [e.g., hypogammaglobulinemia or immunoglobulin A (IgA) deficiency]; and cystic fibrosis.
3. **Clinical features.** Symptoms include a chronic cough productive of purulent sputum, recurrent chest colds or pneumonias, occasional hemoptysis, and pleuritic pain. These symptoms cannot

be differentiated from those of chronic suppurative bronchitis. Progressive dyspnea, cyanosis, digital clubbing, and cor pulmonale are seen in advanced cases.

4. **Diagnosis**
   a. **Physical examination** indicates rales over the area of involvement on repeated examinations.
   b. **Pulmonary function testing** produces normal results in mild cases, but, in moderate or severe cases, it may reveal either restrictive or a mixture of restrictive or obstructive ventilatory patterns.
   c. **Chest radiography** shows peribronchial fibrosis in the involved segment. Segmental lung collapse in areas of bronchiectasis is common.
   d. **Bronchography** can provide a definitive diagnosis if the patient is stable and not actively infected or coughing up blood. Secretions and clots block the entry of contrast medium, and pneumonia causes temporary dilatation of the bronchi.
   e. **Computed tomography (CT) scanning,** particularly **high-resolution computed tomography (HRCT),** can often identify bronchiectasis, eliminating the need for bronchography.

5. **Therapy.** The proper therapy can markedly improve symptoms.
   a. **Medical treatment** is the mainstay and consists of therapy with antibiotics on a frequent or regular basis (e.g., ampicillin, tetracycline, erythromycin, or as indicated by culture and sensitivity testing), postural drainage, and immunization against influenza and pneumococcal pneumonia.
   b. **Surgical resection** generally is not effective for eliminating chronic cough and sputum unless the operation is performed in early childhood for single local airway disease.
   c. **Bronchodilation** may be effective if the obstruction is reversible.
   d. **Oxygen therapy** is appropriate if $Pa{O_2}$ levels are depressed.

B Cystic fibrosis

1. **Definition.** Cystic fibrosis is an autosomal recessive disease characterized by dysfunction of the exocrine glands, leading to obstruction in such organs as the lungs, pancreas, and gastrointestinal tract. In 99% of patients with cystic fibrosis, death is caused by respiratory failure, with portal hypertension secondary to biliary cirrhosis accounting for the remainder of deaths.

2. **Incidence**
   a. An estimated 30,000 individuals with cystic fibrosis patients live in the United States. The disease is most common in whites, occurring in 1 of 2000–2500 births, and 5% of the white population are carriers. Because inheritance is recessive and heterozygotes have no disease, a negative family history does not rule out the disease.
   b. Once thought to be unique to children, cystic fibrosis now is recognized as the most common cause of obstructive airway disease among individuals up to age 30 years. The median age of patients with cystic fibrosis has risen from the teens in the 1960s to approximately 31 years in 1998.

3. **Etiology and pathogenesis.** The genetic abnormality that is responsible for cystic fibrosis has been identified.
   a. Most patients with cystic fibrosis have a deletion at position 508 on the long arm of chromosome 7. This deletion produces an abnormal membrane transport protein called **cystic fibrosis transmembrane regulator (CFTR).**
   b. The abnormality seems to be an electrochemical defect in the epithelial cell that involves chloride impermeability and increased sodium resorption. This abnormality leads to the viscid mucus that is observed and the subsequent obstruction of organs served by exocrine glands.

4. **Clinical features.** The manifestations of cystic fibrosis are varied, with pulmonary abnormalities being the overriding clinical concern.

a. Pulmonary manifestations

(1) The earliest pulmonary manifestation is peripheral airway obstruction resulting from plugged bronchi. Repeated bouts of infection lead to a cycle of obstruction, tissue damage, and infection that ultimately progresses to a loss of pulmonary function.

(2) The predominant organism to colonize the lung is the highly resistant mucoid strain of *Pseudomonas aeruginosa.* Initial infections may be due to *Staphylococcus aureus.* Complete eradication of the organisms is virtually impossible.

(3) Many patients with cystic fibrosis develop sinusitis and nasal polyps, and most have clubbing of the digits.

(4) Older children and adolescents have problems referable to the cardiopulmonary system, but most patients die of respiratory complications.

b. Nonpulmonary manifestations also are common and include meconium ileus, malabsorption, fatty infiltration of the liver, focal biliary cirrhosis, glucose intolerance, sterility in males, and a predilection for heat prostration due to severe salt depletion. As patients live longer, osteoporosis has become a problem in males as well as females. In addition, there appears to be some epidemiologic evidence of an increase in some gastrointestinal cancers.

5. Diagnosis

a. Sweat test. An abnormal sweat test is observed in virtually all cases, and in combination with certain clinical hallmarks, confirms the diagnosis.

(1) The sodium and chloride concentrations in sweat are elevated drastically, whereas normal concentrations of these ions exist elsewhere. The **quantitative pilocarpine iontophoresis sweat test** defines the upper limit of normal as a sweat chloride concentration of 60 mEq/L.

(2) A positive sweat test is diagnostic of cystic fibrosis in the presence of at least one of the following three criteria:

(a) A reliable family history of cystic fibrosis

(b) Obstructive pulmonary disease

(c) Pancreatic insufficiency

b. Pulmonary function testing shows limitation of maximal expiratory flow rate and an elevated RV. The DL_{CO} is usually within normal limits.

c. Chest radiography shows striking manifestations that are more pronounced at the apices, particularly on the right. Findings include hyperinflation, cyst formation, atelectasis, bronchiectasis, and segmental infiltration.

6. Therapy

a. In the **early stages** of the disease, therapy must be individualized according to specific clinical manifestations.

(1) Salt depletion is a potential problem in warmer climates.

(2) Nutritional supplementation and pancreatic enzyme replacement often are indicated.

(3) Pulmonary infections may require hospitalization and vigorous treatment with parenteral antibiotics, hydration, humidification, and supplemental oxygen.

b. In the **late stages** of the disease, therapy is aimed at suppressing infection with specific antibiotics, inducing sputum through physical manipulation, and administering supplemental oxygen as required. Dornase-α, a drug that hydrolyzes extracellular DNA and makes sputum less viscous, has been approved for use in patients with cystic fibrosis. This drug has been shown to decrease respiratory tract infections and increase pulmonary function. Aerosolized tobramycin is the most recent approved agent. The new formulation of this aminoglycoside antibiotic has demonstrated improved pulmonary function and decreased symptoms when used on a chronic basis.

c. In **end-stage** disease, bilateral lung transplantation (the procedure of choice) can be considered. Results are similar to those obtained with bilateral lung transplantation in other end-stage lung diseases.

d. New therapies aimed at counteracting the pathophysiologic process of cystic fibrosis are being tested. These include gene therapy; manipulation of ion transport and protein trafficking; as well as administration of anti-inflammatory agents, antibiotics, and antielastases.

7. **Complications. Cor pulmonale** that is only partially responsive to oxygen therapy develops late in the disease, with all of the manifestations of right-sided heart failure (e.g., hepatomegaly, peripheral edema). Other pulmonary complications of cystic fibrosis include **hemoptysis** and **pneumothorax.**

C Lung abscess (see also Chapter 8 V C 5)

1. **Definition.** A lung abscess is a localized area of infection within the lung parenchyma that develops from an initial pneumonic stage. The center of the infected area first becomes gangrenous, necrotic, and purulent and then becomes well demarcated from the surrounding lung tissue. The wall of the abscess becomes intensely inflamed and lined with fibrous and granulation tissue and abundant blood vessels.
2. **Etiology.** A solitary lung abscess most commonly results from aspiration of secretions in the upper respiratory tract. Other major but less common causes include bronchial obstruction, bacterial pneumonia, pulmonary embolism with infection, spread from transdiaphragmatic infections, chest trauma, and bacteremic infection.
3. **Clinical features**
   a. Initial symptoms are similar to those of acute pneumonia.
   b. Chronically, lung abscess is associated with constitutional symptoms that include weight loss, low-grade fever, fatigue, and malaise.
4. **Diagnosis**
   a. **Physical examination** may reveal relatively normal findings, although clubbing of the nailbeds occasionally is noted. Amphoric breath sounds may be heard over the abscess cavity.
   b. **Pulmonary function testing** usually is not affected by a lung abscess.
   c. **Bronchoscopy** is indicated when an abscess does not resolve completely with antibiotic therapy, or when the possibility of a malignancy or foreign body in the lung must be ruled out.
5. **Therapy.** The treatment of choice is antibiotics, either penicillin or clindamycin. The total duration of therapy may be 4–8 weeks.

V ACUTE RESPIRATORY FAILURE

A Definition

Acute respiratory failure is defined as hypoxemia (i.e., a PaO_2 of < 50 mm Hg) with or without associated hypercapnia (i.e., a $PaCO_2$ of > 45 mm Hg).

B Classification

Acute respiratory failure can be divided into two types.

1. **Type I: respiratory failure without carbon dioxide retention** (i.e., low PaO_2 with low or normal $PaCO_2$). This type of respiratory failure is characterized by marked $\dot{V}/\dot{Q}$ abnormalities and intrapulmonary shunting. **Type I** respiratory failure occurs in such clinical settings as:
   a. *Acute* respiratory distress syndrome (ARDS) [see VI]
   b. Diffuse pneumonia (viral and bacterial)
   c. Aspiration pneumonitis
   d. Fat embolism
   e. Pulmonary edema
2. **Type II: respiratory failure with carbon dioxide retention** (i.e., low PaO_2 with elevated $PaCO_2$). Type II respiratory failure, or **ventilatory failure,** has two basic physiologic abnormalities—$\dot{V}/\dot{Q}$ imbalance and inadequate alveolar ventilation. Patients with type II respiratory failure are divided into two categories.

a. Patients with **intrinsic lung disease** characterized by **both $\dot{V}/\dot{Q}$ imbalance and inadequate alveolar ventilation.** Respiratory failure is precipitated by additional clinical insult, usually infection, which worsens the physiologic abnormalities. Examples of such lung diseases include:
   (1) COPD (chronic bronchitis, emphysema) and cystic fibrosis
   (2) Acute obstructive lung disease (asthma, severe acute bronchitis)

b. Patients **with intrinsically normal lungs** but with **inadequate ventilation** due to:
   (1) Disorders of respiratory control [e.g., as a result of drug overdose, central nervous system (CNS) disease, trauma, or cerebrovascular accident (CVA)]
   (2) Neuromuscular abnormalities (e.g., poliomyelitis, myasthenia gravis, Guillain-Barré syndrome)
   (3) Chest wall trauma, kyphoscoliosis

C Pathophysiologic mechanisms of hypoxemia

1. **$\dot{V}/\dot{Q}$ imbalance,** the most common pathophysiologic cause of hypoxemia, arises when alveolar ventilation decreases with respect to perfusion in the lung. Hypoxemia resulting from a moderate decrease in the $\dot{V}/\dot{Q}$ can be reversed with relatively small increases in the inspired oxygen concentration (i.e., 24%–40% inspired oxygen).

2. **Intrapulmonary shunting** occurs when ventilation approaches or reaches zero in perfused areas (e.g., due to collapsed or fluid-filled alveoli), so that venous blood is shunted directly to the arterial circulation without first being oxygenated. Hypoxemia due to a shunt frequently cannot be corrected, even with 100% inspired oxygen.

3. **Hypoventilation with resulting hypercapnia** may contribute to hypoxemia. This represents type II respiratory failure.

4. **An abnormality in the diffusion of oxygen across the alveolar–capillary membrane** may contribute to hypoxemia during exercise or in conditions of lowered inspired oxygen content [most commonly due to high altitude (e.g., during a commercial airline flight)]. However, the contribution of this mechanism to respiratory failure, if any, is insignificant.

D Therapy

1. **Principles.** Treatment is directed toward the underlying disease as well as toward the ventilatory and hypoxic components. In addition, the acute and chronic aspects of respiratory failure must be considered. Patients with chronic respiratory failure frequently can tolerate a lower $Pa{O_2}$ and a higher $Pa{CO_2}$ than those with acute respiratory failure.

2. **Oxygen therapy**

   a. In **type I respiratory failure,** patients may be given high concentrations of inspired oxygen, because carbon dioxide retention is not a risk. Oxygen may be delivered by mask or nasal cannula. The use of devices to increase end-expiratory lung volumes, such as continuous positive airway pressure (CPAP) or, in more severe cases, intubation with mechanical ventilation (see VI E 1 b), may be required.

   b. In **type II respiratory failure,** treatment depends on the cause.
      (1) When the cause is an exacerbation of COPD, the basis of therapy is controlled administration of oxygen (i.e., low-flow oxygen treatment), with care taken not to increase the $Pa{CO_2}$. Mechanical ventilation may be needed.
         (a) **Noninvasive mask ventilation** with bilevel positive airway pressure (BiPAP) or preset volume ventilation has been used with some success, thus avoiding the need for airway intubation.
      (2) Type II respiratory failure that arises from causes other than COPD usually is an indication for either noninvasive or invasive mechanical ventilation.

VI ACUTE RESPIRATORY DISTRESS SYNDROME (ARDS)

A Definition

1. **Clinical definition.** ARDS is an important form of acute hypoxemic, hypocapnic (i.e., type I) respiratory failure characterized by severe dyspnea, hypoxia, loss of lung compliance, and pulmonary edema. The synonym **"wet lung"** emphasizes the presence of increased extravascular lung water (the basic pathophysiologic mechanism underlying this condition).
2. **Physiologic definition**
   a. The ratio of $Pa{O_2}$ to $F{IO_2}$ is ≤ 200, regardless of the presence or level of positive end-expiratory pressure (PEEP).
   b. There is a finding of bilateral pulmonary infiltrates.
   c. There is pulmonary capillary wedge pressure (PCWP) of ≤ 18 mm Hg or no clinical evidence of elevated left atrial pressure.

B Etiology

ARDS can be initiated by many different events and conditions, including shock, aspiration of fluid, disseminated intravascular coagulation (DIC), bacterial septicemia, trauma, blood transfusion, pancreatitis, smoke inhalation, and heroin overdose.

C Pathogenesis and pathophysiology

1. An insult to the capillary endothelium or alveolar epithelium precipitates ARDS. This insult results in capillary congestion and interstitial edema, leading to disruption of capillary integrity and the extravasation of fluid, fibrin, red blood cells (RBCs), and white blood cells (WBCs) into the lung interstitium, lymphatics, and, ultimately, the alveoli.
   a. Tumor necrosis factor-α (TNF-α) and interleukin-1 (IL-1), "early response" cytokines, are critical for initiating the inflammatory response.
   b. These cytokines then stimulate IL-8, which perpetuates inflammation and coagulation.
2. The severe hypoxemia is caused by extreme $\dot{V}/\dot{Q}$ imbalance and the shunting of blood in the fluid-filled areas of the lung.
3. The lungs stiffen and become less compliant, resulting in difficulty with mechanical ventilation and subsequent high peak airway pressures.

D Clinical features and diagnosis

Symptoms may develop immediately after the insult but usually are delayed 24–48 hours.

1. Progressive tachypnea usually is the earliest sign, followed by dyspnea.
2. Physical findings often are absent or limited to bronchial breath sounds and rales.
3. Pulmonary function and blood gas studies show increased minute ventilation, decreased lung volumes, and acute respiratory alkalosis.
4. Chest radiograph shows patchy, diffuse bilateral, fluffy infiltrates.
5. Cardiac output usually is increased somewhat, although terminally it may decrease and be accompanied by metabolic acidosis and tissue hypoxia.

E Therapy

1. **Oxygenation.** The ultimate goal of therapy is to provide adequate tissue oxygenation. Overall tissue oxygenation can be estimated from the mixed venous oxygen content ($C\bar{v}{O_2}$). In addition, concomitant measurement of cardiac output by thermodilution may aid in the correction of abnormal oxygen transport.
   a. Hypoxemia can be corrected by maintaining the $Pa{O_2}$ at approximately 60–80 mm Hg. This results in approximately a 90% oxygen saturation, which ensures that tissue oxygen needs are met as long as cardiac output and hemoglobin levels are normal.

b. **Mechanical ventilation** is required by most patients with ARDS.

(1) **PEEP** commonly is used to increase lung volume (i.e., FRC), reduce intrapulmonary shunt, and improve $\dot{V}/\dot{Q}$ relationships. PEEP may cause barotrauma or a reduced cardiac output. In patients whose cardiac output is compromised, the PaO_2 increases but oxygen delivery to the tissues may decrease. Therefore, it is important to measure mixed venous PaO_2 (MvO_2) and cardiac output when using PEEP.

(2) A recent large multicentered NIH-supported trial showed that the use of a low tidal volume strategy (e.g., 6 mL/kg) decreased mortality compared with one using a larger tidal volume (12 mL/kg).

(3) Other methods of ventilation such as **inverse-ratio, pressure release,** and **high-frequency ventilation** may be useful in certain situations.

(4) Some studies have demonstrated that placing patients in the prone position or using inhaled nitric oxide may improve oxygenation, but neither treatment improves survival.

2. **Other measures.** The underlying disease process must be treated. In addition, patients who require more than 24–48 hours of mechanical ventilation should receive nutritional support, preferably through the gastrointestinal tract.

3. **Possible new treatments.** Some potential new therapies are undergoing clinical trials. They include surfactant replacement; corticosteroids (given after 3 days); ketoconazole (inhibition of thromboxane synthesis); antiendotoxin antibodies; TNF-α antibodies and IL-1 receptor antagonists; and therapies limiting fluid administration to decrease the development of extravascular lung water.

VII PULMONARY HYPERTENSION

A Definitions

1. Pulmonary hypertension is a condition characterized by chronic elevation of pulmonary artery pressure to >25 mm Hg at rest, or >30 mm Hg with exercise.

   a. The World Health Organization has also recently defined pulmonary hypertension to be present when a systolic pulmonary artery pressure is >40 mm Hg, which corresponds to tricuspid regurgitation on a Doppler echo of 3 to 3.5 m/sec.

2. Pulmonary hypertension is further defined as to whether it is primary or secondary in origin.

   a. **Primary pulmonary hypertension (PPH)** is sustained elevation in pulmonary artery pressure without an identifiable cause.

   b. **Secondary pulmonary hypertension** (also known as ***cor pulmonale***) is sustained elevation of pulmonary artery pressure attributable to an underlying cause, such as emphysema, parenchymal diseases as found in sarcoidosis, idiopathic pulmonary fibrosis, human immunodeficiency virus (HIV) disease, portal hypertension, cocaine inhalation, or use of appetite suppressant drugs.

B Incidence

1. True estimates of the incidence of primary or secondary pulmonary hypertension are difficult to obtain because of the vagueness of patient symptoms, diagnosis made relatively late in the patient's course, and the requirement in some cases for invasive tests to accurately diagnose the disease.

   a. Current data suggest that the incidence of primary pulmonary hypertension in the general population is approximately 1–2 cases per million individuals.

   b. The incidence of secondary pulmonary hypertension is even more difficult to ascertain. In some disorders, such as HIV-related disease, approximately 2% of patients are found to have associated pulmonary hypertension. In patients with pulmonary hypertension, approximately 0.5% of patients are found to have portal hypertension. In patients who use appetite suppressant drugs, the likelihood of developing pulmonary hypertension (odds ratio, 6.3) was much greater if the patients used drugs for more than 3 months.

3. More study is required to estimate the true incidence of secondary pulmonary hypertension, that which is secondary to other disease processes.

C Pathogenesis and Histopathology

1. In patients with primary pulmonary hypertension, three factors contribute to an elevation in pulmonary artery pressure: **vasoconstriction, remodeling of the vascular wall,** and **in situ thrombosis.**
   a. In patients with secondary pulmonary hypertension, these three factors may coexist, in conjunction with a reduction in pulmonary capillary bed size (morbid obesity, massive pleural effusions with volume overload, kyphoscoliosis) or destruction of the underlying lung parenchyma (advanced emphysema, sarcoidosis, and chronic nonresolved thromboembolic disease).
2. Vasoconstriction was first considered to be an important element in the pathogenesis of pulmonary hypertension, because vasodilation was noted in response to administration of acetylcholine. Moreover, evidence of medial hypertrophy of the pulmonary artery wall indicates vasoconstriction inducing arterial smooth muscle proliferation. Other elements considered important in the pathogenesis of vasoconstriction include an imbalance of prostacyclin to thromboxane and impaired synthesis of endothelial-derived nitric oxide, which acts as a local vasorelaxant. As vasoconstriction remains sustained, intimal and adventitial tissue proliferates.
3. Eventually, thrombosis may result from injury to the endothelium, abnormal fibrosis, increased procoagulant activity, and underlying platelet dysfunction.
4. The histopathology of pulmonary hypertension represents a combination of pulmonary artery injury and repair. Although several histopathologic patterns are observed, none appears to be pathognomonic for the entity.
   a. Plexogenic pulmonary arteriopathy is the most common lesion; it is characterized by medial hypertrophy and fibrotic intimal lesions that may contain organized thrombi.
   b. Thrombotic pulmonary arteriopathy is present when organized mural thrombi are seen, causing in situ thrombosis in the setting of an uninvolved arterial wall in a pulmonary artery of normal dimensions.
   c. Increased thickness of the medial smooth wall of the pulmonary artery (e.g., isolated medial hypertrophy) precedes the formation of plexogenic lesions and may be reversible with treatment.

D Epidemiology

1. The mean age of patients developing primary pulmonary hypertension is approximately 36 years of age, with a slight female to male predominance (1.7 vs. 1.0).
2. No racial predilection has ever been found.
3. Investigators speculate that underdiagnosis and underreporting of pulmonary hypertension is probably common and contributes to poor patient outcome by only diagnosing the patient during the later stages of the disease.
4. The International Registry for Primary Pulmonary Hypertension reported that 6% of the enrolled patients had a first-degree relative also afflicted by the disease.
   a. Familial pulmonary hypertension is inherited as an autosomal dominant trait, with variable but low penetrance.
   b. Genetic anticipation (e.g., subsequent generations develop PPH at an earlier age, and greater severity) further affects gene penetrance.
   c. More recently, the gene for familial PPH has been matched to chromosome 2q 31–32.
   d. Furthermore, the bone morphogenetic protein receptor type II gene (BMP R2) has been identified as the actual gene for familial pulmonary hypertension, and its product, transforming growth factor β-receptor, may be important in modulating pulmonary vascular tone.
   e. In a recent study, BMP R2 was found in 26% of patients with sporadic, or nonfamilial, primary pulmonary hypertension, suggesting that a serologic test may identify patients at risk for developing pulmonary hypertension.

E Clinical Features

1. Symptoms associated with pulmonary hypertension are vague and nondescript. This results in most patients having symptoms for approximately 2 years before being diagnosed, although 10% of patients have severe symptoms for 3 years before the diagnosis is actually made.
   a. Fatigue appears to be the most common symptom and affects approximately 60% of individuals.
   b. Dyspnea occurs in 60% of patients when they initially present but is encountered by all as the disease progresses.
   c. Syncope and angina, particularly with exertion, are late manifestations of the disease, suggesting the presence of severe pulmonary hypertension causing reduced cardiac output.

F Diagnosis

1. Pulmonary function tests, electrocardiogram, chest radiograph, echocardiogram, and ventilation–perfusion scan are the important initial diagnostic tests when pulmonary hypertension is suggested. In selected cases, sleep study, chest CT with and without contrast, and right heart catheterization may be required.
   a. Pulmonary function studies are important to evaluate for the presence of other causes contributing to the development of pulmonary hypertension. In patients without underlying parenchymal lung disease who have PPH, there are generally mild restrictive changes but no evidence of obstruction. The diffusing capacity for carbon monoxide ($D_{L_{CO}}$) might be slightly reduced.
   b. The electrocardiogram may indicate right ventricular enlargement or show right ventricular strain.
   c. A chest radiograph may show enlargement of the pulmonary arteries.
   d. The most crucial noninvasive test to document the presence of pulmonary hypertension is an echocardiogram. An echocardiogram can estimate pulmonary artery pressures, show evidence of tricuspid regurgitation, estimate the contractile state of the right ventricular in response to an elevation in right-sided pressures, and also rule out congenital valvular and left ventricular myocardial disease.
   e. Ventilation–perfusion lung imaging is important to exclude chronic unresolved thromboembolic disease. In patients with PPH, it may show a peripheral nonsegmental patchy washout of radioactive tracer.
   f. Chest computed tomography (CT) with intravenous contrast also may be useful in excluding large central artery clot while confirming a cause of secondary pulmonary hypertension (e.g., interstitial lung disease, emphysema).
   g. Serologic studies are also performed to screen for connective tissue diseases. A positive antinuclear antibody test is common in the setting of primary pulmonary hypertension; however, higher titers or specific antibody patterns should raise the index of suspicion for underlying collagen vascular disease that may importantly contribute to the patient's presentation and prognosis.
   h. Right heart catheterization is critical in the evaluation of patients with suspected primary pulmonary hypertension to confirm the presence of the disease, to assess the magnitude of hypertension, and also to evaluate the response of the patient to pharmacologic treatment. It also may be used as a guide in select cases to help decide whether single or double lung transplantation is required in patients whose condition is not responding to pharmacologic therapy.

G Prognosis

1. Historically, the prognosis for patients with PPH has been poor, with an estimated median survival of 2.8 years, as noted in the NIH registry reporting on the use of conventional treatment. In these registry data, survival rates at 1, 3, and 5 years were 68%, 48%, and 34%, respectively.
2. More recent data suggest that anticoagulation may double the 3-year survival rate.

3. In patients whose condition responds to calcium channel blockers, the 5-year survival rate approximates 95%.
4. Five-year survival rates in patients with New York Heart Classifications III and IV who are treated with epoprostenol are equal to those of matched controls.

H Therapy

1. Conventional medical therapy for pulmonary hypertension has centered around the use of diuretics, digoxin, vasodilators, and anticoagulants.
   a. Diuretics are frequently used to treat excessive edema that compromises the patient's condition, especially when hepatic congestion and ascites are present. However, diuretics must be used with caution in patients with higher right-sided pressures to avoid significant reductions in cardiac preload that could further reduce cardiac output.
   b. Anticoagulant therapy is recommended as part of the conventional treatment for patients with pulmonary hypertension. Despite this recommendation, data demonstrating the effectiveness of anticoagulation are limited. One retrospective study and one small prospective trial have shown significant improvements in survival. However, no large, prospective, long-term trial has shown the effectiveness of anticoagulation therapy in a large number of patients. Based on the poor prognosis, and evidence of in situ thrombosis in patients with pulmonary hypertension on histopathologic analysis, anticoagulation is recommended to achieve an international normalized ratio (INR) of 2 to 2.5 times that of normal controls.
   c. Digitalis is recommended by some experts; however, it is somewhat controversial. It is always recommended for use in patients who have pulmonary hypertension with evidence of LV dysfunction. However, its role in patients with isolated RV dysfunction secondary to pulmonary hypertension in the absence of LV dysfunction is unclear.
2. **Vasodilators**

   Vasodilators are the most important new development in the treatment of patients with PPH. The rationale for the use of vasodilators is based on the premise that vasoconstriction is a prominent feature of the disease.
   a. The initial response to a vasodilator may portend a better prognosis and indicate which patients may respond to high-dose calcium channel blockers.
   b. Approximately 10%–25% of patients who present with pulmonary hypertension who show an acute response to either IV adenosine, inhaled nitric oxide, or IV epoprostenol can be effectively treated with high-dose calcium channel blockers.
   c. However, those patients whose condition fails to show an initial favorable response to short-acting agents may show long-term response to epoprostenol, suggesting that factors other than vasoconstriction may be important in the pathogenesis of pulmonary hypertension, or that epoprostenol has an effect other than being a vasodilator, such as antiembolic or anti-inflammatory effects.
3. Long-term oral therapy with calcium channel blockers has produced sustained improvement in pulmonary hypertension in approximately 25%–30% of subjects.
   a. Calcium channel blockers used include nifedipine (dosage range, 30–240 mg/day) and diltiazem (120–900 mg/day).
   b. Caution needs to be exhibited when using these agents because they have durations of 2 to 4.5 hours each, and may precipitously reduce cardiac output.
   c. Side effects include systemic hypotension, edema, and hypoxemia, all of which need to be identified under close administration in a structured setting by experienced clinicians.
4. Epoprostenol has been shown to produce favorable effects on reducing pulmonary artery hypertension, both in the short and the long term.
   a. It must be given by continuous intravenous infusion, because it has a short half-life. It cannot be given orally because it is inactivated by the acidic environment of the stomach.

b. It is administered continuously and intravenously by a portable battery-operated pump connected to a permanent indwelling central venous catheter. In a 3-month prospective, randomized trial, epoprostenol reduced pulmonary artery pressure, increased cardiac output, and improved patients' exercise tolerance, quality of life, and survival, especially in those who had New York Heart Association Class III and IV symptoms. Additionally, beneficial long-term hemodynamic responses have been reported.

c. The major side effects of epoprostenol are related to the complexities imposed by the use of a continuous device and indwelling line and are related to device and line malfunction, bacteremia, thrombosis, and abrupt cessation of drug resulting in rapid return and maybe even rebound of symptoms.

d. Side effects of the drug include jaw pain, flushing, headache, diarrhea, arthralgias, and cardiac arrhythmia.

e. Oral (beraprost) and inhaled (iloprost) analogs of prostacyclin are being studied in an attempt to avoid the complications of continuous administration while maintaining the hemodynamic and survival benefits.

f. Treprostinil is a recent FDA-approved analog of prostacyclin that needs to be administered continuously, but subcutaneously. However, pain and discomfort at the injection site appears to significantly limit the broad application of this drug.

g. A new class of oral agents, endothelin antagonists, shows promise in promoting pulmonary artery vasodilation and decreasing smooth muscle proliferation. A recent placebo-controlled trial showed that the endothelial receptor antagonist bosentan improved exercise tolerance and central hemodynamics in contrast to placebo. Patients administered this drug were able to walk a mean distance of 76 meters further during a 6-minute walk test. The most concerning abnormality associated with bosentan use is a mild but reversible elevation in liver enzymes, which appears to respond to stopping the drug.

5. In patients in whom pulmonary hypertension remains unaffected by the use of the agents described above, lung transplantation is a consideration. Lung transplantation carries with it approximately a 50% 5-year mortality, it is expensive, and it has increased morbidity related to the drugs used for immune suppression, as well as the transplantation procedure itself. However, in selected circumstances, it is an important beneficial therapy.

VIII PULMONARY EMBOLISM

A Definition In pulmonary embolism, a thrombus arises elsewhere in the body and migrates to the pulmonary vascular tree, where it causes obstruction. Nearly all pulmonary emboli derive from deep venous thrombosis (see Chapter 1 VIII A). Rarely (e.g., in sickle cell disease), pulmonary arterial thrombosis occurs as a primary event without discernible clots elsewhere.

B Incidence Acute pulmonary embolism is a major cause of morbidity and mortality in the United States. Fully 50% of cases of deep venous thrombosis are complicated by pulmonary embolism. Each year, as many as 650,000 individuals sustain pulmonary emboli, an estimated 150,000 of whom die as a result. (This mortality figure has not changed during the past 25 years.)

C Etiology

1. **Site of thrombus formation.** Stasis in the **iliofemoral venous system** with subsequent **deep venous thrombosis** is the most common precursor of pulmonary embolism. Other common sites of thrombus formation include the **prostatic and pelvic veins.** Except in drug abusers, pulmonary emboli generally do not originate in the upper extremities.

2. **Predisposing factors.** Conditions that increase a patient's risk of venous thrombosis, and, therefore, pulmonary embolism, are discussed in Chapter 1 VIII A 2.

3. **Precipitating factors.** The factors that control the tethering of a thrombus to the wall of a vein and the dislodging of a thrombus into the circulation are not well understood. However, exercise and straining at defecation, with consequent changes in venous flow and pressure, are well-known precipitating events.

D Pathophysiology

1. **Embolization.** When a thrombus breaks off from its site of origin, it is carried through the inferior vena cava and right ventricle to the pulmonary arteries, where it lodges. Pulmonary emboli may occur singly or multiply and vary in size from microscopic particles to large saddle emboli that completely block the major branches of the pulmonary artery.
2. **Hemodynamic consequences**
   a. Obstruction of the pulmonary arteries by the embolus increases resistance to blood flow through the pulmonary circuit and increases right ventricular afterload. When more than 50%–60% of the pulmonary perfusion is impeded, severe pulmonary hypertension, right ventricular strain, and cardiac failure ensue.
   b. The embolism also may cause intrapulmonary reflexes and the release of humoral substances (e.g., histamine, serotonin, prostaglandins), leading to vasoconstriction throughout the lungs. This vasoconstrictive effect further increases pulmonary vascular resistance and the work of the right ventricle.
   c. Fewer than 10% of cases of pulmonary embolism progress to **pulmonary infarction** because the lung parenchyma has three sources of oxygen (i.e., the airways, the bronchial circulation, and the pulmonary circulation).
   d. Recurrent pulmonary emboli progressively occlude the pulmonary vascular bed and lead to chronic progressive pulmonary hypertension and, ultimately, **cor pulmonale.**
3. **Pulmonary consequences**
   a. The primary pulmonary consequence of an embolism is **$\dot{V}/\dot{Q}$ mismatch.**
      (1) "Wasted" ventilation ("dead space") occurs in the lung segments where the vascular supply is obstructed and perfusion cannot occur.
      (2) Conversely, overperfusion and diminished vascular resistance in other lung segments cause profound right-to-left intrapulmonary shunting, with inadequate oxygenation of a large portion of perfused blood.
   b. Other pulmonary responses include congestive atelectasis of the ischemic segment of the lung, reflex bronchiolar and vascular constriction, and the loss or malfunction of alveolar surfactant.

E Clinical features and diagnosis

1. **Symptoms.** Patients may complain of dyspnea at rest and chest pain resembling that of myocardial infarction (MI). Syncope may occur as cardiac output declines. Pulmonary infarction may cause pleuritic pain and hemoptysis.
2. **Physical examination**
   a. Nearly all patients with pulmonary embolism have tachypnea and tachycardia, and many have a low-grade fever.
   b. In **massive pulmonary embolism,** the severe physiologic consequences are manifested as cyanosis, peripheral venous engorgement, and hepatic congestion; there may be evidence of cor pulmonale. In **submassive pulmonary embolism,** the less profound hemodynamic changes may be transient, so that hypotension, tachycardia, and hypoxia may not be observed at the time of initial examination.
   c. Auscultation indicates percussion dullness and decreased breath sounds over the involved base. Findings are usually normal over the remaining lung segments. Occasionally, a pleural friction rub or wheezing is heard.
   d. Evidence of deep venous thrombosis is seen in 50% of patients.

3. **Chest radiography.** Results are normal in most patients. A few show plate-like atelectasis, a unilaterally high diaphragm, and a small pleural effusion. Occasional findings include a bulging pulmonary artery and a large oligemic lung segment. A wedge-shaped, pleural-based density is typical of a pulmonary infarction.
4. **Electrocardiography.** The electrocardiogram (ECG) usually is not specific but may help differentiate between MI and pulmonary embolism.
   a. The most common finding is sinus tachycardia with or without premature atrial and ventricular contractions. The mean P axis commonly shifts to the right when right-sided pulmonary obstruction is severe and the S wave in lead I and the Q wave in lead III are abnormal.
   b. Right ventricular strain may produce intermittent right bundle branch block, P pulmonale (i.e., "peaked" P waves), and marked clockwise rotation of the ECG.
5. **Blood gas analysis**
   a. ***Hypoxemia*** (indicated by a decrease in **Pa_{O_2}**), hyperventilation (indicated by a decrease in **Pa_{CO_2}**), and a mild acute respiratory alkalosis (indicated by a low Pa_{CO_2} and slightly elevated pH) are the classic changes seen in patients with pulmonary embolism. However, they are **nonspecific** for pulmonary embolism, and pulmonary embolism may occur without these changes.
   b. A more sensitive indicator of abnormal gas exchange is the A-a D_{O_2}; a normal gradient essentially rules out pulmonary embolism.
6. **Pulmonary radioisotope scanning**
   a. In **perfusion scanning,** the patient's blood is labeled with a radioactive tracer. Poorly perfused areas of the lung appear as relatively inactive areas on the scan. However, even though normal results virtually exclude the diagnosis, the test is not specific for pulmonary embolism, because pneumonia and COPD also can produce scanning abnormalities.
   b. In **xenon ventilation scanning,** the patient inhales the radioactive tracer. This procedure often is performed in conjunction with perfusion scanning to increase the specificity of the test. Finding well-ventilated but poorly perfused areas suggests pulmonary embolism; finding areas with both perfusion and ventilation defects suggests parenchymal lung disease rather than pulmonary embolism.
   c. Scanning results must be correlated with the patient's clinical picture and with the results of chest radiography. Diagnostic accuracy may be increased by obtaining ventilation and perfusion scans in four positions and then comparing scanning results with concurrent chest radiographs.
7. Spiral (helical) chest computed tomography with IV contrast is a newer technique to diagnose pulmonary embolism. This technique involves continuous movement of the patient through the scanner with multiple rapid scans of the thorax during a single breath (Figure 2–9). Several studies have reported greater than 95% sensitivity and specificity to diagnose pulmonary embolism; others have reported lower values. Spiral CT is most sensitive for thromboembolism involving the main, lobar, and segmental arteries. Limitations include poor visualization of the peripheral upper and lower lobes, and horizontally oriented vessels in the right middle lobe and lingula. Lymph nodes may result in false-positive studies. New technology using multidetectors and thinner slice images may improve sensitivity and specificity.
8. **Pulmonary angiography** is the time-honored gold standard test for the diagnosis of pulmonary embolism. It is unequivocally diagnostic if emboli are visualized. Although invasive, this test should be performed when ventilation and perfusion scans are equivocal and also when the risks from long-term anticoagulation therapy are greater than usual.
9. When the diagnosis of pulmonary embolism remains in question despite many diagnostic studies, **corroborative evidence** of venous disease in the lower extremities should be sought.
   a. Noninvasive methods include impedance plethysmography, leg and thigh scanning with radioiodinated fibrinogen, and Doppler ultrasonography. However, these techniques can produce false-positive results, and they cannot be used to evaluate pelvic veins.

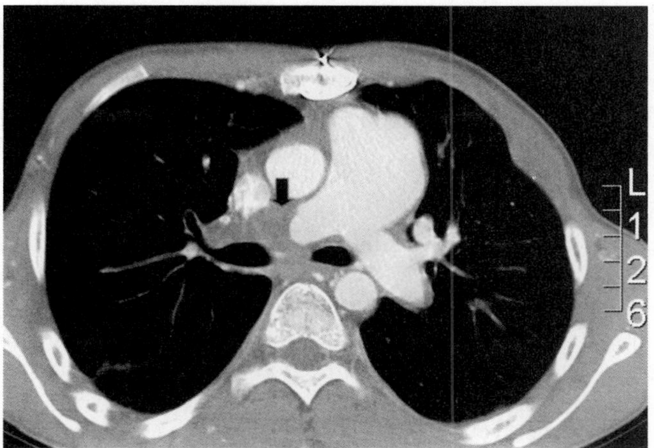

FIGURE 2–9 Spiral CT of the chest with contrast showing large clot (black arrow) obstructing right main pulmonary artery.

b. Contrast venography is helpful in diagnosing occlusion of the pelvic, thigh, and leg veins. This invasive technique is not without morbidity; however; it has been associated with phlebitis, hypersensitivity reactions, and local pain.

c. D-dimer is a degradation product released during endogenous fibrinolysis. Low D-dimer levels are found in < 25% of patients without pulmonary embolism; the negative predictive value of D-dimer has been reported to be 97%–98% in several studies. D-dimer testing is complicated by limitations in assay performance. The enzyme-linked immunosorbent assay (ELISA) is more sensitive but takes longer to perform. Latex agglutination is more rapidly performed, but less reliable. Well-done studies that characterize reliable, rapid performance of the D-dimer assay as well as excluding venous thrombosis or pulmonary embolism, thereby limiting the broad acceptance of D-dimer analysis, are lacking. D-dimer is not considered a standard test for pulmonary embolism.

F Therapy

1. Anticoagulants

a. Unless contraindicated, the drug of choice for documented or suspected pulmonary embolism is **heparin,** given in doses that maintain the partial thromboplastin time (PTT) at 2 to 2½ times normal. It is preferably given by continuous intravenous administration.

b. **Low–molecular-weight heparin** (LMWH) is a type of fractionated natural heparin with a molecular weight of 200–700 daltons (15,000 for standard heparin). It is given subcutaneously. It is an alternative to unfractionated heparin and may enable patients to be discharged earlier, or in some cases, to receive only outpatient therapy.

(1) LMWH has a longer half-life than natural heparin.

(2) LMWH has recently demonstrated efficacy in the prophylaxis and management of venous thrombosis.

c. After anticoagulation with heparin or LMWH has been achieved for a few days, therapy is changed to **warfarin,** given orally, in doses that maintain the prothrombin time (PT) at 2 to 2½ times the normal value or the INR at 2.0–3.0.

(1) The oral anticoagulant is continued for 3–6 months.

(2) **Oxygen** is given routinely to correct hypoxemia, and **bed rest** ordinarily is prescribed until the dyspnea and pain resolve, after which patients may ambulate while remaining on anticoagulant therapy.

2. **Thrombolytic agents.** Fibrinolytic agents are given when rapid lysis of clots is important.
   a. Because thrombolytic agents increase the risk of hemorrhage, they are reserved for use when occlusion has produced right-sided heart failure and hemodynamic instability.
   b. Thrombolytic agents appear to provide long-term physiologic improvement in the pulmonary vascular bed. Newer thrombolytic agents may slightly improve survival in those with submassive thromboembolism and prevent the need for anticoagulant treatment escalation.
3. **Surgery**
   a. Inferior vena caval ligation, clipping, and plication and, more recently, percutaneous "umbrella" insertion, are surgical remedies with modest morbidity that preclude embolic recurrence for a short time.
      (1) Collateral venous channels in the pelvis or lower abdomen may develop in patients with chronic vena caval obstruction and may find routes around the obstruction to the pulmonary artery, eventually negating the effectiveness of the surgical procedure.
      (2) Vena caval occlusion should be reserved for patients in whom embolism recurs, despite adequate anticoagulation therapy, and for patients in whom anticoagulants are contraindicated (e.g., patients with active bleeding).
   b. Embolectomy remains an alternative treatment for patients who cannot maintain effective cardiac output. Occasionally, embolectomy is lifesaving, but the overall survival rate is approximately 10%.
4. **Prophylactic "minidose" heparin therapy.** Giving small doses of heparin prophylactically has been helpful in preventing pulmonary embolism in certain high-risk patients, with little risk of hemorrhage.
   a. "Minidose" heparin prophylaxis is particularly applicable for older patients who undergo lower abdominal or pelvic surgery and who are on bed rest postoperatively. It also is helpful for obese surgical patients. The customary regimen is to give subcutaneous heparin 2 hours before surgery and to continue it after surgery until the patient is ambulatory.
   b. It also is recommended for patients on prolonged bed rest because of stroke, MI, cardiac failure, or cancer.
   c. "Minidose" heparin has not been shown to be effective for major orthopedic, prostatic, ocular, or neurosurgical procedures.

IX DISEASES OF THE PLEURA

A Pleural effusion

1. **Definition.** A pleural effusion is an abnormal accumulation of fluid in the pleural space.
2. **Etiology and pathogenesis**
   a. In healthy patients, the pleural cavity contains a small volume of lubricating serous fluid, formed primarily by transudation from the parietal pleura and absorbed primarily by the capillaries and lymphatics. The balance between formation and removal of this fluid may be compromised by any disorder that increases the pulmonary or systemic venous pressure, lowers the plasma oncotic pressure, increases capillary permeability, or obstructs the lymphatic circulation.
   b. A pleural effusion may be a transudate or an exudate (Table 2–3; see IX A 4 a).
      (1) **Transudates** are caused by elevated venous pressure or by decreased plasma oncotic pressure; the primary pathologic process does not directly involve the pulmonary surface.
      (2) **Exudates** are caused by increased permeability of the pleural surface (due to inflammation, trauma, or disease) or by obstruction of the lymphatics.
   c. A pleural effusion may have a noninflammatory or an inflammatory cause.
      (1) **Noninflammatory pleural effusions** may occur in any condition that causes ascites, obstruction of the venous or lymphatic outflow from the thorax, isolated left- or right-sided congestive heart failure (CHF), or a severe reduction in the plasma protein concentration.

TABLE 2–3 Causes of Pleural Effusions

Causes of exudates
- Malignancy (e.g., bronchogenic carcinoma, lymphoma, metastatic tumor)
- Inflammatory processes
  - Infections (e.g., tuberculosis, pneumonia)
  - Pulmonary embolic disease
  - Collagen vascular disease (e.g., rheumatoid arthritis)
  - Subdiaphragmatic process
  - Asbestosis
  - Pancreatitis
  - Hypothyroidism
- Trauma

Causes of transudates
- Decreased plasma oncotic pressure
- Nephrotic syndrome
- Cirrhosis
- Increased hydrostatic pressure
  - Congestive heart failure

(2) **Inflammatory pleural effusions** result from inflammation of structures adjacent to the pleural surface.

(a) The site of inflammation usually is just beneath the visceral pleura within the lung but occasionally is within the mediastinum, diaphragm, or chest wall. Secondary inflammation of larger areas of the pleural surface may result in rapid outpouring of exudate.

(b) Removal of the fluid by the normal clearing mechanisms may be considerably retarded by inflammatory obstruction of the lymphatics that drain the thorax.

3. Clinical features and diagnosis

a. **Symptoms** result from inflammation of the parietal pleura and compression of the lung.

(1) **Pleuritic pain** occurs most commonly with inflammatory effusions and often is accompanied by a friction rub.

(a) The pain commonly is a sharp, stabbing sensation that is minimal during quiet respiration but intensifies abruptly during full inflation of the lungs.

(b) Pleuritic pain must be differentiated from the pain of rib fracture, costochondritis, compression of intercostal nerve roots, herpes zoster, acute bronchitis, and various cardiovascular and esophageal conditions.

(2) **Dyspnea** can occur if the accumulation of pleural fluid compresses the lung and interferes with the movement of the diaphragm.

b. **Physical signs.** Fluid usually accumulates first at the base of the lung, where the earliest physical signs are noted.

(1) Auscultation usually reveals a dull-to-flat percussion and reduced or absent breath sounds over the area of the effusion. An area of **bronchial breathing** sometimes is heard over the adjacent compressed lung and may be accompanied by an altered voice quality or **egophony.**

(2) The mediastinum usually shifts away from the side of a large effusion unless the mediastinum has become fixed in position by a tumor or a portion of the lung on the affected side has become completely atelectatic.

c. **Radiographic appearance**

(1) **Chest radiography.** The earliest visible signs of effusion on a plain-film radiograph are blunting of the costophrenic angle and blurring of the posterior diaphragm in the lateral

view. A posterior–anterior film may show no abnormality if there is less than 300 mL pleural fluid. A lateral decubitus film may help differentiate free fluid from previous inflammatory adhesions.

(2) **Diagnostic ultrasound** may help localize the effusion more accurately when complete removal by thoracentesis is difficult.

d. Specialized diagnostic procedures

(1) Unless a cause has been established, the presence of fluid in the pleural cavity is an indication for **thoracentesis.**

(a) The fluid should be removed, the gross appearance noted, and specimens sent to the laboratory for examination.

(b) Routine laboratory procedures include measuring the total protein and lactate dehydrogenase (LDH) content and examining the spun specimen for cells. Bacteriologic and cytologic examinations and analysis for glucose, amylase, and pH provide further information.

(2) When an inflammatory effusion is suspected or known to be present, **needle biopsy** may be performed at the time of initial thoracentesis.

(3) When ordinary measures fail to establish a definitive diagnosis and needle biopsy of the pleura is negative, **thoracotomy** or the newer technique of **video-assisted thoracoscopy (VATS)** with exploration of the lung and biopsy of the involved areas of the pleural surface may be essential for accurate diagnosis.

4. Differential diagnosis. Laboratory data can help determine the cause of a pleural effusion.

a. It is useful to establish whether the fluid is an exudate or a transudate (see Table 2–3; IX A 2 c). The following laboratory data indicate the **presence of an exudate:**

(1) Pleural fluid protein > 2.9 g/dL

(2) Pleural fluid:serum protein ratio > 0.5

(3) Pleural fluid LDH > 250 mg/dL

(4) Pleural fluid:serum LDH ratio > 0.6

(5) Pleural fluid cholesterol > 45 mg/dL

(6) Pleural fluid:serum cholesterol ratio > 0.3

b. The presence of **gross blood** in the pleural fluid is most common when the effusion is caused by tumor, trauma, or pulmonary infarction.

c. The pleural fluid:serum **glucose** ratio is rarely low when the effusion is caused by tuberculosis or tumor but usually is very low in effusions that are caused by rheumatoid arthritis.

d. The pleural fluid **amylase** level frequently is elevated when the effusion is attributable to pancreatic disease or rupture of the esophagus, and occasionally is elevated moderately in malignant effusions.

e. The **pH** of pleural fluid usually is 7.3 or greater. Lower values occasionally are seen in tuberculosis and malignant effusions. A pH of less than 7.2 in a parapneumonic effusion suggests an empyema.

5. Therapy

a. Treatment must be directed at the disease causing the effusion. Appropriate therapy may call for chest tube placement, antibiotics, antituberculous therapy, repeated thoracentesis, or chemical pleurodesis to eliminate the pleural space.

b. Dyspnea may be relieved by a thoracentesis, but this procedure carries the risk of pneumothorax (from pleural puncture) or cardiovascular collapse (from removing too much fluid too quickly).

B Empyema

1. Definition and clinical features. An empyema is an accumulation of pus in the pleural space; it is an occasional complication of both bacterial pneumonia and lung abscess. The fluid usually is thick and has the appearance of frank pus. As previously stated, pleural fluid with a pH of less than 7.2 strongly suggests an empyema.

2. **Therapy.** An empyema almost always requires chest tube drainage as well as antibiotic therapy. If the fluid itself is noninfected, with a relatively low WBC count and a pH of more than 7.2, the empyema may resolve with systemic antimicrobial therapy. However, after several days without adequate drainage, most empyemas become loculated, so that tube drainage is not effective and rib resection is necessary to allow open drainage.

C Pneumothorax

1. **Definition.** Pneumothorax is an accumulation of air or gas in the pleural space. If the accumulation is large enough, the underlying lung parenchyma may become collapsed and functionless.
2. **Etiology**
   a. Pneumothorax is a common medical problem, frequently caused by **trauma. Spontaneous pneumothorax** occurs with the rupture of bullae in an upper lobe. It occurs more frequently in men than in women, and especially in men 20–40 years of age.
   b. Pneumothorax also may occur **secondary** to lung involvement in **many diseases** such as tuberculosis, trauma, malignancy, emphysema, histiocytosis X, interstitial pneumonitis and fibrosis, and pulmonary infarction.
3. **Clinical features and diagnosis**
   a. The major **symptoms** of pneumothorax are **pain** and **dyspnea.** The pain may be either sharp and severe or mild and dull.
   b. **Physical examination** shows hyperresonance and decreased breath sounds over the involved side.
   c. **Chest radiographs,** if obtained during expiration, may help demonstrate small pneumothoracic areas, because this technique increases the contrast between the lung and the pleural space.
4. **Therapy**
   a. A small spontaneous pneumothorax often resolves by itself. A more severe or a secondary pneumothorax calls for reexpansion of the lung through placement of an intercostal chest tube and application of appropriate negative pressure. The treatment is continued for 24–48 hours after the lung is reexpanded, so that the pleural space seals and pleural adhesions prevent recurrence. In select cases, smaller, less complicated pneumothoraces can be treated with pneumocentesis (e.g., removal of air during a thoracentesis), without placement of a chest tube.
   b. Spontaneous pneumothorax has a tendency to recur, and surgical treatment should be considered after three or more occurrences on a given side. Surgery involves an open thoracotomy and abrasion of the pleural surfaces, which produces symphysis of the parietal and visceral pleurae.
5. **Complications.** Although pneumothorax is a relatively benign condition, serious complications can result.
   a. **Bilateral simultaneous pneumothorax** is rare but can cause rapid death.
   b. Pneumothorax may be accompanied by hemorrhage into the pleural space, which results in **hemopneumothorax.**
   c. **Tension pneumothorax** is a buildup of positive pressure within the pleural space, which rapidly produces severe respiratory embarrassment. Patients undergoing positive-pressure mechanical ventilation are particularly at risk.
      (1) Tension pneumothorax presumably results from a ball-valve mechanism at the site of the air leak, which allows air to enter but not leave the pleural space.
      (2) This leads to progressive collapse of the lung, a contralateral shift of the mediastinal structures, and reduced blood flow to the right side of the heart, impairing cardiovascular

function as well as lung function. Prompt decompression of the involved pleural space is indicated.

D **Chylothorax** When the thoracic duct is lacerated or obstructed by trauma or tumor, lymph may accumulate in the pleural space. This condition, termed chylothorax, is identified by a murky appearance of the fluid, demonstration of fat droplets on staining with Sudan III, and a total neutral fat content of > 0.5 g/dL.

E **Primary pleural neoplasia**

1. **Localized fibrous mesothelioma.** This uncommon tumor arises from the pleural surface and most commonly is attached to the visceral pleura.
   a. **Symptoms**
      (1) The lesion may cause chest discomfort and dyspnea if it becomes very large. However, most tumors are discovered before these symptoms develop.
      (2) The syndrome of **hypertrophic pulmonary osteoarthropathy,** which is associated with arthralgia of the hands, ankles, wrists, and knees and with clubbing of the fingers, may occur secondary to pleural-based tumors.
   b. **Diagnosis.** Chest radiograph indicates a mass lesion. A pleural effusion occasionally is present.
   c. **Therapy** is surgical resection, which also relieves the symptoms of the hypertrophic pulmonary osteoarthropathy.
   d. **Prognosis.** Most of these tumors are benign, and patients have an excellent prognosis. A few of these tumors are malignant but have favorable courses.
2. **Diffuse malignant mesothelioma**
   a. **Incidence.** This malignant tumor occurs over a wide age range, with the average age at onset being 55 years. The incidence is increased in workers exposed to asbestos; generally, the malignancy develops 20 or more years after exposure.
   b. **Symptoms and diagnosis.** Chest pain and dyspnea are the predominant symptoms. The chest radiograph may show pleural thickening, pleural effusion, or both. The diagnosis is difficult to establish by cytologic examination; open pleural biopsy often is necessary.
   c. **Therapy** involves radiation therapy or chemotherapy; results are uniformly dismal.

X CHEST WALL DISORDERS

A **Etiology** Chest wall disorders may be either mechanical or neuromuscular in origin. They may cause respiratory dysfunction and, in severe cases, respiratory failure.

1. **Mechanical disorders** affecting the chest wall include scoliosis, obesity-associated hypoventilation, fibrothorax, thoracoplasty, ankylosing spondylitis, and chest wall trauma.
2. **Neuromuscular diseases** affecting the chest wall are polyneuropathies, motor system diseases, muscular dystrophies, spinal cord injuries, multiple sclerosis, and myasthenia gravis.

B **Kyphoscoliosis,** the most common and best understood chest wall disease, is used in this discussion as a prototype for the pathophysiology, course, and management of all chest wall disorders.

1. **Definition.** Kyphoscoliosis is a common skeletal abnormality characterized by posterior curvature (**kyphosis**) and lateral curvature (**scoliosis**) of the spine. These processes, alone or in combination, decrease the volume and mobility of the lung and chest wall.
2. **Incidence.** Kyphoscoliosis affects 1% of the United States population and occurs predominantly in females. The deformity is clinically significant in 2.3% of affected individuals.
3. **Etiology** is not clear in 80% of cases. A major known cause is childhood poliomyelitis. Congenital abnormalities with or without bone defects are uncommon.

4. **Pathophysiology**
   a. Lung volume is reduced in kyphoscoliosis because the chest wall is distorted. The distortion also causes stiffness of the chest wall, increasing the work of breathing and causing decreased total respiratory compliance and reduction of FRC. The pressure–volume compliance curve of the lung is nearly normal, and forced expiratory flow is preserved relative to lung volume.
   b. Gas exchange is impaired in marked kyphoscoliosis: alveolar hypoventilation occurs and **Pa_{CO_2}** rises. The A-a D_{O_2} is mildly widened because of $\dot{V}/\dot{Q}$ inequality, which results from the compressive effect of atelectasis and inadequate periodic hyperinflation.
   c. Pulmonary hypertension eventually is present at rest as well as during exercise in patients with moderate chest wall deformity and no clinical signs of cardiac dysfunction.
5. **Clinical features and diagnosis**
   a. **Symptoms**
      (1) **Exertional dyspnea** is the outstanding respiratory symptom. The onset and severity of dyspnea correlate with the degree of the spinal angulation, as measured on the chest film. Hypoventilation supervenes in those patients whose deformity is severe.
      (2) Bronchitic symptoms are unusual unless patients have chronic bronchitis or atelectasis.
      (3) **Sequelae of prolonged arterial hypoxemia,** including pulmonary hypertension, right ventricular dysfunction, and cor pulmonale, may develop as late manifestations.
   b. **Chest radiograph.** Ribs on the convex portion of the spine are widely spaced and rotated posteriorly, causing a characteristic hump. Ribs on the concave aspect are crowded and displaced anteriorly and encroach on the apex of the secondary curve. The degree of kyphoscoliosis is determined by measuring the angle formed by converging line segments drawn on the upper and lower limbs of the primary spinal curves.
6. **Therapy**
   a. Early identification of kyphoscoliosis in adolescence is the key to prevention of symptomatic disease. **Corrective intervention** should be considered when the angulation is greater than 40°. There are two forms of intervention:
      (1) **Mechanical.** A Milwaukee brace can be applied externally during the early stages of the disease.
      (2) **Surgical.** The Harrington procedure, using metal rods and focal spinal fusion, can be performed, after which the patient wears a plaster of Paris jacket cast for several months. Surgery does not improve the maximal breathing capacity but may improve arterial oxygen and oxygen desaturation. At best, surgery appears to preserve whatever pulmonary function is present at the time of intervention.
   b. Periodic hyperinflation with intermittent positive-pressure breathing devices appears to increase lung compliance and **Pa_{O_2}** in outpatients. In patients who develop obstructive sleep apnea because of cervical spine angulation, continuous positive-pressure breathing (CPAP) during sleep is useful. In those who develop chronic hypercapnic respiratory failure, noninvasive positive-pressure ventilation (NPPV) or negative-pressure ventilation may be useful.
7. **Complications.** Respiratory failure and cor pulmonale, the major complications, result from respiratory infections or injudicious use of sedatives, or both.

C Chest trauma

1. **Blunt trauma.** Blunt chest trauma causes injury either by direct application of sudden force to the chest wall and indirect transmission of these forces to the intrathoracic structures or by secondary visceral destruction by chest wall structures.
   a. Injury of extrapulmonary organs often accompanies blunt chest trauma. Disruption of the chest wall may cause rib fractures, hemothorax, pneumothorax, and flail chest. Inertial injury may cause rupture of the bronchial, diaphragmatic, or great blood vessels.

b. **Flail chest** most commonly results from motor vehicle injury or overzealous cardiac resuscitation. The chest wall, or at least one hemithorax, is rendered unstable by multiple fractures of the ribs, sternum, or costochondral joints.
   (1) The injured portion moves **paradoxically,** that is, inward on inspiration as the intrapleural pressure becomes subatmospheric and outward on expiration as the intrapleural pressure increases toward atmospheric.
   (2) Respiratory failure is treated with volume-cycled mechanical ventilation, pain control, and oxygen supplementation.

2. **Penetrating trauma** is characterized by puncture or laceration of the chest wall and intrathoracic fistulae. Vehicular accidents and knife and missile wounds are the usual causes. Exploratory thoracotomies are indicated for persistent hemothorax and sucking chest wounds and to determine the likelihood of mediastinal, diaphragmatic, or cardiac disruption.

XI MEDIASTINAL DISEASES

A Mediastinal masses The mediastinum is divided into three parts: **superior, anterior and middle,** and **posterior.** Mediastinal masses may occur at any age and are characteristic of the mediastinal compartment in which they occur. The lateral chest radiograph often is the most important initial diagnostic measure.

1. **Masses in the superior mediastinum**
   a. **Thymomas** are the most common superior mediastinal masses. **Presentation** frequently involves cough, chest pain, and superior vena caval obstruction. Myasthenia gravis occurs in approximately one third of patients with a thymoma. RBC aplasia and hypogammaglobulinemia are other recognized but rare associations. Surgical excision is recommended.
   b. **Hodgkin's disease** and **non-Hodgkin's lymphomas** rarely manifest as masses in the superior mediastinum.
   c. **Intrathoracic goiters** may occur, particularly in middle-aged women. They usually are asymptomatic but may cause stridor, hoarseness, or dysphagia.
2. **Masses in the anterior and middle mediastinum**
   a. **Dermoid cysts** appear as dense, homogeneous lobular shadows in the anterior mediastinum, often with calcifications in the walls. Teeth may be recognized within the tumor. Dermoid cysts usually are asymptomatic unless infection or malignant change develops.
   b. **Pleuropericardial cysts** occur in the middle mediastinum at the right cardiophrenic angle, characteristically appearing as smooth, sharply demarcated masses of uniform density.
   c. **Bronchogenic cysts** and **reduplication of the esophagus** are rare causes of middle mediastinal masses.
3. **Masses in the posterior mediastinum. Neurogenic tumors** are the most common mediastinal tumors and characteristically occur in the posterior mediastinum along the paravertebral border. These tumors often are asymptomatic in adults but may cause chest pain with stridor, breathlessness, cough, and tracheal compression. Horner's syndrome and spinal cord compression also may occur.
   a. Generalized neurofibromatosis occurs in approximately 25% of patients with a primary posterior mediastinal **neurofibroma.**
   b. Catecholamine secretion may be associated with the rare **pheochromocytoma** in the posterior mediastinum and with other neurogenic tumors.

B Mediastinitis

1. **Acute mediastinitis** is a severe, life-threatening illness that most often follows rupture of the esophagus. It also may follow vomiting, dental work, endoscopy, or other trauma and is characterized by fever, chest pain, and variable mediastinal enlargement. The disease progresses rapidly and requires emergency medical and surgical treatment.

2. **Chronic mediastinitis and mediastinal fibrosis.** *Histoplasma* or, rarely, other fungi or mycobacteria, can produce a chronic granulomatous process in the mediastinum, often with extensive scar tissue that contracts to cause narrowing of the trachea, bronchi, vena cava, pulmonary arteries, and pulmonary veins. Mediastinitis that occurs without any known cause is referred to as **idiopathic mediastinal fibrosis.**

C **Pneumomediastinum** is the presence of air in the mediastinum. Air is presumed to leak from alveoli and to dissect along bronchi to the hilum, from which it may enter the mediastinum. If pressure builds in the mediastinum, air may expand into the neck tissues, producing subcutaneous emphysema. However, if the mediastinal air is confined, the increasing pressure may interfere with circulation. When this occurs, tracheostomy usually is adequate therapy. Intervention is unnecessary in patients without circulatory problems.

XII DIFFUSE INTERSTITIAL LUNG DISEASE

A **Definition** Diffuse interstitial lung disease is a broad term for a group of related disorders, which are all characterized by diffuse inflammatory alveolar infiltration. Regardless of their various causes, these entities share certain clinical, radiographic, pathologic, and physiologic characteristics. All begin acutely and progress to a chronic condition; that is, a potentially reversible interstitial pneumonitis progresses to diffuse pulmonary fibrosis (see Figure 2–10).

B Etiology

1. In approximately 50% of cases, interstitial lung disease occurs spontaneously. The terminology for these diseases is varied. In North America, the term **idiopathic pulmonary fibrosis** is favored, whereas in Great Britain, **cryptogenic fibrosing alveolitis** is preferred.
2. The remaining cases are associated with many known or suspected causes (Table 2–4). Environmental or occupational exposure to a variety of substances is well known to induce interstitial pulmonary fibrosis (see XIII); these substances may act as inciting allergens or directly toxic agents. In other cases, interstitial lung disease is associated with connective tissue disease, sarcoidosis, or chronic hypersensitivity pneumonitis.

C Pathophysiology and histology

1. **Stages.** The pathologic changes in these disorders have a highly variable time course, depending on the degree of exposure and on the type of injurious agent. The clinical course may run from a few weeks to many years.
   a. **Acute stage.** The earliest stage of diffuse interstitial lung disease is characterized by acute damage to capillary and alveolar epithelial cells, leading to interstitial and intra-alveolar edema and subsequent formation of hyaline membranes. This stage may either resolve completely or progress to the stage of acute interstitial pneumonia.
   b. **Chronic stage.** In many patients, the disease progresses to a chronic stage, in which extensive deposition or alteration of collagen results in widespread fibrosis (Figure 2–10). In addition, this stage is marked by smooth muscle hypertrophy and profound disruption of the alveolar spaces, which are lined with atypical cuboidal cells.
   c. **End stage.** The disease eventually progresses until the lung becomes "honeycombed." In this stage, the entire alveolar and capillary network is replaced with fibrous tissue and dilated spaces, the capillary bed is decreased, and the involved lung has no remaining gas exchange function.
2. **Histologic classification**
   a. Several names have been used in an attempt to describe the various pulmonary changes. A common histologic classification consists of the following five categories:
      (1) Usual interstitial pneumonitis (UIP)
      (2) Desquamative interstitial pneumonitis (DIP)
      (3) Lymphocytic interstitial pneumonitis (LIP)

TABLE 2–4 Causes of Diffuse Pulmonary Infiltration

Inhaled substances	**Neoplasia**
Gases (cadmium, mercury)	Bronchoalveolar carcinoma
Mineral dusts (silica, asbestos)	Leukemia
Antigens (bacteria, molds, animal protein)	Lymphoma
Aspirated fluid or foreign body	Lymphangitic spread
Drug therapy	**Metabolic disease**
Busulfan	Uremia
Bleomycin	**Diseases of unknown etiology**
Nitrofurantoin	Sarcoidosis
Gold	Collagen vascular (connective tissue) disease
Cyclophosphamide	Goodpasture's syndrome
Methotrexate	Amyloidosis
Radiation therapy	Idiopathic pulmonary hemosiderosis
Infection	Pulmonary alveolar proteinosis
Recurrent bacterial pneumonia	Bronchiolitis obliterans with organizing pneumonia
Tuberculosis	
Viral infections	

(4) Giant cell interstitial pneumonitis (GIP)
(5) Bronchiolitis obliterans with organizing pneumonia (BOOP)

b. Many authorities believe that these classifications are somewhat artificial and may represent various stages or different pathways in the progression from acute to end-stage pulmonary fibrosis. The histologic pattern observed at biopsy depends largely on the stage of the disease at which the specimen is obtained. In addition, because this is a heterogeneous pathologic process, different areas within a given specimen may show varied stages of anatomic alteration.

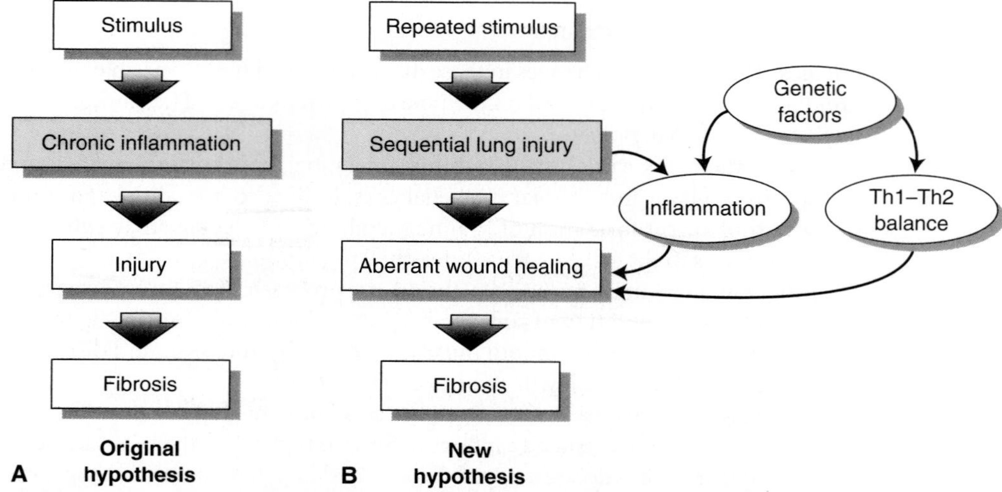

FIGURE 2–10 Original and new hypothesis of idiopathic pulmonary fibrosis pathogenesis. Previously, idiopathic pulmonary fibrosis was seen as a chronic indolent inflammatory response that ultimately leads to chronic lung injury with fibrosis (A). New concept (B) hypothesizes that idiopathic pulmonary fibrosis results from sequential acute lung injuries with the wound healing response culminating in pulmonary fibrosis. Factors that modify the fibrotic response include genetic factors, predominately inflammatory phenotype (TH1-TH2) and environmental factors. Reprinted with request from Gross and Hunninghake. Idiopathic fibrosis. N Engl J Med 2001;345(7):517-525.

3. **Effects on pulmonary function**
   a. In the early stage of disease, hypoxemia and an increase in the A-a DO_2 occur with exercise. As the disease progresses, resting hypoxemia develops. The abnormalities of gas exchange are almost certainly the result of $\dot{V}/\dot{Q}$ abnormalities. Although DL_{CO} usually is decreased as the disease progresses, this becomes significant in causing hypoxemia only during exercise, not at rest.
   b. The ventilatory pattern becomes restrictive late in the disease and is characterized by a decrease in all subdivisions of lung volume. Lung compliance is decreased, shifting the pressure–volume compliance curve downward and to the right. Expiratory flow rates (and hence FEV_1/FVC) usually are well preserved.
   c. The abnormalities in airway function tests that are seen in a number of patients with pulmonary fibrosis indicate that the peripheral airways are significantly involved in this pathologic process.

D Clinical features

1. **Symptoms** of infiltrative lung disease seen most frequently are dyspnea on exertion and nonproductive cough. Increased fatigability, fever, and weight loss also are common.
2. **Physical findings** include tachypnea, digital clubbing, and late inspiratory dry crackles. If the disease is severe, cyanosis and evidence of right ventricular failure also may be present.

E Diagnosis

The clinical, radiographic, and physiologic findings strongly suggest the diagnosis of diffuse infiltrative lung disease. Definitive diagnosis requires tissue confirmation, preferably by open-lung biopsy or VATS.

1. **Laboratory findings,** including pulmonary function studies (see XII C 3), usually are nonspecific. Tests for antinuclear antibodies (ANAs), rheumatoid factor, and immunoglobulins may be positive.
2. **Radiographic findings. Chest radiographs** usually show a diffuse reticulonodular pattern throughout both lung fields that is often more pronounced at the lung bases. Chest CT, especially with high-resolution cuts, provides more extensive data on the extent of lung involvement and whether fibrosis or alveolitis is the predominant process (Figure 2–11). In some cases, however, clinical evidence of disease may exist without radiographic confirmation.

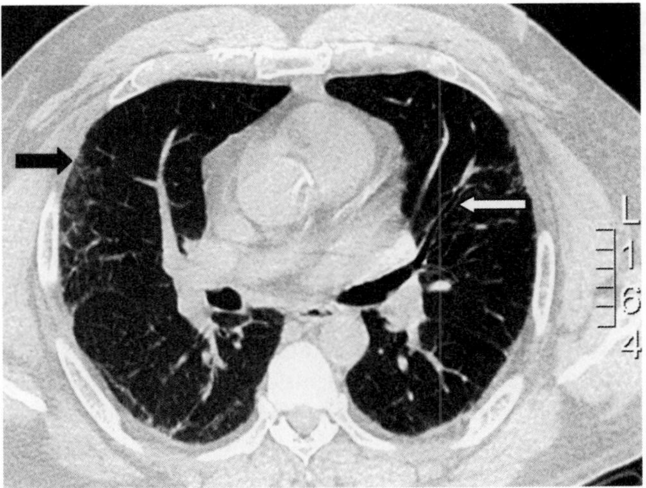

FIGURE 2–11 Chest CT in patients with IPF showing peripheral reticular abnormalities (black arrow) and traction bronchiectasis (white arrow).

3. **Open-lung biopsy** is useful in determining the stage of the disease, the appropriate therapy, and the probable prognosis. Whether the disease responds to therapy appears to correlate well with pathologic evidence of fibrosis. Specimens showing active cellular infiltrates and minimal fibrosis suggest a much better prognosis than those showing extensive fibrosis.
4. Because the histologic changes are heterogeneous, **transbronchial lung biopsy is of limited usefulness** unless there is clear-cut evidence of sarcoid granuloma, infection, or carcinoma.
5. **Bronchoalveolar lavage (BAL),** with analysis of the cellular elements retrieved, is a diagnostic procedure that has been used to differentiate infiltrative lung disease (which is associated with an increased number of polymorphonuclear leukocytes) from hypersensitivity pneumonitis (which is associated with an increased number of lymphocytes). However, it is too nonspecific to be used diagnostically.

F Therapy

1. **Corticosteroids** have been the mainstay of therapy and are clearly indicated when open-lung biopsy shows an active cellular process without extensive fibrosis. Large doses (e.g., prednisone 1 mg/kg/day) may be used initially, and physiologic and radiographic parameters should be monitored closely. If there is improvement after 6 weeks, the dosage should be tapered gradually, with frequent monitoring to detect physiologic relapse.
2. If no improvement occurs with steroids alone, **immunosuppressive agents** may be advisable, either given alone or in combination with steroids. Azathioprine is the most widely used; cyclophosphamide and chlorambucil also have been used. Newer agents that may affect the development of fibrosis, such as interferon gamma, are being investigated.

G Prognosis

Interstitial lung disease has a variable course.

1. Some cases resolve or arrest spontaneously or after removal of a known causative agent (e.g., a drug or environmental factor).
2. However, usual interstitial pneumonitis is a progressive interstitial lung disease that can be an insidious, devastating disease with considerable morbidity and mortality. The average length of survival after diagnosis is 4–5 years.

XIII OCCUPATIONAL LUNG DISEASES

A Introduction

Many respiratory illnesses are caused by inhalation of impure air. To produce lung disease, an injurious inhalant must:

1. Exist in a size and form that is capable of reaching the lower respiratory tract
2. Be deposited on or absorbed into bronchial or alveolar surfaces
3. Remain in the respiratory tract for a sufficient time to produce injury

B Pulmonary responses to mineral dusts

1. **Asbestos-related disease.** *Asbestos* is the term applied to several naturally occurring fibrous silicates, whose fibers may be long, curled, and flexible, or straight and brittle. Asbestos fibers may cause several distinct types of lesions.
   a. **Asbestosis.** This is a diffuse interstitial cellular and fibrotic reaction of the lung to inhaled asbestos fibers. Affected patients complain of breathlessness, and physical signs include digital clubbing and basilar rales. The chest film shows small lungs containing hazy infiltrates composed of small irregular or linear opacities; lower lung zones are more heavily affected. A restrictive ventilatory impairment and a reduced $D_{L_{CO}}$ are the expected abnormalities.
   b. **Nonneoplastic pleural disorders.** Asbestos may cause pleurisy with effusion, pleural plaques, and diffuse pleural thickening.

c. **Cancer.** Many years after exposure (latency period), cancer can develop in persons exposed to asbestos at sufficient concentrations.
   (1) **Bronchogenic carcinoma** is a recognized consequence of asbestos exposure, especially in individuals who smoke.
   (2) **Malignant pleural mesotheliomas** (see IX E 2) are rare tumors. They are usually asbestos-related but are not associated with smoking.

2. **Silica-related disease.** Free silica and silicates are abundant components of the earth's crust. To be injurious to the lungs, these particles must exist as respirable aerosols.
   a. **Silicosis** is a diffuse fibrotic reaction of the lungs to inhalation of free crystalline silica (sand, quartz). Inhaled silica particles are ingested by alveolar macrophages, which soon rupture, releasing cytotoxic enzymes along with the engulfed silica particles. The silica is reingested by other macrophages and the cycle continues, stimulating a local fibrotic reaction. The final result is the formation of the relatively acellular **fibrous silicotic nodule** that characterizes this disease.
      (1) **Simple silicosis.** In this stage, the chest radiograph shows numerous small, rounded opacities (isolated nodules) scattered throughout the lungs. Simple silicosis usually is not associated with ventilatory impairment.
      (2) **Complicated silicosis.** If exposure to silica continues, isolated nodules may coalesce to form larger masses of fibrotic tissue that distort the lungs. This progression also may occur because of mycobacterial or mycotic infections. Complicated silicosis may lead to progressive massive fibrosis (PMF) and often produces a mixture of restrictive and obstructive ventilatory impairment.
   b. **Nonfibrotic effects.** Silicates such as talc, kaolin, fuller's earth, and bentonite can produce simple or complicated **pneumoconiosis,** without diffuse pulmonary fibrosis.

3. **Coal workers' pneumoconiosis (CWP, "black lung")**
   a. Although coal dust is less fibrotic than silica, CWP shares with silicosis the radiographic appearance of small, rounded opacities in the simple stage and large, conglomerate masses in the complicated stage. However, simple CWP only occasionally develops into complicated CWP.
   b. **Simple CWP** has no characteristic functional abnormality. A chronic bronchitis probably accounts for most of the respiratory disability in affected patients. **Complicated CWP** can lead to PMF, with restrictive ventilatory impairment.

4. **Beryllium-related disease.** Beryllium compounds can produce both acute and chronic lung disease. The acute form is a diffuse pneumonitis that can develop into pulmonary edema. The chronic form is strikingly similar to sarcoidosis, with granulomas throughout the body; it causes progressive loss of respiratory function.

5. **Pulmonary response to other mineral dusts.** Some dusts (e.g., tin oxide, iron oxide, barium sulfate), when deposited in the lung, are cleared into aggregations in the pulmonary lobules. These dust collections cause little or no reaction and do not physically interfere with ventilatory function or perfusion.

C Pulmonary response to organic dusts (hypersensitivity pneumonitis, extrinsic allergic alveolitis)

1. **Etiology and pathogenesis.** The inhalation of organic dusts (e.g., fungal spores, thermophilic actinomycetes, and fragments of animal and vegetable matter) causes a diffuse, granulomatous pulmonary parenchymal reaction known as **hypersensitivity pneumonitis** or **extrinsic allergic alveolitis.** Some common examples are listed in Table 2–5. Patients often have antibodies against the offending substances, and the findings suggest a type III hypersensitivity reaction, with tissue damage from the deposition of antigen–antibody complexes. Pathologically, mononuclear interstitial infiltrates and fibrosis predominate.

TABLE 2–5 Selected Examples of Hypersensitivity Pneumonitis (Extrinsic Allergic Alveolitis)

Disorder	Responsible Antigen
Farmer's lung	Spores of thermophilic actinomycetes in moldy hay
Bird fancier's lung	Antigens from feathers, excreta, or serum
Mushroom worker's lung	Spores of thermophilic actinomycetes in compost
Malt worker's lung	Spores of *Aspergillus clavatus* in grain
Grain worker's lung	Dust derived from the grain weevil
Bagassosis	Thermophilic actinomycetes in sugar cane residue
Humidifier (air conditioner) lung	Thermophilic actinomycetes in humidifiers or air conditioners

2. **Clinical features.** Several hours after exposure, patients suffer malaise, fever, and chills, with chest tightness and persistent dry cough. Radiographs obtained during acute attacks show pulmonary infiltrates. Symptoms abate within a few days but recur with subsequent exposures. Repeated exposures may lead to a fixed restrictive lung disease.
3. **Therapy** includes avoidance of exposure and corticosteroid treatment for acute attacks.

D Obstructive airway disease due to inhalants

1. **Occupational asthma.** Exposure to various occupational inhalants can cause occupational asthma, often without a demonstrable immunologic mechanism. Affected individuals usually are not atopic, and the reaction usually occurs several hours after exposure. When asthma results from a single high-level contact inhalation, it is called reactive airways dysfunction syndrome (RADS).
   a. **Etiologic agents**
      (1) Simple inorganic chemicals (e.g., platinum salts)
      (2) Simple organic chemicals (e.g., di-isocyanates, formaldehyde, phthalic anhydrides)
      (3) Detergent enzymes derived from *Bacillus subtilis*
      (4) Wood dust, especially western red cedar
      (5) Fungal antigens and grain weevil antigens
      (6) Animal dander and excretions
      (7) Grain and grain contaminants
   b. **Diagnosis and therapy.** The diagnosis is strongly suggested by a history of coughing fits that occur at 2 A.M. or 3 A.M. on workdays but not on weekends or during vacation from work. Direct confirmation by challenge testing is the most convincing demonstration of the causal relationship. Avoidance of exposure is the most effective treatment. Acute attacks may respond to standard asthma medication.
2. **Byssinosis** is occupational asthma induced by cotton dust; it is seen in textile workers. It is uncertain whether the pathogenic mechanism is immunologic or pharmacologic. At first, the affected worker experiences chest tightness and shortness of breath early in the work week but feels well later in the work week. With years of exposure, the symptoms may last later into the week, until symptoms and signs of chronic fixed airway obstruction finally prevail.
3. **Industrial bronchitis.** When chronic obstructive bronchitis is caused by occupational inhalants, the disorder is hard to recognize because the symptoms of bronchitis (e.g., chronic cough) are so prevalent in the general population. Identification of an occupational inhalant requires careful and extensive epidemiologic studies. Studies linking chronic bronchitis to exposure to inert dust (e.g., coal dust) as well as foundry and gold mine dust have yielded equivocal results.

E Pulmonary response to irritant gases Irritant gases inflame the respiratory tract and can cause upper and lower airway disease. In high concentrations, they can cause pulmonary edema.

1. Such agents include ammonia (NH_3), hydrochloric acid (HCl), sulfur dioxide (SO_2), nitrogen dioxide (NO_2), and phosgene (Cl_2CO).
2. Often, there is a latent period of 12–24 hours before the onset of chest symptoms.
3. The pulmonary edema due to any irritant gas is treated with supportive measures and corticosteroids. In some cases, follow-up shows bronchiolitis obliterans.

XIV PULMONARY DISEASES OF UNKNOWN ETIOLOGY

Except for sarcoidosis, pulmonary diseases of unknown etiology are encountered infrequently by clinicians.

A Sarcoidosis

1. **Definition.** Sarcoidosis is a multisystem disease characterized by the presence of noncaseating granulomas in various organs. The lungs are involved in more than 90% of reported cases. Patients with sarcoidosis usually present with mediastinal or hilar lymphadenopathy with pulmonary infiltration, combined with cutaneous or ocular lesions. Less common but important manifestations include peripheral adenopathy, erythema nodosum, arthritis, splenomegaly, hepatomegaly, hypercalcemia, diffuse or localized CNS involvement, and cardiomyopathy. A consistent immunologic feature is depression of delayed-type hypersensitivity.
2. **Incidence.** Sarcoidosis can occur in either sex at any age but appears most commonly in the third to fifth decades of life. In the United States, the incidence of sarcoidosis is 10- to 18-fold higher in blacks than in whites.
3. **Possible etiologic factors.** The noncaseating epithelioid granuloma of sarcoidosis suggests a tissue response to some focal insult.
   a. **Infectious agents.** Clinical and pathologic similarities have suggested a connection with tuberculosis and other mycobacterial disease. However, a failure to identify any infectious agents consistently and lack of an epidemiologic association have made any infectious cause unlikely.
   b. **Immunologic defects**
      (1) Patients with sarcoidosis show impaired cellular immunity characterized by a complete skin anergy to tuberculin and other common skin antigens. The level of circulating T lymphocytes is decreased, possibly because of sequestration in the lung, because BAL typically shows marked increases in these cells.
      (2) The significance of these immunologic abnormalities is unknown. They may represent a fundamentally abnormal immunologic responsiveness, or it may be that the immunologic changes are secondary phenomena and that the primary pathologic process remains to be discovered.
      (3) Humoral immunity is normal, and susceptibility to infection is not increased.
4. **Pathology**
   a. The fundamental lesion of sarcoidosis is a **noncaseating granuloma.** This cluster of epithelioid cells is indistinguishable from the granulomas occurring in other diseases such as fungal disease, mycobacterial disease, and Hodgkin's disease.
   b. Giant cells frequently are present and contain several types of inclusions. Lymphocytes and rare plasma cells may be present at the periphery of the granuloma; neutrophils and eosinophils are absent.
5. **Clinical features** vary considerably, depending on the site and extent of involvement.
   a. **Pulmonary involvement**
      (1) **Symptoms.** Fatigue and exertional dyspnea are common. Cough, if present, usually is nonproductive. Hemoptysis is rare. Chest pain occurs infrequently, and pleurisy is uncommon.
      (2) **Pulmonary function testing.** Results may be normal but usually show some impairment of gas exchange and some evidence of lung restriction with reduced VC and D_{LCO}. In many cases, small airway function also is abnormal.

(3) **Chest radiography.** Enlarged intrathoracic lymph nodes are seen, particularly early in the course of the disease. Parenchymal manifestations vary from a faint interstitial infiltrate, to well-developed diffuse nodular infiltrates, to varying degrees of lung fibrosis, including "honeycombing." The **radiographic staging** of pulmonary involvement in sarcoidosis is as follows:

(a) **Stage 1:** Bilateral hilar adenopathy and normal lung parenchyma

(b) **Stage 2:** Bilateral hilar adenopathy and interstitial infiltrate

(c) **Stage 3:** Interstitial infiltrate only

(d) **Stage 4:** Fibrosis

b. Systemic involvement

(1) **Uveitis** is a common presentation and may progress to blindness.

(2) A variety of infiltrative **skin lesions** occurs in one third of patients and often portends chronic progressive sarcoidosis. An exception is **erythema nodosum,** which may occur early in the disease and is associated with a good prognosis.

(3) **Bone and joint involvement.** Transient polyarthritis is associated with erythema nodosum; a chronic form of arthritis also occurs. Bone involvement may produce cystic destruction and disability.

(4) **Nervous system involvement** may manifest as Bell's palsy and other cranial neuropathies, peripheral neuropathies, and (rarely) granulomatous meningitis.

(5) **Cardiomyopathy** manifests as arrhythmias and conduction disturbances that carry a high risk for sudden death.

(6) **Liver function abnormalities** may occur.

(7) **Disturbances in calcium metabolism** (e.g., hypercalciuria, renal stones, and hypercalcemia; see Chapter 6 Part I: XII B 4 b) occur in up to 25% of patients.

6. Clinical course and prognosis. The course of sarcoidosis is variable. Granulomas may remain unchanged in tissue for many years, may regress, or may organize, resulting in tissue fibrosis. Chronic inflammation and fibrosis in the lung cause serious structural distortion and loss of function.

a. In most patients, the disease regresses within 2 years and does not recur. Any tissue destruction that occurs is permanent but usually causes no major disability.

b. In approximately 25% of patients, the disease is more progressive and causes serious disability. Multisystem involvement is common, with skin sarcoidosis and hypercalcemia particularly prominent. Approximately 5% of patients die of respiratory failure.

7. Diagnosis

a. Sarcoidosis should be suspected in patients with mediastinal or hilar adenopathy and interstitial lung disease (e.g., pulmonary fibrosis). Erythema nodosum, uveitis, skin lesions, hypercalcemia, multisystem disease, and granulomas of any organ should also suggest sarcoidosis.

b. Diagnostic confirmation requires tissue biopsy showing typical granulomas in a patient with consistent clinical presentations; transbronchial biopsy is often diagnostic. Because sarcoidosis is a diagnosis of exclusion, all tissue samples should be cultured to rule out infectious causes and should be specially stained for identification of fungal disease.

8. Therapy. Corticosteroid administration is the principal treatment for sarcoidosis. However, a decision must be made as to whether a patient's symptoms warrant therapy, which has proved hazardous.

a. Sarcoidosis that carries a threat of disability should be treated. Indications include symptomatic pulmonary disease, uveitis, hypercalcemia, cardiac sarcoidosis, and neurologic sarcoidosis.

b. The patient must be assessed periodically to determine whether continuation of treatment is warranted. Clinical observation, pulmonary function testing, and chest radiography frequently are used to evaluate the effectiveness of the therapeutic regimen. However, serum angiotensin-converting enzyme (ACE) assay and BAL are better indicators of disease activity for use in follow-up.

B Goodpasture's syndrome (see also Chapter 6 Part I: X G)

1. **Definition.** Goodpasture's syndrome is a progressive autoimmune disease of the lungs and kidneys that produces **intra-alveolar hemorrhage** and **glomerulonephritis.** The disease is rare, occurs at all ages, and is predominant in males.
2. **Pathogenesis and pathology**
   - a. Goodpasture's syndrome is caused by an anti–glomerular basement membrane (anti-GBM) antibody, usually IgG, that reacts with glomerular and alveolar basement membranes.
   - b. Linear deposition of the antibody, characteristic of a type II hypersensitivity reaction, occurs along the basement membrane of glomeruli, alveoli, and capillaries.
     - (1) The pathologic result in the lung is diffuse capillary leakage and intra-alveolar hemorrhage but little or no inflammation.
     - (2) The renal lesion is a proliferative glomerulonephritis that progresses to renal failure.
3. **Clinical features.** Patients usually present with hemoptysis and dyspnea. However, renal failure without pulmonary complaints can be an initial finding, and a history of respiratory illness often precedes the onset of pulmonary hemorrhage.
4. **Diagnosis**
   - a. Bilateral alveolar infiltrates on chest radiograph, hypoxemia, and a restrictive pattern on pulmonary function testing are characteristic.
   - b. The diagnosis is confirmed by demonstration of anti-GBM antibody in the serum or in a biopsy specimen from the kidney or lung.
   - c. **Differential diagnosis** includes Wegener's granulomatosis, systemic lupus erythematosus (SLE), and idiopathic pulmonary hemosiderosis.
     - (1) **Wegener's granulomatosis** (see XIV C) usually affects both the upper and lower respiratory tract, and lacks anti-GBM antibody.
     - (2) **SLE** (see Chapter 10 VII) is distinguished from Goodpasture's syndrome by the absence of anti-GBM antibody and the findings of free DNA, various ANAs, and depressed serum levels of complement.
     - (3) **Idiopathic pulmonary hemosiderosis** is characterized by repeated pulmonary hemorrhage but no nephritis. Death caused by massive hemorrhage may occur at any time, but prolonged survival with or without symptoms of pulmonary insufficiency is common. Idiopathic pulmonary hemosiderosis has no known immune mechanisms for pathogenesis, and no successful therapy has evolved.
5. **Prognosis and therapy**
   - a. Untreated Goodpasture's syndrome is rapidly fatal as a result of renal failure or asphyxia from pulmonary hemorrhage.
   - b. Currently, the combination of plasmapheresis to remove circulating anti-GBM antibodies and immunosuppressive therapy with corticosteroids and alkylating agents appears to give the best results. High-dose corticosteroid therapy often controls episodes of lung hemorrhage but not the progressive renal disease. This treatment does not prevent the ultimately fatal outcome.
   - c. Bilateral nephrectomy with hemodialysis or kidney transplantation has been used to control end-stage renal disease.

C Wegener's granulomatosis (see also Chapter 6 Part I: X N 3)

1. **Definition.** This disease is the prototype of a group of rare disorders characterized by granulomatous inflammation and necrosis of the lung and other organs. Individuals of all ages may be affected; males are affected more commonly than females.
   - a. Wegener originally described the syndrome as a destructive granulomatous infiltration of the upper respiratory tract and lung parenchyma combined with glomerulonephritis.

b. Today, the disease is recognized as a systemic vasculitis with a predilection for the respiratory tract and kidney. Other commonly involved sites are the skin, joints, and peripheral nerves. Involvement of the eyes, heart, and CNS also can occur.

c. A variant form affects the respiratory tract, chiefly the lungs, while sparing the kidney.

2. **Pathogenesis and pathology**

a. The pathogenetic mechanism is thought to be an immunologic injury of vessels, with secondary inflammatory changes.

b. The pathologic lesion is an angiitis of small vessels with characteristic tissue necrosis surrounded by mononuclear inflammatory cells, forming noncaseating granulomas.

(1) In the lung, this process commonly results in excavation and destruction of the lung parenchyma, causing hemoptysis and pulmonary insufficiency.

(2) The renal lesion is a focal glomerulonephritis that can progress to renal failure.

3. **Diagnosis.** Wegener's granulomatosis is identified by the classic clinical triad of upper and lower respiratory involvement and glomerulonephritis, supported by a positive antineutrophilic cytoplasmic antibody (ANCA) test and biopsy of the involved tissue.

4. **Prognosis and therapy**

a. The untreated disease is fatal in most patients within 1 month to several years. Some forms of the disease are associated with longer survival rates, particularly those that do not involve active nephritis.

b. Correct diagnosis is critical because of the remarkable efficacy of **cytotoxic therapy.** Cyclophosphamide alone or with corticosteroids produces rapid reversal of the disease, if introduced early in the course.

D Histiocytosis X (eosinophilic granuloma of the lung)

1. **Definition.** Histiocytosis X is a generic term for a group of systemic disorders characterized by various degrees of fibrosis with focal infiltrations of tissue by nonmalignant histiocytes and eosinophils. The disease can be localized to one area (e.g., bone or lung) or it can be widely disseminated. **Eosinophilic granuloma** (of bone or lung) is localized; **Letterer-Siwe disease** and **Hand-Schüller-Christian syndrome** are widespread.

2. **Incidence.** The disease is rare, affects men more commonly than women, and affects children and young adults more commonly than other age-groups. An abnormality of the immune system is suspected.

3. **Pathology.** Proliferating histiocytes show cytoplasmic inclusions, the so-called "X bodies." Pulmonary histiocytosis X produces bilateral, reticulonodular infiltrates, with a predilection for the upper lobes and typical progression to cyst formation, fibrosis, and "honeycombing."

4. **Clinical features and diagnosis**

a. **Findings** may include cough, chest pain, dyspnea, fever, spontaneous pneumothorax, and a "honeycomb" appearance on chest radiography. Lytic bone disease may be present. A triad of diabetes insipidus, exophthalmos, and bone lesions is seen occasionally.

b. **Pulmonary function testing** indicates restriction and impaired gas exchange. In advanced cases, severe obstruction may dominate.

c. **Definitive diagnosis** requires biopsy of involved tissue or electron microscopic demonstration of X bodies in BAL fluid.

5. **Therapy and prognosis.** Corticosteroids are given for pulmonary manifestations, but their efficacy is uncertain. Surgery or radiation therapy is used for localized bone disease. The prognosis is variable—some cases result in death, but spontaneous remissions are common.

E Alveolar proteinosis

1. **Definition.** Alveolar proteinosis is a rare disease characterized by massive accumulations of a phospholipid- and protein-rich substance in alveoli. The interstitium usually is not involved, and

there is no underlying disease or other organ involvement. The disorder is more common in men than in women and has been described in all ages.

2. **Pathology.** The substance in the alveoli is closely related to pulmonary surfactant and probably accumulates as a result of impaired clearance. Macrophages engorged with the substance also are present, but other inflammatory cells are lacking.
3. **Clinical features**
   a. **Findings.** Dyspnea, nonproductive cough, pulmonary rales, and cyanosis are common.
   b. **Clinical course and prognosis**
      (1) Patients are predisposed to lung infection, including nocardiosis and fungal infections, possibly because of a functional impairment of alveolar macrophages.
      (2) The disease may progress to respiratory insufficiency and death, but spontaneous resolution is just as common. Pulmonary fibrosis has been described as a late complication.
4. **Diagnosis.** Pulmonary function testing shows a restrictive ventilatory pattern and hypoxia. Chest radiograph shows an alveolar infiltrate, usually in a bilateral perihilar butterfly distribution similar to the pattern seen in pulmonary edema. Lung biopsy or BAL is necessary to demonstrate the periodic acid–Schiff (PAS)–positive material in the alveoli.
5. **Therapy.** Patients with minimal symptoms require no therapy. For dyspneic patients, whole lung lavage is effective and reverses the physiologic abnormality. Corticosteroids are contraindicated because they increase the risk of infection.

F Bronchiolitis obliterans with organizing pneumonia (BOOP)

1. **Definition and pathology.** BOOP, also called cryptogenic organizing pneumonia (COP), is a clinicopathologic syndrome involving granulation tissue within small airways and alveolar ducts. It is associated with chronic inflammation in the surrounding alveoli.
2. **Etiology.** Viral infection, toxic inhalation, rheumatoid arthritis, and other collagen vascular diseases, as well as drugs, are some of the potential causes of BOOP.
3. **Clinical features**
   a. BOOP affects both men and women. The mean age at presentation is 58 years; patients range in age from 21 to 80 years.
   b. The disease usually presents as a subacute flu-like illness with coughing, fever, malaise, fatigue, and weight loss. Inspiratory crackles are frequently present.
4. **Diagnosis**
   a. **Chest radiography shows** bilateral, peripheral, wedged-shaped alveolar opacities.
   b. **Pulmonary function testing** shows a restrictive defect.
   c. **Lung biopsy** is the definitive way to make a diagnosis.
5. **Therapy.** In two thirds of patients, corticosteroid therapy results in rapid and complete recovery.

XV SLEEP APNEA SYNDROME

A Definition Sleep apnea is a disorder characterized by repetitive periods of **apnea** (i.e., cessation of breathing) occurring during sleep. A period of more than 10 seconds without airflow is considered an apneic episode. Patients with this syndrome can have hundreds of such episodes during the course of one night's sleep. This disorder can be demonstrated in 9% of middle-aged women and 24% of middle-aged men.

B Etiology and pathophysiology Sleep apnea may be obstructive, central, or mixed.

1. In **obstructive sleep apnea,** transient obstruction of the upper airway, usually the oropharynx, prevents inspiratory airflow. The obstruction results from loss of tone in the pharyngeal muscles or the genioglossus muscles (which normally cause the tongue to protrude forward from the posterior pharyngeal wall).

2. In **central apnea,** there is no drive to breathe during the apneic episode; that is, there is no signal from the respiratory center to initiate inspiration. Rarely, the cause is a neurologic disorder. Why the drive is absent in other individuals is not known.
3. In **mixed apnea,** patients have episodes of both obstructive and central apnea.

C Clinical features

1. **Symptoms.** Usually, sleep partners notice patients' problems. **Loud snoring** is prominent, and patients may thrash about during periods of obstructive apnea. During the daytime, they are **overly somnolent** and may show personality changes or slowed mentation.
2. **Physical signs.** In patients with **central** apnea, monitoring of the chest wall motion reveals no movement; this corresponds to cessation of airflow and oxygen desaturation. In patients with **obstructive apnea,** chest wall and abdominal movement can be detected during fruitless attempts to move air through the obstructed airway.

D Therapy

1. **Central apnea.** Treatment involves respiratory stimulants. A phrenic nerve pacemaker may be implanted to stimulate the diaphragm electrically.
2. **Obstructive apnea.** Some patients may respond to respiratory stimulants; others require more drastic measures. In those patients requiring intervention, nasal CPAP is the most common treatment. Oral appliances or surgery to debulk the posterior pharynx may be required on occasion. Rarely, in severe cases, tracheostomy to bypass the upper airway may be required. Weight loss is indicated in most patients, but without bariatric surgery, is rarely successful.

E Complications

Serious complications include cardiac arrhythmias, pulmonary hypertension, and unexplained cor pulmonale.

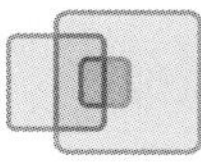

Study Questions

1. A 32-year-old man working on a construction crew falls from the scaffolding and develops multiple long bone fractures. Four hours after presenting to the emergency department, he complains of increased shortness of breath, hypoxemia, and has diffuse infiltrates on his chest radiograph, consistent with development of acute respiratory distress syndrome. Which of the following findings is almost always present in patients who present with ARDS?

- A A small localized mass on chest radiograph
- B Reduced lung compliance
- C Normal oxygenation with impaired minute ventilation
- D Increased arterial P_{CO_2}
- E Pulmonary embolism

2. An 18-year-old girl complains of symptoms of an upper respiratory tract infection for 1 to 2 days, followed by an increase in shortness of breath and greater use of inhaled bronchodilators for treatment of her chronic stable asthma. She presents to the emergency room with increased use of accessory muscles of ventilation, tachypnea, and wheezing. Shortly after the symptoms of her asthmatic attack have resolved, pulmonary function testing is most likely to show which of the following?

- A Normal values for peak expiratory flow
- B Decreased lung compliance
- C Increased residual volume (RV)
- D No change in peak expiratory flow after inhalation of bronchodilator
- E Increased diffuse capacity ($D_{L_{CO}}$)

3. A 16-year-old child presents with recurrent respiratory tract infections, poor weight gain, and breathlessness on exertion. Which of the following combinations of findings would provide a definite diagnosis of cystic fibrosis?

- A A family history of cystic fibrosis: Abnormal pulmonary function
- B Abnormal pulmonary function: Pancreatic insufficiency
- C Pancreatic insufficiency: High electrolyte concentration and sweat
- D High electrolyte, concentration, and sweat: abnormal chest radiograph
- E Abnormal chest radiograph; family history of cystic fibrosis

4. A 65-year-old man with a 35–pack-year history of smoking, complains of increased cough and shortness of breath, with episodic wheezing, Which of the following tests is the best measurement of airflow obstruction?

- A Diffusion capacity ($D_{L_{CO}}$)
- B Residual volume (RV)
- C Forced expiratory volume in 1 sec (FEV_1)
- D Forced expiratory volume in 1 sec: forced vital capacity ratio (FEV_1/FVC)
- E Forced vital capacity (FVC)

5. A 40-year-old woman undergoes a total knee replacement. Her postoperative course is uneventful, and she is discharged from the hospital. Two weeks later, she presents to the outpatient area and complains of increased shortness of breath and leg swelling. Which of the following diagnostic tests is most specific for pulmonary embolism?

- A Pulmonary angiography
- B Ventilation lung scanning

C Perfusion lung scanning
D Arterial blood gas analysis
E Chest radiograph

6. Chronic obstructive pulmonary disease (COPD) is classified as emphysematous or bronchitic, depending on the pathologic changes that occur in the lung. Although these two COPD syndromes rarely exist as pure entities, they may be differentiated on the basis of their clinical presentation. Which of the following clinical features is common to both the emphysematous and bronchitic types of COPD?

A Polycythemia
B Improved airflow with bronchodilators
C Dyspnea
D Chronic cough
E Hypercapnia

7. A 70-year-old man complains of increased shortness of breath after open heart surgery. Chest radiographs show increased bilateral interstitial infiltrates and development of hypoxemia on ambulation. It is considered that the patient may have early manifestations of idiopathic pulmonary fibrosis, or usual interstitial pneumonitis (UIP). Pulmonary function data in this patient would most likely show:

A Low lung volumes
B A decrease in the forced expiratory volume in 1 second: forced vital capacity (FEV_1/FVC) ratio
C An increased vital capacity (VC)
D A decreased diffusing capacity (DL_{CO})
E An increased airways resistance (Raw)

8. A 62-year-old woman with congestive heart failure (CHF) develops pneumonia and a large pleural effusion. Thoracentesis is performed in an effort to establish whether the pleural effusion is due to CHF or pneumonia. Which of the following findings would indicate that the pleural effusion is due to CHF?

A A protein content of 6 g/dL
B A pH of 7.13
C A glucose content of 20 mg/dL
D A lactate dehydrogenase (LDH) content of 100 mg/dL (with a serum LDH level of 420 mg/dL)
E A pleural fluid:serum protein ratio of 0.7

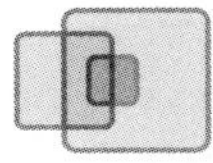

Answers and Explanations

1. The answer is B [VI C–D]. Acute respiratory distress syndrome (ARDS, "wet lung") begins with a disruption of capillary integrity, which leads to extravasation of fluid, fibrin, and protein into the alveoli. As a result, the lungs become wet and stiff (i.e., noncompliant). This condition is characterized by severe hypoxia caused by extreme ventilation–perfusion ($\dot{V}/\dot{Q}$) imbalance and shunting of blood in the fluid-filled areas of the lung. Clinical features include progressive tachypnea; patchy, diffuse, fluffy infiltrates on chest radiograph; increased minute ventilation; and decreased lung volumes. There usually is an absence of specific physical findings.

2. The answer is C [III F 4 a–b]. Patients who have had a recent asthmatic attack, even though asymptomatic, still have residual airflow obstruction that may take a couple of months to disappear. During this time, patients still respond to bronchodilators but show abnormal peak expiratory flow, increased lung compliance, and continued maldistribution of ventilation. Diffusing capacity (DL_{CO}) is decreased in abnormalities of capillary blood volume because of either destruction of the alveolar capillary membrane (e.g., in emphysema) or to a thickened interstitial membrane (e.g., in diffuse interstitial lung disease). Neither of these abnormalities exists in asthma.

3. The answer is C [IV B 5 a (1)–(2) (a)–(c)]. Although chest radiography and pulmonary function testing show abnormalities, the sweat test is the definitive test for cystic fibrosis. In virtually all cases of cystic fibrosis, sodium and chloride concentrations in sweat are increased significantly, while concentrations of these electrolytes are normal elsewhere in the body. To make a diagnosis of cystic fibrosis, this defect must be identified. The diagnosis is confirmed by a positive sweat test combined with any one of the following findings: a family history of cystic fibrosis, obstructive pulmonary disease, or pancreatic insufficiency.

4. The answer is D [I F 1 a]. A decrease in the forced expiratory volume in 1 second/forced vital capacity (FEV_1/FVC) is the hallmark of airflow obstruction. The FEV_1 is the volume of air forcefully expired during the first second after a maximal inhalation, and the FVC is the total volume of air that can be forcibly expelled from the lungs after a maximal inhalation. The FEV_1 is decreased in obstructive as well as restrictive lung disease. The diffusing capacity (DL_{CO}) and the residual volume (RV) do not identify airway obstruction. The DL_{CO} indicates the adequacy of the alveolar–capillary membrane, and the RV is the volume of air remaining in the lungs after a maximal expiratory effort.

5. The answer is A [VIII E 7]. Pulmonary angiography is the standard test for the diagnosis of pulmonary embolism. Algorithms have been developed for patients with appropriate clinical data and high-probability results on ventilation and perfusion lung scanning; in such cases, this combined technique has almost the diagnostic accuracy of pulmonary angiography. Abnormal results on arterial blood gas analysis and chest radiography are too nonspecific to be helpful. When ventilation and perfusion scanning, arterial blood gas analysis, or both produce normal results and the alveolar–arterial PO_2 is normal, pulmonary embolism is extremely unlikely.

6. The answer is C [II E 1, 2 a (1)–(2)]. All patients with chronic obstructive pulmonary disease (COPD) experience dyspnea to some degree. The two classic types of COPD—emphysematous and bronchitic—represent extremes of the spectrum and rarely are encountered in their pure form in clinical practice. By definition, individuals with the emphysematous type of COPD present at a relatively older age (>60 years). This form of disease is characterized by progressive exertional dyspnea, weight loss, little or no cough, mild hypoxia, hypocapnia, and only a mild increase in airway resistance (Raw) that shows little improvement with bronchodilation. Persons with the bronchitic type of COPD present at a relatively young age. This form is characterized by episodic dyspnea, fluid retention, chronic cough, severe hypoxemia, hypercapnia, polycythemia, and an increase in Raw that improves with bronchodilation.

7. **The answer is A** [I F 2]. Restrictive disorders are characterized by low lung volumes. Diffusing capacity (DL_{CO}) may or may not be decreased in pulmonary fibrosis, a type of restrictive disease. A decrease in forced expiratory volume in 1 second/forced vital capacity (FEV_1/FVC) is the hallmark of obstructive, not restrictive, disease. Vital capacity (VC) and airway resistance (Raw) are decreased in restrictive lung disorders.

8. **The answer is D** [IX A 2 (b), 4 (a); Table 2–3]. With the exception of the lactate dehydrogenase (LDH) findings, all of the pleural fluid findings listed indicate the presence of an exudate. Exudates are caused by inflammation or disease of the pleural surface or by lymphatic obstruction (e.g., due to tuberculosis, lung cancer, or pneumonia). Transudates are caused by elevated systemic or pulmonary venous pressure or by decreased plasma oncotic pressure [e.g., due to congestive heart failure (CHF) or nephrotic syndrome]. Therefore, in establishing the etiology of a pleural effusion, it is useful to determine whether the fluid is a transudate or an exudate. This determination often can be made on the basis of a chemical analysis of the pleural fluid. A pleural fluid protein content of more than 2.9 g/dL and an LDH content of more than 250 mg/dL usually indicate the presence of an exudate. In addition, an exudate usually is associated with a pleural fluid:serum protein ratio of less than 0.5 and a pleural fluid:serum LDH ratio of less than 0.6. Pleural fluid pH values below 7.2 and a pleural fluid glucose content of less than 20 mg/dL also are associated with inflammatory effusions (exudates).

chapter **3**

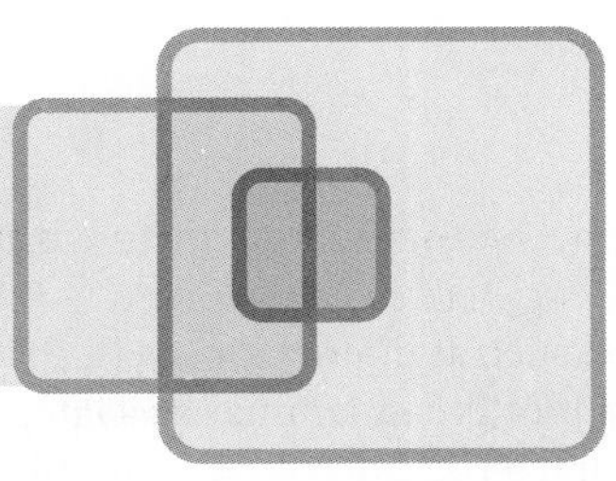

Hematologic Diseases

RONALD N. RUBIN

I RED BLOOD CELL (RBC) DISORDERS

A Anemia caused by abnormal hemoglobin synthesis and iron metabolism Hemoglobin, which represents 95% of the total composition of an RBC, is a mixture of globin and the iron-containing heme compound, **protoporphyrin.** Any abnormality in hemoglobin synthesis or iron metabolism results in hemoglobin-deficient cells. As a rule, such deficient cells exhibit **hypochromia** (i.e., diminished hemoglobin concentration) and **microcytosis** (i.e., diminished size). Both conditions may be detected using the RBC indices available by calculation and the Coulter counter along with an examination of a stained blood smear. Disorders causing this type of anemia fall into four major classes.

1. **Iron deficiency anemia** is the most common form of anemia in the United States, where 20% of adult women are reported to be iron deficient.
   a. **Etiology.** Iron deficiency is most commonly caused by blood loss when the loss of the iron component exceeds dietary intake of iron. Examples include gastrointestinal blood loss from an ulcer or a tumor and menstrual blood loss. Occasionally, in the neonate and young child, new blood formation and subsequent increased iron use exceeds iron intake and results in anemia without concomitant blood loss.
   b. **Clinical manifestations.** The symptoms of iron deficiency anemia, like all anemias, include fatigue and weakness. Symptoms specific to iron deficiency may include epithelial changes such as brittle nails and atrophic tongue. In addition, the underlying pathology may dominate the symptoms (e.g., peptic ulcer).
   c. **Diagnosis.** In the appropriate clinical setting (e.g., in a young woman with excessive menstrual blood loss and anemia), a smear showing hypochromia and microcytosis is adequate for the diagnosis. When more specific tests are needed, a positive diagnosis is made from an absence of marrow iron on bone marrow examination, abnormally low levels of ferritin, and a low serum iron level in association with an elevated total iron-binding capacity.
   d. **Therapy.** Treatment usually involves restoration of the body's iron stores to correct the anemia. As a rule, oral iron in the form of ferrous sulfate suffices; however, for patients who do not tolerate this form, ferrous gluconate and fumarate are available. In difficult cases that are refractory either physiologically or due to an inability to take oral iron, parenteral iron preparations are given. Reticulocytosis occurs 7 days after appropriate treatment; after 3 weeks, the hemoglobin level increases several grams.

2. **Anemia of chronic disease.** This mild-to-moderate anemia is associated with inflammatory diseases such as rheumatoid arthritis, serious infections, and carcinoma.
   a. **Pathophysiology**
      (1) Anemia of chronic disease is characterized by hemoglobin levels of 8–10 g/dL, although lower levels are possible. It is unusual for the hemoglobin level to be less than 7 g/dL.
      (2) Patients with this anemia have plentiful iron but diminished iron utilization by the bone marrow. Therefore, inadequate amounts of iron are available to the bone marrow for RBC formation despite adequate body stores.

(3) Another important mechanism for this anemia is an impaired marrow response to erythropoietin.

(4) Circulating cytokines such as interleukin-6 (IL-6) or tumor necrosis factor (TNF), which are released as a result of the inflammatory state, are involved. These cytokines are able to reproduce the characteristic defective iron utilization and impaired marrow response to erythropoietin both in vivo and in vitro.

b. **Diagnosis** is based on confirmation of the following findings:

(1) The anemia associated with chronic inflammation is of moderate degree and reveals slight hypochromia and microcytosis.

(2) The mean corpuscular volume (MCV) is 80–85 mm^3, and the mean corpuscular hemoglobin concentration (MCHC) is 30%–32%.

(3) If stained, the marrow reveals plentiful iron stores. In addition, serum ferritin levels usually are normal or elevated. Serum iron is lowered as is the total iron-binding capacity, unlike the clinical situation with iron deficiency anemia.

c. **Therapy.** Hematinics, including iron, are not effective treatment for this disorder.

(1) **Correction of the underlying disease** can lead to reversal of the anemia within 1 month.

(2) **Exogenous erythropoietin** is quite effective in certain situations such as perioperatively in rheumatoid patients undergoing joint replacement surgery, AIDS, and inflammatory bowel diseases. Because the inflammatory state induces a relative hyposensitivity to erythropoietin, generous doses may be needed.

3. **Sideroblastic anemias**

a. **Pathophysiology.** These anemias, caused by disorders in the synthesis of the heme moiety of hemoglobin, are characterized by trapped iron in the mitochondria of nucleated RBCs. Many of the enzymes for protoporphyrin synthesis are located in the nucleated RBC mitochondria. Thus, derangements in these pathways cause iron accumulation in the perinuclear mitochondria, which renders this anemia its characteristic morphologic finding of **ringed sideroblasts.** The defective heme synthesis causes diminished hemoglobin levels in these cells; as a result, this cell population is hypochromic and microcytic.

b. **Types.** There are two types of sideroblastic anemias.

(1) **Hereditary sideroblastic anemia.** This X-linked condition is due to an abnormality in pyridoxine (vitamin B_6) metabolism. It is thought to be a congenital defect in the enzyme **δ-aminolevulinic acid (ALA) synthetase.**

(2) **Acquired sideroblastic anemias** are more common than the hereditary type. Lead, alcohol, and the antibacterial drug isoniazid cause sideroblastic anemia by inhibiting enzymes of protoporphyrin synthesis; however, many cases are idiopathic.

c. **Diagnosis.** This anemia may be relatively severe in patients older than 60 years and is characterized by hemoglobin levels of 8–10 g/dL. Coulter counter reveals normocytic or even macrocytic cells, but examination of the blood smear shows a dimorphic population with some very small cells. The bone marrow reveals erythroid hyperplasia, and iron staining demonstrates the ringed sideroblasts. Iron studies show elevated ferritin levels and high serum iron levels with high transferrin saturation. Often, some normal or slightly macrocytic cells are seen intermingling with the hypochromic, microcytic cells, and a blood smear revealing such a condition is diagnostic of this anemia.

d. **Therapy**

(1) If a drug such as isoniazid or alcohol is involved, the anemia and sideroblastic changes regress with discontinuation of the agent.

(2) All patients should be given a trial of **pyridoxine** in high doses; however, in all but the hereditary cases, this usually fails. Often, these patients are transfusion dependent. Acute leukemia develops in a portion (10%) of patients with acquired idiopathic disease. In these patients, the sideroblastic anemia is a preleukemic syndrome, and is classified as a myelodysplastic syndrome.

(3) Efficacy using **exogenous erythropoietin** to treat this condition is approximately 20%, and this therapy should be tried in transfusion-dependent patients.

4. **Thalassemias** are genetic disorders characterized by diminished synthesis of one of the globin chains. These diseases are due to abnormalities in the genes that are responsible for synthesis of the globin portion of the hemoglobin molecule. Thalassemias are named according to the deficient chain.

a. **Types**

(1) **α-Thalassemias.** These disorders are characterized by deficient α-chain synthesis, usually due to deletion of the α-globin gene from the genome. RNA for the α-globin gene is not present in the α-thalassemias. There are four such genes and, thus, four α-thalassemias; these range from a mild, subclinical, asymptomatic anemia to a severe anemia that is fatal in utero. The α-thalassemias are most prevalent in Asian populations.

(2) **β-Thalassemias.** These disorders are due to the absence or malfunction of the β-globin gene. In the latter case, RNA is present but in reduced amounts or in defective forms. The two β-globin genes in the genome result in two different forms of β-thalassemia. **β-Thalassemia major,** or **Cooley's anemia,** is a severe disease that appears in childhood. Such patients are transfusion dependent. Patients with **β-thalassemia minor,** a mild anemia, are not transfusion dependent and can live full, normal lives. The β-thalassemias are most prevalent in individuals of Mediterranean descent, particularly those from Greece and Italy.

b. **Diagnosis.** The thalassemias should be suspected in an anemic patient who reveals marked abnormalities on blood smear. Such abnormalities include microcytosis, hypochromia, and poikilocytosis (i.e., the presence of bizarrely shaped RBCs).

(1) **α-Thalassemia** is most difficult to diagnose when it exists in the carrier state. Patients with the carrier form have a mild microcytic, hypochromic anemia. There is no excess of the non–β-hemoglobins because all chains have α components. Therefore, sophisticated studies are required for definitive diagnosis. In neonates, however, the diagnosis can be made from cord blood tests that show an increase in **Bart's hemoglobin.** With the advent of genetic mapping technology, the presence or absence of α-globin genes can be ascertained to make the diagnosis definitively.

(2) **β-Thalassemia** resembles iron deficiency anemia except that iron is present in the marrow. The diagnosis may be confirmed in several ways.

(a) Measurement of minor hemoglobin chains A_2 and F reveals elevations as the erythron attempts to compensate for the diminished synthesis of β chains by making excessive γ and δ chains instead.

(b) Genetic analysis of hemoglobin mRNA or genetic mapping of the globin genes is now available.

c. **Therapy** includes chronic red cell transfusions and folic acid supplementation. The regular use of ambulatory iron chelation has slowed the development of iron overload in these patients. In selected patients, bone marrow transplantation (BMT) has been curative, and this form of therapy likely will be used more frequently in the future.

B **Macrocytic anemias** are characterized by RBCs that exceed 100 μm in size. Three major mechanisms are linked to the development of macrocytic anemia.

1. **Accelerated erythropoiesis.** Reticulocytes and young erythrocytes are larger than normal; therefore, individuals with large numbers of reticulocytes have large numbers of circulating cells of great size. A reticulocyte count confirms the diagnosis.

2. **Increased membrane surface area.** Patients with excessive plasma lipids absorb these lipids onto RBC surfaces, which creates an enlarged membrane surface area and a macrocytosis in excess of 100 μm. This condition is most common in patients with liver disease and can be diagnosed by a blood smear that reveals the characteristic **target cell** of liver disease (i.e., a round macrocyte

with a redundant membrane). Liver disease causes this by diminished hepatic synthesis of lecithin–cholesterol acetyl transferase (LCAT). Diminished synthesis of LCAT results in excess plasma-free cholesterol, which is absorbed onto RBC membranes.

3. **Defective DNA synthesis** is the main characteristic of the classic **megaloblastic anemias.** In these conditions, RBCs cannot produce nucleic acid, and so nuclear maturation is arrested. Cytoplasmic maturation proceeds, however, resulting in abnormally large cells. These cells are larger than those seen with accelerated erythropoiesis, and they have an increased membrane surface area. An MCV that exceeds 115 mm^3 is not uncommon.
   a. **Etiology.** Megaloblastic anemias usually are caused by a deficiency of either vitamin B_{12} or folic acid.
      (1) **B_{12} deficiency** may result from fish tapeworm infestation, strict vegetarian (vegan) diets, or intestinal blind loops with bacterial overgrowth. The most common cause, however, is a lack of the intrinsic factor necessary for vitamin B_{12} absorption into the terminal ileum. Two forms of atrophic gastritis have been described. Type A is true autoimmune gastritis, involves the fundus and body of the stomach, and has the gastric parietal cell H^-/K^+ ATPase as the molecular target of the autoimmune process. Type B is nonautoimmune, involves the entire stomach, and is associated with *Helicobacter pylori* infection. Pernicious anemia applies to the type A pathophysiology, although both types can cause vitamin B_{12} deficiency.
      (2) **Folic acid deficiency** is caused by dietary deficiency due to inadequate intake, inadequate absorption, or both. This condition is most commonly encountered in alcoholics.
      (3) **Drug-induced disorders of DNA synthesis.** Certain drugs used to treat cancer (e.g., methotrexate), bacterial infections (e.g., trimethoprim), and parasitic infections (e.g., pyrimethamine), as well as phenytoin, interfere with folic acid metabolism and cause megaloblastic anemia and bone marrow changes. These diagnoses can be made easily from patient history.
   b. **Clinical manifestations.** Patients with megaloblastic anemia have varying degrees of anemia associated with large RBCs. Because nucleic acid metabolism is necessary for all cellular elements in bone marrow, white blood cells (WBCs) and platelets are diminished. The ineffective erythropoiesis and intramedullary hemolysis associated with this disorder often result in serum **lactate dehydrogenase (LDH)** levels that exceed 500 units/dL. Both RBCs and WBCs in bone marrow reveal the classic megaloblastic sign of immature, open nuclei in association with mature cytoplasmic components. Blood smear shows characteristic oval macrocytes and hypersegmented polymorphonuclear leukocytes (PMNs).
   c. **Differential diagnosis**
      (1) Serum levels of vitamins as well as RBC folic acid levels should be measured to determine whether the deficiency is in folic acid or vitamin B_{12}.
      (2) Vitamin B_{12} has a neurologic function; therefore, when a macrocytic anemia is associated with neurologic symptoms, particularly posterior column signs and symptoms, vitamin B_{12} deficiency should be suspected. The hallmarks of pernicious anemia are macrocytic anemia, neurologic symptoms and signs, and **atrophic glossitis.**
      (3) The **Schilling test** for the presence of intrinsic factor and intestinal function can be performed to differentiate the cause of vitamin B_{12} deficiency. However, clinicians have become less enthusiastic about this test because of its complexity and occasional inaccuracy. Most practitioners prefer to use more refined biochemical testing of the purine synthetic pathways. Currently, measurement of methylmalonic acid levels (elevated) has replaced the Schilling test as the diagnostic procedure of choice. However, the Schilling test remains useful for study of the physiology of vitamin B_{12}. Serum antiparietal cell antibodies are a relatively specific test finding for the autoimmune type A variant (>90%).
   d. **Therapy.** Specific therapy is determined by the vitamin that is missing. Folic acid alone should never be given in an undiagnosed case of macrocytic anemia; folic acid reverses hematologic signs, but neurologic degeneration continues unabated.

(1) Patients with pernicious anemia due to vitamin B_{12} deficiency require lifelong treatment with parenteral vitamin B_{12}. If reversible causes are found (e.g., intestinal bacterial overgrowth), appropriate measures may reverse the deficiency and obviate the need for permanent vitamin B_{12} therapy.

(2) Folic acid deficiency is treated with oral preparations of folic acid.

C **Normochromic, normocytic anemias** represent a vast array of conditions characterized by normal cell size and hemoglobin concentration. These anemias are not related by common pathogenic mechanisms; **classification is by the degree of marrow response to the anemia.**

1. **Anemia associated with impaired marrow response.** The following anemias are characterized by normal or low reticulocyte counts.
   a. **Hypoplastic, or aplastic anemia,** is an intrinsic marrow disease characterized by an absence of stem cells. All myeloid (derived from the bone marrow) cell lines are involved, with a resultant **pancytopenia.** Severe cases of this serious disease are associated with a high mortality rate. Levels of serum erythropoietin are usually elevated proportionately to the degree of anemia. There is little effective medical treatment. In young patients, BMT techniques are curative in cases in which an appropriate marrow donor is available.
   b. **Disorders characterized by infiltration of bone marrow** (myelophthisic anemias) include myeloma, carcinoma, and leukoerythroblastosis. Disruption of bone marrow architecture is common; a blood smear that reveals immature WBCs and nucleated RBCs is a clue to the presence of these conditions. A bone marrow aspirate and biopsy confirm the diagnosis in such cases.
   c. **Anemia due to diminished erythropoietin secretion** is the anemia of **chronic renal failure.** Erythropoietin is a protein–lipid molecule required by the marrow for adequate RBC formation. With severe kidney disease, the erythropoietin secreted by the kidneys is lost, and anemia ensues. The degree of anemia roughly correlates with the degree of renal failure.
      (1) Proper attention to iron and folic acid stores is important in this group of patients, because deficiencies in these nutrients secondarily complicate the anemia of renal failure.
      (2) Erythropoietin has been uniformly effective in raising the hemoglobin to normal or near normal levels in these patients, and this increase in hemoglobin has translated into an enhanced quality of life.
   d. **Other anemias associated with hypoproliferation of bone marrow** include those associated with hypothyroidism, hypopituitarism, and liver disease.
2. **Anemia associated with appropriately increased RBC production.** The following anemias are characterized by an increased number of reticulocytes.
   a. **Anemia following hemorrhage.** An increased reticulocyte count is the normal marrow response in patients who bleed either overtly (e.g., with surgery) or covertly (e.g., into the gastrointestinal tract) and have adequate iron stores. This condition can be confused with hemolysis; however, the clinical situation of a postoperative patient with a large resolving hematoma confirms the diagnosis of posthemorrhagic anemia.
   b. **Hemolytic anemias** represent conditions in which RBC survival is shortened. In most cases, the marrow is intrinsically normal; thus, adequate new RBCs can be made, and the patients have elevated reticulocyte counts. Diagnostic of these anemias are signs of increased RBC destruction (e.g., shortened RBC half-life, elevated serum LDH, reduced haptoglobin) combined with signs of accelerated marrow activity (e.g., elevated reticulocyte counts and erythroid hyperplasia in the marrow). The diagnosis of hemolysis should be made first, and the specific cause of the hemolysis sought later. Hemolytic anemia exists in hundreds of forms, which are grouped as follows:
      (1) **Hemolytic anemia due to factors extrinsic to the RBC**
         (a) **Autoantibodies** can attach to the RBC and cause its destruction by the reticuloendothelial system. A classic example is **Coombs-positive hemolytic anemia** due to

either warm [immunoglobulin G (IgG)] or cold (IgM) antibodies. This anemia may be idiopathic or may arise as a complication of collagen disease or lymphoma. In severe cases, steroids and splenectomy may be required to control the anemia.

(b) **Exogenous agents** such as malarial organisms can render the RBC liable to hemolysis.

(c) **Abnormalities in the circulation** can cause premature destruction of RBCs. The following are examples of such abnormalities, and disorders associated with each condition are also cited.

(i) Lipid abnormalities (spur-cell anemia in advanced liver disease)

(ii) Fibrin deposition in the microvasculature with shearing of RBCs [disseminated intravascular coagulation (DIC) syndrome]

(iii) RBC damage due to trauma from prosthetic heart valves

(2) **Hemolytic anemia due to factors intrinsic to the RBC.** These disorders involve congenital abnormalities that render the RBC liable to hemolysis.

(a) **Membrane disorders** include such conditions as **hereditary spherocytosis.** In this disorder, a defect in the membrane sodium–potassium–ATPase pump causes RBC swelling. This results in the characteristic finding on blood smear of small, round, hyperchromic RBCs without the usual central pallor (i.e., spherocytes). These cells are osmotically fragile and are destroyed in the spleen. Splenectomy usually controls the anemia, although the RBC defect remains.

(b) **Hemoglobin disorders—hemoglobinopathies.** These diseases, of which more than 250 are known, are caused by point mutations in the DNA code related to variation in a single amino acid in the globin chains. Such amino acid changes cause a variety of structural and functional changes in the RBC. When amino acid changes occur in the inner hydrophobic structural portions of the hemoglobin molecule, unstable hemoglobin disease with low-grade hemolysis can result (e.g., Hb Zurich). Amino acid changes in the heme–oxygen binding areas of the molecule cause changes in oxygen affinity and give rise to the so-called polycythemic hemoglobinopathies (e.g., Hb Potomac). The most commonly encountered hemoglobinopathies involve amino acid changes near the surface of the globular hemoglobin molecule, which predispose the hemoglobin to polymerization. Such polymerization results in the hemoglobin becoming rigid, with subsequent membrane and cell shape changes. These affected RBCs become liable to hemolysis.

(i) **Hemoglobin S (Hb S).** The most common hemoglobinopathy is Hb S, which causes **sickle cell anemia.** This disorder occurs in 1% of African Americans. The disease manifestations result from three major pathophysiologic aspects (Table 3–1). The polymerized hemoglobin severely deforms RBCs and results in **marked, chronic hemolysis.** This manifests as severe, chronic anemia (with hemoglobin in a range from 5–10 g/dL); predisposition to aplastic crises associated with parvovirus and other infections; and elevated bilirubin levels with almost universal gallstone disease and frequent, chronic ulceration of the legs in the ankle area. **Predisposition to infection** has multiple causes, including splenic autoinfarction and diminished synthesis of opsonizing immunoglobulins. This predisposition results in frequent infections, especially with encapsulated microorganisms such as pneumococci and *Haemophilus* and *Salmonella* species. Occasionally, these infections can be overwhelming, causing sepsis and death within hours of onset. Finally, **acute episodes of pain ("painful crises")** are the principal symptom and cause of morbidity in patients with sickle cell disease. Painful crises are thought to be the result of microvascular occlusion with infarction resulting from local hyperviscosity associated with the rigid, deformed and abnormally adhesive sickle cells. Studies have suggested that Hb S reticulocytes and neocytes have abnormally enhanced properties that allow for adhesion to the endothelium, which initiates the sickling process.

TABLE 3–1 Clinical Manifestations of Sickle Cell Anemia

Related to Chronic Hemolytic Anemia	Related to Abnormal Adhesions, Sickling, and Vaso-occlusion	Related to Increased Susceptibility to Infection
Normocytic anemia	Painful crises	Pneumococcal sepsis
Elevated bilirubin and LDH	Cerebrovascular accident	*Salmonella* sepsis
Gallstone disease	Acute and chronic cardiopulmonary disease (e.g., acute chest syndromes, cor pulmonale)	Osteomyelitis
	Priapism	
	Splenic autoinfarction	
	Skeletal changes (e.g., aseptic necrosis of the hip)	

LDH = lactate dehydrogenase.

(ii) Other common hemoglobinopathies that cause less severe sickle syndromes, include hemoglobin C (Hb C), hemoglobin O (Hb O), and mixtures such as hemoglobin SC (Hb SC).

(iii) **Diagnosis** is confirmed by hemoglobin electrophoresis, which demonstrates the characteristic changes in mobility caused by specific amino acid changes.

(iv) **Therapy,** which is still not satisfactory, continues to evolve. **Supportive medical care** remains the cornerstone of effective therapy and includes transfusions when indicated (e.g., during hypoplastic crises), proper fluid management and attention to hydration, and analgesics for the pain of microvascular occlusion.

(v) Studies have demonstrated that specific **complications** are responsible for much of the mortality in sickle cell disease. An important example is the development of **acute chest syndrome.** In this situation, which usually complicates what appears to be a routine painful crisis, the patient develops a fever, frequently manifests an unusually brisk leukocytosis, and then demonstrates profound hypoxia. Soon thereafter, a diffuse chest radiograph infiltrate is evident, and the clinical syndrome evolves into an adult respiratory distress syndrome (ARDS)–like situation. This complication carries a high mortality if not quickly recognized and treated. The syndrome usually responds very well to exchange transfusions to lower Hb S levels to below 50%. Other currently accepted indications for RBC exchange transfusion include stroke and central nervous system (CNS) lesions, priapism, and sickle cell hepatic sequestration crisis. The advent and increasing ease of this therapy has substantially reduced the mortality resulting from these conditions.

(vi) Appropriate **monitoring for** and treatment of the potentially fatal problem of **intercurrent infections** is crucial. In children, prophylactic penicillin has been shown to prevent 80% of potentially lethal cases of pneumococcal bacteremia. Similar generous use of antibiotics and pneumococcal vaccine in adults is recommended as well. Newer directions in therapy have moved toward manipulation of the hemoglobin mix within the cell to diminish the propensity to polymerize. Hb F has been found to have an inhibitory effect on sickling. Certain agents stimulate Hb F production. The cytotoxic agent hydroxyurea has been the most extensively studied, and recent data suggest that enhancing Hb F levels using hydroxyurea results in less painful crises in selected cases. Finally, BMT, which results in phenotypic cure, has been reported in patients with co-existing sickle cell anemia and acute leukemia as well as stand alone cases. As the technology of marrow transplantation evolves and becomes safer, such therapy may become an option. Patients with hemoglobinopathies with significant morbidity and mortality rates (e.g., sickle cell anemia) are candidates for **gene transfer therapy,** a developing technology.

(c) **Disorders of the cytoplasm and enzymes** occur as congenital hemolytic anemias. An RBC lacks a nucleus and mitochondria when it leaves the marrow; therefore, an RBC must survive its 120-day life span with its given complement of enzymes. A deficient cell is hemolyzed earlier than a normal cell.

(i) **Glucose-6-phosphate dehydrogenase (G6PD) deficiency** is an extremely common X-linked disorder; more than 150 subtypes affect more than 100 million individuals worldwide. Deficient individuals are liable to oxidant stress, which occurs with infections and with certain drugs (e.g., sulfa drugs, quinine). Such oxidant stress results in denatured hemoglobin or Heinz bodies, leading to hemolysis of affected RBCs. A deficiency of G6PD also destroys the reducing capacity of the RBCs. It is believed that G6PD protects individuals from falciparum malaria; this disease is most common in endemic areas. **Diagnosis** is made by demonstrating Heinz bodies during an acute hemolytic anemia episode or by measuring abnormally low levels of enzyme in the steady state. Enzyme levels should not be measured during a hemolytic episode, when they may temporarily become more normal as a result of destruction of old, extremely deficient cells and their replacement by relatively G6PD-rich reticulocytes and neocytes.

(ii) **Pyruvate kinase (PK) deficiency** is an autosomal recessive example of an enzymopathy. This deficiency is most common in northern European populations. Patients may benefit from splenectomy.

II HEMATOCRIT DISORDERS

Increases in hematocrit are caused by either **increased RBC mass** or **decreased plasma volume.** The following discussion deals exclusively with disorders associated with abnormal elevation of hematocrit (i.e., hematocrit ≥ 55%).

A Terminology

The term **polycythemia** often is used to describe an increase in the number of RBCs, with no reference to fluctuations in leukocytes and platelets. However, this condition is more accurately termed **erythrocytosis.** [There is a condition called **polycythemia vera** in which leukocytes and platelets also increase in number. See II C 2 b (2) for a discussion of this disorder.] Increased hematocrits occur in two ways.

1. **Relative erythrocytosis** refers to an elevation of hematocrit due to diminished plasma volume; RBC mass remains normal.
2. **Absolute erythrocytosis** refers to an elevation of hematocrit due to a true increase in RBC mass.

B Pathophysiology

Blood flow and viscosity are inversely proportional to hematocrit; therefore, an excessively elevated hematocrit can diminish tissue blood flow, decrease tissue oxygen delivery, and increase cardiac work. In extreme cases, this can result in hyperviscosity syndromes.

C Classification

1. **Relative erythrocytosis** exists in two forms.

   a. **Stress erythrocytosis,** or **Gaisböck's syndrome,** occurs predominantly in middle-aged men. This disorder usually is asymptomatic, although it may be associated with increased cardiovascular disease. It is important to differentiate patients with stress erythrocytosis from those with early and subtle manifestations of the much more serious condition polycythemia vera. Patients with stress erythrocytosis require no treatment.

b. Erythrocytosis occurs secondary to known causes of contracted plasma volume (e.g., excessive diuresis; nasogastric drainage; severe gastroenteritis, especially in infants; burns). These conditions are apparent clinically; therapy includes fluid and plasma replacement with treatment of the underlying condition.

2. Absolute erythrocytosis is classified according to the mechanism responsible for increased RBC mass.

a. Hypoxia

(1) **Etiology.** Causes include severe lung disease, severe heart failure, cyanotic heart disease with right-to-left cardiopulmonary shunts, and abnormal hemoglobins with increased oxygen affinity.

(2) **Pathophysiology.** The RBC mass rises secondary to tissue hypoxia, which causes an increase in renal erythropoietin and subsequent hematocrit elevation.

(3) **Diagnosis** may be apparent clinically, but blood gas analysis showing arterial oxygen saturation less than 92% and P_{50} analysis (i.e., studies of the oxygen-releasing characteristics of hemoglobin) may be required to confirm the diagnosis. As measurement of serum erythropoietin (EPO) becomes more available and more accurate, the finding of a moderately elevated EPO level in a high-hematocrit patient is a useful clue as well.

(4) **Therapy** is somewhat conjectural, but phlebotomy is a favored treatment for patients with hematocrits that are persistently greater than 55%.

b. Neoplasia

(1) **Neoplastic erythropoietin sources** cause the RBC mass to increase.

(a) **Etiology.** Causes include hypernephroma and renal cysts; such renal pathology accounts for more than 90% of this type of erythrocytosis. Other tumors include cerebellar hemangioblastoma, hepatoma, and uterine fibroids.

(b) **Diagnosis** requires radiologic demonstration of the appropriate tumor with intravenous pyelography, computed tomography (CT), or ultrasound techniques. Reasonably accurate assays for erythropoietin are becoming available and demonstrate extremely elevated titers from autonomous erythropoietin secretion by these tumors.

(c) **Therapy.** Removal of the tumor corrects the hematocrit.

(2) **Autonomous bone marrow**

(a) In the condition **polycythemia vera,** the bone marrow becomes autonomous and synthesizes cells independently of erythropoietin levels. (Theoretically, erythropoietin levels should be near zero if measured accurately.) Polycythemia vera represents a true neoplasm of the marrow stem cells.

(i) **Diagnosis.** According to the Polycythemia Vera Study Group, diagnosis is confirmed by the presence of all three of the following **major criteria** or by the first two major criteria and any two of the following **minor criteria.** The **major criteria** are elevated RBC mass, arterial oxygen saturation exceeding 92%, and splenomegaly. The **minor criteria** are leukocytosis, thrombocytosis, elevated leukocyte alkaline phosphatase (LAP), and elevated serum vitamin B_{12} level.

(ii) **Therapy** involves removal of RBCs, suppression of marrow function, or both. **Phlebotomy** removes RBCs and should be performed to lower hematocrit to the 45% range. If used alone, this is the safest therapy. Marrow suppression is needed when hematocrit control requires frequent phlebotomy or when other cell lines are elevated. Interferon α has been shown to be an effective agent to control myeloproliferation and splenomegaly. Radioactive phosphorus, once commonly used to modulate marrow activity, is associated with an increased incidence of leukemia and non-hematologic cancers and is now used only rarely. **Chemotherapy** with the antimetabolite hydroxyurea is used to control many cases of polycythemia vera. Few if any leukemogenic or second malignancy–inducing effects have been encountered with this agent.

(iii) **Survival** is measured in years and is 7–10 years in most studies. With untreated polycythemia vera, however, survival is only 2–3 years. The major causes of morbidity and mortality are thromboembolic and cardiovascular. Leukemic transformation occurs in 5%–10% of patients.

(b) **Myelofibrosis,** a chronic myeloproliferative disorder, is pathophysiologically related. It is characterized by splenomegaly, immature granulocytes and erythrocytes in the blood, distorted tear-drop–shaped RBC forms, and marrow fibrosis. The disease is a **monoclonal stem cell disease** of primitive hematopoietic stem cells. The **fibrosis** is a secondary event.

(i) **Anemia** and signs and symptoms of **massive splenomegaly** are the hallmarks of the disease.

(ii) Most **therapy is supportive.** In selected cases of true hypersplenism and symptoms from massive splenomegaly, splenectomy is beneficial.

D Therapeutic approach (Table 3–2)

TABLE 3–2 Therapeutic Approach to Elevated Hematocrit Levels

Hematocrit	Significance	Comments
55%–60%	Begin to see decreased cardiac output and oxygen delivery; begin to see decreased cerebral blood flow	Consider elective phlebotomy to lower hematocrit
> 60%	Marked increase in blood viscosity; patient may be overtly symptomatic	Clear indication for phlebotomy; in polycythemia vera, marrow suppression therapy

III WHITE BLOOD CELL (WBC) DISORDERS

The WBCs include lymphocytes, monocytes, eosinophils, basophils, and neutrophils (PMNs). Disorders of WBCs can be considered in terms of excessive or reduced numbers of cells and in terms of functional abnormality.

A Lymphocytes

Lymphocytes exist in marrow as well as in the lymphoid tissue of the body. Lymphocyte functions include delayed hypersensitivity, which is performed by T lymphocytes (**T cells**), and antibody production, which is performed by B lymphocytes (**B cells**) and plasma cells.

1. **Lymphopenia** refers to a diminished number of lymphocytes.

a. **Lymphopenia without significant immune deficiency** is seen in many illnesses that cause elevated serum cortisol levels such as acute infections and inflammatory states. Chemotherapy, radiotherapy, and Hodgkin's disease also are associated with lymphopenia. In none of these conditions is antibody production severely affected.

b. **Congenital lymphopenia with immune deficiency** is associated with specific immune deficiency syndromes.

(1) **Varieties**

(a) **B-cell deficiency**

(i) **Bruton's agammaglobulinemia** is an X-linked disease characterized by recurrent infections with encapsulated organisms. It is caused by deficient quantities of opsonizing antibody. Although peripheral lymphocyte counts may be normal, specific counting for B cells shows their absence. In addition, lymphoid follicles reveal no germinal centers, which are the B-cell areas. Therapy consists of exogenous gamma globulin and plasma via transfusion.

(ii) **Other B-cell deficiency states** include common variable hypogammaglobulinemia and IgA deficiency.

(b) **T-cell deficiency. Thymic hypoplasia** (DiGeorge syndrome) is the prototypical T-cell deficiency syndrome. Patients with this condition have variable total lymphocyte counts but low numbers of T cells with absent T-cell function. Recurrent fungal infections are seen in these patients.

(c) **Deficiency of both B and T cells.** Disorders characterized by diminished numbers of both B and T cells include ataxia–telangiectasia syndrome, Wiskott-Aldrich syndrome of immunodeficiency and thrombocytopenia, and severe combined immunodeficiency disease (SCID).

(2) **Diagnosis.** For all of the conditions discussed, diagnosis requires the clinical setting of repeated infections combined with the following findings:

(a) Lymphocyte counts of B and T cells, including surface subset markers

(b) Measurement of specific immunoglobulin levels

(c) Demonstration of the absence of specific B-cell areas (i.e., germinal centers and plasma cells) or T-cell areas (i.e., thymus and lymph node medullary cords)

(3) **Therapy. BMT** has been curative in many of these conditions.

c. **Acquired immunodeficiency syndrome (AIDS).** For a discussion of AIDS, see Chapter 8 C 3.

2. **Lymphocytosis** is defined as an excessive number of lymphocytes (i.e., > 5000/mm^3). The differential diagnosis of absolute lymphocytosis is limited.

a. **Infection.** Certain infections cause lymphocytosis. In children, both pertussis and acute infectious lymphocytosis may cause counts that exceed 50,000/mm^3. In adults, lesser elevations are seen with hepatitis and infectious mononucleosis.

b. **Hematopoietic disorders** associated with lymphocytosis include acute lymphocytic leukemia (ALL), chronic lymphocytic leukemia (CLL), and certain lymphomas.

(1) **CLL.** An adult who is older than 50 years and who manifests a mature lymphocytosis most likely has CLL. The cells associated with CLL are mature lymphocytes that accumulate in the body.

(a) **Diagnosis.** A peripheral blood smear showing a mature lymphocytosis is highly suggestive. Corroborative findings include marrow infiltration by mature lymphocytes, an enlarged spleen, and lymphadenopathy. Lymphocyte markers can also be determined. The technique of flow cytometry is diagnostic.

(b) **Staging.** The CLL tumor burden is related to certain clinical findings, which also have prognostic significance.

(i) **Stage 0** is characterized by peripheral lymphocytosis only. The prognosis for patients with stage 0 CLL is excellent; median survival exceeds 10 years.

(ii) **Stages 1 and 2.** Stage 1 is characterized by peripheral lymphocytosis and lymphadenopathy, and stage 2 by the presence of splenomegaly. Both stages 1 and 2 have intermediate prognoses, with a median survival of 60 months.

(iii) **Stages 3 and 4.** Stage 3 is characterized by the presence of anemia, and stage 4 by the presence of thrombocytopenia. Both stages 3 and 4 signify marrow failure and have poor prognoses, with a median survival < 24 months.

(iv) Other prognostic factors include lymphocyte doubling time, chromosomal and V immunoglobulin gene status, and CD38 expression.

(c) **Therapy** for CLL.

(i) **Early-stage CLL.** As a rule, stages 0, 1, and 2 CLL should not be treated.

(ii) **Late-stage CLL** is treated with an alkylating agent (e.g., chlorambucil), with or without steroids. The purine analog fludarabine is used and has a higher response rate. However, this agent causes a profound and clinically significant reduction in immune function, sometimes resulting in an almost AIDS-like immune deficient state. For example, patients taking fludarabine must receive

Pneumocystis carinii pneumonia (PCP) prophylaxis. Targeted monoclonal antibody therapy (e.g., anti-CD20, rituximab) shows promise.

(2) Certain well-differentiated **lymphomas** also are characterized by an excessive number of lymphocytes in the blood. These disorders are similar to CLL.

(3) **Acute lymphocytic leukemia (ALL)** is characterized by maturation arrest in the lymphoid line with tissue infiltration by lymphoblasts. (This disease is discussed in more detail in IV A.)

3. **Monocytosis and monocytopenia.** Monocytes are **phagocytic cells** that are an important component of the cellular immune system and that secrete many cytokines, including TNF, all of the interferons (IFNs), granulocyte–macrophage colony-stimulating factor (GM-CSF), and granulocyte colony-stimulating factor (G-CSF).

a. **Isolated monocytopenia** does not occur. Monocytopenia in combination with decreases in other cell lines occurs with aplastic anemia, hairy cell leukemia, and steroid use.

b. **Benign monocytosis** can occur in many infectious diseases [e.g., tuberculosis, subacute bacterial endocarditis (SBE), cytomegalovirus (CMV)] and inflammatory diseases (e.g., rheumatoid arthritis, sarcoid). The finding is nonspecific.

c. Monocytosis can accompany essentially all of the hematologic and lymphatic malignancies.

B Basophils, eosinophils, and neutrophils Disorders in these cells also are classified according to fluctuations in cell numbers and to functional deficiency.

1. **Basophils.** An abnormally increased number of basophils is called **basophilia.** This uncommon condition usually is associated with the myeloproliferative syndromes, particularly chronic myelogenous leukemia (CML).

2. **Eosinophils.** An abnormally increased number of eosinophils is called **eosinophilia.** This condition is more common than basophilia and occurs most commonly secondary to other disease processes, including:

a. Neoplasia (e.g., lymphoma, Hodgkin's disease)

b. Addison's disease

c. Allergic and atopic disease (most common cause of eosinophilia)

d. Collagen vascular disease (e.g., necrotizing vasculitis)

e. Parasitic infestation

f. Primary hypereosinophilic symptoms are uncommon. These syndromes are characterized by very high (20,000–50,000) levels of sustained eosinophilia, invasive toxic effects to the heart and lungs, and chromosomal clonal aberrations typical of malignancy.

3. **Neutrophils**

a. **Neutrophilia** is an excessively increased number of neutrophils in the blood. Causes of neutrophilia include the following:

(1) Most cases of neutrophilia result from conditions such as infection, tumor, stress, collagen disorders, and steroids; the underlying disease may not be apparent clinically.

(2) In unusual cases, more than 50,000 neutrophils/mm^3 appear in the blood. These so-called **leukemoid reactions** can be differentiated from the leukemias by the absence of the circulating blast forms and by the finding of elevated LAP values.

(3) Neutrophilia also results from **neoplastic marrow diseases** such as polycythemia vera and CML.

(a) **Diagnosis of CML.** CML is suspected in patients with excessive WBC counts and splenomegaly. Peripheral blood smears reveal a spectrum of cell forms ranging from mature polymorphonuclear neutrophils to immature blasts. Several findings confirm the diagnosis: the presence of an abnormal marker chromosome (the **Philadelphia chromosome**) in the marrow precursor cells and very low LAP levels. The fusion protein of the abnormal gene in CML is detectable, as is the abnormal genetic material itself. The fusion protein results in a functional, mutant tyrosine kinase that results in a lack of control of basic cellular processes such as proliferation rate, adherence, and physiologic death (apoptosis). Affected stem cells manifest a proliferative advantage over normal stem cells, reduced adherence to marrow stroma, and decreased apoptosis.

(i) CML is now diagnosed using polymerase chain reaction (PCR) technology to demonstrate the presence of this abnormal genetic material. PCR is able to reveal the BCR-ABL fusion protein as well as the abnormal chromosomal fusion biochemically, even when the marrow appears normal using morphology and routine cytogenetics.

(ii) Further biochemical studies using these techniques have demonstrated that the fusion of chromosomal material of chromosomes 9 and 22 and its resultant fusion protein cause marrow stem cells to "turn off" the apoptosis pathway of programmed cell death. Thus, these abnormal cells are "immortalized" and create an accumulation of marrow and peripheral blood elements that are clinically recognized as CML.

(b) Prognosis of CML. The median survival rate for CML patients is 3–4 years. Most patients die during the so-called **blast crisis,** when this chronic disorder converts into a highly malignant variety of acute leukemia.

(i) Hydroxyurea is an effective palliative agent that reduces the leukemia cell burden in the chronic phase of CML. Patients obtain a clinical and hematologic remission, but the abnormal cytogenetics and fusion protein remain and are demonstrable on study of marrow and peripheral blood.

(ii) α-Interferon (α-IFN) administered three times weekly also induces remission in 70% of patients. In 40–60% of cases, it can convert the patient's marrow to Philadelphia chromosome–negative status and may be curative in some patients.

(iii) Imatinib mesylate (STI571, Gleevec) is a designed BCR-ABL tyrosine kinase inhibitor that reverses the effects of that fusion protein. It induces remission in > 90% and major cytogenetic reversal in > 50% of cases and has become the initial therapy of choice in CML. Drug resistance over time is a problem (i.e., durability of response), but this agent has become an option to be compared with early transplant in CML. Early results are very favorable.

The elucidation of how abnormal, malignant genetic transformation results in disease and the ability to specifically, pharmacologically intervene in that process marks a milestone in cancer therapeutics.

(iv) Marrow transplantation is curative and is the therapy of choice for younger patients (see IV D 3).

b. Neutropenia is an absolute decrease in the number of circulating neutrophils. Neutropenia occurs rarely as an early manifestation of intrinsic marrow disease (e.g., acute leukemia) but more commonly secondary to exogenous stimuli.

(1) Infections. Certain viral infections (e.g., hepatitis, influenza) and bacterial infections (e.g., typhoid fever) cause neutropenia.

(2) Drugs (e.g., phenothiazines, fluoxetine, antithyroid medications) are associated with neutropenia and, in severe instances, can cause agranulocytosis. Agranulocytosis is characterized by:

(a) Profoundly lowered neutrophil counts (i.e., $< 500/mm^3$)

(b) Severe prostration, high fever, and often a necrotic pharyngitis

(c) Bone marrow showing **maturation arrest** (i.e., large numbers of immature WBC forms in an otherwise normal marrow)

(d) High mortality rates unless treated early and aggressively with supportive measures and potent bactericidal antibiotics. Use of genetically engineered colony-stimulating factor and other marrow growth factors has been encouraging. WBC colony-stimulating factor (G-CSF) have been shown to reduce febrile days and hospital days. Whether they actually reduce mortality remains conjectural, although their use is common in this setting.

(3) The **collagen vascular diseases** [e.g., systemic lupus erythematosus (SLE), rheumatoid arthritis] have been shown to cause neutropenia via immune destruction of WBCs.

(4) **Familial forms of neutropenia** include familial benign chronic neutropenia, cyclic neutropenia, and chronic idiopathic neutropenia. These disorders have good prognoses, although they are associated with increased nuisance infections (e.g., boils) when the neutrophil count is less than 500/mm^3. They respond well to G-CSF.

(5) **Chemotherapeutic agents** used in the therapy of malignant disease are the most common cause of neutropenia. Such agents include alkylating agents (e.g., cyclophosphamide), antimetabolites [e.g., methotrexate, 5-fluorouracil (5-FU), cytosine arabinoside], and tumor antibiotics (e.g., doxorubicin). Chemotherapy-induced neutropenia can be markedly ameliorated in difficult cases by the judicious use of G-CSF.

c. **Functional disorders** of neutrophils involve a compromised ability to fight infection. These conditions are rare; affected individuals have recurrent infections. The following are prototypical examples.

(1) **Chédiak-Higashi syndrome** is an autosomal recessive disorder characterized by albinism and increased pyogenic infection. In addition, neutrophils and other granule-containing cells (e.g., melanosomes) reveal giant, fused, peroxidase-staining granules with decreased ability to kill ingested microbes.

(2) **Chronic granulomatous disease (CGD)** of childhood is an X-linked disorder in neutrophil metabolism characterized by a defect in neutrophil-free radical formation (associated with the oxidative burst and killing activity in neutrophils), resulting in susceptibility to recurrent suppurative infections. This condition often is fatal, and the diagnosis is confirmed by the presence of neutrophils that cannot oxidize nitroblue tetrazolium dye to blue-black from colorless. BMT has been effective in these cases.

IV ACUTE LEUKEMIAS AND MYELODYSPLASIAS

The acute leukemias are disorders in the maturation of hematopoietic tissue that are characterized by the presence of immature leukocytes in the marrow and peripheral blood. The immature cells are arrested in the earliest phases of differentiation and are referred to as **blasts.** Myelodysplasia is a related clonal disorder of the pluripotential stem cells, resulting in inadequate, ineffective erythropoiesis, dysmorphic changes in the marrow, and peripheral cytopenias.

A Acute leukemia classification and epidemiology

It is important both prognostically and therapeutically to distinguish the lymphocytic from the nonlymphocytic (myelogenous) leukemias. Classification of cells involves special histochemical stains (e.g., peroxidase in myelogenous leukemia), marker enzymes (e.g., terminal transferase in ALL), and specific cell-surface antigenic markers; use of these methods in combination allows classification that approaches 95% accuracy. Cytogenetic analysis, marker chromosome defects, and chromosomal banding techniques have even further refined and made more accurate classification of acute leukemias. In addition, such chromosomal groupings appear to identify subgroups within specific leukemia types that have different responses to therapy and different prognoses. Currently, acute leukemias are classified into two major types, acute lymphocytic leukemia (ALL) and acute myelogenous leukemia (AML) [Table 3–3].

1. **ALL** is common in children: 85% of cases of ALL occur in children, and 90% of leukemia that occurs in children is ALL. Conversely, ALL is not a common leukemia in adults. The ALL cell origin is in the lymphoid line. Techniques such as membrane surface markers and antibody detection of surface antigens have enabled investigators to characterize ALL subsets.

TABLE 3–3 Classification of the Acute Leukemias

AML/ALL Subtype	Frequency	Features
Acute Myelogenous Leukemia (AML)		
M1: myeloblastic (without maturation)	Uncommon	
M2: myeloblastic (with maturation)	Common	Most frequent AML
M3: promyelocytic	Uncommon	Blasts with giant granules DIC is a common complication
M4: myelomonocytic	Common	Tissue infiltration
M5: monocytic	Uncommon	Tissue infiltration
M6: erythroleukemia	Rare	Formation of multinucleated RBC blasts in bone marrow
M7: megakaryoblastic	Rare	Acute myelofibrosis
Acute Lymphocytic Leukemia (ALL)		
Acute lymphoblastic leukemia	Common	Classic acute leukemia of childhood B-cell origin
Burkitt's neoplasms (leukemia and lymphoma)	Uncommon	Small, vacuolated blast forms B-cell origin Worse prognosis
Adult T-cell leukemia	Uncommon	Affects young adult men Large mediastinal masses and CNS involvement

CNS = central nervous system; DIC = disseminated intravascular coagulation; RBC = red blood cell.

a. The most common ALL variant (comprising 75% of cases) is of B-cell lineage of null variety (i.e., there is absent rosette formation). This variant also expresses the common ALL antigen (CALLA) on the cell surface.
b. T-cell ALL and other less common varieties constitute the remainder of cases.
c. Most ALL varieties express terminal deoxynucleotidyl transferase (TdT), and staining for this enzyme is useful in differentiating ALL from myelogenous leukemias.
d. Differentiating subtypes has prognostic significance in that, for example, T-cell varieties of ALL are more resistant to therapy and have far worse prognoses than common variety B-cell ALL.

2. **AML,** or **acute nonlymphocytic leukemia (ANLL),** is common in adults, and the incidence increases with age. Specific environmental risks increase AML incidence in populations. They include moderate-to-high doses of ionizing radiation, chemicals such as benzene and petroleum products, and prior exposure to cytotoxic chemotherapy agents such as alkylating drugs (e.g., cyclophosphamide, chlorambucil). The AML cell of origin probably arises at different levels of hematopoiesis in different patients, which accounts for the clinically well-defined subtypes of AML. In most cases, the AML clone arises from multipotential precursors capable of differentiating into granulocyte, erythrocyte, macrophage, or megakaryocyte colony-forming units (CFUs). Therefore, in most patients, lymphoid and erythroid lineages are not involved in the leukemic process.

B **Clinical features** of acute leukemia represent the effects of marrow infiltration by nonmaturing, functionless blast cells, including subsequent bone marrow failure.

1. **Physical findings** include fatigue and pallor (due to anemia); fever and infection (due to neutropenia); petechiae, purpura, and epistaxis (due to thrombocytopenia). Infiltrative symptoms may include splenomegaly, gingival hypertrophy, and bone pain.

2. **Laboratory findings** include almost universal pancytopenia and circulating blast forms. Increased cell turnover results in elevated uric acid levels. In promyelocytic leukemia (M3), DIC is usually present with hypofibrinogenemia and elevated fibrin split products.

C **Diagnosis** The diagnosis of acute leukemia is confirmed by the finding of blast infiltration of the bone marrow. Special histochemical stains (e.g., peroxidase, Sudan black), enzyme markers (e.g., TdT), surface antigenic markers, and chromosome cytogenetic studies are performed to identify the specific subtype of leukemia involved.

D **Therapy** of acute leukemia is complex. **Medical regimens** achieve complete remission in 65%–70% of all patients with de novo AML and appear to cure 25% of these. Therapy carries a 20% early mortality rate and is, therefore, best performed by physicians who are experienced with the drugs used and the supportive care needed to maintain patients through the induction period and to achieve remissions. **Bone marrow transplantation (BMT)** has higher cure rates in patients eligible for this therapy.

1. **Chemotherapy.** Initial therapy consists of chemotherapeutic ablation of the leukemic cell line. In many cases, especially those of AML, it is necessary to ablate all normal marrow as well. Because normal marrow has a shorter generation time than leukemic blasts, recovery with normal marrow tissue is possible. This initial marrow ablation is termed **induction therapy.**
   a. **ALL induction therapy.** ALL blasts are initially more selectively sensitive to chemotherapy than AML blasts. It often is possible to destroy ALL blasts with some sparing of normal marrow. Thus, induction therapy for ALL is associated with lower morbidity and mortality rates than it is for AML.
      (1) Combinations of vincristine, prednisone, anthracyclines, and L-asparaginase are used to obtain initial remissions.
      (2) Consolidation therapy and a period of less intensive maintenance therapy with agents such as mercaptopurine and methotrexate are effective.
      (3) Treatment of potential sanctuary sites such as the CNS is required in many cases of ALL.
      (4) BMT plays a role, usually after initial relapse. Chemotherapy has excellent results in ALL, far superior to those in AML, especially in children younger than 15 years in whom the cure rate approaches 80%. In adults, complete remission rates of 80% can be achieved, usually for longer than 2 years. However, only 15%–20% of these patients remain in remission.
   b. **AML induction therapy** requires ablation of all marrow elements, both blasts and normal tissue. The best available regimen remains cytosine arabinoside and an anthracycline antibiotic. More aggressive administration of cycles of chemotherapy after induction to eliminate residual leukemic cells does prolong the remission duration and is beneficial. Data indicate that:
      (1) Individuals with AML have a 60%–70% complete response rate to induction regimens.
      (2) With varying postinduction regimens, the median response duration is 12–15 months, with 25%–35% of these patients experiencing 24-month disease-free survival.
      (3) Of individuals with AML, 15%–25% are alive 2 years after their diagnosis. Some of these will relapse, and some will be "cured."

2. **Radiotherapy** is used in ALL to sterilize sanctuary sites of late relapse. Such sites are found in the CNS and, possibly, in the testes.

3. **BMT** has emerged as definitive, curative therapy for acute leukemia. BMT usually is used after the first remission has been obtained. The goal of BMT is permanent eradication of the residual leukemia and prevention of relapse. Ultra–high-dose chemotherapy alone or with radiotherapy prior to BMT may be given in doses that are not limited by concerns of toxicity to the marrow, because the subsequent marrow infusion and transplantation "rescues" the patient from the marrow toxicities that these therapies produce.
   a. Suitable donors are a prerequisite for successful BMT. **Allogeneic BMT** uses stem cells obtained from human leukocyte antigen (HLA)–matched donors.

(1) Identical twin donors are optimal but rare. The most common donors (35%) are HLA-matched siblings.

(2) Data continue to show that younger patients do better with BMT, particularly regarding the incidence of graft-versus-host disease (GVHD) and ability to tolerate this effect (see IV D 3 c). Nevertheless, with increasing experience and technological improvements, the upper age limit for BMT continues to rise, and it now exceeds 50 years in many transplant centers.

b. When no matched donors are available, **autologous BMT** using marrow infusion of harvested and stored remission marrow showing improved survival rates has accrued. A recent review demonstrated a 48% survival rate at 4 years in patients undergoing transplantation in first remission. The major cause of failure is recurrent leukemia after transplantation. Various marrow purging techniques to remove leukemic cells are under study.

c. GVHD is a major obstacle encountered in marrow transplantation. This reaction results from the grafting of immunocompetent donor T cells, which respond to alloantigens expressed on host cells.

(1) Major target organs are skin (dermatitis), gastrointestinal tract (diarrhea), and liver.

(2) Therapy may be prolonged and usually consists of some combination of prednisone, cyclosporine, and low-dose azathioprine.

d. Other important post-transplantation factors include the toxicity of the preparative regimens, interstitial pneumonitis, other infections, graft rejection (rare), and hepatic veno-occlusive disease.

4. Supportive therapy is extremely important and serves as a prototype for supportive therapy in other forms of neoplasia. The following principles apply to the use of chemotherapy regimens as well as to bone marrow ablation and transplantation.

a. The **hemoglobin level** should be maintained above 8 g/dL by transfusions of packed RBCs. Leukodepleted and radiated blood is used to avoid allosensitization in the event of later BMT.

b. Hemorrhage is best prevented by prophylactic transfusion of platelet concentrates. Serious spontaneous bleeding is unusual unless the platelet count declines below 10,000/mm^3, and platelet transfusion is used to maintain platelet counts above 10,000/mm^3. This practice has lowered the incidence of fatal hemorrhage in acute leukemia from 80% to less than 20%.

c. Control of infection is a major determinant of survival of patients being treated for the acute leukemia that is caused by drug-induced neutropenia.

(1) **Isolation techniques have been tested as a means of avoiding infection.** Totally protected environments decrease incidence of infections but have little impact on remissions and survival. Such environments feature expensive laminar flow rooms, sterilized food, and gut sterilization by nonabsorbable antibiotics. Many physicians do not use these methods but instead maintain strict hand-washing and skin-care techniques, use long-term central catheters to avoid peripheral indwelling lines, and practice strict rectal care to achieve similar results.

(2) **Infections are treated early and aggressively.** Neutropenic patients (those with PMNs $< 500/mm^3$) are susceptible to all organisms, especially gram-negative rods and fungi (e.g., *Candida, Aspergillus*).

(a) Initial temperature elevations require thorough clinical evaluation, vigorous cultures, and immediate and empiric treatment with broad-spectrum bactericidal antibiotic combinations of cephalosporins aminoglycosides vancomycin, and semisynthetic penicillins (e.g., imipenim).

(b) Secondary temperature elevations that occur after treatment with potent broad-spectrum antibiotics may require the empiric use of antifungal agents (e.g., amphotericin B). Prevention of fungal infections with prophylactic triazoles (e.g., fluconazole) has proved effective and has contributed to diminished morbidity and mortality from fungal infections.

(c) Attention to electrolytes and uric acid is required in those patients with high cell turnover and in those receiving multiple antibiotics.
  (i) Treatment with allopurinol and adequate fluids is required for uric acid control.
  (ii) Electrolyte levels, especially the potassium level, must be maintained in patients being given antibiotics.

d. **Stimulation of marrow recovery** using growth factors made by recombinant DNA technology is finding a role in supportive therapy. Myeloid colony-stimulating factors result in more rapid recovery of PMN counts in AML patients treated with either chemotherapy or BMT. The routine addition of G-CSF to the therapeutic regimen once patients have received and cleared their chemotherapy is a significant advance. This maneuver has resulted in a shortening of the period of severe neutropenia and reduced the morbidity due to infectious disease. In itself, however, such therapy has neither lowered the overall mortality nor raised the successful induction rate in patients with acute leukemia.

E Prognosis

1. The prognosis for children with **ALL is very good;** more than 95% obtain complete remission. Approximately 70%–80% of patients are disease free at 5 years and are likely cured. If relapse occurs, second complete remissions are possible in most cases. Patients in second remissions are candidates for BMT, with 35%–65% probability of long-term survival.
2. The prognosis for patients with **AML is poor.** Among patients receiving the best care, using current chemotherapy regimens, 75% obtain complete remission and 25% die. Furthermore, the usual duration of remission is only 12–18 months. Although some investigators claim 20% cure rates using intensive postremission therapy, there is little common experience with significant cure rates.
   a. In patients younger than 50 years, BMT, both allogeneic and autologous, is the treatment of choice after obtaining a first complete remission (Table 3–4). Current results indicate that 50% of young patients with AML who undergo allogeneic BMT experience prolonged disease-free intervals and may be cured. Similar encouraging results are accruing for autologous BMT rates.

TABLE 3–4 Current Established Indications for Bone Marrow Transplantation (BMT)*
Patients younger than 55 years of age with an HLA-identical sibling and CML (several very large, long follow-up series have reported an overall 10-year survival of 70%, which is by far better than the best interferon or chemotherapy data)
Patients who are otherwise healthy with NHL in the first chemosensitive relapse (a multicenter, prospective, randomized trial favored autologous transplantation)
Patients who are otherwise healthy with myeloma (a multicenter, prospective, randomized trial favored autologous transplantation)
Patients who are otherwise healthy with intermediate or high-risk AML (a majority of several multicenter randomized trials favor transplantation)
Patients who are young and healthy with severe aplastic anemia and an HLA-identical sibling
Patients who are young and healthy with an HLA-identical donor and high-risk ALL (a major review of available trials suggests superior results, although there are no randomized studies as yet).
Patients who are young and healthy with high-risk myelodysplastic syndromes (according to the international MDS risk criteria) and an HLA-identical sibling.

*Data concerning other diseases such as refractory or relapsed Hodgkin's disease, homozygous thalassemia, and sickle cell disease with recurrent stroke or chest syndromes are being gathered, but studies must still be considered experimental.
ALL = acute lymphocytic leukemia; AML = acute myelogenous leukemia; CML = chronic myelogenous leukemia; HLA = human leukocyte antigen; MDS = myelodysplastic syndromes; NHL = non-Hodgkin's lymphoma.

b. As better ways to prevent GVHD appear, the morbidity and mortality rates associated with allogeneic BMT should decline, and curability for patients with AML should increase (see Table 3–4).

F **Myelodysplastic syndrome (MDS) Classification and Epidemiology** The myelodysplasias are clonal disorders characterized clinically and morphologically by defective and ineffective hematopoiesis. They are the result of pathology in the hematopoietic stem cells and are thus characterized by cytopenias of varying degree in red cell, white cell, and megakaryocytic lines. All have a tendency to terminate in AML. A variety of chromosomal abnormalities have been well defined in these syndromes, the most common being loss of chromosome 5 (13%) and chromosome 7 (5%), trisomy 8 (5%), and deletions of parts of chromosomes 17 and 20. Classification schemes are somewhat cumbersome and disputed, but the reasonably established FAB classification is shown in Table 3–5.

G **Clinical features** of the myelodysplasias all relate to bone marrow failure.

1. History and physical findings include anemia features (progressive fatigue, dyspnea on exertion, pallor); neutropenia features (frequent infections); and thrombocytopenia features (bleeding and bruising). MDS particularly affects the elderly (median age of onset is seventh decade), and MDS has replaced iron deficiency as the most frequent cause of anemia in this age-group.
2. Laboratory findings include cytopenias, with anemia being the most frequent presenting feature (90%).

H **Diagnosis** A patient with cytopenia will have normal iron, B_{12}, and folate levels and will be "refractory" to therapy with these hematinics. Peripheral smear demonstrates a variety of abnormalities that are suggestive (teardrop forms, Pelger Huet hypogranulated hypolobular WBC forms, and abnormal platelet forms). Eventually, examination of bone marrow is performed and shows normal or increased cellularity (which in the setting of cytopenias demonstrates ineffective erythropoiesis) and morphologic abnormalities including megaloblastic RBC, asynchronous maturation of cytoplasm and nuclei, ringed sideroblast forms, micromegakaryocytes, and excess blast forms. Detailed, refined cytogenic studies, including polymerase chain reaction analysis, will reveal the frequent chromosomal abnormalities cited above.

I **Therapy** of MDS is complex and relates to the variety of syndromes which have an extremely variable prognosis.

1. Chemotherapy has been quite disappointing in MDS. MDS patients have lower complete remission rates of shorter duration and higher relapse rate than garden-variety AML. Also, the advanced age of most MDS patients makes chemotherapy quite difficult.

TABLE 3–5 FAB Classification of Myelodysplastic Syndromes

Subtype	Peripheral Blood Findings	Marrow Findings
Refractory anemia	Cytopenia of at least one cell line, usually anemia	Normal/hypercellular with dysplastic changes < 5% blasts
Refractory anemia with ringed sideroblasts	Cytopenia of at least one cell line, almost always anemia	Presence of ringed sideroblast forms, more than 15%
Refractory anemia with excess blasts	Cytopenia of at least two cell lines	Dysplastic with 5%–20% blast forms
Refractory anemia with excess blasts in transformation	> 5% blast forms	20%–30% blast forms or presence of Auer rods
Chronic myelomonocytic leukemia (CMML)	Monocytes $>1 \times 10^9$/L	Up to 20% blast forms

FAB = French-American-British.

2. Supportive therapy is the most widely offered strategy. The use of erythropoietin (EPO) and G-CSF to ameliorate anemia and severe neutropenia is supported by evidence-based trials. Because EPO is effective only in the minority, transfusions are used for symptomatic anemia. Aggressive and judicious use of antibiotics and platelet transfusion techniques are similar to those used in AML situations.
3. Novel agents are continuously being evaluated in this difficult patient population. Differentiating agents such as retinoids and arsenic trioxide have shown promise. Immunotherapy with cyclosporin and related products is also being evaluated.
4. In the small subset of high-risk, high-mortality patients of appropriate age-group, BMT has been successfully used and is the only curative therapy available.

J **Prognosis** is variable. As stated, most MDS tends to terminate in AML. Median survivals range from 6 months to 6 years, depending on a complex set of variables, including number and severity of cytopenias; presence or absence of cytogenic abnormalities, and percentage of myeloblasts in the bone marrow. In essentially all subsets, the presence of MDS negatively impacts survival significantly even when MDS is not the primary cause of death.

V DISORDERS OF COAGULATION AND HEMOSTASIS

A **General considerations** Hemostasis requires an intact coagulation system of vascular and tissue components, platelets, and coagulation proteins. Deficiency or disease of any of these components may cause either spontaneous or trauma-related hemorrhage.

1. **History.** A careful history provides clues to the pathogenesis of bleeding. Immediate, mucocutaneous bleeding suggests vascular or platelet disease; delayed deep-tissue bleeding and hemarthrosis suggest coagulation protein deficiency. Genetic transmissions of bleeding disorders (e.g., the X-linked hemophilias) also are elicited by history, as is ingestion of drugs (e.g., aspirin).
2. **Physical findings** aid in differentiation of bleeding syndromes. Mucocutaneous petechiae and purpura suggest platelet disorders; hematomas and hemarthrosis suggest coagulopathy.
3. **Laboratory testing** is vital in the evaluation of bleeding disorders. Single tests rarely provide conclusive results, so various batteries of tests have been developed. The coagulation cascade is shown in Figure 3–1, the interpretation of common tests of hemostasis and blood coagulation is shown in Table 3–6 and the diagnosis of common bleeding disorders based on commonly used tests is shown in Table 3–7.

B **Disorders of blood vessels and vascular tissues** The following bleeding disorders result from pathology in the vessel area itself, with secondary leakage of blood. Most of these disorders have as their hallmark a visible and usually palpable skin lesion. Testing performed on patients with these bleeding disorders reveals normal coagulation and, occasionally, increased bleeding times.

1. **Autoimmune (allergic) purpura (Henoch-Schönlein purpura)** occurs most commonly in children and young adults.
   a. **Etiology.** The syndrome is associated with streptococcal infections and drugs (e.g., penicillin).
   b. **Clinical signs. Perivascular inflammatory lesions** with serosanguinous leakage into the skin, submucosa, and serosa are the hallmark of the disease. The lesions are symmetric and palpable and are usually found on the distal extremities. Bowel lesions may cause gastrointestinal symptoms; joint lesions cause arthritis.
   c. **Therapy and prognosis.** No specific therapy is uniformly helpful. Prognosis is good, except in the 5%–10% of patients who develop glomerulonephritis.
2. **Purpura associated with infections** may be due to embolic occlusion of the microvasculature (e.g., endocarditis) or to endothelial injury by the infectious agent (e.g., *Rickettsia*). Biopsy and culture of the material may be helpful.

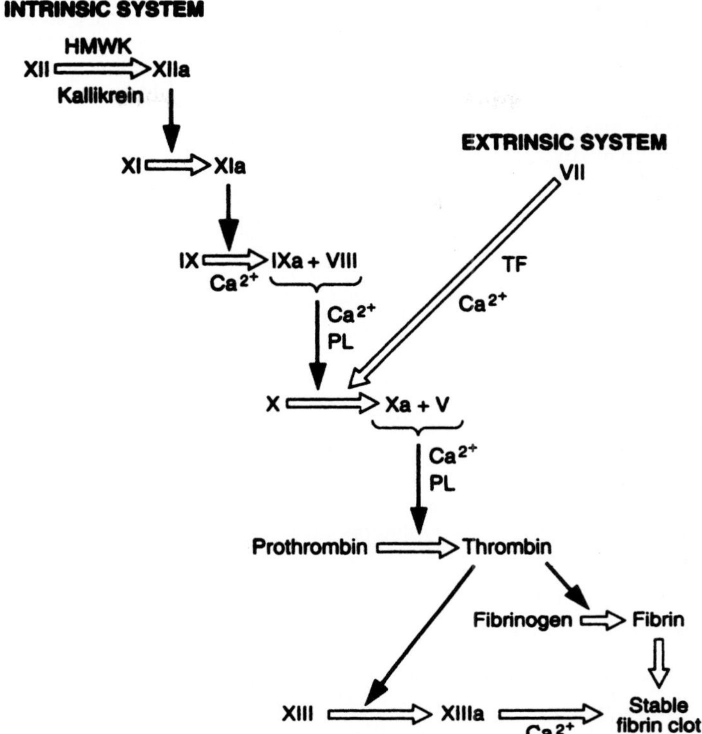

FIGURE 3–1 The coagulation cascade. Each coagulation factor, when activated, activates the next factor in the series. (Factors are numbered in order of their discovery, not in order of activation.) In the intrinsic system, factor XII is initially activated by an unknown mechanism and subsequently by kallikrein during the contact phase. Alternatively, factor VII and tissue factor can initiate the extrinsic system. Intrinsic and extrinsic pathways each end with activation of factor X, setting off a final; common pathway that ends with formation of the fibrin clot. Open *arrows* indicate conversion of a substrate or a reactant to a product. HMWK = high-molecular-weight kininogen; TF = tissue factor; PL = phospholipid.

TABLE 3–6 Interpretation of Common Tests of Hemostasis and Coagulation

Test	Normal Range (± SD)	Causes of Abnormalities
Platelet count	150–450,000/μL	Thrombocytopenia; thrombocytosis
Bleeding time (template method)	2.0–7.5 min	Thrombocytopenia; von Willebrand's disease; platelet dysfunction; vascular disorders
Partial thromboplastin time		Deficiencies or inhibitors of prekallikrein, HMWK; factors VIII, IX, XI, XII; lupus inhibitors; heparin
Standard	60–90 sec	
Activated	30–40 sec	
Plasma prothrombin time	11–14 sec	Deficiencies or inhibitors of factors V, VII, X; prothrombin; lupus inhibitors
Plasma thrombin time	12–20 sec	Hypofibrinogenemia; abnormal fibrinogens; heparin
Fibrinogen assay	160–450 mg/dL	Hypofibrinogenemia; abnormal fibrinogens
Fibrin degradation product assay	<10 μg/mL	DIC; fibrinogenolysis; liver disease

Adapted with permission from Wintrobe MM, et al: *Clinical Hematology,* 8th ed. Philadelphia, Lea and Febiger, 1981, p 1051.
DIC = disseminated intravascular coagulation; HMWK = high-molecular-weight kininogen; SD = standard deviation.

TABLE 3–7 Presumptive Diagnosis of Common Bleeding Disorders by Primary Screening Tests

Platelet Count	Bleeding Time	PTT	PT	Presumptive Diagnosis	Common Etiologies
Decreased	Prolonged	Normal	Normal	Thrombocytopenia	ITP; drugs
Normal	Prolonged	Prolonged	Normal	von Willebrand's disease	. . .
Normal	Prolonged	Normal	Normal	Thrombocytopathy	Drugs; uremia
Normal	Normal	Prolonged	Normal	Coagulopathy of intrinsic pathway	Hemophilia A or hemophilia B; factor VIII and lupus-type inhibitors
Normal	Normal	Prolonged	Prolonged	Coagulopathy of common or multiple pathways	Liver disease; vitamin K deficiency; DIC; heparin
Normal	Normal	Normal	Prolonged	Coagulopathy of extrinsic pathway	Factor VII deficiency
Normal	Normal	Normal	Normal	. . .	Hereditary telangiectasia; allergic purpura

Adapted with permission from Lee GR, et al: *Wintrobe's Clinical Hematology,* 9th ed. Philadelphia, Lea and Febiger, 1993, p 1315.
DIC = disseminated intravascular coagulation; ITP = idiopathic thrombocytopenic purpura; PTT = partial thromboplastin time; PT = prothrombin time.

3. **Structural malformations of vessels and vascular tissues** are associated with the following conditions:
   a. **Scurvy** is caused by vitamin C deficiency; collagen synthesis is impaired as a result of this deficiency. Vessel walls with poor collagen support are pliable and easily ruptured.
      (1) Physical findings associated with scurvy include perifollicular petechiae, gingival bleeding, and subperiosteal hemorrhages. Bleeding time usually is prolonged.
      (2) Therapy with 1 g/day of vitamin C rapidly corrects all bleeding.
   b. **Hereditary hemorrhagic telangiectasia** is an autosomal dominant disorder associated with abnormally thin vessel walls and impaired vascular contractility. Such vessels are markedly friable, liable to burst with trauma, and unable to contract appropriately for primary hemostasis.
      (1) **Physical findings** include small, nodular violaceous lesions on the lips, face, ears, tongue, and gastrointestinal mucosa; these lesions blanch on pressure. Bleeding is common, especially gastrointestinal bleeding and epistaxis, with resultant iron deficiency anemia.
      (2) **Diagnosis** involves the association of three factors: recurrent hemorrhage, multiple telangiectases, and familial occurrence.
      (3) Improvement in supportive measures such as local measures (nasal emollients), EPO, epsilon amino caproic acid, and safer parenteral iron forms have improved quality of life and prognosis in these patients.
   c. **Diminished collagen synthesis** due to **steroid therapy** results in a syndrome of vascular fragility and skin bleeding.
4. **Miscellaneous vascular conditions**
   a. **Paraproteinemias,** including cryoglobulinemias and amyloidosis, are associated with skin bleeding. Diagnosis requires demonstration of the paraprotein.
   b. **Senile purpura** occurs in elderly individuals as a result of degeneration and loss of dermal collagen, elastin, and subcutaneous fat. This disorder, which is thought to be caused by shearing injury to blood vessels from the hypermobility of the skin on the thinned underlying tissue, is characterized by benign purpura of the arms.

C Disorders of platelets Platelets play a role in the primary arrest of bleeding; abnormalities in these hemostatic components result in prolonged bleeding times and lead to hemorrhagic diathesis. Platelet abnormalities are classified according to disorders of number and function.

1. **Thrombocytopenia** (i.e., decreased numbers of platelets) is the **most common cause of abnormal bleeding.**
   a. **General considerations**
      (1) With a platelet count of less than 100,000/mm^3, bleeding time (and clinical bleeding, if the hemostatic system is stressed) begins to prolong. Most individuals experience petechiae or purpura with platelet counts between 50,000 and 20,000/mm^3. More serious spontaneous bleeding (e.g., gastrointestinal, CNS) may occur with platelet counts of less than 10,000/mm^3.
      (2) Thrombocytopenia is frequently an indication for a marrow examination, which reveals the presence of the platelet precursors, **megakaryocytes.** The absence of megakaryocytes indicates platelet production problems. The presence of megakaryocytes indicates either peripheral destruction of platelets or, in the presence of splenomegaly, splenic sequestration of platelets.
   b. **Mechanisms** of thrombocytopenia include impaired platelet production, abnormal platelet pooling, and increased peripheral destruction. Various examples, marrow findings, and therapies are summarized in Table 3–8.
      (1) **Impaired platelet production**
         (a) **Etiology**
            (i) Megakaryocytes may be selectively suppressed by certain agents (e.g., thiazide diuretics, ethanol).
            (ii) A special cause of thrombocytopenia due to impaired platelet production is ineffective thrombopoiesis associated with the megaloblastic hematopoiesis seen in vitamin B_{12} and folate deficiencies as well as in cases of myelodysplastic and preleukemic syndromes. Megakaryocytes are present in marrow but are abnormal (megaloblastic or dysplastic) in morphology and function. Their platelets are abnormal and destroyed in the marrow.
            (iii) Another rare cause is amegakaryocytic thrombocytopenia caused by congenital deficiency of megakaryocyte CFUs.
         (b) **Diagnosis** is confirmed by a bone marrow smear that reveals marrow megakaryocytic hypoplasia.
         (c) **Therapy** involves removal of the offending agent, if possible, or treatment of the underlying disease. Patients have essentially normal platelet half-lives and should be transfused with exogenous platelets if they are thrombocytopenic and bleeding. Unfortunately, such patients cannot be maintained indefinitely because of the eventual emergence of antiplatelet antibodies in multiply transfused patients, which renders further transfusions futile. Special blood bank techniques such as HLA matching of donors and single-donor transfusions can improve and lengthen the efficacy of platelet transfusions. Thrombocytopenia associated with vitamin B_{12} or folate deficiency is rapidly corrected by therapy with the deficient vitamin.
         (d) **Associated conditions**
            (i) Impaired platelet production is associated with aplastic anemia, myelophthisic processes with replacement of marrow by tumor or fibrosis, and certain rare congenital syndromes (e.g., rubella infection with absent radii).
            (ii) Amegakaryocytic thrombocytopenia has responded to therapies directed against the immune system, including antithymocyte globulin and cyclosporine. In these settings thrombocytopenia is associated with pancytopenia.
      (2) **Abnormal platelet pooling** results when platelets are sequestered from the circulation. **Splenic platelet sequestration** is the most common cause of abnormal platelet pooling.

TABLE 3–8 Mechanisms of Thrombocytopenia

Mechanisms	Marrow Findings	Clinical Conditions	Therapy
Impaired production of platelets	Megakaryocytes reduced or absent	Induced chemically or physically (e.g., chemotherapy, radiation)	Removal of offending agents; supportive
		Aplastic anemia, paroxysmal nocturnal hemoglobinuria, leukemia	Marrow transplantation
		Infection (e.g., viral hepatitis, cytomegalovirus, tuberculosis)	Treatment of infection
Ineffective production of platelets	Abnormal and/or dysplastic megakaryocytes	Megaloblastic disorder (vitamin B_{12} deficiency, folate deficiency)	B_{12} or folate supplementation
		Myelodysplasias and myeloproliferative disorders	Treatment of underlying disorder
Enhanced destruction of platelets (immune-mediated)	Increased megakaryocytes	Idiopathic thrombocytopenic purpura	See V C 1 b (3)
		Post-transfusion purpura	Plasmapheresis
		Drug-induced (e.g., rifampin, methicillin, sulfonamides, phenytoin, quinine, quinidine, heparin)	Removal of offending agent
		Lymphomas	Treatment of underlying disorder
		Immune complex disorder (e.g., systemic lupus erythematosus)	Steroids
Enhanced destruction of platelets (not immune-related)	Increased megakaryocytes	Thrombotic thrombocytopenic purpura	Plasmapheresis
		Hemolytic uremic syndrome	Plasmapheresis
		Disseminated intravascular coagulation	Treatment of underlying disorders
		Dilution and cardiopulmonary bypass	Supportive
		Splenomegaly	Usually not required; splenectomy may be necessary occasionally

(a) Pathophysiology. Normally, the spleen holds one-third of the circulating platelet pool. As splenomegaly occurs, higher numbers of platelets are sequestered and, thus, are unavailable for hemostasis. In very large spleens, as much as 90% of the platelet pool may be sequestered; however, platelets in the peripheral circulation do have normal survival times.

(b) Diagnosis of hypersplenism is suggested by a moderate thrombocytopenia (platelet counts of < 40,000/mm^3 are unusual), a bone marrow smear that reveals adequate marrow megakaryocytes, and evidence of significant splenic enlargement.

(c) Clinical features in such cases are dominated by the underlying illness causing the splenomegaly (e.g., cirrhosis with portal hypertension).

(d) Therapy usually is not required, although splenectomy may correct the problem. Transfused platelets are sequestered in the same ratio and are less effective than in hypoactive marrow states.

(3) **Increased peripheral destruction** of platelets is the **most common form of thrombocytopenia.** Conditions involving increased platelet destruction are characterized by shortened platelet survival and increased numbers of marrow megakaryocytes. **Idiopathic thrombocytopenic purpura (ITP)** is the prototypical immune-mediated thrombocytopenia; no apparent exogenous causes for platelet destruction exist.

(a) **Clinical features.** The **acute variant** of ITP occurs in children between the ages of 2 and 6 years and often occurs after a nonspecific viral illness. The **chronic variant** occurs in young adults, more commonly in young women. All ITP patients show varying degrees of thrombocytopenia, which in some acute cases is severe (i.e., associated with platelet counts of < $1000/mm^3$), and all show increased megakaryocytes. Other blood findings and cell lines are normal. Patients have mucocutaneous bleeding with petechiae, purpura, mucosal bullae, and excessive bleeding after trauma.

(b) **Diagnosis** requires exclusion of associated illnesses (e.g., SLE) and thrombocytopenia that is induced by drugs (e.g., quinidine). Platelet antibody techniques are available but remain nonspecific and are not as helpful either diagnostically or as disease monitors as had been hoped.

(i) In patients who are younger than 60 years of age with otherwise normal blood counts, bone marrow examination is no longer required. The clinical diagnosis of ITP can be made as long as splenectomy is not contemplated (in which case a confirmatory marrow examination is performed).

(ii) In patients older than 60 years, a marrow examination should be performed because of the increasing incidence of myelodysplasia in such patients.

(iii) New epidemiologic studies have shown a high incidence of HIV and hepatitis C as causes of thrombocytopenia, and many authorities suggest testing for them in ITP patients. If appropriate on clinical grounds, lupus testing also should be performed. These conditions can manifest as apparently isolated thrombocytopenia.

(c) **Clinical course.** The acute childhood variant often runs its course and resolves within 4–8 weeks; the adult form is more chronic and demonstrates relapses and remissions.

(d) **Therapy** for the acute childhood form usually involves protection from trauma and, in some cases, a short course of steroids. Treatment of adult ITP is more complex and protracted.

(i) **High doses of steroids** produce complete remission and remain the core therapy for chronic ITP.

(ii) Steroids induce remissions in approximately two thirds of cases and in 35% result in sustained remissions requiring no further treatment.

(iii) **Splenectomy** may be necessary in resistant cases and is associated with complete remission. The need for splenectomy has diminished in recent years.

(iv) **Refractory patients** may require **immunosuppressive therapy** (e.g., with azathioprine and cyclophosphamide). Although **platelet transfusions** should not be withheld in ITP patients who are bleeding, such exogenous transfusions are less efficacious than in other thrombocytopenic states because of the same short survival of the platelets.

(vi) An effective therapy that can temporarily elevate platelet counts in an acute crisis is **infusion with intravenous IgG.** The infused IgG apparently competes for and saturates reticuloendothelial binding sites, making fewer of them available for platelet binding and destruction. This maneuver has also gained popularity as a preoperative therapy in ITP patients who require surgery. **Hyperimmune anti-Rh(D) globulin** (e.g., such as that given to women after giving birth to Rh-positive infants) has been found to act in a like manner as an urgent therapy in ITP and can be used in similar settings (i.e., prior to surgery or when thrombocytopenia is extreme) with excellent results. These maneuvers have become the initial therapy in most cases of acute and severe ITP.

(e) **Prognosis.** The overall prognosis is good; only 2%–3% of ITP patients die after 5 years.

2. **Thrombocytopathia** involves platelets that are adequate in number but unable to function properly in hemostasis and in the primary arrest of bleeding.
   a. **Description.** Thrombocytopathia is characterized by:
      (1) Platelet-type mucocutaneous bleeding
      (2) Normal platelet counts but prolonged bleeding times
      (3) Demonstrate abnormalities in platelet function testing (e.g., aggregometry)
   b. **Etiology**
      (1) **Drug-related platelet dysfunction** is the most common cause of abnormal platelet function.
         (a) **Aspirin** permanently acetylates platelet membranes, impairing the platelet prostaglandin synthesis [e.g., impairing synthesis of thromboxane A_2 (TXA_2)] required for proper platelet function. Such impaired platelets may prolong bleeding times and cause bruising and increase hemorrhage with trauma. The aspirin-induced platelet lesion permanently alters circulating platelets and lasts until the platelets are replaced by new unaffected ones, usually in 3–7 days.
         (b) Clopidogrel (Plavix) is a new and powerful antiplatelet agent that selectively inhibits platelet receptor binding of adenosine diphosphate (ADP) and subsequent activation of the IIB/IIIA complex. Like aspirin, the effect is irreversible and lasts for the remainder of the exposed platelet's life span.
         (c) **Other anti-inflammatory drugs** (e.g., indomethacin) cause similar dysfunction but differ from aspirin in that their effects are not permanent and disappear when the agent is withdrawn.
      (2) **Uremia-associated dysfunction** is caused by uremic plasma disaggregation of high–molecular-weight polymers of factor VIII that are required for proper platelet function.
         (a) **Therapy.** In bleeding uremic patients, dialysis may evoke a response. Maneuvers to restore normal–molecular-weight forms of factor VIII may temporarily correct this dysfunction. These maneuvers include administering factor VIII exogenously as cryoprecipitate and eliciting endogenous increases in factor VIII by giving desmopressin (dDAVP).
      (3) **Congenital forms of platelet dysfunction** include Glanzmann's thrombasthenia (an intrinsic platelet disorder) and von Willebrand's disease (vWD; a congenital absence of the high–molecular-weight forms of factor VIII required for platelet aggregation). Many deficiencies in platelet prostaglandin pathway enzymes have been elucidated in recent years. These are rare autosomal recessive syndromes characterized by bleeding and prolonged bleeding times with normal platelet counts. Refined platelet studies are required for diagnosis. Most show some response to dDAVP. In serious bleeding situations, transfusion of platelets may be needed.

D **Disorders of the coagulation system** may be classified as hereditary or acquired. The hereditary forms usually result from deficiency of a single coagulation protein. Although greatly variable in degree, the clinical manifestations of these disorders are somewhat similar. The acquired forms, which are more complex than the hereditary forms, usually result from multiple and mixed deficiencies in the coagulation proteins.

1. The **hereditary coagulopathies** are best exemplified by the disorders of factor VIII.
   a. **Hemophilia A** is the most common hereditary coagulopathy, accounting for 68%–80% of such conditions.
      (1) **Pathogenesis.** Genetically, hemophilia A is transmitted as a classic X-linked recessive trait—the disorder is carried by females and manifested in males. Bleeding results from

the absence of VIII^{pro}, the low–molecular-weight, or **procoagulant, portion** of the factor VIII molecule. The large **antigenic portion** of the molecule, VIII^{ag}, is present in normal amounts. The genetic locus for hemophilia has been elucidated and studied. The milder forms (Table 3–9) are characterized by lesser changes (i.e., single amino acids) that result in synthesis of abnormal factor VIII^{pro}, antigenically recognizable but functionally defective. Such patients do not make antibodies to factor VIII^{pro} in response to concentrate therapy. Severe forms (<1%) are characterized by gene deletion, which results in absent antigenically recognizable factor VIII protein material. Exogenous factor VIII given as treatment is seen as foreign protein and is problematic. Anti-VIII^{pro} antibodies form in 20%–25% of cases.

(2) **Clinical features** vary with the degree of deficiency and are summarized in Table 3–9. The nature of hemorrhage is deep-tissue bleeding with deep hematomas, hemarthrosis, and significant bleeding after stress such as trauma and surgery. Repeated hemarthrosis results in severe disabling arthropathy, which is the clinical hallmark of severe hemophilia A.

(3) **Diagnosis.** The constellation of spontaneous or unexpected hemorrhage, especially hemarthrosis, in a male patient with an appropriate family history is suggestive. Laboratory tests reveal a prolonged **partial thromboplastin time (PTT),** which is indicative of deficiencies in the intrinsic thromboplastin system; other coagulation tests are normal. The diagnosis is confirmed by factor assay demonstrating low levels of VIII^{pro} and normal levels of VIII^{ag}. Detection of the abnormal gene itself is now possible and clinically available.

(4) **Therapy** is with VIII^{pro} transfusion in the form of either cryoprecipitate or factor VIII concentrates. Traditional multiple-donor VIII concentrates were associated with an unacceptably high incidence of transmitted hepatitis and human immunodeficiency virus (HIV). Newer pasteurized preparations and genetically engineered preparations, which obviate these problems, are widely available. These forms of therapy have markedly reduced the mortality and morbidity rates associated with hemophilia A. The formation of VIII^{pro} antibodies is a difficult complication in patients with severe hemophilia.

b. von Willebrand's disease is a heterogeneous disorder that also involves the factor VIII molecule.

(1) **Pathophysiology.** Genetically, its transmission is variable, but in its most common form, vWD is transmitted as an autosomal dominant trait with variable penetrance. This

TABLE 3–9 Clinical and Laboratory Findings in Hemophilia A and Hemophilia B

Severity	Level of Factor VIII or IX (U/dL)	Partial Thromboplastin Time	Clinical Picture
Severe	0–2	Very prolonged	Hemarthrosis and spontaneous bleeding severe and frequent; crippling common
Moderate	2–5	Prolonged	Hemarthrosis and spontaneous bleeding infrequent; disability uncommon; severe bleeding from injuries and surgery
Mild	5–25	Variable	Hemarthrosis and spontaneous bleeding very unusual; unsuspected and severe bleeding from injuries and surgery
Subclinical	25–49	Usually normal	Bleeding after major trauma or surgery possible; diagnosis often missed

Adapted with permission from Lee GR, et al: *Wintrobe's Clinical Hematology,* 9th ed. Philadelphia, Lea and Febiger, 1993, p 1428.

disorder involves hereditary deficiency or derangement of VIII^{ag} and VIII^{pro}. Because VIII^{ag} serves as a cofactor for platelet adhesion, patients manifest both coagulopathy and abnormal platelet function.

(2) **Clinical features** include immediate, mucocutaneous (i.e., platelet-type) bleeding due to VIII^{ag} deficiency and delayed, deep-tissue, post-trauma (i.e., coagulation-type) bleeding due to VIII^{pro} deficiency. As with hemophilia A, the clinical picture for vWD varies with the degree of deficiency.

(3) **Diagnosis** is suggested by abnormal bleeding of a mixed nature in an individual with an appropriate family history. Laboratory tests show prolonged bleeding time due to decreased platelet function and a frequently prolonged PTT due to VIII^{pro} deficiency. Measurements of factor VIII demonstrate either a combined and equivalent deficiency of VIII^{ag} and VIII^{pro} or a derangement in multimer mixtures of VIII^{ag}. Ristocetin-induced platelet aggregation is abnormal in vWD. Other tests of platelet aggregation are normal.

(4) **Therapy** requires the replacement and coordination of both the antigenic and procoagulant portions of factor VIII. Concentrates are rich in VIII^{pro} but low in VIII^{ag}; therefore, either cryoprecipitate or plasma, which contain both, may be used in vWD. A variety of concentrates rich in VIII^{ag} and von Willebrand's factor have been developed. They can be virally cleansed by pasteurization of detergent techniques and have volume advantages when a vWD patient needs more intense or prolonged therapy. In mild cases, increased secretion of VIII can be induced by giving DDAVP.

c. **Other hereditary coagulation disorders** are uncommon. Diagnosis requires factor analysis to demonstrate the specific deficiency.

(1) **Hemophilia B (factor IX deficiency)** is identical to hemophilia A in its genetic features and clinical manifestations. Therapy differs in that either plasma or a purified prothrombin complex (which contains concentrated factors II, VII, IX, and X) is used as a source for factor IX.

(2) **Factor XI deficiency** is an autosomal recessive coagulopathy with milder clinical manifestations than those of the hemophilias. PTT is prolonged due to low factor XI levels. Plasma serves as adequate replacement therapy.

(3) **Factor XII, prekallikrein,** and **high–molecular-weight kininogen deficiencies** are unique in that they cause significant prolongation of PTT yet no predisposition to hemorrhage. Diagnosis is suggested by abnormal PTT with no history of bleeding, even with trauma. Factor analysis is necessary to demonstrate the deficient factor.

(4) **Deficiencies of all other factors** have been described but are rare.

2. The **acquired coagulation disorders** are more complex than the hereditary forms. The acquired coagulopathies usually involve multiple and mixed factor deficiencies and often are complications of other diseases. Coagulation testing shows abnormalities in multiple pathways; often the bleeding severity correlates poorly with coagulation abnormalities seen in laboratory testing.

a. **Vitamin K–dependent factor deficiency**

(1) **Etiology**

(a) This coagulopathy occurs with **liver failure** when hepatocyte dysfunction is sufficient to impair the synthesis by the liver of factors II, VII, IX, and X. In such cases, evidence of liver disease is present (i.e., jaundice, transaminase elevation) in addition to the coagulopathy.

(b) **Malabsorption** of vitamin K can occur with biliary obstruction as well as with intestinal disease (e.g., sprue). Again, coagulopathy merely complicates the obvious clinical picture.

(c) Particularly in intensive care units, **nutritional deficiency** occurs in patients with poor oral intake of vitamin K and in those in whom antibiotics have removed the gastrointestinal flora that serve as an alternate source of vitamin K.

(d) **Drugs** can interfere with vitamin K metabolism, most specifically, the vitamin K antagonist **coumarin,** which is used to treat thrombotic diseases.

(2) **Pathophysiology.** The liver synthesizes factors II, VII, IX, and X. The final post-translational step in their synthesis renders these proteins functional and requires γ-carboxylation of a minimum of 10 terminal glutamic acid residues, with vitamin K as a cofactor. Interference in this mechanism causes functional deficiency of these clotting proteins, particularly impairing Ca^{++} binding of the proteins at the clot site.

(3) **Diagnosis.** Because many clotting factors are deficient, laboratory testing shows **prolonged PTT** and **prothrombin time (PT).** Specific measurements demonstrate the deficiency of factors II, VII, IX, and X.

(4) **Therapy** for vitamin K–related coagulopathy varies with its cause.

(a) In cases of malabsorption and nutritional deficiency, supplemental (often parenteral) vitamin K corrects the coagulopathy.

(b) In cases of excess coumarin, withdrawal of the offending drug with supplemental vitamin K is efficacious.

(c) In bleeding patients or patients with liver dysfunction who cannot respond to vitamin K, the deficient factors must be administered in the form of plasma.

(d) Recent clinical studies of the use of vitamin K to reverse coumarin excess have shown that, in patients with normal GI function, oral administration is more effective (speed and extent of recovery) than SQ administration. Furthermore, small doses in the 1–3-mg range can be used.

b. Disseminated intravascular coagulation (DIC)

(1) **Etiology.** DIC is a common acquired coagulopathy that occurs secondary to other disease processes such as the following:

(a) Activation of the intrinsic coagulation pathway by endothelial damage (e.g., in gram-negative sepsis, meningococcemia, and viremia)

(b) Activation of the extrinsic pathway by abnormal entry of tissue thromboplastins into the circulation (e.g., in obstetric complications, carcinomatosis, and massive trauma)

(2) **Pathophysiology.** DIC is initiated by stimuli in the systemic circulation that activate the coagulation mechanism and cause the abnormal formation of excessive systemic thrombin. The thrombin, in turn, causes extensive activation of coagulation in the microcirculation, which consumes many coagulation moieties and activates the fibrinolytic system secondarily. Current literature stresses the role of tissue factor in more cases of DIC.

(3) **Clinical features** vary depending on the balance between intravascular coagulation and fibrinolysis and factor depletion.

(a) In florid acute cases (e.g., amniotic fluid embolism), the coagulopathy is dominant, and the major symptoms are bleeding and shock.

(b) In more chronic cases (e.g., carcinomatosis), thrombosis and clotting may predominate.

(c) Many cases of DIC involve abnormal coagulation parameters but no bleeding or clotting, whereas other cases have a mixture of both bleeding and clotting complications.

(4) **Diagnosis.** Laboratory tests reveal a complicated picture. Many coagulation factors are consumed in the diffuse clotting process; these factor deficiencies prolong both PT and PTT. Platelet consumption results in thrombocytopenia. Fibrinogen deficiency arises from thrombin-mediated clotting as well as plasmin-mediated fibrinolysis. The secondary fibrinolysis is demonstrated by the presence of high titers of fibrin degradation products (FDP), increasingly being measured by d-dimer assays.

(5) **Therapy** is controversial; however, it is unanimously agreed that addressing the underlying "trigger" disease is paramount. The role of both factor replacements and anticoagulants to impair the ongoing thrombin production is less clear. The author prefers to administer platelets and plasma to bleeding patients with markedly lowered levels and to

reserve heparin for patients with thrombotic complications (e.g., skin infarction, acral gangrene, recognizable vessel thromboses). Many patients require no specific coagulation therapy.

c. **Liver disease** results in a complex coagulopathy involving many aspects of clotting.

(1) Liver disease results in impaired synthesis of vitamin K–dependent clotting proteins, fibrinogen, antithrombin III, plasminogen, and other protein moieties.

(a) Studies have shown that there is a hierarchy of coagulation function deficits. Prognostic data also relate to specific defects in coagulation function encountered in liver disease.

(i) The earliest, most sensitive, most reversible defect is the lowering of vitamin K–dependent factors such as factor VII. As hepatocellular function deteriorates further, fibrinogen levels become quantitatively lower and at times even qualitatively abnormal (dysfibrinogenemia).

(ii) The most severe situation, which correlates well with poor regenerative capacity and overall mortality, is the lowering of factor V to levels less than 50%. Many liver transplant centers strongly emphasize factor V levels in transplant decisions.

(b) These studies can be used to rate severity of disease, prognosis, and urgency for liver transplantation.

(2) Impaired clearance of FDPs and activated coagulation factors may result in a mild DIC-type condition.

(3) Portal hypertension may result in splenomegaly and excessive platelet pooling with thrombocytopenia.

(4) The accumulation of FDPs causes impaired platelet function (thrombocytopathia).

(5) **Therapy.** Sustaining coagulation function and controlling hemorrhage in advanced liver disease patients is one of the most difficult situations in coagulation medicine. The number of deficient proteins and the short half-lives of some (e.g., factor VII, 4–6 hours) render most concentrates non-effective. Fresh frozen plasma (FFP) has been used traditionally, but, because of volume complications and short T½, the results are poor. Recently, concentrates of genetically engineered factor VII^{A} have been introduced and may prove more efficacious and useful.

d. **Pathologic inhibitors of coagulation**

(1) The **lupus-type inhibitor** is the most common coagulation inhibitor. Although first described in patients with SLE, lupus inhibitors most often occur with other conditions or idiopathically.

(a) The inhibitor is an antiphospholipid that has inhibitory activity at the prothrombin–platelet membrane complex (see Figure 3–1). Although these inhibitors have activity in vitro (i.e., often prolonging the PTT and sometimes the PT as well), they rarely, if ever, cause in vivo coagulopathy despite the abnormal laboratory tests.

(b) Clinical testing reveals prolonged PT and more commonly PTT but little evidence of bleeding. The diagnosis is suggested by demonstrating that patient plasma causes similar abnormalities when mixed with normal plasma, unlike deficiency states in which such mixtures correct the abnormality. The diagnosis can be confirmed by a positive thromboplastin tissue inhibition (TTI) test and antiphospholipid assays.

(c) Therapy should be directed toward the underlying disease. These patients do not bleed and need not receive coagulation therapy. Thrombosis is a more common complication. In fact, lupus inhibitors may be the most common acquired causes of so-called hypercoagulable states, or the tendency to manifest abnormal thrombosis.

(i) In patients suspected of hypercoagulability (e.g., unusual or recurrent thrombosis), measurement of anticardiolipin antibodies and testing for the presence of a lupus inhibitor is indicated whether or not the PTT is prolonged.

(ii) Such patients often require anticoagulation chronically, although the precise duration and intensity of anticoagulation in the lupus inhibitor hypercoagulability state remain somewhat controversial.

(2) **Specific inhibitors** of coagulation are antibodies with specificity for single coagulation proteins. The most common inhibitor is factor VIII antibody, which arises in 20% of patients with hemophilia who have received factor therapy. The idiopathic variety occurs in patients older than 65 years and presents as an explosive coagulopathy in a previously normal person.

(a) Clinically, such antibodies cause profound bleeding dyscrasias of similar severity to congenital deficiency.

(b) Diagnosis is made by demonstrating a specific factor deficiency that is not corrected by administration of normal plasma (abnormal mixing study).

(c) Therapy is difficult because the antibody also inactivates exogenously administered factors. Steroids and immunosuppressive agents have been used with limited success. The new VII^{A} preparations have been used with success.

e. **Other acquired coagulation disorders.** Coagulopathy has been associated with amyloidosis (factor X deficiency), nephrotic syndrome (due to renal wasting of coagulation proteins, especially factor IX), extracorporeal circulation (thought to activate the coagulation system partially and cause low-grade DIC), and massive transfusions (the patient hemorrhages normal blood, but it is replaced with blood bank–derived blood that is poor in coagulation factors and platelets).

VI ABNORMALITIES RELATED TO HYPERCOAGULABILITY AND INCREASED TENDENCY TO THROMBOSIS

A Anatomic abnormalities of vessels and blood flow Disorders that predispose the patient to thrombosis related to anatomic abnormalities of vessels and blood flow, not to intrinsic abnormalities in the blood itself, include the following:

1. **Stasis** can occur in conditions such as postoperative states, orthopedic injury, and neurologic diseases. Pathogenetic factors include venodilation and localized areas of reduced clearance of activated procoagulant factors.
2. **Turbulence** (e.g., associated with aneurysms) can damage vascular endothelium and expose blood to the interior of the vessel wall, facilitating endothelial–platelet–coagulation protein interaction.
3. **Trauma** to blood vessels can damage and disrupt vessel walls. Tumors can directly invade blood vessels or indirectly render the endothelium procoagulant. The vasculitic syndromes are another example.

B Intrinsic blood disorders Disorders predispose to thrombosis related to intrinsic blood disorders that are associated with abnormalities of platelets.

1. Epidemiologic evidence suggests that shortened platelet half-life, platelet activation, and enhanced incidence of thrombosis exist in certain common thrombotic medical conditions including **diabetes, atherosclerosis,** and **hypercholesterolemia.** Affected patients clearly have enhanced thrombotic tendency. It remains unclear, however, whether this tendency results from increased platelet activation or whether the platelet activation is a secondary event resulting from disease-related vascular abnormality.
2. Specific disorders in which primary abnormalities of platelets result in thrombotic tendency include the following:
   a. **Myeloproliferative diseases** such as polycythemia vera and essential (hemorrhagic) thrombocythemia, especially when the platelet count exceeds $10^6/mm^3$
   b. **Paroxysmal nocturnal hemoglobinuria (PNH),** which is associated with enhanced platelet reactivity and unusual thromboses involving abdominal hepatic veins

c. **Heparin-induced thrombocytopenia (HIT) syndrome,** which is associated with thrombosis of venous and arterial sites in patients using heparin. This syndrome has become more commonly recognized.

(1) Incidence is 1%–5% of patients on heparin therapy. Most data suggest that this is more common in settings such as CABG and other intense vascular manipulation situations.

(2) Pathogenesis involves heparin-dependent antiplatelet IgG antibody. The platelet undergoes an "activating event" (as with vascular surgery), which results in expression of PF4 on its membrane. The heparin binds to the PF4, creating a neoantigen to which an IgG heparin-dependent antibody is made. The antibody activates platelets and causes release of platelet microparticles into the circulation, resulting in dual hypercoagulability, platelet hyperreactivity, and plasma hypercoagulability.

(3) Diagnostic testing is suboptimal. Thus, HIT remains a clinical diagnosis that must be managed when there is a strong clinical suspicion. More sensitive and specific enzyme-linked immunoadsorbent assay (ELISA) techniques are available but have a high false-positive rate. Older serotonin release assays are more specific but have 30% false negatives. Thrombocytopenia usually precedes thrombosis, so platelet counts should be monitored in heparin patients and heparin discontinued if the platelet count significantly declines. Once thrombosis occurs, the mortality rate can range from 10%–50%.

(4) The newer low–molecular-weight heparins (LMWHs) are less likely to induce HIT in heparin-naive patients. They do cross-react in patients with established HIT and thus must not be considered an effective substitute for standard heparin. The US Food and Drug Administration (FDA) has approved the use of recombinant hirudins, which are derived from extracts of leech salivary glands, for HIT. Because these substances are excreted solely by the kidney, extreme caution is required in the setting of elevated creatinine and renal failure. Furthermore, unlike the heparins, protamine is not an effective antidote in these patients. Argatroban, a computer-designed small peptide that inhibits the thrombin catalytic site, has also been approved for HIT. Because it is excreted solely by hepatic metabolism, caution is required in the setting of liver dysfunction and elevated bilirubin. As with hirudin, there is no antidote. These agents have markedly improved the management and prognosis of HIT.

C **Specific hereditary disorders of enhanced thrombosis associated with abnormalities of plasma proteins** include:

1. **Abnormal fibrinogens** (dysfibrinogens) that are too sensitive to thrombin or that clot too tightly and do not allow for physiologic lysis by plasmin and **abnormal plasminogens** that are unable to dissolve clots physiologically are rare.

2. **Deficiencies of coagulation inhibitors**

a. **Antithrombin III deficiency** can be quantitative or qualitative. The defect has variable phenotypic penetrance but often causes recurrent venous thrombosis in young patients.

b. **Protein C deficiency.** Protein C is a vitamin K–dependent factor synthesized by the liver, which inhibits factors VIIIa and Va. The homozygotic condition causes purpura fulminans in neonates. The heterozygotic condition results in enhanced venous thrombosis and a possible predisposition to skin necrosis when placed on warfarin without concomitant heparin.

c. **Activated protein C resistance [Factor V (Leiden)]** is a genetic defect in factor V, which renders it refractory to the inhibitory activity of protein C. This condition is now known to be the most common congenital hypercoagulable state. Some studies report a 20% incidence in hypercoagulable state workups. A substrate abnormality, rather than a lack of agonist, causes the "deficiency" and disease. Data now demonstrate that this lesion alone frequently is not sufficient to cause thrombosis, and approximately 50% of known heterozygotes never experience thrombosis. The heterozygous condition acts as a comorbid risk factor with other events such as childbirth, long bone fracture, and surgery to cause thrombosis. This "multiple hit" pathophysiology appears to be common in most hypercoagulable situations.

d. **Protein S deficiency.** Protein S is a cofactor that facilitates factors VIIIa and Va inhibition by protein C. Its deficiency results in a thrombotic diathesis syndrome similar to protein C deficiency.

e. **Abnormal prothrombin variant** (G20210A) levels and elevated homocysteine also increase thrombosis.

D Specific acquired disorders of enhanced thrombosis associated with abnormalities of plasma proteins

1. **Pregnancy and oral contraceptive agents** are associated with statistically increased incidence of stroke, acute myocardial infarction (MI), and venous thrombosis. Pregnancy and oral contraceptives cause elevation in most procoagulant proteins and diminution of most fibrinolytic and inhibitor proteins, thus altering the hemostatic balance in favor of clotting. In a small but significant subpopulation, an additional lesion (e.g., factor V Leiden, lupus inhibitor) will be found.
   a. **Therapy.** Heparin therapy is used in pregnancy. Warfarin must be avoided, because it crosses the placenta and is teratogenic. Lower-molecular-weight heparins are quite effective and are more convenient to use. The anticoagulation period must extend through to the peripartum period, because the month after delivery may be the period of highest risk.

2. **Nephrotic syndrome** is associated with urine wasting of antithrombin III and, more importantly, hypoalbuminemia, which may result in enhanced platelet aggregation.

3. **Lupus inhibitor syndrome.** The presence of the so-called lupus inhibitor, antiphospholipid antibody syndrome is associated with increased thrombosis, especially in patients with SLE. This association probably also exists in non-SLE patients. Most cases, however, are not associated with SLE or other underlying conditions. It remains unclear whether the presence of the inhibitor is causative or merely a marker. Lupus inhibitor is becoming one of the more common diagnosable conditions related to hypercoagulability, with an incidence of thrombotic complications ranging from 9% to 28% in affected patients.
   a. **Pathophysiology.** The lupus inhibitor, or antiphospholipid antibodies, or both, interact with the coagulation pathway at the X–V–Ca complex.
   b. **Clinical manifestations.** Despite prolonged laboratory clotting times, thrombosis (both arterial and venous), placental dysfunction, and recurrent miscarriage are major symptoms and signs of this disorder. Abnormal bleeding does not occur.
   c. **Diagnosis.** Laboratory findings include prolongation of the PT and more commonly the PTT that does not reverse when patient plasma is mixed with normal plasma. Diagnosis is confirmed by further demonstrating the inhibitor reaction within the clotting system using the thromboplastin tissue inhibition (TTI) test and dilute Russell's venom viper assays.
   d. **Therapy. Aggressive anticoagulation** initially with heparin and followed by warfarin is indicated in cases of lupus inhibitor syndrome accompanied by clinical thrombosis. Warfarin anticoagulation to an international normalized ratio (INR) of 2.0–3.0 has recently been shown to be adequate.

4. **Thrombotic thrombocytopenic purpura (TTP)** is associated with apparent premature release of macroaggregated VIII^{ag} into plasma by damaged endothelial cells. In many patients, defective or deficient cysteine protease, such that macro-aggregated factor VIII^{ag} cannot be properly metabolized, has been found. These large-molecular-weight forms cause hypernormal platelet adhesion.
   a. This abnormal protein causes excessive platelet–endothelial binding, with microthrombi seen in most vascular beds. Plasmapheresis, which removes much of this abnormal protein, is an effective therapy.
   b. The initial lesions of TTP involve abnormal platelet aggregation and deposition, with resultant microangiopathy. Renal, CNS, and febrile responses follow. A smear must be examined in suspect cases, and it may be abnormal for quite some time before the morbid events develop.

c. Plasmapheresis therapy apparently adds cysteine protease and also removes factor VIII^{ag} macroaggregates. Pheresis has resulted in a reversal in mortality from 80+% before pheresis to <20% now.

d. **TTP syndrome** occurs idiopathically but is also seen as a complication of advanced AIDS, drugs (e.g., antirejection drugs, cyclosporin, or infections, e.g., toxigenic *Escherichia coli 0157*).

5. **Malignancy associated with chronic DIC (Trousseau's syndrome)** causes enhanced thrombosis of many varieties. The mechanism for enhanced thrombosis is chronic DIC initiated by tumor cells releasing either thromboplastic substances, activating factor XII, or both.
   a. Migratory thrombophlebitis of superficial veins is uniformly associated with chronic DIC in classic Trousseau's syndrome. Common neoplasms are adenocarcinomas of lung, pancreas, stomach, and prostate. This condition requires heparin therapy for control.
   b. Marantic endocarditis is another DIC variant; it results in fibrin vegetation in the heart and recurrent embolization.
   c. Routine deep vein thrombosis and pulmonary embolism are also statistically associated with malignancy. In one large study, 7% of patients with idiopathic disease developed neoplasia at 2 years compared with 2.5% in age-matched controls.

E Diagnostic and therapeutic approach to hypercoagulability

1. **Diagnostic approach**
   a. Clinical settings in which investigation for a hypercoagulable state is indicated include:
      (1) Family history of documented thromboembolic events
      (2) Age younger than 40 years at onset of thromboembolic events
      (3) Recurrent thromboembolic events
      (4) Unusual sites of thrombosis (e.g., mesenteric or cerebral veins)
      (5) Resistance to standard therapy for thrombosis
   b. Table 3–10 summarizes several causes of hypercoagulability.
2. **Treatment depends on the underlying cause.**
   a. In myeloproliferative disorders, platelet counts should be lowered to less than $10^6/mm^3$. Hydroxyurea and anagrelide are effective. Occasionally, plateletpheresis is needed.

TABLE 3–10 Hypercoagulable Syndromes

Inherited Forms	
Relatively Common	Rare
Factor V (Leiden) and protein C resistance	Abnormal fibrinogens
Antithrombin III deficiency	Plasminogen deficiency
• Quantitative	• Qualitative
• Qualitative	• Quantitative
Protein C deficiency	Decreased release of plasminogen activator
Protein S deficiency	Increased levels of histidine-rich glycoprotein
Prothrombin variant (G20210A)	
Hyperhomocysteinemia	
Acquired Forms	
Pregnancy (especially postpartum period)	
Oral contraceptive and estrogen use	
Lupus anticoagulants and anticardiolipin antibodies	
Malignancy (chronic DIC)	
Myeloproliferative diseases (*P. vera,* ET) and PNH	
Nephrotic syndrome	
Heparin-induced thrombocytopenia syndrome	

TABLE 3–11 Management of Hypercoagulable States According to Venous Thromboembolism (VTE) Risk Stratification

Moderate Risk
- Carriers of inherited thrombophilias who have never experienced a thrombotic event
- Patients with an acquired thrombophilia who have not experienced a thrombotic event (e.g., antiphospholipid antibodies, malignancy)
- Patients with one thrombotic event associated with a provocative reversible comorbid stimulus (e.g., leg casting, hormonal therapy)

Aggressive VTE prophylaxis when exposed to high risk situations (e.g., pregnancy, prolonged immobility)

High Risk
- Two or more documented VTE events
- One VTE event of life-threatening nature (e.g., massive PE)
- One documented VTE event plus
  - ➢ presence of multiple inherited defect
  - ➢ presence specifically of AT III deficiency, protein C/S deficiency
  - ➢ presence of antiphospholipid antibody syndrome or active malignancy
  - ➢ idiopathic VTE event (?)

Indefinite anticoagulation using an accepted regimen

b. Vessel abnormalities can be surgically repaired if found at angiography.

c. Most congenital protein deficiency states, including protein C, are managed with lifelong warfarin therapy once a thrombotic event has occurred. No treatment is given to asymptomatic carriers, because at least 50% of these individuals never develop a thrombosis. Such individuals should be given aggressive prophylaxis, however, when in high-risk situations such as fracture or surgery.

d. Lupus-inhibitor patients who have manifested thrombosis are managed with warfarin as long as the inhibitor is present. The amount of warfarin anticoagulation continues to be controversial.

e. Hypercoagulability associated with cancer usually requires long-term subcutaneous heparin therapy, because warfarin does not control the thrombotic diathesis in these cases. When effective therapy for the tumor is available, as it is for prostate cancer, it temporarily resolves the coagulopathy.

f. TTP requires plasmapheresis to remove the abnormal factor VIII protein.

g. Table 3–11 summarizes therapeutic principles for the common hypercoagulable states.

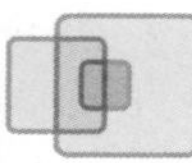

Study Questions

1. An 83-year-old received a hip replacement in her left leg 2 months previously. At that time, a mild anemia of 10.0 g/dL was noted, and she had been started on iron therapy by her primary care physician. She has mild hypertension. There was remote gastric surgery for unknown reasons 40 years ago. She denies symptoms of weakness or fatigue as well as shortness of breath with exertion. However, her ambulation has been somewhat limited by her hip surgery. Her appetite is "good," but her family reports her oral intake has been poor for some time. She denies all other symptoms.

   Physical examination reveals a thin-appearing female in no distress. There is pallor of her conjunctival and oral mucous membranes. The tongue is papillated except for the lateral edges, which are smooth. Heart examination reveals regular rhythm 96 beats/min with a Grade II systolic murmur along the left sternal border. Abdomen is soft without masses or hepatosplenomegaly. A well-healed midline laparotomy incision is present. Neurologic examination results were normal. Stool was hemoccult negative.

   Complete blood count revealed WBC of 5.8K/mm^3; platelets 190K/mm^3. However, hemoglobin is 8.2 g/dL (hematocrit 25%) with an MCV of 111 mm^3. Reticulocytes were 25,000/mm^3 (1.4%). An outpatient iron panel obtained after her hip surgery admission showed serum iron 80, transferrin 360, and ferritin of 50 μg/dL.

   Which of the following is the most appropriate management for this patient?

   A Increase the iron dosage and add vitamin C to her regimen.
   B Obtain vitamin B_{12} and folic acid levels and initiate therapy with both, pending results.
   C Initiate a course of parenteral iron therapy.
   D Obtain a bone marrow aspirate and initiate erythropoietin therapy for myelodysplasias.

2. A 61-year-old woman is admitted for urgent cardiac catheterization. The patient had experienced ischemic cardiac pain at an outside hospital and was treated in standard fashion including IV heparin, but she continued to decompensate. She was transferred for cardiac catheterization, which demonstrated triple-vessel coronary artery disease. She received full-dose intravenous heparin as well as nitrates for 3 days then was taken to the OR for CABG. The patient had nonremarkable preoperative blood counts. On the third postoperative day, she was found to have right lower extremity venous thrombosis and was restarted on IV heparin with rapid attainment of therapeutic PTT. The next day, the right foot became cool, cyanotic, and painful. Doppler study demonstrated extensive DVT in right proximal venous system and arterial occlusion in the right iliac artery. Blood studies showed hemoglobin 12.0 g/dL, WBC 21K, and platelets 33K. Blood smear was nonremarkable save for decreased platelets.

   Which of the following is the most likely diagnosis for these events?

   A Inadequate heparin dosage with recurrent thrombosis
   B Thrombotic thrombocytopenic purpura (TTP)
   C Heparin-induced thrombocytopenia syndrome (HIT)
   D Cardiac embolism
   E Homocysteinemia

3. A 20-year-old African American man is admitted for management of sickle cell anemia. He started to experience pain in his joints and lower back, consistent with his usual sickle cell pain pattern, about 48 hours before admission. He has Percocet at home for such episodes, but has not received much relief from them. He does well with his sickle cell anemia, requiring hospital admission about

2–3 times per year for pain management. He holds a full-time job in retail and is engaged to be married. His CBC in the receiving ward showed hemoglobin 7.9 g/dL and WBC 24,000/mm^3, which compare to known baseline levels of 7.8 and 14,000, respectively. Chest film was scheduled for first thing in the morning.

You examine him on morning rounds and find him to be in mild respiratory distress. He has developed moderate pleuritic pain. Vital signs are temperature 38.6°C; blood pressure 110/70 mm Hg; pulse 110 beats/min and respirations 24 breaths/min. He has mild scleral icterus. Chest examination shows a few rales in both bases without signs of consolidation.

Morning laboratory findings demonstrate a hemoglobin of 7.2 g/dL with a reticulocyte count of 230,000/mm^3 and a WBC of 33,000/mm^3 with a left shift. Bilirubin is 4.0 mg/dL, but other liver functions are normal. The chest film shows small, bilateral infiltrates in the bases. An O_2 saturation on room air is 90%.

What is the most appropriate definitive management for this patient?

A Arrange for an exchange transfusion.
B Perform an ultrasound and CT scan of the abdomen to exclude ascending cholangitis.
C Initiate heparin for acute pulmonary embolism.
D Initiate antibiotics with specific pneumococcus and salmonella coverage.
E Initiate hydroxyurea 1000 mg/day

4. A 19-year-old man experiences moderate trauma while playing in an intramural football game. That evening he experiences worsening pain and swelling in the left thigh. On evaluation, he manifests marked swelling in the left thigh, hemoglobin of 9 g/dL, and PTT 56 seconds. MRI shows a large hematoma. The most likely diagnosis is which of the following?

A Uremia
B Hemophilia A
C Therapy with aspirin
D Factor XII deficiency
E Idiopathic thrombocytopenic purpura (ITP)

5. A 29-year-old woman presents with new purpura and petechiae on both lower legs. She has also experienced menorrhagia in her last two menstrual cycles. On examination in addition to the purpura and petechiae above, several petechiae are noted on her tongue and hard palate. Blood count reveals hemoglobin 12 g/dL WBC 8000/cc, and platelets 9000/cc. Which of the following is an expected part of her diagnostic evaluation or management?

A Bone marrow megakaryocytes are generally decreased.
B Platelet-associated immunoglobulin G (IgG) is diagnostic.
C Splenomegaly and other cytopenias are usually present.
D The platelet life span is prolonged.
E IVIg is an effective therapy.

6. You admit a 27-year-old man to your service with acute myelogenous leukemia (AML), with the intention of initiating induction phase therapy. Which of the following maneuvers is least effective in this setting?

A Empiric, aggressive use of broad-spectrum antibiotics
B Maintenance of platelet counts in excess of 10,000–15,000/mm^3
C Stimulation of marrow recovery by growth factors
D Vaccination with pneumococcal vaccine and use of immunoglobulins
E Isolation techniques of varying intensity

7. A 28-year-old Caucasian woman is in the 30th week of gestation and notes persistent swelling and discomfort in the right calf. She is previously healthy without prior major medical problems. She has used carrier contraception before her pregnancy. There is no family history of venous thromboembolism (VTE). A Doppler study confirms DVT of the right lower extremity. Which of the following is most likely in this patient?

A Antithrombin III deficiency
B Protein C deficiency
C Factor V (Leiden) deficiency
D Hemophilia A
E Trousseau's syndrome

8. In which of the following clinical situations associated with bleeding does laboratory testing reveal a normal bleeding time?

A A 58-year-old man with renal failure who requires hemodialysis
B A 50-year-old woman with rheumatoid arthritis on chronic aspirin therapy
C A 30-year-old man with endocarditis who requires high doses of penicillin
D A 5-year-old boy with hemophilia and active hemarthrosis
E An 18-year-old woman with von Willebrand's disease (vWD) and menorrhagia

9. A 62-year-old man has had an elevated hematocrit for at least 3 years. His past medical history and review of systems are negative, except for mild, well-controlled hypertension. His latest complete blood count reveals: hemoglobin, 18 mg/dL; hematocrit, 56%; and WBC count, 17,500 mm^3, with platelets, 800,000 mm^3. On further investigation, which of the following findings is the most typical and expected?

A Ringed sideroblasts on bone marrow examination
B Arterial blood oxygen saturation less than 88%
C Presence of a Philadelphia chromosome on cytogenetic testing
D Very low to absent erythropoietin titer
E Many Pelger-Huët cells on peripheral blood smear

The response options for Items 10–13 are the same. You will be required to select one answer for each item in the set.

QUESTIONS 10–13

A Protein C deficiency
B Paroxysmal nocturnal hemoglobinuria (PNH)
C Lupus inhibitor syndrome
D Trousseau's syndrome

Match each of the following clinical vignettes with the most likely diagnosis.

10. A 30-year-old woman with a history of rash and arthritis has deep vein thrombosis; in addition, she has had a problem with recurrent abortions.

11. A 45-year-old man, who has been followed by his physician for 4 years for chronic iron deficiency anemia with unknown source of blood loss, has portal vein thrombosis.

12. A 60-year-old man had deep vein thrombosis of his left leg last month and is being appropriately managed with warfarin. He has symptoms of new clot formation in the right leg as well as a clot in his left forearm.

13. A 67-year-old woman with mitral stenosis is started on warfarin by her cardiologist. On the third day, painful red areas appear on her thigh and breast.

The response options for Items 14–17 are the same. You will be required to select one answer for each item in the set.

QUESTIONS 14–17

- A Aggressive, marrow ablative chemotherapy
- B Interferon (IFN)
- C Bone marrow transplantation (BMT)
- D Supportive therapy such as transfusions of cellular components and erythropoietin

Match each of the following clinical situations with the initial therapy that is most appropriate.

14. A 37-year-old man has Philadelphia chromosome–positive chronic myelogenous leukemia (CML).

15. A 9-year-old girl has pancytopenia and marrow findings consistent with standard risk acute lymphocytic leukemia (AML).

16. A 23-year-old man has severe aplastic anemia.

17. A 73-year-old man has pancytopenia, Pelger-Huët–type cells on peripheral smear, ringed sideroblasts, and increased immature forms in his marrow specimen.

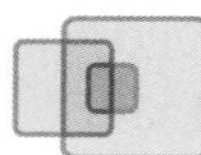

Answers and Explanations

1. The answer is B [I B 3 d]. The patient's findings suggest the presence of at least one of the common nutritional anemias—iron deficiency, folate deficiency, or B_{12} deficiency. Her diet seems poor. In addition, there is a history of and evidence for some type of a gastric surgery—either total or partial resection in the past. The most common anemia after gastric resection is iron deficiency that results from removal of acid-secreting cells, which are needed to reduce iron to its ferrous form, the absorbable form of iron. In addition, loss of absorptive surface and the presence of stomal erosions and bleeding also contribute to this pathophysiology. However, this patient's serum ferritin does fall within the normal range, which strongly suggests that the lack of iron is not what is interfering with blood formation in this patient at this time. Furthermore, the patient is displaying marcrocytic indices with an MCV of 111 mm^3, which again almost assuredly means that iron-deficient erythropoiesis characterized by deficient hemoglobin synthesis and microcytosis are not the driving force of the anemia in this situation. Thus, answer A, increasing iron dosage and adding ascorbic acid to facilitate absorption, although based on sound physiologic principles in this instance, might not be expected to reverse this anemia. Answer C is another iron maneuver that can sometimes be required in true malabsorptive situations. The newer parenteral forms are less allergenic than traditional preparations and have made this therapy safer. However, this still requires a time-consuming infusion, and all avenues of oral iron therapy should be employed before resorting to this. In this case, data do not point to iron deficiency as the primary lesion here.

Myelodysplasia (MDS) has become the most common cause for anemia in the geriatric population and is an important consideration in this setting. Typically, patients with MDS manifest a slight macrocytosis but only rarely to the degree seen here. MDS can be classified by studying bone marrow findings, and in approximately 25% of cases the anemia responds to pharmacologic doses of EPO. However, before the diagnosis of MDS can be made, reversible causes of marcrocytic anemia such as B_{12} and folic deficiency *must* be excluded, so answer D is not appropriate for this patient.

The appropriate management for this patient is answer B, obtaining B_{12} and folic acid levels and initiating therapy pending results. Her significant macrocytosis and subtle physical findings of tongue atrophy suggest B_{12} deficiency, including true type A autoimmune gastritis involving the fundus and body of the stomach, which is the classical Addisonian pernicious anemia. This patient had some form of gastric surgery and a history of PUD. Thus, she may have B_{12} deficiency associated with total gastric resection, which, although less common than iron deficiency, affects patients having had that operation about a decade later, or type B *H. pylori*–associated atrophic gastritis (which affects fundus, body, and antrum) related to her PUD. A variety of excellent biochemical tests can determine whether there is B_{12} deficiency (serum B_{12} level by radioimmune assay, methylmalonic acid levels) and whether there is true autoimmune pernicious anemia and its causes (the presence of circulating intrinsic factor autoantibodies). Because there is a possibility of folate deficiency, a folic acid level should be obtained. Because ongoing B_{12} deficiency–related neurologic morbidity can progress and become irreversible, therapy can and should be initiated with parenteral B_{12} while waiting for the biochemical confirmation. Thus, answer B is the most appropriate course of management here.

2. The answer is C [VI B 2 c]. This explosive situation is typical of the heparin-induced thrombocytopenia (HIT) with thrombosis syndrome. Heparin is a widely used anticoagulant across many indications. In approximately 3% of cases, patients develop a clinically and biologically active antibody to a heparin–PF4 neo-antigen on the platelet, which in the further presence of heparin causes platelet activation, aggregation, thrombocytopenia, and release of tissue factor. If the heparin is still continued, paradoxical thrombosis associated with massive platelet aggregates ("white clot") may ensue. The time course is usually with 5–10 days of heparin exposure, although in patients with prior exposure to heparin, HIT may occur much faster. There is a hierarchy of incidence risk with full-dose intravenous use causing more HIT than subcutaneous and other less intense regimens. However, all forms and routes can elicit the reaction. In studies, low-molecular-weight heparin (LMWH) forms less commonly incite HIT. However, LMWH will cross react and trigger HIT in sensitized patients. When HIT proceeds into thrombosis, both arterial and venous thrombosis can occur and can be limb- and life-threatening in up to 50% of cases. When HIT is suspected, all heparins by all routes (including dialysis) must be discontinued. Alternative anticoagulants (hirudin, Argatroban) are now available for patients who require ongoing anticoagulation. HIT is frequently a clinical diagnosis initially—the development of thrombocytopenia without other obvious cause in a patient on heparin. There are confirmatory laboratory tests such as the ELISA HIT antibody assay.

Thrombosis can propagate or recur in heparinized patients (answer A). However, the development of a significant new thrombocytopenia in association with the clots would not be expected and is more typical of HIT. TTP (answer B) does manifest the combination of thrombosis and thrombocytopenia. However, the thrombotic aspects of TTP are in the microcirculation rather than in large arteries or veins; and a cardinal finding is microangiopathic hemolysis with RBC fragmentation and schistocytes, which were absent here. Cardiac embolism (answer D) would not be expected to involve the venous system. Homocystineimia (answer E) is a hypercoagulable syndrome that indeed can involve both arterial and venous circulations with premature and recurrent thrombotic events. This patient's presentation should elicit a homocysteine measurement. However, thrombocytopenia would not be expected as part of homocysteinemia.

3. The answer is A [I C (2) b i–vi]. This patient is manifesting clear findings consistent with the acute chest syndrome, the leading cause of death and second most common cause for hospitalization in patients with sickle cell anemia. Typical findings demonstrated here include fever, shortness of breath, tachypnea, striking leukocytosis, chest infiltrates, and hypoxemia. Initiating events can be both infectious or noninfectious (e.g., bone marrow embolism from vasoocclusive events), but once established, the pathophysiology seems similar to acute respiratory distress syndrome (ARDS). The syndrome can result in respiratory failure with requirement for ventilation and mortality in as many as 9% of cases. The acute chest syndrome (ACS) is one of the accepted criteria for exchange transfusion of red cells, and that is the most appropriate choice here. The procedure is usually easily performed in the ICU setting and has excellent results, with an 81% recovery even after mechanical ventilation, which is far superior to that of other patients with ARDS. Simple transfusion may be adequate in mild cases, but exchange is preferred in rapidly deteriorating cases as seen here. Other accepted indications for exchange transfusion in sickle cell patients include neurologic complications such as stroke, priapism, and the less common hepatic sequestration crisis, which causes exquisitely tender and massive hepatomegaly and extreme elevations of bilirubin.

The patient has had cholecystectomy, which is usual for an adult sickle cell patient. These patients have lifelong hemolysis and universally form bilirubin gallstones. The prior cholecystectomy, absence of abdominal symptoms, normal liver function studies, and only minimally elevated bilirubin are strong negatives for the diagnosis of ascending cholangitis. The bilirubin elevation is quite consistent with the hemolytic anemia present. Thus, answer B would not be the initial diagnostic or therapeutic pathway of choice.

Although newer studies have indicated that ACS can be caused frequently by bone marrow fat emboli from infarcted marrow, which occurs during an initial painful crisis, the pathophysiology of ACS is quite different from that of traditional thromboembolism. The emboli are small fat emboli, not clots, and initiate ARDS via cytokine and surfactant mechanisms. In the absence of DVT, which was not suspected epidemiologically or clinically here, heparin (choice C) would not be the preferred therapy.

Patients with homozygous sickle cell anemia have been shown to be predisposed to serious infections from encapsulated organisms, particularly the *Pneumococcus* and *Salmonella* species. These patients have increased incidence and severity from such infections, which should be in the differential of a febrile sickle cell patient. However, this patient also displays the entire spectrum of ACS findings, so is past the point of using antibiotics alone for therapy. He requires aggressive pulmonary measures (oxygen, bronchodilators, etc.) and a transfusion maneuver in addition to any antibiotics. Furthermore, recent studies have expanded the universe of infectious agents seen with ACS and suggest the addition of a macrolide in such cases. Answer D is inadequate on many counts as therapy in this situation.

Hydroxyurea has been used *chronically* in selected homozygous sickle cell anemia patients. Earlier theories suggested that its ability to raise HbF levels and reduce sickling were the basis for its use. More recent data suggest that its role is much more complex and involves lowering WBC (an independent mortality predictor in sickle cell patients) and modulating cytokine levels in patients, which may be as important as or more so than HbF levels. Nonetheless, hydroxyurea requires weeks to have effect and thus is not an appropriate acute therapy.

4. The answer is B [V D 1 a]. Hemophilia A involves coagulation factor VIII^{pro}; platelet function is not affected in this disease. This results in a coagulation-type bleeding syndrome with delayed, deep tissue–type bleeding. Although the exact mechanism is unclear, uremia is believed to cause platelet dysfunction by toxins that alter the factor VIII antigen polymers required for normal platelet function. Aspirin causes thrombocytopathia by inhibiting synthesis of thromboxane A_2 (TXA_2), a strong inducer of platelet aggregation. Factor XII deficiency results in prolongation of the PTT but is not associated with abnormal bleeding.

5. The answer is E [V C 1 b (3)]. Except when thrombocytopenia has caused chronic bleeding with iron deficiency anemia, isolated thrombocytopenia is the rule in idiopathic thrombocytopenic purpura (ITP). Splenomegaly and other cytopenias are not part of ITP, and their presence should bring the diagnosis into doubt. ITP is the prototypical thrombocytopenia due to increased peripheral destruction. Platelet life span is markedly shortened, and, in response, the bone marrow megakaryocytes are increased. Platelet-associated antibodies can usually be found on platelets and in plasma, although their significance remains controversial. Long-term therapy involves IVIg, particularly in the acute setting, corticosteroids, and splenectomy. Immunosuppression may be required in refractory cases.

6. The answer is D [I C 2 b (2) (b) (iv); IV D 4 b, c, d]. Pneumococcal vaccine and exogenous immunoglobulins have been shown to diminish infectious morbidity and mortality in certain hematologic patients (i.e., patients who are postsplenectomy or have sickle cell anemia or chronic lymphocytic anemia), but their role in acute leukemia is limited at best. Humoral immunity is well maintained in patients with acute myelogenous leukemia (AML) and partly, if ever, requires such exogenous support. The therapy for AML, or acute nonlymphocytic leukemia (ANLL), is aggressive and difficult. It involves the ablation of leukemic tissue but invariably results in ablation of normal marrow tissue as well. Profound and prolonged pancytopenia results. The functions of marrow elements must therefore be supported. The empiric use of broad-spectrum antibiotics in febrile patients with polymorphonuclear leukocytes (PMNs) less than 500/mm^3 and the use of prophylactic platelet transfusion to maintain platelet counts greater than 10,000/mm^3 have markedly diminished the incidence of early mortality from infection and bleeding, respectively. Early studies using genetically engineered growth factors indicate their ability to hasten marrow recovery and resolution of cytopenias with similar lessening of infectious and hemorrhagic morbidity. Isolation techniques play a role in lowering the incidence of infection, but the combination that is most effective remains controversial.

7. The answer is C [VI E 2; Table 3–9]. One of the newer developments in hypercoagulability has been the finding of a situation in which the defect for the coagulation inhibitor agonist protein C is located in the receptor molecule rather than in the amount of function of protein C itself. The defective factor V molecule, which is named for the place it was discovered—Leiden, Belgium, is the abnormal protein that is insensitive to the physiologic inhibition by protein C.

Most experts agree that this factor V defect may be the most common diagnosable inborn defects associated with a hypercoagulable state; some studies found an incidence as high as 20% in hypercoagulability workups. A common setting for VTE associated with Leiden is a comorbid risk factor such as pregnancy or use of oral contraceptives. Protein C and antithrombin III deficiencies are traditional defects in the inhibitors themselves, either due to qualitative defects in the inhibitor or quantitative deficiency of the molecules. They have been found to have a higher VTE potential than V Leiden and are less commonly associated with a second risk factor. Trousseau's syndrome is another known hypercoagulable state, but it is acquired rather than genetic. The condition is the result of a form of disseminated intravascular coagulation (DIC) caused by carcinoma, especially mucin-producing adenocarcinoma. Hemophilia, although hereditary and caused by a variety of molecular lesions, is associated with profound bleeding rather than clotting.

8. The answer is D [V C 2 b (1)–(3)]. Hemophilia is an essentially pure coagulation defect and thus clinically results in delayed and deep-tissue bleeding such as hemarthroses. Platelet function is normal, and this is reflected in the normal bleeding time.

All of the other conditions listed result in defects in platelet function. Although platelet counts may be normal, immediate and mucocutaneous platelet-type bleeding (e.g., epistaxis) is encountered clinically and is demonstrable in the laboratory by prolongation of the template bleeding time. Uremia is an acquired condition where the uremic plasma breaks down factor VIII–von Willebrand factor (vWF) multimers into smaller forms that are nonfunctional (with regard to platelet adhesion), resulting in a defect in platelet function. Aspirin acetylates the platelet membrane and diminishes its cyclo-oxygenase pathway, thus reducing the ability of the platelets to make thromboxane A_2, which renders them dysfunctional. This leads to platelet-type bleeding and a prolonged bleeding time. High doses of penicillins such as those used in the therapy of endocarditis also can interfere with platelet function, with similar results. Finally, in von Willebrand's disease (vWD), an inborn deficiency or defect in the previously mentioned factor VIII–vWF protein results in insufficient function of these molecules for physiologic platelet function—specifically adhesions to endothelium. Affected patients may manifest platelet-type bleeding with prolonged bleeding times, as well as coagulation-type bleeding from diminished levels of factor VIII itself.

9. The answer is D [II A 1; C 1, 2]. The very elevated hemoglobin and hematocrit, which strongly correlate with true elevations in red blood cell (RBC) mass rather than plasma contraction, are consistent with polycythemia. Polycythemia then is broken down into autonomous or primary polycythemia vera, a stem cell disease, where the marrow is autonomously creating too many cells, versus reactive or secondary forms, where the marrow is responding to increased erythropoietin from some alteration of normal physiology. The elevations of the other cell lines suggest polycythemia vera, because this stem cell disease involves all marrow cell lines. Ringed sideroblasts and Pelger-Huët cells are seen in myelodysplasia, which is another condition resulting from abnormal marrow clonal stem cells. However, in this condition, cytopenias rather than increases in counts are expected. On occasion, chronic myelogenous leukemia (CML), another marrow stem cell clonal proliferative disease, may manifest with elevated counts—specifically the white blood cell (WBC) count and to a lesser extent, platelets. In CML, a hemoglobin and hematocrit elevated to this degree would be unusual and are much more typical of polycythemia vera.

High hemoglobins and hematocrits from secondary causes such as tissue hypoxia (as with certain cardiac and pulmonary diseases) result from physiologic increases in erythropoietin seen in these states or (as with renal tumors) spectacularly, pathologically elevated levels seen in paraneoplastic cases of high hematocrits. The low oxygen saturation could cause a secondary elevated hemoglobin, but not the elevations in the other cell lines manifested by this patient.

10–13. The answers are: 10-C [VI D 3], **11-B** [VI B 2 b], **12-D** [VI D 5], **13-A** [VI C 2 b]. The lupus inhibitor is found in one third of patients with systemic lupus erythematosus (SLE). In these patients, the association with thrombosis risk is 10%–15%. In patients without SLE who display a similar inhibitor-type antibody, there is less risk of thrombosis, but the risk is still far in excess of normal.

Paroxysmal nocturnal hemoglobinuria (PNH) is a difficult diagnosis to make, and the disorder can masquerade as chronic iron deficiency (due to urine losses), chronic hemolysis, or both. PNH is associated with increased thrombotic risk and has a tendency to involve intra-abdominal veins.

Recurrent thrombosis associated with adequate warfarin anticoagulation, especially when migratory and involving superficial veins, suggests the presence of chronic disseminated intravascular coagulation (DIC) with an occult adenocarcinoma (Trousseau's syndrome).

Warfarin can, in the early phases of administration, lower the vitamin K–dependent, short half-life protein inhibitor protein C more rapidly and create an imbalance with coagulation factors II, VII, IX, and X, thus affecting the hemostatic balance toward clotting. Characteristically, it occurs soon after the initiation of warfarin without concomitant administration of heparin.

14–17. The answers are: 14-C [Table 3–4], **15-A** [Table 3–4], **16-C** [Table 3–4], **17-D** [Table 3–4]. These questions relate to current indications for bone marrow transplantation (BMT). Although this technology continues to develop, clinical trials have confirmed that BMT is superior to other available therapies in several specific situations.

Because the 37-year-old man is under age 55 years and has CML, he is a candidate for BMT. The 23-year-old man with severe aplastic anemia also satisfies the indications for BMT.

The 9-year-old girl should initially undergo chemotherapy, however. Most authorities try to induce remission in standard-risk children with acute lymphocytic leukemia (ALL) with chemotherapy, because these patients have a 70%–80% cure rate. In most cases of childhood ALL, transplantation is used after a first relapse.

BMT is inappropriate for the 73-year-old man because he is too old, and the toxicities of graft-versus-host disease (GVHD) and prolonged cytopenia cannot be tolerated. In this common clinical situation, supportive therapy remains the standard of care.

chapter **4**

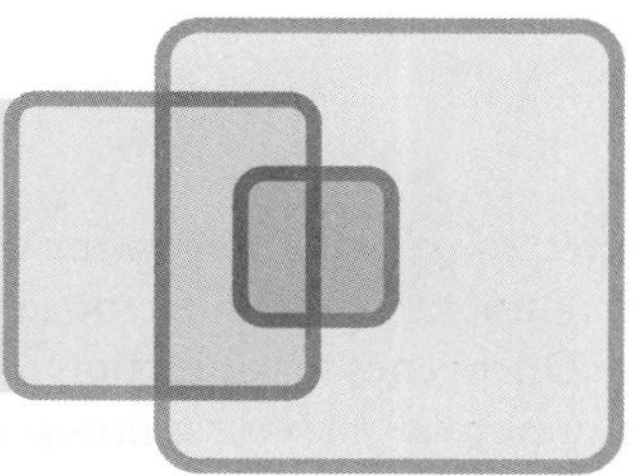

Oncologic Diseases

HOSSEIN BORGHAEI, LOUIS M. WEINER

I TUMOR GROWTH

Uncontrolled growth distinguishes malignant from normal cells. Malignant cells are characterized by a loss of responsiveness to growth-inhibitory signals. More rapidly growing tumors may be more poorly differentiated, but they may be more sensitive to certain kinds of chemotherapy treatments.

A Patterns of tumor growth

Cancer growth follows two general patterns.

1. **Direct invasion** of the tissue in which the cancer arose
2. **Metastasis** (dissemination) to distant organs via the bloodstream, lymphatic system, or by intracavitary extension
   a. Different types of **tumors vary in metastatic potential.** For example, primary brain cancers tend to remain localized and rarely spread to distant foci. However, many carcinomas such as small-cell lung cancer (SCLC) are already widely disseminated in most patients at the time of diagnosis.
   b. Each cancer also exhibits a distinct **pattern of spread** dictated by the biology of the tumor cell–host interaction. For example, common sites of metastases in colon cancer include the liver, lungs, and peritoneal cavity, and common sites in SCLC include the lungs, liver, bones, and neuraxis.

B Tumor growth rate and prognosis

Growth rate and patterns of spread are important determinants of prognosis in the absence of treatment and in the response to particular therapeutic modalities such as surgery, chemotherapy, or radiation therapy.

1. **Rapidly growing neoplasms** such as acute leukemias, SCLC, and lymphomas are generally highly responsive to chemotherapy and radiation therapy. However, there are numerous exceptions.
2. **Slow-growing tumors** such as low-grade sarcomas are less responsive to systemic treatment modalities. Surgical resection and radiation therapy are more effective treatment options for such neoplasms.
3. Growth rates can be estimated using **flow cytometry** to determine the percentage of tumor nuclei in the S phase of the cell cycle. Immunohistochemistry can be used to determine Ki-67, another reflection of cell proliferation. S-phase determination may help predict the prognosis and potential need for adjuvant chemotherapy in early-stage breast cancer.

C Genetic changes and cancer

1. **Cancers are genetic diseases characterized by mutations or overexpression of genes that regulate vital cell processes. Oncogenes** (cancer-promoting genes) interfere with the regulatory controls of the cell. Most oncogenes are derived from **proto-oncogenes,** normal genes that ordinarily regulate cell growth processes.

a. Oncogenes modify the affected cell, resulting in the acquisition of malignant characteristics such as changes in shape, autocrine growth factor secretion, loss of contact inhibition, and anchorage independence. Oncogenes may function in a number of ways:
   (1) They may cause the tumor cell to secrete mitogenic growth factors that then stimulate growth of the same cell, leading to autostimulation of cell growth, or **autocrine growth.**
   (2) They may affect growth factor–induced signal transduction.
      (a) Typically, cell surface receptors engaged by their respective ligands transmit signals through a series of defined intracellular pathways that culminate in the regulation of DNA synthesis or transcription.
      (b) Mutations or altered gene expression in any of these pathways may disturb such regulated signaling, leading to a loss of regulated cell growth or function. The protein products of some oncogenes such as *ras* mutate so that they constitutively promote cell growth in the absence of growth factor interactions with their receptors.

b. Single oncogenes typically do not induce the transformation of fully normal cells into fully malignant cells. Each oncogene **induces only a subset of changes** associated with full malignancy. A series of genetic changes is typically required.

c. **Activation of proto-oncogenes**
   (1) **Point mutations.** A point mutation is a single-base change in a gene. A single mutation in codon 12 of the *ras* gene causes activation of *ras,* the most commonly activated oncogene in solid malignancies.
   (2) **Gene fusion.** In chronic myelogenous leukemia (CML), the *abl* proto-oncogene is typically fused with a fully unrelated gene, the BCR gene. The protein encoded by the BCR-*abl* hybrid (p210) has a novel structure and function.
   (3) **Amplification.** Differences in the level of expression of encoded proteins also can cause proto-oncogenes to become oncogenic. For example, in childhood neuroblastoma, the amount of the N-*myc* gene is increased from a diploid number to many dozens per cell. N-*myc* gene amplification is associated with a poor prognosis and is a significant factor in the aggressiveness of this tumor.

2. **Tumor suppressor genes** function in the normal cell to restrict or repress cellular proliferation. The inactivation of tumor suppressor genes can promote tumorigenesis.
   a. Inactive alleles of tumor suppressor genes may be acquired in two ways:
      (1) Somatic mutation
      (2) Incorporation in the germ line to create a congenital predisposition to cancer (e.g., as in retinoblastoma)
   b. Inactivation of tumor suppressor genes is associated with neuroblastoma, SCLC, kidney cancer, colon carcinoma, Wilms' tumor, bladder cancer, osteoblastoma, and liver cancer, among other malignancies.
   c. Specific mutations in the BRCA1 gene in affected women increase the risk of early-onset breast cancer. Research has recently shown that the BRCA1 gene, a heritable somatic gene prevalent in Ashkenazi Jews, is normally involved in estrogen receptor (ER) function.

II CANCER STAGING

Conventional tumor–node–metastasis (TNM) staging systems define a series of categories or stages, each of which defines a prognostic stage of a tumor.

A Objectives of staging

1. **Estimating prognosis.** Higher stages are associated with progressively poorer prognoses.
2. **Determining the best course of therapy.** Accurate staging is necessary to determine the appropriate sequence of local, regional, and systemic treatment approaches.

3. **Facilitating investigation.** Staging provides a uniform classification system to develop uniform treatment criteria and to evaluate the clinical trials literature.

B Staging systems

Staging systems for all solid tumors are based principally on the **anatomic extent of disease.** Differences in tumor biology preclude a universal staging system applicable to all cancers.

1. The **TNM classification system** is the most widely used staging system for carcinomas and sarcomas. This system assigns the tumor to a **T level,** which corresponds to the size and extent of the primary tumor; an **N level,** which describes the degree of regional nodal involvement; and an **M level,** which describes the presence and extent of distant metastases. Site-specific definitions of TNM stages have been compiled for a wide range of neoplasms.
2. Older classification systems still are frequently used to stage lymphomas and carcinomas of the colon, rectum, prostate, and testicle.

C Staging procedures

The American Joint Committee on Cancer (AJCC) has defined the following three levels of staging information.*

1. **Clinical staging** uses all available **pretreatment data,** including diagnostic data obtained from physical examination, radiologic or nuclear imaging techniques, laboratory tests, and endoscopy or other invasive procedures.
2. **Pathologic staging** is based on data obtained during surgery and from pathologic examination of the resected specimen.
3. **Retreatment staging** may be used to restage the tumor before additional therapy, after failure of initial treatment.

III TREATMENT MODALITIES

A General principles

1. Cancer treatment may be either **curative** or **palliative** in intent.
   a. **Curative** treatments aim to permanently eradicate the tumor.
   b. **Palliative** treatments seek to optimize quality of life and, when possible, to prolong life when cure cannot be achieved.
2. Successful treatment programs typically include one or more of the following components: surgery, radiation therapy, chemotherapy, and other noncytotoxic systemic therapies.
3. Therapy must be customized to meet the specific needs of individual patients. In many disease presentations, a multidisciplinary approach that coordinates the efforts of the pathologist, surgical oncologist, medical oncologist, radiation oncologist, and other specialists is desirable.
4. **Clinical trials,** which are essential to progress in cancer therapy, are integrated into the routine care of many cancer patients. Trials can be conducted to identify new treatment options in patients for whom no effective therapy is available or to further refine existing effective treatment strategies. The clinical trial process typically involves three distinct types of trials.
   a. **Phase I trials** use new agents or new combinations of agents to identify toxicities and **maximally tolerated doses,** to establish a working dose for further studies, and to determine the disposition (**pharmacokinetics**) and biologic effects as they relate to disposition (**pharmacodynamics**). When possible, studies should provide a proof-of-concept that the agent has the desired effects on its putative target at doses to be used in phase II studies. For each drug tested, phase I trials typically involve fewer than 25 patients with advanced disease.

*For full staging information, please see the most recent edition of the AJCC Cancer Staging Handbook. At press time, the most recent edition is American Joint Committee on Cancer: AJCC Cancer Staging Handbook, 6th edition. New York, Springer-Verlag, 2002.

b. **Phase II trials** are designed to evaluate the efficacy of new agents or drug combinations in a particular stage of disease. Usually, phase II trials are conducted in 30–50 patients, with early stopping rules if the new treatment proves ineffective.

c. If phase II trials yield encouraging results, randomized **phase III trials** are conducted to compare the new treatment with the existing standard of care. Phase III trials typically require hundreds to thousands of patients.

B **Radiation therapy** Fifty percent of all cancer patients require radiation therapy at some point during the course of their disease.

1. **Applications**
   a. Radiation therapy, either alone or in conjunction with chemotherapy and surgery, is curative in some cancers (e.g., Hodgkin's disease, head and neck cancer, cervical cancer, rectal cancer).
   b. Radiation therapy also has important palliative applications (e.g., relief from metastatic bone pain in advanced breast cancer).

2. **Uses.** Radiation therapy can be used alone or in combination with chemotherapy or surgery.
   a. **Before radiation therapy. Chemotherapy** may be used concurrently with or before radiation to enhance efficacy.
      (1) For example, the pyrimidine analog 5-fluorouracil (5-FU), the alkylating agent cisplatin, gemcitabine, a nucleoside analog that primarily kills cells undergoing DNA synthesis (S-phase) and blocks the progression of cells through the G1/S-phase boundary, and the microtubule stabilizer paclitaxel (Taxol) all act as radiation sensitizers when administered concurrently with radiation therapy.
      (2) However, combined-modality therapy also can contribute to severe toxicity reactions. The **radiation recall effect,** an enhanced or reactivated response in a previously irradiated area precipitated by the concurrent administration of doxorubicin or methotrexate, is a classic example.
   b. **Surgery.** Radiation therapy may be used **before surgery** to induce tumor regression and facilitate the surgical procedure. Radiation also may be used **postoperatively** to reduce the risk of local recurrence. In most cancers, the optimal timing of adjunctive radiation therapy (e.g., preoperative versus postoperative) has not been determined.

3. **Side effects.** Radiation therapy is associated with local side effects, especially in patients who are receiving curative-intent high-dose radiation (e.g., for the treatment of head or neck cancer).
   a. **Time course**
      (1) **Acute effects,** principally inflammation, may occur within days or weeks of treatment.
      (2) **Chronic effects** such as fibrosis and scarring may not be apparent until months or even years after therapy.
   b. The **severity** of adverse reactions is a function of the treatment site, the size of the radiation port, the amount of radiation energy, and dosage variables (e.g., total dose, radiation dose per fraction, dose rate). The toxicity of high-dose radiation therapy may be reduced by the use of tailored, conformal radiation fields. Side effects can be minimized by:
      (1) Accurately targeting the tumor area by using sophisticated radiologic techniques [e.g., computed tomography (CT), magnetic resonance imaging (MRI)]
      (2) Directing radiation to avoid critical organs with low tolerance to radiation (e.g., the spinal cord)
      (3) Blocking normal tissue from radiation
      (4) Reducing the treatment field over the course of therapy
   c. **Systemic effects** of radiation therapy include malaise, fatigue, anorexia, and depressed blood count. These generalized symptoms are especially common in patients treated concurrently with radiation and chemotherapy.

d. Skin reactions occur after high-dose therapy directed to sites on or near the skin surface (e.g., chest wall after mastectomy) or female reproductive organs (e.g., vulva). Such reactions are less common after high-energy photon beam therapy. Retreatment or the use of overlapping fields may result in severe and persistent skin reactions.

(1) **Acute reactions** consist of erythema, dry desquamation with pruritus, and moist desquamation.

(2) The affected area should be kept as clean and dry as possible. Additional treatment measures include:

(a) Topical application of vitamin A and D ointment, baby oil, or cornstarch

(b) Cleansing the area with a 1:1 solution of hydrogen peroxide and normal saline

(c) Topical application of corticosteroids

(3) Patients should avoid irritating clothing and direct exposure to the sun.

e. Reactions of the **oral cavity and pharynx** such as mucositis, pain, anorexia, xerostomia, and dental caries occur after high-dose radiation to the head or neck area.

(1) Strict attention to dental hygiene, topical anesthetics, artificial saliva preparations, and nutritional counseling may be helpful.

(2) Severe cases of nausea or gastrointestinal intolerance may require insertion of a gastric feeding tube or percutaneous gastrostomy.

f. Gastrointestinal reactions occur with cumulative radiation doses exceeding 4000–5500 cGy.

(1) **Esophagitis** usually subsides in 7–10 days but predisposes patients to superimposed *Candida* infections. Treatment measures include use of antacids, a bland diet, and topical anesthetics.

(2) **Radiation gastritis** or **enteritis** may manifest as nausea, vomiting, diarrhea, abdominal pain, anorexia, or bleeding. Treatment measures include:

(a) Antiemetics (e.g., prochlorperazine, trimethobenzamide)

(b) Antidiarrheals (e.g., diphenoxylate hydrochloride-atropine sulfate, loperamide hydrochloride)

(c) A bland, low-fat, low-residue, high-gluten diet

(d) Dietary supplements

(3) **Rectal inflammation** may result in bleeding or pain. A low-residue diet, stool softeners, or steroid enemas may give relief.

g. Radiation pneumonitis, characterized by cough, dyspnea, and chest pain, usually occurs 2–3 months after delivery of radiation to a significant lung volume. Corticosteroids are usually effective. Steroids should be discontinued gradually to avoid recurrence of symptoms.

h. Central nervous system (CNS) symptoms may occur during therapy or may not appear until weeks or months later.

(1) **Acute symptoms** accompanying intracranial irradiation include headache and signs of increased intracranial pressure (ICP); gastrointestinal symptoms (i.e., nausea and vomiting) also may occur. Dexamethasone usually provides rapid relief.

(2) **Delayed symptoms** include short-term memory loss, visual memory disturbances, and white matter abnormalities such as calcifications and ventricular dilatation. These toxicities are particularly common in patients undergoing prophylactic cranial radiation for limited-stage SCLC.

(3) **A somnolence syndrome** characterized by hypersomnia and fatigue has been observed several weeks or months after intracranial irradiation, especially in patients who are receiving concurrent intrathecal chemotherapy.

i. Bone marrow suppression may follow the large-field irradiation used in the treatment of Hodgkin's disease or pelvic malignancies, especially if patients are receiving concurrent chemotherapy. Leukopenia or thrombocytopenia may require suspension of therapy; however, anemia is rare. Hemoglobin values below 9 g/dL may require transfusion.

j. In Hodgkin's disease, mediastinal irradiation is associated with long-term toxicities such as hypothyroidism and coronary artery disease.

4. **Newer Techniques**

   Intensity modulated radiation therapy (IMRT) and stereotactic radiation therapy are newer modalities that minimize damage to normal tissue while delivering higher doses of radiation to the target organs.

C Chemotherapy

1. **General comments.** Practitioners have used chemotherapeutic agents for over 50 years, ever since the introduction of nitrogen mustard in the late 1940s.
   a. Combinations of chemotherapy agents used in conjunction with other cytoreductive treatment modalities may increase cure rates in patients with colorectal neoplasms, esophageal cancer, and breast cancer.
   b. Chemotherapy plays an important role in the palliative treatment of patients with advanced or metastatic cancers. In this setting, the sequential use of modestly active single agents may be preferable to the use of more active, but more toxic, combinations.
   c. Recent improvements in drug development and the screening of new agents have led to the introduction of numerous new agents, offering patients more treatment options. These advances have been coupled with an increased understanding of tumor biology.
2. **Assessment of treatment outcome.** Chemotherapy should be used only when patients benefit from the treatment. When cure is the objective, complete responses are generally required, and considerable host toxicity is acceptable [e.g., the use of bone marrow transplantation (BMT) for patients with acute leukemias]. However, when palliation is the goal, acceptable toxicity must be coupled with an absence of disease progression. In general, individuals who exhibit an objective (e.g., complete or partial) response to chemotherapy live better and longer than do those with stable or progressive disease. Disease may be defined as **measurable** (e.g., at least 1 cm in each perpendicular dimension) by a radiographic or reliable physical examination or **evaluable** [not meeting the criteria for measurable disease but with clear evidence of active cancer (e.g., malignant pleural effusion)]. Some of these guidelines may require alteration if noncytotoxic agents that inhibit cell growth are part of the therapeutic armamentarium.
   a. A **complete response** is defined as the complete disappearance of all known malignant disease without development of any new malignant lesions. This state must persist for at least two consecutive evaluations at least 1 month apart.
   b. A **partial response** is achieved when the overall area of measurable tumor (e.g., the sum of the greatest length multiplied by the greatest perpendicular width for all lesions) reduces by more than 50% from baseline, for at least two consecutive evaluations at least 1 month apart. No new lesions may appear, and no individual lesion may increase in size (as defined above) by more than 25%.
   c. **Stable disease** implies either a decrease of less than 50% or an increase of less than 25% in size of all measurable tumor masses.
   d. **Progressive disease** implies a 25% or greater increase in the size of all measurable lesions or the development of a new lesion considered to represent metastatic disease.
3. **Combination chemotherapy.** This approach has revolutionized the treatment of potentially curable or highly chemotherapy-responsive cancers. In general, combinations of active agents are required to cure patients with advanced, chemotherapy-sensitive diseases such as acute leukemia and testicular cancer. Such combination regimens contain effective drugs with high response rates for the particular tumor type being treated.
   a. Combinations are selected based on evidence of therapeutic synergy or additivity with acceptable host toxicity. When possible, highly active agents with nonoverlapping toxicity profiles are chosen.

b. Combinations of marginally active chemotherapeutic agents tend to be relatively inactive but more toxic than the use of single agents with comparable efficacy profiles. However, in chemotherapy-sensitive cancers, combination chemotherapy is usually far more effective than single-agent therapy.

c. Combination chemotherapy may prevent or delay the development of drug resistance that commonly develops when malignant cells are exposed to a single agent over a given period.

4. Drug resistance. This phenomenon may be either **innate** or **acquired.** Certain malignancies (e.g., pancreatic cancer, hepatocellular carcinoma), which rarely respond to conventional chemotherapy agents, exhibit innate drug resistance. Other cancers (e.g., SCLC, ovarian cancer, breast cancer) initially respond well to chemotherapy before the emergence of drug-resistant variants, leading to disease progression. Several mechanisms of drug resistance have been identified.

a. Inhibition of drug accumulation or active drug efflux. Multidrug resistance mediated by the MDR1 gene, which encodes the p-glycoprotein transporter, exemplifies this phenomenon. MDR1 promotes the efflux of a variety of structurally unrelated natural products such as doxorubicin, etoposide, taxanes, and vinca alkaloids. The MRP gene member of the c-MOAT transporter family appears to be another example of this phenomenon. Some agents such as methotrexate require polyglutamylation to be retained intracellularly.

b. Overexpression of the drug target. This type of drug resistance is specific to such common drugs as the antimetabolite methotrexate, in which resistance to the antimetabolite can result from gene amplification of the drug's target, the enzyme dihydrofolate reductase. Similarly, overexpression of the enzyme ara-CTP deaminase can account for resistance to cytosine arabinoside in acute leukemia. These factors form the basis for high-dose therapy with methotrexate and cytosine arabinoside; the object is to saturate the overexpressed enzymes.

c. Accelerated repair of chemotherapy-induced cellular damage. Alkylating agents cross-link with DNA to induce potentially lethal cellular damage. This damage stimulates the activity of DNA repair enzymes, which can repair lesions. Accelerated expression or activity of these repair enzymes may promote alkylator drug resistance.

d. Inhibition of cell death (apoptosis) pathways. Evidently, cell damage activates programmed cell death (apoptosis) to protect the organism. In many malignant cells, apoptosis pathways are dysregulated, sometimes because of overexpression of a particular antiapoptotic pathway component, or by the loss of a proapoptotic element. The existence of such "common pathways" for response (or lack of response) to lethal cellular injury may explain the innate drug resistance seen in many malignancies.

5. Commonly used chemotherapeutic agents. The most often used chemotherapeutic drugs and their mechanisms of action, therapeutic uses, and toxicities are discussed in the following sections (Table 4–1).

6. Types of chemotherapeutic agents

a. Alkylating agents. Chemical classes include nitrogen mustards, platinum analogs, nitrosoureas, alkyl sulfonates (busulfan), ethylenimines and methylmelamines, and triazenes (dacarbazine).

(1) Mechanism of action

(a) Alkylating agents react strongly with nucleophilic substances and form covalent linkages. The platinum complexes of the platinum analogs bind to DNA, forming intrastrand cross-links. In addition, the platinum analogs also bind to nuclear and cytoplasmic proteins. Cisplatin behaves as a bifunctional alkylating agent.

(b) The toxic effects of alkylating agents are believed to be related to free radical formation and alkylation of the components of DNA, RNA, and cellular proteins. These reactions have profound effects on DNA replication and transcription and may cause cytotoxicity, mutagenesis, and carcinogenesis.

TABLE 4–1 Classes of Common Chemotherapeutic Agents Used in Oncologic Disease

Alkylating Agents	**Antibiotics**
Nitrogen mustards	Daunorubicin
Mechlorethamine	Doxorubicin (Adriamycin)
Cyclophosphamide	Mitoxantrone
Ifosfamide	Mitomycin-C
Melphalan	Bleomycin
Chlorambucil	**Antimetabolites**
Platinum analogs	Methotrexate
Cisplatin	5-Fluorouracil (5-FU)
Carboplatin	Floxuridine (FUDR)
Oxaliplatin	Fludarabine
Nitrosoureas	Mercaptopurine (6-MP)
Carmustine (BCNU)	Cytarabine (Ara-C)
Lomustine (CCNU)	Thioguanine (6-TG)
Streptozocin	Pentostatin
Alkyl sulfonates	**Topoisomerase Inhibitors**
Busulfan	Topoisomerase I
Ethylenimines and methylmelamines	Irinotecan
Thiotepa	Topotecan
Hexamethylmelamine	Topoisomerase II
Triazenes	Etoposide
Dacarbazine (DTIC)	**Miscellaneous Agents**
Microtubule Inhibitors	Procarbazine
Vinca alkaloids	
Vincristine	
Vinblastine	
Vinorelbine	
Taxanes	
Paclitaxel	
Docetaxel	
Estramustine	

(c) Alkylation can take place in proliferating and nonproliferating cells. Therefore, alkylating agents are not cell cycle–specific. The proliferating compartment is more sensitive to the killing effects of these drugs.

(2) **Drug resistance** to alkylating agents may occur because of decreased drug accumulation by resistant cells, increased pharmacologic inactivation of alkylating agents, increased repair of alkylating agent–induced damage, and increased intracellular sulfhydryl groups (e.g., free thiols), which compete with other targets (e.g., DNA) to neutralize the drug intracellularly. Patients who fail treatment with one alkylating agent often respond to another.

(3) **Therapeutic uses and toxicities** are summarized in Tables 4–2 through 4–7.

b. Microtubule inhibitors

(1) Mechanism of action

(a) **Vinca alkaloids** interfere with the function of microtubular spindle proteins, leading to an arrest of the cell cycle in mitosis.

(b) **Podophyllotoxins** cause metaphase arrest by exerting a macromolecular effect on DNA synthesis. They can induce strand breaks in DNA by interacting with topoisomerase II.

TABLE 4–2 Nitrogen Mustards

Drug	Therapeutic Uses	Common Toxicities
Mechlorethamine (nitrogen mustard)	Hodgkin's disease; sclerosing agent for pleural effusions; topical dilute solution in mycosis fungoides	Bone marrow suppression; nausea; vomiting; alopecia; infertility; sclerosing agent
Cyclophosphamide (Cytoxan)	Hodgkin's disease; lymphomas; chronic lymphocytic leukemia (CLL); multiple myeloma; breast cancer; small-cell lung cancer; ovarian cancer; pediatric tumors; bone marrow transplantation	Bone marrow suppression; infertility; alopecia; nausea; vomiting; hemorrhagic cystitis (which is prevented by high fluid intake)
Ifosfamide (Ifex)	Soft tissue sarcomas; testicular cancer; ovarian cancer; cervical cancer; lymphomas	Bone marrow suppression; infertility; alopecia; vomiting; central nervous system (CNS) toxicity (which may be reduced by limiting high single doses, reducing narcotic use, reducing antinausea agents, and other CNS active drugs)
Melphalan (Alkeran)	Myeloma; macroglobulinemia; formerly used in ovarian and breast cancer	Bone marrow suppression; infertility; nausea; alopecia
Chlorambucil (Leukeran)	CLL; macroglobulinemia; lymphoma	Bone marrow suppression; nausea; alopecia (rare); infertility; skin rash; rarely hepatic toxicity

TABLE 4–3 Platinum Analogs

Drug	Therapeutic Uses	Common Toxicities
Cisplatin (Platinol)	Testicular, ovarian, head and neck, lung, bladder, cervix, and esophageal cancer; lymphoma; a radiation sensitizer	Renal toxicity; vomiting; hearing loss; myelosuppression; tinnitus; peripheral neuropathy; hair loss
Carboplatin (Paraplatin)	Ovarian and lung cancer; other cisplatin-sensitive tumors	Myelosuppression; vomiting; much less nephrotoxicity, neuropathy, and ototoxicity than cisplatin
Oxaliplatin	Colorectal cancer	Neuropathy

TABLE 4–4 Nitrosoureas

Drug	Therapeutic Uses	Common Toxicities
Carmustine (BCNU)	Brain tumors; Hodgkin's disease; multiple myeloma; bone marrow transplantation	Bone marrow suppression; nausea; vomiting; mild and reversible liver toxicity; rare lung and kidney damage
Lomustine (CCNU)	Lymphoma; brain tumors; colon cancer	Bone marrow suppression; nausea; vomiting; dermatitis; alopecia; transient hepatotoxicity (usually rare and mild)
Streptozocin (Zanosar)	Pancreatic islet cell tumors; carcinoids	Nausea; vomiting; duodenal ulcers; renal toxicity; mild bone marrow suppression; glucose intolerance due to islet cell damage; mild hepatic toxicity

TABLE 4–5 Alkyl Sulfonates

Drug	Therapeutic Uses	Common Toxicities
Busulfan (Myleran)	Chronic myelogenous leukemia; bone marrow transplantation	Bone marrow suppression; infertility; pulmonary fibrosis; skin hyperpigmentation

(c) **Taxanes** stabilize microtubule polymerization and lead to a breakdown of mitotic spindle formation.

(2) **Therapeutic uses and toxicities** are summarized in Table 4–8.

c. **Antibiotics**

(1) **Mechanism of action.** Antitumor antibiotics are natural substances that inhibit DNA and RNA synthesis. They behave as both phase-specific and phase-nonspecific agents and exhibit a variety of effects on different phases of the cell cycle.

(2) **Therapeutic uses and toxicities** are summarized in Table 4–9.

d. **Antimetabolites**

(1) **Mechanism of action.** Most antimetabolites are phase-specific and act during the S phase of the cell cycle. Antimetabolites interact with cellular enzymes by:

(a) Substituting some metabolite that is normally incorporated into a key molecule such as DNA or RNA, thus interfering with cellular function

(b) Competing with a normal metabolite for occupation of the catalytic site of a key enzyme

(c) Competing with normal metabolites that act as important enzyme regulatory sites or other important receptors

(2) **Therapeutic uses and toxicities** are summarized in Table 4–10.

e. **Topoisomerase I inhibitors**

(1) **Mechanism of action.** These agents inhibit the function of topoisomerase I, an enzyme that regulates the unwinding of supercoiled DNA.

(2) **Therapeutic uses and toxicities** are summarized in Table 4–11.

f. **Miscellaneous agents.** Procarbazine is in this category (Table 4–12).

D **Biologic response modifiers** are agents that alter the growth characteristics or antigenicity of a tumor, resulting in a therapeutic enhancement of host response. The mechanism of action may be immunologic or nonimmunologic.

1. **Classification.** Biologic response modifiers are classified according to the following functional categories.

TABLE 4–6 Ethylenimines and Methylmelamines

Drug	Therapeutic Uses	Common Toxicities
Thiotepa (TSPA)	Lymphoma; superficial bladder cancer; breast cancer; ovarian cancer; bone marrow transplantation; intrathecal therapy for carcinomatous meningitis	Bone marrow suppression; infertility; nausea and vomiting (rare with low doses)
Hexamethylmelamine (Hexalen)	Ovarian cancer; small-cell lung cancer; lymphoma; endometrial cancer; cervical cancer	Nausea; vomiting; bone marrow suppression; infertility; mood changes; peripheral neuropathy; paresthesias; ataxia

TABLE 4–7 Triazenes

Drug	Therapeutic Uses	Common Toxicities
Dacarbazine (DTIC)	Melanoma; sarcomas; Hodgkin's disease	Nausea; vomiting; malaise; low-grade fever; flu-like syndrome; bone marrow suppression; rare hepatic toxicity and diarrhea

TABLE 4–8 Microtubule Inhibitors

Drug	Therapeutic Uses	Common Toxicities
Vinca alkaloids		
Vincristine (Oncovin)	Acute lymphocytic leukemia; Hodgkin's disease; lymphoma; Kaposi's sarcoma	Neurotoxicity (the first signs are loss of deep tendon reflexes, decreased distal sensation, and paresthesias); sclerosing agent; alopecia; constipation
Vinblastine (Velban)	Hodgkin's disease; lymphoma; testicular cancer; non–small-cell lung cancer; Kaposi's sarcoma	Bone marrow suppression; nausea; peripheral neuropathy; constipation; a sclerosing agent
Vinorelbine (Navelbine)	Non–small-cell lung cancer; breast cancer; lymphoma	Bone marrow suppression; peripheral neuropathy; mild alopecia; sclerosing agent
Taxanes		
Paclitaxel (Taxol)	Ovarian, breast, lung, and head and neck cancer	Allergic reactions (which may be prevented by premedication with dexamethasone, Benadryl, and cimetidine); myelosuppression; alopecia; myalgias; flu-like syndrome
Docetaxel (Taxotere)	Ovarian, breast, lung, and head and neck cancers	Myelosuppression, alopecia, peripheral edema requiring corticosteroid prophylaxis
Estramustine (Emcyt)	Prostate cancer	Myelosuppression, nausea and vomiting

TABLE 4–9 Antibiotics

Drug	Therapeutic Uses	Common Toxicities
Daunorubicin	Acute myelogenous leukemia (AML)	Bone marrow suppression; nausea; vomiting; alopecia; sclerosing agent; infertility; cardiomyopathy
Doxorubicin (Adriamycin)	Breast cancer; lymphomas; sarcomas; lung cancer; stomach cancer; thyroid cancer	Bone marrow suppression; nausea; vomiting; mucositis; gastrointestinal toxicity; alopecia; infertility; cardiomyopathy; sclerosing agent
Mitoxantrone (DHAD)	Breast cancer, lymphoma; AML	Myelosuppression; rarely nausea; vomiting; alopecia; elevated liver function tests; occasionally blue urine; cardiotoxicity
Mitomycin (Mutamycin)	Breast cancer; cancer of the stomach, pancreas, colon, cervix, and lung; used as a radiosensitizer with 5-fluorouracil for anal cancer	Bone marrow suppression; sclerosing agent; lung, hepatic, and kidney damage; infertility; hemolytic–uremic syndrome; cardiotoxicity
Bleomycin (Blenoxane)	Testicular cancer; head and neck cancer; lymphomas; Hodgkin's disease; cervical cancer	Mild myelosuppression; fever; allergic reactions; lung toxicity; skin changes; alopecia; rarely hypotension; sclerosing agent

TABLE 4–10 Antimetabolites

Drug	Therapeutic Uses	Common Toxicities
Methotrexate	Acute lymphocytic leukemia (ALL); osteogenic sarcoma; lymphoma; breast, head, neck, gastric, and bladder cancers; choriocarcinoma; intrathecal use for carcinomatous meningitis	Bone marrow suppression; mucositis; diarrhea; nausea; rare kidney and liver damage. (Toxicities are increased when used with other highly protein-bound drugs. High doses should be given with intravenous leucovorin, hydration and alkalinization of the urine.)
5-Fluorouracil (5-FU)	Cancers of the breast, colon, stomach, pancreas, head and neck, esophagus, and anus; antitumor activity is increased when it is given with leucovorin	Bone marrow suppression; mucositis; diarrhea; hyperpigmentation; rare cerebellar ataxia; myocardial ischemia
Floxiuridine	Colon cancer; regional perfusion with hepatic artery	Biliary sclerosis
Fludarabine (Fludara)	Chronic lymphocytic leukemia; lymphoma	Myelosuppression; flu-like syndrome; nausea; alopecia
Mercaptopurine (6-MP)	Maintenance therapy for acute leukemia	Bone marrow suppression; nausea; stomatitis; rarely rash; liver toxicity; intrahepatic cholestasis
Cytarabine (ara-C)	Acute myelogenous leukemia (AML); ALL; blastic phase of chronic myelogenous leukemia; preleukemia	Bone marrow suppression; nausea; anorexia; stomatitis; flu-like syndrome; liver toxicity; cerebellar dysfunction
Thioguanine (6-TG)	AML	Bone marrow suppression
Pentostatin (Nipent)	Lymphoma; hairy cell leukemia	Bone marrow suppression; increased renal toxicity; conjunctivitis; fever; hepatotoxicity

TABLE 4–11 Topoisomerase Inhibitors

Drug	Therapeutic Uses	Common Toxicities
Etoposide (VP-16)	Testicular cancer, small-cell lung cancer, non–small-cell lung cancer, lymphomas, sarcomas, (pediatric and Kaposi's)	Delayed leukopenia, mild thrombocytopenia, rare nausea anorexia, diarrhea, rare hypotension with rapid infusions
Irinotecan (Camptosar)	Colorectal cancer, non–small-cell lung cancer	Diarrhea, myelosuppression, alopecia
Topotecan (Hycamtin)	Ovarian cancer, small-cell lung cancer	Myelosuppression, anemia

TABLE 4–12 Miscellaneous Agents

Drug	Therapeutic Uses	Common Toxicities
Procarbazine (Matulane)	Hodgkin's disease; lymphoma	Neurologic symptoms; hypotensive reactions with tricyclic antidepressants and substances with high tyramine contents; disulfiram-like reaction with alcohol and drugs in nose drops, cough preparations, and local anesthetics; bone marrow depression; nausea; vomiting; peripheral neuropathy; lethargy; rash; central nervous system toxicity

a. Agents that **restore, augment,** or **modify host immunologic mechanisms** thought to be critical for tumor growth and metastasis [e.g., bacille Calmette-Guérin (BCG), interferon-α (IFN-α)]

b. Cells or cellular products that have direct **cytotoxic** or **cytostatic** effects (e.g., donor lymphocyte infusions)

c. Agents that alter **metastatic potential** or that affect the **initiation** or **maintenance of neoplastic transformation** (e.g., retinoids, matrix metalloproteinase inhibitors, angiogenesis inhibitors, cyclooxygenase-2 inhibitors, signal transduction inhibitors)

2. **BCG.** An attenuated strain of *Mycobacterium bovis,* BCG has demonstrated activity when administered locally in direct contact with tumor cells.

a. **Therapeutic indications.** BCG therapy is **used successfully in the treatment of recurrent superficial bladder cancers.** Direct instillation of BCG into the bladder after transurethral resection or fulguration of visible lesions significantly reduces the incidence of recurrent tumors as well as the number of patients ultimately requiring cystectomy for invasive bladder cancer.

b. **Toxicity.** Local irritation and a flu-like illness, consisting of fever and malaise, is common in the first 24 hours after administration.

3. **Hematopoietic growth factors.** This family of proteins regulates the proliferation, differentiation, maturation, and function of blood cells.

a. The **interleukins IL-1, IL-3, and IL-6** affect totipotential **stem cells,** or immature hematopoietic precursors. In addition, these cytokines have widespread physiologic effects on lymphocytes and other organs.

b. **Colony-stimulating factors** act primarily on differentiated cells. These factors include erythropoietin (EPO), granulocyte colony-stimulating factor (G-CSF), granulocyte macrophage colony-stimulating factor (GM-CSF), macrophage colony-stimulating factor (M-CSF), flt-3 ligand, and thrombopoietin.

(1) **EPO,** synthesized by the kidney, is a major regulatory factor of red blood cell (RBC) production. Intravenous administration of EPO results in a marked increase in reticulocyte number and the hematocrit.

(a) **Therapeutic indications.** Anemia attributable to chronic illness such as renal disease and acquired immunodeficiency syndrome (AIDS) as well as myelodysplastic syndromes and anemia from chemotherapy are associated with decreased EPO production.

(b) **Side effects.** Rarely, EPO administration is associated with an increase in diastolic blood pressure.

(2) **GM-CSF** primarily stimulates the production of neutrophils, eosinophils, granulocytes, and monocytes, whereas G-CSF stimulates neutrophils and granulocytes.

(a) **Therapeutic indications.** Both G-CSF and GM-CSF reduce and shorten granulocyte nadirs from chemotherapy, hasten recovery after BMT, and help restore bone marrow function in disease-related or iatrogenic neutropenia. As a result, patients experience fewer febrile episodes and a reduced requirement for antibiotics after chemotherapy and BMT.

(b) **Side effects.** G-CSF may produce mild-to-moderate bone or muscle pain or alterations in blood chemistry values. A few patients may develop splenomegaly, headache, flushing, chest discomfort, cutaneous reactions, or hypotension.

4. **Interferons (IFNs)** are glycoproteins that possess antiviral and antiproliferative activities. They also enhance T-cell and macrophage activity, stimulate the expression of tumor-specific cell surface antigens, modify oncogene expression, and promote cellular differentiation.

a. Two types of IFN-α have been approved for the treatment of hairy-cell leukemia and Kaposi's sarcoma. IFN-α has also been used in CML, non-Hodgkin's lymphoma, renal cell cancer, mycosis fungoides, melanoma, carcinoid tumors, and myeloma.

b. Toxic reactions include a flu-like illness, with fever, chills, malaise, mild leukopenia, and elevation of hepatic enzymes.

5. **IL-2,** a lymphokine secreted by activated T lymphocytes, modifies the proliferation and function of T and B cells and is essential for the growth of T cells and peripheral blood lymphocytes.
   a. IL-2 is occasionally effective in patients with advanced melanoma and renal cell carcinoma. In rare instances, these responses are complete and very durable. High-dose therapy with IL-2, although very toxic (see III D 5 d), is required to achieve these durable complete responses.
   b. The mechanisms underlying these responses appear to be the activation and expansion of T cells reactive with cancer cell–specific antigens, leading to the establishment of an effective adaptive antitumor immune response. IL-2 therapy also stimulates the production of activated natural killer (NK) cells, termed **lymphokine-activated killer (LAK) cells,** which mediate broad, non–major histocompatibility complex (MHC)–restricted tumor lysis. However, the therapeutic relevance of these cells, which rarely infiltrate tumors, is unclear.
   c. **Indications.** IL-2 therapy is indicated in patients with advanced renal cell carcinoma and melanomas.
   d. **Side effects.** High-dose IL-2 therapy is associated with severe toxicity, including a capillary leak syndrome, fluid retention, renal failure, pulmonary edema, severe neurologic symptoms, shortness of breath, elevations in serum creatinine and bilirubin, anemia, thrombocytopenia, diarrhea, skin rashes, and fever. Although high-dose therapy frequently requires intensive care unit–based management, lower doses of IL-2 can be effectively administered in an outpatient setting with equivalent overall clinical activity, but fewer durable complete remissions.
6. **Monoclonal antibodies** directed against tumor antigens can be produced by conventional hybridoma technology or by recombinant engineering. Targets for monoclonal antibodies include antigens that are **selectively expressed** by malignant cells [e.g., carcinoembryonic antigen (CEA)] or that exert important **functional effects** on malignant cell growth or viability when they are engaged (e.g., HER2/*neu,* epidermal growth factor receptor).
   a. **Diagnostic uses.** Monoclonal antibodies targeting differentiation antigens or other cancer-related extracellular or intracellular structures facilitate histopathologic diagnosis. They have particular value in staging leukemias and lymphomas and in identifying the origin of poorly differentiated tumors.
   b. **Therapeutic uses.** Recent years have witnessed the emergence of several monoclonal antibodies for the treatment of various malignancies. As the concept of targeted therapy gains more momentum, more monoclonal antibodies and "small molecules" against specific targets have become available. Two antibodies have had the greatest impact on the treatment of patients with cancer thus far.
      (1) Trastuzumab (Herceptin™), a monoclonal antibody directed against the extracellular domain of HER2/*neu* oncogene–derived protein, directly inhibits breast cancer cell growth and potentiates the effects of cytotoxic chemotherapeutic agents such as taxanes and platinum compounds. Herceptin has been approved by the Food and Drug Administration (FDA) for the treatment of metastatic breast cancer patients whose tumors overexpress HER2/*neu,* either as a single agent or in conjunction with traditional chemotherapeutic agents.
      (2) Rituximab (Rituxan™) is a chimeric monoclonal antibody against the CD20 antigen on the surface of mature B lymphocytes. This agent is approved by the FDA for the treatment of patients with B cell non-Hodgkin's lymphoma (NHL). Clinical trials have shown that, even in previously treated patients, single-agent Rituximab is effective in inducing remissions. However, there is no evidence that the overall survival of patients with B cell NHL is improved by the use of this antibody. Rituximab in conjunction with chemotherapy is

now the standard of care in the management of patients with intermediate and high-grade lymphoma.

(3) Other antibodies are emerging as well. Bevacizumab (Avastin™) is a recombinant humanized monoclonal antibody against the vascular endothelial growth factor (VEGF). This anti-angiogenesis target has been shown to be effective in the treatment of a number of malignancies, including kidney, colorectal, and lung cancers. In combination with chemotherapy, it is expected to be approved by the FDA for the treatment of advanced colorectal cancer based on recently reported studies. This novel approach carries the promise of depriving the tumor of the essential blood supply it needs for its growth and perhaps metastases. The mechanisms underlying the efficacy of these antibodies are under investigation but include the following possibilities:

(4) Immunologic destruction of tumor cells via complement-mediated cytotoxicity and antibody-dependent cell-mediated cytotoxicity

(5) Direct inhibition of tumor growth via engagement of cell surface ligands to perturb signal transduction pathways

c. Other uses

(1) Antibodies may be used ex vivo to purge autologous bone marrow of residual tumor cells before reinfusion after high-dose cytotoxic chemotherapy.

(2) Antibodies also have potential utility as vehicles for the delivery of radioisotopes and chemotherapeutic agents.

(a) **Radiolabeled Monoclonal Antibodies**

Two radiolabeled antibodies have recently been approved by the FDA for the treatment of patients with low-grade, refractory NHL. Ibritumomab tiuxetan (Zevalin™) and tositumomab (Bexxar™) are capable of delivering lethal radiation doses to lymphoma cells. Both agents exhibit high levels of anti-tumor activity in heavily pretreated patients. Zevalin™ uses ^{90}Yttrium and Bexxar™ uses ^{131} Iodine as the sources of radiation. Both can be given on an outpatient basis with minimal risk to other patient contacts.

(b) **Chemoimmunoconjugates** that contain an antibody reactive with CD33 and the drug calicheamicin exhibit significant activity in chemotherapy-refractory acute myelogenous leukemia (AML).

(c) **Immunotoxins** that contain antibody-binding domains and catalytic toxins such as ricin A chain or *Pseudomonas* exotoxin have undergone extensive clinical testing.

(3) **Anti-idiotypic antibodies** induce the production of host antibodies that mimic and ultimately recognize tumor-associated cell-surface antigens. These agents are being investigated as possible **tumor vaccines.**

7. Cancer vaccines may result from new understanding of tumor immunology and the components and regulation of the human antitumor immune response. Modern molecular biology and progress in genetic engineering have generated interest in these vaccines.

a. Tumor cell vaccines, usually lethally irradiated and then administered with various immunologic adjuvants, have not proved consistently beneficial but continue to be actively studied, particularly as adjuvant therapy in high-risk colon cancer. Genes for cytokines such as **GM-CSF** or **IL-2** or immune costimulatory molecules such as **B7.1** have been introduced into **genetically modified tumor cell vaccines** to stimulate local immune responses and break immunologic tolerance to otherwise cryptic tumor antigens. Purified or recombinantly produced tumor antigens can be admixed with adjuvants to induce specific immunity to those antigens.

b. Typically, the goal of cancer vaccine efforts has been to induce **T cell–mediated cytotoxic immune responses,** because these seem to be the most relevant to cancers based on preclinical models. To this end, **peptide vaccines** have been developed; the peptides bind to class I MHC molecules and are recognized by defined T-cell receptors whose engagement mediates tumor regression. These peptides can be mixed in conventional adjuvants or can be directly loaded onto professional antigen-presenting cells such as **dendritic cells.** T-cell recognition epitopes from a variety of antigens identified to be targets in regressing melanomas have been prepared as peptide vaccines, and peptide vaccines have been prepared from other potential tumor antigens in other diseases. Dendritic cells also can be directly loaded with whole proteins, or even transduced with the genetic material from a defined gene or malignant cell to stimulate a class I–dependent immune response.

c. Vaccines designed to stimulate antibody responses are under active investigation as well in a number of disease settings, using defined immunogens as well as the anti-idiotype approach [see III D 6 c (3)].

8. **Angiogenesis inhibition,** which is based on the observation that neovascularization is a necessary component of cancer growth, has become an exciting area of cancer investigation, culminating in the development of Bevacizumab™ (see section 6.b). Accordingly, inhibition of the normal host response to angiogenic factors (e.g., vascular endothelial growth factor, basic fibroblast growth factor, angiogenin) elaborated by tumor cells should exert a profound antiproliferative effect. In preclinical models, a number of strategies have exhibited promise, and early clinical trials are being conducted to identify the most promising strategies for future implementation.

IV LUNG CANCER

A Incidence The frequency of lung cancer is increasing rapidly. Originally a disease that primarily afflicted men older than age 60 years, lung cancer has become the second most common cause of cancer in women. It is the leading cause of cancer death in both men and women.

B Etiology Epidemiologic studies have linked lung cancer to the following factors:

1. **Cigarette smoking.** Research has demonstrated a direct correlation between smoking and lung cancer, with increases in daily cigarette consumption leading to increases in cancer incidence. "Passive smoking" is associated with a small but significant increase in the incidence of lung cancer.
2. **Industrial carcinogens.** Exposure to beryllium, radon, and asbestos has been linked to lung cancer. Cigarette smoking exacerbates the risk associated with such exposure. Smoking and asbestos exposure increase the risk 53-fold.
3. **Air pollutants** (e.g., diesel exhaust, pitch, tar, arsenic, chromium, cadmium, nickel) increase the risk of lung cancer.
4. **Existing lung damage.** Adenocarcinomas of the lung may develop in areas scarred by **tuberculosis** or other lung conditions associated with **fibrosis.** These tumors are called **scar carcinomas.**
5. Patients with **lymphoma** or **malignancies of the head, neck,** and **esophagus** have an increased incidence of lung cancer.

C Pathology There are four major varieties of lung cancer: three types are commonly described as non–small-cell lung cancer (non-SCLC), and one is termed small-cell lung cancer (SCLC).

1. **Squamous cell carcinomas** (non-SCLC) were once the most common type of non-SCLC, but they have become less common than adenocarcinomas. Squamous cell tumors tend to arise centrally near the hilum, where they present as endobronchial disease or as a peripheral lesion.
2. **Adenocarcinoma** (non-SCLC) is increasing in frequency, especially in women. These lesions are often peripheral, occurring in more distal airways. **Bronchoalveolar cell cancer,** a variant of adenocarcinoma, arises in the alveoli and causes lobular consolidation on the chest radiograph.

3. **Large-cell undifferentiated cancers** (non-SCLC) account for 5%–10% of all lung cancers. These tumors are usually peripheral lesions.
4. **Small-cell lung carcinoma** (SCLC) arises from neural crest neuroendocrine or amine precursor uptake and decarboxylation cells and progresses rapidly without treatment. The average survival time in the absence of treatment is only 2–4 months.

D Clinical features

1. **Local symptoms** of intrathoracic disease include cough, hemoptysis, obstructive pneumonia (due to endobronchial tumors), chest pain, pleural effusion, hoarseness (due to recurrent laryngeal nerve compression by a mediastinal tumor), and superior vena cava syndrome (due to obstruction of the vessel by a mediastinal tumor). Patients with bronchoalveolar cell cancer may have a severe cough productive of clear sputum.
2. **Systemic manifestations** include:
   a. Anorexia and weight loss
   b. Bone pain from distant metastases
   c. Hepatomegaly, tenderness, and fever caused by liver involvement
   d. CNS signs or seizures from brain metastases or carcinomatous meningitis
   e. Hypercalcemia from bone metastases or other humoral substances
3. Patients with SCLC may present with symptoms of ectopic hormone production or other **paraneoplastic syndromes.**
   a. **Ectopic adrenocorticotropic hormone (ACTH) secretion** causes hypokalemia and muscle wasting.
   b. **Syndrome of inappropriate antidiuretic hormone secretion (SIADH)** results in hyponatremia.

E Diagnosis

1. **Sputum cytology or bronchoscopy** confirms the diagnosis in patients with endobronchial disease. Bronchoscopy also assesses proximal endobronchial tumor extension and the status of the contralateral lung. It should be performed in all patients with centrally located tumors and in selected patients with peripheral tumors, especially if they are potential surgical candidates.
2. **Transthoracic needle biopsy,** guided by radiography or CT, is often necessary for the diagnosis of peripheral lesions. The false-negative rate is 15%.
3. **Transbronchial needle aspiration** of mediastinal nodes may obviate the need for more invasive procedures.
4. **Thoracotomy** or **mediastinoscopy** is required in approximately 5%–10% of patients. These invasive procedures are especially useful in the diagnosis of SCLC, which grows centrally in the mediastinum rather than endobronchially. Mediastinoscopy or mediastinotomy also can be used to assess the resectability of mediastinal and hilar nodes.
5. **Video-assisted transthorascopic surgery (VATS)** is less invasive than thoracotomy. VATS involves three or four incisions (1–2 cm) in the chest wall, diaphragm, lung parenchyma, and mediastinal structures. Visible lesions may be removed by biopsy.
6. **Node biopsy** is used to evaluate suspicious supraclavicular or neck lymph nodes.
7. **CT scans** of the chest, liver, brain, and adrenal glands can establish the **extent of metastatic disease** and can provide important information about mediastinal node involvement and chest wall invasion.
8. **Radionuclide bone scans** may be used to rule out metastatic disease.
9. **MRI** of the chest is most useful for evaluating spread to cardiovascular organs (e.g., heart, aorta, superior vena cava).

10. **PET Scan** (Positron Emission Tomography) is now widely used in the initial staging of patients with non-small-cell lung cancer (IVc). It provides better information regarding the involvement of medistinal nodes and can therefore affect the staging of patients. It also plays a role in post-treatment and follow-up phases of patient care.

F Staging **Please refer to the most recent edition of the American Joint Committee on Cancer (AJCC) Manual of Cancer Staging Table for complete staging information of all cancers discussed in this chapter.***

1. **Non-SCLC.** Because **surgery is the only curative option,** the goals of staging are to evaluate tumor resectability and to determine the extent of disease spread beyond the hemithorax.
2. **SCLC**
   a. Staging aims to differentiate between limited and extensive disease.
      (1) **Limited disease** is that which is confined to one hemithorax; the entire tumor can be encompassed in a single radiation therapy portal.
      (2) **Extensive disease** is characterized by distant metastases, supraclavicular node involvement, or pleural effusions.
   b. Staging procedures include chest radiography; CT of the chest, liver, and brain, followed by bone scans with plain film radiography of suspicious areas; and bilateral bone marrow biopsies or aspirates.

G Therapy

1. **Non-SCLC**
   a. **Pretreatment considerations**
      (1) A tumor is resectable if **thoracotomy** demonstrates that all of the tumor can be completely excised with pathologically negative margins.
      (2) Mediastinoscopy or mediastinotomy should be used only if positive findings will prevent a curative thoracotomy.
   b. **Therapeutic modalities**
      (1) **Surgery**
         (a) **Operable tumors.** If cardiopulmonary status is compatible with lung resection, surgical options include lobectomy or pneumonectomy, depending on the extent of disease. The surgeon should aim to remove the tumor completely with adequate margins of resection while conserving as much normal lung tissue as possible.
         (b) **Advanced local cancer.** Selected patients may undergo surgical resection with or without chest irradiation.
            (i) Patients with small tumors in the ipsilateral mediastinal nodes or large primary tumors without mediastinal node involvement have 5-year survival rates as high as 35% with a combination of surgery and radiation therapy.
            (ii) **Pancoast's tumor** or tumors of the superior sulcus also may be cured by a combination of surgery and radiation therapy.
      (2) **Radiation therapy**
         (a) Radiation therapy reduces local recurrences in operable stage II tumors.
         (b) Patients who cannot tolerate surgery because of insufficient cardiopulmonary reserve should receive chest irradiation. Survival rates at 5 years range from 5% to 20%.
         (c) **Definitive radiation therapy** is often used in patients with **unresectable but localized cancers,** with less than 5% long-term survival. **Palliative radiation therapy** can relieve the symptoms of pain, hemoptysis, superior vena cava syndrome, or pneumonitis that are associated with obstructive lesions. Selected patients with metastatic disease may also be treated with palliative radiation.

*For full staging information, please see the most recent edition of the AJCC Cancer Staging Handbook.

(3) **Chemotherapy**

(a) The benefit of adjuvant chemotherapy in patients with resected tumors was demonstrated in an international study of over 1800 patients with non-SCLC who were treated with up to 4 cycles of a platinum-based combination chemotherapy after resection of their primary tumors. Results of this study showed a 5% improvement in overall survival. Several studies have shown that neoadjuvant chemotherapy improves survival in stage III patients. In one study, researchers found that two courses of cisplatin and vinblastine before radiation therapy in stage III unresectable patients was superior to radiation alone. The survival rates were 55% (versus 40%) at 1 year, 26% (versus 13%) at 2 years, and 23% (versus 11%) at 3 years. In addition, several studies have shown that concurrent chemo-radiation therapy is superior to sequential treatment.

(b) Combination chemotherapy has a response rate of approximately 10%–30% **in patients with metastatic non-SCLC.** Response rates double in ambulatory patients who have not lost weight. The most commonly used drug combinations include:

(i) Carboplatin and paclitaxel
(ii) Cisplatin and etoposide
(iii) Gemcitabine and cisplatin or carboplatin
(iv) Irinotecan and cisplatin
(v) Vinorelbine and cisplatin
(vi) Docetaxel and carboplatin

2. SCLC

a. **Pretreatment considerations.** With **limited disease,** the highest long-term survival rates (10%–50%) are obtained with **concurrent radiation therapy and chemotherapy.** Hyperfractionated radiation therapy combined with chemotherapy may improve treatment outcome.

b. **Therapeutic modalities**

(1) **Chemotherapy** (mainstay of treatment). For **extensive disease,** single-agent or **combination chemotherapy** is standard.

(a) **Commonly used regimens** include etoposide plus cisplatin or carboplatin.

(b) Other active drugs include ifosfamide, vincristine, paclitaxel, topotecan, and irinotecan. Combination chemotherapy with cisplatin and irinotecan has shown promise in a recent phase II trial.

(2) **Radiation therapy. Prophylactic cranial irradiation** should be considered in responsive patients with limited disease. Radiation therapy has only palliative benefit in patients whose condition has failed to respond to chemotherapy or who have brain metastases.

H Prognosis

1. **Non-SCLC.** Key prognostic factors include the **extent of tumor dissemination, performance status,** and **weight loss.**

a. Survival rates range from 40% to 50% in stage I disease and from 15% to 30% in stage II disease.

b. Higher rates are observed in patients who undergo extensive mediastinal node sampling.

c. Patients with metastatic disease have median survivals of under 1 year.

2. **Limited SCLC.** Long-term survival rates in patients with **limited SCLC** vary from 10% to 50% after combined chemotherapy and radiation therapy. Extensive disease is not curable, however, and median survival does not exceed 1 year, despite initial responsiveness to chemotherapy.

I Mesothelioma

This is a neoplasm that arises from the mesothelial lining of the pleural and peritoneal cavities. It has a very poor prognosis, with a median survival of 6–18 months, and so far no effective treatments have been identified. A very select group of patients is surgically treated, and even then the overall survival is poor. There is a high association between asbestos exposure and the development of this disease. Smoking and asbestos exposure increases the risk of development of lung cancer by 90-fold. Several chemotherapeutic agents have been evaluated for the treatment of this condition. These include Doxil, gemcitabine, cisplatin, and carboplatin. Most recently, multi-targeted antifolate pemetrexed (Alimta™) has received much attention as a possible new and effective agent in the treatment of mesotheliomas. The combination of this agent with a platinum agent is superior to the use of platinum alone.

V BREAST CANCER

A Incidence Breast carcinoma has increased in frequency over the last decade. As many as one in nine women will develop breast cancer during her lifetime.

B Risk factors

1. **Family history.** At least two hereditary patterns are characteristic of breast cancer.
   a. **Familial aggregation** is associated with a modest increase in risk and is relatively common. The risk is markedly increased among first-degree relatives.
   b. **True genetic pattern.** Linkage to a specific gene with high penetrance accounts for fewer than 5% of all cases of breast cancer. Cancer tends to occur at a younger age and is more likely to be bilateral. Multiple family members over three or more generations are affected.
      (1) **p53** is a tumor suppressor gene that appears in carriers and patients in Li-Fraumeni families. The gene is located on chromosome 17.
      (2) Mutations in the **BRCA1 gene,** located on chromosome 17q, are seen in some patients with a family history of breast and ovarian cancer. Mutations in the BRCA2 gene also confer increased risk for breast cancer.
2. **Early menarche**
3. **Late menopause**
4. **Nulliparity or a first pregnancy after age 30 years**
5. **Fibrocystic breast disease**
6. **Prior history of invasive or noninvasive breast cancers** [intraductal or lobular carcinoma in situ (CIS)]
7. **Age**
8. **Estrogen replacement therapy (ERT)** is associated with a modest relative risk of breast cancer.
9. **Prolonged use of oral contraceptives** before the first pregnancy
10. **Dietary factors** [e.g., high-fat diet (unproven), alcohol consumption]

C Pathology Breast cancers are adenocarcinomas.

1. **Classification.** Most breast cancers are irregular masses or areas associated with microcalcifications.
   a. **Papillary carcinomas** (1% of breast cancers) are low-grade, noninvasive intraductal lesions.
   b. **Medullary carcinomas** (5%–10% of breast cancers) are large bulky tumors that have a low-grade infiltrating tendency and are surrounded by lymphocytes.
   c. **Inflammatory carcinomas** (5% of breast cancers) invade the dermal lymphatics and cause skin redness, induration, warmth, and an erysipeloid margin.
   d. **Infiltrating ductal carcinomas** (70% of breast cancers) are characterized by nests and cords of tumor cells surrounded by a dense collagenous stroma.
2. **Hormone receptor status.** Breast cancer can be classified according to the presence or absence of ERs, which are cellular proteins found in hormone-responsive tissues. Receptor status can change over the course of the disease. The 20%–30% of breast cancer patients with HER2/*neu*

oncogene gene amplification and overexpression have more aggressive cancers and may have greater drug resistance.

a. **ER-positive** tumors are more common in postmenopausal patients. Approximately 60% of primary breast cancers have detectable ER.

b. **ER-negative** tumors are common in premenopausal patients. One third of patients with ER-negative primary breast cancers develop recurrent tumors that are ER-positive.

D Diagnosis

1. **Early detection.** Routine breast self-examination and screening mammography have led to earlier detection of curable breast cancers.
   a. **Breast self-examination.** All women should be taught the technique of breast self-examination. Such examinations are best performed monthly after the menstrual period, when breast swelling and fibrocystic changes are less likely to interfere with the detection of a lump or mass. More than 80% of breast cancers occur as painless masses.
   b. **Mammography.** All women between 35 and 40 years of age should have a baseline mammogram.
      (1) Depending on the presence of known risk factors, patients should undergo mammography either yearly or every other year between age 40 and 50 years, and yearly after age 50 years.
      (2) Women with risk factors for breast carcinoma should have a yearly mammogram at an earlier age.
2. **Pretreatment evaluation**
   a. In addition to a **medical history, physical examination, chest radiograph,** and **routine laboratory tests** (e.g., blood count, liver and renal function values, and serum calcium), all women with newly diagnosed breast cancer should have a **mammogram to detect multicentricity** or **bilateral involvement.**
   b. **Radiologic tests** may include a bone scan and, in advanced breast cancer, a CT or MRI scan of the liver, as dictated by clinical presentation. If a bone scan shows evidence of metastatic disease and radiographs are negative, a CT scan or MRI scan of the bone or a bone biopsy should be performed to determine the correct therapy.
   c. **Excisional biopsy** is indicated for patients who are good candidates for lumpectomy and breast preservation. **Needle biopsy** also may be helpful for diagnostic purposes before excisional biopsy.
   d. Patients with metastatic disease may have elevation in CA 15–3 or CEA **tumor markers.** The value of these markers to monitor disease status remains controversial.

E Staging.*

F Therapy

The primary goal of local therapy is to provide optimal control of the disease in the breast and regional tissues while providing the best possible cosmetic result. Systemic therapy should be given to patients at high risk for metastatic disease to eradicate micrometastases. Patients should be seen by a medical oncologist, radiation therapist, and surgeon to determine the best course of treatment, which may include surgery, radiation therapy, adjuvant chemotherapy, adjuvant endocrine therapy, or a combination of modalities.

1. **Surgery**
   a. The optimal surgical **approach** is determined by the following factors.
      (1) Disease stage
      (2) Tumor size
      (3) Tumor location
      (4) Breast size and configuration
      (5) Number of tumors in the breast

*For full staging information, please see the most recent edition of the AJCC Cancer Staging Handbook.

(6) Available surgical and radiotherapeutic techniques
(7) Patient preference concerning breast conservation

b. **Procedures.** In the past, most patients underwent modified radical mastectomy. Recent data indicate that breast conservation procedures such as lumpectomy plus radiation allow adequate local control of the tumor and improve cosmetic outcome in selected cases; however, not all patients are suitable candidates for breast conservation (see Table 4–13)

(1) **Modified radical mastectomy** entails removal of the breast and axillary contents with preservation of the pectoral muscles. Patients may undergo breast reconstruction during surgery or at a later time.

(2) **Partial mastectomy,** or **lumpectomy,** involves excision of the tumor and an adjacent rim of normal tissue.

(a) **Level I or II axillary dissection** is performed for adequate staging and local control. **Sentinel node biopsy** has emerged as a useful means for limiting lymph node dissection.

(b) **Level III dissection** should be considered in patients with clinically positive lymph nodes.

(c) After surgery, external beam radiation is used in some patients with multiple positive lymph nodes, with a boost to the local tumor site.

2. **Radiation therapy**

a. **Patients treated with lumpectomy and axillary dissection** should receive definitive radiation therapy to the breast. Patients with positive lymph nodes should receive radiation to the lymphatic bed.

b. **Patients undergoing mastectomy** should be considered for postoperative radiation if they have any of the following risk factors for local recurrence.

(1) Primary tumor > 4 cm
(2) More than three positive axillary nodes
(3) Tumors involving the margin of surgical resection, invasion of pectoral fascia or muscle, or extranodal extension into the axillary fat

c. In **patients at high risk for distant metastases,** radiation therapy can be given concurrently or delayed until the completion of adjuvant chemotherapy. The risk of ipsilateral arm lymphedema is increased by postoperative axillary radiation.

3. **Adjuvant chemotherapy.** This technique delays or prevents recurrence and improves survival in patients with positive axillary nodes as well as in some patients with negative axillary nodes. Premenopausal patients with positive axillary nodes are most likely to benefit from chemotherapy; such patients experience a 25%–30% reduction in mortality.

a. **Combination chemotherapy.** This approach is commonly used in the high-risk adjuvant setting, and 4–6 months of treatment are usually sufficient to obtain maximal benefit. In patients

TABLE 4–13 Contraindications for Breast Conservation Surgery

Large tumor in a small breast (increases likelihood of poor cosmetic results)
Subareolar primary tumors
More than one tumor in the breast
Contraindications to radiation therapy
Advanced disease (i.e., beyond stage II)
Large areas of intraductal disease or microcalcifications
Tumors with an extensive intraductal component (i.e., >25% of the primary tumor is in situ and there is at least one focus of breast cancer that is in situ in normal breast tissue and is separate from the breast primary)

with metastatic breast cancer, the use of effective single agents may be as effective as the use of more active but more toxic combination chemotherapy regimens. High-dose therapy with autologous stem cell rescue, which does not improve treatment outcomes in women with metastatic disease, is not standard therapy in the high-risk setting. Four to six cycles of therapy (depending on the regimen employed) over 3 to 6 months are as effective as longer treatment periods.

b. Drug regimens. Maximally tolerated doses should be used unless significant toxicity develops.

(1) The most commonly used adjuvant therapy regimens contain some combination of the agents doxorubicin, cyclophosphamide, methotrexate, and 5-FU. In hormone receptor–positive cancers, tamoxifen or other hormonal agents are widely used as well. Taxanes are now important components of adjuvant therapy in patients with node-positive disease. The anti HER2-*neu* antibody, Herceptin™, is still under investigation for use in the adjuvant setting.

(2) Patients at higher risk for developing recurrent or metastatic disease are typically offered doxorubicin- or taxane-containing regimens.

(3) Other **active chemotherapeutic agents** may be used to palliate patients with metastatic disease. These include the taxanes [paclitaxel (Taxol) or docetaxel (Taxotere)], the anti-HER2/*neu* antibody trastuzamab (Herceptin), vinblastine, vinorelbine, gemcitabine, and oral formulations of 5-FU.

4. Adjuvant endocrine therapy

a. Hormonal therapy

(1) **Postmenopausal patients with positive hormone receptors.** The estrogen antagonist tamoxifen is the preferred agent. In these patients, tamoxifen delays recurrence and improves survival.

(a) The benefit of tamoxifen in premenopausal patients with ER-positive tumors is less clear.

(b) Patients with ER-negative tumors exhibit little or no response.

(2) **Hormonal therapy for metastatic breast cancer**

(a) Hormonal therapy is appropriate for patients with subcutaneous metastases, lymph node involvement, pleural effusions, bone metastases, and nonlymphangitic lung metastases. Most patients with liver metastases, lymphangitic disease of the lung, pericardial metastases, or other potentially life-threatening metastases are treated initially with chemotherapy to obtain a rapid response, but such treatment decisions must be customized.

(b) Patients with ER-positive primary tumors exhibit response rates of at least 30% to hormone therapy. If the tumor contains both positive estrogen and progesterone receptors, response rates are higher.

(c) Postmenopausal patients whose hormone receptor status is unknown may respond to hormone therapy.

(d) Patients with a previous response to hormonal therapy may respond to discontinuation of the original agent and substitution of a second agent.

(e) Other hormonal therapies include megestrol (Megace), anastrozole (Arimidex), fluoxymesterone (Halotestin), aminoglutethimide, and luteinizing hormone–releasing hormone (LH-RH) antagonists.

b. The results of studies of **ovarian ablation by radiation, oophorectomy,** or **chemical ablation** in premenopausal patients have been mixed. Certain subgroups may gain long-term benefits.

5. Other types of breast cancer and treatment recommendations

a. Intraductal breast cancer. Because the tumor is noninvasive (i.e., confined to the ducts), careful pathologic review can exclude any risk of lymph node involvement or distant metastases. The prognosis is excellent.

(1) Patients may be treated by total mastectomy or by lumpectomy followed by radiation, although this procedure is associated with a slightly higher incidence of second breast primaries.

(2) Axillary node dissection is controversial; most experts believe it is unnecessary.

(3) Ductal carcinoma in situ (CIS) may require definitive surgery. Tamoxifen is widely used in the postoperative setting.

b. **Lobular CIS.** Patients with this noninvasive lesion are at high risk for development of invasive cancer in both breasts. Treatment options include bilateral mastectomy, rigorous observation and follow-up, and tamoxifen therapy.

c. **Stage I and stage II disease.** Most patients have the option of either modified radical mastectomy or breast conservation with lumpectomy, axillary dissection, or postoperative radiation therapy. Adjuvant therapy should be offered to high-risk stage I patients and all stage II patients.

d. **Stage III disease.** Treatment options are determined by tumor resectability.

(1) **Patients with operable tumors** are generally treated with modified radical mastectomy and postoperative radiation therapy. These patients frequently receive preoperative or postoperative adjuvant chemotherapy.

(2) **Patients with inoperable stage III disease** have a high rate of local and distant recurrence and poor survival rates.

(a) A combined-modality approach, using systemic chemotherapy in addition to surgery and radiation, is required.

(b) In most cases, aggressive combination chemotherapy is initiated after biopsy to reduce tumor bulk, facilitate local treatment, and treat distant micrometastases.

e. **Cord compression.** This is an oncologic emergency and represents metastatic disease. Metastatic disease to the vertebrae could impinge upon the spinal cord. Pain is the usual symptom at the level of involvement. Neurologic symptoms could range from mild difficulty ambulating to loss of bowel and urinary bladder function., depending on the location of the lesion. Prompt intervention with high dose steroids and immediate radiation therapy is indicated.

G Prognosis Approximately 50% of patients with operable breast cancer develop recurrent disease unless they receive adjuvant chemotherapy or hormone therapy. Prognostic factors include:

1. **Tumor size.** This factor is the most important predictor of recurrence and survival. Tumors larger than 5 cm are associated with a decreased survival rate and an increased risk of recurrence.
2. **Axillary node status.** Seventy percent of patients with negative nodes are disease-free at 10 years. This figure declines to 40% of patients with no more than three positive nodes and 15%–25% of patients with four or more positive nodes.
3. **Histopathology.** Poorly differentiated tumors with high nuclear grades have higher recurrence rates.
4. **Hormone receptor status.** Of primary breast cancers, 60%–70% express ERs, and 40%–50% express progesterone receptors. Patients with hormone receptor–positive tumors have lower rates of recurrence and prolonged survival rates compared with those with receptor-negative tumors.
5. **S-phase fraction and DNA index.** The S-phase fraction (i.e., the percentage of tumor cells in the S phase of the cell cycle) is proportional to the tumor growth rate. Patients with aneuploid tumors or high S-phase fractions, as determined by flow cytometry, have a poor prognosis compared with those with slow-growing diploid tumors.
6. **Oncogenic expression.** Expression of the HER-2/*neu* oncogene is associated with a poor prognosis.
7. **Other prognostic factors.** In some studies, the following prognostic factors have been associated with a poorer prognosis: cathepsin-D, mutated p53, epidermal growth factor receptor, and tumor growth factor-β (TGF-β).

VI GASTROINTESTINAL CANCERS

A Carcinoma of the colon, rectum, and anus

1. **Incidence.** Cancers of the colon and rectum occur in 132,000 individuals annually in the United States and account for 56,000 deaths each year.
   a. All adults older than 40 years with signs or symptoms consistent with colorectal neoplasms should undergo testing to exclude the presence of a mass lesion in the colon or rectum.
   b. All adults aged 50 years or older should undergo regular digital rectal examinations and stool occult blood testing, along with less frequent flexible sigmoidoscopy, barium enema, or colonoscopy.

2. **Etiology.** Genetic and epidemiologic studies have linked colon and rectal cancer to the following factors:
   a. **Inherited predisposition.** Familial syndromes such as adenomatous polyposis coli (APC), an autosomal dominant disorder caused by mutations in the FAP gene on chromosome 5, may lead to an increased risk of colon cancer. In APC, cancers commonly develop in adolescence and young adulthood, and the incidence of colorectal neoplasms is nearly 100% by age 50. Hereditary nonpolyposis colon cancer (HNPCC), which is also familial, is associated with a lower but significant risk of cancer of the colon and rectum. Mutations in tumor suppressor genes such as MCC, DCC, BRCA1, and p53 also confer higher risks for colorectal neoplasms.
   b. **Somatic mutation.** The well-established genetic changes that accompany the progression from epithelial hyperplasia through polyp formation and eventual cancer development form a continuum. These changes indicate an association among inherited predispositions (e.g., mutated p53) and acquired mutations in either tumor suppressor genes such as DCC or in oncogenes such as *ras.*
   c. **Dietary influence.** The higher incidence of colorectal neoplasms in industrialized western societies has led to hypotheses that high-fat, low-fiber diets that are deficient in calcium, selenium, and other trace elements predispose individuals to the development of colorectal neoplasms.
   d. **Preexisting inflammatory disease.** Inflammatory bowel disease, particularly ulcerative colitis with pancolitis, is associated with a higher incidence of colorectal neoplasms.

3. **Pathology**
   a. The large majority of colorectal neoplasms are **adenocarcinomas,** and most are well or moderately differentiated. Poorly differentiated neoplasms are associated with poor prognosis.
   b. **Squamous cell carcinomas** can arise in the anus. Such neoplasms differ from adenocarcinomas in terms of biology and therapy.

4. **Clinical features**
   a. **Local symptoms** include a change in bowel habits that may involve constipation, diarrhea, a change in stool caliber, crampy abdominal pain, and rectal bleeding. Signs of obstruction may occur. Tenesmus may be present in rectal primaries. Patients with locally advanced rectal carcinoma may present with symptoms of perineal pain.
   b. **Systemic manifestations** are uncommon in individuals with localized neoplasms. When the cancer has metastasized to distant organs, the most common manifestations are:
      (1) Anorexia and weight loss
      (2) Hepatomegaly, pain, or fever due to liver involvement

5. **Diagnosis**
   a. **Barium enema, flexible sigmoidoscopy, or colonoscopy** are usually required to identify a suspicious mass lesion.
   b. **Biopsy** of suspicious lesions is needed to establish a diagnosis.
   c. When a diagnosis of colorectal neoplasia has been established, additional studies may be necessary both to evaluate the extent of local disease and to screen for metastatic disease.

(1) **CT scans of the pelvis** and **endorectal ultrasound** may be appropriate for rectal neoplasms.

(2) **CT scans of the chest and abdomen** can screen for the presence of intraabdominal (e.g., mesenteric or retroperitoneal lymph node enlargement), hepatic, or pulmonary metastases.

6. **Staging.*** Cure rates for $T_1N_0M_0$, $T_2N_0M_0$, and $T_3N_0M_0$ lesions are greater than 90%, 85%, and 70%, respectively. If primary cancers involve regional lymph nodes, cure rates with surgery alone are 35%–40%. These rates decrease with increasing numbers of involved lymph nodes or increasing T stage.

7. **Therapy**

a. **Colorectal cancer**

(1) **Surgery**

(a) **Colon cancer.** Treatment of cancers above the peritoneal reflection usually involves **partial colectomy,** unless the extent of metastatic disease and the absence of colonic obstruction necessitate systemic chemotherapy [see VI A 7 a (3)]. Principles of surgical oncology, including the establishment of wide surgical margins, should be followed to optimize patient outcome. In experienced hands, laparoscopic partial colectomy is acceptable.

(b) **Rectal cancer.** Treatment involves either abdominoperineal resection or, if the lesion is in the high rectum, low anterior resection that preserves sphincter function and does not require colostomy. Experimental approaches for low rectal tumors include preoperative chemotherapy and radiation followed by segmental rectum resection with formation of a coloanal anastomosis.

(2) **Radiation therapy**

(a) **Colon cancer.** Prospective randomized trials have not established the value of adjunctive radiation for enhancement of surgical cures. Nevertheless, adjunctive radiation, frequently in combination with chemotherapy, is commonly offered to patients with T_4 lesions or those with positive operative margins.

(b) **Rectal cancer. Adjunctive radiation, in conjunction with chemotherapy,** enhances cure rates in patients with transmural or lymph node–positive rectal neoplasms.

(3) **Chemotherapy. 5-FU** has long been the mainstay of chemotherapy for colorectal neoplasms. Biochemical modulation of 5-FU to enhance its mechanism of action can be achieved either by administering the agent by continuous intravenous infusion, or by coadministering calcium leucovorin. **Calcium leucovorin** enhances the binding of the primary 5-FU metabolite, 5-fluorodeoxyuridine (5-FUDR) to its substrate, thymidylate synthase, which is required for pyrimidine synthesis. Recently, another agent, **irinotecan,** has been approved for use and appears to have a degree of efficacy similar to that of 5-FU. Another new agent, **oxaliplatin,** also shows promise. Newly available oral formulations based on 5-FU such as **capecitabine** offer greater ease of administration and continuous exposure to the drug, which maximizes antitumor properties.

(a) **Adjuvant therapy for colon cancer.** Surgery cures only 35%–40% of patients with lymph node–positive (e.g., any T, N_1 or N_2, M_0) colon cancer. Cure rates increase to approximately 50% when such patients are treated for 6 months with 5-FU plus calcium leucovorin. Continuous infusional (CI) 5-FU regimens are being increasingly used based on ongoing clinical data from several studies, which show superiority of this treatment approach to the bolus administration.

(i) However, **the role of adjuvant chemotherapy in the management of patients with lymph node–negative (e.g., $T_3N_0M_0$) lesions remains controversial.**

*For full staging information, please see the most recent edition of the AJCC Cancer Staging Handbook.

Adjuvant chemotherapy is not indicated in patients with nontransmural cancers in the absence of regional lymph node involvement. Recent preliminary results from clinical trials suggest a benefit to the use of chemotherapy in the adjuvant setting.

(ii) The effectiveness of newer agents such as irinotecan, oxaliplatin, or capecitabine has not yet been proved in the adjuvant therapy setting.

(b) Adjuvant therapy for rectal cancer. The combined administration of radiation therapy and 5-FU improves cure rates. Typically, combined-modality therapy is administered postoperatively, followed by an additional 4 months of chemotherapy alone. Excellent results are also obtained when the chemoradiation precedes surgery.

(c) Pseudoadjuvant therapy following the resection of metastases. Rarely, individuals present with metastases that are solitary or restricted to a solitary organ and are amenable to either resection or some ablative procedure such as cryosurgery. In patients who undergo hepatic lobectomies to resect metastases, the combined use of a systemic 5-FU–based compound and intrahepatic arterial FUDR is associated with a survival benefit compared with surgery alone.

(d) Disseminated metastatic disease. Most commonly, metastases are disseminated, and chemotherapy is offered with palliative intent. Biochemically modulated 5-FU (e.g., continuous infusion or 5-FU plus calcium leucovorin) is the standard of care for patients with previously untreated metastatic disease. Chemotherapy with oxaliplatin or irinotecan is more active than 5-FU alone. Infusional 5-FU–based schedules are better tolerated and are at least as active as bolus 5-FU–based schedules and are emerging as the preferred schedules of administration. The angiogenesis inhibitor bevacizumab (Avastin™) improves both the response rate and overall survival in patients with newly diagnosed metastatic colon cancer, in conjunction with contemporary chemotherapy regimens.

(i) Capecitabine alone, or **irinotecan in combination with 5-FU and calcium leucovorin,** improves response rates and survival. In metastatic disease that is refractory to chemotherapy with 5-FU plus calcium leucovorin, irinotecan treatment improves response rates, time to progression, survival, and quality of life in comparison with either no therapy or continuous-infusion 5-FU. **Oxaliplatin** promises to add another option.

(ii) Other agents that are infrequently used include continuous infusions of **5-FU,** or single-agent administration of **mitomycin-C** or **nitrosoureas.**

b. Anal cancer. Combined-modality chemotherapy and radiation therapy for localized cancers usually involve **5-FU and mitomycin-C.** The majority of patients with localized cancers are cured, and function of the anal sphincter is preserved.

8. Prognosis

a. Colorectal cancer. Key prognostic factors include the **extent of tumor invasion, lymph node involvement,** and **the presence or absence of distant metastases.** Mutations in p53 result in an adverse prognosis, as does clinical presentation of bowel obstruction.

b. Anal cancer. Long-term survival rates in patients with **localized squamous cell carcinoma of the anus** are approximately 80% after combined chemotherapy and radiation therapy. However, metastatic disease is not curable, despite the initial responsiveness of this cancer to chemotherapy.

B Carcinoma of the pancreas

1. Incidence. Cancers of the pancreas occur in approximately 28,000 individuals annually in the United States and account for more than 27,000 deaths each year.

2. Etiology. Although scientists have found mutations in some putative tumor suppressor genes, the causes of pancreatic cancers remain unknown. Neither pancreatitis nor diabetes increases the risk of pancreatic cancer. Caffeine intake remains controversial as a cause of pancreatic cancer. Causes may include:

a. **Cigarette smoking**
b. **Dietary carcinogens**
c. **Environmental carcinogens**

3. **Pathology.** The vast majority of pancreatic neoplasms are adenocarcinomas. Most are poorly or moderately differentiated.
   a. **Adenocarcinomas** can arise in the head, body, or tail of the pancreas.
   b. **Neuroendocrine tumors** such as carcinoid tumors or islet cell tumors are less common but may be associated with hepatic metastases. In contrast to exocrine tumors, these malignancies may have relatively indolent natural histories. These tumors may produce hormones that induce **carcinoid syndrome,** which is characterized by flushing, hypotension, diarrhea, and valvular heart disease.

4. **Clinical features**
   a. **Local symptoms** may include painless jaundice, epigastric fullness, or symptoms of gastric outlet obstruction. When adjacent nerves are involved, patients commonly complain of abdominal pain that radiates into the back.
   b. **Systemic manifestations** are common and may include:
      (1) Anorexia, weight loss
      (2) Hepatomegaly, pain, or fever attributable to liver involvement
      (3) Bleeding (disorder) manifested by either recurrent superficial thrombophlebitis (Trousseau's syndrome), deep thrombophlebitis, or disseminated intravascular coagulation (DIC)

5. **Diagnosis.** Pancreatic cancer is notoriously difficult to diagnose, and patients frequently present when the cancer is not resectable for cure. Frequently used diagnostic modalities include the following:
   a. **CT scanning** may identify a suspicious mass lesion.
   b. **Biopsy** of suspicious lesions is needed to establish a diagnosis. This may be accomplished by endoscopic retrograde cholangiopancreatography (ERCP), fine-needle aspiration, or exploratory laparoscopy or laparotomy. Some authorities have expressed concern that fine-needle aspiration tracks may be sites of tumor implantation.
   c. When a diagnosis of pancreatic cancer has been established, additional studies may be necessary to evaluate the extent of local disease and to screen for metastatic disease.
      (1) Patients who are potential candidates for curative-attempt surgery frequently undergo **CT scans of the chest and abdomen,** along with **angiography or MRI-based imaging techniques** to assess patency and integrity of key vascular structures such as the superior mesenteric artery.
      (2) **Bone scans and brain imaging are not indicated** in patients with no symptoms of brain or bone metastases.

6. **Staging.***

7. **Therapy**
   a. **Localized disease**
      (1) **Surgery.** Surgery is the treatment of choice for patients with localized pancreatic cancer. With an experienced surgeon, the Whipple procedure may be performed with acceptable operative morbidity and mortality. However, only a small fraction of patients who undergo this operation or total pancreatectomies are cured of pancreatic cancer.
      (2) **Adjuvant chemotherapy and radiation therapy.** Postoperative radiation therapy administered in conjunction with **5-FU–based chemotherapy** has been shown to improve cure rates.

*For full staging information, please see the most recent edition of the AJCC Cancer Staging Handbook.

b. **Metastatic disease**
   (1) The approach to metastatic disease is purely palliative. Narcotic analgesics or celiac plexus blocks may palliate pain. Either operative bypass or the placement of biliary stents or catheters may palliate obstructive jaundice.
   (2) Chemotherapy using the antimetabolite **gemcitabine** improves quality of life and survival, but few patients with metastatic pancreatic adenocarcinoma survive beyond 1 year. 5-FU has less palliative benefit than does gemcitabine.

c. **Neuroendocrine tumors.** Many patients present with metastatic disease to the liver. **Carcinoid tumors** may have an indolent natural history, and patients may be followed for years before needing therapeutic intervention. Chemotherapy with **5-FU and streptozocin** can provide palliation. **Locoregional approaches** to liver metastases such as chemoembolization or intrahepatic arterial chemotherapy may be appropriate in selected patients. Metastatic **islet cell tumors** are responsive to chemotherapy with **streptozocin** and **doxorubicin.** Patients with **carcinoid syndrome** may benefit from treatment with **somatostatin analogs.**

8. **Prognosis**
   a. **Surgically resectable cancer.** Studies have found that patients who undergo surgery followed by adjuvant chemoradiation may have long-term survival as high as 40%.
   b. **Locally advanced, unresectable cancer.** These patients cannot be cured, but the use of chemotherapy plus radiation therapy increases average survival to approximately 1 year.
   c. **Metastatic cancer.** The survival of untreated patients averages about 3 months. This increases to almost 6 months when gemcitabine chemotherapy is used. Long-term survival is exceedingly rare.

C Carcinoma of the stomach

1. **Incidence.** Cancers of the stomach occur in approximately 23,000 individuals annually in the United States, and account for approximately 14,000 deaths each year. Striking decreases in the incidence of gastric adenocarcinomas have been noted in the United States since the early part of the twentieth century; the causes of this change are not known.

2. **Etiology.** The etiology of stomach cancers remains largely unknown. Some tumors are associated with infections by *Helicobacter pylori.*

3. **Pathology.** The vast majority of stomach neoplasms are adenocarcinomas. Most are poorly or moderately differentiated.
   a. **Adenocarcinomas** may originate in any part of the stomach. In the past few decades, there has been a rise in the incidence of adenocarcinomas arising in or near the gastroesophageal junction.
   b. **Lymphomas** may arise in the stomach.

4. **Clinical features**
   a. **Local symptoms** may include gastrointestinal bleeding, dyspepsia, dysphagia, odynophagia, or symptoms of gastric outlet obstruction.
   b. **Systemic manifestations** are common and may include:
      (1) Anorexia, weight loss
      (2) Fatigue due to anemia
      (3) Pain due to bone metastases
      (4) Hepatomegaly, pain, or fever due to liver involvement
      (5) Bleeding (disorder) manifested by either recurrent superficial thrombophlebitis (Trousseau's syndrome), deep thrombophlebitis, or DIC

5. **Diagnosis.** Patients with gastric cancer may present with **ulcers** or **gastrointestinal bleeding.** Cancers must be diagnosed and staged.
   a. An **upper gastrointestinal series or upper gastrointestinal endoscopy** establishes the presence of a mass. Occasionally, gastric cancer manifests as **linitis plastica,** without an obvious epithelial lesion, but with a submucosal tumor infiltrating the organ.

b. **Biopsy** should be performed in all gastric ulcers, even those that appear to be benign (if deemed safe). Ulcers should be followed carefully to ensure that complete healing occurs. Typically, endoscopic biopsy diagnoses the presence of a gastric cancer.

c. Commonly used **staging procedures** include the following:

(1) **CT scanning** may identify perigastric or celiac lymph node involvement. In addition, it can identify the presence of pulmonary, mediastinal, liver, retroperitoneal lymph node, or pelvic metastases.

(2) **Laparoscopy** may be used preoperatively to evaluate the omentum, which is a common site of metastasis that is poorly visualized on CT scans.

(3) **Bone scans and brain imaging are not indicated** in patients with no symptoms of brain or bone metastases.

6. **Staging.***

7. **Therapy**

a. **Surgery.** Surgery is the treatment of choice for patients with localized gastric cancer. The **probability of surgical cure is directly related to the stage of the cancer.** Patients with transmural, lymph node–involved cancers have surgical cure rates of only 15%.

(1) Because gastric cancer is typically diagnosed at relatively advanced stages in the United States, relatively few patients are cured. More extensive surgery, pioneered in Japan, has not been definitively shown to improve outcomes in patients with localized but advanced-stage cancers.

(2) **Adjuvant chemotherapy and chemotherapy.** Postoperative radiation therapy has not been shown to improve surgical outcomes in patients who have undergone surgery with curative intent. However, adjuvant therapy with radiation therapy plus 5-fluorouracil chemotherapy improves survival.

b. **Palliative approach to metastatic disease.** Narcotic analgesics or celiac plexus blocks may reduce pain. Either operative bypass or the placement of biliary stents or catheters may palliate obstructive jaundice. Although chemotherapeutic agents such as 5-FU, doxorubicin, mitomycin-C, etoposide, methotrexate, paclitaxel, docetaxel, or cisplatin have modest single-agent activity and may provide palliation of symptoms, they have no meaningful impact on survival. Combination therapy with two or more of these agents may improve quality of life and survival, but the overall impact is not great.

c. **Additional use of chemotherapy.** The treatment of **gastric lymphomas** typically involves chemotherapy. Aggressive chemotherapy of tumors that respond rapidly may result in gastric perforation, however.

8. **Prognosis**

a. **Surgically resectable cancer.** Cures result in the majority of patients who undergo surgery for early (e.g., $T_1N_0M_0$) lesions, but surgical cure rates decline rapidly with advancing disease stage.

b. **Metastatic cancer.** The average survival of untreated patients is approximately 6 months, and treatment with combination chemotherapy increases this time by only several months.

D Carcinoma of the esophagus

1. **Incidence.** Cancers of the esophagus occur in approximately 12,000 individuals annually in the United States and account for more than 11,000 deaths each year. Striking increases in the incidence of esophageal adenocarcinomas have been noted in the United States since the early part of the twentieth century; the causes of this change are not known.

2. **Etiology.** The etiology of esophageal cancers remains largely unknown. Most **adenocarcinomas** arise in **Barrett's esophagus,** but relatively few individuals with Barrett's esophagus develop esophageal malignancies. **Alcohol abuse** and **tobacco use** predispose individuals to squamous cell carcinomas.

*For full staging information, please see the most recent edition of the AJCC Cancer Staging Handbook.

3. **Pathology.** The vast majority of esophageal adenocarcinomas are poorly or moderately differentiated. **Adenocarcinomas** typically arise in or near the gastroesophageal junction in Barrett's esophagus. In the past few decades, the incidence of adenocarcinomas arising in or near the gastroesophageal junction has increased.
4. **Clinical features**
   a. **Local symptoms** most commonly include dyspepsia, dysphagia or odynophagia, and occasionally gastrointestinal bleeding.
   b. **Systemic manifestations** are common and may include:
      (1) Anorexia, weight loss
      (2) Fatigue due to anemia
      (3) Pain due to bone metastases
      (4) Hepatomegaly, pain, or fever due to liver involvement
5. **Diagnosis**
   a. Barium swallow or upper gastrointestinal endoscopy establishes the presence of a mass lesion.
   b. Typically, **endoscopic biopsy** diagnoses the presence of a gastric cancer.
   c. Commonly used **staging studies** include the following:
      (1) **CT scanning** may identify mediastinal or celiac lymph node involvement. It can identify the presence of pulmonary, liver, retroperitoneal lymph node, or pelvic metastases.
      (2) **Endoscopic ultrasound** may define the extent of tumor invasion in the esophagus and the presence of periesophageal lymph node enlargement.
      (3) **Laparoscopy** may be used preoperatively to evaluate the omentum, which is a common site of metastasis that is poorly visualized in CT scans.
      (4) **Bone scans and brain imaging are not indicated** in patients with no symptoms of brain or bone metastases.
6. **Staging.***
7. **Therapy**
   a. **Localized cancer**
      (1) **Surgery.** Cure may result from either surgery alone, chemotherapy and radiation therapy, or chemotherapy and radiation therapy followed by surgery. Surgery, either alone or preceded by chemotherapy and radiation therapy, is the most commonly used curative treatment modality in esophageal disease. The probability of surgical cure relates directly to the stage of the cancer. A minority of patients with transmural or lymph node–involved cancers are cured by esophagectomy. A curative approach is not usually taken for supraclavicular or celiac lymph node metastases.
      (2) **Preoperative chemotherapy and radiation therapy.** Preoperative chemotherapy with 5-FU and cisplatin in conjunction with radiation therapy has been shown to improve surgical outcomes in patients who have undergone surgery with curative intent. When used alone, neither chemotherapy nor radiation therapy improves surgical outcome in either preoperative or postoperative settings.
   b. **Metastatic disease.** Treatment is palliative.
      (1) **Radiation therapy in conjunction with chemotherapy** with agents such as 5-FU or cisplatin may palliate local symptoms caused by esophageal obstruction.
      (2) **Esophageal stents and feeding tubes** may maintain enteral nutrition and reduce the risks of aspiration of esophageal contents.
      (3) **Narcotic analgesics** may palliate pain.
      (4) **Other chemotherapeutic approaches** may be useful. **Single-agent chemotherapy** with agents such as 5-FU, etoposide, irinotecan, paclitaxel, docetaxel, or cisplatin may display moderate activity and may provide palliation of symptoms but without meaningful

*For full staging information, please see the most recent edition of the AJCC Cancer Staging Handbook.

impact on survival. **Combination chemotherapy** with two or more of these drugs may improve quality of life but has minimal overall impact on survival.

8. **Prognosis**
   a. **Surgically resectable cancer.** Most patients who undergo surgery for early (e.g., $T_1N_0M_0$) lesions are cured, but surgical cure rates decrease rapidly as the stage of cancer increases.
   b. **Metastatic cancer.** The survival of untreated patients averages about 6 months, and chemotherapy increases average survival by several months in responsive patients.

E Carcinoma of the hepatobiliary system

1. **Incidence.** Hepatobiliary cancers occur in approximately 20,000 individuals annually in the United States and account for more than 16,000 deaths each year.
2. **Etiology. Hepatocellular carcinoma** is associated with diseases that cause chronic liver injury such as **chronic active hepatitis** caused by **hepatitis B (HBV), hepatitis C (HCV), alcoholic cirrhosis, hemochromatosis,** dietary iron overload, and Wilson's disease. Biliary tract neoplasms such as **cholangiocarcinoma** and **gallbladder cancer** have increased incidence in individuals with inflammatory bowel disease.
3. **Pathology.** Most hepatobiliary neoplasms are adenocarcinomas.
4. **Clinical features**
   a. **Local symptoms** of **hepatocellular carcinoma** include **pain** resulting from distention of the liver capsule. **Obstructive jaundice** is a characteristic presentation for **cholangiocarcinoma.** Jaundice may be a manifestation of **gallbladder cancer.**
   b. **Systemic manifestations** are common and may include:
      (1) Signs and symptoms of liver failure such as jaundice, edema, ascites, and portal hypertension
      (2) Anorexia and weight loss
      (3) Fatigue due to anemia
      (4) Pain due to bone metastases or peritoneal metastases
      (5) Dyspnea or cough due to pulmonary metastases
      (6) Hepatomegaly, pain, or fever due to liver involvement
5. **Diagnosis. Hepatocellular carcinoma** may be initially suspected in at-risk individuals by a rise in **the α-fetoprotein (AFP) serum tumor marker** or by the presence of mass on a screening liver **ultrasound.** On occasion, **gallbladder carcinoma** is discovered at cholecystectomy for symptomatic, apparently benign gallbladder disease.
   a. **CT scans** and **MRI imaging** may identify a mass or masses in the liver. Typically, the diagnosis of hepatocellular carcinoma is established by a CT-guided or ultrasound-guided fine-needle aspiration biopsy.
   b. In patients who present with right upper quadrant **pain** or **jaundice, CT scan** or **ERCP** may detect either a mass, obstruction of biliary flow, or a filling defect in a major biliary radicle. Either fine-needle aspiration biopsy or ERCP-guided biopsy can establish a diagnosis of **cholangiocarcinoma.**
   c. **Commonly used staging studies** include the following:
      (1) **CT scanning** may identify mediastinal or celiac lymph node involvement. It can identify the presence of pulmonary, liver, retroperitoneal lymph node, or pelvic metastases.
      (2) **Bone scans and brain imaging are not indicated** in patients with no symptoms of brain or bone metastases.
6. **Staging.***
7. **Therapy**
   a. **Localized cancer**
      (1) **Surgery**

*For full staging information, please see the most recent edition of the AJCC Cancer Staging Handbook.

(a) In **localized hepatobiliary neoplasms,** surgery alone may provide a cure in some instances. Some patients with technically unresectable but liver-confined neoplasms may be candidates for **liver transplantation.** Radiation therapy and standard chemotherapy have no defined roles in the management of hepatocellular carcinoma, although chemotherapy is occasionally used to reduce tumor size and facilitate curative-attempt surgery.

(b) In **biliary tract neoplasms,** adjunctive 5-FU–based chemotherapy plus external beam or high dose-rate intraluminal radiation is commonly used, although prospective, randomized clinical trials have not validated its utility.

(2) **Other locoregional approaches.** Patients with small but unresectable lesions may benefit from the instillation of **intralesional alcohol** or **chemoembolization,** which involves injection of a slurry of chemotherapeutic agents in an oil emulsion directly into the vessel supplying the neoplastic lesion. Neither of these extensively used approaches has been validated in randomized clinical trials. Radio-frequency ablation of lesions and instillation of radiolabeled microspheres in the hepatic tumors are two promising newer techniques that are under investigation.

(3) **Metastatic disease.** Standard chemotherapeutic agents are ineffective in patients with advanced hepatocellular carcinoma. Administration of chemotherapy is complicated by comorbidities associated with liver failure. **No one chemotherapeutic agent or regimen has emerged as a standard of care in biliary neoplasms, but several agents have antitumor effects, and patients with metastatic disease may be treated with palliative intent.** In addition, **stenting** of obstructed bile ducts, when feasible, can palliate jaundice. **Narcotic analgesics** may palliate pain.

8. **Prognosis**
   a. **Surgically resectable cancer.** Surgical cure rates decrease rapidly with increasing disease stage.
   b. **Metastatic cancer.** The average survival of untreated patients is approximately 6 months.

VII GYNECOLOGIC MALIGNANCIES

A Ovarian cancer

1. **Incidence.** Ovarian cancer develops in 1 in 70 women and is the most common cause of death from gynecologic malignancy. Incidence rates are highest in industrialized nations.

2. **Risk factors** for ovarian cancer include:
   a. Nulliparity
   b. Fewer than average number of pregnancies or a history of miscarriage
   c. Family history of ovarian cancer
   d. History of endocrine disorders

3. **Diagnosis.** Ovarian cancer is rarely diagnosed before the disease has reached an advanced stage.
   a. **Early detection.** Women with average risk for ovarian cancer should obtain routine gynecologic examinations. No existing diagnostic modality exhibits sufficient sensitivity and specificity to permit the reliable early detection of surgically curable cancers.
      (1) **Pelvic ultrasound** detects small lesions in the ovary, even those that cannot be palpated during bimanual examination.
      (2) Determination of levels of the **tumor marker CA 125** and an annual **pelvic ultrasound** are recommended for patients with a family history of ovarian cancer.
   b. **Pretreatment evaluation**
      (1) All patients with a new diagnosis of ovarian cancer should undergo abdominal and pelvic CT scanning and a pelvic ultrasound. Chest radiography, barium enemas, cystoscopy, and flexible sigmoidoscopy may be considered, depending on the presentation of the disease.
      (2) Routine blood chemistries, including albumin, magnesium, and renal and liver function testing, should be performed. An elevated CA 125 is found in 80%–85% of patients with disease that is not localized to the ovaries. If a germ cell tumor is suspected, the following

tumor markers should be drawn: lactate dehydrogenase (LDH), AFP, and human chorionic gonadotropin (hCG).

(3) A careful laparotomy establishes the stage and extent of the disease and may permit the reduction of tumor masses.

(a) The entire abdominal contents should be explored, and any suspicious lesions should be removed or examined by biopsy.

(b) In addition to checking the primary tumor for rupture or adherence, the surgeon should note the amount and type of ascites (if present). Samples of fluid should be collected for cytologic analysis by peritoneal washing.

(c) The para-aortic nodes in the region of the renal hila should be examined by biopsy.

(d) The diaphragmatic surfaces should be carefully explored.

4. **Staging.***

5. **Therapy**

a. **Surgery**

(1) **Procedures**

(a) Most patients undergo **bilateral salpingo-oophorectomy** and **transabdominal hysterectomy.** All gross residual disease should be resected if possible. In most cases, if a patient has metastatic disease outside the abdominal and pelvic areas, debulking surgery is not indicated.

(b) Because ovarian cancer frequently spreads throughout the peritoneal cavity and usually is associated with omental and peritoneal seeding, the entire abdominal and pelvic cavities should be explored, a **partial omentectomy** performed, and the paracolic gutters inspected.

(2) **Adjuvant therapy and follow-up**

(a) Patients with stage IA or stage IB disease with well-differentiated or moderately differentiated tumors require no additional adjuvant therapy after surgery. Otherwise, patients should receive adjuvant therapy, which usually consists of **chemotherapy.** Alternatives include **total abdominal radiation therapy or intraperitoneal radioisotopes.** Advanced ovarian cancer (i.e., stages III or IV) is not curable by surgery alone. However, **reduction** of bulky cancer is associated with an improved response to either radiation or chemotherapy, if the largest residual mass is reduced to less than 2 cm in diameter. Less extensive reductions are not beneficial, even if large amounts of the tumor are removed.

(b) **Second-look surgery.** Surgical reexploration at the conclusion of chemotherapy can detect remission, assess response, and allow further cytoreductive surgery in an attempt to prolong survival. Approximately 50% of patients with clinically complete responses have surgically documented complete remissions. The value of the routine use of this procedure has not been established.

b. **Chemotherapy.** Systemic chemotherapy results in high response rates in patients with ovarian cancer and increases the likelihood of a cure in patients with resectable disease.

(1) **Drug regimens.** The most commonly used agents are paclitaxel, cyclophosphamide, cisplatin, and carboplatin. Few data support the use of doxorubicin-based regimens. In the past, standard therapy consisted of cyclophosphamide and carboplatin or cisplatin, but contemporary regimens commonly use paclitaxel in conjunction with carboplatin or cisplatin.

(a) Carboplatin (dose-adjusted for renal function to area-under-the-curve) is equivalent in efficacy to cisplatin and is associated with less emesis, peripheral neuropathy, and ototoxicity, although it has an increased rate of bone marrow toxicity compared with cisplatin. Because carboplatin can be administered easily in the outpatient setting, it is generally preferred over cisplatin to treat ovarian cancer.

*For full staging information, please see the most recent edition of the AJCC Cancer Staging Handbook.

(b) Taxanes are associated with approximately 30% response rates in patients who have failed to respond to other therapies. Taxane–platinum combinations induce complete clinical remission in more than 60% of women with previously untreated stage III ovarian cancer.

(2) **Treatment of residual disease after induction chemotherapy.** Radiation therapy has consistently failed to prolong survival and is associated with unacceptable rates of bowel toxicity.

(a) **Intraperitoneal chemotherapy** is based on the slow peritoneal clearance of many chemotherapeutic agents relative to total body clearance. Some studies demonstrate that intraperitoneal chemotherapy is advantageous compared with systemic chemotherapy in the treatment of ovarian cancer.

(i) Drugs are administered in large volumes (1–2 L) through semipermanent systems (e.g., catheters).

(ii) Agents that have been used intraperitoneally in ovarian cancer include methotrexate, 5-FU, carboplatin, and cisplatin.

(b) **Salvage chemotherapy** options include the agents topotecan, gemcitabine, and hexamethylmelamine. Both topotecan and gemcitabine are active agents undergoing testing in patients with chemotherapy-naive disease. High-dose therapy with autologous stem cell rescue is feasible, but it has failed to show significant improvement over conventional dosing.

(c) **Radiation therapy.** For patients with advanced disease, radiation therapy is an option for palliation of symptoms. Success is directly related to the location and volume of disease at the time of therapy.

6. **Prognosis**

a. The **stage of disease** is the most important prognostic factor.

(1) Patients with distant metastases are rarely cured, even after combination chemotherapy.

(2) Patients with disease limited to the ovary may be cured with surgery alone.

(3) Patients with minimal stage III disease have an excellent prognosis with debulking surgery followed by combination chemotherapy, especially if the residual tumor masses measure less than 2 cm in diameter.

b. **Histologic grade** has greater prognostic significance than type. Borderline tumors, which display nuclear characteristics of malignancy but lack stromal invasion, behave in an indolent fashion and are not responsive to chemotherapy.

B Cervical cancer

1. **Incidence.** Carcinoma of the cervix was once one of the most common causes of death from cancer, but incidence rates have decreased by one-half in the past 30 years.

a. This decline in mortality rate is largely attributable to the introduction of the Papanicolaou (Pap) smear for the diagnosis of dysplasia or CIS.

b. Invasive cancer is most frequently seen in patients between 45 and 55 years of age from lower socioeconomic groups.

2. **Etiology**

a. **Risk factors** for cervical cancer include:

(1) Early initial sexual activity

(2) Multiple sexual partners

(3) Early age at first pregnancy and multiple pregnancies

(4) History of venereal infection

(5) Oral contraceptive use

b. Recent studies have implicated infection with human papillomavirus (HPV), which causes common genital warts, in the progression of cervical cancer. Several oncogenes have been implicated as well, including c-*myc* and *ras*.

3. **Pathology**
   a. **Squamous metaplasia** is the precursor of **cervical intraepithelial neoplasia (CIN),** which is subdivided into three grades according to severity.
      (1) Grade I (mild-to-moderate dysplasia)
      (2) Grade II (moderate-to-severe dysplasia)
      (3) Grade III (severe dysplasia and CIS)
   b. CIS exhibits cytologic evidence of neoplasia without invasion of the basement membrane. This stage can persist as long as 3–10 years before progressing to invasive cervical carcinoma.
4. **Diagnosis**
   a. **Early detection**
      (1) The **Pap smear** is useful for detecting early lesions and has a sensitivity of 90%–95%.
         (a) As a preventive measure, women over 20 years of age should have two consecutive yearly smears; if results are negative, the test should be repeated every 3 years until age 65.
         (b) Hemorrhage, inflammatory reactions (e.g., a fungating mass), or invasive cancer may result in false-negative smears.
      (2) Women with epithelial abnormalities in the Pap smear should undergo **cervical biopsy.** Visible lesions necessitate biopsy, regardless of Pap smear findings. If there are no visible lesions, colposcopy (using a binocular microscope and light source) reduces the need for cervical conization.
   b. **Pretreatment evaluation** should include chest radiograph, CT scans of the abdomen and pelvis, complete blood count (CBC), liver and renal function studies, and a barium enema in patients with symptoms involving the colon or rectum.
      (1) Because of the possibility of upper extension of the tumor, **curettage** of the endocervical canal and endometrium is recommended during the initial evaluation.
      (2) A **pelvic CT scan** can define the extent of pelvic disease.
      (3) **Cystoscopy** and **rectosigmoidoscopy** are performed in selected patients with advanced disease.
5. **Staging.*** Clinical staging is often inaccurate, and staging laparotomy studies have shown that approximately 30% of patients have more extensive disease than is suggested by clinical staging procedures.
6. **Therapy.** Cervical cancer in most patients is treated with **surgery, radiation therapy,** or a **combination of both.** Chemotherapy with cisplatin also may be prescribed as a radiation sensitizer. Cisplatin has documented activity as a single agent.
   a. **Total abdominal hysterectomy** is the usual treatment for CIS and CIN. In women who wish to bear children, management with cervical conization and careful follow-up may be appropriate. Therapy for stage I microinvasive cancer (i.e., an invasion of < 3 mm in depth) is identical to that for CIS. The risk of central recurrence and lymph node metastasis is increased when the tumor exceeds 3–5 mm in depth; in these cases, hysterectomy and pelvic lymphadenectomy are indicated.
   b. **Radical hysterectomy, pelvic lymphadenectomy, and radiation therapy** have similar results in stage IB and stage IIA cancers. Because of the 15%–25% incidence of lymph node metastases, treatment consists of radical hysterectomy and bilateral pelvic lymphadenectomy.
      (1) Postsurgical complications include bladder and urethral dysfunction or fistulas.
      (2) Radiation therapy (brachytherapy and external beam radiation) may be administered after surgery. Adjuvant radiation is indicated after surgery if there is microscopic parametrial extension, lesions of more than 4 cm, nodal metastases, lymphatic or vascular invasion, positive margins, or grade III lesions.

*For full staging information, please see the most recent edition of the AJCC Cancer Staging Handbook.

c. **Radiation therapy or surgery** is appropriate for patients with invasion beyond the cervix but without distant metastatic involvement. If there is parametrial spread (i.e., the tumor extends through the pelvic wall or into the vagina), radiation therapy may be preferred.

7. **Prognosis.** The 5-year survival rate for stage I cervical cancer is 75%–90%; for stage II, 50%–70%; for stage III, 30%–35%; and for stage IV, 10%–15%.
   a. **Tumor volume** is an important prognostic factor within stages. Both the grade and tumor volume within a given grade have prognostic significance. Histologic type has little significance, except for some unusual variants.
   b. **Lymph node metastases** are associated with a poor prognosis. Other poor prognostic factors include **tumor grade, depth of invasion,** and **lymphovascular space invasion.**

C Endometrial cancer

1. **Incidence.** Carcinoma of the endometrium is the most common gynecologic malignancy, accounting for 9% of all malignant tumors in women. The incidence of endometrial cancer has been steadily increasing since the 1970s. Approximately 34,000 new cases are diagnosed annually, resulting in approximately 3000 deaths.
2. **Risk factors**
   a. **Obesity, diabetes, hypertension, polycystic ovarian disease, late onset of menopause,** and **increasing age** are associated with an increased risk of endometrial cancer.
   b. **Unopposed estrogen therapy** also poses an increased risk. Progesterone decreases the risk associated with the use of postmenopausal estrogens. Use of combination oral contraceptives appears to decrease risk.
   c. Other risk factors include tamoxifen, chronic anovulation, and irregular menses.
3. **Pathology.** Most endometrial cancers are **adenocarcinomas.** Sixty-seven percent are characteristic endometrial adenocarcinomas, 20% are endometrial adenocarcinomas with focal areas of benign squamous metaplasia, and 13% are adenosquamous carcinomas.
4. **Clinical features and diagnosis**
   a. Most women with endometrial cancer have abnormal uterine bleeding.
   b. Only 15%–20% of cases of endometrial cancer are identified by Pap smear. Diagnostic procedures include biopsy, fractional dilatation and curettage (D&C), endometrial brush, and jet-wash techniques.
   c. **Pretreatment evaluation** includes routine hematologic and blood chemistries, urinalysis, chest radiograph, and occasionally, hysteroscopy or hysterography.
      (1) **CT** and **cystoscopy** should be performed if there is evidence of bladder dysfunction.
      (2) Patients with lower gastrointestinal symptoms should undergo **proctosigmoidoscopy** and **barium enema.**
      (3) **Lymphangiography** may be used to define involvement of the para-aortic nodes in high-risk patients. It is performed uncommonly.
5. **Staging.*** Seventy-four percent of patients who are seen have stage I disease; 13%, stage II disease; 9%, stage III disease; and 3%, stage IV disease.
6. **Therapy**
   a. Treatment measures include **surgery, radiation therapy, hormone therapy,** and, occasionally, **chemotherapy.**
      (1) Synthetic progestogens are the most commonly used hormone therapy agents, with response rates of approximately 35%. The probability of response depends on the histologic grade of the tumor and the presence of progesterone receptors. Well-differentiated tumors have the highest response rates.

*For full staging information, please see the most recent edition of the AJCC Cancer Staging Handbook.

(2) Chemotherapy is of little benefit, but some activity has been seen with cyclophosphamide, 5-FU, doxorubicin, and cisplatin.

b. Specific treatment recommendations

(1) Adenomatous hyperplasia can be treated with hysterectomy or hormone therapy, depending on the patient's desire for children.

(a) Continuous combination estrogen and progesterone contraceptive agents or high-dose progestogens are used in hormone therapy. Ovulation can be induced with clomiphene.

(b) Patients maintained on hormone therapy should be carefully monitored and undergo routine endometrial sampling.

(2) Patients with uncomplicated endometrial carcinoma are treated with total abdominal hysterectomy and bilateral salpingo-oophorectomy. Radiation therapy is sometimes considered for high-risk patients.

(3) In patients with stage IB disease, preoperative intracavitary radiation therapy is followed by total abdominal hysterectomy. High-risk patients also may receive postoperative radiation therapy.

(4) Patients with stage II disease and extensive cervical involvement should be managed with intracavitary brachytherapy, external beam radiation therapy, extrafascial hysterectomy, and bilateral salpingo-oophorectomy.

(5) Patients with pelvic involvement are treated with surgery and radiation therapy.

7. Prognosis

a. **Stage at diagnosis** is the most important prognostic factor. Five-year survival rates range from 76% in stage I disease to 9% in stage IV disease.

b. Other important prognostic factors include the **extent of cervical and myometrial invasion, lymph node involvement** (especially pelvic or para-aortic nodes), and **histologic grade.** Of lesser importance are uterine size, positive peritoneal cytology, cell type, and patient age.

VIII CANCER OF UNKNOWN PRIMARY SITE (CUPS)

A Incidence

Patients with CUPS have metastatic carcinoma in the absence of a demonstrable primary site. Approximately 2%–10% of new cancer patients have CUPS. Even at autopsy, the primary site remains obscure in 15%–20% of these patients.

B Pathology

1. Histologic subtypes

a. Adenocarcinoma is the most common subtype, occurring in 40%–77% of patients.

b. Squamous cell carcinomas are present in 5%–15% of patients.

c. Other cell types include lymphomas, germ cell tumors, melanomas, and sarcomas.

(1) **Lymphoma** can sometimes be distinguished from undifferentiated carcinoma by special immunohistochemical stains for leukocyte markers such as leukocyte common antigen.

(2) **Metastatic small-cell endocrine tumors** can be identified by staining for S-100 or neuron-specific enolase.

(3) **Germ cell tumors** may stain positive for AFP or hCG.

2. Light microscopy, electron microscopy, and immunohistochemical techniques may be useful in identifying the histologic subtype or tissue origin.

a. Visualization of the cellular architecture by **light microscopy** may identify adenocarcinomas, squamous cell carcinomas, melanoma, sarcoma, or lymphoma. However, because CUPS is often anaplastic, differentiation by light microscopy is not always possible.

b. **Immunohistochemical markers** are important pathologic tools. For example, a positive keratin stain implies that the tumor is of epithelial origin. Table 4–14 lists the immunohistochemical markers that correspond to various cell types.

c. **Electron microscopy** detects **intercellular bridging,** characteristic of squamous cell carcinomas; **neurosecretory granules,** characteristic of neuroendocrine tumors; **melanosomes,** characteristic of melanoma; and **intracellular structures** such as myofibrils, characteristic of sarcomas.

TABLE 4–14 Tumor Markers for Identifying Tissue Origin in Cancer of Unknown Primary Site (CUPS)

Marker	Cell or Tumor Type
Immunohistochemical	
Keratin	Epithelial
Mucin	Adenocarcinoma
Estrogen or progesterone receptors	Breast, endometrium, ovary
Acid phosphatase	Prostate
Thyroglobulin	Thyroid
Gremilius	Neuroendocrine
s-100	Sarcoma, melanoma
Vimentin, desmin	Sarcoma
Lymphocyte common antigen	Lymphoma
Serum markers	
Human chorionic gonadotropin (β-hCG)	Germ cell tumor
α-fetoprotein (AFP)	Germ cell tumor, hepatomas
Prostate-specific antigen (PSA)	Prostate
Carcinoembryonic antigen (CEA)	Gastrointestinal malignancies
CA 125	Ovary
CA 15-3	Breast

C Diagnosis Because pancreatic, lung, and colon cancers are the most likely primary sources of undifferentiated adenocarcinoma, routine diagnostic procedures include a chest radiograph, fecal occult blood test (accompanied by colonoscopy in positive cases), and abdominal CT.

1. **Women** should also undergo **mammography, pelvic examination,** and **pelvic ultrasound.**
2. **Prostate-specific antigen (PSA) levels** should be determined in **men.**
3. Patients with suspected germ cell carcinomas should also undergo β-hCG and AFP determinations.

D Therapy Individuals, particularly men, with CUPS presenting with midline-dominant lesions (e.g., para-aortic lymphadenopathy, mediastinal lymphadenopathy) and pulmonary nodules should be treated for poor prognosis nonseminomatous germ cell tumors. Treatment varies according to the suspected primary site but typically includes palliative radiation therapy or chemotherapy.

1. **Slow-growing tumors** may merely be monitored at 4- to 8-week intervals.
2. Chemotherapy is an experimental option for **adenocarcinoma.** Women with suspected adenocarcinoma in an axillary node should be considered to have stage II breast cancer and be treated accordingly.
3. Patients with **squamous cell carcinoma metastatic to the neck** from an unknown primary site, but no distant metastases, should be treated with neck dissection and radiation therapy to the neck.
4. Young men with **anaplastic tumors of the mediastinum or retroperitoneum** may respond to treatment modalities used for germ cell tumors of the testis, especially if AFP or β-hCG levels are elevated.

E Prognosis Median survival is only 5–6 months after diagnosis, although the range is broad; 3%–5% of patients may be alive after 5 years.

IX CANCERS OF THE KIDNEY, BLADDER, AND PROSTATE

A Renal cell cancer

1. **Incidence.** Cancer of the kidney (hypernephroma) accounts for 2%–3% of all cancers. The ratio of affected men to women is 2:3, with an average age of 55–60 years at presentation.

2. **Risk factors.** Patients with von Hippel-Lindau disease or acquired polycystic kidney disease have a higher incidence of renal carcinoma. Familial types of renal cell carcinoma have been associated with abnormalities of chromosome 3 and the *p53* gene.

3. **Pathology**
   a. Most renal tumors are clear-cell carcinomas (adenocarcinomas); however, granular cell tumors, mixed tumors, and aggressive carcinosarcomas (adenocarcinomas with sarcomatous degeneration) also occur. Rarely, tumors arise in renal cysts.
   b. Renal cancers are usually **extremely vascular, readily metastasizing** to the lung, bone, liver, brain, and other sites. Dissemination also may occur when tumor emboli enter the renal vein and inferior vena cava or by nodal spread in the para-aortic, paracaval, hilar, and mediastinal areas.

4. **Clinical features**
   a. Hematuria (40%–70% of patients)
   b. Abdominal mass with flank pain (20%–40% of patients)
   c. Weight loss (30% of patients)
   d. Fever, malaise, night sweats, or anemia (15%–30% of patients)
   e. Paraneoplastic syndromes, including hypercalcemia, polycythemia, or hypertension

5. **Diagnosis.** In the past, diagnostic procedures included hematologic studies, intravenous pyelography (IVP), renal ultrasound, and, in some cases, a selective renal arteriogram or venacavogram. Now, chest radiographs, abdominal CT, and radionuclide bone scans are used to detect the presence of metastases. CT scans are adequate for initial diagnosis and staging. MRI scans are superior for visualizing tumor or clot in the renal vein and vena cava.

6. **Staging.***

7. **Therapy**
   a. **Surgery**
      (1) **Radical nephrectomy** with lymph node dissection is the treatment of choice for stage I, stage II, and stage III renal cell carcinomas. Nephrectomy should also be considered for patients with disseminated disease to relieve hematuria, flank pain, or paraneoplastic syndromes.
      (2) In certain cases, **selective renal arterial embolization** permits surgical resection or halts life-threatening hematuria.
      (3) Patients with one or two metastatic lesions, indolent tumor growth, and no evidence of progressive metastasis may be candidates for aggressive **surgical resection of metastases.**
   b. **Radiation therapy** has only limited value, because most tumors are relatively radioresistant. However, radiation therapy offers the best palliative options for painful bone metastases or nerve root compressions.
   c. **Chemotherapy** is also relatively ineffective, with transient tumor regression occurring in fewer than 5% of patients. Targeted therapy with agents directed against the intracellular tyrosine kinases are under active investigation. One agent in particular, SU 011248, which targets PDGFR, VEGFR, KIT, and FLP-3, demonstrates promising efficacy in preliminary studies.
   d. **Biologic response modifiers**
      (1) **IFN-α** yields response rates of 13%–20% in patients with soft tissue or lung metastases.
      (2) High-dose **IL-2** therapy yields partial or complete tumor regression in approximately 15% of cases. However, the treatment is extremely toxic and requires a high level of supportive care. Although most responses are limited in duration, complete responses tend to be durable.

8. **Prognosis.** Radical nephrectomy yields a 5-year survival rate in 75% of patients with localized tumors. However, patients with high-grade stage III lesions with invasion of major vascular structures have an overall survival rate of only 30%–40%.

*For full staging information, please see the most recent edition of the AJCC Cancer Staging Handbook.

B Urothelial (transitional cell) carcinomas (bladder, ureter, and renal pelvis)

1. **Incidence.** These tumors account for approximately 3% of the cancer deaths in the United States. Bladder carcinomas are three times more common in men than in women and usually occur in patients who are 50–70 years of age. The total incidence of approximately 50,000 cases per year includes 80%–85% that involve presentation as superficial (e.g., T_a, T_{1s}, T_1) tumors without muscle wall invasion at diagnosis.
2. **Etiology.** Bladder cancers have been related to **tobacco** as well as to certain chemical and biologic carcinogens.
   a. **Occupational carcinogens** in the rubber, dye, printing, and chemical industries have been implicated in bladder carcinoma.
   b. **Saccharin** has been proved to cause bladder tumors in animals, but its role in humans is unproven.
   c. Schistosomiasis of the bladder has been strongly correlated with squamous cell carcinoma.
   d. Other etiologic agents include **cyclophosphamide, phenacetin, renal stones,** and **chronic infection.**
   e. **Molecular alterations** in the **p53** and **Rb** tumor suppressor genes are involved in 20%–40% of tumors, depending on the stage and grade of the primary tumor. The prognosis worsens when one or more of these genes is mutated.
3. **Pathology.** Bladder tumors are generally of transitional cell origin, with the exception of the schistosome-related variant, which is of squamous cell origin.
4. **Clinical features.** Seventy-five percent of bladder cancer patients present with **hematuria. Bladder irritability** and **infection** are the presenting symptoms in the remaining 25%.
5. **Diagnosis**
   a. **Cystoscopy,** with bimanual palpation and subsequent biopsy, is the definitive diagnostic procedure. This technique is nearly 100% accurate.
   b. **Radiologic procedures** include pelvic and abdominal CT scans, chest radiograph, bone scan, and retrograde pyelography for renal pelvic or ureteral tumors.
   c. **Laboratory tests** include a CBC and chemistry profile as well as urine cytology and flow cytometry for high-risk patients.
6. **Staging.***
7. **Therapy**
   a. **Surgery**
      (1) **Superficial lesions** (stages T_a, T_1, and sometimes T_{2a}) are treated with **endoscopic resection** and **fulguration,** followed by cystoscopy every 3 months. Recurrent or multiple lesions are treated with intravesicular instillation of thiotepa, mitomycin, or bacille Calmette-Guérin (BCG).
         (a) The recurrence rate after transurethral resection (TUR) is 50%–70%. The recurrence rate is higher if the size of the tumor is greater than 3 cm, if it is multifocal and associated with CIS, or if it is a high-grade T_1 lesion.
         (b) Even with BCG prophylaxis after TUR, most patients develop recurrences, and some progress to muscle-invasive disease.
      (2) **Recurrent cancer, diffuse transitional cell CIS,** or **stages T_2 and T_3 invasive cancers** are treated with **radical cystectomy.**
      (3) Tumors of the renal pelvis or ureter are treated by **removal of the affected kidney or ureter.**
   b. **Combination chemotherapy**
      (1) In randomized studies, combination chemotherapy with gemcitabine and cisplatin has been shown to be as effective and much less toxic and better tolerated than MVAC

*For full staging information, please see the most recent edition of the AJCC Cancer Staging Handbook.

[methotrexate-vinblastine-doxorubicin (Adriamycin)-cisplatin] in patients with advanced disease. However, these studies were not powered to detect a survival benefit with this regimen.

(2) Newer combination regimens under investigation include gemcitabine plus paclitaxel, cisplatin plus paclitaxel, and paclitaxel plus carboplatin.

C Prostate carcinoma

1. **Incidence.** Cancer of the prostate accounts for 18% of all new cancers in the United States (approximately 75,000 cases). Incidence rates are higher among blacks and increase with age. The disease is much less common in Asian men. At autopsy, the incidence among men older than age 50 years ranges from 14% to 46%. In the United States, the risk of death is approximately 3%.

2. **Pathology.** Nearly all prostate cancers are adenocarcinomas.
   a. Prostate adenocarcinomas are classified as **well-, moderately well-,** or **poorly differentiated,** according to the **Gleason prognostic classification system,** which assigns a grade between 0 and 5 to the primary and secondary differentiation patterns.
   b. Most prostatic tumors originate in the peripheral zone; only 25% originate in the central zone.
   c. More than 90% of distant metastases involve bone, but soft tissue metastases also can occur in the nodes, lung, and liver.

3. **Clinical features.** Presenting characteristics once included a palpable nodule (in >50% of patients), dysuria, urinary retention, terminal hematuria, and urinary dribbling, frequency, or urgency. Currently, when PSA levels influence diagnosis, nonpalpable (T_{1c}) tumors are more common.

4. **Diagnosis**
   a. **Screening and diagnosis**
      (1) **Digital rectal examination** remains the diagnostic gold standard for prostate carcinoma, even though only 10% of the prostatic tumors found as nodules on rectal examination are sufficiently localized for cure.
      (2) **Pathologic examination** of tissue removed for treatment of obstructive prostatic hypertrophy shows that 10% of cases are malignant. The remaining cases, when found, are in advanced stages; often these cancers are **revealed in investigations for metastatic bone disease.**
      (3) **PSA** is an established diagnostic marker, but false-positive values may occur. If the PSA is more than 10 ng/mm^3, then 66% of the prostate biopsies indicate prostate cancer. If the PSA is between 4 and 10 ng/mm^3, then 22% of the biopsies will be positive. The percentage of free PSA (e.g., unbound to plasma α_1-antichymotrypsin) may increase diagnostic specificity, but this occurs at the cost of overall sensitivity.
      (4) **Transrectal ultrasonography (TRUS)** is most useful for evaluation of prostate size and for the precise biopsy of lesions that are not palpable. However, as a sole diagnostic tool, it is insensitive and nonspecific.
   b. **Confirmation**
      (1) **Needle biopsy,** obtained via the rectum, perineum, or urethra, confirms the diagnosis.
      (2) **Laboratory studies** are used to assess renal function, whereas bone scans, radiographs, and pelvic or abdominal CT confirm the presence of metastatic disease.

5. **Staging.*** Staging techniques are used along with the histologic grade and the PSA level to determine the probability that carcinoma limited to the prostate is curable by surgery or radiation. Clinical staging alone is not accurate.
   a. **Stage T_{1A} and T_{1B} tumors** are unsuspected clinically and are found at autopsy or by examining tissue removed for alleged benign disease. **T_{1A} (well-differentiated** with three or fewer foci) tumors have better prognoses than **T_{1B}** (**poorly differentiated,** or more than three foci)

*For full staging information, please see the most recent edition of the AJCC Cancer Staging Handbook.

tumors. **T_{1C}** tumors, which are nonpalpable, are detected by elevated PSA levels. Prostate cancers are most commonly diagnosed at the T_{1C} stage.

b. **Stage T_2 tumors** are **neoplasms that are confined to the prostate gland.** These are the classic nodules found on rectal examination, which theoretically are curable by surgery. Clinically palpable lesions in the prostate are stage **T_{2A}** (involving one lobe) and stage **T_{2B}** (bilateral).

c. **Stage T_3 tumors** are cancers that have spread beyond the prostate capsule or to the seminal vesicles, but not to distant sites. These usually cannot be cured by surgery.

d. **Stage T_4 tumors** are cancers that have spread from the prostate area to pelvic lymph nodes, bone, or elsewhere. Approximately 50% of newly diagnosed cases are stage IV on presentation.

6. **Therapy and prognosis** are determined by the clinical stage of disease, PSA level, and histologic (Gleason) grade at diagnosis. Comorbidities and life expectancies also factor into treatment decisions.

   a. **Early disease** is treated with radical prostatectomy, external beam radiation, or interstitial implantation radiation therapy. In selected cases, no treatment (e.g., expectant management) is appropriate.

      (1) **Prostatectomy** is performed in patients with at least a 10-year life expectancy. Patients with cancers of stage T_{1B}, T_{2A}, and T_{2B}, and younger patients with T_{1A} disease are candidates for surgical cure. Up to 16% of patients presenting with T_{1A} disease, who are thought to have benign disease, progress.

      (2) **Nerve-sparing radical prostatectomy** is appropriate for patients with small lesions. This surgical approach preserves sexual functioning in some men but is associated with a 5%–15% rate of postsurgical urinary incontinence and depends on the expertise and training of the surgeon.

      (3) **Radiation therapy** is used for older patients, those with other medical disorders or large prostatic lesions precluding surgery, and for men who wish a better chance to retain normal sexual activity. With modern techniques, including conformal radiation therapy, 70–75 Gy provides good local control with acceptable morbidity. External beam radiation is useful in palliating metastatic bone disease. Strontium-89 or samarium-153 may be useful when administered intravenously to palliate pain in patients with widespread bone disease. Novel techniques such as IMRT are used in select centers to deliver high radiation dose with improved normal tissue tolerance. Diarrhea, rectal bleeding, and proctitis are sometimes associated with this form of treatment.

   b. **Stage IV tumors** cannot be cured, but survival may be long (>5 years) in subgroups of patients with low-grade tumors. The early use of androgen suppression also may improve survival.

      (1) **Endocrine therapy** is generally the initial mode of treatment.

         (a) In the past, **orchiectomy** and **exogenous estrogens** were used interchangeably.

            (i) Orchiectomy is preferred in patients with cardiovascular or thrombotic risk.

            (ii) Postsurgical administration of exogenous hormones such as diethylstilbestrol (DES; 1–3 mg daily) further suppresses testosterone levels.

         (b) More recent approaches have focused on the LH-RH analog **leuprolide** (Zoladex), either alone or in combination with an antiandrogen (**flutamide,** bicalutamide, or nilutamide). **Aminoglutethimide or ketoconazole plus a corticosteroid** are options for patients who fail to respond to primary hormone treatment.

            (i) These hormonal manipulations induce remissions in approximately 50%–80% of patients, although cures are rare.

            (ii) Typically, prostate and soft tissue lesions regress, acid phosphatase and PSA levels decline toward normal values, and bone pain decreases.

            (iii) The average duration of the initial hormone response is 9–18 months.

         (c) Other hormonal manipulations may produce transient responses.

      (2) **Chemotherapy** has improved and is destined to be used in earlier stages of disease. The most frequently used agents are estramustine plus either vinblastine, paclitaxel, docetaxel,

or etoposide. Mitoxantrone plus a corticosteroid has established palliative value beyond that of corticosteroids alone, and the U.S. Food and Drug Administration (FDA) has approved the use of this combination in hormone-refractory prostate cancer. Doxorubicin and cyclophosphamide also may produce palliation. Treatment options may be limited for metastatic hormone refractory prostate cancer because of advanced age and additional co-morbidities.

X TESTICULAR CANCER

A Incidence Testicular cancer is the most common malignancy in young men and accounts for 1% of all male cancers. The average age at diagnosis is 32 years. Because this cancer can be cured with vigilant monitoring and meticulous therapy, appropriate management is especially imperative.

B Risk factors The presence of a **cryptorchid testicle** and a **prior history** of testicular cancer present a risk.

C Pathology Testicular tumors are classified as **seminomatous** or **nonseminomatous.**

1. **Seminomas** may be further subclassified as **classical, anaplastic,** or **spermatocystic.**
2. Four histologic types of **nonseminomatous tumors** are recognized.
   a. **Embryonal carcinoma**
   b. **Teratoma**
   c. **Yolk sac carcinoma** (also known as **endodermal sinus tumor**)
   d. **Choriocarcinoma**

D Clinical features

1. More than 90%–95% of patients have a **painless, solid testicular swelling.** Occasionally, patients with painful testicular masses are erroneously diagnosed as having epididymitis or orchitis.
2. Para-aortic lymph node involvement can manifest as **ureteral obstruction,** back pain, or new-onset varicocele.
3. Patients also may have **abdominal complaints** from an abdominal mass or **pulmonary symptoms** from multiple nodules.
4. **Gynecomastia and hyperthyroidism** may occur in patients with elevated β-hCG levels. Unilateral gynecomastia may occur after successful treatment as a consequence of testicular failure and low testosterone levels after chemotherapy.

E Diagnosis

1. **Scrotal ultrasound** may show a suspicious intratesticular echogenic focus. Ultrasound can also define penetration of the spermatic cord, epididymis, and scrotum.
2. **Radiologic tests** may include:
   a. **Chest radiograph**
   b. **CT scans** of the chest, abdomen, and pelvis, as well as the brain (in patients with neurologic symptoms)
   c. **Excretory urography** (to determine the course of the ureter)
   d. **Venacavogram**
   e. **Bone scan** (if there is skeletal pain)
3. **Inguinal exploratory surgery,** including high ligation of the spermatic cord and orchiectomy, is necessary for patients with suspicious scrotal masses and no confirmed diagnosis.
   a. Vascular control must be achieved before manipulation of the tumor.
   b. Open biopsy and scrotal exploration are contraindicated because of the possibility of tumor spread.

4. **Elevated blood levels of AFP or β-hCG** are diagnostic for nonseminomatous germ cell tumors. However, levels are normal in many patients with seminomas.

F Staging

1. **Anatomic staging.** The TNM classification for primary testicular tumors, nodal involvement, and distant metastases can be found in the AJCC Staging Handbook.
2. An older, alternative staging system is outlined below.
   a. **Stage A** tumors are confined to the testis.
   b. **Stage B_1** exhibits minimal retroperitoneal nodal involvement (less than six positive nodes and no nodes > 2 cm in diameter).
   c. **Stage B_2** is characterized by moderate retroperitoneal adenopathy (more than six positive nodes or any one node between 2 and 5 cm in diameter).
   d. **Stage B_3** tumors have massive retroperitoneal nodal involvement or a nodal mass greater than 5 cm.
   e. **Stage C** involves metastasis to nodes above the diaphragm or to distant sites.

G Therapy

1. **Nonseminomatous tumors.** In the absence of advanced metastases requiring immediate chemotherapy, most patients undergo orchiectomy for definitive treatment and histologic analysis of the primary tumor. Approximately 30% of these patients with clinical stage I nonseminomatous germ cell tumors have occult retroperitoneal lymph node metastases. The risk is higher (approximately 50%) if the primary tumor is predominantly embryonal carcinoma and shows vascular invasion.
   a. **Clinical stage I disease** (limited to the testis) may be managed in several ways:
      (1) **Retroperitoneal lymph node dissection,** which may be unilateral and thus nerve-sparing with preservation of ejaculatory function, if nodes are negative, may be necessary. Otherwise, a bilateral procedure is performed. Observation with rigorous follow-up, including CT imaging and marker studies, may be appropriate.
      (2) Primary chemotherapy with two cycles of chemotherapy with bleomycin, etoposide, and cisplatin, which effectively prevents relapse, "overtreats" approximately 50% of patients.
      (3) The treatment chosen depends on several factors, including patient age, reliability, feasibility of close follow-up, risk of relapse (as estimated from primary tumor histologic features and CT scan), and need to maintain fertility.
         (a) In TN_1-, TN_2-, or M_0-staged patients with nonseminomatous cancer, those with seminomas and elevated AFP levels, or seminomas with persistent β-hCG elevation after orchiectomy, a bilateral retroperitoneal lymph node dissection is performed.
         (b) Observation is an option for clinical N_0 patients.
   b. **Stage II disease** involves surgery or chemotherapy.
      (1) Patients with tumors less than 3 cm in diameter may be treated with node dissection for curative intent.
      (2) Patients with retroperitoneal tumors more than 5 cm in diameter should receive chemotherapy.
      (3) Adjuvant chemotherapy after complete resection is optional. Patients who have proven extranodal extension, any node more than 2 cm in diameter, or at least six positive nodes have a relapse rate after node dissection of greater than 50%. With adjuvant chemotherapy (e.g., two cycles of etoposide plus cisplatin), however, the relapse rate approaches zero.
2. **Seminomatous tumors**
   a. **Stage I seminomas** are treated with retroperitoneal and pelvic radiation therapy. In recent years, the pelvic field has not been used for this purpose at some centers, and observation only, with no radiation, has been feasible in selected patients. Using this approach, approximately 15% of

patients relapse, but salvage therapy using chemotherapy or radiation therapy is effective in almost all cases. In the United States, radiation therapy remains the standard approach. After treatment, patients should be reevaluated every month for the first year and every 2 months for a second year.

b. **Stage II seminomas.** All patients with stage II seminoma have retroperitoneal node metastases.
   (1) **Radiation therapy** is the treatment of choice for patients with N_1 and N_2 disease. Because of bone marrow toxicity from mediastinal radiation therapy, prophylactic radiation to the mediastinum is no longer indicated.
   (2) Patients with N_3 retroperitoneal adenopathy have a high relapse rate after radiation therapy. Thus, these patients should receive **chemotherapy** instead. Either three cycles of bleomycin plus etoposide plus cisplatin or four cycles of etoposide plus cisplatin may be used.

c. **Stage III or IV seminomas (and nonseminomatous germ cell tumors)** are generally treated with cisplatin in combination with etoposide and bleomycin at 3-week intervals for 3–4 cycles. Four cycles of etoposide plus cisplatin have been shown to be equivalent to three cycles of bleomycin plus etoposide plus cisplatin. Patients with AJCC stage IIIB or stage IIIC disease should receive four cycles of bleomycin plus etoposide plus cisplatin.
   (1) Other chemotherapeutic options for patients with recurrent disease include ifosfamide, paclitaxel, and vinblastine.
   (2) Surgical removal of residual masses postchemotherapy is usually recommended. Such masses contain viable cancer in 10%–15% of cases, fibrosis or necrosis in 40%–45%, and teratomas in 40%. Radiologic studies cannot reliably distinguish between these possibilities. Patients with viable residual tumors should receive two additional cycles of chemotherapy. Surgery also may be considered as a "salvage" therapy for patients who are refractory to cisplatin-based chemotherapy, if disease is confined to one anatomic site and is deemed resectable.
   (3) High-dose chemotherapy with carboplatin, etoposide, and oxazophosphamide may be combined with an autologous BMT or peripheral blood stem cell support in selected patients with chemotherapy-sensitive relapses.

H Prognosis

1. **Seminomatous tumors.** Patients with stage A and stage B (mass < 5 cm) disease have cure rates of greater than 90% after radiation therapy. Chemotherapy results in complete response rates of approximately 90% for advanced [e.g., > N_3 (> 5-cm node)] disease.
2. **Nonseminomatous germ cell tumors.** Complete remission can be obtained in 50%–70% of patients with metastatic disease after chemotherapy alone. Another 10%–15% are disease-free after surgical removal of residual tumor. Relapses occur in 10%–20% of patients within the first 2 years of initial diagnosis and treatment. Patients should be followed indefinitely at 6- to 12-month intervals, because late relapses occur in 3%–5% of those in complete remission.
3. The probability of complete response to chemotherapy depends on the location and bulk of metastatic disease, and patients can be divided into three prognostic groups: good, intermediate, and poor. In the **good prognosis** group, 5-year survival rates in patients with nonseminomatous tumors (56% of patients with nonseminomas) are 92%. These patients have no nonpulmonary visceral metastases, AFP < 100 ng/mm^3, hCG less than 1000 ng/mm^3 (e.g., < 5000 IU/L), and LDH less than 1.5 times the upper limit of normal. In the **poor prognosis** group, 5-year survival rates in patients in the poor prognosis group (16% of patients with nonseminomas) are only 48%. These patients have a mediastinal primary or nonpulmonary visceral metastasis, AFP greater than 10,000 ng/mm^3, hCG over 50,000 IU/L, or an LDH greater than 10 times the upper limit of normal.
4. **Mediastinal seminoma** is highly curable with four cycles of etoposide plus cisplatin or three cycles of bleomycin plus etoposide plus cisplatin.

5. **Mediastinal nonseminomatous germ cell tumors** have poor prognosis as well as a different biology and natural history than other nonseminomatous tumors, with an association with hematologic malignancies. Patients are customarily treated with bleomycin plus etoposide plus cisplatin for four cycles, followed by resection, but the prognosis remains poor.

XI HEAD AND NECK CARCINOMAS

A Incidence Head and neck carcinomas account for 5% of the cancers reported each year in the United States. These tumors occur three times more frequently in men than in women. Patients are typically between 50 and 60 years of age. The most frequently affected sites are the oral cavity (40%), larynx (25%), oropharynx and hypopharynx (15%), and salivary gland (10%).

B Risk factors The following factors have been associated with an increased incidence of head and neck carcinomas.

1. **Tobacco use.** Cigarette smoking is the major cause of head and neck cancer, and relative risk increases with the number of cigarettes smoked per day. Chewing tobacco is responsible for a recent increase in the incidence of oral cancer among young adults.
2. **Alcohol consumption** works in combination with cigarette smoking to increase the incidence of head and neck cancer 10- to 40-fold.
3. **Nickel exposure** increases the risk of cancers of the nasal cavity and paranasal sinus.
4. **Syphilis** is associated with an increased incidence of cancer of the tongue.
5. **Prolonged sun exposure** increases the incidence of lip cancer.
6. The **Epstein-Barr virus** and certain **food dyes** have been linked to nasopharyngeal cancers in Asians.

C Pathology Most of these tumors (95%) are squamous cell carcinomas, which vary from well-differentiated varieties to invasive, poorly differentiated or undifferentiated varieties. Nodal involvement is a factor of the primary tumor site, size, and degree of differentiation.

1. **Tumors of the salivary gland** are most commonly of the mixed type, although adenoid cystic carcinomas are not uncommon.
2. **Nasopharyngeal cancers** may be squamous cell cancers, lymphoepitheliomas, or lymphomas.

D Clinical features Common symptoms include dysphagia, hoarseness, head or neck pain, ear pain, and neck or head swellings. Affected patients with large lesions may present with ulcerations or white patches. Some patients present with adenopathy in the absence of an obvious primary source.

E Diagnosis

1. **Detection**
   a. **Tissue diagnosis** relies on biopsy of the non-necrotic portion of the tumor, tumor edge, and adjacent normal mucosa. Open biopsy of the neck nodes should be avoided if head and neck cancer of the squamous cell type is suspected.
   b. **Radiologic studies** may include:
      (1) Radiographs of the mandible, sinus, or nasopharynx
      (2) CT and MRI scans to evaluate the nasopharynx, thymus, oral cavity, and oral pharynx, and to check nodal involvement
      (3) Barium swallow (in patients with evidence of tumor encroachment on the cervical esophagus)
2. **Pretreatment evaluation**
   a. A thorough **dental evaluation** is necessary before radiation therapy to help decrease the risk of osteoradionecrosis.

b. If a mutilating surgical procedure is anticipated, a **prosthodontist** should be consulted to plan reconstructive cosmetic surgery.
c. Many patients with head and neck cancer are malnourished because of their inability to swallow and chew. All patients should therefore undergo a complete **nutritional assessment,** and every attempt should be made to bring the patient into positive nitrogen balance to reduce the complications of treatment.

F Therapy Small lesions can be treated with curative surgery and radiation therapy. Patients with advanced, unresectable disease can benefit from radiation therapy or combined-modality approaches.

1. **Surgery**
   a. Primary tumors should be excised with negative margins, which may require skin flaps.
   b. Patients with neck lymph node involvement require **radical neck dissection** (i.e., dissection of the superficial and deep cervical fascia and close lymph nodes; sternocleidomastoid muscles; internal, external, and jugular veins; spinal accessory nerve; and submandibular glands).
   c. Patients with cancers of the oral cavity, oral pharynx, or supraglottic larynx, and no evidence of nodal involvement are treated with a **functional neck dissection** for better functional and cosmetic results.
   d. Surgery is often associated with **morbidity,** including cosmetic deformities, speech impediments, aspiration pneumonia, shoulder droop, and pain.
2. **Radiation therapy.** Most patients are treated with radiation over a 5- to 6-week interval. Side effects include dry mouth, loss of taste, mouth ulcers, osteoradionecrosis of the mandible (which can be prevented by appropriate dental extractions, antibiotics, and fluoride administration), laryngeal edema, and, rarely, hypothyroidism.
3. **Chemotherapy** for locally unresectable or metastatic disease may include cisplatin, infused 5-FU, methotrexate, and taxanes.
   a. New drugs such as irinotecan, pemetrexed, epidermal growth factor receptor antagonists, and P53 gene therapy (e.g., taxanes) are being tested in clinical trials and show promise.
   b. **Combination chemotherapy regimens** have reported high response rates in patients with unresectable disease. These patients exhibit response rates as high as 90% after administration of cisplatin and a continuous infusion of 5-FU.

XII SARCOMAS

A Incidence Approximately 7000 new sarcomas are diagnosed in the United States each year, constituting 1% of adult malignancies.

B Risk factors

1. Exposure to **radiation**
2. Exposure to **chemicals** (e.g., wood preservatives, herbicides, or asbestos)
3. **Genetic abnormalities.** For example, patients with von Recklinghausen's disease have a 10% lifetime risk of development of a neurofibrosarcoma.
4. **Preexisting bone disease.** Osteosarcomas occur in 0.2% of patients with Paget's disease; however, most osteosarcomas occur in patients younger than 20 years of age.

C Clinical features

1. **Soft tissue sarcomas** often manifest as a **mass, swelling,** or **pain** in the trunk or extremities.
2. Patients with **retroperitoneal tumors** generally experience **weight loss** or **deep-seated pain.**
3. **Bleeding** is the most common presenting feature of **gynecologic** and **gastrointestinal sarcomas.**
4. Most patients with osteosarcomas present with either **pain,** a **mass, or both.**

D Diagnosis

1. **Biopsy**
   a. A rapidly growing mass or one that exceeds 5 cm in diameter should be regarded with suspicion, especially if it is firm, deep, or fixed.
   b. These lesions require a generous incisional biopsy or an excisional biopsy; needle biopsy is usually inadequate.
   c. The biopsy site must be selected carefully to allow for the possibility of limb-sparing surgery.
2. **Imaging procedures** include radiographs, MRI, CT, and bone scans.
   a. For soft tissue sarcomas, MRI is superior to CT, providing better definition of soft tissue planes and tumor margins.
   b. MRI or CT and bone scanning are preferred for evaluating bony involvement.
   c. MRI or CT scans of the liver identify hepatic metastases in those patients with visceral sarcomas and in those with extremity sarcomas accompanied by evidence of abnormal hepatic function.

E Therapy

Surgery is the mainstay of therapy, supplemented with radiation therapy or chemotherapy.

1. **Surgery**
   a. **Definitive resection** may consist of extensive surgical excision, including a 2- to 4-cm pathologically documented margin of normal tissue, or conservative resection with documented tumor-free margins, supplemented with radiation therapy. Re-excision should be considered after biopsy if microscopically involved margins are demonstrated.
   b. **Limb-sparing surgery** can be considered in the majority of patients with extremity sarcomas.
      (1) This procedure is associated with a 90% local control rate and an overall disease-free survival rate of 60%, a success rate that is similar to that found with amputation or radical resection procedures.
      (2) Preoperative intra-arterial chemotherapy and radiation therapy may facilitate limb-sparing surgery in borderline resectable tumors.
   c. Surgeons should avoid seeding the entire surgical field during the procedure. If such seeding occurs, wide excision should be followed by 6600 cGy radiation therapy.
   d. Surgery offers the chance of a cure for patients with few (i.e., no more than 10–15) pulmonary metastases.
2. **Radiation therapy** may be used when the tumor margins are less than 2–4 cm or if tumor seeding has occurred. Studies have shown that a combination of limb-sparing surgery and radiation therapy is as effective as amputation.
3. **Chemotherapy**
   a. **Adjuvant chemotherapy** has no clear benefit except in young patients with osteosarcoma and adults with extremity sarcomas. A few studies have reported an increase in disease-free survival rates and overall survival rates with the use of doxorubicin-based combination regimens in extremity sarcomas. Doxorubicin alone appears ineffective.
   b. **Advanced sarcomas.** Previously treated patients may respond to doxorubicin (15%–35%), dacarbazine (17%), or ifosfamide (20%–40%). Some studies suggest that combination chemotherapy, particularly with doxorubicin and ifosfamide, may yield improved results. The combination of gemcitabine plus taxotere is highly active in patients with leiomyosarcomas.

F Prognosis

Histologic grade and tumor size are the most important prognostic factors.

1. **Histologic grade** is determined by the mitotic rate, nuclear grade, extent of necrosis, nuclear morphology, and cellularity.
2. **Tumor size** is an independent prognostic factor. Small (< 5 cm), completely excised, low-grade lesions rarely recur locally and have a low metastatic rate.

3. **Other factors.** Multivariant analysis identified the following factors as being associated with an increased risk of local recurrence: age older than 53 years; presentation with recurrent disease; high-grade, painful mass; limb-sparing surgery; and inadequate surgical margins.

XIII MULTIPLE MYELOMA (see Chapter 6 Part I: X P)

A Incidence

Myeloma is a neoplasm of the plasma cells that are derived from B lymphocytes. It is an uncommon neoplasm, accounting for less than 1%–2% of the adult cancers in the United States. The incidence of myeloma increases with advancing age and is twice as common in blacks.

B Etiology

1. Although no specific underlying causes have been proven, chronic stimulation to the immune system may play a role in the pathogenesis of myeloma. Interestingly, IL-6 can promote the growth of myeloma cells in vitro.
2. Genetic factors, as well as exposure to petroleum, asbestos, laxatives, and radiation, also may be important factors.
3. Benign monoclonal gammopathies are suspected precursors of multiple myeloma.

C Clinical features

With the advent of automated laboratory blood testing, myeloma may be detected earlier.

1. The **major feature** of myeloma is the demonstration of an abnormal monoclonal protein (**M protein**) in the **blood, urine,** or **both.** This M protein usually consists of either one or a combination of heavy chains (IgG and IgA) and light chains (κ and λ).
   a. M proteins consisting of the whole immunoglobulin molecules IgG and IgA account for 50% and 25% of the cases, respectively.
   b. M proteins consisting of only light chains account for 25% of cases. In these cases, the M protein is found only in the urine.
2. **Complications** include:
   a. Infiltration of the marrow by large numbers of plasma cells, which are usually abnormal
   b. **Weakness, fatigue, infection,** and **bleeding** due to marrow failure
   c. **Osteolytic lesions** resulting from myeloma-induced bone resorption with subsequent pain and fracture
   d. **Renal abnormalities** due to myeloma infiltration of the kidney, hypercalcemia, toxic effects of light chains on tubules, amyloid deposition, and hyperuricemia
   e. **Recurrent infections** due to acquired hypogammaglobulinemia and leukopenia
   f. **Hypercalcemia** due to myeloma-stimulated osteoclast activity
   g. **Hyperviscosity** due to a high concentration of the M protein, which tends to aggregate

D Diagnosis

The following features must be demonstrated.

1. **An abnormal M protein level** (i.e., > 3.5 g/dL) in the serum, urine, or both
2. **Marrow infiltration** by plasma cells (i.e., > 30% plasma cells on bone marrow biopsy)
3. **Additional supportive findings,** including anemia, osteolytic skeletal lesions, renal abnormalities, and hypercalcemia. The once-common symptoms of **anemia** and **bone pain** are seen less frequently.
4. **Plasmacytoma** on tissue biopsy. Because marrow plasmacytosis occurs in many chronic infections or inflammatory processes without an M component, the major difficulty in differential diagnosis is distinguishing myeloma from monoclonal gammopathy of unknown significance (MGUS).

E Staging

The linear relationship between the easily measured M protein and the cellular tumor burden forms the basis for staging myeloma.

1. **Stage I** (low tumor burden). Patients have normal calcium and bone films as well as the following blood data:
   a. Hemoglobin level > 10 g/dL
   b. IgG level < 5 g/dL
   c. IgA level < 3 g/dL
2. **Stage II** (intermediate tumor burden). Patients have the following blood data:
   a. Hemoglobin level β 8.5–10 g/dL
   b. IgG level = 5–7 g/dL
   c. IgA level = 3–5 g/dL
3. **Stage III** (high tumor burden). Patients have hypercalcemia and osteolytic lesions as well as the following blood data:
   a. Hemoglobin level < 8.5 g/dL
   b. IgG level > 7 g/dL
   c. IgA level > 5 g/dL

F Therapy

1. Patients in whom a differential diagnosis of MGUS cannot be excluded and patients with very low-grade **smoldering myeloma** should be examined only at 3- to 6-month intervals for evidence of disease progression.
2. Therapy should be given to patients with bone pain, hypercalcemia, renal failure, bone marrow suppression, and spinal cord compression. Responses are obtained in approximately two thirds of patients.
   a. **Chemotherapy**
      (1) **Agents**
         (a) Classically, **alkylating agents** (e.g., **melphalan**) and **prednisone** are used, although some physicians advocate more aggressive regimens that also contain **doxorubicin, vincristine,** and **nitrosoureas.** The superiority of multiple drug regimens over melphalan and prednisone has not been demonstrated.
            (i) The **vincristine–doxorubicin (Adriamycin)–dexamethasone (VAD) regimen,** in which vincristine and doxorubicin are administered as a continuous infusion with pulse dexamethasone, can be used as a primary or salvage therapy.
            (ii) Thalidomide, with or without dexamethasone, has been shown to be effective in the treatment of multiple myeloma. For patients who are not candidates for therapy with VAD, thalidomide and dexamethasone is a reasonable alternative. Recently the FDA approved the use of a proteasome inhibitor, bortezomib (Velcade), in patients with multiple myeloma who had failed at least two prior therapies.
         (b) **IFN** has been used for maintenance therapy.
      (2) **Toxicity.** Therapy damages marrow and leads to leukemias and excessive secondary marrow diseases in long-term survivors.
      (3) **Evaluation of effectiveness.** When therapy is effective, the M protein levels decline. Therapy can be stopped if the M protein levels become normal or stabilize at 75% below initial levels. Therapy can be resumed when disease progression occurs, although results with retreatment are not as good as those with initial therapy.
   b. **Autologous transplantation** has been performed in many patients, most of whom have been reinfused with unpurged marrow. The complete remission rate is 20%–30%; 50% of patients who achieve a complete remission are disease-free at 4 years.
   c. **Supportive therapy** is extremely important in the management of myeloma and includes:
      (1) **Radiation therapy** for local bone disease
      (2) **Hydration** and proper **management of hypercalcemia**

(3) **Orthopedic support** and care
(4) **Plasmapheresis** for hyperviscosity syndrome.

G Prognosis This clearly depends on the extent of myeloma at presentation. Patients with smoldering or stage I myeloma may go many years without a need for therapy, whereas patients with stage III myeloma and renal and orthopedic complications do poorly. Mean survival for patients requiring therapy is 2–3 years.

XIV HODGKIN'S DISEASE

A Incidence In the United States, 7000–7500 new cases of Hodgkin's disease are reported each year. This neoplasm has a characteristic **bimodal age distribution.**

1. A **young adult peak** occurs between the ages of 10 and 25 years and is characterized by equal incidence in men and women, a preponderance of nodular sclerosis pathology, and a more benign clinical course.
2. A **second adult peak** occurs after age 50 years and is characterized by high incidence among men, a preponderance of mixed cellularity, and a more aggressive clinical course.

B Etiology

1. Clustering of cases in time and place occurs in Hodgkin's disease, suggesting that **viruses or environmental factors may play a role.** However, this clustering is sporadic and has not been substantiated by firm evidence. Studies have suggested an association with **Epstein-Barr virus** infection.
2. Statistical evidence links early-onset Hodgkin's disease with **higher socioeconomic class,** and an increased incidence of Hodgkin's disease among family members suggests a **genetic predisposition.**

C Pathology There are four major histologic variants of Hodgkin's disease. Of interest, however, is the fact that the precise nature of the truly malignant cell (the binucleate giant cell called the **Reed-Sternberg cell**) remains a point of controversy, despite new techniques that indicate that this cell is more likely derived from the mononuclear phagocyte system than from transformed lymphocytes.

D Clinical features and staging Hodgkin's disease tends to spread in an orderly fashion from node group to node group. This contiguous nature is in marked contrast to non-Hodgkin's lymphomas, which are multicentric early in their development.

1. The modified **Ann Arbor classification** is used for **staging Hodgkin's disease.***
   a. Hodgkin's disease patients, especially young patients, usually have **asymptomatic swelling of a lymph node.** The B subclassification implies, however, that Hodgkin's disease may present with such **systemic symptoms** as **fever, weight loss,** and **drenching sweats.**
   b. Workup is based on the principle that **early-stage** Hodgkin's disease **can be treated locally** but **late-stage** Hodgkin's disease **requires systemic therapy.** Therefore, patients are aggressively staged to include or exclude stage $IIIA_2$, stage IIIB, and stage IV disease. (This staging is far more extensive than staging for non-Hodgkin's lymphomas.)
2. **Staging procedures** include:
   a. Thorough history and physical examination
   b. Chest radiographs, CT scans of the chest, abdomen, and pelvis.
   c. Percutaneous bilateral bone marrow biopsies
   d. PET Scan

E Therapy Treatment of Hodgkin's disease continues to evolve. However, certain principles have been established and should be firmly adhered to, because **even advanced disease is curable.** Indi-

*For full staging information, please see the most recent edition of the AJCC Cancer Staging Handbook.

vidual variations in treatment should be avoided and, if used, should be limited to well-controlled clinical trials.

1. **Stage I** or **II** disease is treated with **extended-field radiation therapy.**
2. **Stage IIIA$_1$ disease (pathologically staged) is treated with total nodal radiation therapy.** Patients who relapse after radiation therapy can be successfully given **chemotherapy.** More than 50% of such patients have long-term disease-free survival when such techniques are used. Clinical stage IIIA$_1$ disease (e.g., no staging laparotomy) is usually treated with chemotherapy.
3. **Stage IIIA$_2$, IIIB,** or **IV** disease requires **systemic chemotherapy.** BMTs have been used in cases of relapse.
   a. **Regimens**
      (1) Many regimens are available. The classic **mechlorethamine–vincristine (Oncovin)–procarbazine–prednisone (MOPP) regimen,** which is given for at least six cycles plus two additional cycles after complete remission, is documented, was the first curative regimen. However, The **doxorubicin (Adriamycin)–bleomycin–vinblastine–dacarbazine (DTIC) [ABVD] regimen** is currently the first line combination chemotherapy of choice. This regimen has been shown to be more effective and less toxic than MOPP and as effective as and less toxic than the MOPP/ABVD combinations.
      (2) Other regimens such as Stanford V, which uses a combination of multiple chemotherapy agents and radiation treatment to bulky (>5 cm) lymph nodes, are also in use. A randomized trial of ABVD versus Stanford V is underway.
   b. **Principles**
      (1) Combined chemotherapy and radiation therapy should not be used routinely until further clinical trials prove the effectiveness of such a regimen.
      (2) Unless chemotherapeutic agents are given in full doses and according to prescribed schedules, their effectiveness can be significantly compromised.
   c. **Side effects.** Both chemotherapy and total nodal irradiation are difficult, toxic, and have many side effects, including severe nausea and vomiting, hypothyroidism, sterility (in some cases), and development of secondary marrow problems, including acute leukemia.

F Prognosis Outcome varies mainly with the stage of disease and, to a lesser extent, with histology. Overall, there is a 55%–60% 5-year survival rate with all cases of Hodgkin's disease.

1. Patients with stage I or stage II disease have a 5-year disease-free survival rate exceeding 80%.
2. Patients with stage IIIA disease have roughly a 67% rate of 5-year disease-free survival.
3. Patients with stage IIIA$_2$, stage IIIB, or stage IV disease, if treated with chemotherapy, obtain remissions in 80%–95% of cases, with more than 50% of these patients achieving prolonged (i.e., > 5 years) disease-free survival.

XV NON-HODGKIN'S LYMPHOMA

A Incidence More than 45,000 patients are diagnosed with non-Hodgkin's lymphoma in the United States each year. An increased incidence in older people is attributable to a rising incidence in diffuse large-cell lymphoma. Non-Hodgkin's lymphomas (especially CNS lymphomas) are more common in patients with acquired immunodeficiency states and in patients receiving immunosuppressive drugs such as those with kidney and heart transplants.

B Etiology

1. **Cytogenetic abnormalities** such as chromosome translocations are commonly observed in lymphoma cells.

2. **Viral infection**
   a. The **Epstein-Barr virus** has been linked to **Burkitt's lymphoma,** a disease usually found in Africa.
   b. An aggressive T-cell leukemia or lymphoma occurs in Japan and the Caribbean and is associated with human T lymphotropic virus type I **(HTLV-I) infection.**

C Pathology A number of histologic classification schemes are in use; the one most widely used in the clinical literature is the World Health Organization (WHO) classification system. The WHO classification for lymphoid neoplasms is found in the AJCC Cancer Staging Handbook.*

1. The **low-grade lymphomas** are predominantly B-cell tumors. The **intermediate-grade lymphomas** include both B- and some T-cell lymphomas, whereas **immunoblastic lymphomas** are predominantly B-cell tumors, and **lymphoblastic lymphomas** are T-cell types. Most B-cell tumors are monoclonal and produce either a κ or a λ light chain immunoglobulin.
2. **Follicular small-cleaved cell lymphomas** are the most common histologic type, accounting for approximately 40% of cases. These patients have predominantly stage III or stage IV disease with a high incidence of bone marrow involvement and an indolent course, evolving over many years.
3. **Follicular mixed small-cleaved and large-cell lymphomas** represent 20%–40% of patients. Large cells may account for as much as 25% of the cell population. The lymph node architecture shows distinct nodules, which are usually present throughout the node. Marrow involvement is common. This subtype is indolent but more aggressive than follicular small-cleaved cell lymphoma.
4. **Diffuse large-cell lymphomas** are characterized by large malignant lymphocytes with increased nuclear diameters. These cells have cytologic features of large cleaved or noncleaved follicular cells, with nucleoli, abundant cytoplasm, and frequent mitoses.
5. **Immunoblastic lymphomas** and other high-grade non-Hodgkin's lymphomas include **plasmacytoid, clear-cell,** and **polymorphic** categories. These subtypes are rapidly fatal unless effective treatment is administered promptly.

D Clinical features

1. Most patients are **asymptomatic.** Twenty percent of patients have **fever, night sweats,** or **weight loss.**
2. Patients with indolent lymphomas may have **waxing and waning adenopathy** for several months before diagnosis, although **persistent nodal enlargement** is more common. Extranodal disease most often involves the stomach, lung, and bone, resulting in symptoms characteristic of the affected organ.

E Staging and diagnosis

1. The Ann Arbor staging system used to classify Hodgkin's disease is also used to stage non-Hodgkin's lymphomas (see the AJCC Cancer Staging Handbook*).
2. **Staging procedures** include:
   a. An adequate surgical lymph node **biopsy,** examined by an experienced pathologist
   b. **Hematologic studies,** including a CBC, differential, platelet count, liver and kidney function studies, and uric acid level studies. Serum protein electrophoresis rules out hypogammaglobulinemia or a monoclonal gammopathy.
   c. A complete **history** and **physical examination,** with particular emphasis on all lymph node–bearing areas, including Waldeyer's ring, as well as liver and spleen size
   d. **Bone marrow biopsies** and **aspirates**
   e. **Radiologic studies,** including chest radiography; CT of the chest, abdomen, and pelvis.

F Therapy Treatment usually requires a multidisciplinary approach. Radiation therapy and chemotherapy after surgical biopsy are the most common treatment modalities.

1. **Radiation therapy.** Non-Hodgkin's lymphomas are very radiosensitive.
   a. In localized disease, radiation should be targeted to the affected site (4000 cGy to the involved field). The nodal site and draining lymphatics should be included in the radiation field.
   b. Radiation therapy is used **palliatively** in disseminated disease or to "consolidate" a complete response to chemotherapy in areas of bulky disease.
   c. **Electron beam therapy** has been used in the management of cutaneous lymphomas such as the early stages of mycosis fungoides.
   d. **Stage I indolent lymphomas.** Long-term patient follow-up after involved or extended field radiation therapy for localized stage I and stage II low-grade lymphoma reveals a 10-year relapse-free survival rate of greater than 50%, especially in younger patients.
2. **Chemotherapy**
   a. **Low-grade indolent lymphomas** may not require treatment for many years. When therapy is indicated, **chlorambucil** or **cyclophosphamide,** with or without prednisone, is the agent of choice. Initial results with high-dose chemotherapy followed by autologous marrow transplantation are favorable, but success needs to be measured by long-term follow-up because these patients generally have long-term survival rates, even with less toxic treatment. The anti-CD20 antibody, rituximab, is useful in relapsed patients, as is the nucleoside analog, fludarabine.
   b. **Stage I or II intermediate and high-grade lymphomas** often respond to combination chemotherapy and rituximab, with or without radiation therapy. Cure rates approach 80%–90%.
   c. **Aggressive intermediate or high-grade lymphomas** (e.g., lymphoblastic or Burkitt's lymphoma) require immediate combination chemotherapy with protocols similar to those used in the treatment of acute lymphoblastic leukemia (ALL). Prophylactic intrathecal chemotherapy may also be given for high-grade lymphomas. **Salvage combination chemotherapy** produces second complete or partial remissions but is rarely curative unless the patient undergoes BMT.
      (1) The **most common regimen involves cyclophosphamide–doxorubicin–vincristine (Oncovin)–prednisone (CHOP) plus rituximab.** Aggressive chemotherapy with autologous stem cell support may improve survival in newly diagnosed high-risk patients.
      (2) Because of encouraging results with combination chemotherapy in patients with stage III and stage IV disease followed by radiation therapy, randomized clinical trials are underway to compare chemotherapy alone and chemotherapy followed by radiation therapy.
      (3) **Colony-stimulating factors** hasten granulocyte recovery and may permit higher doses and better cure rates.
      (4) **Radiolabeled monoclonal antibodies** Zevalin™ and Bexxar™ are now approved for salvage therapy in patients who have failed rituximab and conventional chemotherapy.

G **Prognosis** Many patients who achieve a complete response, particularly those with diffuse large-cell lymphoma, remain disease-free for an extended period and will be cured. Aggressive combination chemotherapy regimens containing doxorubicin have high complete response rates ranging from 40% to 80%. Prognostic factors (International Prognostic Indicators) for large-cell lymphoma include increasing patient age, stage, LDH level, performance status, and in older patients, the presence or absence of extranodal disease.

XVI PARANEOPLASTIC SYNDROMES

A **Endocrine syndromes** resulting from ectopic polypeptide hormone production are the most common and best understood of the paraneoplastic processes. Many tumors produce more than one biologically active hormone, leading to multiple endocrine paraneoplastic syndromes.

1. **Criteria** for establishing ectopic hormone secretion by tumor cells include:
   a. **Increased hormone levels,** as evidenced by radioimmunoassay or other techniques. However, some patients with elevated hormone levels do not have clinical symptoms.

b. **Decreased hormone levels after removal or treatment of the tumor**
c. **Persistent hormone elevation after removal of the normal gland** that secretes the normal hormone
d. An **arteriovenous gradient for hormone levels** across the tumor vascular bed

2. **Types**
a. **Ectopic growth hormone secretion** has been detected in patients with **lung and gastric carcinomas.** The elevated hormone levels may lead to hypertrophic pulmonary osteoarthropathy. Organomegaly may occur with slow-growing carcinoid tumors.
b. **Ectopic ACTH secretion** was the first paraneoplastic endocrine syndrome described in the literature.
(1) The most common **tumors associated with ectopic ACTH production** are **small-cell lung cancer** and **atypical carcinoids.** High cortisol levels have also been described in patients with adenocarcinoma and large-cell carcinoma of the lung, other carcinoid tumors, thymoma, neural crest tumors, medullary carcinoma of the thyroid, and bronchial adenomas.
(2) **Clinical features.** Most patients have **hypokalemia** and **metabolic alkalosis.**
(a) Patients rarely live long enough for frank Cushing's syndrome to develop. However, diabetes, hypertension, edema, muscle wasting, central obesity, moon facies, and striae may develop in those with extremely high cortisol levels.
(b) Alterations in mental status, fatigue, and anorexia caused by opiate-like peptide fragments are rare symptoms.
(3) **Diagnosis** is confirmed by a plasma ACTH level of more than 200 pg/mm^3, a plasma cortisol level of more than 40 mg/dL without diurnal variation, or a positive dexamethasone suppression test.

B **Hematologic syndromes** may affect cellular blood elements, the coagulation system, or circulating immunoglobulins.

1. **Paraneoplastic syndromes of cellular blood components**
a. **Erythrocytosis** occurs in renal cancer and hepatoma.
b. **Pure red cell aplasia.** Severe anemia due to a complete lack of RBC production is uncommon. However, 50% of patients with pure red cell aplasia have **thymoma.** Many patients with pure red cell aplasia also have other immunologic abnormalities such as hypogammaglobulinemia, paraproteinemia, positive antinuclear antibodies, or autoimmune hemolytic anemia.
(1) **Etiology.** The cause may relate to effects of suppressor T cells on RBC production, leading to a severe reticulocytopenic anemia.
(2) **Therapy.** In thymoma, surgery or radiation therapy is not uniformly successful in reversing the anemia. **Corticosteroids, splenectomy,** and **immunosuppressive therapy** with cyclophosphamide may be useful.
c. **Autoimmune hemolytic anemia, or cold agglutinin disease,** is usually caused by an immunoglobulin produced by lymphoma or chronic lymphocytic leukemia cells.
(1) **RBC** indices may be high or low depending on the reticulocyte response. If the reticulocyte count is high, due to normal marrow function, the indices are normal or high. If immune hemolysis is present, multiple spherocytes are present.
(2) **Therapy** with **prednisone** (1.0–1.5 mg/kg/day) is often effective. **Splenectomy** is also occasionally useful. In most cases, however, neither splenectomy nor corticosteroids are effective for long periods unless the underlying malignancy is effectively treated.
d. **Microangiopathic hemolytic anemia** occurs with mucin-producing adenocarcinomas, especially gastric cancer.
(1) **DIC** can be diagnosed by measurement of fibrinogen and fibrin split products.
(2) There is no effective **treatment** except treating the underlying tumor. Heparin should not be used unless there is concomitant DIC.

e. **Granulocytosis** occurs even in the absence of bone marrow involvement. Other causes of inflammation or infection must be excluded. The most common malignancies associated with granulocytosis include gastric, lung, and pancreatic carcinoma; melanoma; CNS tumors; Hodgkin's disease; and large-cell lymphomas.

f. **Thrombocytosis** occurs in as many as one third of all cancer patients. If essential thrombocythemia is present, hydroxyurea should be given to keep the platelet count below 500,000/mm^3.

g. **Thrombocytopenia** is often due to secondary effects of chemotherapy, bone marrow involvement, or radiation therapy, but is also seen in severe microangiopathic hemolytic anemia and DIC. A syndrome resembling autoimmune thrombocytopenia has been described in Hodgkin's disease, lymphoma, some types of leukemia, and certain solid tumors. This form of idiopathic thrombocytopenic purpura (ITP) is treated with corticosteroids, splenectomy, or immunosuppressive drugs.

2. **Paraneoplastic syndromes of the coagulation system**

a. **Primary DIC** occurs most frequently with mucin-producing adenocarcinomas such as pancreatic, gastric, lung, prostate, and colon cancers. Both acute and chronic DIC are associated with thrombophlebitis, arterial emboli, endocarditis, circulating inhibitors of coagulation, and abnormal circulating proteins that may precipitate hemorrhagic complications.

(1) **Acute DIC** is often observed in acute promyelocytic leukemia, as the result of the release of a procoagulant contained in the abnormal granules of the leukemia promyelocyte.

(a) **Clinical features.** Elevation of the prothrombin time (PT) is one of the earliest detectable symptoms along with elevation of fibrin split products and lowered fibrinogen levels. Further decreases in fibrinogen levels and an increase in the partial thromboplastin time (PTT) occur in more severe cases.

(b) **Therapy.** Improved management of acute DIC has led to a better short-term prognosis for most patients.

(i) Measures include **aggressive transfusion support** to maintain the platelet count between 35,000 and 50,000/mm^3, **intravenous vitamin K,** and **clotting factor replacement** with fresh-frozen plasma or cryoprecipitate if the fibrinogen level is less than 75 mg/dL.

(ii) **Heparin** is controversial but can be administered cautiously to **refractory patients.**

(2) **Chronic DIC** is most common in patients with adenocarcinomas.

(a) **Clinical features** include mild prolongations of the PT, high fibrinogen levels, and elevation of the fibrin split products. Patients often have thrombophlebitis or pulmonary emboli.

(b) **Heparin** is the treatment of choice; **thrombolytic therapy** also may be considered if there are no contraindications.

b. **Syndromes associated with paraproteins**

(1) **Coagulopathy.** Abnormal hemostasis and coagulation may develop in patients with plasma cell dysplasias such as multiple myeloma as a result of the effects of paraproteins on normal clotting factors and platelet receptor function. Paraproteins can also inhibit fibrin monomer aggregation and act as inhibitors of factor VIII. If patients have intractable bleeding, plasmapheresis may be required in combination with chemotherapy.

(2) **Hyperviscosity.** In multiple myeloma and macroglobulinemia, patients with a serum viscosity greater than 4.0 (relative to water) may have signs of decreased blood flow, including headaches, dizziness, epistaxis, seizures, hearing loss, altered mental status, and cardiac disease. Treatment consists of prompt plasmapheresis to remove the excessive paraprotein and avoid dehydration, as well as treatment of the underlying plasma cell dyscrasia.

C CNS syndromes are rare The most common (and the malignancies associated with them) are listed in Table 4–15.

TABLE 4–15 Central Nervous System Paraneoplastic Syndromes and Associated Malignancies

Syndrome	Associated Malignancy
Limbic encephalitis	Small-cell lung cancer
Subacute cellular degeneration	Small-cell lung cancer, ovarian cancer
Subacute motor neuropathy	Lymphoma
Subacute sensory neuropathy	Small-cell lung cancer
Sensorimotor polyneuropathy	Small-cell lung carcinoma, Hodgkin's disease
Eaton-Lambert myasthenia	Lung cancer, ovarian cancer
Polymyositis or dermatomyositis	Varied; breast, lung, gastrointestinal, and ovarian carcinomas are most common

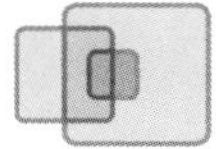

Study Questions

1. A 55-year-old, postmenopausal woman presents for a yearly visit. A 1-cm nodule is palpated in the upper, outer quadrant of her right breast. Her most recent mammogram 6 months ago was negative. Her family history is significant for her mother and a sister both diagnosed with breast cancer in their early to mid 50s. She has hypertension and hypercholesterolemia. What is the most appropriate next step in her management?

   A Repeat mammogram and ultrasound now
   B Repeat mammogram in 6 months
   C Repeat clinical examination in 1 month and refer to mammography if there is an increase in the size of the nodule
   D Begin tamoxifen
   E Refer her to a surgeon

2. The yearly mammogram in a 65-year-old postmenopausal woman shows an irregular area of microcalcification, which has grown in size compared with her mammogram from 2 years ago. She missed her mammogram last year. Physical examination is unrevealing, without lymphadenopathy or any nodularity in the breasts. You refer her to a surgeon. Eventually a 2-cm invasive ductal carcinoma is removed from her left breast. Sentinel lymph node biopsy shows two positive lymph nodes, and axillary lymph node dissection indicates 5 more positive lymph nodes. The tumor expresses the estrogen receptor (ER+). Which of the following interventions would increase her chance of cure?

   A Chemotherapy followed by hormonal therapy
   B Radiation therapy
   C Total mastectomy
   D Hormonal therapy alone
   E High-dose chemotherapy with stem cell support

3. An 18-year-old boy presents with swollen lymph nodes in his neck for 2 weeks. He has been treated with antibiotics for 10 days, but the lymph nodes continue to grow. He has had a 10-lb. weight loss in the past 2 months and is experiencing drenching night sweats. He reports fatigue and inability to play basketball like he used to. He has not been sexually active in the past 1 year. The next best course of action is

   A Changing the antibiotics
   B CT scan of the chest
   C Refer to a surgeon for lymph node biopsy
   D Check the HIV status of this patient
   E Assure him that he has a self-limiting viral illness

4. Eventually he is diagnosed with nodular sclerosing Hodgkin's disease. His bone marrow biopsy is negative, and he is found to have disease in both sides of the diaphragm (Stage III). Treatment of choice in the United States is:

   A Chemotherapy with the ABVD regimen
   B Radiation to all the affected lymph nodes

C Surgical resection of all the affected lymph nodes
D Treatment with rituximab
E High-dose chemotherapy with stem cell support

5. The most serious long-term side effect of this treatment is

A Congestive heart failure
B Peripheral neuropathy
C Myelodysplastic syndrome/acute myelogenous leukemia
D Early myocardial infarction
E Early-onset cataract

6. A 55-year-old African-American man is seen in the emergency room with a 2-day history of hematuria, back pain, double vision, and altered mental status. He is an engineer with an office-based occupation with no exposure to chemicals or radiation. Family history is positive for an uncle with "bone cancer." He smokes half pack of cigarettes a day but does not drink alcohol. Laboratory evaluation in the ER shows an elevated total protein of 22 mg/dL, elevated gamma globulins, a serum creatinine of 2.5 mg/dL, and a hemoglobin of 9.0 g/L. Blood smear shows roulette formation. You suspect:

A Acute renal failure of unknown etiology
B Hyperviscosity syndrome secondary to multiple myeloma
C A genitourinary malignancy
D Drug toxicity
E Intravascular hemolysis

7. Best management option at this point is

A Plasmapheresis
B Transfusion of red blood cells
C Hemodialysis
D Broad-spectrum antibiotics
E Supportive care

8. To establish a diagnosis, you should

A Obtain bone marrow biopsies and a skeletal survey
B Obtain a CT scan of chest, abdomen, and pelvis
C Perform an ultrasound of the kidneys
D Perform a bone scan
E Perform a kidney biopsy

9. A 50-year-old executive undergoes his first screening colonoscopy. He has been constipated for 1 year, relieved by laxatives. There has been no blood in his stools. A fungating mass is seen in the sigmoid colon. Subsequent surgery shows a lesion that has penetrated through the muscularis propria. Three regional lymph nodes are positive for adenocarcinoma. His best chance for cure would occur with which form of therapy?

A No further therapy needed
B Adjuvant chemotherapy
C Radiation treatment
D Concurrent chemotherapy and radiation therapy
E Immunotherapy

10. Patient completes a course of adjuvant chemotherapy. Further follow-up should consists of:

- A Periodic evaluations, initially every 3 months, with history and physical and liver function tests.
- B Option A plus CEA level
- C Option B plus CT scans of chest, abdomen, and pelvis
- D All of the above plus a PET scan
- E Yearly pan-endoscopy

11. A 57-year-old postmenopausal woman has completed her adjuvant treatment for a Stage II, ER-/PR-positive breast cancer. She is presenting for a discussion regarding initiation of hormonal treatment with tamoxifen. The optimal duration of treatment with this agent is:

- A 10 years
- B 5 years
- C 2 years
- D Lifetime
- E Intermittent treatment for 5 years

12. A 67-year-old man with a significant smoking history has had a persistent right upper lobe infiltrate. A CT scan shows a 3-cm solitary lesion with irregular borders. A fine-needle aspiration shows adenocarcinoma. Appropriate staging workup at this point includes:

- A Bone marrow biopsy
- B PA and lateral chest radiograms
- C Lymphangiogram
- D CT scans of the chest, abdomen, and pelvis and a PET scan
- E Video-assisted thoracic surgery (VATS)

13. A 48-year-old woman, smoker, with a history of Hodgkin's disease at the age of 29, treated with chest radiation, has developed a squamous cell carcinoma of the lung. Staging workup shows only a 2.5-cm solitary lesion in the left upper lobe. Her FEV1 and FVC are 70% of the predicted values, respectively. The best treatment option for her is:

- A Radiation
- B Chemotherapy with carboplatin and Taxol
- C Lobectomy
- D Concurrent chemotherapy and radiation
- E Radiation followed by surgery

14. A 55-year-old postmenopausal woman presents with a 2-month history of lower back pain. Further questioning indicates bony pain involving the left arm and leg. Radiographic imaging shows multiple punched-out lesions throughout the skeleton. Serum calcium is elevated, and she is anemic. The most likely diagnosis is:

- A Osteoporosis
- B Metastatic breast cancer
- C Multiple myeloma
- D Lymphoma
- E Sarcoma

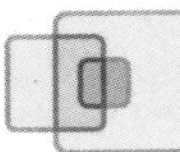

Answers and Explanations

1. **The answer is A** [V D 1]. A palpable mass during the physical examination warrants an immediate evaluation. Even though she had undergone a mammography 6 months ago, most oncologists, radiologists, and surgeons would repeat this study. In addition, an ultrasound evaluation might reveal whether this is a cyst or a more solid mass. Repeating the mammogram in 6 months is not a good option, because this will delay treatment if the abnormal finding is in fact a malignancy. The same is true for answer C. Virtually no one will begin therapy without a firm diagnosis; therefore, answer D is incorrect.

2. **The answer is A** [V F 3]. This patient is in high risk of recurrence by virtue of having disease in her lymph nodes. Radiation therapy or surgical excision of the breast cancer usually provide local control and provide adequate protection against recurrence of disease in the tumor bed. However, micrometastatic disease can only be addressed through the administration of systemic therapy such as cytotoxic chemotherapy. In patients with hormonally sensitive tumors (e.g., estrogen receptor positive), hormonal therapy has been shown to be very effective in the prevention of disease recurrence after chemotherapy and can be used as a sole treatment option in selected patients. Randomized clinical trials have shown that lumpectomy and radiation therapy is equal to a total mastectomy in terms of overall survival. For tumors that can be removed totally with adequate margins (>10 mm), lumpectomy offers better cosmetic and psychological results. It is a less invasive surgery and allows for faster recovery time.

3. **The answer is C** [XIV D 1]. Any lymph node that does not respond to the usual treatment, such as two courses of different antibiotics, should raise the suspicion of the treating physicians. For easily accessible lymph nodes, the preferred method of investigation is a full excisional biopsy. The examination of an intact lymph node allows pathologists to examine the lymph node architecture and arrive at a definitive diagnosis. Although a CT scan might eventually be needed, it should not be the first choice. Also, the HIV status of a patient with high-risk behavior needs to be determined, but there is no indication from the case presentation that this patient falls in this category and it should not be the first choice.

4. **The answer is A** [XIV E 3 a]. This combination chemotherapy is the treatment of choice in most parts of the United States. Other multi-agent chemotherapy regimens are also acceptable. Ongoing clinical trials are comparing effective regimens to determine whether there are superior alternatives to the ABVD regimen. There is no indication that the removal of all involved lymph nodes is surgically feasible or therapeutic. Disseminated Hodgkin's lymphoma is a systemic disease and should be treated as such. Also, radiation therapy is reserved for cases in which either there is bulky disease or a focal area of the body is involved. Delivery of radiation to multiple sites is generally not feasible because of the toxicity of this approach. Choice D, treatment with rituximab, is for non-Hodgkin's lymphomas.

5. **The answer is C** [XIV E 3 c]. Cytotoxic chemotherapy could lead to various chromosomal abnormalities that could result in acute leukemia or myelodysplastic syndrome. The risk of secondary myeloid malignancies approaches 2% with the ABVD regimen, and increased incidence of non-Hodgkin's lymphoma is noted as well. A number of chemotherapeutic agents that alkylate DNA are thought to be involved in this process. In general, high-dose therapy with any of these agents is associated with the development of AML/MDS. Congestive heart failure as a result of exposure to doxorubicin (Adriamycin) is known to occur. However, usually this toxicity is seen with doses exceeding 480 mg/m^2. The risk of myocardial infarction at a young age should not be an issue if radiation to the chest and thorax is not needed. Peripheral neuropathy is also a manageable toxicity seen with vinca alkaloids such as vincristine.

6. **The answer is B** [XIII C 2]. This challenging case requires a close examination of the laboratory results and of the patient presentation in an attempt to arrive at a unifying diagnosis that explains all of the

observed abnormalities. The elevated total protein and the presence of roulettes in the blood smear are classic signs of paraproteinemia. The history of change in mental status and double vision, in a patient with elevated total protein, should raise concerns for the development of hyperviscosity syndrome. Once the presence of anemia and renal insufficiency has been established, the diagnosis of multiple myeloma should strongly be considered. A GU malignancy usually does not lead to an elevated total protein or changes in the blood smear as discussed in this case.

7. The answer is A [XIII F c (4)]. Plasmapheresis offers the only option for reducing the amount of protein in the circulation to alleviate some of the symptoms. Blood transfusions could be detrimental until the hyperviscosity has been improved, because blood transfusions will raise blood viscosity. The other two options would not address the issue with high protein content in the circulation.

8. The answer is A [XIII D 2]. Bone marrow biopsy will determine the percentage of plasma cells in the bone marrow, which is required to establish the diagnosis of multiple myeloma. A skeletal survey will enumerate the extent of bone involvement and is useful in staging, which can guide therapy and establish a prognosis. The level of paraprotein in the blood, the number of bone lesions, the level of hemoglobin, and renal functions are used to establish the stage of the disease. Additional blood studies to determine the isotype of the paraprotein (IgG, IgA) and the light chain usage (κ or λ) can provide additional useful information. A bone scan would not be helpful in this case because bony lesions in this disease are not blastic and therefore would not be seen on a bone scan. CT scans are usually negative in this disease, and renal ultrasounds will not help in establishing the diagnosis.

9. The answer is B [VI 7 3 a]. Of the options presented, only adjuvant chemotherapy would increase the likelihood of cure for a patient who has had resection of stage III (e.g., lymph node metastasis positive, T_{any}, $N_{1 \text{ or } 2}$, M_0) adenocarcinoma of the colon. This has been repeatedly demonstrated in a number of clinical trials. Once cancer has been found in the lymph nodes, the patient has a high rate of systemic dissemination. The guidelines are less clear for the management of patients with transmurally invasive cancers that do not metastasize to regional lymph nodes (e.g., stage II, $T_3N_0M_0$). Although meta-analysis suggest a very small advantage for the use of 5-fluorouracil–based adjuvant chemotherapy, most authorities based treatment recommendations on the balance of anticipated benefit with patient fitness and treatment preferences. The preliminary results of a randomized clinical trial employing multi-agent chemotherapy with 5-fluorouracil and oxaliplatin shows a survival advantage for the combination in patients with both stage II and stage III disease, and may change the adjuvant therapy paradigm in the future.

10. The answer is A [VI 7 3 a]. Periodic evaluation with history, physical examination, and laboratory studies is the optimum approach. The CEA marker, although widely used, is insufficiently sensitive to detect metastases when they are still localized. CT scans should be reserved for patients who have either concerning symptoms or abnormal liver function tests. Endoscopies would not delineate metastatic lesions.

11. The answer is B [V 4 a]. The optimal duration of treatment with tamoxifen is 5 years. Large randomized clinical trials have proved that shorter treatment duration is not as protective as 5 years of treatment. Also, longer duration of treatment (10 years) is associated with more side effects such as thromboembolic phenomenon.

12. The answer is D [IV E]. The appropriate staging of a patient with a diagnosis of lung cancer requires all the tests mentioned in this answer. The goal is to rule out the presence of gross disease in all the areas where lung cancer can potentially metastasize. This includes liver, the adrenal glands, mediastinal lymph nodes, and contralateral chest. Routine chest films are not sensitive enough to detect smaller lymph nodes in the hilar region. Neither bone marrow biopsies nor lymphangiograms are indicated for staging of lung cancer. In fact, lymphangiograms are no longer routinely performed. PET scans are increasingly used in the initial staging of patients with lung cancer because of their sensitivity in detecting minimal disease. Accurate staging information has a major impact on the choice of therapy for this disease. A patient who, based on initial CT scans, is considered to be a candidate for potentially curative surgery might be found to have metastatic disease by PET scan and therefore be a candidate for palliative chemotherapy.

13. The answer is C [IV G 1]. Treatment of choice for stage I lung cancer is surgical resection of the tumor. This can be accomplished by a lobectomy or a wedge resection of the involved lung segment. Surgical resection for stage I or II non–small cell lung cancer is potentially curative, with 5-year survival of close to 70%. Neither chemotherapy alone nor concurrent chemoradiation therapy is appropriate for a young otherwise healthy patient with early stage lung cancer.

14. The answer is C [XIII C 2 c]. The appearance of punched-out lesions (lytic lesions) is pathognomonic for multiple myeloma. In fact, the presence of more than one lytic lesion signals the presence of higher tumor burden. Although a patient with osteoporosis could have anemia and hypercalcemia due to other causes, the general radiographic appearance of the bones is one of osteopenia and not punched-out lesions. Metastatic breast cancer usually is not associated with purely lytic lesions, and the case presentation is not consistent with this disease. The presence of anemia, hypercalcemia, and lytic lesions is indicative of multiple myeloma.

chapter **5**

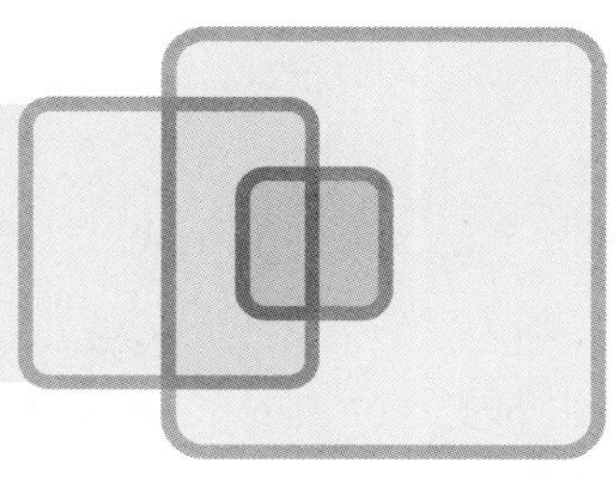

Gastrointestinal Diseases

ANTHONY J. DIMARINO, JR.

I DISEASES OF THE ESOPHAGUS

The esophagus is basically an organ of transport, with no significant absorptive or secretory function.

A Features common to clinical disorders

1. **Dysphagia,** or difficulty in swallowing, is a symptom often described as a **sticking sensation.**
   a. **Dysphagia for solids** indicates an esophageal obstruction as a result of:
      (1) Carcinoma
      (2) An esophageal web or ring
      (3) Benign esophageal stricture
      (4) Dysphagia lusoria, which occurs when an anomalous blood vessel (usually the right subclavian artery) crosses behind the esophagus
   b. **Dysphagia for solids and liquids** indicates an esophageal abnormality as a result of motor dysfunction, such as:
      (1) Scleroderma
      (2) Achalasia
      (3) Symptomatic diffuse esophageal spasm (SDES)
   c. **Transfer dysphagia** indicates a difficulty in initiating swallowing and is often associated with a neuromuscular disorder of the pharynx or proximal esophagus (e.g., after a cerebrovascular accident), proximal muscle weakness of the pharynx or esophagus (e.g., polymyositis), or other neuromuscular disorders (myasthenia gravis, myotonia dystrophica, or Parkinson's disease).
2. **Odynophagia,** or pain on swallowing, may be due to:
   a. **Motor disorders** of the esophagus, especially achalasia and diffuse esophageal spasm
   b. **Mucosal disruption** caused by ingestion of lye or other caustic agents, severe peptic esophagitis, severe infections of the esophagus [e.g., human immunodeficiency virus (HIV), candidal esophagitis, herpetic esophagitis, cytomegalovirus (CMV), and *Mycobacterium avium-intracellulare* (MAI)], drug-induced esophagitis (see I B 4 f), and radiation esophagitis
3. **Heartburn** is a substernal burning sensation that radiates in an orad direction and may be initiated by bending forward. This is a specific symptom of gastroesophageal reflux.

B Specific disorders

1. **Reflux esophagitis** is caused by the recurrent reflux of gastric contents into the distal esophagus.
   a. **Etiology and pathogenesis**
      (1) **Lower esophageal sphincter (LES) dysfunction.** Normally, the LES blocks reflux of gastric juice into the esophagus. Reflux esophagitis is thought to stem from a defect in this LES mechanism, such as:
         (a) Decreased resting LES pressure
         (b) Prolonged or repeated intermittent transient relaxation of the LES
         (c) Transient increase in abdominal pressure

(2) **Secondary causes** of reflux esophagitis should always be suspected and corrected if possible. The following conditions appear to decrease LES pressure:

(a) **Pregnancy.** Especially during the last trimester, heartburn may be severe and probably is caused by progesterone's inhibitory effects on the LES.

(b) **Drugs.** Medications that may decrease the LES pressure as a side effect of smooth muscle relaxation include:

(i) Anticholinergic agents

(ii) β_2-Adrenergic agonists and theophylline used to treat asthma and chronic bronchitis

(iii) Calcium channel–blocking agents and nitrates

(c) **Scleroderma.** Weakening of the esophageal smooth muscle and the LES region causes severe reflux esophagitis.

(d) **Surgical vagotomy.** This procedure also may produce anatomic alterations that lead to reflux esophagitis.

b. Clinical features

(1) **Heartburn or acid regurgitation** is a specific symptom of gastroesophageal regurgitation.

(2) **Dysphagia** in the esophagitis patient generally is for solids and may indicate a developing stricture.

(3) **Anemia** may occur if recurrent esophageal bleeding is present.

(4) **Extraesophageal manifestations** include recurrent laryngitis, reflux-induced asthma, cough, **atypical chest pain,** or hiccups.

c. Diagnosis. Several tests have been proposed for the diagnosis of reflux esophagitis.

(1) **Barium swallow and upper gastrointestinal series.** This is the least sensitive test. Generally, it is positive only in severe gastroesophageal reflux with a very weakened LES or in the presence of esophageal ulceration.

(2) **Acid-perfusion test (Bernstein test).** This test is intended to reproduce the pain associated with reflux and involves esophageal perfusion of 0.1 *N* HCl alternately with normal saline solution.

(3) **Twenty-four hour pH monitoring.** This measures the number of episodes and length of time that the distal esophageal pH is less than 4.0.

(4) **Scintigraphy.** This technique involves the introduction of technetium 99 (^{99}Tc) into the stomach followed by abdominal compression and radiographic counting over the esophagus. This noninvasive technique can demonstrate reflux as well as provide a useful quantitative measure of its presence.

(5) **Endoscopy with biopsy.** This procedure is especially helpful in ruling out associated Barrett's esophagus (see B 1 e 5). However, erosive changes are seen in only a minority of patients who undergo endoscopy. A squamous papilloma is a small benign polyp at the end of the esophagus, thought to be secondary to chronic reflux esophagitis.

(6) **Esophageal manometry.** This procedure is useful in evaluating LES pressure. Pressures consistently measured at less than one third of the lower limit of normal usually are associated with significant reflux. This technique is especially useful in the preoperative evaluation of esophageal reflux when a fundoplication is contemplated.

d. Therapy

(1) **Increasing the reflux barrier** may be accomplished by:

(a) Lifestyle modification such as elevating the head of the bed 4–6 inches, avoiding eating for 3 hours before bedtime, and avoiding fatty or large-volume meals.

(b) Administration of alginic acid and antacid combinations

(c) Administration of drugs that increase LES tone (e.g., bethanechol, metoclopramide, domperidone, cisapride).

(d) Antireflux surgery, especially Nissen fundoplication

(2) **Decreasing gastric acid effects** may be accomplished by:
(a) Administration of antacids
(b) Administration of histamine$_2$ (H_2)-receptor antagonists (e.g., cimetidine, famotidine, ranitidine, nizatidine)
(c) Administration of hydrogen/potassium (H+/K+) proton pump adenosine triphosphatase (ATPase) blockers (proton pump inhibitors) such as omeprazole, lansoprazole, pantoprazole, esomeprazole, rabeprazole.

(3) **Maintaining LES pressure.** The following agents decrease LES pressure and should be avoided:
(a) Anticholinergic agents
(b) β-Adrenergic drugs
(c) Calcium channel–blocking agents
(d) Chocolate
(e) Fats
(f) Nicotine (smoking)
(g) Nitrates
(h) Xanthine and its derivatives (e.g., caffeine)
(i) Peppermint

e. **Complications**

(1) **Benign esophageal stricture** probably occurs in a small portion of all reflux esophagitis cases and is best diagnosed by a bolus barium swallow, endoscopy with biopsy, or cytology.

(2) **Esophageal ulceration** may be accompanied by hemorrhage. However, the primary symptom is severe and unrelenting pain.

(3) **Reflux-induced laryngitis** is a common cause of recurrent hoarseness in adults.

(4) **Pulmonary aspiration** is a serious sequela of reflux esophagitis. Patients older than 30 years of age who develop repeated pneumonia or asthma should be evaluated for esophageal reflux.

(5) **Barrett's esophagus** refers to a condition in which columnar epithelium replaces the normal squamous epithelium of the esophagus, possibly as a result of continuous inflammation. This is considered a premalignant state, with a 40-fold increased risk of adenocarcinoma, and is probably responsible for the increased incidence of adenocarcinoma of the esophagus.

2. **Obstructive esophageal conditions**

a. **Carcinoma**

(1) **Epidemiology.** In the United States, the incidence of adenocarcinoma of the esophagus is equivalent to that of squamous cell carcinoma of the esophagus. Carcinoma occurs predominantly in men and with varying incidence throughout the world. The population of the United States is considered at low risk; esophageal cancer occurs in only 4 of 100,000 individuals.

(2) **Etiology.** Certain factors appear to increase the risk of esophageal cancer.
(a) **Tobacco smoking,** which increases the risk of squamous cell carcinoma twofold to fourfold
(b) **Alcohol consumption,** which has been shown to increase the risk up to 12 times in France. Alcohol and tobacco appear to have an additive effect.
(c) **Geographic factors.** Incidence levels, which were found to be 400 times greater in certain regions in China and Iran, may be attributable to a diet that includes increased amounts of pickled food, nitrosamines, and molds as well as decreased amounts of selenium, fresh fruits, and vegetables.
(d) **Vitamin deficiency,** especially of vitamins A and C, which may be associated with an increased risk for esophageal cancer

(e) **Lye ingestion,** which is associated with the development of esophageal cancer many years after exposure

(f) **Achalasia,** which may be associated with a 10% risk of subsequent carcinomas

(g) **Barrett's esophagus** [see I B 1 e (5)]. Adenocarcinoma eventually may develop in 10% of patients with this condition.

(h) **Tylosis–hyperkeratosis of the palms and soles.** More than 80% of patients with this autosomal dominant condition develop squamous cell carcinoma of the esophagus.

(i) **Celiac sprue**

(j) **Esophageal dysplasia** associated with human papilloma virus (HPV)

(3) **Clinical features**

(a) **Progressive dysphagia for solids** indicates the presence of an ongoing obstructive lesion. Usually, when the esophageal lumen narrows to 1.2 cm or less, a **persistent dysphagia** for solid food is observed.

(b) **Pain** usually signifies extension of the tumor beyond the wall of the esophagus.

(c) **Dysphagia for liquids, cough, hoarseness,** and **weight loss** generally are symptoms of advanced esophageal carcinoma.

(4) **Diagnosis**

(a) **Barium radiograph** with a barium-coated bolus (e.g., bread or a marshmallow) should be performed when obstructive dysphagia is suspected.

(b) **Endoscopy with biopsy and cytologic study,** if performed together, establishes a diagnosis in approximately 90% of cases and is the diagnostic procedure of choice.

(c) **Computed tomography** (CT) and **bronchoscopy** should be used to evaluate the presence and extent of nodal metastases and bronchial invasion.

(d) **Endoscopic ultrasound (EUS)** is useful for staging esophageal carcinomas.

(5) **Therapy** (see Chapter 4 VI D 7, 8)

b. **Benign esophageal stricture** may be a sequela of prolonged reflux esophagitis. Heartburn may lessen as solid-food dysphagia worsens with progression of the stricture. Diagnosis is established by a bolus barium swallow and endoscopy. Treatment generally is with tapered bougies or with balloon dilatation catheters.

c. **Esophageal webs** seen in the upper one-third of the esophagus may be caused by a failure of complete embryologic recanalization. Webs in this area also may be associated with iron deficiency anemia in the **Plummer-Vinson (Paterson-Kelly) syndrome.** Effective treatment of this syndrome includes administering iron for the anemia and using an esophageal bougie to fracture the webs.

d. **Esophageal rings** most commonly occur at the squamocolumnar junction and are called **Schatzki's rings.** Dysphagia for solids often is intermittent in this condition, especially if the narrowest point of the esophagus measures between 1.2 and 2 cm. Esophageal bougienage often is effective therapy.

3. **Esophageal motor disorders**

a. **Oropharyngeal dysphagia (transfer dysphagia)** is a descriptive term applied to a disorder of the neuromuscular apparatus of the distal pharynx and upper esophagus. Symptoms include difficulty in initiating swallowing, nasal regurgitation, and cough with pulmonary aspiration. The types of disorders associated with oropharyngeal dysphagia include:

(1) **Cerebrovascular accident (CVA),** which may be the most common of these disorders and usually is attributable to transient brain stem edema

(2) **Myasthenia gravis**

(3) **Myotonic dystrophy**

(4) **Polymyositis**

(5) **Bulbar poliomyelitis**

(6) **Parkinson's disease**

(7) **Multiple sclerosis (MS)**

(8) **Amyotrophic lateral sclerosis**
(9) **Hypothyroidism**

b. SDES [I A 1 b (3)]

(1) **Pathology.** Although occasional reports have described an esophageal muscular hypertrophy, these are not consistent. Most investigators think that a neural defect exists. LES abnormalities (similar to achalasia), with incomplete relaxation, have been described in 30% of cases, and documented progression to classic achalasia lends credence to a neural pathogenesis.

(2) **Clinical features**
(a) **Dysphagia** for both solids and liquids occurs.
(b) **Odynophagia** may occur, especially after ingestion of extremely hot or cold solids or liquids.
(c) **Spontaneous chest pain** similar to angina pectoris may be evident. Nocturnal pain, which is often described, is relieved by the smooth muscle relaxant nitroglycerin (the same treatment prescribed for anginal pain). The ability of nitroglycerin to provide relief may further confuse the diagnosis.

(3) **Diagnosis.** Clinical evidence is the basis of diagnosis.
(a) **Radiography** may reveal a corkscrew-shaped esophagus.
(b) **Esophageal manometry** should reveal:
(i) High-amplitude, repetitive, simultaneous contractions in approximately 30% of the basal state or after ergonovine or edrophonium stimulation (not a routinely performed test). (In a variant of SDES called the **nutcracker esophagus,** high-amplitude prolonged contractions may be associated with chest pain.)
(ii) Several normal peristaltic sequences to differentiate SDES from achalasia
(iii) Incomplete relaxation of the LES in approximately 30% of patients
(c) **Balloon distention of the esophageal lumen** can be used as a stimulus. A smaller-than-normal amount of air or water insufflation of the balloon indicates a lower threshold for pain.

(4) **Therapy** (successful in approximately 50% of cases)
(a) Anticholinergic agents
(b) Nitrates (short- or long-acting)
(c) Calcium channel–blocking agents
(d) Esophageal bougienage
(e) Hydralazine to decrease peristaltic amplitude
(f) Surgery with a longitudinal esophageal myotomy (in severe, incapacitating cases only)

c. Achalasia

(1) **Epidemiology.** Achalasia occurs in approximately 1 in 100,000 individuals in the United States and equally in both sexes. The most common age of onset is between 20 and 40 years.

(2) **Pathology.** A neural defect is suggested by decreased ganglion cells, with fibrosis and scarring in Auerbach's plexus. **Wallerian degeneration** is suggested by examination of vagal esophageal fibers. The dorsal vagal nucleus also is abnormal. Supersensitivity to cholinergic stimulation and exogenous gastrin is described.

(3) **Clinical features**
(a) Dysphagia for solids and liquids in 95%–100% of patients
(b) Weight loss in 90% of patients
(c) Chest pain, which is severe in approximately 60% of patients
(d) Nocturnal cough in approximately 30% of patients, indicating possible overflow aspiration of unemptied esophageal contents and, in such cases, the need for immediate treatment
(e) Recurrent bronchitis or pneumonia, both of which are serious complications, in approximately 7%–8% of patients

(4) **Diagnosis.** Diagnosis involves excluding malignancy (i.e., carcinoma or lymphoma) at the esophagogastric junction, which may mimic achalasia ("secondary achalasia"). Secondary achalasia may be characterized by greater weight loss, shorter duration of symptoms, and less esophageal dilatation in an older person.

(a) **Radiography** may reveal a flaccid, dilated, fluid-filled esophagus with a beak-like tapering over the LES region. A CT scan of the chest and abdomen or an endoscopic ultrasound of the esophagogastric junction may be needed to rule out secondary (often malignant) achalasia.

(b) **Manometry** is the most sensitive diagnostic method and should reveal:

(i) Absence of normal peristalsis in the entire esophagus

(ii) Elevated LES pressure

(iii) Incomplete relaxation of the LES, which probably accounts for the major clinical findings because there is a persistent obstructing barrier after swallowing

(5) **Therapy**

(a) **Drugs** such as nitrates, anticholinergic agents, β_2-adrenergic agonists, and calcium channel-blocking agents are effective in less than 50% of patients.

(b) **Pneumatic dilation** is effective in 70%–90% of patients, has a mortality rate of approximately 0.2%, and has a perforation rate of roughly 2%–3%.

(c) **Endoscopic injection of botulinum toxin** into the LES results in decreased LES pressure and decreased dysphagia in 70%–80% of patients. Repeated injections may be necessary, and long-term efficacy is noted in less than 50% of patients.

(d) **Surgical therapy.** The favored procedure is a **Heller myotomy,** which has a 65%–90% success rate and a 3%–4% surgical complication rate. For operations that do not incorporate an antireflux procedure, the rate of postoperative reflux may increase to 25%–30% after several years. Laparoscopic techniques are favored.

d. Systemic sclerosis (scleroderma) is a systemic collagen vascular disease involving the skin in 98% of cases. The esophagus is found to be abnormal in 75% of autopsies and in 80% of cases studied manometrically.

(1) **Pathology.** The early esophageal effects are thought to be neural because no anatomic abnormality of the smooth muscle can be identified at a time when marked weakness of the esophagus is noted. The strong association with Raynaud's phenomenon, which also is believed to have a neural basis, is consistent with this theory. A late defect may include a disuse type of atrophy of the circular smooth muscle elements of the esophagus; the longitudinal muscular layers remain intact.

(2) **Clinical features**

(a) Dysphagia for solids and liquids

(b) Severe heartburn in approximately 50% of patients

(c) Esophageal stricture in approximately 25% of long-term survivors

(3) **Diagnosis**

(a) **Radiography.** Supine esophagography may indicate poor esophageal emptying because of an absence of peristalsis.

(b) **Manometry.** This procedure, which is the most reliable diagnostic technique, reveals:

(i) Decreased LES pressure

(ii) Very weak, low-amplitude peristaltic contractions in the distal smooth muscle portion (lower two thirds) of the esophagus

(4) **Therapy.** The esophageal disorder is treated with antireflux measures (see I B 1 d).

4. Other esophageal disorders

a. Diverticula

(1) **Zenker's diverticulum** is a mucosal herniation (not a true diverticulum) above the cricopharyngeal region. Obstructive symptoms may occur if there is incomplete emptying of this diverticulum. Large diverticula are treated surgically.

(2) **Traction diverticula** occur in the mid and distal regions and are thought to be secondary to an adjacent inflammatory process such as tuberculosis.

(3) **Epiphrenic diverticula** occur in the distal esophagus, above the LES, and often are asymptomatic.

b. Infections. Bacterial and viral sources of esophageal infection are common, but several infectious agents are of particular interest.

(1) **Candidal esophagitis** usually occurs in diabetic patients, immunocompromised hosts (e.g., patients infected with HIV or patients undergoing cancer chemotherapy or steroid treatment), and in those with poor esophageal emptying (e.g., patients with achalasia or severe stricture). Odynophagia is a major symptom, and diagnosis is made by endoscopy and cytologic studies. Treatment is with nystatin, ketoconazole, fluconazole, or, in resistant cases, low doses of amphotericin B.

(2) **Herpes simplex virus (HSV)** may cause esophagitis in immunocompromised hosts. The esophagitis is characterized by relatively small, isolated ulcers. Biopsy of the ulcerating edges may show characteristic multinucleated cells with nuclear inclusions. Treatment is with vidarabine or acyclovir.

(3) **CMV** infection of the esophagus is often seen in immunocompromised patients and may produce very large ulcerations of the esophagus. Intranuclear inclusion bodies are observed on biopsy. Treatment is with ganciclovir.

(4) **HIV esophagitis** may result in a diffuse inflammatory esophagitis. Treatment of isolated acquired immunodeficiency syndrome (AIDS) esophagitis is with steroids.

c. Esophageal burns. Ingestion of caustic agents (i.e., strong alkali or acid) can cause serious esophageal burns. Ingestion of lye or detergents such as chlorine bleach is a common suicidal gesture in adults and a common accident in children. Emergency endoscopy should be performed to assess the extent of damage. Steroids and broad-spectrum antibiotics are recommended initially in management of esophageal burns. Long-term sequelae in survivors may include esophageal stricture and esophageal carcinoma.

d. Esophageal tears. These conditions are seen most commonly after vomiting (75% of cases), straining, or coughing.

(1) A mucosal tear **(Mallory-Weiss syndrome)** produces significant hematemesis after an initial nonbloody vomitus. Surgery is required in less than 10% of these cases.

(2) A rupture of the esophagus **(Boerhaave's syndrome)** usually occurs above the esophagogastric junction. Air in the left mediastinal region suggests the diagnosis, and immediate surgical intervention is necessary if the patient is to survive.

e. Paraesophageal hernia. Unlike the much more common and clinically insignificant hiatal hernia, a paraesophageal hernia may lead to gastric vascular compromise. The esophagogastric junction traverses the diaphragm in the appropriate location. The body of the stomach then travels above the diaphragm, and gastric volvulus with incarceration may occur. Surgery may be necessary to alleviate symptoms of pain, upper gastrointestinal bleeding, and ischemia.

f. Pill-induced esophagitis. This condition is often caused by medications such as **oral bisphosphonates,** aspirin and other nonsteroidal anti-inflammatory drugs (NSAIDs), potassium chloride tablets, iron preparations, quinidine, and tetracyclines and other antibiotics. These medications are often temporarily lodged in the esophagus because of either inadequate liquid with swallowing or a relative narrowing of the esophagus. Severe erosions and strictures may develop in a minority of cases. Treatment is symptomatic.

II DISEASES OF THE STOMACH

A Gastritis

1. **Acute gastritis** is an inflammation of the gastric mucosa, which may be diffuse or localized and usually is self-limited.

a. **Etiology**
   (1) **Drugs** that can damage the mucosal barrier and lead to back-diffusion of acid and pepsin include:
      (a) Aspirin and similar NSAIDs
      (b) Alcohol, which may produce an additive effect with aspirin
   (2) **Accidental ingestion of caustic substances** such as strong alkali (e.g., lye), strong acid [e.g., sulfuric acid (H_2SO_4), HCl], or fixatives [e.g., formaldehyde, trinitrophenol (picric acid)] can be fatal. Patients who survive the ingestion of such corrosives sustain injuries that leave considerable scars and subsequent antral narrowing.
   (3) **Stress** related to severe illness, especially illness involving many organ systems, causes acute gastritis. Ischemia and gastric acid, even at normal levels, may be involved. Antacids, H_2-receptor antagonists, proton pump inhibitors, and cytoprotective agents (e.g., sucralfate, prostaglandins) may be effective as prophylactic or therapeutic agents in cases of stress-induced gastritis.
   (4) **Infections**
      (a) *Helicobacter pylori* infectious gastritis (see III C 4)
      (b) **Phlegmonous gastritis,** bacterial invasion of the stomach wall, is a rare but fatal condition most commonly caused by streptococci; however, it also has been associated with staphylococci.
      (c) **Infections with CMV, herpesvirus, MAI, *Candida, Treponema pallidum,*** and ***Mycobacterium tuberculosis*** have been associated with gastritis, especially in immunocompromised patients.

b. **Clinical features** (present in 70% of patients)
   (1) **Epigastric burning** and **pain, nausea,** and **vomiting**
   (2) **Gastrointestinal bleeding,** which may be severe and associated with hematemesis and shock

c. **Diagnosis.** In most cases, diagnosis is made on the basis of endoscopic visualization with or without biopsy. Congestion, friability, superficial ulceration, and petechiae frequently are seen in the gastric mucosa.

d. **Therapy.** Treatment begins with removal of offending agents. Antacids, antiviral and antifungal agents, H_2-receptor antagonists, proton pump inhibitors, and surface-acting agents (e.g., sucralfate) are useful as well. Patients with acute hemorrhagic gastritis usually respond to fluid or blood replacement combined with a regimen of antacids, H_2-receptor antagonists, and omeprazole or lansoprazole, which keep the gastric pH above 3.5. Surgery rarely is necessary for these patients and is associated with high morbidity and mortality rates.

2. **Chronic gastritis** is characterized by a superficial lymphocyte infiltrate in the lamina propria.
   a. **Etiology.** Chronic gastritis can be caused by:
      (1) Prolonged use of alcohol, aspirin, and other irritating drugs
      (2) Radiation or thermal injury
      (3) Immunologic factors
      (4) Infections (e.g., *H. pylori*)
   b. **Types**
      (1) **Chronic type A gastritis** involves the fundus and body of the stomach; the antrum is spared. This type of gastritis is associated with parietal cell antibodies, high serum gastrin levels, and pernicious anemia.
      (2) **Chronic type B gastritis** involves the antrum of the stomach; the body and fundus are relatively spared. Gastrin cell antibodies have been detected in some patients with this gastritis. More commonly, reflux of duodenal or biliary secretions or *H. pylori* infections are linked causatively to type B gastritis.
   c. **Clinical features.** Clinical evidence may be limited in patients with chronic gastritis. Type A gastritis is associated with hypochlorhydria or achlorhydria, whereas type B gastritis is asso-

ciated with normal acid levels. Hypothyroidism, diabetes mellitus, and vitiligo occur more frequently with type A than with type B gastritis.

d. **Clinical course.** Data suggest that these lesions may remain unchanged for several years. Gastric atrophy develops in approximately 50% of patients with superficial gastritis over 10–20 years. There is an increased association with gastric polyps, gastric ulcer, and gastric cancer in both types of chronic gastritis, with type B being associated with a higher incidence of gastric cancer than type A.

e. **Therapy.** Treatment usually is unnecessary; however, conditions associated with gastritis (e.g., pernicious anemia, *H. pylori* infections, hypothyroidism, diabetes) should be treated accordingly. Some authors suggest yearly gastric cytologic analysis as a means of diagnosing an early cancer in affected patients.

3. **Special types of gastritis**

a. ***H. pylori*** infectious gastritis is caused by a gram-negative, spiral-shaped bacterium that survives in the acidic milieu of the stomach by producing urease, which liberates ammonia. Chronic gastritis involving *H. pylori* has been associated with 80%–90% of duodenal ulcer patients (see III C 4) and with 60%–70% of gastric ulcer patients. In addition, it has been associated with mucosa-associated lymphatic tissue (MALT)–type gastric lymphoma and implicated in adenocarcinoma of the stomach.

b. **Eosinophilic gastroenteritis** refers to the infiltration of eosinophils into the gastric antrum, small bowel, or both. This infiltration, which is believed to be immunologically mediated, causes thickening of the intestinal wall with subsequent antral obstruction. **Peripheral edema due to protein-losing enteropathy may occur.** Peripheral eosinophilia **is common.** Differentiation from other infiltrative diseases (e.g., tuberculosis, sarcoidosis, lymphoma, syphilis, histoplasmosis, Crohn's disease, carcinoma) may be difficult and depends on endoscopic biopsy. Corticosteroid therapy has been successful in providing prolonged remission.

c. **Granulomatous gastritis** is an infiltrative disease characterized by noncaseating granulomas, with or without giant cells. Crohn's disease, sarcoidosis, beryllium poisoning, or idiopathic causes may result in granulomatous gastritis. Gastric outlet obstruction is common. Treatment with steroids or surgery is often required.

d. **Hypertrophic gastritis** is an uncommon condition associated with massive enlargement of the gastric folds.

(1) **Clinical features.** In its most extreme form (i.e., Ménétrier's disease), there is hyposecretion of gastric acid, protein loss from the stomach, peripheral edema, weight loss, and abdominal pain.

(2) **Diagnosis.** Endoscopy and biopsy, often with a suction apparatus, provide the diagnosis.

(a) On biopsy, gastric mucous cells are hyperplastic, and inflammatory cells are present in some patients.

(b) Lymphoma, amyloid infiltration, carcinoma, and Zollinger-Ellison syndrome also can cause large rugal folds and should be excluded.

(c) A type of hypersecretory hypertrophic gastritis is similar to Ménétrier's disease but is associated with high acid output and hyperplasia of parietal gastric cells.

(3) **Therapy.** Treatment includes anticholinergic agents, which appear to close the tight junctions between cells and decrease protein loss, H_2-receptor antagonists, and steroids. Surgery (gastric resection) is reserved for intractable cases.

B Gastric neoplasms

1. **Gastric carcinoma**

a. **Epidemiology.** Formerly the most common cancer in the United States, gastric carcinoma continues to decline in incidence in this country. The incidence of gastric cancer remains high, however, in Japan and eastern Europe, and it appears to be inversely related to the incidence of carcinoma of the colon. Recently, there has been an increased incidence of fundic gastric adenocarcinoma associated with young, middle-class, white men. Gastric carcinoma is twice as common in men as it is in women and usually occurs in patients who are 50–75 years of age. Antral gastric carcinoma is highest among individuals of lower socioeconomic class.

b. **Pathogenesis.** Although the cause of gastric carcinoma is unknown, certain relationships have been observed. A 20% higher incidence of gastric cancer among family members and a higher incidence among individuals with blood group A suggest that a genetic component may be present. Tobacco use, vitamin C deficiency, and consumption of preserved foods (especially salted or smoked foods) and nitrosamines also are thought to play etiologic roles. Premalignant conditions include:
   (1) Pernicious anemia
   (2) Atrophic gastritis
   (3) Postgastrectomy, especially 10–20 years after Billroth II resection
   (4) Gastric polyps, which have approximately a 40% incidence of malignancy if they are adenomatous and larger than 2 cm in diameter*
   (5) Immunodeficiency disorders, especially common variable immunodeficiency†
   (6) *H. pylori* infection

c. **Clinical features**
   (1) **Weight loss** and **anorexia** are observed in approximately 70%–80% of patients.
   (2) **Epigastric pain** is described by approximately 70% of patients.
   (3) Several other symptoms may be noted, including early satiety, vomiting, and weakness and fatigue secondary to chronic blood loss and anemia.
      (a) Early satiety is particularly common in patients with **linitis plastica,** because the gastric wall does not distend normally.
      (b) Vomiting often is a result of pyloric obstruction by the tumor mass but also may result from impaired gastric motility.
      (c) Gross gastrointestinal bleeding is rare in gastric carcinomas, occurring in less than 10% of patients. Dysphagia may occur if the lesion is near the esophagogastric junction.
      (d) A palpable, left supraclavicular (Virchow's) node may indicate metastatic disease.

d. **Diagnosis.** The following procedures may be used to establish the diagnosis.
   (1) **Upper gastrointestinal series** can reveal a mass, ulcer, or thickened, nondistensible "leather bottle" stomach (linitis plastica). The simultaneous use of air contrast techniques enhances the diagnostic accuracy of radiographs.
   (2) **Endoscopy** with biopsy and brush cytology has a 95%–99% accuracy rate in diagnosing gastric cancer.
   (3) **Increased serum carcinoembryonic antigen (CEA) levels** as well as elevated 2-glucuronidase levels in gastric secretions may be seen in gastric carcinoma patients. Achlorhydria in response to maximum stimulation and in the presence of a gastric ulcer almost always indicates malignant ulceration.

e. **Therapy** (see Chapter 4 VI C 7, 8)

2. **Lymphomas**

   a. **True gastric lymphoma** usually occurs as a bulky mass associated with large, thickened gastric folds. Pain is the most common presenting symptom. Histologic examination usually shows diffuse histiocytic non-Hodgkin's lymphoma, but non-Hodgkin's lymphomas of all types are more common than Hodgkin's disease in the stomach. Gastric lymphoma, especially of the MALT type, has been strongly associated with *H. pylori* infection.
      (1) **Diagnosis.** Gastric lymphoma should be differentiated from Ménétrier's disease, Zollinger-Ellison syndrome, and hypertrophic gastritis. Diagnosis is confirmed by biopsy, either at endoscopy with a suction apparatus or at surgery.

*Most gastric polyps are hyperplastic and not thought to be malignant.
†In one series, 33% of patients developed gastric cancer.

(2) **Therapy.** Surgery and localized radiation therapy are the generally accepted forms of therapy, with 5-year survival rates approaching 50% in non-Hodgkin's lymphoma patients whose lymphoma is confined to the stomach. Chemotherapy is valuable in patients with systemic disease. If *H. pylori* lymphoma is identified, treatment of the *H. pylori* alone may lead to resolution.

b. **Gastric pseudolymphoma** is a condition that may occur after therapy with certain drugs, especially phenytoin. Often associated with gastric ulceration and granulation, it does not usually perforate. No mass is noted, and the lymphocytic infiltrate has germinal centers.

3. **Other gastric tumors**

a. **Gastrointestinal stromal tumors (GISTS).** The stomach is the most common site for GISTS, with the small bowel being the second most frequent location. GIST tumors constitute 1%–3% of all gastric tumors and develop from the interstitial cells of Cajal (or pacemaker cells). These tumors express CD 117 and are C-KIT positive on histologic staining. They may be benign or malignant and present with GI bleeding (40%), abdominal mass (40%), or abdominal pain (20%). Malignancy is often determined by the size (>4 cm), or the number of mitotic figures seen in a high-power field (HPF) (>25). Treatment is with surgery or a tyrosine kinase inhibitor such as imatinib mesylate (Gleevec).

b. **Gastric malignancies** such as **fibrosarcomas, neurogenic sarcomas, carcinoids,** and **metastatic carcinomas** (especially from breast and lung carcinomas and melanoma) must be differentiated from primary gastric carcinoma.

C Disorders of gastric emptying

1. **Pyloric stenosis**

a. **Acquired pyloric stenosis** occurs transiently, as the result of edema from peptic ulcer disease, or chronically, as the result of pyloric scarring from recurrent ulcer disease or neoplasm.

b. **Congenital pyloric stenosis** usually manifests in infancy.

(1) **Incidence.** Congenital pyloric stenosis occurs in approximately 2–4 of 1000 births and usually is seen in firstborn male children. There is a familial incidence.

(2) **Clinical features.** Postprandial projectile vomiting of nonbilious material, dehydration, and weight loss may occur. Visible peristalsis may be noted, with a mass palpated in the epigastrium.

(3) **Diagnosis.** Radiographic evidence is the basis of diagnosis. A plain film shows air in the stomach, and a barium swallow confirms the diagnosis.

(4) **Therapy.** Treatment is surgical (Ramstedt operation) and consists of a myotomy of the circular muscle of the pylorus.

2. **Gastric bezoars** are collections of nondigestible substances that sometimes form and cannot pass through the pylorus. Trichobezoars are composed of hair, and phytobezoars are composed of plant fibers. Bezoars generally are seen in patients who have undergone previous gastric surgery or in mentally retarded individuals who consume nondigestible substances. The symptoms include those of gastric outlet obstruction and bleeding from superficial ulcerations. It is important to exclude a gastric mass or cancer, and the diagnosis can be established endoscopically. Bezoars sometimes can be enzymatically dissolved with papain, acetylcysteine, or cellulase; otherwise, endoscopic or surgical removal is necessary.

3. **Gastric diverticula** occur on the posterior wall of the stomach in approximately 75% of cases and usually are within 2 cm of the esophagogastric junction. Unless they bleed or perforate, these congenital lesions are asymptomatic. **Pseudodiverticula,** seen most commonly in the antrum, are scarred remnants of previous peptic disease.

4. **Gastric volvulus** may occur as a result of weak ligamentous attachments or may be secondary to a paraesophageal hernia, an intrinsic gastric lesion, or an adjacent mass. Diagnosis is supported by the finding of two separate fluid levels in the left upper quadrant and by a lack of barium

passage into the pylorus. Therapy consists of temporary nasogastric suction. Recurrent or acute volvulus with gastric vascular compromise may require surgery.

5. **Gastroparesis** is a disorder of gastric emptying that is not caused by an obstruction. The diagnosis should be made by a nuclear solid-phase gastric emptying study after mechanical obstruction has been ruled out by an upper gastrointestinal series or by endoscopy. Gastroparesis most frequently is caused by type 1 (insulin-dependent) diabetes mellitus of longer than 10 years' duration. Other conditions associated with gastroparesis include systemic sclerosis, postvagotomy states, and therapy with anticholinergic agents or narcotics. In diabetes, loss of gastric phase III activity is noted on electrical recordings, with other signs of diabetic visceral neuropathy often being seen as well. Treatment with prokinetic agents such as metoclopramide, domperidone, or erythromycin has been effective. Electrical gastric pacing may be necessary in resistant cases.

III PEPTIC ULCER DISEASE

A Introduction Peptic ulcer disease refers to a group of disorders of the gastrointestinal tract. The disorders are similar in that they all involve areas of discrete tissue destruction caused by acid and pepsin. Peptic ulcers occur most commonly in the stomach or proximal duodenum, less commonly in the distal esophagus, and rarely in the small intestine. (Peptic ulcers in the distal small intestine usually are associated with a Meckel's diverticulum that contains gastric mucosa.) In general, the clinical features and treatment of peptic ulcer disease are similar regardless of location, although peptic esophagitis caused by reflux of gastric contents has some unique features (see I B 1).

B Incidence Peptic ulcer disease occurs more commonly in men than in women. Duodenal ulcers are three times more common than gastric ulcers and occur approximately 10 years earlier; the peak incidence for duodenal ulcers is at approximately 40 years of age, as opposed to 50 years of age for gastric ulcers. Duodenal ulcers have a 1-year relapse rate of approximately 80% (much lower if associated with *H. pylori* that has been eradicated). Patients with gastric ulcers have a 33% chance of developing subsequent duodenal ulcers.

C Pathogenesis Acid and pepsin are necessary for development of ulcers. However, several factors, especially *H. pylori* infection, are thought to contribute to the pathogenesis.

1. **Social factors**
   a. **Tobacco smoking** increases the risk of development of peptic ulcer disease. Smoking also raises the morbidity and mortality rates and lowers the healing rate for peptic ulcers. The mechanism may be a decrease in pancreatic bicarbonate secretion and, therefore, a lowered alkaline level in the duodenum, an increase in gastric emptying with a lowered duodenal pH, an increase in serum pepsinogen I secretion, or a decrease in pyloric sphincter pressure with an increased reflux into the stomach.
   b. **Drugs** such as NSAIDs are implicated in ulcer disease, with an antiprostaglandin effect suggested as an underlying factor. Ulcers develop in approximately 30% of arthritis patients who take high doses of aspirin. Steroids also are thought to break the mucosal barrier and may double the risk of peptic ulcer disease.
   c. **Alcohol** compromises the mucosal barrier and increases gastric acid secretion.
2. **Physiologic factors**
   a. **Gastric acid,** although essential for ulcer production, generally is measured at normal or decreased levels in gastric ulcer patients. Many investigators attribute this to an increase in the back-diffusion of hydrogen ion (H^+) into the mucosa or submucosa. Slightly elevated levels of gastric acid are noted in the basal and stimulated states in duodenal ulcer patients.
   b. **Serum gastrin** levels are normal during fasting and increased in the postprandial state in duodenal ulcer patients. Both fasting and postprandial levels of serum gastrin are higher than normal in gastric ulcer patients.

3. **Genetic factors**
   a. **First-degree relatives** of gastric ulcer patients have three times the risk of development of gastric ulcers as the general population. Similarly, the risk of duodenal ulcer is increased in the first-degree relatives of duodenal ulcer patients.
   b. An increased incidence of duodenal ulcer has been documented among individuals with blood group O, those who demonstrate elevated serum levels of pepsinogen I, and those who are nonsecretors of blood group substances.

4. **Infectious etiology**
   a. **Microbiology.** *H. pylori* has been identified on cultures of the gastric antrum in 90% of patients with duodenal ulcer disease or antral type B gastritis, and the association for patients with gastric ulcer disease is 60%–70%. In addition, the association between *H. pylori* infections of MALT lymphomas of the stomach and gastric cancer is increased.
   b. **Pathophysiology.** *H. pylori* is found on gastric epithelium and does not penetrate the cell. It has secretory immunoglobulin A (IgA) and host immunoglobulin (IgG) specificity. If it is a primary offender, it may act as a "barrier breaker," allowing acid back-diffusion and peptic ulcer disease to develop. *H. pylori* elaborates ammonia, which damages cell surfaces, and liberates a number of other inflammatory cell recruiting factors and adhesion molecules.
   c. **Diagnosis.** *H. pylori* liberates urease, and a biopsy of the gastric antrum may change a pH color monitor. A urea breath test using carbon 13 (^{13}C)- or ^{14}C-labeled urea measures exhaled labeled carbon dioxide. Supplemented culture medium (starch, blood, or charcoal) may be optimal under microaerophilic conditions at 37°C. Warthin-Starry silver, Giemsa, or hematoxylin and eosin stains may show the organism in an extracellular location. Antibodies to *H. pylori* detected by enzyme-linked immunosorbent assay (ELISA) indicate active or prior infection.
   d. **Therapy.** Treatment is usually with amoxicillin, doxycycline with metronidazole, or clarithromycin in combination with a proton pump inhibitor and a bismuth preparation for 2 weeks.
   e. **Outcome.** Studies have shown a decreased relapse rate in duodenal ulcers treated with antibiotics and bismuth as compared with H_2 blockers.

5. **Associated diseases**
   a. Some patients with **multiple endocrine neoplasia, type I (MEN I)**, present with gastrin-secreting tumors. This probably accounts for the reported association of duodenal ulcer disease with hyperparathyroidism.
   b. **Antral atrophic gastritis** may be caused by back-diffusion of bile through the pylorus. This condition is associated with a high incidence of gastric ulcers.
   c. Patients with **rheumatoid arthritis** have an increased risk of ulcer disease, which probably is secondary to the drugs used for treatment.
   d. **Chronic obstructive pulmonary disease (COPD)** has been found in a significant number of gastric ulcer patients.
   e. **Hepatic cirrhosis** and **chronic renal failure** are associated with an increased risk of duodenal ulcer.

6. **Psychosomatic factors** include chronic anxiety and "type A" personality.

D Clinical features

1. **Pain** is the predominant symptom, although it may be absent in 25% of gastric ulcer patients. The pain characteristically is described as an epigastric burning sensation and may be accompanied by bloating or nausea. Eating may exacerbate the pain in gastric ulcer patients, whereas in duodenal ulcer patients, the pain usually is diminished by eating, only to recur 2–3 hours later. Pain may awaken patients from sleep, especially those with duodenal ulcers.
2. **Upper gastrointestinal hemorrhage** may be the presenting sign of peptic ulcer disease, and anemia from chronic blood loss may be seen.

3. **Less common symptoms**
   a. **Repeated vomiting,** which may indicate gastric outlet obstruction
   b. **Weight loss,** which is somewhat more common with gastric ulcer

E Diagnosis Because affected patients may complain of only vague symptoms, a high index of suspicion is needed.

1. **Radiography** is a useful screening tool; however, an upper gastrointestinal series may miss up to 30% of gastric ulcers, and scarring of the duodenal bulb from chronic or recurrent ulcer disease may make radiographic interpretation difficult. Double-contrast techniques may improve diagnostic accuracy. Duodenal ulcers always are benign; however, gastric ulcers may be benign or malignant. Radiographic criteria for benign gastric ulcers include:
   a. Ulcer crater extending beyond the gastric wall
   b. Gastric folds radiating into the base of the ulcer
   c. Thick radiolucent collar of edema (Hampton's line) surrounding the ulcer base
   d. Smooth, regular, round or ovoid ulcer crater
   e. Pliable and normally distensible gastric wall in the area of the ulcer
2. **Endoscopy** may be used as the primary diagnostic maneuver or to confirm a radiographic diagnosis. Because 5% of gastric ulcers that occur in the United States are malignant, many authors advocate endoscopy with multiple biopsies at the margin of the ulcer and simultaneous cytologic brushings for the evaluation of all gastric ulcers, with subsequent endoscopy in 6–8 weeks to document healing.
3. **Gastric acid analysis** may help distinguish benign from malignant gastric ulcers. Because benign ulcers rarely exist in the setting of achlorhydria, the absence of acid should prompt further workup with gastric biopsies and cytologic studies. Although gastric ulcers in the presence of achlorhydria nearly always are malignant, most malignant ulcers occur in stomachs with normal acid secretion.

F Therapy Treatment is virtually the same for esophageal, gastric, and duodenal ulcers.

1. **Intensive antacids,** while they have been shown to promote the healing of gastric and duodenal ulcers, are generally of historical significance only. More potent acid suppressive agents in the form of H_2-receptor antagonists or proton pump inhibitors are favored, particularly in combination with therapy for *H. pylori,* because this bacteria has been seen in most patients with both gastric and duodenal ulcers.
2. **H_2-receptor antagonists (cimetidine, ranitidine, famotidine, and nizatidine),** and **proton pump inhibitors (omeprazole, esomeprazole, pentoprazole, lansoprazole, and rabeprazole)** are the mainstay of treatment because of patient convenience, sustained acid reduction, and increased healing rates with diminished relapse rates—**particularly in combination with antibiotics if *H. pylori* is present.**
   a. **Side effects** are few. Cimetidine affects the cytochrome P-450 system, so decreased dosages are advised for patients taking warfarin, diazepam, theophylline, and other drugs that affect the cytochrome P-450 system. Compared with other H_2-receptor antagonists, large doses of cimetidine may slightly increase the risk of central nervous system (CNS) side effects or gynecomastia. Proton pump inhibitors have minimal effects on drug metabolism. Both H_2-receptor antagonists and proton pump inhibitors have been released for over-the-counter use.
3. **Antibiotics** are used to treat *H. pylori* infection. Regimens typically involve combinations of an antibiotic (e.g., metronidazole, amoxicillin, tetracycline preparations, clarithromycin), a bismuth-containing product, and a proton pump inhibitor (double or triple therapy). Treatment is for approximately 2 weeks, with a 70%–90% response rate, depending on the regimen selected.
4. **Anticholinergic agents** have a limited therapeutic role because they decrease meal-stimulated acid secretion by only approximately 30%. These agents may be used to delay gastric emptying

of antacids, especially at night. More selective anticholinergic agents such as pirenzepine may be more useful.

5. **Dietary factors** may be of some importance. There is no proof that bland diets promote healing in peptic ulcer disease. In fact, milk may be harmful because it increases acid secretion, probably by calcium- and protein-stimulated gastrin release. Caffeine and alcohol stimulate gastric acid secretion and, therefore, should be restricted in acute cases. Decaffeinated coffee also may stimulate acid release. Ulcer patients who smoke should be urged to decrease or stop smoking.

6. **Other therapeutic agents**
   a. **Sucralfate** is a nonsystemic agent that, in the presence of an acid pH, coats the ulcer bed and promotes healing. Sucralfate is as effective as H_2-receptor antagonists and antacids and has no significant side effects.
   b. **Bismuth** has both ulcer-insulating and pepsin-inactivating properties but does not decrease gastric acid production. Healing rates are slightly better in gastric than in duodenal ulcer patients, and the overall rate of adverse reaction is low. In *H. pylori*–associated disease, bismuth may cause the organisms to dislodge from gastric epithelial cells. Milk and antacids may interfere with its action and should be avoided for 1 hour before and after ingestion of bismuth.
   c. **Prostaglandin E_2 (PGE_2)** and **PGF_2** may have a cytoprotective effect on gastric mucosa. These agents also increase gastric blood flow and decrease gastrin-stimulated acid secretion. A PGE_2 analog, **misoprostol,** has been shown to be effective in treating peptic ulcer disease and has been released for use in preventing gastric ulcers in patients taking NSAIDs. The major side effects of prostaglandins are diarrhea and nausea.
   d. **Tricyclic antidepressants** (e.g., doxepin) have proved effective in treating peptic ulcers, probably because of their H_2-receptor antagonist effects.
   e. **Proton pump inhibitors** (e.g., omeprazole, lansoprazole) are approved for treatment of reflux esophagitis and duodenal ulcers. These compounds irreversibly block proton pump function and markedly decrease acid production. This class of powerful drugs has been shown to cause carcinoid tumors in rats given very high doses of these drugs for more than 2 years.

7. **Gastric irradiation** decreases acid production for approximately 1 year and may play a role in treating recurrent disease in elderly patients who cannot tolerate drugs or surgery.

8. **Surgery** is effective therapy for peptic ulcer disease and reduces recurrence rates to a low percentage.
   a. **Procedures.** The most commonly performed operation is **distal subtotal gastrectomy,** with wedge resection of a gastric ulcer if one is present. **Vagotomy with drainage (V + D)** and **vagotomy with antrectomy (V + A)** are the usual procedures for complicated peptic ulcer disease. V + D is associated with a higher recurrence rate (approximately 7%–15%) than V + A (3%), but it is associated with less postoperative weight loss. A proximal selective vagotomy appears to lessen postoperative complications.
   b. **Indications.** The high incidence of postoperative complications, regardless of the type of procedure, has limited the role of surgery to **treatment of complications** (including acute emergencies) and **intractable cases.**

G Complications

1. **Hemorrhage** occurs in 20% of patients and is the most serious complication, having a 10% mortality rate. If blood requirements exceed 3 U in 24 hours for longer than 48–72 hours or if in-hospital rebleeding occurs, surgical intervention is indicated. Repeated bleeding episodes occur in approximately 30%–40% of cases and may require surgery.

2. **Perforation** occurs in approximately 5%–10% of all peptic ulcers and is far more common with duodenal ulcers than with gastric ulcers. Of ulcers that perforate, 10% bleed simultaneously. Symptoms and signs include intense pain, a rigid abdomen, decreased bowel sounds, and direct or rebound tenderness. This catastrophic complication is confirmed in approximately 75%–85%

of cases by an erect abdominal radiograph showing free air under the diaphragm. Most cases require immediate surgical intervention, but selected patients have been treated successfully with nasogastric suction and antibiotics.

3. **Gastric outlet obstruction** occurs in approximately 5%–10% of ulcer patients. Of these, 80% of the cases are caused by recurrent duodenal ulcer disease, with prepyloric or pyloric channel ulcers being less common causes. Early satiety, epigastric fullness, nausea, and vomiting of undigested food (frequently ingested several hours earlier) suggest the diagnosis. Weight loss is common. Physical examination may show a succussion splash. The diagnosis is confirmed by aspiration of greater than 300 cc of gastric contents more than 3 hours after a meal or by a positive saline load test. Treatment consists of nasogastric aspiration for at least 72 hours, with close attention to replacement of H^+, Na^+, chloride ion (Cl^-), and potassium ion (K^+). Approximately 25%–40% of patients require surgery because 20%–40% of medically treated patients have recurrent obstruction.

4. **Penetration** into an adjacent organ usually is a complication of posterior duodenal ulcers, with penetration into the pancreas. Pain usually is sudden in onset and radiates to the back. Serum amylase and lipase levels frequently are elevated. Treatment is surgical.

H Postsurgical complications

1. **Stomal ulceration** after surgery may indicate an unrecognized hypersecretory state (e.g., Zollinger-Ellison syndrome, retained gastric antrum, or incomplete vagotomy). The diagnosis of a stomal ulcer is best made by endoscopy. Treatment is with long-term proton pump inhibitors, and repeat surgery may be necessary.

2. **Afferent loop obstruction** is a rare complication. The patient usually complains of bloating and vomiting of a clear or bilious material approximately 30–60 minutes after eating. The diagnosis is suggested by the failure of orally ingested barium to enter the loop or by the retention inside the loop of technetium-iminodiacetic acid (Tc-HIDA), which is cleared by the liver and biliary system after intravenous injection but does not enter the gastrointestinal tract. Bacterial overgrowth can occur, and surgical revision of the afferent loop may be necessary.

3. **Alkaline gastritis** often is seen endoscopically in patients who have undergone antrectomy or subtotal gastrectomy. Gastritis often is asymptomatic but may cause nausea, vomiting, weight loss, and epigastric pain. Diagnosis may be aided by measurement of HIDA-labeled bile refluxing back into the stomach. Because the gastritis is secondary to this increased reflux of duodenal secretions into the stomach, patients may require surgery (a Roux-en-Y anastomosis) to divert these secretions further down the gastrointestinal tract. Some cases may be treated effectively with substances that bind bile acids (e.g., aluminum-containing antacids and cholestyramine) or with sucralfate.

4. **Dumping syndrome** is a nonspecific term that refers to a variety of postprandial symptoms.
   a. **Early dumping syndrome** occurs approximately 30 minutes after a meal and is associated with dizziness, flushing, diaphoresis, and palpitations. These symptoms have been ascribed to osmotic shifts of fluid or release of massive amounts of intestinal hormones as food empties rapidly from the stomach. The early dumping syndrome can be minimized by decreasing the carbohydrate content of meals and by avoiding liquids with meals. Synthetic somatostatin has been used in resistant cases.
   b. **Late dumping syndrome** occurs several hours after a meal and is characterized by dizziness, weakness, and drowsiness. This syndrome may be caused by reactive hypoglycemia.

5. **Nutritional problems**
   a. **Anemia** occurs in approximately 25% of patients after surgery for peptic ulcer disease. Factors that may contribute to iron deficiency include low-grade blood loss from alkaline pouch gastritis, diversion of iron away from its preferential absorption site (i.e., the duodenum), and lack of gastric acid needed for conversion of iron to the preferred form for absorption (i.e., Fe^{3+}). A lack of intrinsic factor leads to vitamin B_{12} deficiency in patients who have undergone a substantial gastric resection.

b. **Weight loss** occurs in approximately 50% of postoperative patients but is not severe unless a large gastric resection has been performed.
c. **Significant steatorrhea** usually indicates a secondary problem (e.g., bacterial overgrowth or unmasked celiac disease), although 50% of patients have an increase in stool fat secondary to rapid transit and poor mixing of food with bile salts and pancreatic enzymes.
d. **Bone thinning** may be due to decreased absorption of vitamin D and calcium.

6. **Gastric pouch cancer** rates are two to four times greater in ulcer patients who have undergone surgery than in patients whose ulcers are treated medically, especially 15–20 years after Billroth II gastric resection.

I **Zollinger-Ellison syndrome** refers to a non–β islet cell tumor that produces gastrin and is associated with gastric acid hypersecretion and peptic ulcer disease. The tumors are biologically malignant in 60% of cases and most commonly involve the pancreas. Other tumor sites include the stomach, duodenum, spleen, and lymph nodes. Tumor size varies from 2 mm to 20 cm. Approximately 10% of the patients with Zollinger-Ellison syndrome have a resectable lesion.

1. **Clinical features**
   a. **Pain** from peptic ulcer disease is common in Zollinger-Ellison syndrome. In approximately 75% of cases, the ulcers are located in the duodenal bulb. The remaining cases involve ulcers in the distal duodenum or jejunum or ulcers in multiple locations.
   b. **Diarrhea** occurs in approximately 50% of cases because of gastric acid hypersecretion. The high acid levels may damage the small intestinal mucosa, inactivate pancreatic lipase, and precipitate bile acids, causing steatorrhea. The high gastrin levels cause incomplete Na^+ and water absorption and increase intestinal motility. In addition, the volume of gastric secretion alone may cause diarrhea.
   c. **Endocrine abnormalities.** Zollinger-Ellison syndrome commonly is associated with other endocrinopathies. Approximately 20% of these patients have hyperparathyroidism. Pituitary, adrenal, ovarian, and thyroid tumors also have been reported with Zollinger-Ellison syndrome. A distinct syndrome of pancreatic, pituitary, and parathyroid tumors (i.e., MEN I) shows an autosomal dominant pattern of inheritance.

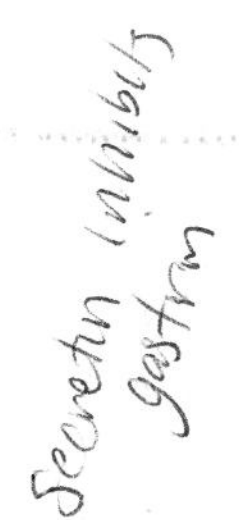

2. **Diagnosis**
   a. **Gastrin levels.** Patients demonstrate elevated basal-state gastrin levels that do not increase 1 hour after a meal. Gastrin levels increase (rather than decline) by 200 U after intravenous secretin administration and rise markedly (rather than modestly) after intravenous calcium administration.
   b. **Gastric acid output.** Patients with Zollinger-Ellison syndrome often have basal gastric acid output rates of more than 10 mEq/hr and basal-to-peak output ratios of greater than 0.6.
   c. **Angiography.** Because gastrin-secreting tumors may be highly vascular, angiography may be helpful.
3. **Therapy**
   a. **Surgical treatment**
      (1) **Total gastrectomy** is the traditional therapy. The 10-year survival rate of 50% with this procedure is thought to be attributable primarily to the slow-growing nature of this lesion. Most of the late deaths are caused by metastatic disease.
      (2) **Tumor localization,** which involves sampling gastrin levels through cannulation of multiple pancreatic and abdominal veins, may be useful. This technique offers the hope of surgical cure in cases of multiple primary tumors and in cases involving a tumor that is too small to be visualized by ordinary means.
   b. **Medical treatment**
      (1) **Proton pump inhibitors** are the medical treatment of choice and may require high-dose therapy, depending on the response to acid-suppressive therapy using gastric analysis for documentation of acid suppression.

(2) H_2-receptor antagonists in combination with **anticholinergic agents** have been used, especially in conjunction with a V + D procedure. Patients who have been unresponsive to H_2-receptor blockade may become responsive as a result of surgery.

J Other disorders of the stomach

1. **Portal hypertensive gastropathy** is the term given to diffuse submucosal dilatation of gastric vessels that may rupture. It accounts for upper gastrointestinal bleeding in approximately 10% of patients with portal hypertension. A diffuse but irregular pattern of red spots or linear streaks produces a characteristic pattern at endoscopy. Treatment with β-blockade or bicap (electrocautery) or laser therapy to the gastric wall may decrease rebleeding.
2. **Dieulafoy's ulcer** is a difficult-to-diagnose vascular lesion generally seen in the gastric fundus. This ulcer may be a cause of significant recurrent upper gastrointestinal bleeding. Men older than 50 years of age are most commonly affected. The lesion appears as an exposed arterial defect with no or minimal mucosal ulceration. Endoscopy with laser or bicap treatment is effective in stopping the bleeding, but angiography or surgery is often necessary because of the difficulty of identifying the small vascular defect during endoscopy.

IV DISEASES OF THE SMALL INTESTINE

A Intestinal obstruction is a term used to denote failure of passage of intestinal contents and may be due to mechanical obstruction or adynamic ileus.

1. **Mechanical obstruction**
   a. **Etiology**
      (1) **Extrinsic causes**
         (a) Adhesions from prior surgery
         (b) Incarcerated hernia
         (c) Metastatic tumors
         (d) Volvulus
         (e) Endometriosis
         (f) NSAID-induced strictures (often multiple)
      (2) **Intramural causes**
         (a) Hematomas from trauma
         (b) Strictures
         (c) Intramural tumors
      (3) **Intraluminal causes**
         (a) Epithelial tumors (especially colonic)
         (b) Intussusception
         (c) Foreign bodies
   b. **Clinical features**
      (1) Crampy pain that waxes and wanes in intensity
      (2) High-pitched bowel sounds with rushes and tinkles
      (3) Constipation and obstipation
      (4) Vomiting, which is more prominent in proximal intestinal obstruction
      (5) Distention, which is more prominent in distal intestinal obstruction
      (6) Intestinal ischemia, leading first to edema, then to petechial hemorrhages, and finally to necrosis and gangrene*

*This is secondary to increased intraluminal pressure occurring after 6–12 hours of obstruction, when absorption ceases and secretion commences.

c. **Diagnosis** usually is made with plain and upright abdominal radiographs. Characteristic air-fluid levels exist above the area of obstruction, and no air is seen in the rectum. A barium enema may be useful in diagnosing colonic obstruction. Reflux of barium into the small bowel also may be helpful in the diagnosis of low small bowel obstruction.

d. **Therapy**
   (1) Replacement of fluid and electrolytes
   (2) Intestinal decompression with nasogastric suction or small bowel intubation
   (3) Surgery, which usually is required for definitive treatment of the underlying problem

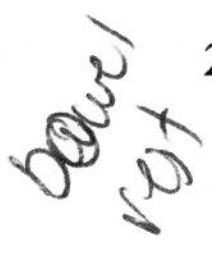

2. **Adynamic,** or **paralytic, ileus** is a nonobstructive lack of propulsion through the intestinal tract.
   a. **Etiology.** Adynamic ileus commonly is linked to the following conditions:
      (1) Recent abdominal surgery, which results in ileus that usually is transient (lasting 2–3 days)
      (2) Electrolyte imbalance, especially hypokalemia
      (3) Chemical or bacterial peritonitis
      (4) Severe intra-abdominal inflammation such as pancreatitis and cholecystitis
      (5) Systemic illness such as pneumonia
   b. **Clinical features.** Physical examination shows a distended abdomen and diminished bowel sounds.
   c. **Diagnosis.** Radiographs show diffuse intestinal gas and air in the rectum.
   d. **Therapy**
      (1) Bowel rest (i.e., nothing by mouth) and placement of a nasogastric tube
      (2) Correction of underlying causes, **especially hypokalemia.**
      (3) Intravenous neostigmine (with careful cardiac monitoring) may be used in resistant cases with careful cardiac monitoring.

B **Intestinal pseudo-obstruction** is a rare but important entity characterized by apparently recurrent episodes of mechanical obstruction but with no demonstrable source of obstruction.

1. **Classification.** Pseudo-obstruction may exist with or without an underlying condition.
   a. **Secondary pseudo-obstruction.** Pseudo-obstruction occurs secondary to many conditions that affect either the smooth muscle of the gastrointestinal tract or the neurologic and hormonal control of intestinal motility.
      (1) Underlying diseases that involve the smooth muscle include collagen vascular disease (especially scleroderma), amyloidosis, and myotonic dystrophy.
      (2) Underlying neurologic diseases include Chagas' disease, Parkinson's disease, and Hirschsprung's disease.
      (3) Underlying endocrine disorders include hypothyroidism, diabetes mellitus, hypoparathyroidism, and pheochromocytoma.
      (4) Drugs that depress intestinal smooth muscle function include phenothiazines, tricyclic antidepressants, ganglionic blockers, and clonidine.
      (5) Nontropical sprue and ceroid deposits in the bowel (mahogany bowel) are rare causes of pseudo-obstruction.
   b. **Primary pseudo-obstruction.** There are two forms of this condition.
      (1) Hereditary **hollow visceral myopathy** is a vacuolization and atrophy of intestinal smooth muscle. This disorder, which is transmitted as an autosomal dominant trait, also affects esophageal and urinary tract smooth muscle.
      (2) An **autonomic nervous system abnormality** has been described in some families with primary pseudo-obstruction. There may be a decrease in total myenteric plexus neurons or neuronal eosinophilic intranuclear inclusions. Possible symptoms include orthostatic hypotension, ataxic gait, dysarthria, and absent deep tendon reflexes.

2. **Diagnosis.** Rigorous exclusion of causes of mechanical obstruction with documentation of abnormal motility is necessary.

a. **Esophageal manometry** showing normal or low LES pressure with decreased amplitude of peristalsis distally indicates the smooth muscle vacuolization type of pseudo-obstruction. Incomplete relaxation of the LES with absent peristalsis and repetitive esophageal contractions may indicate an autonomic nervous system abnormality.
b. **Radionuclide gastric emptying scans** may show delayed emptying.
c. **Barium studies** yield nonspecific findings. Most patients show dilated areas of the intestine.

3. **Therapy.** Treatment is supportive during acute exacerbations. Cholinergic agents and prokinetic agents have been used with limited success, and surgery should be avoided. Home parenteral hyperalimentation may be required for nutritional support. Intestinal stasis with bacterial overgrowth should be treated with antibiotics.

C Small bowel diverticula

1. **Duodenal diverticula** usually are found incidentally during an upper gastrointestinal series, at endoscopy, or at autopsy. They occur most frequently in the proximal duodenum, within 1–2 cm of the ampulla of Vater, and are asymptomatic in most patients, although duodenal diverticula may rarely cause upper gastrointestinal bleeding. In some cases, the common bile duct empties directly into the diverticulum, and common bile duct obstruction may occur because of anatomic interference with emptying.

2. **Jejunal diverticula** probably are acquired rather than congenital and usually are asymptomatic. Jejunal diverticula may lead to malabsorption secondary to bile salt deconjugation when stasis is sufficient to allow an increase in small bowel bacteria. This leads to diarrhea, steatorrhea, weight loss, and anemia. Hypochlorhydria or achlorhydria also may be present. Continuous or alternating antimicrobial therapy often corrects malabsorption, although surgical removal of multiple diverticula or of a single large diverticulum may be necessary in refractory cases.

3. **Meckel's diverticulum** is a common congenital structural defect that represents the remnant of the vitelline duct. It is found in approximately 2% of autopsies and usually is located in the terminal ileum within 60 cm of the ileocecal valve. Meckel's diverticula average 5–7 cm in length and may be quite large. Approximately one third of Meckel's diverticula contain gastric mucosa, which may produce acid. Diverticulitis, ulceration, bleeding, perforation, and obstruction are complications that require surgical intervention and frequently mimic the symptoms of acute appendicitis. Because of the presence of gastric mucosa, the diagnosis sometimes can be made by means of pertechnetate scanning after H_2-receptor blockade.

D **Diarrhea** is defined as an increase in stool frequency and volume. The stool usually is liquid, and 24-hour output exceeds 250 g. Patients may experience lower abdominal crampy pain and fecal urgency.

1. **Classification.** Pathophysiologic criteria are used to classify diarrhea as one of three distinct types.
   a. **Secretory diarrhea**
      (1) **Pathophysiology.** Secretory diarrhea occurs when the secretion of fluid and electrolytes is increased or when the normal absorptive capacity of the bowel is decreased. In some cases, increased secretion is caused by activation of the adenyl cyclase–cyclic adenosine 3',5'-monophosphate (cAMP) system in mucosal cells.
         (a) Agents that activate the adenyl cyclase–cAMP system include cholera toxin, heat-labile *Escherichia coli* toxin, *Salmonella* enterotoxin, and vasoactive intestinal peptide (VIP).
         (b) Agents that probably do not activate the adenyl cyclase–cAMP system include heat-stable *E. coli* toxin, a variety of other bacterial enterotoxins (e.g., those produced by *Clostridium perfringens, Pseudomonas aeruginosa,* and *Klebsiella pneumoniae*), castor oil, and phenolphthalein.
         (c) Chronic secretory diarrhea is seen in the pancreatic cholera syndrome with VIP secretion, in medullary carcinoma of the thyroid gland with calcitonin secretion, in carcinoid syndrome with serotonin secretion, and in villous adenoma of the rectum.

(2) **Diagnosis.** Persistent diarrhea in the absence of food intake and by the lack of a gap between total stool osmolarity and two times the sum of stool Na^+ and K^+ concentrations should be demonstrated.

(3) **Therapy.** Fluid and electrolyte support should be given while the cause of the diarrhea is being determined. In general, diarrhea secondary to bacterial enterotoxin is self-limited. Any contributing exogenous agent (e.g., phenolphthalein and castor oil) must be withdrawn.

b. **Osmotic diarrhea** is caused by the presence of nonabsorbable substances in the intestine, with the secondary accumulation of fluid and electrolytes. Such nonabsorbable substances include lactose in a patient with lactase deficiency, laxatives (e.g., magnesium citrate, sodium phosphate), and foodstuffs in a patient with malabsorption. The diagnosis is suggested by the absence of diarrhea after a 48- to 72-hour fast (with concurrent intravenous fluid replacement). There is a gap of greater than 50 between total stool osmolarity and two times the sum of stool Na^+ and K^+ concentrations.

c. **Abnormal intestinal motility** causes or contributes to the diarrhea seen in diabetes, irritable bowel syndrome, postvagotomy states, carcinoid syndrome, and hyperthyroidism. Mechanisms of abnormal intestinal motility include the following:

(1) If small bowel peristalsis is too rapid, an abnormally large amount of fluid and partially digested foodstuffs may be delivered to the colon.

(2) Extremely slow peristalsis may allow bacterial overgrowth to occur and bile salt deconjugation to cause secondary malabsorption.

(3) Rapid colonic motility may not allow adequate time for the colon to absorb fluid delivered to the cecum. (Normally, 90% of the fluid is absorbed.)

2. **Diagnosis**

a. **Tests** performed on stool samples include:

(1) **Culture and sensitivity testing** to detect a pathogenic bacterial strain. A positive stool culture is found for 40% of patients who have white blood cells (WBCs) in the stool and fever.

(2) **Microscopic examination** to identify ova and parasites (three samples should be sent to increase yield)

(3) **Guaiac testing** to detect occult blood

(4) **Sudan staining** to detect fat droplets

(5) **Wright** or **methylene blue staining** to detect WBCs, which are indicative of invasive infectious causes of diarrhea*

(6) Testing for the presence of **Clostridium difficile** in stool

b. **Proctosigmoidoscopy** also is performed, especially to exclude or confirm a diagnosis of inflammatory bowel disease.

3. **Other causes of persistent diarrhea**

a. **Irritable bowel syndrome (IBS)** is an intestinal motor disorder of unknown cause.

(1) **Pathophysiology.** Studies of colonic myoelectric activity show an increased incidence of three cycles per minute of slow-wave activity among patients with irritable bowel syndrome (i.e., 40% as compared with 10% in normal individuals). Intestinal contractions after a meal or a cholecystokinin injection are more likely to be in the three–cycle per minute range when compared with the intestinal contractions of normal individuals. The colonic spike activity is delayed from 40 minutes to 70–90 minutes postprandially. The abnormal slow-wave activity may indicate an intrinsic myogenic defect, and the prolonged postprandial spike and contractile activity may indicate a neural or hormonal

*Toxigenic *E. coli*, viruses, Norwalk agent, and *Giardia lamblia* are not invasive. Irritable bowel syndrome, malabsorption syndrome, and laxative abuse do not cause pus in the stool. *Staphylococcus aureus*, *C. perfringens*, and *Entamoeba histolytica* also may be present with fecal leukocytes.

abnormality. Irritable bowel syndrome is six to eight times more common in women than men, which also suggests a hormonal mechanism. Visceral hypersensitivity to afferent stimuli also has been described.

(2) **Clinical features.** Signs and symptoms include alternating diarrhea and constipation with postprandial pain but usually no weight loss, gastrointestinal bleeding, protracted nausea, vomiting, or fever. Diarrhea, if present, generally is characterized by a 24-hour output of less than 500 cc. Neither pain nor diarrhea awakens the patient from sleep.

(3) **Diagnosis.** Exclusion of other gastrointestinal conditions with appropriate tests, including blood studies, stool analysis, guaiac testing, and radiography or colonoscopy, is the basis of diagnosis. Celiac disease, which may have similar symptoms to diarrhea-predominant IBS, should be eliminated with celiac antibody testing or small bowel biopsy.

(4) **Therapy.** Treatment includes stool bulking agents, antispasmodics, and patient reassurance. For diarrhea-predominant IBS, the serotonin $5HT_3$-antagonist alosetron is effective, and in constipation-predominant IBS, the $5HT_4$-partial agonist tegaserod has also been shown in blinded clinical trials to be efficacious.

b. **Disaccharidase deficiency** (i.e., deficiency of the enzymes required to split nonabsorbable disaccharides into absorbable monosaccharides) is a cause of osmotic diarrhea.

(1) **Sucrase** and **isomaltase deficiencies** are rare, occurring in 0.2% of the population. These deficiencies usually present as watery diarrhea in infancy.

(2) **Lactase deficiency** usually is not complete (i.e., patients have some enzyme activity), and presenting symptoms occur after puberty. It affects 60%–80% of blacks and occurs to a lesser extent in Asian and Mediterranean populations. Symptoms of lactase deficiency include abdominal bloating, cramping, and watery diarrhea after milk ingestion. Diagnosis can be made by measuring the increase in serum glucose in response to orally administered lactose, with an increase of 20 mg/dL expected after an oral lactose intake of 50–100 mg. Lactose breath tests measure increased H^+ excretion from colonic bacterial digestion of lactose. A relative lactase deficiency may occur after an acute episode of viral enteritis or in association with celiac disease, Whipple's disease, or cystic fibrosis.

c. **Incontinence** is a disturbing symptom that patients may find difficult to discuss with a physician. It is often not true diarrhea but is associated with inflammatory diseases of the anal canal (e.g., acute gonococcal proctitis, Crohn's disease, ulcerative colitis) or with systemic neuromuscular diseases (e.g., diabetes mellitus, scleroderma). Incontinence also may be a complication of anal surgery (e.g., fistulectomy, hemorrhoidectomy).

d. **Laxative abuse,** which may be associated with psychiatric problems and a desire to lose weight, is an increasing cause of diarrhea. The type of laxative ingested determines the clinical features. Magnesium sulfate, nonabsorbable sugars (e.g., lactulose), and sodium phosphate result in osmotic diarrhea. Dihydroxy bile salts, castor oil, and dioctyl sodium sulfosuccinate (docusate sodium) cause secretory diarrhea. (These secretory agents as well as bisacodyl and phenolphthalein may increase PGE synthesis, thereby reducing or reversing water flux from the intestinal lumen into the blood.) Surreptitious laxative use is difficult to document except in cases of phenolphthalein use, in which alkalinization of a stool or urine sample by the addition of sodium hydroxide causes the color of the sample to change to pink.

e. **Systemic mastocytosis** is characterized by mast cell proliferation in the skin, bones, lymph nodes, and parenchymal organs. Eighty percent of affected patients have gastrointestinal symptoms that include nausea, vomiting, and recurrent episodes of diarrhea and abdominal pain. Pruritus, flushing, tachycardia, hypotensive episodes, and headaches also may be seen on an episodic basis. Heparin, also liberated from mast cells, can contribute to gastrointestinal hemorrhage from peptic ulcer disease, which is related to histamine-induced hyperchlorhydria.

(1) **Diagnosis** is suggested when jejunal biopsies show large numbers of mast cells in the lamina propria, muscularis mucosa, and submucosa with normal or mild villous atrophy.

The classic dermatologic finding is that of urticaria pigmentosa associated with systemic mastocytosis.

(2) **Therapy** has been with agents to block both H_1 and H_2 receptors, anticholinergics, and, occasionally, steroids.

4. **Infectious causes** of diarrhea include the bacteria listed in Table 5–1, which cause food poisoning. Some organisms, such as *C. difficile* and *Entamoeba histolytica,* primarily attach to the colon and rectum, respectively.
   a. ***E. coli*** is the most common cause of **traveler's diarrhea,** which is the often severe diarrhea that occurs within 2 weeks of a visit to a tropical area. Traveler's diarrhea usually is self-limited.
      (1) A toxigenic, heat-labile *E. coli* can activate cAMP or cyclic guanosine 3',5'-monophosphate (cGMP) to cause a secretory diarrhea that may be bloody. Species of *Shigella, Salmonella,* and *Campylobacter* as well as *E. histolytica* and *Giardia lamblia* are other known causes of traveler's diarrhea.
      (2) Trimethoprim–sulfamethoxazole combinations, bismuth subsalicylate, quinolone antibiotics, and oxytetracycline preparations have been shown to be effective in prevention and treatment.
   b. ***G. lamblia,*** a flagellate protozoan, is the most common cause of **water-borne infectious diarrhea** in the United States. It also is common in developing nations because of sewage contamination of drinking water. Infected patients may be asymptomatic, have mild diarrhea, or have a prolonged illness characterized by malabsorption, diarrhea, bloating, and crampy abdominal pain. Because the organism preferentially resides in the upper small intestine, the diagnosis can be made by demonstration of trophozoites in duodenal aspirates, although examination of stools for cysts and trophozoites is a good screening test. Treatment with metronidazole or quinacrine usually is successful.
   c. **Viruses** commonly cause **acute self-limited diarrhea.** Although many different viruses may cause gastroenteritis, causes of viral gastroenteritis that can be identified with certainty are the **Norwalk agent** (a parvovirus) and the **rotavirus.**
   d. ***Salmonella* infection,** or salmonellosis, may be highly variable in its presentation. Gastroenteritis, the most common form of salmonellosis, is an acute self-limited diarrheal syndrome with crampy abdominal pain and fever. Enteric fever is a severe illness primarily caused by *Salmonella typhi* or *Salmonella paratyphi* but also is seen with infection by other types of salmonella. Clinical manifestations include prolonged fever, abdominal pain, rash, and diarrhea. Salmonella septicemia may be seen in patients with osteomyelitis, mycotic aneurysms, or abscesses with no evidence or history of gastrointestinal disease. Salmonellosis is diagnosed using stool and blood culturing techniques. Because a prolonged carrier state may be induced, patients with gastroenteritis are not given antibiotics. In severe infection, ampicillin, trimethoprim–sulfamethoxazole, or chloramphenicol is used.
   e. ***Shigella*** infection, or shigellosis, is characterized by acute diarrhea with fever and crampy abdominal pain. If left untreated, the disease progresses to a chronic bloody diarrhea without fever but with weight loss and debilitation, which may last for weeks. Diagnosis is made by positive stool culture. In contrast to that for salmonellosis, antibiotic therapy for shigellosis offers symptomatic improvement, with decreased duration of excretion of the organism.
   f. ***Campylobacter*** infection is the most common cause of bacterial diarrhea in the United States. Symptoms include diarrhea, which may be bloody, and fever. Diagnosis is made by positive stool culture but requires special media and handling. Treatment is with erythromycin because the organism is resistant to most other commonly used antibiotics.
   g. ***Cryptosporidium*** infection, or cryptosporidiosis, is a protozoal infection seen commonly in immunocompromised patients such as those with AIDS. This diarrheal syndrome rarely occurs in normal individuals, except in a self-limited fashion, particularly in animal (calf) handlers. The diarrhea is watery, profuse, and debilitating. Diagnosis is made by a modified

TABLE 5–1 Bacterial Food Poisoning Syndromes

Organism	Incubation Period	Symptoms	Sources of Contamination	Pathogenic Mechanisms	Comments
Staphylococcus aureus	2–8 hours	SP, SV, D	Meat and dairy food	Toxin	Sudden onset; intense vomiting; no therapy needed in most cases
Bacillus cereus	2–8 hours	SP, SV, SD	Reheated fried rice	Tissue invasion	Early vomiting, later diarrhea; recovery within 24 hours
Clostridium perfringens	8–14 hours	V, SD	Reheated meat	Toxin	Profuse diarrhea
Vibrio parahaemolyticus	6 hours–4 days	V, SD, F	Saltwater seafood	Toxin; tissue invasion	Outbreaks usually associated with ingestion of oysters, clams, and crabs
Salmonella species	8–48 hours	V, SD, F, H, systemic disease	Food	Mild tissue invasion; possible toxin	Diarrhea with low-grade fever; carrier state possible; should not be treated
Pathogenic *Escherichia coli*	1–3 days	SD	Food and water	Toxin; tissue invasion	Traveler's diarrhea; prophylaxis or therapy with trimethoprim–sulfa combinations, bismuth subsalicylate, or doxycycline
Hemorrhagic *E. coli*, serotype 0157:H7	1–7 days	SP, SD, B	Raw beef; unprocessed milk; water	Toxin; tissue invasion	Severe pain and bloody diarrhea; may be associated with hemolytic–uremic syndrome or TTP; high mortality rate; therapy with amoxicillin or quinolones
Vibrio cholerae	1–3 days	V, SD	Poor hygiene	Toxin	Life-threatening diarrhea; therapy is intravenous replacement of fluid and electrolytes; epidemic occurrence
Shigella species (mild cases)	1–3 days	SD, F, B	Fecal–oral spread; flies	Toxin; tissue invasion	Therapy with ampicillin, trimethoprim–sulfamethoxazole, or chloramphenicol
Clostridium botulinum	1–4 days	V, H, RE	Canned foods	Toxin	Severe CNS symptoms; ventilatory support needed; high mortality rate
Campylobacter jejuni	2–8 days	SD, B	Fecal–oral spread; pets	Tissue invasion	Bloody diarrhea, especially in children; therapy with erythromycin
Clostridium difficile	?	SD, F, B	Fecal–oral spread	Toxin	Postantibiotic diarrhea; therapy with vancomycin or metronidazole
Yersinia enterocolitica	24–48 hours	SP, SD, B	Fecal–oral spread; pets	Tissue invasion; possible toxin	May be seen with polyarthritis in children; therapy with tetracycline

S = severe; P = abdominal pain; V = vomiting; D = diarrhea; F = fever; B = blood in stool; H = headache; RE = respiratory embarrassment; CNS = central nervous system; TTP = thrombotic thrombocytopenic purpura.

acid-fast stain of stool. No effective therapy is available, although spiramycin may provide temporary relief.

h. ***Isospora belli*** infection occurs similarly to cryptosporidiosis. Treatment is with trimethoprim–sulfamethoxazole.

i. ***E. histolytica*** causes bloody dysentery with fever. Diagnosis is by serologic and stool analysis. Treatment is with metronidazole or iodoquinol.

j. **Hemorrhagic *E. coli* serotype 0157:H7** produces Shiga toxin and causes bloody diarrhea. Hemorrhagic *E. coli* serotype 0157:H7 infection may be associated with hemolytic–uremic syndrome or thrombotic thrombocytopenic purpura (TTP). Transmission may occur through ingestion of poorly cooked beef, unprocessed milk, or apple cider made in mills where poorly washed fruit is contaminated with infected animal feces.

5. **Nonbacterial food poisoning**

a. **Fish poisoning** is caused by ichthyosarcotoxins (toxins found in the flesh of poisonous fish).

(1) **Ciguatera poisoning** is acquired from certain bottom-dwelling fish found in temperate and tropical coastal zones. Ingestion of such fish is followed in 30 minutes to 30 hours by nausea, vomiting, diarrhea, and paresthesia or numbness of the lips, tongue, and limbs. Treatment is supportive.

(2) **Scombroid poisoning** is acquired from certain fish species (usually tuna, mackerel, bluefish, herring, and bonito) that are susceptible to the production of a heat-stable toxin by the action of *Proteus morganii.* Symptoms resemble those of a histamine reaction and include flushing, headache, dizziness, abdominal cramping, vomiting, and diarrhea. The symptoms appear soon after ingestion and last 4–6 hours. Cooking does not inactivate the toxin once it is formed. Antihistamines may be used for symptomatic relief.

(3) **Tetraodon poisoning** may result from consumption of **puffer fish.** These fish produce a neurotoxin termed tetrodotoxin, which may cause paresthesia of the face and extremities with nausea, vomiting, and diarrhea. Ventilator support may be necessary.

b. **Mushroom poisoning** occurs after ingestion of any of the 50 species of mushrooms known to be toxic to humans. *Amanita verna, Amanita virosa,* and *Amanita phalloides* account for most cases of mushroom poisoning. Nausea, vomiting, fever, diarrhea, and abdominal pain develop 6–24 hours after ingestion; 1–4 days later, hepatic and renal insufficiency may develop with subsequent coagulopathy, heart failure, convulsions, and coma. Mushroom poisoning has a mortality rate of 40%–90%.

(1) **Diagnosis** is made by history of ingestion or by detection of mushroom toxins in the gastric aspirate.

(2) **Therapy** is supportive. Thioctic acid may be curative and should be administered promptly.

E **Malabsorption** of food or nutrients results from a defect at any step of the digestive process or in any of the organs that participate in normal digestion. The clinical features vary widely because malabsorption may involve a single nutrient or multiple nutrients.

1. **Etiology**

a. **Maldigestion** refers to a defect either in intraluminal hydrolysis of triglycerides or in micelle formation, which results from the following conditions:

(1) **Pancreatic insufficiency** caused by chronic pancreatitis, pancreatic carcinoma, or cystic fibrosis

(2) **Deficiency of conjugated bile salts** because of cholestatic or obstructive liver disease (e.g., cholangiocarcinoma)

(3) **Bile salt deconjugation** attributable to bacterial overgrowth in blind loops (after Billroth II gastrectomy) or in jejunal diverticula or in association with enterocolonic fistulae or motility disorders (e.g., scleroderma, pseudo-obstruction)

(4) **Inadequate mixing of gastric contents with bile salts and pancreatic enzymes** as a result of previous gastric surgery, especially Billroth II gastrectomy

b. Intrinsic small bowel disease

(1) **Celiac disease** causes flattening of the villi and inflammatory cell infiltration in the lamina propria (see IV E 4 c).

(2) **Whipple's disease,** a systemic disease that is infectious in origin, causes mucosal damage and lymphatic obstruction (see IV E 4 d).

(3) **Collagenous sprue** refers to the deposition of a collagenous substance in the lamina propria in a patient who otherwise has the clinical and histologic features of celiac disease. Fifty percent of cases of collagenous sprue are responsive to steroids.

(4) **Nongranulomatous ulcerative ileojejunitis** is a rare condition of unknown cause characterized by fever, weight loss, crampy abdominal pain, bloating, and diarrhea. Intestinal ulcerations may occur, and splenomegaly is noted in 20% of cases. Despite therapeutic attempts with steroids and immunosuppressive drugs or surgery, the clinical course often is relentless and the prognosis poor.

(5) **Eosinophilic gastroenteritis** is characterized by peripheral eosinophilia and infiltration of the wall of the stomach, small intestine, or colon by mature eosinophils. Many patients present with a specific food allergy and other allergic disorders such as asthma, eczema, and allergic rhinitis, and some patients show symptoms of gastritis. Diagnosis is made by biopsy of the gastric antrum or small bowel, which shows the eosinophilic infiltration. Steroid therapy may induce a prolonged remission. Elimination diets to remove possible allergens have been successful in some patients.

(6) **Amyloidosis** (either primary or secondary) may affect the small intestine in 70% of cases by amyloid infiltration of the submucosa. Altered motility that allows bacterial overgrowth also may contribute to malabsorption. Gastrointestinal bleeding (occult) may be observed in approximately 25% of cases. Diagnosis is made by biopsy (usually of a rectal valve or stomach) with special stains (e.g., Congo red). Treatment primarily is supportive. A trial of antibiotics for bacterial overgrowth may be given.

(7) **Crohn's disease** may cause malabsorption by mucosal damage, by multiple strictures with bacterial overgrowth, or as a result of the need for multiple bowel resections (see IV G).

c. Inadequate absorptive surface results from extensive small bowel resection, usually for Crohn's disease or vascular compromise of the small intestine.

(1) Resection of up to 50% of the small intestine is well tolerated if the remaining bowel is normal, and survival is possible after more extensive resection but requires careful management. If the proximal small bowel is resected, calcium, folic acid, and iron may not be absorbed; tetany may result. If the ileum is removed, bile acid and vitamin B_{12} absorption is impaired greatly. Hepatic dysfunction, oxalate kidney stones, and increased gastric acid secretion are common complications of extensive bowel resection. D-Lactic acidosis is a rare but life-threatening complication.

(2) Initial therapy includes intravenous fluid and electrolyte administration or parenteral hyperalimentation. Oral feedings should include medium-chain triglycerides (MCT oil), fat-soluble vitamins, and iron. Intramuscular vitamin B_{12} injections and antidiarrheal agents (to slow the transit time) may be needed. Cholestyramine resin may bind nonabsorbed bile salts and lessen the diarrhea; however, this drug also depletes the total body bile salt pool and usually is not used if more than 100 cm of distal ileum has been resected.

d. Lymphatic obstruction

(1) **Intestinal lymphangiectasia** may be primary (congenital) or secondary to intestinal tuberculosis, Whipple's disease, trauma, neoplasia, or retroperitoneal fibrosis. In advanced disease, dilated lymphatic channels rupture and leak into the intestinal lumen, causing lymphopenia, low serum protein levels, and massive peripheral edema. Small bowel biopsy reveals the characteristic dilated lymphatics. Treatment is with low-fat diet and MCT supplementation.

(2) **Intestinal lymphoma** may mimic Crohn's disease or adult celiac disease both clinically and radiographically. Clues to the differential diagnosis include persistent fevers and a short duration of symptoms. Enlarged lymph nodes or hepatosplenomegaly may be found on physical examination, and CT may show enlarged retroperitoneal nodes. Diagnosis often is made only after surgical biopsy. Therapy includes local resection and radiation therapy. Chemotherapy is used for disseminated disease.

e. **Multiple defects** contribute to malabsorption in the following settings:

(1) **After gastrectomy.** Malabsorption can result after Billroth II gastrectomy, when poor mixing of gastric contents with pancreatic enzymes and stasis in the afferent loop with bacterial overgrowth are present. Therapy includes surgical correction of the afferent loop and broad-spectrum antibiotics.

(2) **Radiation enteritis.** This condition interferes with the blood supply to the intestine. Bacterial overgrowth also may occur secondary to the radiation-induced intestinal stricture. Lymphatic obstruction due to edema or fibrosis also may be a part of the syndrome.

(3) **Diabetes mellitus.** Altered gut motility from diabetic neuropathy, bacterial overgrowth, and exocrine pancreatic insufficiency all have been implicated as mechanisms of diabetes mellitus–induced malabsorption.

f. **Other causes of malabsorption**

(1) **Abetalipoproteinemia** is a rare disease with neurologic manifestations (e.g., ataxia, nystagmus, incoordination, retinitis pigmentosa), morphologically abnormal "spiny" red blood cells (RBCs), low serum cholesterol and triglyceride levels, and low serum betalipoprotein levels. Steatorrhea occurs because apoprotein B, which is necessary for normal chylomicron formation, is lacking in intestinal cells. Fat is found in the epithelial cells on small bowel biopsy. Treatment with MCT oil bypasses the absorption defect. Fat-soluble vitamin supplementation also may be required.

(2) **Infections** can cause malabsorption and may be viral, bacterial, or parasitic.

(a) **Viral** and **bacterial enteritis** may cause temporary malabsorption secondary to disaccharidase deficiency, mucosal damage, or both.

(b) **Tropical sprue** is an endemic malabsorption disorder occurring in the tropics. It is thought to have an infectious etiology because travelers are susceptible to the disease, and treatment with tetracycline usually is effective.

(c) Other infectious causes of malabsorption include hookworm, tapeworm, strongyloidiasis, and *Capillaria philippinensis* (roundworm) infection, which are common outside the United States, and giardiasis, which is relatively common in the United States.

(3) **Chronic intestinal ischemia** may cause malabsorption when two of the three major intestinal vessels—the celiac artery, superior mesenteric artery, and inferior mesenteric artery—are occluded (as can be shown angiographically). Symptoms usually are weight loss and crampy postprandial pain, with occasional bloody diarrhea. Vascular surgery may result in improvement.

(4) **Hypogammaglobulinemia** may cause malabsorption, especially if it is associated with serum IgA, serum IgG, or intestinal IgA deficiency. Intestinal and serum IgM also may be increased. Small bowel biopsy shows absence of plasma cells. Nodular lymphoid hyperplasia may be seen in the distal small bowel on radiograph, and *G. lamblia* may be detected in stool or duodenal aspirate. There is an increased risk of intestinal lymphomas and gastric cancer in affected patients. Treatment of giardiasis with metronidazole or quinacrine may improve absorption. Common variable immunodeficiency is treated with intravenous gammaglobulin, which may result in a decrease in intestinal infections.

(5) **Metastatic carcinoid syndrome** is associated with an increased production of 5-hydroxytryptamine (serotonin), which causes increased gastrointestinal motility. Methysergide, cyproheptadine, or somatostatin may be used for therapy if surgical resection is not possible.

(6) **Hypoparathyroidism** may manifest as steatorrhea. The mechanism by which parathormone affects fat absorption is unknown, but vitamin D–dependent calcium absorption may play a role.

(7) **Drugs** that may cause malabsorption include neomycin, kanamycin, and bacitracin. Phenytoin causes a selective folic acid malabsorption.

2. **Clinical features** are variable. Patients may present with some or all of the following clinical manifestations:
   a. Passage of abnormal stools, which are greasy, soft, bulky, and foul smelling and may float in the toilet because of their increased gas content; a film of grease or oil droplets may be seen on the surface of the water
   b. Weight loss, which may be severe and involve marked muscle wasting
   c. Edema and ascites secondary to hypoalbuminemia
   d. Anemia secondary to altered absorption of iron, vitamin B_{12}, folate, or a combination of these
   e. Bone pain or fractures from vitamin D deficiency
   f. Paresthesias or tetany from calcium deficiency
   g. Bleeding from vitamin K deficiency

3. **Diagnosis** is based on clinical evidence, with confirmation by laboratory tests.
   a. **Stool fat analysis.** This test may be qualitative or quantitative. A positive Sudan stain indicates excretion of greater than 15 g fat per day in the stool. A 72-hour fecal fat collection can be used to quantify the amount of fat absorption. Normally, an individual absorbs 93%–95% of all dietary fat ingested. Pancreatic disease often is associated with fecal fat excretion in excess of 20–30 g/day on a diet of 100 g/day of fat.
   b. **D-Xylose absorption testing.** Because D-xylose, a five-carbon sugar, does not require enzymatic degradation or micelle formation for absorption, it can be used to measure intestinal mucosal integrity. After a 25-g oral dose, a 5-hour urine collection should contain at least 4–5 g D-xylose. Alternatively, a 2-hour serum sample may be used.
   c. **Testing for unabsorbed carbohydrate.** Lowered stool pH occurs when unabsorbed carbohydrates reach the colon and bacterial fermentation occurs. This is particularly common in lactase deficiency but also may be seen in celiac disease and short bowel syndrome.
   d. **Pancreatic function testing.** Testing involves measuring the bicarbonate and total fluid output from the duodenum after secretin stimulation or using pancreatic chymotrypsin (the bentiromide test) to release *para*-aminobenzoic acid (PABA), which is excreted in the urine. Less than 60% urinary excretion of PABA suggests pancreatic insufficiency.
   e. **Measurement of serum carotene levels.** Because vitamin A is fat-soluble and the serum carotene level is a reflection of vitamin A metabolism, a low serum carotene level with normal vitamin A intake may be a useful screening test for fat malabsorption.
   f. **Bacterial overgrowth testing**

      (1) **Direct culture** of jejunal aspirates yielding greater than 10^5 organisms/mm^3 of aspirate is considered abnormal. The diagnosis is strongly suggested by the presence of fastidious anaerobes (clostridia and bacteroides), facultative anaerobes (lactobacilli and enterococci), or coliforms.

      (2) **Bile acid breath tests** are becoming more popular. The tests are based on the fact that bacteria deconjugate ^{14}C-labeled glycine-cholate before it can be absorbed. ^{14}C-glycine then is metabolized to $^{14}CO_2$, which is exhaled and measured in the breath of patients with bacterial overgrowth.

      (3) **Measurement of tryptophan metabolites.** Elevated urinary levels of indican and 5-hydroxyindoleacetic acid are caused by increased metabolism of tryptophan. This test is not specific, however, because abnormal levels of tryptophan metabolites also are obtained in carcinoid syndrome and Whipple's disease.
   g. **Small bowel radiography.** This procedure, especially using the intubated air contrast technique, may be useful. Pooling or flocculation of barium does not occur as frequently as with

previous barium techniques but, if noted, suggests celiac disease. Thick folds may be seen in Whipple's disease, lymphoma, amyloidosis, radiation enteritis, Zollinger-Ellison syndrome, and eosinophilic enteritis, and a pseudo-Whipple's appearance is observed in patients with AIDS enteropathy.

h. Schilling test. This technique is used to diagnose vitamin B_{12} malabsorption.

(1) An abnormal first-stage Schilling test (administration of radiolabeled vitamin B_{12} only) with a normal second-stage Schilling test (administration of a complex of vitamin B_{12} and intrinsic factor) indicates gastric defects such as pernicious anemia and lack of intrinsic factor caused by gastric resection. The second-stage test may be abnormal because of bacterial overgrowth or resection or inflammation of the terminal ileum, which is the site of absorption. Severe celiac disease also may cause an abnormal second-stage test.

(2) In severe pancreatic insufficiency, pancreatic proteases are not present in sufficient quantity to cleave B_{12} from gastrin R proteins. In the third stage of the test, labeled B_{12} absorption is improved after pancreatic enzymes are given orally to the patient at the time of the testing procedure.

i. Small bowel biopsy. This procedure is essential for the diagnosis of many cases of malabsorption. In properly prepared specimens, normal villous crypt ratios are 3:1 or 4:1. Flattening of the villi with inflammatory cell infiltration is characteristic of celiac disease, but flattened villi alone may be seen in infectious enteritis, giardiasis, lymphoma, and bacterial overgrowth.

4. Characteristics and management of specific causes of malabsorption

a. Pancreatic insufficiency may be caused by chronic pancreatitis, pancreatic carcinoma, or cystic fibrosis. Bentiromide test or pancreatic secretin test results may be abnormal. Treatment is pancreatic enzyme replacement. H_2-receptor antagonists may increase the potency of enzymes when given 1 hour before meals because acid may inactivate the exogenous enzymes.

b. Bacterial overgrowth may be attributable to altered motility (e.g., in diabetes, amyloidosis, intestinal pseudo-obstruction), small bowel diverticula, strictures (e.g., in lymphoma and Crohn's disease), or blind loops after Billroth II gastrectomy. Surgical correction of the anatomic problems may be considered, but treatment with antibiotics frequently is successful. Ampicillin, amoxicillin and clavulanate potassium, tetracycline, or chloramphenicol may be used. Some patients require continuous therapy, and in these cases, antibiotics should be rotated.

c. Celiac disease (nontropical sprue)

(1) Although the **etiology** and **pathogenesis** are not fully understood, it is clear that an abnormal sensitivity to gluten, a protein component of wheat, causes damage to the intestinal mucosa of these patients. The importance of genetic factors is demonstrated by abnormal small bowel biopsies in 10%–15% of first-degree relatives of patients. Previously thought to be present in only 1 in 10,000 Americans, recent studies have indicated that even in nonaffected relatives, the incidence may be as high as 1 in 120 to 1 in 150 of the United States population. Nearly all celiac patients (approximately 98%) have HLA DQ_2 or DQ_8 human leukocyte antigens, compared with 20%–30% of the general population. Together, these factors may contribute to a binding of gliadin—the offensive protein component in gluten—to intestinal epithelial cells and, hence, to the immunogenicity of the bound product. Celiac patients have proximal intestinal involvement with a relative sparing of the distal ileum.

(2) **Clinical features** include diarrhea, steatorrhea, weight loss, and abdominal bloating. Symptoms may begin in childhood and then lessen, only to reappear in the third to sixth decade of life. Only 30%–40% of adult patients will present with the classic symptoms of diarrhea, abdominal bloating, weight loss, and steatorrhea. Most of the patients will have insidious presentations including osteoporosis, anemia, autoimmune diseases such as type I diabetes mellitus, rheumatoid arthritis or systemic lupus erythematosus, and so forth. Iron deficiency anemia unassociated with gastrointestinal blood loss may be seen because iron is preferentially absorbed in the more severely involved proximal small

intestine. Unexplained central nervous system symptoms such as depression, neurologic deficit, or even seizures may be more common in celiac patients.

(3) **Diagnosis** requires small bowel biopsy, which shows villous atrophy, crypt hypertrophy, and cuboidal change in the epithelial cells. Inflammatory cell infiltration in the lamina propria at endoscopy may show "scalloped folds" in the proximal duodenum. Antigliadin antibodies (IgG, IgA) are elevated in 90% of patients, especially in those who have not received treatment. Antireticulin and antiendomysial antibodies may be more specific, although less sensitive for celiac disease. Anti-tissue transglutaminase antibody (IgA) is currently the diagnostic antibody of choice with the highest sensitivity and specificity for celiac disease. All antibodies may decrease or disappear with treatment. Because approximately 5%–7% of patients with celiac disease may be IgA deficient, a total IgA level may be necessary if one is relying on IgA celiac antibodies for diagnostic purposes.

(4) **Therapy** is based on withdrawal of gluten from the diet by eliminating wheat, rye, barley, and oats. Only corn and rice flour are permitted. Although clinical response to gluten withdrawal often is dramatic and may be seen in a few days, histologic recovery demonstrated on repeat small bowel biopsy may be delayed for months and, in up to 50% of patients, may never be demonstrated. In severely ill patients, steroids may be of short-term benefit.

(5) **Complications**

(a) **Lymphoma** or **carcinoma** (especially esophageal) occurs with increased incidence. Lymphoma (especially T cell lymphoma) may be increased 30-to 50-fold, particularly if patients are noncompliant with a gluten-free diet.

(b) **Intestinal ulcers** or **strictures** may be late complications in some patients with celiac disease.

(c) **Dermatitis herpetiformis** is a skin lesion characterized by papular vesicular eruptions and pruritus. Most patients have an abnormal intestinal biopsy showing villous atrophy, and the skin lesions may respond to gluten withdrawal.

(d) **Collagenous sprue** may develop with a thick band of collagen (>10–15 μm in diameter) in the lamina propria and is extremely resistant to medical therapy.

(e) **The incidence of autoimmune diseases is increased in celiac patients.**

d. **Whipple's disease** is a systemic disorder most commonly occurring in middle-aged men.

(1) The **etiology** and **pathogenesis** of Whipple's disease have recently been elucidated. Numerous small gram-positive cocci are seen in macrophages in individual organs, and the organism *Tropheryma whippelii* has been isolated as the infectious agent.

(2) **Clinical features** depend on organ involvement. In the intestine, periodic acid–Schiff (PAS)–positive macrophages (i.e., macrophages that contain bacilli) are found in the lamina propria. The mesenteric lymph nodes, heart, spleen, lungs, and CNS also may be involved. Malabsorption is caused by mucosal damage and lymphatic obstruction. Fever occurs in one third to one half of patients. Arthralgia and arthritis are present in 60% of patients and may precede the gastrointestinal symptoms.

(3) **Diagnosis** is made by intestinal biopsy with a PAS stain. A small bowel radiograph may show thickened folds. In rare cases, the disease is focal and the biopsy specimen is normal.

(4) **Therapy** with penicillin, ampicillin, or tetracycline is required for at least 4–6 months and may be continued intermittently (i.e., every other day) thereafter. The relapse rate is approximately 10%.

F **Protein-losing enteropathy (PLE)** refers to the excessive loss of serum proteins into the gastrointestinal tract. Three types of disorders may cause PLE.

1. **Mucosal ulceration** causes leakage of protein at the ulcer site and results from the following conditions:

a. Malignant disease involving the gastrointestinal tract
b. Multiple peptic ulcers
c. Nongranulomatous ileojejunitis

2. **Mucosal disease without ulceration** but with altered metabolism or cell turnover leads to increased permeability to protein. Such diseases include:
   a. Ménétrier's disease (giant hypertrophic gastritis)
   b. Celiac disease
   c. Whipple's disease
   d. Infectious enteritis
3. **Lymph flow obstruction** causes increased lymphatic pressure and protein leakage. Lymphatic obstruction results from the following conditions:
   a. Lymphoma
   b. Intestinal lymphangiectasia
   c. Cardiac disease such as constrictive pericarditis and tricuspid valve disease
   d. *C. philippinensis* infection

G **Crohn's disease (regional enteritis)** is a chronic granulomatous disease that may occur anywhere in the gastrointestinal tract from the mouth to the anus. The ileum most often is involved, with ileocolitis in more than 50% of patients. The first peak of incidence occurs between the ages of 12 and 30 years; a secondary peak occurs at age 50 years.

1. **Etiology**
   a. **Genetic factors** appear to play a role, with an increased incidence of disease noted in monozygotic twins and siblings. Approximately 17% of patients with Crohn's disease have first-degree relatives with the disease. Men are affected more often than women, and the disease is more common among Jews. Compared with the general population, Jewish men have six times the risk for development of Crohn's disease. An abnormality in chromosome 16—the NOD-2 gene—has been associated with fibrostenosing small bowel Crohn's disease.
   b. **Infectious agents** have been postulated but never identified as a cause of Crohn's disease. An inflammatory response can be induced in the footpads and intestinal walls of mice by injecting an extract of Crohn's disease tissue, and this may reflect a small transmissible agent such as an RNA virus or a cell wall–defective bacterium. A mycobacterium has been proposed as an etiologic agent.
   c. An **immunologic mechanism** is the most prominent theory. Abnormal numbers, subsets, and functions of T cells have been identified in cases of Crohn's disease. Hyperresponsive immune function, rather than abnormal function, is characteristic of an unrestricted response to inflammation. Recently, a defect in the ability of intestinal epithelial cells to produce normal amounts of suppressor T (Ts) cells (CD8 cells) has been noted.
2. **Pathologic features**
   a. Marked thickening of the involved intestinal wall with transmural inflammation
   b. Enlarged and matted mesenteric lymph nodes
   c. Focal granulomas in 50% of specimens
   d. Deep serpiginous or linear ulcerations leading to cobblestoning and fistula formation
   e. Stricture formation secondary to scarring
   f. Alternating areas of normal and involved mucosa
3. **Clinical features** are characterized by periodic exacerbations and remissions.
   a. **Pain** often is colicky, especially in the lower abdomen, and may be increased after meals because of the obstructive nature of the pathologic process.
   b. **Systemic symptoms** are common and include fever, weight loss, malaise, and anorexia.
   c. **Diarrhea** is the usual presenting symptom.

d. **Intestinal obstruction** is the presenting symptom in approximately 25% of cases. Massive gastrointestinal bleeding may be a presenting symptom in 2%–3% of cases.

e. **Extraintestinal manifestations** are numerous.

(1) Anemia as well as growth or sexual retardation probably are attributable to inadequate caloric intake.

(2) Hepatobiliary disorders include fatty liver, pericholangitis, nonspecific hepatitis, cirrhosis, and sclerosing cholangitis. There is an increased risk of gallstones. Liver enzyme or liver biopsy abnormalities occur in 50%–70% of Crohn's disease patients.

(3) Renal disorders include right ureteral obstruction secondary to contiguous bowel involvement and nephrolithiasis. An increase in calcium oxalate stones is caused by increased oxalate absorption, and an increase in uric acid stones is ascribed to increased cell turnover and a concentrated acid urine.

(4) Peripheral arthritis occurs in 10%–12% of patients and ankylosing spondylitis in 2%–10%.

(5) Skin problems include erythema nodosum and, rarely, pyoderma gangrenosum.

(6) Episcleritis or uveitis may occur in 3%–10% of patients.

f. **Fistulas** to the skin or other organs occur in approximately 20% of patients. Perianal fistulas or abscesses are especially common in Crohn's colitis. Perianal skin tags are characteristic of colonic Crohn's disease.

4. **Diagnosis** is based on clinical signs and symptoms combined with characteristic radiographic findings, including deep (collar button) ulcerations, long strictured segments (string sign), and skip areas. Colonoscopy may be helpful when there is colonic involvement, and biopsies may show granuloma formation. Laboratory studies are not specific but may show multifactorial anemia, leukocytosis, an increased sedimentation rate, and evidence of malabsorption or protein loss. The differential diagnosis includes lymphoma, tuberculosis, radiation enteritis, and *Yersinia* infection (especially in acute enteritis).

5. **Therapy** is symptomatic. No specific therapy or cure exists.

a. **Supportive measures** include short-term, broad-spectrum antibiotics; antidiarrheal agents; bowel rest with intravenous fluid support (i.e., nothing by mouth); enteral nutrition with tube feedings; total parenteral nutrition; and vitamin supplementation.

b. **Medical treatment**

(1) **Sulfasalazine** or 5-aminosalicylic acid preparations in doses of 3–4 g/day may be used alone or in combination with corticosteroids to treat acute disease. This may be more effective in Crohn's colitis. Ethyl cellulose–coated oral 5-aminosalicylic acid preparations may be useful in small bowel disease.

(2) **Vitamin B_{12}** injections are indicated when ileal disease causes malabsorption of this vitamin.

(3) **Increased oral calcium, vitamin D,** or **both** may be helpful in patients with calcium oxalate stones by binding oxalate in the bowel and decreasing urinary oxalate.

(4) **Metronidazole, oral quinolone antibiotics,** or **both** may be effective in treatment of perineal and perianal fistulas.

(5) **Corticosteroids** have been proven effective by the National Cooperative Crohn's Disease Study, especially in patients with small bowel disease. When remission is obtained, the dosage should be tapered gradually.

(6) **6-Mercaptopurine, azathioprine,** and **methotrexate** also have been used. **Cyclosporine** may be useful as a down-regulator of the immune system.

(7) **Infliximab,** a chimeric antibody that binds tumor necrosis factor (TNF) [an important proinflammatory cytokine in Crohn's disease], is an effective treatment method. Administration of this agent results in a dramatic decrease in Crohn's disease activity index (CDAI) in two thirds of patients and remission in one third of all patients. These results may be observed within just 4–6 weeks of therapy. Natalizumab is a monoclonal antibody against alpha-4 integrin and may be helpful as an immune modulating agent.

c. **Surgery** may be necessary for recurrent intestinal obstruction, enterocutaneous fistulas, and perforation as well as for growth retardation that does not respond to increased caloric intake. The recurrence rate after initial resection may be as high as 80% within 15 years, especially with initial small bowel involvement.

H Small bowel tumors

1. **Malignant tumors** of the small intestine are rare and include **adenocarcinomas, carcinoid tumors, lymphomas, and leiomyosarcomas.** (GISTs—see 5II-B3)
   a. **Etiology and pathogenesis.** Some small bowel malignancies arise de novo, but many are related to underlying conditions such as Crohn's disease and celiac disease. Rarely, these malignancies arise from the polyps of Peutz-Jeghers syndrome, familial polyposis, and Gardner's syndrome. A particular type of lymphoma called Mediterranean lymphoma is endemic to the Middle East. Patients with celiac disease may have a 10%–15% incidence of small bowel malignancy, usually lymphoma.
   b. **Pathology.** Adenocarcinoma, the most common small bowel tumor, is especially common in the proximal small bowel; lymphomas and carcinoid tumors primarily occur in the appendix and ileum. Small bowel tumors may be metastatic from the breast, kidney, ovary, and testis as well as from melanoma.
   c. **Clinical features.** Bleeding, obstruction, and malabsorption may occur. Carcinoid tumors of the appendix may occur as acute appendicitis but usually are asymptomatic. Rarely, appendiceal carcinoid tumors are metastatic to the liver and, in such cases, may cause carcinoid syndrome, which is characterized by flushing and diarrhea.
   d. **Therapy and prognosis.** Surgery is the treatment of choice, but the prognosis is poor, especially for adenocarcinomas. Lymphomas and leiomyosarcomas have a better prognosis if they are localized to a small segment of the bowel. Radiation therapy and chemotherapy are used postoperatively to treat systemic lymphomas. Carcinoid tumors grow slowly, and patients may survive for many years even if the disease is metastatic. Foregut carcinoids respond to streptozocin in approximately 50% of cases. Somatostatin often decreases the flushing and diarrhea in metastatic carcinoid tumors.
2. **Benign tumors** of the small intestine include **adenomas, lipomas,** and **leiomyomas,** which may be associated with obstruction or bleeding but usually are asymptomatic.

I Acute appendicitis is a common and curable cause of an acute abdomen. Appendicitis develops at any age and in both sexes but most often occurs in males between 10 and 30 years of age.

1. **Pathogenesis.** It is believed that the primary event is an obstruction of the appendiceal lumen by a fecalith, inflammation, foreign body, or neoplasm. After obstruction of the lumen, increased intraluminal pressure and infection may cause appendiceal necrosis and perforation.
2. **Clinical features.** Appendicitis is characterized by pain in the right lower quadrant, which initially is vague but becomes localized to McBurney's point, peritoneal signs, fever, and leukocytosis in the range of 10,000–20,000/mm^3. Rectal tenderness is common in pelvic appendicitis, and retrocecal appendicitis causes psoas muscle pain on hip extension. Patients at the extremes of age, greatly obese patients, and patients taking corticosteroids may have nonspecific complaints and a relatively benign physical examination. A high index of clinical suspicion must be maintained in these cases.
3. **Diagnosis**
   a. **Differential diagnoses.** Possible diagnoses include acute gastroenteritis, mesenteric adenitis, Meckel's diverticulum, and Crohn's disease. In young women, ovarian torsion, ruptured ovarian cyst, and pelvic inflammatory disease (PID) should be considered. In elderly patients, diverticulitis, cholecystitis, incarcerated hernia, cecal carcinoma, and mesenteric thrombosis should be ruled out.

b. **Diagnostic modalities.** In difficult-to-diagnose cases, a **barium enema** may be used to identify lack of filling of the appendix. A **CT scan** shows a mass-like effect in the right lower quadrant. On **ultrasound,** a classic "bull's-eye" appearance of the right lower quadrant is believed to be relatively diagnostic of appendicitis.

4. **Therapy. Surgery** should be performed as early as possible to prevent perforation.

V DISEASES OF THE COLON

A Constipation

1. **Simple constipation** is the result of delayed transit of intestinal contents. The highly refined, low-fiber diets of western nations probably contribute to this problem. Although the epidemiologic definition of constipation is less than three stools per week, individual differences exist. Treatment of simple constipation is directed toward increasing intestinal bulk by increasing dietary fiber content with fruits, vegetables, and bulking agents such as psyllium hydrophilic colloids, which trap water and electrolytes within the bowel lumen. Long-term use of potent laxatives should be avoided because they may result in destruction of colonic intramural nerve plexuses and cathartic colon.

2. **Constipation** may occur with a variety of diseases, including ulcerative proctitis, rectal fissures or abscesses, and rectal strictures as well as the varied causes of diffusely decreased intestinal activity discussed in IV A and B. Irritable bowel syndrome, which may present as either constipation or diarrhea, is discussed in IV D 3 a.

3. **Colonic inertia** is a motility disorder of the colon characterized by poor propulsion and ineffective mixing. When radiopaque markers are given to patients, they often remain in the colon for several days. These markers are distributed throughout the colon, indicating poor total colonic motility. **Outlet obstruction** usually occurs when a problem with internal or external sphincteric relaxation develops; when Sitz-Marks studies are given to affected patients, the markers collect in the rectum before defecation.

B Colonic diverticula

Colonic diverticula are outpouchings of the mucosa only and, therefore, are not true diverticula. In the United States, colonic diverticula occur in approximately 50% of individuals older than 60 years of age.

1. **Pathogenesis.** In western nations, colonic diverticula have been linked to low-fiber diets. Diets low in fiber and bulk are thought to cause an increased intraluminal pressure, particularly in the narrow sigmoid colon. (This belief is based on LaPlace's law, which states that the smaller the radius of a cylinder, the greater the pressure generated at a given tension.) Eventually, the increased intraluminal pressure causes a mucosal herniation at the site of a perforating arteriole carrying blood from the serosal surface to the mucosa.

2. **Clinical features.** Symptoms often are absent in uncomplicated colonic diverticula; however, patients may complain of crampy abdominal pain in the left lower quadrant, with alternating diarrhea and constipation. Often, there is relief of these symptoms after bowel movement.

3. **Therapy.** Treatment is aimed at increasing stool bulk, thereby decreasing intraluminal pressure with high-fiber foods and hydrophilic colloids. Often this results in symptomatic improvement, probably by regulating bowel frequency. Anticholinergic agents sometimes are used but have not been proven effective.

4. **Complications**

   a. **Diverticulitis** occurs in approximately 25% of patients with diverticulosis. Generally, there is a microperforation (rarely a free perforation) with peridiverticular abscess. Symptoms include left lower abdominal pain, fever, and constipation. Because of the characteristic leukocytosis and left lower abdominal tenderness on physical examination, this condition sometimes is called **left-sided appendicitis.** Treatment with antibiotics, intravenous fluids, and bowel rest (i.e., nothing by mouth) is effective in most cases. Metronidazole, ciprofloxacin, or ampicillin sodium/sulbactam sodium are used most commonly. Severely ill or toxic patients may require additional antibiotics for adequate coverage of *Pseudomonas* and anaerobes. If an abscess occurs, a fistula to the bladder or vagina may develop.

b. Bleeding occurs in approximately 20%–25% of cases and usually is brisk, painless, and not associated with straining. Blood transfusion may be necessary. In most cases, bleeding stops spontaneously with only supportive therapy. Arteriography or rapid-sequence nuclear scanning using technetium sulfur colloid or technetium-labeled erythrocytes may localize the bleeding portion of the colon and allow segmental surgical resection, if necessary.

C **Hirschsprung's disease** is a congenital cause of megacolon. This condition occurs in 1 of 5000 live births and is more common in males.

1. **Etiology.** Hirschsprung's disease is caused by incomplete caudad migration of neural crest cells, which renders the internal anal sphincter and a variable segment of the rectum and sigmoid without innervation. The involved segment constitutes a functional obstruction, and the normal proximal colon becomes dilated.
2. **Clinical features.** The disease may occur in infancy as meconium ileus, intestinal obstruction, or severe constipation, or it may develop in later life with milder symptoms.
3. **Diagnosis.** Physical examination indicates the absence of stool in the rectum, and barium enema shows a narrowed (diseased) segment with a dilated proximal colon (normal segment) in approximately 75% of cases. Anal manometry is a good screening test for this disease and indicates a lack of reflex relaxation in the internal anal sphincter on rectal distention. The absence of ganglion cells on a full-thickness rectal biopsy is diagnostic.
4. **Therapy.** Treatment is surgical.

D **Ulcerative colitis** is a chronic inflammatory disease of the colonic mucosa and submucosa. Ulcerative colitis and Crohn's disease share some features and, despite their dissimilarities, often are placed together under the generic heading of inflammatory bowel disease. Ulcerative colitis occurs in 2–7 of 100,000 individuals, and females are affected more commonly than males. The major peak of incidence occurs between the ages of 15 and 30 years, with a lesser peak between the ages of 50 and 65 years.

1. **Etiology and pathogenesis** are similar to those of Crohn's disease (see IV G). Family members have an increased risk for the development of inflammatory bowel disease; approximately 15%–17% of patients have a first-degree relative with inflammatory bowel disease. Viral, bacterial, and immunologic theories (similar to those for Crohn's disease) have been proposed, and the incidence is increased twofold to fourfold in Jews. Whereas smoking increases the risk for the development of Crohn's disease, it decreases the risk of the development of ulcerative colitis to approximately half that of the general population. There is an increased risk of the development of ulcerative colitis in patients who have recently discontinued smoking. Ulcerative colitis patients who are HLA-B27 positive have a strong association with arthritis, and especially with ankylosing spondylitis.
2. **Pathology.** The hallmarks of ulcerative colitis are the microabscesses of the crypts of Lieberkühn, which are seen in approximately 70% of cases. The inflammatory response generally is limited to the mucosa. Macroscopic ulcerations are noted with confluence of the inflammatory response. Pseudopolyps occur when normal mucosa is isolated by severe ulcerations, but there are no skip areas. The rectum and distal colon are involved most commonly. Pancolitis is seen in 25% of cases. Ulcerative colitis with rectal sparing is extremely uncommon.
3. **Clinical features** are mild when the disease is limited to the rectum (ulcerative proctitis). Moderate-to-severe symptoms may occur with extensive disease, particularly pancolitis, and include bloody diarrhea, weight loss, fever, left lower abdominal cramping pain, and nocturnal passage of a small

volume of blood and mucus. Fulminant disease occurs in 15% of cases. Extraintestinal manifestations, especially Crohn's colitis, are similar to those of Crohn's disease and are evident in 10%–15% of patients. Extraintestinal signs and symptoms include nonsymmetrical large joint arthritis, sacroiliitis (especially in HLA B27 patients), erythema nodosum, pyoderma gangrenosum, sclerosing cholangitis, and uveitis.

4. **Diagnosis** is based on clinical presentation along with the exclusion of infectious, parasitic, and neoplastic etiologic factors. Serologic analysis for perinuclear antineutrophil cytoplasmic antibody (p-ANCA) may aid in differentiation between ulcerative colitis and Crohn's disease (see IV G). These antibodies occur in 60%–85% of patients with ulcerative colitis and may be found in 60%–80% of patients with Crohn's disease.
   a. **Stool examination** reveals mucus, blood, and white blood cells without parasites or bacterial pathogens. It is important to rule out the usual causes of dysentery, including *Salmonella, Shigella, Campylobacter,* pathogenic *E. coli* (especially *E. coli* 0157:H7), amebiasis, or *C. difficile* infection.
   b. **Colonoscopy or proctosigmoidoscopy** reveals friability, edema, and hyperemia of the mucosa. Ulcerations and a mucopurulent exudate may be present. Islands of normal tissue may have the appearance of pseudopolyps. Numerous biopsy samples should be obtained.
   c. **Barium enema** should not be performed in severely ill or toxic patients. If the symptoms are subacute, a barium radiograph after minimal preparation may show a lack of haustral markings, fine serrations (compatible with small ulcerations), large ulcerations, and pseudopolyps.
5. **Therapy** varies with the severity and extent of disease.
   a. In acute flares, **bowel rest with intravenous fluids** (i.e., nothing by mouth) may be useful for short periods. Total parenteral nutrition allows prolonged bowel rest (i.e., nothing by mouth) with repletion of vitamins, minerals, electrolytes, and calories in the form of carbohydrate, protein, and fat.
   b. **5-Aminosalicylic acid and sulfasalazine** have been shown to induce remission and decrease relapse rates in ulcerative colitis patients. The active moiety may be the antiprostaglandin substance 5-aminosalicylic acid, which is released in the colon by bacteria. Side effects include headache, nausea, rash, and agranulocytosis. 5-Aminosalicylic acid enemas are effective in left-sided colitis.
   c. **Corticosteroids,** which are administered by enema (especially in distal disease such as ulcerative proctitis) or systemically, may be effective in inducing remission. Prednisone is given orally in doses of 20–60 mg/day, and adrenocorticotropic hormone is administered in doses of 40–80 U/24 hr. Budesonide, a corticosteroid that is inactivated by first-pass metabolism through the liver, minimizes systemic side effects while maintaining efficacy.
   d. In mild-to-moderate cases, **antidiarrheal agents, anticholinergic agents,** and **sedation** may be used cautiously.
   e. **Immunomodulating agents** such as 6-mercaptopurine, azathioprine, cyclosporine, methotrexate, and hydroxychloroquine have been tried in the hopes of avoiding or delaying emergent surgery or as a steroid-sparing agent in steroid-resistant patients. Biologic therapy including infliximab may be effective in select cases and continues to be evaluated in large clinical trials.
   f. **Surgery** requires the removal of the entire colon with the creation of an ileostomy or with mucosectomy and creation of an ileal J-pouch with ileoanal anastomosis. Surgery is generally reserved for the following conditions:
      (1) Toxic megacolon that is unresponsive to 24–72 hours of intensive conservative medical measures
      (2) Perforation
      (3) Massive hemorrhage that is unresponsive to conservative treatment (rare)
      (4) Carcinoma
      (5) Suspected carcinoma in colonic strictures

(6) Growth failure in adolescents, which is unresponsive to conservative treatment

(7) Dysplasia noted on biopsy at the time of sigmoidoscopy or colonoscopy, which should be performed routinely for screening in long-standing diseases

(8) Cure, especially after 10 years of disease because of the increased risk of cancer. The ileoanal anastomotic procedure that strips the colonic mucosa and avoids the need for a permanent colostomy has become widespread.

6. **Complications.** The systemic complications noted for Crohn's disease (see IV G 3 e) often occur in ulcerative colitis. Additional complications occur with ulcerative colitis, which usually are not seen in Crohn's disease.
   a. **Toxic megacolon** refers to an acute dilatation of the colon (usually the transverse portion) to a diameter in excess of 6 cm. This complication of ulcerative colitis probably is attributable to severe inflammation, which affects large segments of the colonic musculature as well as neural control of the colon. Anticholinergic and antidiarrheal medications also may contribute. Patients usually are severely ill, with high fever, abdominal pain, and a marked leukocytosis. Treatment is intensive medical therapy for 48–72 hours. Patients who do not respond should undergo an emergency total colectomy.
   b. **Carcinoma** of the colon is associated with long-standing disease of great extent (usually pancolitis). At 10 years, the risk of carcinoma is 10% and may increase to 20% at 20 years and 40% at 25–30 years. The malignancies often are multicentric and aggressive. Strictured areas of the colon present a particularly difficult problem because of the difficulty in differentiating intensive inflammatory disease from ischemic narrowing or carcinoma. Yearly colonoscopic examinations with biopsy samples obtained every 10–20 cm should be performed in patients who have had ulcerative colitis for longer than 8–10 years. If high-grade dysplasia is noted, a prophylactic total colectomy should be considered.
7. **Prognosis.** Mortality rates are approximately 20% in toxic megacolon, with higher rates noted in patients older than 60 years. Approximately 10% of patients do not experience a recurrent attack after the initial onset of disease. Continuous symptoms occur in 10% of patients. Approximately 70%–80% of patients have recurrent remissions and relapses, and approximately 20% of patients eventually require total colectomy. Surveillance colonoscopy with biopsy to evaluate for dysplasia should be performed every 1–2 years after 8–10 years of pancolitis or 12–15 years of left-sided disease.

E **Angiodysplasia** refers to small vascular abnormalities, which usually are seen in the ascending colon or cecum in patients older than 60 years of age. Involvement of the small bowel or stomach also has been reported but is less common. Associations with aortic stenosis and chronic renal insufficiency have been reported.

1. **Pathogenesis.** Angiodysplasia is believed to result from obstruction of intestinal capillaries and venules as these vessels pass through the muscularis.
2. **Clinical features.** Most patients are asymptomatic, but the abnormal vessels are a common cause of painless lower gastrointestinal bleeding in older individuals.
3. **Diagnosis.** Angiographic or colonoscopic demonstration of intraluminal extravasation of blood during the acute episode may be used to make the diagnosis.
4. **Therapy.** Bleeding usually can be managed conservatively with colonoscopic heater probe or laser treatment, but a right colon resection occasionally is needed for recurrent or massive bleeding. Estrogen treatment has decreased bleeding in some patients.

F **Endometriosis** involves the colon in approximately 10% of cases. Symptoms include pain or rectal bleeding during menses. A barium enema often reveals extrinsic compression of the rectosigmoid or descending colon. Treatment is hormonal. Rarely, surgery is necessary to alleviate obstruction, pain, or recurrent bleeding.

G Tumors of the colon

1. **Benign tumors.** There are several histologic types of benign colonic polyps. **Adenomatous polyps** are considered to be precursors of adenocarcinoma, and the risk for adenocarcinoma increases when the polyps are larger than 2 cm, villous rather than tubular, and sessile rather than pedunculated. Approximately 5%–10% of individuals older than age 40 years have colonic polyps, but most of these polyps are small hyperplastic lesions that carry no malignant potential. Other benign tumors include leiomyomas, lipomas, and fibromas.
   a. **Clinical features.** Rectal bleeding occurs and may be microscopic or macroscopic. Large polyps may cause symptoms of an incomplete intestinal obstruction with occasional crampy abdominal pain.
   b. **Diagnosis.** Diagnosis involves use of an air contrast barium enema, endoscopic visualization of the colon, or both.
   c. **Therapy**
      (1) Therapy for pedunculated lesions is colonoscopic removal with snare electrocautery. Sessile lesions may require surgical excision.
      (2) Because carcinoma occurring in an adenomatous polyp may be focal, careful histologic sectioning of the entire polyp, not just a biopsy, is necessary to exclude carcinoma. If malignancy invades the stalk of a polyp, a segmental resection of the colon is indicated to rule out lymphatic spread.
      (3) Synchronous polyps occur in 20% of cases, and metachronous lesions occur in approximately 30% of cases. Therefore, an air contrast barium enema, full colonoscopy, or both should be performed at the time a polyp is first identified and every 3 years thereafter. A yearly stool Hemoccult test also should be performed.
      (4) First-degree relatives of a patient with colonic polyps or carcinoma have approximately a fourfold to fivefold increased risk of development of a similar lesion. The daily use of aspirin or other NSAIDs may be associated with decreased polyp formation.
2. **Hereditary polyposis syndromes**
   a. **Familial adenomatous polyposis (FAP)** is an autosomal dominant syndrome characterized by adenomas of the colon. Allelic loss in chromosome 5q21-q22 was named the adenomatous polyposis coli (*APC*) gene and can be detected in peripheral blood leukocytes of patients with familial polyposis of the colon.
      (1) Hundreds of adenomatous polyps of the large intestine or cancer of the periampullary region of the small bowel is noted in patients and should be evaluated periodically with esophagogastric duodenoscopy.
      (2) When osteomas or soft tissue tumors (lipomas, fibromas, desmoid tumors of the mesentery) are present, this condition is called **Gardner's syndrome.**
      (3) Colonic malignancy develops by age 40 years in 80%–90% of patients. A subtotal resection of the colon with close subsequent observation should be performed by age 30 years. Sulindac therapy has led to regression of polyps in several patients.
   b. **Peutz-Jeghers syndrome** is an autosomal dominant polyposis syndrome with mucocutaneous pigmentation, particularly of the buccal mucosa. The polyps are hamartomas, not adenomas, which carry a low risk for malignant transformation and may be present in the stomach and small bowel as well as in the colon. Patients may have recurrent gastrointestinal bleeding.
   c. **Turcot syndrome** refers to pancolonic adenomas with malignant CNS tumors. This autosomal dominant polyposis syndrome has a high risk of malignancy.
   d. **Juvenile polyposis** is an autosomal dominant syndrome with gastrointestinal bleeding from polyps of the colon, small bowel, and stomach. The risk of malignancy is slightly increased in later life.
   e. **Cronkhite-Canada syndrome** is a rare association of intestinal polyps with alopecia, hyperpigmentation, and a lack of fingernails. No conclusive inheritance pattern has been noted.

f. **Cowden's disease** is a rare autosomal dominant condition characterized by multiple hamartomas of the face, other parts of the skin (acral keratoses), or mouth. Breast lesions (fibrocystic disease or cancer) occur in approximately 50% of patients. Thyroid abnormalities, including goiter or cancer, occur in 10%–15% of patients. There is no increased risk of cancer associated with the gastrointestinal hamartomatous polyps.

3. **Adenocarcinoma** of the colon. This type of cancer has been steadily increasing in frequency in the United States and ranks second to lung cancer in men and third to breast cancer and lung cancer in women (overall second in men and women) as the major life-threatening malignancy.

a. **Epidemiology.** The incidence of colorectal carcinomas is increased in developed countries, especially those with a diet high in red meat and low in fiber. In the United States, the incidence is decreased in Seventh-Day Adventists who practice strict vegetarianism, which also suggests an association with diet. The incidence of colorectal carcinomas is higher in asbestos workers, machinists, and factory woodworkers than in the general population. Increased calcium and folic acid intake in men and women, as well as postmenopausal hormone therapy in women, may be protective. Daily use of aspirin or other NSAIDs also may guard against the development of colon cancer.

b. **Etiology**

(1) **Dietary factors.** Diet has been the focus of most etiologic studies. The increased amounts of red meat and animal fat in the diet in the United States promote the growth of bacterial strains that produce carcinogens in the colonic lumen. Bile salts also may contribute to this process. Vitamins A, C, and E in certain foods may inactivate the carcinogens, and broccoli, turnips, and cauliflower induce benzpyrene hydroxylase, which also may inactivate ingested carcinogens.

(2) **Genetic factors.** The role of genetic factors is demonstrated by familial polyposis syndromes and by the fact that first-degree relatives of patients with carcinoma or polyps have a threefold to fivefold increased risk of development of colorectal carcinoma. Familial adenomatous polyposis (FAP) accounts for approximately 1% of colorectal cancer and is an abnormality in chromosome 5q21-q22 (see V G 2). Hereditary non-polyposis colorectal cancer (HNPCC) family syndromes account for 5%–10%. HNPCC is an autosomal dominant syndrome characterized by an abnormality in mismatch repair genes, especially due to a loss of hMSH2 and hMLH1 genes. hPMS1 and hPMS2 are also involved to a lesser extent. Suspect a genetic cause of colorectal cancer if the patient is younger than age 50 or has a first-degree relative with colon or associated colon cancer syndromes.

(a) **HNPCC type I** is an autosomal dominant inherited condition characterized by cancer of the colon in younger patients. HNPCC often develops before patients reach 45 years of age and frequently involves the ascending colon.

(b) **HNPCC type II** is associated with carcinoma of the endometrium, ovary, ureter, renal pelvis, stomach, pancreas, and biliary tree and otherwise is similar to HNPCC type I.

(3) **Other risk factors**

(a) Ulcerative colitis, especially pancolitis and disease of greater than 10 years' duration (10% risk)

(b) History of colon cancer or adenoma (10% risk)

(c) Familial polyposis syndrome

(d) History of female genital or breast cancer

(e) History of juvenile polyps

(f) Family cancer syndromes

(g) Immunodeficiency diseases

c. **Clinical features.** Signs and symptoms vary, depending on the location and size of the tumor. Tumors in the left colon, especially those in the distal 25 cm, may manifest as obstruction. Right colon tumors frequently occur as iron deficiency anemia and fatigue. Other common symptoms include a change in bowel habit, a decrease in stool size, obvious blood in the stool, and crampy abdominal pain. Metastatic disease usually involves the liver; however, the bone, lung, and brain also may be affected.

d. Screening (see Table 5–2)*

e. Diagnosis

(1) Diagnosis is made by colonoscopy or air contrast barium enema demonstration of polyps or tumors followed by endoscopic visualization with biopsy and cytologic study. The air contrast barium enema is far more sensitive than the single contrast examination. Despite these techniques, it can be difficult to differentiate the tumor from diverticulitis, benign stricture, and Crohn's disease.

(2) High-risk patients should have frequent stool guaiac testing and thorough evaluation of unexplained blood loss.

(3) CEA determinations, although not useful for screening purposes, may be used for periodic follow-up in patients with a history of carcinoma of the colon, with an increasing titer being indicative of recurrent or metastatic disease.

f. Therapy (see Chapter 4 VI A 7)

g. Prognosis. The overall 10-year survival rate is 45% and has not changed significantly over the past several years.

(1) **Dukes' classification A and B.** Cancer confined to the mucosa is often detected by Hemoccult testing or sigmoidoscopy and is associated with an 80%–90% survival rate.

(2) **Dukes' classification C.** Cancer that is limited to the regional lymph nodes is associated with a 50%–60% survival rate.

TABLE 5–2 Colorectal Cancer Screening Recommendations

Risk for CRC	Recommendations
Average risk patients	FOBT (×3) yearly after age 50 Flex sig or BE q 3–5 yrs after age 50 Colonoscopy q 10 yrs after age 50
Increased risk patients	FAP Flex sig q 1 yr after puberty (consider total colectomy) Genetic counseling for patient and family
HNPCC	Colonoscopy q 1–2 yrs after age 20 or 10 yrs earlier than the youngest age of colon cancer diagnosis in the family (genetic counseling for patient & family)
Ulcerative colitis	Colonoscopy q 1–2 yrs after 8 yrs of disease in patients with pancolitis or colonoscopy q 1–2 yrs after 15 yrs in patients with left-sided colitis
1st-Degree relatives with colon cancer	Same screening as average risk patients, except begin at age 40 or 10 yrs earlier than the 1st-degree relative's diagnosis
History of adenomatous polyps (variable)	• Colonoscopy in 1–3 yrs if multiple (>3) adenomas or advanced adenoma • 1 small (<1 cm) tubular adenoma—colonoscopy at 5 yrs
Adenomatous polyps	• Patients with advanced large (>1 cm) villous or noninvasive malignant—colonoscopy in 1–3 yrs (multiple >3) • Patients with 1 small (<1 cm) tubular adenoma—colonoscopy in 3–5 yrs

FOBT = fecal occult blood testing; FAP = familial adenomatous polyposis; HNPCC = hereditary nonpolyposis colorectal cancer syndrome; Flex sig = flexible sigmoidoscopy; CRC = colorectal cancer.

* "Virtual colonoscopy" is a radiographic computerized colonography often using three-dimensional techniques and may become an accepted screening method.

(3) **Dukes' classification D.** Cancer that has metastasized to distant organs is associated with a survival rate of less than 25%.

H **Collagenous colitis** is a recently described syndrome of chronic watery diarrhea, especially seen in middle-aged women. Laboratory data are usually normal, except 50% of patients may have an increase in erythrocyte sedimentation rate. Hypoalbuminemia and mild steatorrhea have been reported. Colonoscopic examination findings are normal, but biopsy indicates a thick layer of subepithelial collagen deposition, which is greater than 15 μm in thickness (normal collagen deposition is less than 5 μm). Treatment is with antidiarrheal agents, sulfasalazine, steroids, or all three. **Microscopic colitis,** marked by a lymphocytic infiltrate, is probably an early stage of collagenous colitis.

I **Pseudomembranous colitis** is an acute, potentially severe disease of the colon characterized by exudative plaques that cover the intestinal mucosa.

1. **Pathogenesis.** The disease is caused by an enterotoxin produced by *C. difficile,* an anaerobic bacterium. It is thought that antibiotic therapy may "select out" the *C. difficile* organism, allowing proliferation and toxin production. Symptoms begin 3 days to 4 weeks after initiating antibiotic therapy. Virtually all antibiotics have been associated with this disease, but clindamycin, ampicillin, and the cephalosporins are the most common offenders.
2. **Clinical features.** Signs and symptoms include watery diarrhea, crampy abdominal pain, lower abdominal tenderness, and fever. Leukocytosis is common. Dehydration and electrolyte disturbances may develop in severely ill patients. Toxic megacolon and colonic perforation are rare but are serious complications that may require surgical intervention. Approximately 20% of patients have a relapse after primary treatment.
3. **Diagnosis.** Demonstration of *C. difficile* toxin in the stool or by sigmoidoscopic visualization of the characteristic yellow-white plaques in an erythematous and edematous mucosa suggests the diagnosis. Biopsy of the plaques shows a mucinous, fibrinous, polymorphonuclear exudate. Most patients have disease throughout the colon; however, the disease may be confined to the right colon, and in such cases sigmoidoscopic findings are negative.
4. **Therapy.** The first step in treatment is to discontinue unnecessary antibiotics, which results in improvement in most patients. Cholestyramine may be used to bind the toxin. The organism is sensitive to vancomycin, bacitracin, and metronidazole.

J **Cloacogenic carcinoma** accounts for 2.5% of all anorectal carcinomas. It is a carcinoma of the transitional epithelium of the region of the dentate line in the anal canal. It occurs at the junction of the ectoderm and entodermal cloaca—the blind caudal extension of the hindgut. It is more common in women, with a 3:1 ratio, and it is most common in the 55- to 70-year-old age group. Treatment is with radiation and then surgery.

K **Volvulus of the colon** generally involves either the sigmoid colon (slightly more common) or the cecal region. Sigmoid volvulus usually occurs in individuals older than 60 years of age who live in nursing homes, have CNS disease, or take antimotility drugs. Men are more susceptible, especially those with chronic constipation. Cecal volvulus commonly follows previous surgery. Acute cases require emergency colonoscopy or barium enema. Surgical resection may be necessary in 70%–90% of cases.

L **Cytomegalovirus (CMV) colitis** is often seen in patients with AIDS, severe diabetes, renal failure, or inflammatory bowel disease. Bloody diarrhea may occur because of a deeply ulcerated colon. Intranuclear inclusion bodies may be noted on biopsy. The ulcers of CMV colitis may lead to perforation. Ganciclovir has been used for treatment in some cases.

M **Diversion colitis** is colitis that develops in segments of the colon that have been diverted from the fecal stream. The diverted colon is erythematous, friable, and may be associated with bleeding.

Although the gross endoscopic appearance mimics that of ulcerative colitis, histologic differentiation from ulcerative colitis may also be difficult. Treatment of diversion colitis has included short-chain fatty acids or replacement of the colon in continuity with the fecal stream. Differentiation between diversion colitis and ulcerative colitis is necessary, because the latter condition often flares up when reanastomosis occurs.

VI DISEASES OF THE RECTUM AND ANUS

A Ulcerative proctitis is a localized form of ulcerative colitis, which has a better prognosis and a greatly decreased risk of malignancy.

1. **Clinical features.** Symptoms include diarrhea, rectal bleeding, and tenesmus; only rarely do fever, weight loss, and the systemic complications of ulcerative colitis occur.
2. **Diagnosis.** Other causes of proctitis, especially infection, should be ruled out. The absence of inflammation above the rectum should be verified by sigmoidoscopy.
3. **Therapy.** Sulfasalazine, rectal corticosteroids, and 5-aminosalicylic acid enemas often are effective treatment.
4. **Outcome.** In approximately 15%–20% of cases, ulcerative proctitis progresses to diffuse ulcerative colitis.

B Infectious proctitis

1. **Venereal diseases** that cause infectious proctitis include syphilis, gonorrhea, lymphogranuloma venereum, and herpes simplex. These diseases are especially common in homosexual men, who may have multiple simultaneous infections (see Chapter 8 VI D).
   a. **Syphilis** of the rectum almost always is primary syphilis. The chancre, which is painless, appears 10–90 days after exposure. Diagnosis is made by dark-field examination of discharge from the chancre and by serologic testing, although the Venereal Disease Research Laboratories (VDRL) test does not become positive until 1–2 weeks after the appearance of the chancre.
   b. **Gonorrhea** may be asymptomatic or may cause rectal bleeding and diarrhea. Diagnosis is made by culturing the organism.
   c. **Lymphogranuloma venereum** is caused by one strain of *Chlamydia trachomatis*, a gram-negative obligate intracellular bacterium. When left untreated, the acute proctitis may develop into a chronic destructive inflammation with late stricture formation. The organism is difficult to culture, although culture in yolk sacs and tissue cultures are possible. Serologic diagnosis generally is more available. Titers of greater than or equal to 1:16 are highly suggestive of current infection.
   d. **Herpes simplex** may cause constipation, hematochezia, severe anorectal pain, tenesmus, and mucopurulent discharge from the rectum. Bladder dysfunction with impotence may be present. Rectal biopsy shows intranuclear inclusions. The symptoms subside spontaneously but may recur.
2. **Amebiasis** (i.e., infection with *E. histolytica*) may present as a diffuse colitis or extraintestinal disease (e.g., meningitis, liver abscess), or it may be confined to the rectosigmoid colon, especially in homosexual men. Symptoms range from mild diarrhea to bloody dysentery. Diagnosis is made by demonstrating the organism in the stool or in sigmoidoscopic biopsy specimens of the characteristic flask-shaped ulcers. Treatment with metronidazole or iodoquinone may be useful.

C Solitary rectal ulcer is a syndrome consisting of a superficial ulceration of unknown cause combined with passage of mucus or blood and dull rectal pain. The ulcers usually are 2 cm in diameter on the anterior rectal mucosal wall and located 7–10 cm from the anal verge. They are multiple in 25% of patients. A weakness in the rectal sling musculature may be a contributing cause. Diagnosis is made by excluding other causes of rectal ulcers, including infections, inflammatory bowel disease, and carcinoma. Treatment is supportive.

D **Hemorrhoids** are dilated internal or external veins of the hemorrhoidal plexus located in the lower rectum. In the United States, 60%–70% of the population experience symptoms of hemorrhoids at some time. Signs and symptoms include perianal pruritus, rectal bleeding (especially small amounts on the toilet tissue or bright droplets into the toilet bowl), anal pain, and a palpable mass in the anal region. The diagnosis is made by anoscopy or sigmoidoscopy. Treatment is with stool softeners, supportive care with heat or antiedema measures, or surgery. Internal hemorrhoids may be tied with rubber banding or resected with laser or bicap electrocautery techniques.

E **Anal fissures, abscesses, and fistulas** are tears, infections, and hollow channels from the rectum to the perianal skin, respectively. Locally applied heat, sitz baths, and antibiotics may be effective. However, surgical drainage or excision of an abscess or a fistulous tract is necessary occasionally.

F **Pruritus** of the perianal skin has many causes, including infection (bacterial, fungal, or parasitic), localized anorectal disease (e.g., fistulas, fissures), dermatologic diseases (e.g., psoriasis, eczema), poor hygiene, diarrhea, and systemic diseases such as diabetes mellitus. The underlying condition should be treated. In addition, local care with careful cleaning following defecation and nightly application of hydrocortisone cream may be helpful in controlling symptoms.

G **Squamous cell carcinoma** of the anus is a rare malignancy that manifests as bleeding, pain, a mass, and change in bowel habits. Treatment is surgical, and the 5-year survival rate is 60%.

H **Cloacogenic carcinoma** is described in V J.

VII DISEASES OF THE PANCREAS

A Acute pancreatitis

1. **Etiology**
   a. **Common causes.** Approximately 70% of cases of acute pancreatitis that occur in the United States are attributable to either alcohol abuse or gallstones.
      (1) In alcoholic pancreatitis, proteinaceous plugs develop in the pancreatic ducts and calcify in the body of the pancreas, leading to stasis and atrophy of distal segments. Alcoholic pancreatitis is most common in men who have ingested large amounts of alcohol over at least 10 years.
      (2) In gallstone pancreatitis, the passage of a common duct stone (or multiple small stones, or even microlithiasis) may initiate reflux of biliary or intestinal contents into the pancreatic gland.
   b. Less common causes of acute pancreatitis
      (1) Postoperative pancreatitis, which may be severe and is especially common after hepatobiliary tract surgery
      (2) Abdominal trauma
      (3) Hyperlipidemia, types I and V (increased chylomicrons). Dietary and medical treatment of hypertriglyceridemia reduces recurrences.
      (4) Drugs such as azathioprine, 6-mercaptopurine, estrogens, thiazides, furosemide, sulfonamides, tetracyclines, corticosteroids, valproic acid, pentamidine, 2–3 dideoxyinosine, octreotide, and 5-aminosalicylic acid.
      (5) Hypercalcemia
      (6) Uremia
      (7) Peptic ulcer disease, with penetration into the pancreas
      (8) Cystic fibrosis (in rare cases)
      (9) Endoscopic retrograde cholangiopancreatography (ERCP)
      (10) Viral infections, especially mumps, coxsackievirus B
      (11) Vascular insufficiency

(12) Pancreatic cancer, probably by localized ductal obstruction
(13) Hereditary pancreatitis, which may be inherited in an autosomal dominant pattern and carries an increased risk for development of pancreatic carcinoma
(14) Ampullary lesions or duodenal disease involving the ampulla and periampullary regions
(15) Pancreas divisum, in which the main portion of the pancreas drains into the smaller accessory duct (see VII B 1 c)
(16) The bite of a certain scorpion (*Tityus trinitatis*), which causes increased pancreatic enzyme secretion and may be associated with pancreatitis
(17) Idiopathic causes

2. **Clinical features**
   a. **Abdominal pain,** which often is a steady or severe pain in the periumbilical region and may radiate to the back
   b. **Nausea and vomiting,** which occur in 70% of cases
   c. **Abdominal tenderness,** usually without guarding or rebound
   d. **Diminished or absent bowel sounds**
   e. **Epigastric fullness or mass,** which usually is found late in the course of the disease
   f. **Retroperitoneal bleeding,** causing a hematoma at the umbilicus (**Cullen's sign**) or flank (**Turner's sign**), which is seen in hemorrhagic pancreatitis
3. **Diagnosis** usually is based on characteristic clinical presentations, especially in patients with a history of previous pancreatitis.
   a. Elevated serum amylase levels almost always exist during an acute attack but also may be caused by perforated ulcer, intestinal infarction, obstruction, ruptured ectopic pregnancy, amylase-producing tumors, salivary gland disease, and decreased amylase clearance attributable to amylase–globulin complexes (macroamylase) or renal disease. All amylase-producing tumors (e.g., lung and ovary) are salivary-amylase–type tumors. Amylase may be falsely low in hyperlipidemic pancreatitis.
   b. Elevated serum lipase levels also are found in acute attacks. Increased serum trypsinogen levels may be helpful in difficult-to-diagnose cases.
   c. The amylase:creatinine clearance ratio may be elevated above the normal range of 1%–4% in acute pancreatitis. However, this ratio also is elevated postoperatively, in diabetic ketoacidosis, and in burn patients.
   d. Abdominal radiographs may show a localized ileus (sentinel loop) in the small bowel region adjacent to the pancreas. CT scanning is very helpful for diagnosis and staging of the disease. The severity of the pancreatitis can be differentiated into edematous and necrotizing pancreatitis on the basis of the CT scan.
4. **Therapy** is supportive and includes intravenous administration of fluids and analgesics and bowel rest (i.e., nothing by mouth). Morphine may cause sphincter of Oddi spasm and should be avoided. Nasogastric suction often is used to drain gastric secretions and thereby limit pancreatic stimulation; however, the effectiveness of this procedure has not been proved. Intravenous hyperalimentation, which does not stimulate exocrine pancreatic release, may be used in protracted illness. If an impacted gallstone causes pancreatitis, then ERCP, sphincterotomy, and stone removal is the treatment of choice.
5. **Complications** account for the 10% mortality rate associated with acute pancreatitis.
   a. **Hemorrhagic pancreatitis** is considered an extension of edematous pancreatitis caused by chemical mediators (e.g., elastase), which leads to retroperitoneal hemorrhage and widespread tissue necrosis. Hemorrhagic pancreatitis is more common after trauma, postoperative pancreatitis, and the initial attack of acute pancreatitis and may require peritoneal lavage or surgical intervention for placement of drains. Blood may be present in the peritoneal cavity. The diagnosis is suggested by a declining hematocrit in a severely ill patient. An elevated methemalbumin level also may be observed.

b. **Acute respiratory distress syndrome** (ARDS) is caused by increased alveolar capillary permeability and may cause severe hypoxia requiring mechanical ventilation.
c. **Pancreatic abscess** is suggested when high fever, elevated serum amylase levels, and leukocytosis persist beyond 7–10 days. Gas shadows in the region of the pancreas may be visualized by an abdominal flat plate or by CT. Treatment includes surgical drainage and antibiotics.
d. **Pancreatic pseudocyst** refers to a collection of fluid and debris within the pancreas or in a space lined by the pancreas and other adjacent structures. Diagnosis is made by ultrasonography. Approximately 50% of pseudocysts (usually smaller ones) resolve spontaneously. Those persisting beyond 6–10 weeks require drainage to avoid potentially serious complications such as hemorrhage and rupture.
e. **Pancreatic ascites** may occur because of a leaking pseudocyst with pancreatic ductal destruction. The diagnosis is suggested by very high serum amylase levels in peritoneal fluid. Conservative therapy with total parenteral nutrition and repeated paracentesis may lead to resolution, but pancreatic resection may be necessary in intractable cases.

B **Chronic pancreatitis** results in permanent structural damage of pancreatic tissue.

1. **Etiology.** Most of the causes of acute pancreatitis in the United States also can result in chronic pancreatitis. A notable exception is gallstones, which cause only recurrent acute attacks of pancreatitis.
   a. Alcohol abuse accounts for 90% of cases of chronic pancreatitis in adults.
   b. Cystic fibrosis is the most common cause of chronic disease in children.
   c. In pancreas divisum, which results from a congenital failure of the dorsal and ventral pancreas to fuse (approximately 5% of individuals), the main portion of the pancreas may drain through the small accessory duct of Santorini, not the large duct of Wirsung. Chronic obstruction to drainage and pancreatitis may occur in approximately one third of patients with this drainage. Pancreas divisum remains controversial as a cause of chronic pancreatitis.
2. **Clinical features**
   a. **Pain,** the usual presenting symptom, typically occurs in the epigastrium after eating and radiates to the back.
   b. **Malabsorption** occurs in association with **steatorrhea** and **weight loss.**
   c. **Jaundice** occurs because of edema and fibrosis in the pancreatic head and causes obstruction of the pancreatic portion of the common bile duct.
   d. **Diabetes** is common; however, ketoacidosis, nephropathy, and diabetic vascular disease rarely occur.
3. **Diagnosis.** The development of continuous pain and signs of pancreatic insufficiency in a patient with known recurrent pancreatitis, especially when attributable to alcohol ingestion, is suggestive. Specific tests include:
   a. Abdominal radiographs, which show pancreatic calcification in 30%–40% of cases
   b. Secretin-stimulation testing with duodenal intubation and aspiration, which indicates a low bicarbonate concentration in the pancreatic secretion and low enzyme output
   c. ERCP, which shows diffuse ductal dilatation with an irregular, beaded ("chain of lakes") appearance
4. **Therapy.** Treatment is aimed at controlling the manifestations of the disease because the underlying damage to the gland is permanent. In addition, agents that may promote further damage (e.g., alcohol) should be withdrawn.
   a. Control of pain may require narcotic analgesics, but care must be taken to avoid addiction. With abstinence from alcohol over time, some patients experience a lessening of pain.
   b. Replacement of pancreatic enzymes may be indicated for the treatment of steatorrhea or for the relief of pain. Antacids or H_2-receptor antagonists may increase the effectiveness of oral enzyme preparations.

c. Insulin may be needed in advanced cases.
d. MCTs, which are more easily absorbed than longer-chain fatty acids, are often given.
e. Treatment of pancreas divisum may involve enlargement of the accessory duct surgically or endoscopically with a sphincterotomy or pancreatic stent.
f. Surgery is a last resort and generally is used for severe pain or recurrent, severe attacks. Subtotal (80%) pancreatectomy and the Puestow procedure (i.e., anastomosis of the pancreatic duct lengthwise to a loop of the jejunum) are used most commonly.

C **Neoplastic cystic lesions** of the pancreas include serous and mucinous cystadenomas and adenocarcinomas. These lesions are true cysts of the pancreas, with multiple small cysts (serous) or large cysts (mucinous). These are not seen to communicate with the pancreatic duct on ERCP. They do not contain amylase, and the serum amylase level is usually normal (as discussed, the serum amylase level is elevated in approximately 60%–75% of cases of pseudocysts). These lesions are more common in women, and most affected individuals experience weight loss and have no history of pancreatitis. Angiography usually shows hypervascularity, and treatment is surgical removal—often with complete cure.

D **Adenocarcinoma** of the pancreas accounts for more than 90% of pancreatic malignancies.

1. **Epidemiology.** The adenocarcinoma is pancreatic ductal in approximately 95% of patients. This tumor, which increased in incidence during the twentieth century, is second to colon carcinoma as the leading cause of gastrointestinal cancer–related death. Men are affected more commonly than women, and the average age at presentation is 55–65 years. Seventy percent of adenocarcinoma of the pancreas occurs in the head of the pancreas, with 30% occurring in the body or tail.
2. **Etiology.** The risk of pancreatic carcinoma is significantly increased in patients with hereditary pancreatitis, **obese individuals, smokers, patients with chronic pancreatitis,** and the risk is slightly increased in individuals with diabetes mellitus. A recent study suggests that long-term exposure to the insecticide dichlorodiphenyltrichloroethane (DDT) may be associated with an increased risk of pancreatic cancer. Chronic pancreatitis is also a known predisposing cause for pancreatic cancer.
3. **Clinical features**
   a. **Common symptoms.** Approximately 75% of patients have pain that has been present for 3–4 months by the time of diagnosis. The pain typically is postprandial epigastric or periumbilical discomfort, which radiates to the back and is relieved by sitting up or bending both knees. Jaundice is present in approximately 65% of patients, and weight loss occurs in 60% of patients. Diarrhea and steatorrhea also are somewhat common. The gallbladder may be palpable (Courvoisier's sign) in some patients. A palpable epigastric mass may be found on physical examination.
   b. Less common symptoms include unexplained thrombophlebitis (Trousseau's sign), depression, the new onset of diabetes mellitus, or acute pancreatitis.
4. **Diagnosis.** A high index of suspicion in patients with constant epigastric or periumbilical distress often is required.
   a. **Laboratory tests** indicate an elevated serum alkaline phosphatase level in 80% of patients, which often is attributable to hepatic metastasis but may be caused by compression of the pancreatic portion of the common bile duct. Elevated levels of CEA, lactate dehydrogenase (LDH), and aspartate aminotransferase (AST) also are common. Jaundice is found in 65% of patients, and 25% of patients have high serum amylase levels. CA 19–9, a tumor marker, has been associated with carcinoma of the pancreas. Although not useful as a screening test, it has an approximate 80% sensitivity and 90% specificity for carcinoma of the pancreas and may be a marker for recurrent diseases or metastasis after primary resection.
   b. An **upper gastrointestinal series** may reveal a widened loop or an "inverted 3 sign" due to indentation by the pancreas along the medial aspect of the duodenum.

c. **Spiral CT, magnetic resonance imaging (MRI), or ultrasonography** of the pancreas demonstrate a mass in 75%–80% of patients.
d. **ERCP** is abnormal in approximately 85%–90% of patients and generally shows a discrete stricture in the main pancreatic duct with proximal dilatation.
e. **EUS** may be more sensitive than extracorporeal ultrasound.
f. **Angiography** may show displacement or encasement of the pancreatic or duodenal arteries. The venous phase may be especially useful if the superior mesenteric vein or splenic vein is occluded.
g. **Secretin-stimulation testing** may indicate a decrease in the volume of pancreatic secretion but normal enzyme and bicarbonate concentrations.
h. **Chiba (skinny) needle biopsy** under the guidance of CT or ultrasonography may be used to obtain cytologic specimens and is positive for malignancy in 80%–90% of patients.

5. **Therapy and prognosis** (see Chapter 4 VI B 7, 8)

E **Islet cell tumors** account for 5% of pancreatic adenocarcinomas. They may be multicentric and tend to grow more slowly than tumors of ductular origin. Islet cell tumors frequently are associated with endocrine adenomas in the pituitary and parathyroid glands (e.g., in MEN I syndrome).

1. **Gastrinoma** causes the Zollinger-Ellison syndrome (see III I).
2. **Insulinoma** is characterized by inappropriately high insulin levels in the presence of hypoglycemia. Because only 10%–15% of insulinomas are malignant, surgical resection is the treatment of choice. Synthetic somatostatin may be an effective treatment.
3. **Glucagonoma** is found in patients with a syndrome of diabetes mellitus, weight loss, anemia, and a characteristic rash (migratory necrolytic erythema). Most glucagonomas are malignant, but surgical debulking may provide symptomatic improvement. Streptozocin is the most commonly used chemotherapeutic agent. Somatostatin may be used.
4. **Somatostatinoma** usually occurs in association with the triad of diabetes, steatorrhea, and gallstones. Approximately 50% of patients have a positive family history of islet cell tumors. The diagnosis usually is made either incidentally at surgery for another problem (e.g., cholecystitis) or late in the course of the disease when metastatic disease is present. Streptozocin therapy has been effective in a small number of patients.
5. **VIPoma** (also called **pancreatic cholera, Verner-Morrison syndrome,** and the **watery diarrhea, hypokalemia,** and **achlorhydria syndrome**) is a tumor of non-α, non-β islet cells that secrete VIP, which causes watery diarrhea. Solitary lesions may be cured by surgical resection. Some individuals are responsive to corticosteroids, and streptozocin has been used successfully in patients with metastatic disease. Synthetic somatostatin also may be used.

VIII DISEASES OF THE BILIARY TRACT

A **Gallstones** are extremely common, occurring in 15%–20% of the population of the United States.

1. **Types**
   a. **Cholesterol gallstones.** Most gallstones that occur in western populations are composed primarily of cholesterol, which is thought to precipitate from supersaturated bile, especially at night when bile is concentrated in the gallbladder. For women, the risk of cholesterol gallstones increases with age, use of oral contraceptives (at least during the first 5 years of use), or pregnancy. Rapid weight loss; family history of diabetes mellitus; ileal disease (Crohn's disease) or ileal resection resulting in a decreased bile salt pool; the use of drugs such as clofibrate, ceftriaxone, or octreotide; or total parenteral nutrition all may increase the risk of cholesterol gallstones.
   b. **Pigmented gallstones.** Composed primarily of calcium bilirubinate, pigmented gallstones are found in patients with chronic hemolysis (e.g., sickle cell disease) as well as in Asian populations.

In Asia, biliary infection with β-glucuronidase–producing organisms leads to increased amounts of poorly soluble deconjugated bilirubin in bile.

2. **Therapy.** One third to one half of patients with gallstones are asymptomatic and should be treated expectantly. Surgical removal of asymptomatic gallstones is unnecessary, except in diabetic patients, in whom the risk of acute cholecystitis with complications is high.

B Acute cholecystitis

1. **Etiology.** In 90%–95% of cases, acute cholecystitis is caused by obstruction of the cystic duct by an impacted gallstone, which leads to edema of the gallbladder wall with submucosal hemorrhage and mucosal ulceration. Polymorphonuclear infiltration is a later event and probably is attributable to the low bacterial count of the obstructed gallbladder. Acalculous cholecystitis may occur secondary to salmonellosis, polyarteritis nodosa, sepsis, and trauma.
2. **Clinical features**
   a. An attack of acute cholecystitis starts with crampy pain in the epigastrium or right upper quadrant, which may radiate to the back near the right scapular tip (biliary colic). The pain is thought to be generated by ductal obstruction and often is postprandial, typically subsiding within several hours.
   b. An elevated temperature or WBC count, fever, nausea, vomiting, and ileus also may be present.
   c. Right upper quadrant tenderness precipitated by deep inspiration during palpation of the right upper quadrant is known as **Murphy's sign.**
   d. Jaundice occurs in 20% of patients and is thought to be attributable to common duct stones or edema of the common bile duct.
3. **Diagnosis.** The characteristic clinical picture, especially in a patient known to have gallstones, suggests the diagnosis.
   a. Most gallstones consist of cholesterol and are radiolucent; 10%–15% of gallstones contain enough calcium to appear radiopaque.
   b. Although gallbladder ultrasonography can show the presence of stones (i.e., the fluid-filled gallbladder appears lucent, whereas the stones within it are sono-opaque and cast shadows), this test cannot be used to demonstrate cystic duct obstruction.
   c. Failure to visualize the gallbladder during radionuclide scanning after an intravenous injection of iminodiacetic acid (HIDA scanning) strongly suggests cystic duct obstruction.
   d. Cystic duct obstruction is also suggested when oral cholecystography fails to visualize the gallbladder, but cholecystography is not as reliable as HIDA scanning.
4. **Therapy**
   a. **Supportive treatment** should be provided initially, with intravenous fluid replacement and nasogastric suction for 24–48 hours. Later, the gallbladder may be removed surgically.
   b. **Dissolution** may be used to dissolve cholesterol stones in patients who are not surgical candidates. **Ursodeoxycholic acid** or **chenodeoxycholic acid** may be used. If several small stones are present and floating, a 50%–70% chance of dissolving the stones may be expected over a period of 12–24 months.
   c. **Lithotripsy** may be tried if the gallbladder is functional, the stone mass is less than 3.0 cm, and the patient has no acute symptoms (approximately 20%–25% of patients).
   d. **Percutaneous introduction of methylterbutaline ether** also has been used in patients who refuse cholecystectomy.
   e. **Laparoscopic cholecystectomy** may allow gallbladder removal on a "same-day surgery" basis in many cases.
5. **Complications.** Surgical intervention generally is required.
   a. **Empyema** refers to a pus-filled gallbladder. Patients may be toxic and are at high risk for perforation.

b. **Perforation**

(1) Localized perforation occurs several days to 1 week after the onset of acute cholecystitis and leads to a pericholecystic abscess.

(2) Free perforation into the abdominal cavity, which has a 25% mortality rate, occurs early in the clinical course, probably because inflammation in the early stages is insufficient to wall off the abscess.

(3) Perforation into an adjacent organ may involve the duodenum, jejunum, colon, or stomach. If a large stone is passed into the lumen, intestinal obstruction (gallstone ileus) may result.

c. **Emphysematous cholecystitis** is caused by gas-forming bacteria (often clostridia, *E. coli,* or streptococci) in the gallbladder lumen and wall. Men are affected more commonly than women, and 20%–30% of patients have diabetes mellitus. Early surgical intervention is indicated to prevent perforation.

d. **Postcholecystectomy syndrome** refers to abdominal pain that persists after cholecystectomy. The usual cause is an initially mistaken diagnosis, with pain persisting from the underlying process (e.g., pancreatic disease, irritable bowel syndrome). Some patients may have common duct stones.

C **Chronic cholecystitis** is a clinical term used to describe a condition of recurrent subacute symptoms caused by gallstones. Patients with chronic cholecystitis show wide variability in the thickening and fibrosis of the gallbladder wall and in the inflammatory infiltrate. The diagnosis is based on failure to visualize the gallbladder with oral cholecystography. After other sources of chronic abdominal pain (e.g., peptic ulcer disease, pancreatitis, irritable bowel syndrome) are ruled out, a cholecystectomy may be performed to relieve symptoms.

D Choledocholithiasis

1. **Pathophysiology.** Choledocholithiasis usually occurs when a gallstone is passed into the common duct from the gallbladder or when a gallstone that was missed during operative cholangiography or common duct exploration is retained. Occasionally, a stone forms de novo in the common duct, especially when there is stasis from ductal obstruction.
2. **Clinical features.** Symptoms frequently are intermittent and include colicky pain in the right upper quadrant, fever, chills, and jaundice accompanied by elevated serum levels of alkaline phosphatase and the transaminases. Sepsis may result from ascending cholangitis, which is a closed-space infection.
3. **Therapy.** Antibiotics are given as needed to control infection, but definitive treatment consists of surgical removal of the stone or endoscopic sphincterotomy and stone extraction. Patients who are poor surgical risks and in whom there is access to the biliary tree (i.e., with a T tube) may be treated by infusion of mono-octanoin to dissolve the stones or by extracorporeal shock wave lithotripsy.

E **Biliary dyskinesia** is a clinical syndrome of right upper quadrant symptoms, and it is similar to chronic calculous cholecystitis, although not associated with the structural abnormality of the biliary tree often seen after cholecystectomy.

1. **Pathophysiology.** An abnormality of biliary motor function is proposed, and manometric findings may indicate elevated basal sphincter of Oddi pressure (usually 40 mm Hg greater than intraduodenal pressure), a paradoxical contraction of the sphincter of Oddi after cholecystokinin injection, or both.
2. **Therapy.** Patients may respond to smooth muscle relaxants (e.g., nitrates, calcium channel-blocking agents) or to endoscopic or surgical sphincterotomy of the sphincter of Oddi.

F Biliary stricture

1. **Pathophysiology.** Biliary stricture is a narrowing of the common bile duct generally caused by surgical injury or scarring subsequent to exploration of the common bile duct. Rarely, trauma or choledocholithiasis may result in a biliary stricture.
2. **Clinical features.** Patients usually have intermittent obstructive jaundice several weeks to months after biliary tract surgery. Cholangiography demonstrates the presence of a smooth concentric narrowing of the duct, with proximal dilatation being a common finding.
3. **Therapy.** The usual treatment is surgical anastomosis of the dilated proximal end of the bile duct to the intestine, but some patients may undergo percutaneous transhepatic or endoscopic balloon dilatation with biliary stent placement.

G Sclerosing cholangitis, a rare disease that causes progressive narrowing of the bile ducts, generally is diagnosed in the third or fourth decade of life and is three times more common in men than in women.

1. **Clinical features.** Approximately 70% of patients have inflammatory bowel disease (usually ulcerative colitis), but the biliary and intestinal diseases have independent clinical courses. The usual presenting symptom is pruritus. There is an increased risk of cholangiocarcinoma in such patients.
2. **Diagnosis.** Early diagnosis is possible in asymptomatic patients who show marked elevation of serum alkaline phosphatase levels on routine biochemical screening. ERCP or percutaneous cholangiography should establish the diagnosis.
3. **Therapy**
   a. **Medical treatment.** Corticosteroids, ursodeoxycholic acid, methotrexate, long-term antibiotics, or varying combinations of these medications have been used with varying success. ERCP with balloon dilatation or stent placement may be used if a dominant stricture is identified.
   b. **Surgical treatment.** Surgical anastomosis of the diseased duct to the intestine may be difficult or impossible, but liver transplantation is a consideration in many patients. Endoscopic or percutaneous dilatation of strictures is possible in some cases.

H Oriental cholangitis is a disease of Asian populations or first-generation immigrants from Asia. Incidence rates for men and women are equal. The etiologic factors may be bile stasis (often associated with parasitic infestation) and a low-protein diet. The disease is characterized by recurrent right upper quadrant pain, fever, jaundice, and bile duct–pigmented stones. Infected bile is often found at surgery. Treatment is with surgery and surgical drainage of the bile ducts.

I Cystic malformation of the bile ducts

1. **Choledochal cysts** may present as jaundice, cholangitis, or a large cyst filled with numerous stones. Diagnosis may be made by cholangiography. Surgery is used to excise the cyst or to anastomose the cyst to the intestine.
2. **Caroli's disease** is characterized by saccular dilatation of the intrahepatic ducts, which may be associated with right upper quadrant pain, cholangitis, or both because of ductal stone formation. Hepatic fibrosis with portal hypertension may develop, especially in patients with medullary sponge kidney. Recently, cholangiocarcinoma has been reported in congenital biliary cysts (up to 30%), especially if stones are present in the cyst. Surgical decompression occasionally is helpful, and antibiotics are used during acute episodes of cholangitis.

J Tumors of the gallbladder

1. **Adenocarcinoma** of the gallbladder is a disease of older women. The tumor affects three times as many women as it does men, and the average age at diagnosis is 65–75 years. Although most patients have associated gallstones, cancer develops in less than 1% of all patients with stones. Symptoms generally mimic those of acute or chronic cholecystitis. On physical examination, a

mass may be palpable in the right upper quadrant, and obstructive jaundice may be seen secondary to local spread of the tumor to the common bile duct. A calcified gallbladder may be seen on abdominal radiographs. An operation consisting of cholecystectomy, lymph node dissection, and removal of a small portion of the adjacent liver is indicated if no obvious metastatic disease is found, but prognosis generally is poor.

2. **Benign tumors** of the gallbladder include abnormalities of the mucosal lining (e.g., adenomatous hyperplasia, cholesterolosis, cholesterol polyps), cystic changes in the glands, and papillary adenomas. These lesions usually are asymptomatic. In some patients with no other demonstrable causes for abdominal pain, however, cholecystectomy has provided relief of symptoms.

K **Tumors of the bile duct** Adenocarcinoma of the bile duct (cholangiocarcinoma) is a disease of older men and is not associated with gallstones.

1. **Etiology.** An increased risk is observed in patients with ulcerative colitis who have sclerosing cholangitis and in patients exposed to benzene or toluene derivatives. Parasitic infection, especially with *Clonorchis,* of the biliary system has been linked to the high rate of cholangiocarcinoma in Asian populations.
2. **Pathology.** Most tumors are of the scirrhous or papillary type. An extensive desmoplastic reaction may make diagnosis difficult. Two thirds of the tumors are located in the common bile duct or at the bifurcation of the common hepatic duct **(Klatskin tumors).**
3. **Clinical features.** Jaundice, with or without pain, is present in most patients, and weight loss also is common. Pruritus may be severe. Common duct tumors causing obstruction distal to the cystic duct result in a palpable gallbladder that is not tender.
4. **Laboratory data.** Serum alkaline phosphatase levels are markedly increased, as are direct and total bilirubin levels. Serum transaminase levels show smaller increases and generally are less than 200 mg/dL.
5. **Diagnosis.** Dilatation of the intrahepatic ducts is shown by ultrasonography or CT, and percutaneous cholangiography or ERCP findings generally suggest the diagnosis. The differential diagnosis includes pancreatic carcinoma, choledocholithiasis, biliary stricture, and sclerosing cholangitis.
6. **Therapy** (see Chapter 4 VI E 7, 8)

IX DISEASES OF THE LIVER

A **Acute liver disease** (Table **5–3**)

1. **Acute viral hepatitis,** one of the most common health problems in the world, is caused by any one of several viruses.
   a. **Etiology**
      (1) **Hepatitis A** (HAV) is an RNA virus transmitted primarily by the fecal–oral route. The incubation period is 2–6 weeks. Acute infection is anicteric in 50% of cases. HAV does not lead to chronic disease or to a carrier state.
      (2) **Hepatitis B** (HBV) is a DNA virus transmitted parenterally. Individuals at high risk include intravenous drug abusers, homosexual men, and those exposed to blood and blood products (e.g., patients and health care professionals in dialysis units). The incubation period ranges from 1 to 6 months. Chronic HBV disease or a persistent carrier state develops in approximately 10% of patients.
      (3) **Hepatitis C** (HCV) is an RNA virus that **formerly accounted for** 90% of post-transfusion hepatitis. The modes of transmission (parenteral, sexual, and perhaps perinatal) are similar to those of HBV. The incubation period is 2 weeks to 6 months. Chronic hepatitis develops in up to 85% of patients. Cirrhosis may develop in 20% of patients, with an

TABLE 5–3 Comparison of Viral Hepatitis Types

	Hepatitis A	Hepatitis B	Hepatitis C	Delta Agent (Hepatitis D)	Hepatitis E	Hepatitis G
Type of virus	RNA	DNA	RNA	RNA (hepatitis B required for replication)	RNA	RNA
Incidence of positive antibody in the United States (%)	40	10	2–3	Low	Very low	Low
Incidence after blood transfusion (%)	0 to extremely rare	10–20	60–90	?	. . .	. . .
Incubation period	2–6 weeks	1–6 months	2–24 weeks	1–6 months	2–8 weeks	2–24 weeks
Infectivity stage	Last 3 weeks of inoculation to 1–2 weeks after jaundice occurs	During hepatitis B surface antigen positivity	?	?	?	?
Complications	Fulminant hepatitis (rare)	Fulminant hepatitis (rare but more common than with hepatitis A); chronic active hepatitis	Fulminant hepatitis (rare but more common than with hepatitis A); chronic active hepatitis	Present in 20%–50% of cases of fulminant hepatitis and/or chronic active hepatitis	Fulminant hepatitis in pregnant women with 10%–20% mortality	Chronic carrier states; fulminant hepatitis
Mechanism of spread	Fecal–oral	Parenteral	Parenteral	Parenteral	Fecal–oral	Parenteral
Prevention	Pooled immune serum globulin; vaccination	Hepatitis B immune globulin; vaccination	Pooled immune serum globulin	?	Good hygiene	?
Carrier State	Rare, if ever	1%–2%	Yes (50% of patients)	?	?	Yes

increased risk of hepatocellular carcinoma. Genotype I accounts for most hepatitis C patients in the United States and may not respond as readily to antiviral/interferon therapy as other genotypes.

(4) **Non-A, non-B, non-C hepatitis** may be caused by more than one virus. The incubation period is similar to that of HCV (2 weeks to 6 months). Most cases previously designated as non-A, non-B hepatitis are designated as HCV. Cases that are not accounted for by HCV, and so are designated as non-A, non-B hepatitis, may progress to chronic hepatitis, as occurs in HCV.

(5) **Delta hepatitis** [**hepatitis D (HDV)**] is caused by a small, defective RNA virus (delta agent) that is infectious only in the presence of HBV infection, because it relies on HBV proteins for replication. It therefore can complicate acute HBV infection but is seen more commonly as a "superinfection" with an increase in abnormal liver function tests in a patient with chronic HBV. HDV generally has a chronic, severe clinical course.

(6) **Hepatitis E** is a small RNA virus (possibly a calicivirus) that has been described in cases of acute hepatitis in Mexico, Asia, and Africa. It has a short incubation period and is probably waterborne. The mortality rate in pregnant women may be 10%–20%. Cholestasis is relatively common.

(7) **Hepatitis G** is an RNA virus with a genomic organization similar to that of HCV. Hepatitis G is transmitted parenterally and accounts for approximately 15% of non-A, non-B, non-C cases of chronic hepatitis. It is found more frequently in intravenous drug abusers and patients on hemodialysis.

(8) **Other viruses** that can cause acute hepatitis include the Epstein-Barr virus, CMV, HSV, and those causing yellow fever and rubella.

b. Pathology. The lesions of acute viral hepatitis are similar regardless of etiology and include mononuclear cell infiltration, cellular ballooning and necrosis, and condensed cytoplasm with pyknotic nuclei (acidophilic bodies).

c. Clinical features

(1) Malaise, anorexia, and fatigue

(2) Arthritis and urticaria, which are especially common in HBV, are ascribed to circulating immune complexes. Polyarteritis nodosa or glomerulonephritis may be seen in HBV patients.

(3) Influenza-like syndrome, which is especially common in HAV

(4) Jaundice (with dark urine or light stools), which is seen in 50% of cases

(5) Hepatic enlargement or tenderness

(6) Splenomegaly, which occurs in 20% of patients

(7) HCV only: concomitant porphyria cutanea tarda, **lichen planus,** mixed cryoglobulinemia, **thyroiditis,** or membranoproliferative glomerulonephritis. Immune complex disease is relatively common in HCV patients.

d. Diagnosis. Acute viral hepatitis is diagnosed based on clinical features as well as such laboratory findings as elevated levels of the transaminases [i.e., aspartate aminotransferase (AST), alanine aminotransaminase (ALT)], serum bilirubin, and serum alkaline phosphatase. The increase in bilirubin exceeds the increase in alkaline phosphatase.

(1) In HAV, the IgM antibody is elevated early in the course, followed by an elevation of the IgG antibody in 2–3 months.

(2) In HBV, a positive surface antigen usually is diagnostic. However, because this is an early finding, it may be necessary to follow the increase of IgM anticore and later of antisurface antibodies to document acute infection (Figure 5–1).

(3) HCV can be diagnosed by using techniques that detect viral RNA.

(4) HDV may be diagnosed by an elevated delta antibody titer, often with the disappearance of B surface antigen from the serum. A persistently high or slowly falling hepatitis delta antibody is seen in chronic states.

(5) Hepatitis E serologic testing is also available.

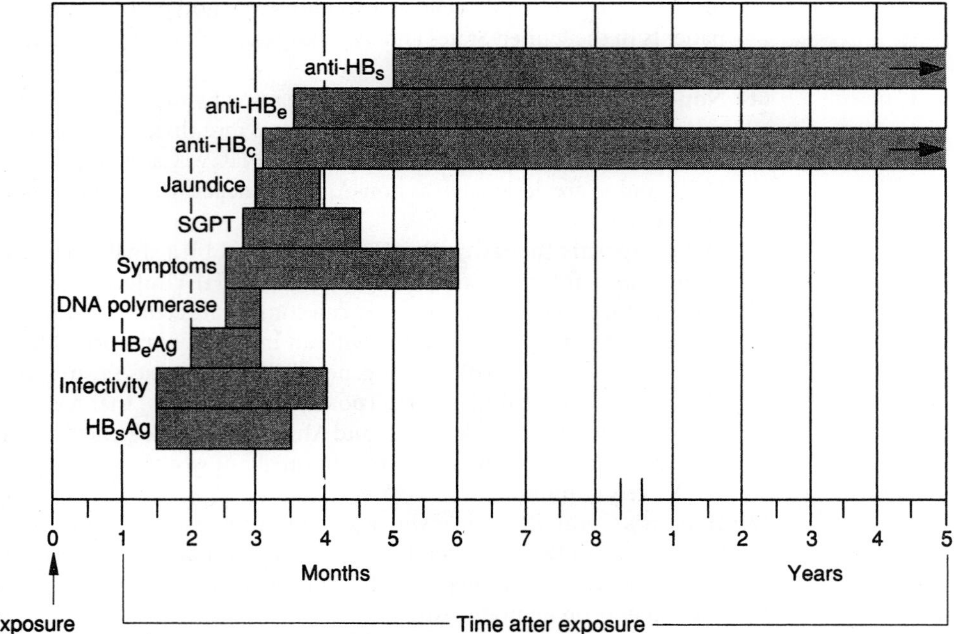

FIGURE 5–1 Typical clinical course of acute hepatitis B (HBV). Recombinant and pooled-plasma vaccines against HBV do not transmit active hepatitis B surface antigen (Hb_sAg) and do not contain hepatitis B e antigen (Hb_eAg) or hepatitis core antigen. Consequently, the serologic profile of a vaccinated individual consists of hepatitis B surface antibody (anti-HB_s) only. SGPT = serum glutamic–pyruvic transaminase (ALT); anti-HB_c = hepatitis B core antibody; anti-HB_e = hepatitis B e antibody.

e. **Therapy.** Treatment for acute or active disease is supportive and includes intravenous fluids to provide hydration, correct electrolyte abnormalities, and provide caloric intake if nausea and vomiting are present. Vitamin K should be given if the prothrombin time (PT) is elevated. For chronic cases of HBV, the protease inhibitor lamivudine or adefovir has been effective in clearing active viral replication. Some viral mutations have been noted with chronic lamivudine treatment. For chronic HCV, pegulated interferon (PEG-IFN), generally in combination with ribavirin, results in sustained viral clearing rates between 30% and 70%, depending on the viral load and the genomic identity of the virus (genotype I responds less favorably).

f. **Clinical course and complications.** Nearly all cases of acute viral hepatitis are benign, with most patients showing normal results on liver function testing by 8–10 weeks. However, complications may occur.

(1) **Fulminant hepatitis,** a rare complication of HAV and HCV, occurs in 1%–2% of patients with HBV. It is an especially common complication of delta agent superinfection in patients with chronic hepatitis B antigenemia. Patients usually have progressive jaundice, hepatic encephalopathy, and ascites. Hepatorenal syndrome is common. Elevated PT is an early sign. The initially elevated serum transaminase levels later decline, and liver size decreases as a result of necrosis of the liver parenchyma. The mortality rate varies with age and approaches 90%–100%, especially in patients older than 60 years of age.

(2) **Chronic hepatitis** is a complication of HBV and HCV, in which serum transaminase levels are elevated for more than 6 months. Fifteen percent of patients with chronic HCV may have hepatitis C antibody but no actively replicating virus; they are individuals who have recovered from acute and chronic HCV infection.

(a) Pathologically, inflammation, necrosis, and fibrosis bridging portal areas or between portal areas and central veins occurs. The disease may progress to cirrhosis. On physical examination, patients may have splenomegaly, spider angiomata, caput medusae, and other signs of chronic liver disease. Liver biopsy is necessary for diagnosis.

(b) Therapy for HBV involves **antiviral agents** such as lamivudine or adefovir. Treatment for HCV involves the use of PEG-IFN plus ribavirin. Treatment should be given to nondecompensated patients. Cirrhosis may be noted in approximately 5% of patients with long-term chronic HBV, or 10%–20% of patients after chronic hepatitis C. There is an increased risk of cirrhosis if there are coexistent illnesses such as HIV or alcoholism.

(3) A **chronic carrier state** for hepatitis B surface antigen exists in 0.2% of the population of the United States. A carrier state also exists for HCV, because blood donated by apparently normal individuals may transmit this disease when transfused. Carriers of HBV or HCV may have an increased risk of hepatoma.

(4) **Cholestatic hepatitis** may occur, particularly with hepatitis E and rarely with HAV and HCV. This condition is characterized by the alkaline phosphatase level elevated disproportionately to the transaminase level. The clinical course is typical of acute viral hepatitis, but the presentation must be differentiated from biliary tract obstruction.

(5) **Aplastic anemia** is seen rarely after acute viral hepatitis. The mortality rate is high, and no treatment has proved effective.

g. Therapy of acute disease. PEG-IFN alone or in combination with ribavirin may clear hepatitis C virus after acute infection (such as parenteral exposure, blood transfusion, etc.)

h. Prevention

(1) **Immune serum globulin** is effective when administered after exposure to HAV and also may be partially protective against HBV and HCV.

(2) **Hepatitis B immune globulin,** which is immunoglobulin that contains high titers of antibody to HBV, conveys passive immunity and is recommended after confirmed exposure to HBV (e.g., from skin puncture by a contaminated needle).

(3) **Vaccines**

(a) **HAV vaccine.** An effective vaccine for prevention of HAV is available. It is particularly recommended for individuals who travel to endemic areas or who have other forms of chronic liver disease. The vaccine also may be effective for secondary prevention in HAV household contacts.

(b) **HBV vaccine.** This preparation of the hepatitis B surface antigen conveys active immunity. It is recommended for individuals at high risk such as dialysis patients, medical personnel with frequent exposure to blood products, and individuals who are hepatitis B antibody–negative and who have had confirmed exposure to HBV. Infants are routinely vaccinated.

2. Drug-induced liver disease may follow exposure to virtually any drug and manifests as a variety of clinical syndromes and histologic findings (Table 5–4). Any drug may induce liver disease that overlaps two or more categories of disease mechanisms.

a. Direct toxicity by a chemical (e.g., carbon tetrachloride) or a metabolite (e.g., acetaminophen) usually represents a dose-related injury. Niacin may cause a dose-related toxicity at greater than 3 g/day in crystalline form or 1–2 g/day in sustained-release form. Acetaminophen overdose can be treated with *N*-acetylcysteine, which binds to the toxic metabolite and provides cysteine for glutathione synthesis, or intravenous cimetidine, which decreases cytochrome P-450 activity and prevents conversion of acetaminophen to its toxic metabolite. Small doses of acetaminophen (3–14 g) ingested with alcohol may induce hepatic necrosis marked by high levels of hepatic aspartate aminotransferase (3000–24,000 IU). Such cases have a high mortality rate.

b. Indirect toxicity may result from interference with the metabolism of bilirubin (e.g., by estrogens and androgens) or with protein synthesis (e.g., by intravenous tetracycline, which causes microvesicular fat accumulation in hepatocytes).

TABLE 5–4 Agents of Drug-Induced Liver Disease

		Drugs Causing Immune-Mediated Reactions			
Drugs Causing Direct Toxicity	**Drugs Causing Altered Metabolism**	VIRAL HEPATITIS-LIKE	GRANULOMATOUS HEPATITIS	INFLAMMATORY CHOLESTASIS	CHRONIC ACTIVE HEPATITIS
Acetaminophen	Androgens	Halothane	Allopurinol	Chlorpromazine	Acetaminophen
Amiodarone	Corticosteroids (?)	Isoniazid	Hydralazine	Chlorpropamide	Aspirin
Aspirin	Estrogens	Oxacillin	Phenylbutazone	Erythromycin estolate	Isoniazid
Alcohol	Ethanol	Phenytoin	Phenytoin	Propylthiouracil	Methyldopa
Carbon tetrachloride	Intravenous tetracycline	Sulfonamides	Quinidine	Thiazides	Nitrofurantoin
Heavy metals		Valproic acid	Sulfa drugs		Oxyphenisatin
Methotrexate					
Mushroom toxins (phalloidin and phallin)					
Niacin					
Phosphorus					

c. **Immunologic drug reactions** can cause a variety of syndromes, including cholestatic jaundice (a syndrome that mimics acute viral hepatitis), a condition with a histologic picture indistinguishable from chronic active hepatitis, and granulomatous hepatitis. Skin rashes, eosinophilia, and fever may be present. In some cases, it has been postulated that a drug or metabolite binds to the liver cell membrane and acts as a **hapten.**
   (1) **Isoniazid** causes a clinical condition similar to viral hepatitis and has been shown to be related to a metabolite.
   (2) **Halothane** and other fluorinated anesthetics frequently cause only mild hepatitis or postoperative fever after first exposure but may cause fulminant hepatitis and death on reexposure.
   (3) **Chlorpromazine** and **chlorpropamide** cause cholestatic jaundice. An inflammatory infiltrate that frequently includes eosinophils is shown on liver biopsy.
   (4) **Diphenylhydantoin** causes a serum sickness–like syndrome, which may result in massive hepatic necrosis and death.
   (5) **Methyldopa** may cause the clinical and histologic findings of chronic active hepatitis, and some authors believe that a metabolite is responsible.
   (6) **Excess intake of vitamin A** (20,000–40,000 U/day) for years may cause cholestatic hepatic injury. Vitamin A is deposited in the Ito cells of the liver, and large deposits compress the sinusoids. Serum bilirubin and alkaline phosphatase levels may be elevated, prothrombin time may increase, and hepatic enzyme activity may be relatively normal. Over time, cirrhosis may result.

3. **Alcoholic liver disease** refers to the group of liver disorders caused by acute and chronic alcoholism. Acute effects include alcoholic fatty liver and alcoholic hepatitis. Chronic alcoholism is a major cause of cirrhosis of the liver, which is discussed in IX B 2 b. In the United States, alcoholic liver disease represents the fourth most common cause of death of adults 35–55 years of age. It appears that alcohol consumption of less than 80 g/day in men and 40 g/day in (nonpregnant) women generally is not associated with alcoholic liver disease.
   a. **Alcoholic fatty liver** occurs because alcohol alters normal lipid metabolism. Most patients have hepatomegaly but otherwise are asymptomatic unless they have other systemic problems related to alcohol use (e.g., pancreatitis, delirium tremens). Laboratory abnormalities include

increases in γ-glutamyl transpeptidase, serum transaminases, and alkaline phosphatase. Histologic examination shows large-droplet fatty change in the liver. The prognosis is excellent for patients who completely abstain from alcohol consumption.

b. **Alcoholic hepatitis** is an acute syndrome that generally occurs in the setting of heavy alcohol consumption. Many patients are reported to have ingested more than 100 g alcohol daily for more than 1 year. (Approximately 100 g alcohol are contained in 8 ounces of 100-proof whiskey, in 30 ounces of wine, and in eight 12-ounce cans of beer.) The role of decreased vitamin and protein intake is controversial.

(1) **Clinical features** include fever, jaundice, hepatomegaly, and liver tenderness. Ascites, encephalopathy, and variceal bleeding occasionally are present.

(2) **Laboratory data** include leukocytosis, increased AST (usually < 350 IU/mm^3), elevated serum bilirubin, decreased serum albumin, and a modest increase in serum alkaline phosphatase. Occasionally, a cholestatic phase is present with marked elevations in the alkaline phosphatase and direct bilirubin. The ALT almost always is lower than the AST because of decreased pyridoxine intake and conversion to pyridoxal phosphate. Alcohol-induced thrombocytopenia is present in 10% of patients.

(3) **Diagnosis** is based on liver biopsy that shows large-droplet fatty liver, polymorphonuclear infiltration, alcoholic hyaline (Mallory bodies), hepatocyte necrosis, and, occasionally, sclerosis of central veins.

(4) **Therapy** is supportive and includes a daily diet of 2500–3000 kcal with supplemental B vitamins (especially thiamine) and folate. Absolute abstinence from alcohol is crucial. Propylthiouracil (PTU) and corticosteroids have a controversial therapeutic role but may be useful in severe cases.

4. **Nonalcoholic fatty liver disease (NAFLD)** is often associated with obesity, diabetes mellitus, **hyperlipidemia,** intravenous hyperalimentation, or jejunoileal bypass surgery and is the third leading cause of cirrhosis in the United States. The liver is fatty on biopsy, and Mallory bodies are occasionally observed. There is a modest increase in transaminase levels (twofold to fourfold above normal). Although initially thought to be benign, prolonged steatohepatitis may lead to cirrhosis. Treatment involves removal of the offending agent or use of insulin-sensitizing medications, or in the case of obesity, weight loss. Loss of approximately 10% of body fat may result in decreased hepatic enzyme elevation.

B Chronic liver disease

1. **Chronic hepatitis** most commonly is caused by viral infection or drugs. When not associated with either of these etiologies, chronic active hepatitis generally is thought to be immunologically mediated, although an immunologic mechanism has not been proved. This form of chronic active hepatitis sometimes is called lupoid hepatitis (but idiopathic autoimmune hepatitis is the more appropriate term), because the typical patient is a young woman with a positive antinuclear antibody (ANA).

a. **Clinical features** include malaise, fatigue, and vasculitis. As the disease progresses, manifestations of chronic liver disease, including ascites, encephalopathy, and variceal bleeding, dominate the clinical picture.

b. **Diagnosis** is based on liver biopsy that shows piecemeal necrosis and bridging fibrosis. The serum transaminases are persistently elevated to levels that often are 10 times the normal levels. Positive ANA is present in 50% of patients, and anti–smooth muscle antibody is found in 75%.

c. **Therapy** with high-dose corticosteroids, azathioprine, or both is beneficial in the immune-mediated type of chronic hepatitis but usually not in the drug- and virus-associated diseases. IFN (3–5 million U three times weekly) has been shown to decrease evidence of HBV and HCV activity in 30%–60% of cases. Lamivudine may eliminate or decrease HBV activity, but recurrence may occur after withdrawal of therapy. Studies with ribavirin and IFN-α are ongoing.

Treatment of the idiopathic autoimmune type of chronic active hepatitis is continued until the serum transaminase levels decline to less than twice the normal levels and a repeat liver biopsy shows resolution of the inflammation (generally after more than 1–2 years).

2. **Cirrhosis of the liver**
   a. **Overview of pathology.** Two basic types of liver cirrhosis occur, but the sine qua non of all cirrhotic liver disease is the presence of fibrosis with the formation of nodules that lack a central vein.
      (1) **Chronic sclerosing cirrhosis** is characterized by minimal regenerative activity of the hepatocytes, resulting in fibrosis without substantial nodule formation. The liver is small and hard.
      (2) **Nodular cirrhosis** is characterized by regenerative activity and the appearance of numerous fine nodules. The liver initially may be quite large.
   b. **Alcohol-induced cirrhosis.** Chronic alcohol abuse causes cirrhosis of the liver (Laennec's cirrhosis), which, in most cases, is thought to be a sequela of alcoholic hepatitis. The clinical features of alcohol-induced cirrhosis reflect impaired blood flow through the liver caused by obstruction by fibrotic bands, resulting in portal hypertension, and by a decrease in hepatocytes available for metabolic functions. Long-term alcohol use also may be directly toxic to the testis, resulting in testicular atrophy and impotence. These effects are compounded in men by increased peripheral levels of estrogens, which cause spider angiomata, gynecomastia, and palmar erythema. Complications of alcohol-induced cirrhosis include the following conditions:
      (1) **Ascites**
         (a) **Pathogenesis.** Increased back-pressure into capillaries as well as decreased oncotic pressure as the result of decreased albumin synthesis allow accumulation of a transudative fluid in the peritoneal cavity. In addition, increased circulating aldosterone (possibly secondary to altered liver metabolism) contributes to Na^+ and water retention.
         (b) **Diagnosis.** If fluid accumulation is large, diagnosis may be obvious on physical examination. Ultrasonography is effective for detecting small amounts of fluid. Paracentesis, which may require guidance through ultrasonography, yields a straw-colored fluid with less than 2.5 g/dL protein, a WBC count of less than 300/mm^3 (usually mononuclear), a normal glucose level, and a low serum amylase level. A serum albumin–ascites gradient (SAAG) greater than 1.1 g/dL is indicative of portal hypertension.
         (c) **Therapy.** Treatment is based on sodium restriction (usually 500 mg/24 hr) and bed rest (to decrease endogenous aldosterone production). Fluid restriction may be necessary if hyponatremia develops. Aldosterone antagonists (e.g., spironolactone) and other mild diuretics are used if initial measures fail. Large-volume paracentesis can be used, and 10 g albumin should be replaced intravenously for each 1 L of ascitic fluid removed. Because peritoneal lymphatics have a limited ability to mobilize ascites, weight loss should be limited to 2 lb/day unless peripheral edema exists. Surgical shunting (Le Veen or Denver shunt) may be useful in recalcitrant cases, but bacteremia and disseminated intravascular coagulation (DIC) are potential complications of these shunts. Placement of a **transjugular intrahepatic portosystemic shunt (TIPS)** to connect the hepatic and portal veins can reduce portal hypertension and relieve ascites.
         (d) **Complications.** Respiratory compromise and rupture of an umbilical hernia may occur in cases of massive ascites. Infection of even a small amount of fluid (e.g., due to spontaneous bacterial peritonitis) can be fatal.
      (2) **Varices** occur as a result of the development of collateral vessels that bypass the obstructed liver. Varices are common in the esophagus and somewhat less common in the stomach, duodenum, and hemorrhoidal plexus. **Portal hypertensive gastropathy**

involves dilatation of venous and capillary vessels in the mucosa and submucosa with minimal inflammatory infiltrate (see III J 1). Affected patients may suffer bleeding from the mucosal lining of the stomach itself. In most patients, portal decompression results in a decrease of portal hypertensive gastropathy and cessation of bleeding.

(a) **Diagnosis** of esophagogastric varices may be suggested by an upper gastrointestinal series but is best made by endoscopy. Endoscopy is essential in the acutely bleeding patient because the mortality rate is high (40%–50% for each episode of bleeding), and early treatment can be lifesaving.

(b) **Short-term therapy** with vasopressin by continuous intravenous infusion (usually in conjunction with nitroglycerin to decrease complications) is effective in 60% of patients. Somatostatin given by continuous intravenous infusion is also effective in 60%–70% of cases. Balloon tamponade with a Sengstaken-Blakemore tube controls bleeding in 80% of patients but is associated with a risk of aspiration and esophageal rupture. Emergency surgery has a 50% mortality rate. Endoscopic sclerotherapy or endoscopic rubber banding is effective in approximately 80%–90% of acute cases. A TIPS can stop variceal bleeding.

(c) **Long-term therapy** to reduce the chance of rebleeding includes multiple endoscopic sclerotherapy or variceal rubber banding procedures to obliterate all varices and non-selective β-adrenergic blockers (e.g., propranolol, nadolol) to reduce portal pressure. Surgical portal decompression does not increase survival rates because there is increased encephalopathy and liver failure. In Japan, devascularization of the distal esophagus and proximal stomach (Sugiura procedure) has been effective. Liver transplantation is reserved for good-risk alcohol-abstinent individuals.

(3) **Portosystemic encephalopathy** is a reversible neurologic syndrome characterized by mood changes, confusion, drowsiness, disorientation, and coma.

(a) **Etiology.** The primary cause of hepatic encephalopathy is unclear. Elevated ammonia levels are found in the blood. However, more recently, false neurotransmitters and elevated levels of mercaptans and fatty acids have been implicated. Increased levels of endogenous benzodiazepine substances may be noted. In addition, increased levels of aromatic amino acids and decreased levels of branched-chain amino acids are found in the blood, brain, and urine. Secondary causes of hepatic encephalopathy are thought to include:

(i) Azotemia, due to increased nitrogen load

(ii) Constipation, which causes increased ammonia production and absorption because of prolonged contact of intestinal contents with the gastrointestinal tract

(iii) Increased dietary protein, which causes increased production of ammonia and other nitrogenous wastes

(iv) Gastrointestinal bleeding, which delivers a protein load to the gastrointestinal tract

(v) Hypokalemia

(vi) Alkalosis, which together with hypokalemia leads to impaired renal excretion of ammonia and to increased transfer of ammonia across the blood-brain barrier

(vii) Infection, which leads to increased tissue catabolism and increased protein load

(viii) Sedatives, whose direct depressant effect on the brain is compounded by decreased hepatic catabolism of the drugs

(b) **Therapy.** Treatment includes reversal of any of the secondary causes. In addition, the following measures may be effective.

(i) Lactulose effectively decreases colonic pH and traps ammonium ion (NH_4^+) in the gastrointestinal tract. It also is an effective cathartic.

(ii) Neomycin decreases intestinal flora that convert gastrointestinal proteins into ammonia.

(iii) Dietary protein should be limited to less than 40 g/day.
(iv) The use of branched-chain amino acids, although academically appealing, may not improve encephalopathy.
(v) Predisposing factors (e.g., hypokalemia, constipation, alkalosis) should be corrected.

(4) **Hepatorenal syndrome** is a progressive renal failure that occurs in patients with severe liver disease. It is a functional renal failure because the kidneys are morphologically normal and function well when transplanted into normal recipients. The mortality rate is 90%–100%.

(a) **Etiology.** Although the exact mechanism of hepatorenal syndrome is not known, several factors are implicated, including:
(i) Afferent arteriolar vasoconstriction, which leads to increased renal vascular constriction
(ii) Relative shunting of blood from the cortex to the medulla of the kidney
(iii) Decreased glomerular filtration rate (GFR)
(iv) Decreased renal blood flow

(b) **Diagnosis.** The combination of oliguria (i.e., urine output < 300 mm^3/24 hr) with increasing blood urea nitrogen (BUN) and creatinine concentrations in a patient with severe liver disease is suggestive. Additional laboratory findings include urinary Na^+ concentration of less than 10 mEq/L and benign urine sediment. It is important to rule out other causes of oliguria [e.g., acute tubular necrosis (ATN), hypovolemia, urinary tract obstruction].

(c) **Therapy.** Generally, treatment is unsuccessful. A fluid challenge should be given to all patients to rule out hypovolemia. Success occasionally has been reported with Le Veen or Denver shunts, portacaval shunts, or liver transplantation. No drugs have been shown to be beneficial.

(5) **Coagulation defects** usually are attributable to decreased hepatic synthesis of clotting factors. In addition, splenomegaly may contribute to thrombocytopenia.

(6) **Hepatopulmonary syndrome** is a hypoxic state most likely caused by intrapulmonary vascular shunting (effectively, a right-to-left shunt). Exercise or standing-induced hypoxia is noted, and clubbing may occur in severe cases. This syndrome is probably present in 30% of patients with cirrhosis and may be severe in 10% of patients.

c. **Nonalcoholic cirrhosis** may be caused by a variety of disease processes and toxins but, in general, has clinical features that are similar to those of alcohol-induced cirrhosis.

(1) **Primary biliary cirrhosis** is a disease of unknown etiology. The usual patient age at diagnosis is 40–60 years, and 90% of patients are women.

(a) **Pathogenesis,** which is thought to be immunologic, involves inflammatory destruction of small intrahepatic biliary ducts. Early histologic changes include lymphocytic infiltration and periductal granuloma formation. Later in the disease process, the portal areas may show an absence of ducts.

(b) **Clinical features**
(i) There is a lack of symptoms early in the course of this disease. However, an early diagnosis often is suspected on the basis of a marked increase in the alkaline phosphatase level noted on routine biochemical screening.
(ii) The first symptom usually is **pruritus,** which may be devastatingly severe, especially at night.
(iii) **Jaundice** occurs in later stages of the disease, as do **osteopenia** (in 25% of patients) and **xanthomas** (in approximately 10% of patients).
(iv) In addition, primary biliary cirrhosis is associated with such conditions as Sjögren's syndrome (in 75% of patients), the presence of antithyroid antibody (in 25% of patients), rheumatoid arthritis (in 5% of patients), and the CREST

syndrome (calcinosis, Raynaud's phenomenon, esophageal motility dysfunction, sclerodactyly, and telangiectasia) [in 3% of patients].

(c) **Diagnosis** is made by the constellation of increased serum cholesterol, markedly increased alkaline phosphatase (four to six times the normal level), increased direct bilirubin, and the presence of a positive antimitochondrial antibody, which is found in more than 90% of patients. The liver biopsy shows characteristic changes. Extrahepatic biliary obstruction must be ruled out.

(d) **Therapy** is supportive and includes administration of antipruritic agents and supplementation of vitamins D and K and calcium, as well as aminobisphonates for prevention of osteoporosis. MCTs, which do not require bile salt micelles for adsorption, may be used as a dietary supplement. The pruritus may respond to cholestyramine, which binds bile salts in the intestine. Results have been achieved with certain drugs (i.e., azathioprine, chlorambucil, colchicine, methotrexate). Perhaps the most promising medical treatment is ursodeoxycholic acid, which may improve hepatic structure and function if initiated before advanced stages of the disease. Intravenous naloxone therapy may be useful for severe pruritus. Standard definitive surgery is liver transplantation, with 5-year survival rates of 70% in most series.

(2) **Secondary biliary cirrhosis** usually occurs after several years of biliary tract obstruction.

(a) **Etiology** includes common bile duct stones, common duct strictures, cholangiocarcinoma, ampullar carcinoma, sclerosing cholangitis, and chronic pancreatitis with compression of the common duct as it traverses the pancreatic head.

(b) **Clinical features** are similar to those of primary biliary cirrhosis but may be superseded by manifestations of the underlying disease. In addition, patients may develop cholangitis with shaking chills, fever, leukocytosis, and jaundice. Antimitochondrial antibodies usually are not present.

(c) **Therapy** is aimed at relieving the obstruction and includes surgery, external drainage, and placement of an indwelling stent.

d. **Cardiac cirrhosis** is a rare, late manifestation of severe prolonged right ventricular failure, which is most often seen with rheumatic heart disease (either mitral or aortic stenosis with tricuspid regurgitation). Constrictive pericarditis and severe cardiomyopathy also may be associated with cardiac cirrhosis. Clinical features include an enlarged liver, ascites, and splenomegaly. PT often is prolonged and precludes the use of anticoagulants in treatment of the valvular lesion. Prognosis depends on the course of the cardiac disease.

e. **Other causes of cirrhosis** include Wilson's disease, α_1-antitrypsin deficiency, hemochromatosis, drug-induced liver disease, NAFLD (see 5 IX A 4), or virus-induced cirrhosis of the liver.

f. **Vascular problems that mimic cirrhosis**

(1) **Budd-Chiari syndrome,** or **hepatic vein thrombosis,** is associated with hypercoagulable states, pregnancy, tumors, abdominal trauma, and use of oral contraceptives. Patients usually have ascites, and liver biopsy shows centrilobular congestion. Doppler ultrasound examination may show decreased or absent flow in the hepatic vein. Attempts to catheterize the hepatic vein often are unsuccessful, and the mortality rate is 50%–90%. In acute Budd-Chiari syndrome (within 1 week of onset), treatment with streptokinase or thromboplastin-activating factor may be beneficial. Side-to-side portacaval shunts may prolong survival. Liver transplantation may be required.

(2) **Splenic vein thrombosis** is due to abdominal trauma, pancreatitis, and tumor. Although the portal vein remains patent, gastric varices develop as splenic vein collaterals. Both esophageal and gastric varices develop in 15% of cases. Diagnosis is made by angiography, and therapy with splenectomy is curative.

(3) **Veno-occlusive disease,** a disease of small hepatic vessels, may follow hepatic radiation (>3500 cGy), azathioprine therapy, or ingestion of certain types of Jamaican tea. After bone

marrow transplantation (BMT), veno-occlusive disease is seen in approximately 20% of patients.

g. **Nodular transformation of the liver** is a noncirrhotic cause of portal hypertension characterized by the unexplained development of small nodules, especially in the perihilar area. Recurrent variceal bleeding may occur.

3. **Liver abscess**

a. **Amebic liver abscess.** Of the six *Entamoeba* species found in the human colon, *E. histolytica* is the only true pathogen. In the United States, homosexual men and institutionalized individuals are at greatest risk for amebic liver abscess. This disease also is common where diarrheal disease due to *E. histolytica* is endemic.

(1) **Clinical features.** Right upper quadrant pain and fever may be present. Pleuritic pain, chills, and night sweats also may be noted. There is a history of intestinal amebiasis in 50% of patients.

(2) **Laboratory data.** More than 50% of patients have elevated WBC counts (>20,000/mm^3), serum transaminase levels, and serum bilirubin levels. Serum alkaline phosphatase levels are abnormal in approximately 80% of affected individuals.

(3) **Diagnosis.** Demonstration of a filling defect in the liver through the use of ultrasonography, CT, or MRI is suggestive of the diagnosis. Aspiration of a cystic cavity may reveal "anchovy paste" fluid with trophozoites. Serologic tests (e.g., indirect hemagglutination inhibition and gel diffusion tests) are positive in 95% of cases.

(4) **Therapy.** Amebicides (e.g., metronidazole, chloroquine, diiodohydroxyquin) may be effective alone or may be combined with CT or ultrasound-directed aspiration of the abscess cavity. Liver scanning should be continued until healing occurs.

(5) **Complications.** Rupture of the cyst into the pleural space, lung, bowel, and retroperitoneum may occur. Rarely, a cyst extends to the body surface.

b. **Pyogenic liver abscess** usually is due to biliary tract disease, including acute cholecystitis and cholangitis. Other infections (e.g., appendicitis, diverticulitis) as well as intrinsic hepatic lesions also are important causes. In 10% of cases, the causative factor cannot be determined. Approximately 70% of abscesses contain mixed flora; the most commonly found organisms are anaerobes, *E. coli, Klebsiella* species, *Staphylococcus aureus,* and streptococci.

(1) **Clinical features.** Fever, chills, right upper quadrant pain, anorexia, and nausea may be present. Pleuritic pain occasionally occurs, and weight loss is common. Tender hepatomegaly is present in 50% of cases. The alkaline phosphatase level is elevated in approximately 80% of patients, jaundice is present in approximately 33%, and blood cultures are positive in 40%. CT combined with liver scanning, ultrasonography, or both can be used to detect an abscess greater than 2 cm.

(2) **Diagnosis.** The clinical presentation suggests the diagnosis, which can be confirmed by CT- or ultrasonography-guided aspiration.

(3) **Therapy.** Antibiotics, with or without external drainage, frequently are successful and necessary for multiple small abscesses. Treatment usually is continued for 4–6 weeks. Occasionally, surgical drainage is required.

c. **Focal hepatic candidiasis** is an entity consisting of hepatic and splenic granulomas containing *Candida albicans* hyphae in immunocompromised hosts. Most patients have previously received cytosine arabinoside for acute leukemia.

(1) **Clinical features** include a fever of unknown origin in immunocompromised hosts. Signs of oropharyngeal candidiasis may be present, and there may be right upper quadrant pain or tenderness.

(2) **Diagnosis** is made by **liver biopsy.** At laparotomy or laparoscopy, small white nodules less than 5 mm in width are seen. Liver function abnormalities include modest bilirubin and enzyme elevation with an increase in alkaline phosphatase.

(3) **Therapy** involves systemic amphotericin B, often in conjunction with fluconazole.

4. **Hepatic cysts**
   a. **Solitary cysts,** generally found in the right lobe of the liver, usually are asymptomatic but may cause pain and fever secondary to bleeding, infection, or rupture.
   b. **Polycystic liver disease** is the presence of multiple cysts that range from several millimeters to greater than 10–15 cm in diameter. Like solitary cysts, most cysts in polycystic liver disease are asymptomatic except in cases involving hemorrhage, infection, or rupture. Renal cysts are found in 50% of patients; cysts also may be found in the pancreas, spleen, and lungs. Results of liver function testing usually are normal, although mild elevation of serum alkaline phosphatase levels may be seen. Surgical aspiration or decompression occasionally is necessary.
   c. **Hydatid cysts** are most common in individuals who live in Greece, France, Italy, the Middle East, South America, and Iceland. This disease may be found elsewhere in the descendants of individuals from these regions.
      (1) **Etiology.** Hydatid cysts are formed when the infecting organism (i.e., *Echinococcus granulosus* or *Echinococcus multilocularis*) is ingested and travels through the portal circulation to the liver.
      (2) **Clinical features.** The cyst usually enlarges for 10–20 years after the initial infection before becoming symptomatic. There is calcification of a solitary cyst (seen in 50% of patients) and the presence of daughter cysts within a larger cyst.
      (3) **Diagnosis.** Diagnosis is made by positive complement fixation or indirect hemagglutination tests. Eosinophilia is occasionally seen. Liver biopsy and aspiration are not suggested because leakage may cause fatal anaphylaxis.
      (4) **Therapy.** Treatment may be surgical. Recently, ultrasound-guided injection of alcohol into cyst cavities has been used.
      (5) **Complications.** Rupture, infection, hemorrhage, and slow leakage causing allergic manifestations may develop.
   d. **Peliosis hepatitis** is a rare condition involving multiple blood-filled hepatic cysts. The liver often has a mottled blue appearance. Rupture with bleeding may be fatal. There is an association between this condition and tuberculosis, therapy with androgenic steroids, and the use of oral contraceptives. There is also an association with AIDS patients, especially those with angiomatosis (*Rochenellia*). Progressive hepatomegaly with liver failure may occur. CT scanning may show multiple defects. Percutaneous liver biopsy shows characteristic changes but is dangerous because of the vascular nature of the lesions.

5. **Granulomatous hepatitis**
   a. **Etiology.** Granulomatous hepatitis most often is secondary to systemic infections (e.g., tuberculosis), sarcoidosis, fungal infections, syphilis, and viral infections (e.g., infectious mononucleosis, CMV infection, varicella). Q fever, parasitic diseases, MAI (especially in HIV-infected patients), Hodgkin's disease, and beryllium toxicity also may cause granulomatous hepatitis. In addition, granulomatous hepatitis may be a manifestation of drug reactions involving phenylbutazone, sulfa drugs, hydralazine, or allopurinol. Occasionally, no cause can be found.
   b. **Clinical features.** Symptoms include weakness, fatigue, markedly increased erythrocyte sedimentation rate, and fever.
   c. **Diagnosis.** Liver biopsy is used to make the diagnosis.
   d. **Therapy.** Treatment of the secondary form includes withdrawal of the offending agent and treatment of the underlying lesion. The idiopathic form may respond to corticosteroid therapy.

C Systemic diseases with prominent liver involvement

1. α_1-Antitrypsin deficiency is a genetic defect of the glycoprotein that normally inhibits proteolytic enzymes such as trypsin, chymotrypsin, and elastase. There are 24 alleles in the protease inhibitor (Pi) system. Ninety percent of the population of the United States is genotype PiMM. The 22 genotype is homozygous for the disease state, and patients have less than 20% of normal serum levels of α_1-antitrypsin. Individuals with genotype PiMZ have approximately

50%–60% of normal levels. Homozygotes (PiZZ) usually have liver disease in childhood. Liver disease may develop in PiSZ or PiMZ heterozygotes, especially those who smoke, and COPD may develop in them as adults (see Chapter 2 II B). Disease does not develop in all individuals with the abnormal genotypes. Diagnosis is made based on a decreased α_1-globulin level observed on a protein electrophoresis, a decreased α_1-antitrypsin level in the serum, and by Pi typing. Liver biopsy shows diastase-resistant PAS-positive globules in portal areas. There is no effective therapy. Liver transplantation may be used in advanced cases.

2. **Amyloidosis** involves the liver in 50% of cases. Patients have hepatomegaly on physical examination but usually are asymptomatic. Results of liver function testing often are normal but may indicate a marked elevation of serum alkaline phosphatase.

3. **Hemochromatosis** is an inherited disorder (thought to be autosomal recessive) in which increased absorption of iron leads to iron deposition in the liver, heart, pancreas, and other organs. Men are more commonly affected than women (at a ratio of 8:1). In the United States, approximately 8%–9% of the population are heterozygotes and 1 in every 220 are homozygotes, making hemochromatosis one of the most common genetic liver diseases.
   a. **Clinical features.** Hepatomegaly, hyperpigmentation, and abnormalities of the cardiac conduction system, testes, and joints may occur. Fifty percent of the patients have abdominal pain. Cirrhosis and diabetes also may develop.
   b. **Laboratory findings.** Elevated levels of serum transaminases, increased serum iron with elevated percent saturation (generally > 80%), and high serum level of ferritin are seen. The HFE gene is linked to HLA-A_3 locus on chromosome 6. Approximately 85% of patients with hemochromatosis have this C282Y mutation. Liver biopsy shows iron deposits in both hepatocytes and Kupffer cells. This finding rules out secondary iron overload (hemosiderosis) in which iron is deposited in Kupffer cells alone. A skin or intestinal biopsy as well as an analysis of family members for elevated iron, total iron-binding capacity, or ferritin levels also may be helpful in the differential diagnosis. Screening family members for the elevated HLA haplotypes may be used. CT or MRI of the liver shows characteristic changes.
   c. **Therapy.** Repeated phlebotomy (usually once or twice weekly for several months or years) decreases total body iron stores, which may be at 10 times the normal level. Phlebotomy is continued until anemia develops or serum iron and ferritin levels normalize. Untreated patients have an increased risk of hepatoma.
   d. **Prognosis.** If hemochromatosis is diagnosed before cirrhosis develops, the prognosis with treatment is good (80% survival at 15 years). If cirrhosis or diabetes mellitus is present at the time of diagnosis, or if the iron stores do not decrease to normal levels after 18 months of treatment, the prognosis is not as favorable. Patients with hemochromatosis and cirrhosis have approximately a 220-fold increased risk of liver cancer.

4. **Sarcoidosis.** Approximately 70% of patients with sarcoidosis have granulomas in the liver. Patients usually do not have symptoms referable to the liver but may have increased serum alkaline phosphatase levels. Forty percent of patients have hepatomegaly. A liver biopsy showing noncaseating granulomas may aid in the diagnosis.

5. **Wilson's disease** is an autosomal recessive disease characterized by excessive copper deposition, which, if untreated, may lead to fulminant hepatic failure. Copper also is deposited in the brain, kidney, and cornea; copper depositions in the cornea cause **Kayser-Fleischer rings.** CNS disease may be prominent if the diagnosis is made in adulthood. Diagnosis is suggested by decreased serum ceruloplasmin levels, and increased urinary copper excretion (> 100 μg/24 hr); it is confirmed by an increased hepatic copper concentration in a liver biopsy sample. Treatment is with D-penicillamine, trientine, or zinc in combination with a low-copper diet. Hepatic transplantation has been used for fulminant hepatic failure.

6. **Liver disease of pregnancy**
   a. **Cholestasis** usually is seen in the last trimester of pregnancy and is benign. Patients may complain of pruritus and jaundice, and all symptoms disappear rapidly after delivery. The syndrome

is thought to be mediated by estrogens, progesterone, or both, and subsequent use of oral contraceptives or pregnancy may cause a recurrence of symptoms. Recently, ursodeoxycholic acid therapy has relieved pruritus and allowed the delay of delivery for greater fetal maturity.

b. **Acute fatty liver** is a severe disease usually occurring in a primigravida in the last trimester of pregnancy. Fulminant liver failure may develop, and an association with toxemia has been reported. Prognosis is poor but is improved by prompt delivery. Pathologic changes in the liver include small-droplet fatty change similar to that seen in fatty liver induced by tetracycline and valproic acid.

c. **HELLP syndrome** (hemolysis, elevated liver enzymes, low platelet count) is often seen in the third trimester of pregnancy. This condition is associated with toxemia in approximately 50% of patients. Abdominal pain and vomiting may be severe. Treatment is delivery of the infant.

d. **Hepatic rupture** rarely occurs after necrosis of the liver in eclamptic patients in their last trimester. Patients with hepatic rupture have generally been older and multiparous.

D Inherited disorders of bilirubin metabolism

1. **Gilbert's syndrome** is an essentially benign condition that occurs in approximately 7% of the population of the United States. Decreased uridine diphosphate (UDP) glucuronyl transferase activity leads to mild unconjugated hyperbilirubinemia (usually < 3 mg/dL), which increases after fasting.

2. **Crigler-Najjar syndrome** exists in two forms:

   a. **Type I** is rare and is characterized by an absence of hepatic UDP glucuronyl transferase activity. Patients usually die in infancy.

   b. **Type II** also is rare and is characterized by markedly diminished hepatic UDP glucuronyl transferase activity, leading to unconjugated hyperbilirubinemia in the range of 5–25 mg/dL. Phenobarbital may be used to induce microsomal enzyme activity. In most cases, there are no clinical sequelae.

3. **Rotor's syndrome** is a rare autosomal recessive condition. Impaired transport of conjugated bilirubin out of the hepatocyte leads to conjugated hyperbilirubinemia in the range of 2–10 mg/dL. Liver biopsy is normal, and the clinical course is benign.

4. **Dubin-Johnson syndrome** is similar to Rotor's syndrome, except that liver biopsy shows the accumulation of a dark pigment within hepatocytes. The elevated serum bilirubin may respond somewhat to phenobarbital therapy.

5. **Alagille's syndrome** is one of various types of familial intrahepatic cholestasis syndromes. Alagille's syndrome is an autosomal dominant syndrome that is generally identified in infants younger than 3 months of age. It is associated with congenital heart disease (ventricular or atrial septal defects), bony defects (butterfly vertebra or spina bifida), and renal or biliary tree anomalies. There are classic cholestatic laboratory test findings, and few bile ducts are seen on liver biopsy. Most patients have mild disease, but cirrhosis develops later in approximately 10% of these patients.

E Tumors of the liver

1. **Benign tumors**

   a. **Hepatic adenomas** usually occur in women of childbearing age and are more common in those who use oral contraceptives.

      (1) **Clinical features** may be completely absent. Some patients report right upper quadrant fullness. Occasionally, spontaneous rupture of the adenoma leads to intra-abdominal hemorrhage, which is fatal in 25% of patients.

      (2) **Diagnosis** is made by demonstration of a hepatic mass by CT and a cold spot through liver scanning. Results of liver function testing are normal, and serum α-fetoprotein (AFP) is normal. Because the tumors are hypervascular, liver biopsy is not suggested.

      (3) **Therapy** includes discontinuing the use of oral contraceptives and monitoring tumor size to document regression. If regression does not occur, the tumor should be removed surgically to prevent rupture.

b. **Focal nodular hyperplasia** also occurs primarily in women; the theory that this lesion is associated with oral contraceptive use is controversial. The lesion is composed of central connective tissue with radiating septa, which divide the mass into nodules. Liver scanning may not show an abnormality because all the elements of liver tissue, including Kupffer cells, are present. However, CT and angiography demonstrate a hypervascular mass. The clinical course is benign. There is no potential for malignant transformation, and hemorrhage, rupture, and necrosis are rare.

c. **Hemangiomas** are the most common benign tumors of the liver and are found at autopsy in 5%–7% of patients. Women are affected more commonly than men.

(1) **Clinical features** usually are absent. Large lesions may be associated with thrombocytopenia and hypofibrinogenemia, especially in infants. Hemangiomas also may be associated with telangiectasia of other organs.

(2) **Diagnosis** is made by angiography, rapid-sequence CT, MRI, or single-photon emission computed tomography (SPECT) liver scan. Abdominal radiographs may show calcification. Liver scanning shows a cold spot, which ultrasonography shows to be a solid mass. Hemangiomas usually are single but may be multiple.

(3) **Therapy** usually is not necessary. However, corticosteroid therapy, radiation therapy, and embolization all have been shown to be effective in decreasing the size of large hemangiomas.

2. **Malignant tumors** (see Chapter 4 VI E)

X DISEASES OF THE PERITONEUM, MESENTERY, AND ABDOMINAL VASCULATURE

A Diseases of the peritoneum

1. **Ascites** refers to the accumulation of fluid in the peritoneal cavity.

a. **Pathogenesis.** The following mechanisms lead to ascites formation:

(1) **Increased hydrostatic pressure,** which may be due to:
- (a) Cirrhosis
- (b) Hepatic vein occlusion (Budd-Chiari syndrome)
- (c) Inferior vena cava obstruction
- (d) Constrictive pericarditis
- (e) Congestive heart failure (CHF)

(2) **Decreased colloid osmotic pressure,** which may result from:
- (a) End-stage liver disease with poor protein synthesis
- (b) Nephrotic syndrome with protein loss
- (c) Malnutrition
- (d) Protein-losing enteropathy (PLE)

(3) **Increased permeability of peritoneal capillaries,** which may result from:
- (a) Tuberculous peritonitis
- (b) Bacterial peritonitis
- (c) Malignant disease of the peritoneum

(4) **Leakage of fluid into the peritoneal cavity,** leading to:
- (a) Bile ascites
- (b) Pancreatic ascites (usually secondary to a leaking pseudocyst)
- (c) Chylous ascites (secondary to lymphatic duct disruption due to lymphoma or trauma)
- (d) Urine ascites

(5) **Miscellaneous causes,** including:
- (a) Myxedema
- (b) Ovarian disease (Meigs' syndrome)
- (c) Chronic hemodialysis

b. Diagnosis. The presence of ascites usually is indicated on physical examination by abdominal distention, a fluid wave, or shifting dullness. Abdominal ultrasonography can reliably detect small amounts of fluid. Paracentesis can be performed with or without guidance by ultrasonography, and the ascitic fluid should be analyzed.

(1) From measurement of the albumin concentration in the ascitic fluid and the serum albumin concentration, a SAAG can be determined.

(a) If the SAAG is greater than 1.1 g/dL, the patient has portal hypertension (accuracy of approximately 97%), with cirrhosis, cardiac ascites, Budd-Chiari syndrome, portal vein thrombosis, veno-occlusive disease, or fatty liver of pregnancy.

(b) If the SAAG is less than 1.1 g/dL, the patient may have peritoneal carcinomatosis, infection (e.g., peritonitis or tuberculosis), nephrotic syndrome, or pancreatic or biliary ascites.

(2) The amylase concentration is elevated in pancreatic ascites.

(3) The triglyceride concentration is elevated in chylous ascites.

(4) Cytologic findings are frequently positive in malignancy.

(5) An absolute WBC count [generally polymorphonuclear leukocytes (PMNs)] greater than $250/mm^3$ is suggestive of infection. When mononuclear cells predominate, tuberculosis or fungal infection is likely.

(6) An RBC count greater than $50,000/mm^3$ denotes hemorrhagic ascites, which usually is due to malignancy, tuberculosis, or trauma. Hemorrhagic pancreatitis, a ruptured aortic aneurysm, and a ruptured hepatic adenoma may cause frank bleeding into the peritoneal cavity.

(7) Gram staining and culture document bacterial infection.

(8) A pH of less than 7 suggests bacterial infection.

c. Therapy. Treatment depends on the underlying cause. Transudative ascites may be treated with bed rest, Na^+ restriction, and careful use of diuretics. Paracentesis of up to 1 L of fluid may provide relief of acute respiratory embarrassment secondary to tense ascites. Removal of more than 1 L at a time may lead to hypovolemia and shock, unless 10 g albumin is replaced intravenously for each 1 L ascitic fluid removed. A Le Veen or Denver shunt may be used for intractable or malignant ascites, but these shunts introduce high risks of infection and DIC. The TIPS procedure also has been shown to be useful in treating refractory ascites.

2. Bacterial peritonitis

a. Pathogenesis

(1) **Primary** or **spontaneous bacterial peritonitis** usually develops in the setting of preexisting ascites.

(2) **Secondary** or **acute bacterial peritonitis** usually results from a perforated viscus, a ruptured appendix, an intestinal infarction, or ulcerative colitis.

b. Clinical features

(1) Abdominal pain, with or without guarding and rebound

(2) Fever

(3) Leukocytosis

(4) Paralytic ileus

c. Diagnosis

(1) **Paracentesis** aids in determining whether the fluid is exudative or transudative, has an elevated WBC count (a predominance of PMNs is diagnostic), and can be cultured to identify the infecting organism. Inoculating an anaerobic culture tube with freshly drawn ascitic fluid (i.e., at the patient's bedside) and inoculation of blood culture bottles are often useful. If the initial ascitic fluid total protein content is less than 1.0 mg/dL, patients have an increased risk for spontaneous bacterial peritonitis.

(2) **Radiographic examination** indicates free air under the diaphragm in the presence of a perforated viscus, may show a nonspecific ileus, or may show a hazy appearance consistent with ascites.

d. **Therapy**
   (1) Supportive measures include intravenous administration of fluids, correction of electrolyte abnormalities, and nasogastric suction.
   (2) Antimicrobial therapy for spontaneous bacterial peritonitis includes a third-generation cephalosporin to cover gram-negative organisms, pneumococcus, other streptococci, and anaerobic organisms.
   (3) Surgical intervention is necessary in cases of secondary bacterial peritonitis.

3. **Other causes of peritonitis**
   a. **Bile peritonitis**
      (1) **Pathogenesis.** Bile spillage into the peritoneal cavity (e.g., from a ruptured gallbladder or gallbladder puncture during liver biopsy) results in a chemical peritonitis.
      (2) **Clinical features.** Severe abdominal pain and shock secondary to exudation of fluid from the damaged peritoneum may occur.
      (3) **Therapy.** Treatment is surgical after patients have been stabilized with intravenous volume replacement and correction of electrolyte abnormalities.
   b. **Starch peritonitis**
      (1) **Pathogenesis.** Approximately 2–4 weeks after abdominal surgery, granulomatous peritonitis develops if the peritoneal cavity has been contaminated with surgical glove powder (starch), lint from surgical drapes, particles of suture material, or talc.
      (2) **Clinical features.** Abdominal pain, distention, tenderness, and fullness may be present.
      (3) **Diagnosis.** Examination of the ascitic fluid under a polarized microscope shows starch granules termed **maltese crosses.** Laparoscopy shows studding of the peritoneal surface.
      (4) **Therapy.** Corticosteroids or NSAIDs are appropriate.
   c. **Gonococcal peritonitis (Fitz-Hugh–Curtis syndrome)** usually is seen in young women and is caused by an ascending infection originating in the pelvis. Chlamydia recently has been reported to cause an identical syndrome.
      (1) **Clinical features.** Signs and symptoms, which mimic those of acute cholecystitis, include abdominal pain, fever, and right upper quadrant peritoneal signs. Occasionally, a hepatic friction rub is present.
      (2) **Diagnosis.** Laboratory tests show an elevated WBC count and mild abnormalities in liver function. Pelvic examination may indicate adnexal tenderness, and culture of cervical mucus usually is positive. Laparoscopy shows **violin-string adhesions** from the liver to either the right adnexa or the abdominal wall.
      (3) **Therapy.** Ceftriaxone is administered. If chlamydia also is present, tetracycline is given.

4. **Subphrenic abscess** refers to a collection of pus located inferior to the diaphragm and above the liver, spleen, or stomach.
   a. **Pathogenesis.** Abscess formation usually is a complication of diverticulitis, a ruptured appendix, a perforated ulcer, or an abdominal wound with peritoneal soiling. Occasionally, an abscess is seen after uncomplicated abdominal surgery.
   b. **Clinical features.** Fever, leukocytosis, and abdominal and shoulder pain may occur.
   c. **Diagnosis.** A radiograph showing elevation of one hemidiaphragm may suggest the diagnosis, which usually requires demonstration of the abscess cavity by CT or ultrasonography.
   d. **Therapy.** Treatment involves surgical drainage and broad-spectrum antibiotics to combat gram-negative as well as anaerobic organisms.

5. **Tumors of the peritoneum**
   a. **Metastatic lesions** are the most common peritoneal tumors. The primary lesion usually is adenocarcinoma of the gastrointestinal tract, pancreas, or ovary. However, sarcomas, lymphomas, leukemias, and carcinoid tumors all may involve the peritoneum.
      (1) **Diagnosis.** Paracentesis showing an exudative fluid with a moderately increased lymphocyte count and positive cytologic findings are diagnostic. Needle biopsy of the peritoneum also may be used.

(2) **Therapy.** Treatment is directed at the underlying malignancy. Intraperitoneal injection of a sclerosing agent occasionally may be palliative.

b. **Mesothelioma** is seen most commonly in men older than 50 years of age and is associated with asbestos exposure.

(1) **Clinical features** include abdominal distention, abdominal pain, nausea, vomiting, and weight loss.

(2) **Diagnosis** requires demonstration of malignant cells through paracentesis with cytologic testing, needle biopsy, or laparotomy with biopsy.

(3) **Therapy** includes radiation therapy, chemotherapy, or both, but patient response usually is poor.

c. **Pseudomyxoma peritonei** is a rare condition characterized by the presence of thick gelatinous material in the peritoneal cavity.

(1) **Pathogenesis.** This condition results from the rupture of either an appendiceal mucocele or an ovarian mucinous cystadenoma. Some authors have reported the presence of low-grade malignancy in a high percentage of the underlying tumors.

(2) **Clinical features.** Increasing abdominal girth without shifting dullness in an otherwise healthy individual may occur.

(3) **Diagnosis.** Laparotomy is often required.

(4) **Therapy.** Treatment involves surgical removal of the mucinous material and underlying tumor.

B Diseases of the mesentery

1. **Mesenteric panniculitis (mesenteric Weber-Christian disease)** is a rare condition usually seen in older men, which causes inflammation and fibrosis of the mesentery.

a. **Pathogenesis** is thought to involve overgrowth of normal fat tissue in the mesentery with subsequent degeneration, necrosis, and progression to fibrosis and scar formation. The initiating event may be ischemia, infection, or trauma.

b. **Clinical features** include crampy abdominal pain, fever, weight loss, nausea, and vomiting. Lymphatic obstruction may develop with resultant ascites, steatorrhea, and PLE.

c. **Diagnosis** requires laparotomy, which shows a thickened fibrotic mesentery with fat necrosis and infiltration by foamy macrophages.

d. **Therapy** with corticosteroids or immunosuppressive drugs has varying results. In many patients, the process appears to be self-limited, and the prognosis is excellent.

2. **Mesenteric cysts** are congenital anomalies of the mesenteric lymphatic system, which occur as slowly enlarging, painless, round, smooth, mobile masses. Treatment is drainage or excision. Mesenteric cysts are benign but rarely may cause symptoms because of rupture, bleeding, or torsion.

3. **Mesenteric adenitis** generally is seen in children and young adults and mimics acute appendicitis.

a. **Etiology** usually involves a viral infection. However, many cases are caused by *Yersinia.*

b. **Clinical features** are abdominal pain (which may be severe), nausea, vomiting, and fever. Some patients have additional evidence of a viral infection (e.g., pharyngitis and myalgia).

c. **Diagnosis** usually is made at laparotomy for presumed appendicitis.

d. **Therapy** includes antibiotics, if *Yersinia* is identified, and supportive care.

C Diseases of the abdominal vasculature

1. **Abdominal aortic aneurysm** usually manifests as an asymptomatic pulsatile mass, but some patients have abdominal pain, back pain, and leg ischemia. The cause usually is atherosclerosis. Leakage of blood into surrounding tissues with associated abdominal, back, or flank pain may precede overt rupture by several weeks. Rupture into the duodenum—occurring as massive gastrointestinal hemorrhage—or into the abdomen may be catastrophic. Treatment is surgical, with replacement of the aneurysm with an aortic graft made of Dacron or some other synthetic

material. Postoperative aortoenteric fistulas with erosion of the graft into the duodenum (usually in the setting of an infected graft) may be seen several years after aneurysmectomy and may result in fatal bleeding if not recognized early.

2. **Acute mesenteric ischemia** is a classic syndrome of decreased blood supply, usually involving the superior mesenteric artery. Patients have advanced arteriosclerotic cardiovascular disease, often with a history of CHF, acute myocardial infarction (MI), cerebrovascular disease, or peripherovascular disease. Many patients have taken splanchnic constricting agents such as digoxin. Embolic disease (which affects 25% of patients) often is associated with unstable cardiac rhythms. Thrombosis and nonocclusive mesenteric ischemia are the leading causes of acute mesenteric ischemic syndromes, each accounting for 25% of cases. Mesenteric venous infarction and inferior mesenteric arterial disease account for the rest of the cases.
   a. **Clinical features.** Sudden severe periumbilical pain is the most common symptom. A benign but hypoperistaltic abdomen is observed. Anteroposterior (flat plate) radiograph of the abdomen often shows normal findings, but may show separation of bowel loops or "thumbprinting" (submucosal hemorrhage and edema).
   b. **Diagnosis.** An increased WBC count (often > 20,000/mm^3) supports the diagnosis, which is confirmed by abdominal angiography. Doppler ultrasonography also may show decreased flow through the superior mesenteric arterial or celiac tree.
   c. **Therapy.** Treatment is surgical removal of the embolus or thrombus, although occasionally antithrombotic agents, balloon angioplasty of narrowed vessels, or bypass surgery is used.

3. **Chronic mesenteric ischemia** usually is seen only when there is significant occlusion of two of the three major splanchnic arteries. The syndrome usually is seen in older patients with a history of cardiovascular disease.
   a. **Clinical features** include intermittent crampy abdominal pain occurring 15–30 minutes after eating and lasting several hours. Because of the association of pain with eating, patients characteristically become fearful of eating and decrease their intake to the point of substantial weight loss. Physical examination frequently discloses evidence of peripheral vascular disease, but there are no specific findings indicating intestinal ischemia. The presence or absence of an abdominal bruit is not helpful.
   b. **Diagnosis** is difficult and must be based on strong clinical suspicion combined with angiographic demonstration of significant narrowing (> 50%) of two of the three major splanchnic arteries.
   c. **Therapy** is surgical vascular reconstruction. Vasodilators have not been shown to be effective.

4. **Ischemic colitis** is due to a lack of arterial blood to the colon. Although any portion of the colon may be affected, the most common site is the left colon and, in particular, the so-called "watershed area" at the splenic flexure. This area is vulnerable because it is the site where the superior mesenteric arterial supply ends and the inferior mesenteric arterial supply begins. The rectum usually is spared because it has a generous dual blood supply.
   a. **Clinical features** include bloody diarrhea, lower abdominal pain, and occasional vomiting. Infarction rarely occurs. The older adult who has a history of heart disease or abdominal aortic aneurysm surgery (with ligation of the inferior mesenteric artery) is particularly susceptible.
   b. **Diagnosis** is suggested by negative findings for other causes of bloody diarrhea in the elderly population (i.e., polyp, carcinoma, diverticulosis, and angiodysplasia). The WBC count may be elevated to approximately 20,000/mm^3. A flat-plate radiograph of the abdomen may show thumbprinting. A barium enema is a safe study and may show diffuse submucosal change. Generally, sigmoidoscopy shows only bloody fluid.
   c. **Therapy** is supportive with NPO (i.e., nothing by mouth), intravenous fluids, blood replacement, and antibiotics to prevent secondary invasion.
   d. **Prognosis** generally is good. Late strictures may develop, which could require balloon dilation or surgery.

5. **Vasculitis.** Involvement of the mesenteric vessels by polyarteritis nodosa, lupus erythematosus, or rheumatoid vasculitis mimics arterial embolization (causing bowel infarction) or chronic mesenteric ischemia. The diagnosis is suggested by the systemic features of the disease. Surgery is required for acute infarction. Otherwise, medical treatment with corticosteroids, immunosuppressive agents, or both, frequently is effective.
6. **Splenic infarction** is characterized by severe abdominal pain in young patients (<40 years) who have primary hematologic disease (sickle cell disease, leukemia, lymphoma), or in older patients (≥ 40 years) who have embolic diseases. An abscess may develop with hemorrhage or rupture. Diagnosis is suggested by CT or spleen scan with ^{99}Tc. Treatment is surgical.

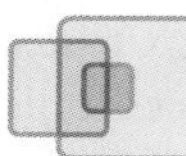

Study Questions

1. A 30-year-old man has had difficulty swallowing for both solids and liquids over the past 6 months. What is the most likely diagnosis?
   - A Esophageal carcinoma
   - B Achalasia
   - C Schatzki's rings
   - D Benign esophageal stricture
   - E Barrett's esophagus

2. A 52-year-old man with a history of heartburn was diagnosed with carcinoma of the esophagus. What is the most likely cell type of this tumor?
   - A Squamous cell
   - B Oat cell
   - C Transitional cell
   - D Adenocarcinoma
   - E Primary esophageal melanoma

3. An 84-year-old woman was found to have an esophageal web in the distal esophagus (Plummer-Vinson syndrome). Which one of the following statements is correct?
   - A They are caused by folate deficiency.
   - B They are located in the distal esophagus.
   - C They cause gastroesophageal reflux.
   - D Treatment includes esophageal bougienage.
   - E They result in elevated iron stores in the blood.

4. A 54-year-old obese woman has chronic gastroesophageal reflux. Which of the following drugs are known to exacerbate her reflux esophagitis?
   - A Chlorpropamide
   - B Metoclopramide
   - C Theophylline
   - D Acetaminophen
   - E Omeprazole

5. A 32-year-old man with HIV has pain on swallowing. Which of the following is the most likely cause?
   - A Scleroderma
   - B Esophageal varices
   - C Herpes simplex virus (HSV) infection
   - D Achalasia
   - E Schatzki's rings

6. A 23-year-old woman reports a 2–3-year history of postprandial lower abdominal discomfort and bloating with no specific food predilection. Physical examination and laboratory studies are normal. Celiac antibodies were negative. Which of the following statements concerning the most likely diagnosis is correct?
   - A Lactase deficiency is the preferred term.
   - B An underlying neuromuscular or hormonal defect is likely with visceral hypersensitivity.

C An underlying immunologic defect is likely.
D The syndrome may be a premalignant state.
E Incontinence is a common clinical feature.

7. A 29-year-old internal medicine resident who had received recombinant hepatitis B vaccine most likely had which of the following immunologic markers?

A Hepatitis B surface antigen (HB_sAg)
B Hepatitis B core antibody (anti-HB_c)
C Hepatitis Be antibody (anti-HB_e)
D Hepatitis B surface antibody (anti-HB_s)
E Anti-HB_c and anti-HB_s

8. A 51-year-old man with recurrent peptic ulcer disease had a fasting gastrin level of 1000. A presumptive diagnosis of Zollinger-Ellison syndrome was made. Which of the following organs is the most common site of origin of the tumor associated with this syndrome?

A Stomach
B Duodenum
C Lymph nodes
D Spleen
E Pancreas

9. A 79-year-old male smoker with a history of coronary artery disease and peripheral vascular disease developed bloody diarrhea. No infectious pathogens were identified. Which part of the colon is most vulnerable to ischemic insult?

A Splenic flexure
B Cecum
C Rectum
D Sigmoid colon
E Hepatic flexure

10. A 63-year-old diabetic man with cholelithiasis and steatorrhea was found to have a positive octreotide abdominal scan. Which of the following neuroendocrine tumors is the most likely etiology?

A Gastrinomas
B Somatostatinomas
C VIPomas
D Glucagonomas
E Insulinomas

11. A 42-year-old IV drug abuser was found to have both hepatitis B and hepatitis C with chronic elevations of his hepatic transaminases. Which of the following epidemiologic statements is most appropriate?

A Chronic hepatitis will develop in approximately 30%–50% of such patients.
B There is a high 1-year mortality rate after active infection.
C Vaccine protection is available to protect against both diseases.
D The coexistence of HBV and HCV is rare in intravenous drug abusers.
E There is an increased risk for hepatoma.

12. A 32-year-old man recently returned from a ski vacation in New England. Nonbloody diarrhea developed toward the latter stages of his trip. Stool samples tested for fecal leukocytes were negative. Which of the following is the most likely diagnosis?

A *Shigella* infection
B *Escherichia coli* serotype 0157:H7 infection
C Ulcerative colitis
D *Giardia lamblia* infection
E Colonic ischemia

13. A 22-year-old woman with changes in her bowel habits was found to have multiple discrete polyps. On family history, two first-degree relatives were noted to have colon cancer. In which of the following conditions are multiple polypoid lesions highly associated with malignancy?

A Ulcerative colitis
B Crohn's disease
C Gardner's syndrome
D Peutz-Jeghers syndrome
E Juvenile polyposis

14. A 32-year-old woman was found to have severe iron deficiency anemia. An upper endoscopy, colonoscopy, and video endoscopy were all normal. Family history revealed osteoporosis in her 39-year-old brother, which is currently being investigated. Her only GI symptoms were those of occasional postprandial abdominal bloating with episodes of diarrhea, previously diagnosed as irritable bowel syndrome. Her mother has a known diagnosis of rheumatoid arthritis. All laboratory studies are normal. Which of the following is the most likely diagnosis?

A Ulcerative colitis
B Crohn's disease
C Lactose intolerance
D Irritable bowel syndrome
E Celiac disease

15. Which of the following findings is likely to be found in this patient?

A Prominent villi on small intestine biopsy
B 3 g of D-xylose in a 5-hour urine collection
C High carotene level with normal vitamin A intake
D Four grams of fat on a 72-hour fecal fat collection
E Negative Sudan stain

16. A 22-year-old college student was found to have right lower quadrant pain, fever, leukocytosis, and localization to McBurney's point. On rectal examination, he was tender in the right lower quadrant. The most likely diagnosis is:

A Diverticulitis
B Ulcerative colitis
C Appendicitis
D Tubo-ovarian abscess
E Cholecystitis

17. A 78-year-old woman was found to have a hemoglobin of 9 g with hematocrit of 29%. During evaluation of her anemia, an upper endoscopy indicated gastritis in the proximal half of the stomach. The most likely associated abnormalities would include:

A Parietal cell antibody
B Decreased serum gastrin level
C *Helicobacter pylori* infection
D Antral involvement
E Nonsteroidal anti-inflammatory drugs (NSAIDs)

18. A 48-year-old woman was referred to GI clinic for recurrent nausea with occasional episodes of diarrhea alternating with constipation. A solid-phase gastric emptying study indicated markedly delayed gastric emptying. The most likely explanation for gastroparesis in this setting is:

A Cholinergic drug therapy
B Duodenal ulcer
C Diabetes insipidus
D Scleroderma
E Gastric varices

19. A fourth-year medical student rotating on a radiology elective was presented an x-ray of the abdomen, which showed multiple air–fluid levels with dilated loops of small bowel, paucity of air in the colon, and no air in the rectum. The radiology attending turned to the fourth-year medical student and asked which of the following clinical features would most likely be found in this patient.

A Hypoactive bowel sounds
B Pain out of proportion to physical examination
C Crampy abdominal pain that waxes and wanes
D Diarrhea
E A flat, rigid abdomen

20. A 50-year-old man undergoing screening colonoscopy with no associated symptoms was found to have a single small colonic polyp. Inquiring about his risk of cancer, which of the following circumstances indicates the greatest risk for cancer in an individual polyp?

A When they are of tubular histology
B When they are associated with active bleeding
C When they are larger than 2 cm in diameter
D When they are pedunculated
E When patients are younger than 50 years of age

21. A 56-year-old patient with advanced alcoholic cirrhosis and known ascites is found to have abdominal pain, fever to 102°, and a peripheral white blood cell count of 17,000 with a shift to the left. Which of the following statements regarding the primary diagnosis is correct?

A It is more likely when ascitic fluid total protein exceeds 1.0 mg/dL.
B It develops in the setting of preexisting ascites.
C The ascitic polymorphonuclear count is less than 100 cells/mm^3.
D It is often associated with aspergillosis.
E It is associated with a perforated viscus.

22. A 76-year-old man with a history of an acute myocardial infarction and peripheral vascular disease is seen in the emergency department for very severe abdominal pain, out of proportion to clinical findings. On physical examination, his abdomen is soft with hypoactive bowel sounds. Which of the following is associated with the most likely diagnosis?

A A normal white blood cell (WBC) count
B Involvement of the inferior mesenteric artery
C Constipation
D A definitive clinical presentation
E Lack of a significant medical history

23. A 32-year-old woman with Raynaud's phenomenon has had heartburn and regurgitation for 2 years. What is the most likely mechanism for these symptoms in this case?

A Presence of *Helicobacter pylori* in the gastric mucosa
B Decreased lower esophageal sphincter (LES) pressure

C Increased gastric acid secretion
D Decreased peristalsis in the upper third of the esophagus
E Esophageal muscular spasm

24. A 52-year-old man developed dysphagia for solids. An upper GI series showed a mass lesion in the distal esophagus. Endoscopy confirmed the presence of adenocarcinoma of the esophagus. Which of the following is the most important predisposing factor in his disease?

A Achalasia
B Palmoplantar keratosis (tylosis)
C Barrett's esophagus
D Celiac sprue
E Alcohol intake

25. A 38-year-old man from Taiwan recently moved to this country and was found to have hepatitis B (HBV) on blood studies. Which of the following laboratory tests most reliably distinguish a chronic healthy carrier state from chronic active hepatitis B disease?

A Serum hepatitis B surface antigen (HB_sAG)
B Serum hepatitis B core antibody (anti-HB_c)
C Serum anti–smooth muscle antibody
D Liver biopsy
E Serum α-fetoprotein (AFP)

26. A 35-year-old man with acquired immunodeficiency syndrome (AIDS) with a CD4 count of 150 cells/mm^3 has had jaundice and fever for 1 month. Liver function tests indicate the following:

Total bilirubin: 3.2 mg/dL

Direct bilirubin: 2.7 mg/dL

Alkaline phosphatase: Elevated (three times normal)

AST and ALT: Normal

Liver ultrasound shows hepatomegaly with normal caliber biliary ducts, and liver biopsy indicates granulomatous liver disease. Which of the following is the most likely diagnosis?

A Polycystic liver disease
B Hepatitis C (HCV)
C *Mycobacterium avium-intracellulare* (MAI)
D Sclerosing cholangitis
E Hepatitis B (HBV)

27. Results of hepatitis serology are as follows:

Positive hepatitis A IgG antibody

Negative hepatitis A IgM antibody

Positive hepatitis B surface antibody (anti-HB_e)

Negative hepatitis B core antibody (anti-HB_c)

Negative hepatitis C antibody

Which of the following is the most likely diagnosis?

A Acute hepatitis A (HAV)
B Acute hepatitis B (HBV)

C Immunity against hepatitis C (HCV)
D Previous vaccination against hepatitis B (HBV)
E Past exposure to hepatitis B (HBV)

28. A 35-year-old man with a history of IV drug abuse was found to have chronic fatigue and AST elevated 4 times with an ALT elevated at fivefold normal. Polyarteritis was subsequently diagnosed by vascular biopsy. The most likely diagnosis is:

A Hepatitis B
B Hepatitis C
C Hepatitis A
D Hepatitis E
E Hepatitis G

29. Which of the following is indicative of active viral replication in the above patient?

A Hepatitis B DNA level
B Hepatitis C DNA level
C Hepatitis C RNA level
D Hepatitis B RNA level
E Hepatitis C antibody

30. The best means to protect his first-degree relatives in the absence of any prior evidence of hepatitis would be:

A Vaccination
B Pooled immune globulin (gamma globulin)
C Avoidance of household contact
D Avoidance of shellfish ingestion
E Hepatitis immunoglobulin

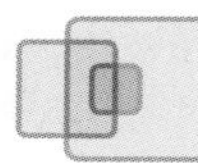

Answers and Explanations

1. The answer is B [I A 1 b (2), B 2 c]. Esophageal motor disorders such as achalasia are characterized by dysphagia for both solids and liquids. Obstructive esophageal conditions such as carcinoma, stricture, and Schatzki's rings cause dysphagia for solids but allow free passage of liquids. The dysphagia associated with Schatzki's rings is intermittent; in carcinoma and stricture, however, the dysphagia is constant. Barrett's esophagus is the replacement of normal squamous epithelium with columnar epithelium; there is no dysphagia unless an ulceration or stricture complicates this condition.

2. The answer is D [I B 2 a (1)]. Adenocarcinoma of the esophagus has been the second fastest rising cancer in the United States, second only to malignant melanoma. Primary cell type in a 52-year-old gentleman with a history of reflux places him at great risk for adenocarcinoma. Oat cell and transitional cell carcinomas are not primary malignancies of the esophagus, and malignant melanoma would be a metastatic lesion that, in this setting, would be considered unlikely.

3. The answer is D [I B 2 c]. Esophageal webs are seen in the upper third of the esophagus and may be caused by failure of complete embryologic recannulation or by mucosal proliferation secondary to iron deficiency—the Plummer-Vinson (Paterson-Kelly) syndrome. Because of the associated iron deficiency, treatment includes iron supplementation in addition to fracturing the webs with an esophageal bougie.

4. The answer is C [I B 1 a (2)]. Theophylline, a β-adrenergic drug used as a bronchodilator for treating asthma and chronic bronchitis, is a smooth muscle–relaxing agent that exacerbates reflux esophagitis. Other smooth muscle–relaxing agents that can exacerbate gastroesophageal reflux disease include diltiazem, isosorbide dinitrate, and atropine. Chlorpropamide, an oral hypoglycemic agent, has no effect on the lower esophageal sphincter (LES). Metoclopramide is a prokinetic agent that has constricting effects on the LES and improves gastric emptying. Acetaminophen has no direct irritating effects on gastrointestinal mucosa. Omeprazole, a proton pump inhibitor, is helpful in the management of resistant gastroesophageal reflux disease.

5. The answer is C [I A 2, B 4 b]. Odynophagia, or pain on swallowing, may be caused by motor disorders of the esophagus (e.g., diffuse esophageal spasm) or mucosal disruption (e.g., as a result of infection or drug-induced esophagitis). The most important infectious agents are *Candida,* herpes simplex virus (HSV), cytomegalovirus (CMV), and human immunodeficiency virus (HIV), infections that are commonly seen in immunocompromised hosts. Severe gastroesophageal reflux with ulcerative esophagitis and radiation esophagitis can lead to severe odynophagia as well. Drugs that may cause mucosal disruption include potassium chloride tablets, tetracycline preparations, clindamycin, quinidine, ascorbic acid, and iron sulfate. Scleroderma is a motor disorder that affects the smooth muscle portion of the esophagus, causing weak, simultaneous, ineffective peristalsis. Dysphagia is usually the only symptom. Esophageal varices caused by portal hypertension are generally found incidentally at the time of upper endoscopy or when acute upper gastrointestinal bleeding is present. Schatzki's rings are benign esophageal strictures primarily seen in the distal esophagus, in which dysphagia is the only symptom present.

6. The answer is B [IV D 3 a]. Irritable bowel syndrome, a common cause of alternating diarrhea and constipation, is a functional disorder of motility that probably involves a neuromuscular or hormonal defect. Lactase deficiency is a separate entity that may contribute to irritable bowel syndrome but also may be totally unrelated. There is no evidence of an immunologic defect, and the syndrome is not considered a premalignant state. Incontinence is a symptom of altered anorectal physiology that is seen with inflammatory diseases of the anal canal and with systemic neuromuscular disorders such as diabetes or scleroderma. Although incontinence occasionally occurs with explosive diarrhea, incontinence is not a common feature of irritable bowel syndrome and should suggest a systemic disorder.

7. The answer is D [IX A 1 d; Figure 5–1]. The vaccine against hepatitis B (HBV), in either the recombinant or the pooled plasma form, does not contain hepatitis B e or hepatitis B core antigen (HB_eAg or HB_cAg, respectively). Therefore, the antibody produced is simply that against hepatitis surface antigen (HB_sAG). Because no active HB_sAg is transmitted, tests for hepatitis B surface antigenemia are negative.

8. The answer is E [III I]. The Zollinger-Ellison syndrome is a non–β islet cell tumor that produces gastrin and is associated with gastric acid hypersecretion and peptic ulcer disease. Tumors are biologically malignant in 60% of cases, and the most common site involved is the pancreas. Tumor size ranges from 2 mm to 20 cm.

9. The answer is A [X C 4]. Ischemic colitis is caused by a lack of arterial blood supply to the colon. Although any portion of the colon may be affected, the most common site is the left colon, particularly the so-called "watershed" area at the splenic flexure.

10. The answer is B [VII E 4]. Somatostatinomas are associated with three clinical features—diabetes, steatorrhea, and gallstones. Gastrinomas, which cause Zollinger-Ellison syndrome, are associated with recurrent peptic ulcer disease, diarrhea, and multiple endocrine neoplasia, type I (MEN-I), syndrome in 20% of patients. VIPoma (pancreatic cholera, Verner-Morrison syndrome, and the watery diarrhea, hypokalemia, and achlorhydria syndrome) is a non-α, non-β islet cell tumor that secretes vasoactive intestinal peptide (VIP), leading to watery diarrhea. Glucagonomas are characterized by a syndrome of diabetes mellitus, weight loss, anemia, and a rash (migratory necrolytic erythema). Insulinomas are characterized by high insulin levels in the presence of hypoglycemia.

11. The answer is E [IX A 1]. Patients who are chronic carriers of hepatitis B (HBV) and those with chronic active HBV and hepatitis C (HCV) infection are at increased risk for developing hepatoma. HBV is parenterally transmitted, putting intravenous drug abusers, homosexual men, and those exposed to blood or blood products at risk. There is a 10% risk of chronic disease or becoming a chronic carrier. HCV is transmitted through parenteral, sexual, and perhaps perinatal methods and accounts for 90% of cases of posttransfusion hepatitis. Approximately 30%–50% of patients develop chronic hepatitis. Fulminant HBV is associated with a high mortality rate, whereas fulminant HCV rarely occurs. Vaccination provides adequate protection against HBV; however, currently there is no HCV vaccine.

12. The answer is D [IV D 4 b, e, j; V D; X C 4; Table 5–1]. *Giardia lamblia* is the most common cause of waterborne infectious diarrhea in the United States. The organism preferentially resides in the upper small intestine, and infected patients may be asymptomatic, have mild diarrhea, or develop a prolonged illness characterized by malabsorption, diarrhea, bloating, and crampy abdominal pain. Organisms such as *Shigella* and *Escherichia coli* serotype 0157:H7 are invasive pathogens that can cause fever, crampy abdominal pain, and bloody diarrhea. Ulcerative colitis is an inflammatory bowel disease characterized by bloody diarrhea. Colonic ischemia is characterized by the acute onset of crampy abdominal pain and bloody diarrhea caused by a low-flow state to the colon.

13. The answer is C [V G 2]. Gardner's syndrome, characterized by familial adenomatous polyposis associated with osteomas or soft tissue tumors, has an extremely high risk for the development of colorectal cancer. Peutz-Jeghers syndrome is characterized by mucocutaneous pigmentation of the buccal mucosa and hamartomatous polyps in the stomach, small bowel, and colon. These polyps carry a very low risk for malignant transformation. Both ulcerative colitis and Crohn's disease do carry an increased risk of colon cancer, but these disorders are not associated with adenomatous colonic polyps. If multiple colonic polyps are seen in ulcerative colitis, they are generally pseudopolyps and are not neoplastic. Juvenile polyposis commonly leads to gastrointestinal bleeding from polyps of the colon, small bowel, and stomach, and the risk of malignancy is slightly increased later in life.

14. The answer is E [IV E 4 c]. Celiac (nontropical) sprue is a disease characterized by abnormal sensitivity to gluten, a protein component of wheat. Celiac patients have proximal intestinal involvement with relative sparing of the distal ileum. Iron is absorbed in the duodenum, and, therefore, iron deficiency anemia not due to blood loss is common in this setting. Crohn's disease and ulcerative colitis are active inflammatory diseases that would be associated with changes on intestinal visualization. Lactose intolerance would not be associated with iron deficiency anemia. A coexisting autoimmune disease in her mother (rheumatoid arthritis) and osteoporosis in a young male are clues that she most likely has associated family members with either celiac disease or other autoimmune disorders.

15. The answer is B [IV E 3 a, b, e, i]. After a 25-g oral dose of D-xylose, a 5-hour urine collection should contain at least 5 g D-xylose. The finding of less than 4–5 g D-xylose in the stool is indicative of the malabsorption syndromes seen with celiac disease. Flat villi with inflammatory cell infiltration on small bowel biopsy are characterized by celiac disease. The serum carotene level is a reflection of vitamin A metabolism. Because vitamin A is a fat-soluble vitamin, a low serum carotene level with normal vitamin A intake may be useful in screening for fat malabsorption. A positive Sudan stain is indicative of an underlying malabsorptive process. However, the gold standard test for fat malabsorption is a 72-hour stool collection for fecal fat. The coefficient of fat absorption in the small intestine is 7%. As a result, a patient consuming a 100-g fat diet should have no more than 7 g fat in the stool each day; more than 7 g fat would be consistent with a malabsorption syndrome.

16. The answer is C [IV I]. Acute appendicitis most often occurs in males between the ages of 10 and 30 years. Clinical features include right lower quadrant (McBurney's point) pain, fever, and leukocytosis. Differential diagnoses include acute gastroenteritis, mesenteric adenitis, Meckel's diverticulum, Crohn's disease, ovarian torsion, ruptured ovarian cyst, pelvic inflammatory disease (PID), and, in elderly patients, diverticulitis, cholecystitis, incarcerated hernia, and mesenteric thrombosis.

17. The answer is A [II A 2 b (1)]. The most likely diagnosis is chronic type A gastritis, which is immunologically mediated, an assumption that is based on the serologic finding of parietal cell antibody. Parietal cells are gastric acid–producing cells located in the body and fundus (but not the antrum) of the stomach. As a result of parietal cell damage, chronic type A gastritis is characterized by hypo- or achlorhydria. Because there is little or no gastric acid to shut down production of gastrin, serum gastrin levels are high. In addition, intrinsic factor is produced by parietal cells and, therefore, vitamin B_{12} deficiency is common in affected patients. Vitamin B_{12} deficiency accounts for the common finding of pernicious anemia in chronic type A gastritis. Type B gastritis predominantly involves the antrum and is most often caused by *Helicobacter pylori* infection and chronic administration of nonsteroidal anti-inflammatory drugs (NSAIDs).

18. The answer is D [II C 5]. Gastroparesis is a disorder of gastric emptying and is not associated with mechanical obstruction. It is most frequently associated with a greater than 10-year history of type 1 (insulin-dependent) diabetes mellitus. Other conditions associated with gastroparesis include systemic sclerosis, postvagotomy states, and the use of anticholinergic agents. Prokinetic agents (e.g., metoclopramide, domperidone, erythromycin, cisapride) have been used to treat gastroparesis. Gastric varices have no effect on gastric emptying.

19. The answer is C [IV A 1 b]. The patient has a mechanical intestinal obstruction, as the description of the air–fluid levels indicates a mechanical intestinal obstruction. Mechanical intestinal obstruction may be the result of extrinsic, intramural, or intraluminal causes. Symptoms include crampy abdominal pain that waxes and wanes, obstipation or constipation, nausea and vomiting, and abdominal distention. Physical examination of the abdomen reveals high-pitched bowel sounds and rushes and tinkles, as well as marked abdominal distention and tympany on percussion. Pain out of proportion to the physical examination is most suggestive of acute mesenteric ischemia.

20. The answer is C [V G 1]. Adenomatous polyps that represent an increased risk for adenocarcinoma are greater than 2 cm in diameter, villous rather than tubular, and sessile rather than pedunculated. There is no association with increased risk related to bleeding or patient age.

21. The answer is B [X A 2]. The clinical features of spontaneous (primary) bacterial peritonitis, which develops in a setting of preexisting ascites, include abdominal pain, fever, leukocytosis, and paralytic ileus. The initial ascitic fluid total protein count is less than 1.0 mm^3/dL. The absolute polymorphonuclear count in the ascitic fluid is generally greater than 250 cells/dL. Bacterial peritonitis associated with a perforated viscus is secondary bacterial peritonitis.

22. The answer is D [X C 2]. This patient has acute mesenteric ischemia, which is a classic syndrome characterized by decreased blood supply; usually the superior mesenteric artery is involved. In general, patients have comorbid conditions such as atherosclerotic cardiovascular disease, congestive heart failure (CHF), acute myocardial infarction (MI), cerebrovascular disease, or peripheral vascular disease. Clinical presentation is the basis of diagnosis. Symptoms include sudden, severe periumbilical pain with a benign physical examination (symptoms are out of proportion to the physical examination). Abdominal radiographs may show separation of bowel loops or “thumbprinting.” The leukocyte count is generally greater than 20,000 cells/mm^3, and metabolic acidosis is present.

23. The answer is B [I B 3 d]. The most likely mechanism for gastroesophageal reflux in patients with scleroderma is decreased lower esophageal sphincter (LES) pressure. Presence of *Helicobacter pylori* in gastric mucosa is not a predisposing factor for gastroesophageal reflux. Although increased gastric acid secretion may cause and aggravate gastroesophageal reflux, it is not the mechanism in this case. Decreased esophageal peristalsis can be observed in patients with scleroderma but occurs in the lower third of esophagus. Esophageal muscle spasm is not associated with gastroesophageal reflux.

24. The answer is C [I B 2 a]. Barrett’s esophagus is the major predisposing factor in patients with adenocarcinoma of the esophagus. Smoking, alcohol ingestion, geographic factors, achalasia, and tylosis are important predisposing factors for squamous cell carcinoma of the esophagus. Achalasia and celiac sprue are associated with squamous cell carcinoma of the esophagus.

25. The answer is D [IX A 1 f]. The characteristic histologic findings in patients with chronic hepatitis are inflammation of portal triad with piecemeal necrosis. Chronic healthy carriers of hepatitis B (HBV) have normal liver histology. Hepatitis B surface antigen (HB_sAG) and core antibody (anti-HB_c) are detected in healthy carriers and patients with chronic hepatitis. Anti–smooth muscle antibody and α-fetoprotein (AFP) are not markers for HBV.

26. The answer is C [IX B 5]. In immunocompromised patients, *Mycobacterium avium-intracellulare* (MAI) can cause fever. Presence of granuloma is highly suggestive of mycobacterial infection. Polycystic liver disease generally does not cause increased liver tests. Hepatitis B (HBV) and hepatitis C (HCV) cause necroinflammatory parenchymal liver disease, and patients present with elevated aspartate aminotransferase (AST) and alanine aminotransferase (ALT). Although sclerosing cholangitis may occur in patients with acquired immunodeficiency syndrome (AIDS), granuloma is not the usual histologic finding in these individuals.

27. The answer is D [IX A 1 d]. The presence of hepatitis B surface antibody (anti-HB_s) in the absence of hepatitis B core antibody (anti-HB_c) indicates previous vaccination against hepatitis B (HBV). Patients with acute hepatitis A (HAV) have hepatitis A IgM antibody, and those with acute HBV are positive for hepatitis B surface antigen (HB_sAg).

28. The answer is A [IX A]. **Hepatitis B**

29. The answer is D [IX A]. **Hepatitis B RNA level**

30. The answer is A [IX A]. **Vaccination**

Polyarteritis nodosa or glomerulonephritis may develop in patients with hepatitis B (HBV). HBV places intravenous drug abusers, homosexual men, and individuals exposed to blood and blood products at high risk for HBV, a DNA virus. Hepatocellular carcinoma, cirrhosis, and chronic hepatitis may develop in patients in HBV, HCV, and hepatitis D (HDV). HDV is a small, defective RNA virus (delta agent). Cryoglobulinemia occurs in patients with HCV only and not those with other forms of hepatitis. Fulminant hepatitis develops in HAV, HBV, and HCV. With hepatitis E, the mortality rate in pregnant women may be 10%–20%. Vaccines for the prevention of both HAV and HBV are available, which are far more effective in preventing transmission than recommendations to avoid contact or exposure to hepatitis patients. Hepatitis B immune globulin (HBIG) has been shown to decrease the severity of hepatitis B but is not as effective as vaccination in preventing hepatitis B.

chapter 6

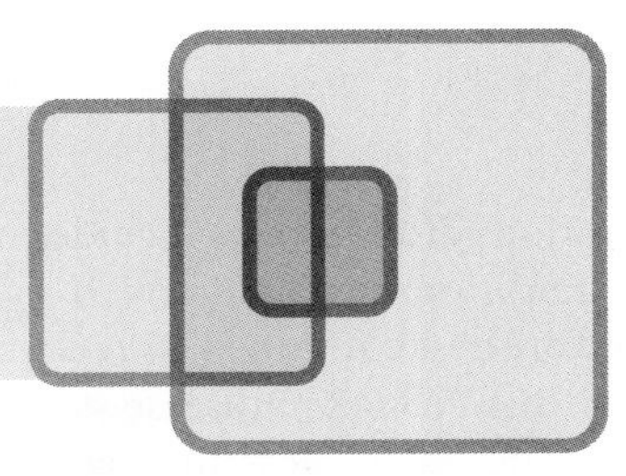

Renal Diseases, Fluid and Electrolyte Disorders, and Hypertension

FUAD N. ZIYADEH, STANLEY GOLDFARB

PART I: RENAL DISEASES

I CLINICAL ASSESSMENT OF RENAL FUNCTION

A Urinalysis

1. **Color.** Urine normally is yellow.
   a. **Darkening** on standing may be seen with some diseases (e.g., porphyria) and with certain drugs (e.g., methyldopa).
   b. **Red–orange–brown urine** may be seen with hematuria, hemoglobinuria, and myoglobinuria and with certain drugs (e.g., phenothiazines).
2. **Chemistry.** Qualitative chemical analysis of urine is performed with commercially available **dipsticks.**
   a. **Blood** usually is not present in normal urine. Intact erythrocytes, hemoglobin, and myoglobin all produce positive test results.
   b. **Glucose** usually is not present in normal urine above 0.3 g/24 hr.
   c. **Ketone bodies** are present in the urine of healthy individuals only during fasting. Sodium nitroprusside reagent detects acetoacetate but not β-hydroxybutyrate.
   d. **Protein** usually is not present in normal urine above 150 mg/24 hr. The dipstick detects only albumin, not immunoglobulins or light-chain polypeptides, which must be assayed using acid precipitation.
   e. **Bilirubin** is not present in normal urine. If elevated in blood, water-soluble conjugated bilirubin is filtered and present in urine.
   f. **Urine pH** can be maximally acidified below a pH of 5.0 and maximally alkalinized above a pH of 7.5.
3. **Concentration and dilution.** These values are measured by either specific gravity (normal = 1.000–1.025) or osmolality (normal = 50–1000 mOsm/kg urine). Many factors can affect urine concentration and dilution.
4. **Urinary sediment** of formed elements is prepared by centrifugation of urine at 2000 rpm for 10 minutes. The sediment from 12 mL of urine is resuspended in 1 mL of supernatant and is examined microscopically.
   a. **Crystals** that are seen in acid urine include cystine and uric acid; those found in alkaline urine include calcium phosphate and calcium oxalate.

b. **Cells** that are found in various disease states include erythrocytes, leukocytes, and epithelial cells (i.e., renal tubular, transitional, or squamous).

c. **Bacteria** may be seen and are best confirmed with Gram staining of the sediment.

d. **Casts** are cylindrical elements formed in disease states associated with low intrarenal urine flow or heavy proteinuria. The cast is a protein coagulum, which is formed in the renal tubule and traps any tubular luminal contents within its matrix. Casts are named for the elements recognized within them such as:

(1) Red blood cell (RBC) cast
(2) White blood cell (WBC) cast
(3) Renal tubular cell cast
(4) Granular cast
(5) Hyaline cast
(6) Waxy cast

B Renal function testing

1. **Glomerular filtration rate (GFR)** is a measure of the amount of plasma ultrafiltrate derived from blood in a specified period. (A normal GFR is 115–125 mL/min.) In most kidney diseases, the GFR is an accurate index of overall renal function.

2. **Urine concentrating ability** is determined by measuring urine osmolality after 18–24 hours of water deprivation and again after the administration of 5 units of **vasopressin.** Under these conditions, urine reaches an osmolality of 900 mOsm/kg (or a specific gravity of 1.023) in 90% of normal individuals.

3. **Urine diluting ability** is determined by measuring urine osmolality and volume 5 hours after a water load of 20 mL/kg body weight. In normal individuals, urine reaches an osmolality of 100 mOsm/kg (or a specific gravity of 1.003), and urine volume exceeds 80% of the water load.

4. **Renal urine acidification** can be tested by administering 100 mg ammonium chloride/kg body weight to decrease plasma bicarbonate concentration below 20 mEq/L. Urine normally acidifies (i.e., urine pH drops below 5.5) under these conditions. Fasting urine pH normally is below 5.5.

C Radiography

1. Plain film radiography, ultrasonography, and computed tomography (CT) are useful noninvasive techniques for determining renal size and the presence of obstruction, stones, or mass lesions.

2. Newer modalities such as Doppler ultrasonography may be useful for determining both vascular flow rates and urine flow. Magnetic resonance arteriography (MRA) is another newly developed method that allows noninvasive assessment of arterial function.

3. Intravenous urography and arteriography may also help define intrarenal morphology.

D Renal biopsy

1. **Indications** include acute renal failure of unknown etiology or abnormal course, delayed recovery from acute renal failure, and a poorly functioning or deteriorating renal allograft. Also, renal biopsy occasionally may be indicated in cases of nephrotic syndrome, acute glomerulonephritis, and in defining the progression of lupus nephritis.

2. **Contraindications** include diastolic blood pressure exceeding 100 mm Hg, infection at the biopsy site, and abnormal blood coagulation.

II ACUTE RENAL FAILURE

This sudden, rapid, but potentially reversible deterioration in renal function is sufficient to cause nitrogenous waste accumulation in body fluids.

A Etiology Causes may be prerenal, postrenal, or parenchymal (Table 6–1).

B Clinical features

1. **Azotemia.** Rising blood urea nitrogen (BUN) and serum creatinine levels are the most readily available laboratory signs of a decrease in GFR. These biochemical changes may be independent of clinical symptoms. Confounding variables that influence BUN and creatinine must be considered before renal failure is confirmed.
   a. BUN level is affected by rates of urea production, a function of the amount of dietary protein or protein breakdown (e.g., catabolic drugs or tissue injury), and by resorption of gastrointestinal or soft-tissue hemorrhage.
   b. Creatinine level is affected by endogenous creatinine production (increased by breakdown of muscle tissue), by renal creatinine secretion (which is blocked by such drugs as cimetidine and trimethoprim), and by noncreatinine chromogens (usually drugs) that cause measurement errors.
2. **Derangement of urine volume**
   a. **Anuria** (i.e., urine output of < 100 mL/day). Usually an ominous sign, anuria often indicates either complete arterial occlusion or severe renal injury. However, urine volume per se confers very little diagnostic specificity.
   b. **Oliguria** (i.e., urine output < 500 mL/day). Such output is insufficient to excrete the daily osmolar load. Although most patients with acute renal failure are oliguric, 25%–50% of such patients are not and produce more than 800 mL of urine daily.
   c. **Polyuria.** Patients may have acutely rising BUN and serum creatinine levels yet produce more than 3 L of urine daily. This condition may represent a less severe form of acute renal failure, with preservation of small amounts of glomerular filtration in the presence of tubular damage. Patients with partial urinary tract obstruction frequently present with polyuria.

C Diagnosis

1. **Patient history.** Acute renal failure usually results from several, often synergistic, renal injuries. A history should include information concerning:

TABLE 6–1 Causes of Acute Renal Failure

Classification	Pathophysiology	Example
Prerenal	Severe extracellular volume depletion	Gastrointestinal bleeding
	Decreased renal perfusion	Congestive heart failure
	Renal arterial obstruction	Renal embolus
Postrenal*	Intratubular obstruction	Acute urate nephropathy
	Intrarenal pelvic obstruction	Staghorn calculus
	Ureteropelvic obstruction	Kidney stone
	Ureteral obstruction	Stone, clot, compression by extrarenal lymph nodes
	Bladder outlet obstruction	Prostatic hypertrophy
Renal parenchymal	Acute tubular necrosis	Sepsis
	Nephrotoxicity	Aminoglycoside antibiotics, radiocontrast dyes
	Intrinsic renal diseases	
	Glomerulonephritis	Poststreptococcal glomerulonephritis
	Tubulointerstitial nephritis	Drug-induced
	Vasculitis	Wegener's granulomatosis

*Must be bilateral, except in patients with only one kidney when it is unilateral.

a. Recent surgical and radiographic procedures
b. Past and present use of medications
c. Allergies
d. Underlying chronic renal disease
e. Family history of renal disease
f. History of voiding difficulties (suggestive of obstructive uropathy)

2. **Physical examination.** The physical examination should be organized to parallel the differential diagnosis.
   a. **Prerenal failure** is suggested by clinical signs of:
      (1) Intravascular volume depletion (e.g., orthostatic changes in blood pressure and pulse, poor skin turgor)
      (2) Congestive heart failure (CHF)
   b. **Acute allergic interstitial nephritis** is suggested by eosinophilia, eosinophiluria, fever, and maculopapular rash.
   c. **Lower urinary tract obstruction** is suggested by a suprapubic or flank mass or symptoms of bladder dysfunction (e.g., hesitancy, urgency).

3. **Urinalysis**
   a. **Sediment.** Microscopic examination of urinary sediment provides information for the differential diagnosis.
      (1) The presence of few formed elements or only **hyaline casts** is suggestive of prerenal or postrenal failure.
      (2) An abundance of **erythrocytes** is uncommon in the absence of calculi, trauma, infection, or tumor.
      (3) An abundance of **leukocytes** may signify infection, immune-mediated inflammation, or an allergic reaction somewhere in the urinary tract.
      (4) **Eosinophiluria** occurs in up to 95% of patients with acute allergic interstitial nephritis. Hansel's stain often is needed to distinguish eosinophils from neutrophils in urine.
      (5) **Brownish pigmented cellular casts** and many renal tubular epithelial cells are observed in 75% of patients with acute tubular necrosis (ATN). Pigmented casts without erythrocytes in the sediment from urine with a positive dipstick for occult blood indicate either hemoglobinuria or myoglobinuria.
      (6) **RBC casts** suggest the possibility of acute glomerulonephritis.
   b. **Culture.** Urine culture should be performed in all patients.
   c. **Urine and blood chemistries.** Several biochemical indices aid in evaluation. Mainly, these tests distinguish acute oliguria due to prerenal azotemia from that due to parenchymal renal disease (ATN), on the basis that renal tubular function is preserved in the former condition and severely disturbed in the latter.
      (1) The **renal failure index** is the ratio of the urine sodium concentration to the urine-to-plasma creatinine ratio expressed as a percentage $[U_{Na}/(U_{Cr}/P_{Cr}) \times 100]$. Generally, values below 1% are consistent with prerenal failure but may be seen in ATN following cardiac surgery, and values above 1% indicate ATN.
      (2) The **fractional excretion of sodium** is the ratio of the urine-to-plasma sodium ratio to the urine-to-plasma creatinine ratio expressed as a percentage $[(U_{Na}/P_{Na})/(U_{Cr}/P_{Cr}) \times 100]$. Values below 1% suggest prerenal failure, and values above 1% suggest ATN.
      (3) **Abnormal blood chemistries** occasionally aid in the diagnosis of renal failure. A BUN-to-serum creatinine ratio above 20 is common in prerenal azotemia.

4. **Radiography**
   a. **Ultrasonography** is the method of choice for identifying the presence of two kidneys, for evaluating kidney size and shape, and for detecting **hydronephrosis** or **hydroureter.** Kidneys measurements are 10%–20% smaller with ultrasonography than with intravenous urography.

Renal calculi, abdominal aneurysms, and renal vein thrombosis sometimes are detected by ultrasonography.

b. **Isotopic flow scans** are marginally useful for evaluating the degree of renal perfusion and the presence of obstructive uropathy. Particularly useful is the radiopharmaceutical agent **diethylenetriamine pentaacetic acid (DTPA),** which is excreted only when there is free flow. Scanning using **hippurate** is useful in assessing whether tubular function is intact. Isotopic scans are most helpful in evaluating the function of the renal allograft.

c. **CT** scans are especially useful in evaluating the nature of **cystic masses** (i.e., benign or malignant).

d. **Retrograde pyelography** is performed by injecting contrast material into the ureteral orifice during cystoscopic examination. Specific indications include certain cases of suspected obstructive uropathy in which intervention to relieve the obstruction is contemplated.

5. **Biopsy** is relevant in only a select group of candidates, because the histologic severity and clinical course of acute renal failure usually do not correlate well. It is reserved for patients in whom the cause of nephrotic syndrome is sought or in whom an acute inflammatory lesion such as vasculitis is suspected and requires cytotoxic therapy for treatment. (Patients who follow a classic laboratory and clinical course of ATN usually do not benefit from renal biopsy.)

6. **Cystoscopy** is indicated in all cases of urethral obstruction and in some cases of ureteral obstruction.

D Clinical course

1. **Stages.** Acute renal failure due to ATN typically occurs in three stages: **azotemic, diuretic,** and **recovery.** The initial, azotemic stage can be either oliguric or nonoliguric.

2. **Morbidity and mortality.** The occurrence of oliguria affects morbidity and mortality rates.
   a. Gastrointestinal bleeding, septicemia, metabolic acidemia, and neurologic abnormalities are more common in patients with oliguria.
   b. The risk of mortality is more than two times greater in patients with oliguria, although other factors such as concomitant respiratory or cardiac failure also increase mortality dramatically.

3. **Prognosis.** Both the severity of the underlying disease and the clinical setting in which acute renal failure occurs affect outcome. For example, the mortality rate among patients with ATN is 60% when ATN is a result of surgery or trauma, 30% when it occurs as a complication of medical illness, and 10%–15% when pregnancy is involved. Ischemia-associated ATN has nearly twice the mortality risk of nephrotoxic ATN. In patients with no complicating factors who survive an episode of acute renal failure, the chance of complete recovery of kidney function is 90%. Recent data suggest that the use of certain types of dialyzers in patients who require dialysis may also influence prognosis (see Part I: I E 4).

E Therapy

1. **Preliminary measures**
   a. **Exclusion of reversible causes.** Obstruction should be relieved, nephrotoxic drugs should be withdrawn, infection should be treated, and electrolyte derangements should be corrected.
   b. **Correction of prerenal factors.** Intravascular volume and cardiac performance should be optimized.
   c. **Maintenance of urine output.** Although the prognostic importance of oliguria is debated, management of patients without oliguria is clearly easier than management of patients with oliguria. Hemodynamic parameters and intravascular volume should be optimized. Loop diuretics may be useful to convert the oliguric form of ATN to the nonoliguric form. Sustained infusions of loop-active diuretics rather than bolus infusions are the most effective mechanism for increasing urine flow.

2. **Conservative measures**
   a. **Fluid and electrolyte management.** Patients with acute renal failure are catabolic and usually lose 0.3 kg of body weight daily. Weight gain or stability usually indicates salt and water retention.
      (1) Total oral and intravenous water administration should equal daily **sensible losses** (via urine, stool, and nasogastric or surgical tube drainage) plus estimated **insensible** (i.e., respiratory and dermal) losses, which usually equal 600–800 mL/day.
      (2) Combined dietary and intravenous sodium and potassium intake should not exceed the measured 24-hour urinary losses of these electrolytes.
      (3) Sodium bicarbonate should be administered if acidemia becomes severe (i.e., if serum bicarbonate concentration drops below 16 mEq/L).
      (4) Oral phosphate-binding antacids (e.g., **calcium acetate**) should be given if the serum phosphate concentration exceeds 6.0 mg/dL.
      (5) Magnesium-containing drugs (e.g., magnesium citrate, magnesium hydroxide–containing antacids) should be withheld.
   b. **Dietary management.** Adequate caloric intake is essential for patients with renal failure. Generally, sufficient calories reflect a diet that provides 40–60 g of protein and 35–50 kcal/kg lean body weight. In some patients, severe catabolism occurs, and protein supplementation to achieve 1.25 g of protein/kg body weight is required to maintain nitrogen balance.
3. **Drug usage.** Patients who develop renal failure abruptly show only a 1.0 mg/dL/day increase in serum creatinine because endogenous creatinine production remains constant. Therefore, it is impossible to calculate appropriate drug doses based on serum creatinine level until a new steady state is achieved. Measurement of serum drug levels often is necessary for safe drug use.
4. **Dialysis.** This procedure is indicated in the management of progressive renal failure that leads to severe uremia, intractable acidemia, hyperkalemia, or volume overload. Clinical research has demonstrated that the use of artificial **biocompatible membranes** improves the mortality of patients with acute renal failure who require dialysis. In addition to hemodialysis and peritoneal dialysis, **chronic arteriovenous hemofiltration with or without dialysis (CAVH or CAVHD)** or the more commonly used **chronic venovenous hemofiltration (CVVH or CVVHD)** are highly effective forms of renal replacement therapy. These modalities utilize highly permeable membranes, which allow the dialysis or filtration processes to occur at very low hydrostatic pressures and flows. Thus, the patient's own blood pressure **(CAVH) or simple blood pumps (CVVH)** can provide the driving force.

F Complications

1. **Intravascular overload** involves weight gain, hypertension, elevated central venous pressure (as indicated by internal jugular vein distention), and pulmonary or peripheral edema.
2. **Hyperkalemia** (i.e., serum potassium concentration > 5.5 mEq/L) develops as a result of decreased renal excretion combined with tissue necrosis or hemolysis.
3. **Hyponatremia** (i.e., serum sodium concentration < 135 mEq/L) results from excessive water intake in the face of excretory failure.
4. **Hyperphosphatemia** (i.e., serum phosphate concentration > 5.5 mg/dL) results from ongoing phosphorus intake in the face of excretory failure or tissue necrosis.
5. **Hypocalcemia** (i.e., serum calcium concentration < 8.5 mg/dL) results from decreased 1,25-hydroxy vitamin D levels, hyperphosphatemia, or hypoalbuminemia.
6. **Hypercalcemia** (i.e., serum calcium concentration > 10.5 mg/dL) rarely occurs during the recovery phase following rhabdomyolysis-induced acute renal failure.
7. **Acidemia** (i.e., arterial blood pH < 7.35) is associated with sepsis or severe heart failure.

8. **Hyperuricemia** does not require therapy unless the serum uric acid concentration exceeds 15 mg/dL.
9. **Bleeding** may occur secondary to platelet dysfunction and coagulopathy associated with sepsis.
10. **Seizures** are related to uremia.
11. **Chronic renal failure** may occur. A modest decline in filtration may exist in 10% of patients for several months following acute renal failure. In patients with underlying renal disease who experience acute renal failure, progression to chronic renal failure is relatively likely. The majority of patients who survive acute renal failure recover from the acute insult. However, surviving patients with **diabetes mellitus** are more likely to develop chronic renal failure that requires dialysis.

III CHRONIC RENAL FAILURE

This substantial and irreversible reduction in renal function develops over a period of months or years to less than 20% of normal.

A Etiology

1. **Prerenal causes** include severe, long-standing renal artery stenosis and bilateral renal arterial embolism.
2. **Renal causes** include chronic glomerulonephritis, chronic tubulointerstitial nephritis, systemic lupus erythematosus (SLE), diabetes mellitus, amyloidosis, hypertension, cystic diseases, neoplasia, and radiation nephritis.
3. **Postrenal causes** derive from long-standing urinary obstruction.

B Clinical features

Presenting manifestations are highly variable. The following constellation of signs and symptoms is referred to as **uremia.**

1. **Neurologic signs** of lethargy, somnolence, confusion, and neuromuscular irritability develop either gradually or abruptly. Asterixis is a typical finding.
2. **Cardiovascular signs** of hypertension, CHF, and pericarditis also may be precipitous.
3. **Gastrointestinal signs,** particularly anorexia, nausea, vomiting, and a metallic taste, are very common.
4. **Metabolic signs** can either be nonspecific (e.g., fatigue, pruritus, sleep disturbances) or be referable to a specific defect (e.g., bone pain from secondary hyperparathyroidism).

C Diagnosis

The important aim of the diagnostic approach is to establish the chronicity of the renal disease as well as the potential etiologies. Specific approaches are provided in the discussions of specific etiologies.

D Therapy

1. **Dietary restrictions** are vital to the proper care of patients to reduce symptoms and, possibly, retard the progression of renal failure. Dietary protein is restricted to 0.6 g/kg lean body weight, and dietary sodium is restricted to 4 g/day unless residual urine output obligates greater daily losses. (In these cases, urine sodium excretion should be measured and replaced, but not exceeded, in the diet.) Dietary intake of potassium, magnesium, and phosphorus is restricted, and a fluid intake limit is established based on daily losses. It should be noted that most patients with chronic renal failure who do not yet require dialysis do not need severe fluid restriction.
2. **Renal replacement therapy** is necessary for maintenance care of end-stage renal disease.
   a. **Indications** include clinical uremia, severe azotemia (i.e., GFR < 15 mL/min), intractable hyperkalemia or acidemia, and intravascular volume overload.
   b. **Modalities** include hemodialysis, peritoneal dialysis, and renal allograft transplantation.

E Complications Various disorders arise in the course of chronic renal failure and during long-term renal replacement therapy. (A more detailed discussion of renal replacement therapy and complications associated with its treatment appears in Part I: IV.)

1. **Hematologic disorders** include severe anemia and bleeding.
2. **Cardiovascular disorders** include hypertension, pericarditis, cardiomyopathy, arrhythmias, and CHF.
3. **Neuromuscular disorders** include generalized seizures, confusion, lethargy, emotional lability, myopathy, peripheral neuropathy, and syndromes related to nerve compression (e.g., carpal tunnel syndrome).
4. **Gastrointestinal disorders** include ulcers, gastroduodenitis, colitis, and angiomas of the entire gastrointestinal tract.
5. **Endocrine disorders** include secondary hyperparathyroidism, clinically euthyroid hypothyroxinemia, hyperprolactinemia, altered pituitary and gonadal function (amenorrhea and impotence), and gynecomastia.
6. **Immune system disturbances** include lymphocytopenia, anergy, increased serum anticomplement activity, and abnormal monocyte motility. Whether patients may have increased vulnerability to infectious diseases remains unproven.
7. **Metabolic disorders** include renal osteodystrophy (osteitis fibrosa and osteomalacia) and altered drug metabolism.

IV MEDICAL COMPLICATIONS OF RENAL REPLACEMENT THERAPY

A Introduction Renal replacement therapy in patients with chronic renal failure is indicated for uremia (especially pericarditis, neuropathy, and osteodystrophy); intractable hyperkalemia, acidemia, and CHF; extracellular fluid volume overload that is unresponsive to diuretics; and certain intoxications and poisonings. The choice of modality (i.e., hemodialysis, peritoneal dialysis, or renal transplantation) and the timing of initiation of renal replacement therapy are based on patient age, underlying diseases, complicating medical conditions, patient preference and motivation, and practical considerations relating to donor availability and to available sites of peritoneal or vascular dialysis access.

B Hemodialysis This type of renal replacement therapy involves **extracorporeal circulation** of blood through a dialysis membrane–containing unit via a surgically constructed vascular fistula or a temporary or permanent external catheter. Percutaneous puncture and cannulation of the vascular access are required at each treatment. Blood and dialysate are separated by the semipermeable membrane, which allows solutes and water to move from blood to dialysate along electrochemical, hydrostatic and osmotic pressure gradients. Complications of hemodialysis, with various manifestations and etiologies, can develop at any stage of the procedure (Table 6–2).

C Peritoneal dialysis This type of renal replacement therapy involves instillation of 1–3 L sterile dialysate into the peritoneal cavity via a surgically implanted catheter and drainage of the dialysate after a specified **dwell period.** Frequent, brief exchanges (i.e., forty-eight 1-hour exchanges) may be performed weekly in-center. Longer exchanges (i.e., four 6-hour exchanges) also are effective and may be done on a continuous ambulatory basis daily. **Even more frequent exchanges may be performed at night with an automated cycler.** Maintenance peritoneal dialysis is associated with specific complications.

1. **Excessive removal of fluid** may result in hypotension, light-headedness, weakness, or syncope.
2. **Catheter-related complications** include occlusion (usually by fibrinous debris), infection, malposition, and, rarely, fracture.

TABLE 6–2 Complications of Dialysis—Their Manifestations or Etiologies

Acute Complication	Manifestations or Etiologies
Improper dialyzer preparation	Contamination by preservative (formalin), air bubbles, or bacteria, embolism, sepsis, or membrane rupture
Improper water treatment	Excess calcium, magnesium, aluminum, fluoride, or copper; improper cleansing of municipal water supplies, which may lead to chloramine poisoning and severe hemolysis
Equipment failure	Power failure, air leaks, blood loss from line separation, hypo- or hyperthermia due to improperly warmed dialysate
Allergic reactions	Urticaria, anaphylaxis in response to material in tubing or dialyzer (e.g., sterilants)
Vascular access problems	Bleeding from puncture sites, suture lines, aneurysmal dilatation, endovascular infection
Anticoagulant complications	Local access bleeding, gastrointestinal bleeding
Transfusion complications	Hemosiderosis, hepatitis
Hypotension	Induced by acute volume shifts or true volume depletion; acetate in dialysis fluid, which may induce vasodilatation; autonomic dysfunction secondary to uremic neuropathy
Cardiac arrhythmias	During and following treatment; premature ventricular contractions are commonest form
Dialysis dysequilibrium	Headache, nausea, vomiting, muscle aches, and cramps

3. **Dialysate-related complications** that develop if dialysate is too rapidly infused or inadequately warmed include abdominal or back pain, nausea, and vomiting.
4. **Peritonitis** is the most serious complication occurring in chronic peritoneal dialysis patients. Infection develops by inoculation through or around the catheter or by contamination of dialysate.
   a. Recurrent peritonitis is associated with high morbidity rates, frequent hospital stays, and considerable expense. Peritoneal fibrosis and loss of dialysis efficiency can complicate multiple recurrent infections and may constitute criteria for withdrawal from this form of therapy.
   b. Treatment of peritonitis is with parenteral and intraperitoneal antibiotics.
   c. Newer catheter configurations (y sets) have markedly reduced the incidence of dialysis-induced peritonitis.

D **Renal allograft transplantation** This procedure may be performed from a donor to a recipient if these individuals are **histocompatible.** Histocompatibility is measured by determination of **human leukocyte antigen (HLA)** types, **mixed lymphocyte reactivity (MLR),** and **blood group** types. Donor kidneys may be from a living relative or from a cadaver with no evidence of infectious disease, specifically, bacteremia, hepatitis, acquired immunodeficiency syndrome (AIDS), cytomegalovirus (CMV), syphilis, or malaria. Transplant recipients are given maintenance immunosuppressive agents (e.g., **prednisone, azathioprine, mycophenolate mofetil, cyclosporine, tacrolimus,** or **rapamycin**) to prevent graft rejection. Complications of transplantation originate from several sources.

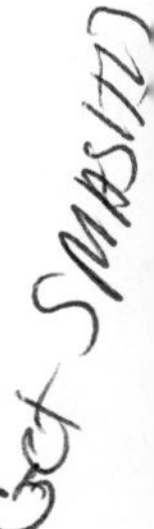

1. **Immunosuppressive disorders** include leukopenia (alkylating agents), hepatitis and vaso-occlusive disease (azathioprine), diarrhea (mycophenolate mofetil), diabetes, obesity, cataracts, and, possibly, peptic ulcer disease, avascular necrosis of bone, and pancreatitis (prednisone). Nephrotoxicity, tremors, hirsutism, and hypertension may result from use of cyclosporine and tacrolimus. Diabetes mellitus is reported with tacrolimus. Hyperlipidemia is common with rapamycin.
2. **Secondary hypertension** may develop from extracellular fluid overload (prednisone), high renin secretion from native kidneys, vascular stenosis of the graft from anastomotic stricture or extrinsic

compression by lymphocele or urinoma, rejection, recurrent glomerular disease, ureteral obstruction, or hypercalcemia. Coincident primary (essential) hypertension also may develop.

3. **Infection** may occur at any time following transplantation by common pathogens as well as by opportunistic organisms.
   a. Common infections include urinary tract infection (60% of patients), pneumonia (20% of patients), wound or cannula infection, hepatitis, and sepsis.
   b. Uncommon infections encountered in transplant recipients include CMV-associated pneumonia, hepatitis, retinitis, encephalitis, or mononucleosis syndrome; *Cryptococcus* infection; *Listeria monocytogenes* meningitis (usually occurring 6 months post-transplantation); *Pneumocystis carinii* infection, and *Legionella pneumophila* infection.
4. **Rejection** may be **hyperacute** (immediate and intraoperative), **acute** (occurring 4–60 days following transplantation), or **chronic** (occurring > 60 days following transplantation).
   a. **Acute rejection** is associated with fever, decreased creatinine clearance, oliguria, sodium retention, graft enlargement and tenderness, hypertension, and proteinuria. Treatment for acute rejection may include high-dose corticosteroids, antilymphocyte globulin, monoclonal antibodies directed against cytotoxic lymphocytes, and, occasionally, transplant (graft) nephrectomy.
   b. **Chronic rejection,** which is clinically less dramatic, can be suspected on the basis of decreased creatinine clearance, increased proteinuria, hyperchloremic metabolic acidosis, hypertension, oliguria, weight gain, and edema. About 5% of allografts are lost due to chronic rejection that occurs within 5 years of transplantation. Chronic rejection occurs in the majority of grafts with time, and there is no therapy.
5. **Malignancy** develops in 2%–7% of transplant recipients, a rate that is 100 times greater than the malignancy rate in healthy, age-matched individuals.
   a. The majority of tumors (in order of frequency) involve cancer of the skin and lips, lymphomas [especially of the central nervous system (CNS)], cervical carcinoma, lung carcinoma, head and neck cancer, and colon carcinoma.
   b. The average time for malignancy to develop is 40 months but may range from 1–158 months. Lymphomas develop sooner (within 27 months of transplantation).

V PROTEINURIA

A Definition

Normal adults excrete less than 150 mg of protein in a 24-hour period; **small–molecular-weight proteins** are the major component. Urinary protein excretion exceeding 300 mg/24 hr is termed **proteinuria.** Albumin normally is excreted in the urine at a rate of less than 25 mg/day. Higher rates suggest an abnormality in glomerular barrier function, which normally precludes the albumin molecule from crossing the glomerular basement membrane (GBM). **Macroalbuminuria** refers to an excretion rate of albumin greater than 300 mg/day, a condition detectable with routine screening methods. **Microalbuminuria** refers to a urine albumin excretion rate that exceeds 20 μg/min but is less than 200 μg/min (i.e., 30–300 mg/24 hr). Small–molecular-weight proteins are excreted at an increased rate if proximal reabsorptive function is impaired (as in **tubular proteinuria**).

B Etiology

1. **Orthostatic proteinuria** refers to an increase in urinary protein that is detectable only when the patient has been standing. The 24-hour urinary protein output tends to remain constant at about 0.5–2.5 g/24 hr, renal function remains normal, and the prognosis is excellent.
2. **Tubulointerstitial nephritis** involves the excretion of tubular proteins such as **Tamm-Horsfall protein and β_2-microglobulin** in addition to albumin. Tubulointerstitial nephritis is typically seen in patients with drug-induced disease, chronic inflammatory disease (e.g., sarcoidosis), or analgesic nephropathy.

3. **Glomerulonephritis** typically produces albuminuria (> 2 g/24 hr). Nephrotic syndrome (hypoalbuminemia, edema, and hyperlipidemia) occurs when protein excretion exceeds 3 g/24 hr.

C Diagnosis

1. **Urinalysis**
   a. Screening tests for proteinuria include urine dipstick (albumin only) and **sulfosalicylic acid precipitation** (albumin, paraproteins, immunoglobulins, and amyloid).
   b. Quantitative, 24-hour testing for urinary protein is essential, particularly in low-volume/high-concentration states (e.g., CHF). However, an early morning single urine specimen in which albumin concentration is factored for creatinine concentration (gram of protein per gram of creatinine) is a convenient screening assay. A ratio > 0.3 is indicative of significant proteinuria. The diagnosis of **microalbuminuria** requires a sensitive radioimmunoassay on first morning (early morning) voided urine and also should be factored for creatinine to correct for problems of varying urinary concentration. Microalbuminuria is present when the albumin-to-creatinine ratio is between 30 and 300 mg per g creatinine.
   c. Lipiduria is suggested by oval fat bodies on microscopic study.
2. **Urine and blood chemistries** in patients with macroalbuminuria should include quantitative protein measurement and urine protein electrophoresis. Elevated blood lipids and hypoalbuminemia support a diagnosis of nephrotic syndrome.
3. **Biopsy** is indicated in the evaluation of patients with significant proteinuria and nephrotic syndrome when no obvious cause is identified by noninvasive means. Pathologic study should include electron microscopy, immunofluorescence, and the use of special stains (e.g., Congo red for amyloid).

D Therapy

1. **Orthostatic proteinuria.** Treatment is not required.
2. **Tubulointerstitial proteinuria.** The underlying disorder must be identified and treated.
3. **Glomerulonephritic proteinuria.** The underlying disorder should be treated. Angiotensin-converting enzyme (ACE) inhibitors are useful for controlling proteinuria associated with glomerular disease. Supportive therapy includes diuretics, lipid-lowering agents, and dietary protein restriction.

E Complications

The consequences of hyperlipidemia (atherosclerosis and coronary artery disease), vitamin D deficiency (bone disease), urinary loss of certain proteins impeding spontaneous coagulation (thrombosis), and marked salt retention (massive edema, or anasarca) may result. It has been suggested that patients with nephrotic syndrome are more susceptible to bacterial infections, particularly spontaneous bacterial peritonitis secondary to pneumococcus in children.

VI HEMATURIA

A Definition

Normal adults excrete 500,000–2,000,000 erythrocytes/24 hr, which amounts to less than three erythrocytes per high-power field of resuspended urinary sediment.

B Etiology

Causes of hematuria are summarized in Table 6–3.

C Diagnosis

1. **Urinalysis**
   a. Dipstick testing cannot differentiate hematuria from pigmenturia (i.e., hemoglobinuria or myoglobinuria). A positive **orthotolidine test** in the absence of microscopically detected erythrocytes practically confirms the diagnosis of pigmenturia.
   b. Urine culture should be performed routinely.

TABLE 6–3 Causes of Hematuria

Etiology	Clinical Features
Glomerulonephritis Diffuse (e.g., SLE, vasculitis)	Gross or microscopic hematuria, abnormal proteinuria, red blood cell casts, dysmorphic red cells by phase-contrast microscopy
Focal (e.g., I_gA nephritis, thin basement membrane disease)	Gross or microscopic hematuria without proteinuria, dysmorphic red cells by phase-contrast microscopy
Vascular disease	Gross or microscopic hematuria without proteinuria, isomorphic red cells by phase-contrast microscopy
Tumors (e.g., hypernephroma, bladder cancer)	Isomorphic red cells by phase-contrast microscopy
Trauma	Isomorphic red cells by phase-contrast microscopy
Kidney stones	Isomorphic red cells by phase-contrast microscopy
Systemic coagulopathies	Isomorphic red cells by phase-contrast microscopy

SLE = systemic lupus erythematosus.

2. **Radiography**
   a. Intravenous urography can demonstrate renal masses, cysts, vascular malformations, papillary necrosis, ureteral stricture or obstruction by calculus, bladder tumor, and ureteral deviation. CT scanning is the preferred modality for assessment of renal masses or cysts for malignant characteristics.
   b. Special studies (e.g., angiography, nuclear scanning) occasionally are of value in delineating mass lesions.
3. **Biopsy** occasionally may assist in making a diagnosis of **renal hematuria with thin basement membranes** or in characterizing the lesion of a primary glomerular disease.
4. **Cystoscopy** is indicated in the evaluation of hematuria when physical examination, urinalysis, and other imaging studies fail to reveal the cause.

D Therapy

1. The underlying disorder must be identified and treated.
2. Urine volume should be maintained to prevent clots and obstruction in the lower urinary tract.

E Complications

1. **Iron deficiency anemia** rarely may complicate chronic, significant hematuria.
2. **Lower urinary tract clots** can induce obstruction.

VII NEPHROLITHIASIS

A Definition **Renal calculi** or **stones** arise due to papillary calcification or precipitation in urine of organized crystalline bodies of calcium salts, uric acid, cystine, or struvite. The etiologies of nephrolithiasis are given in Table 6–4.

B Clinical features Signs and symptoms may vary considerably.

1. **Occult passage** of small, asymptomatic stones may occur. More frequently, however, asymptomatic renal stones are identified radiographically during evaluation for other, unrelated conditions.
2. **Hematuria** virtually always accompanies stone movement within the urinary tract and may be microscopic or gross. Hematuria may occur with or without pain.

TABLE 6–4 Etiology of Nephrolithiasis

Stone Type	Etiology or Associated Condition
Calcium phosphate stones	Hyperparathyroidism, distal renal tubular acidosis, idiopathic hypercalciuria, and medullary sponge kidney
Calcium oxalate stones	Idiopathic hypercalciuria, excess diet oxalate, vitamin C abuse, small bowel diseases, primary hyperoxaluria, and hypercalcemia; 50% of patients have no identifiable abnormality
Uric acid stones	Persistently concentrated and acid urine, hyperuricosuria, hyperuricemia (in gout), and excess dietary purine
Cystine stones	Cystinuria
Struvite stones (triple phosphate, or magnesium–ammonium–calcium phosphate)	Urinary tract infection (chronic or recurrent) by urease-producing bacteria such as *Proteus, Providencia, Klebsiella, Pseudomonas, Serratia,* and *Enterobacter* species

3. **Frequency** and **dysuria** are common complaints of patients with stones lodged in the intravesical segment of the distal ureter and may be mistaken for the symptoms of **cystitis.** Dysuria also occurs during the passage of **sludge.**
4. **Abdominal pain, tenesmus,** and **rectal pain** may occur with a stone in the renal pelvis and often are accompanied by nausea and vomiting.
5. **Renal colic,** with flank pain radiating to the inguinal ligament, urethra, labia, testis, or penis, is typical of a stone in the midureter.
6. **Acute obstruction** by a stone may occur, generating renal colic. **Subacute obstruction** may occur with few or no symptoms.
7. **Infection** often complicates stone disease and usually produces flank or back pain, fever, and chills, particularly with urinary obstruction.

C Diagnosis

1. **Patient history** should identify other family members with stone disease as well as the patient's past and present use of drugs and vitamins (particularly vitamins A, C, and D).
2. **Physical examination** is necessary to differentiate acute renal colic from other causes of abdominal, pelvic, and back pain.
3. **Urinalysis** provides data in all cases.
   a. Urine pH is inappropriately high in renal tubular acidosis, favoring calcium phosphate stone formation. Low urine volume with low urine pH is a risk factor for uric acid stones.
   b. Crystals often are found appropriate to urine pH, with **acid urine** containing crystals of uric acid and cystine and **alkaline urine** containing crystals of calcium phosphate and struvite.
   c. Bacteriuria may signal infection-related stones; in such patients, urine culture should be performed.
4. **Urine** and **blood chemistries** are critical to the metabolic evaluation of the patient with nephrolithiasis.
   a. A blood sample should be examined for levels of electrolytes, creatinine, BUN, calcium, phosphate, and uric acid.
   b. A 24-hour urine collection should be studied for urine volume and pH as well as levels of calcium, phosphate, uric acid, oxalate, creatinine, sodium, citrate, and cystine.
5. **Radiography**
   a. **Plain abdominal films** are useful for identifying the composition of renal stones. Calcium stones are intensely radiopaque; cystine, struvite (infection-induced), and mixed uric acid–

calcium stones are moderately radiopaque. Abdominal films also help localize stones, and serial films indicate disease activity as reflected by increases in stone size and number.

b. **Intravenous urography** is necessary for evaluating radiolucent stones (uric acid) and obstruction of urine flow.

c. **Ultrasonography** and **CT** may be useful in some cases. Spiral (helical) CT, which has been shown to provide highly sensitive and specific information regarding the presence of kidney stones, is often the imaging modality of choice for the diagnosis of nephrolithiasis.

6. **Cystoscopy** is indicated for the detection and removal of bladder calculi and for the removal of ureteral stones lodged near the ureterovesical junction.

7. **Stone analysis** is the definitive tool for ascertaining the status of the stone (passed or retained) and its composition. All efforts should be made to strain urine and capture stones for chemical analysis.

D Therapy

1. **Medical therapy** is predicated on the identified metabolic disorder. In all circumstances, however, a urine volume of more than 2 L/day should be achieved.

a. **Calcium phosphate stones.** Primary hyperparathyroidism necessitates prompt treatment with parathyroidectomy, distal tubular acidosis requires independent evaluation, and idiopathic hypercalciuria requires diuretics (thiazides or amiloride) or oral neutral potassium phosphate.

b. **Calcium oxalate stones.** Therapy includes dietary restriction of oxalate-rich food, elimination of large doses (i.e., > 500 mg/day) of ascorbic acid, and administration of hypocalciuric diuretics (thiazides or amiloride) or oral neutral potassium phosphate. Oral administration of potassium citrate may be useful in increasing the urinary excretion of citrate, a major urinary chelator of ionized calcium and an inhibitor of calcium oxalate crystal growth.

c. **Uric acid stones.** Therapy includes administration of oral sodium bicarbonate to maintain an alkaline urine (i.e., pH > 6) and, in selected patients, restriction of dietary purine or administration of allopurinol.

d. **Cystine stones.** Sodium bicarbonate is administered to keep urine pH above 7.5, and acetazolamide is given at bedtime to maintain urine alkalinity during the night. Urine output should be maintained at more than 4 L/day. Noncompliant patients and those with severe or refractory stone disease may be candidates for oral D-penicillamine or intrarenal stone dissolution by alkaline or acetylcysteine irrigation.

e. **Struvite stones.** Treatment is aimed at maintaining urinary asepsis, which may require antibiotics.

2. In **extracorporeal shock wave lithotripsy,** electrically induced shock waves generated in a water bath are focused on the stone, leading to its in situ dissolution. This technique is safe and effective; moreover, it does not involve surgery. Its use in very large staghorn calculi may be somewhat limited because percutaneous extraction may be required to augment the noninvasive lithotripsy approach. Recent advances involving in situ lithotriptic techniques have broadened the scope of this approach.

3. **Surgical removal** is rarely required but is indicated for obstructing stones if there is infection proximal to the stone or if radiographic views indicate that the stone is too large to pass spontaneously. Staghorn calculi should be removed if renal function is in jeopardy.

VIII URINARY TRACT OBSTRUCTION

A Introduction An obstruction in the urinary tract may occur at any point between the renal tubules and the urethra. Urinary obstruction may be acute or chronic, unilateral or bilateral, and partial or complete. Chronic urinary obstruction often is partial and may be asymptomatic, particularly in slowly progressive cases. The consequences of urinary obstruction include structural changes in the lower urinary tract as a result of increases in pressure opposing normal urine flow (**obstructive uropathy**), gross dilatation of the calyces and collecting system of the affected kidney (**hydronephrosis**), and, ultimately, renal parenchymal damage (**obstructive nephropathy**).

B Etiology The causes of urinary obstruction can be divided into **mechanical** causes, which may be intrinsic or extrinsic, and **functional** causes.

1. **Intrinsic mechanical causes**
   a. **Intrarenal tubular obstruction** results from precipitation of uric acid, sulfonamide, or paraprotein crystals. Drugs such as indinavir, which are used in the treatment of human immunodeficiency virus (HIV), may lead to intratubular precipitation of crystals.
   b. **Extrarenal pelvic** or **ureteral obstruction** is caused by calculus, thrombus, papillary necrosis, or tumor.
   c. **Structural lesions of the ureter or bladder** include stricture, tumor, urethral valves, ureteroceles, and foreign body.
2. **Extrinsic mechanical causes**
   a. **Compression** may be caused by:
      (1) Prostatic hypertrophy or carcinoma
      (2) Uterine prolapse or tumor
      (3) Ovarian abscess, cyst, or tumor
      (4) Endometriosis
      (5) Pregnancy
      (6) Enlarged or aneurysmal pelvic vessels
      (7) Retroperitoneal tumor, infection, lymphadenopathy, or fibrosis
   b. **Surgical misadventures** include accidental ureteral ligation.
3. **Functional causes.** Ureteral or bladder dysfunction results from myelodysplasia; injury or congenital defect of the spinal cord; tabes dorsalis; diabetes mellitus; multiple sclerosis (MS), and autonomic neuropathy, including drug-induced neuropathy (e.g., due to disopyramide).

C Clinical features Signs and symptoms vary depending on the site of the obstruction and the speed with which the obstruction develops.

1. **An absence of symptoms** often occurs in chronic, slowly advancing obstructive disease. The clinical picture often is overshadowed by signs of the primary disease (e.g., in a case of metastatic tumor or surgical complications) until biochemical evidence of renal impairment develops.
2. **Pain and renal enlargement** (abdominal or flank mass) usually are present in acute obstruction. The pain characteristically is a steady crescendo, is most severe in the flank, and radiates toward the ipsilateral testis or labium.
3. **Urinary symptoms** predominate in obstructive disease of the bladder or urethra. Hesitancy, decreased force of urinary stream, urinary frequency, and dribbling are common in the context of obstruction.
4. **Renal functional impairment** typically is expressed as tubular defects in acid and potassium transport as well as defective tubular responsiveness to hormone action. Clinically, hyperkalemia, mild acidemia, and polyuria precede azotemia, which may progress to renal failure.

D Diagnosis

1. **Urinalysis** varies but may reveal inappropriately dilute urine, hematuria (in cases of obstruction due to calculus or tumor), or bacteriuria. Because infection often complicates obstruction, causing serious detriment to renal function, urine culture is essential. Examination of the urinary sediment often shows no abnormality but may reveal crystals of uric acid or sulfonamide.

2. **Blood chemistries** usually are not diagnostic but are helpful in assessing the severity of impaired renal function.

3. **Radiography** provides the clinical essential evidence of obstruction. Ultrasonography or CT reliably detects evidence of hydronephrosis such as calyceal blunting and dilatation of the renal pelvis, ureter, or both. Doppler ultrasonography may be effective in demonstrating the rate of urine flow from each ureter. Intravenous urography may fail to visualize the kidneys if the GFR is decreased substantially. Retrograde urography occasionally may help identify unilateral (particularly partial) ureteral obstruction. Nuclear scanning of the kidney often is specific enough to confirm the diagnosis.

E Therapy

1. **Relief of obstruction** is paramount and should be appropriate to the structural nature of the occluding lesion. Methods include surgery, percutaneous nephrostomy, ureteral stent, and nephroscopic stone removal.

2. **Medical management** following relief of obstruction is aimed at correcting postobstructive diuresis. Contributing factors include the excretion of solute (urea) that was retained during the period of obstruction and the impaired concentrating ability that usually exists in the recently obstructed kidney. Management involves careful, adequate fluid replacement with frequent assessment of body weight, intravascular volume, and blood and urine electrolyte concentration.

F Complications

1. **Infection,** particularly in the context of obstructing calculi, must be detected and promptly treated to prevent extensive pyelonephritis, perirenal abscess, and sepsis. A destructive process termed **xanthogranulomatous pyelonephritis** rarely may result from delay in treatment of the infected, obstructed kidney (see Part I IX F 2).

2. **Hypertension** occurs secondary to both intravascular volume expansion and ischemic stimulation of renin secretion.

3. **Polycythemia** has been reported in association with hydronephrosis and is purportedly due to increased erythropoietin release.

4. **Persistent tubular defects** may continue beyond 1 year following relief of obstruction. Impaired concentrating ability and limited excretion of a potassium load are the most common defects.

5. **Chronic renal failure** can develop from obstructive disease, most commonly with longstanding obstruction or with complicating urinary tract infection.

IX URINARY TRACT INFECTION

A Definition

Urinary tract infections are defined in terms of the involved urinary structures such as:

1. **Cystitis:** inflammation of the bladder
2. **Urethritis:** inflammation of the urethra
3. **Pyelonephritis:** inflammation of renal tubules and interstitium
4. **Prostatitis:** inflammation of the prostate gland

B Etiology

A clinical urinary tract infection occasionally develops from simple inoculation of the lower urinary tract during instrumentation or sexual intercourse. More commonly, however, other risk factors are present and increase the likelihood that inoculation will progress to clinical infection.

1. **Agents of infection**
   a. **Common agents** include *Escherichia coli, Proteus, Klebsiella, Enterobacter, Pseudomonas, Serratia,* enterococci, *Candida, Neisseria gonorrhoeae, Trichomonas vaginalis,* and herpes simplex virus (HSV).

b. **Uncommon agents** include *Staphylococcus* and mycobacteria that cause tuberculosis.
c. **Rare agents** include *Nocardia, Actinomyces, Brucella,* adenovirus, and *Torulopsis.*

2. **Routes of inoculation**
   a. **Urethral inoculation.** This route is very common in women, particularly those with vaginal and periurethral colonization by virulent bacteria. Local trauma, either mechanical (e.g., intercourse) or biologic (e.g., vaginitis, intertrigo), can predispose to superinfection of the periurethral mucosa. Surgery, particularly cystoscopy, can contaminate the bladder urine.
   b. **Hematogenous spread.** It is extremely unusual for gram-negative bacterial sepsis to induce pyelonephritis in the absence of other risk factors.

3. **Risk factors**
   a. **Obstruction** that induces urinary stasis and impairs host defenses (i.e., via decreased renal blood flow and decreased delivery of leukocytes and antibodies) is a crucial predisposing factor.
   b. **Vesicoureteral reflux** may promote ascending infection in several ways, including increased delivery of bacteria, increased size of the inoculum, incomplete bladder emptying, altered renal hemodynamics, and, possibly, altered host defenses.
   c. **Instrumentation,** particularly the use of urinary drainage (Foley) catheters, frequently is associated with significant bacteriuria.
   d. **Pregnancy** is clearly associated with altered ureteral smooth muscle function and a higher incidence of asymptomatic bacteriuria. The asymptomatic bacteriuria seen in pregnant women is more likely to progress to pyelonephritis than it is in nonpregnant women.
   e. **Diabetes mellitus** is associated with a high rate of infection. Part of this risk involves neurogenic bladder disturbances.
   f. **Immune deficiency,** whether congenital, acquired, or drug-induced, increases the risk of urinary infection in concert with generally increased patient susceptibility.

C Clinical features

1. **Lower tract infection.** Symptoms include urinary frequency, dysuria, burning, suprapubic pain, malodorous or cloudy urine, and continence difficulties. These symptoms (in any combination) are most common in urethritis, prostatitis (with or without perineal pain and ejaculatory pain), and cystitis.
2. **Acute pyelonephritis** (parenchymal renal infection). Symptoms include flank pain, fever, malaise, and any symptoms of lower tract infection.
3. **Septic shock.** Presenting signs of this condition, which is frequently seen in elderly or institutionalized patients, include hypothermia, mental status alterations, syncope, and coma.

D Diagnosis

1. **Urinalysis** of fresh, unspun urine should be performed. Dipstick tests that demonstrate the presence of enzymes such as the leukocyte esterases may be useful; sensitivity is over 90%. The identification of 1 bacterium per high-power field (400×) is indicative of a colony growth on culture of more than 10^5 colonies/mL. Analysis of the centrifuged sediment usually reveals leukocyturia (neutrophils) and bacteriuria. Gram staining of the urinary sediment is routine and may additionally characterize the offending organism, allowing more specific therapy before culture results are known. Microscopic hematuria is common.
2. **Routine urine culture** is the definitive method of diagnosis. A clean-catch, midstream specimen should be submitted for plating within 3 hours; the specimen should be refrigerated if any delay is anticipated. Unquestionably, the growth of more than 10^5 colonies/mL in the presence of symptoms signifies infection worthy of treatment. The diagnostic significance of culture growth below this level is debated. However, a growth of less than 10^5 colonies/mL may warrant therapy under appropriate clinical circumstances such as severe symptoms, a history of partial antibiotic treatment, known recurrent infections, any suspicion about the accuracy of the laboratory report,

and the presence of renal calculi. In some women, a count of 10^2 colonies/mL may indicate significant infection if accompanied by fever and pyuria. In men, in whom the likelihood of contamination is lower, 10^2 colonies/mL likely indicates infection.

3. **Special urine cultures** must be specifically ordered.
   a. In patients with typical symptoms but repeatedly negative routine cultures (**urethral syndrome**), infection with *Ureaplasma* or *Chlamydia* should be suspected and the laboratory instructed to search for these organisms.
   b. **HSV** requires special culture methods, and ***N. gonorrhoeae*** requires immediate inoculation on Thayer-Martin (chocolate agar) media and carbon dioxide incubation.
   c. Sterile pyuria, even in asymptomatic patients, should arouse suspicion of **renal tuberculosis.** A first morning urine specimen is best for detecting this condition.
4. **Blood chemistries** provide little information but occasionally demonstrate leukocytosis.
5. **Radiographic procedures** such as intravenous urography are helpful in the evaluation of infection complicating chronic vesicoureteral reflux, obstruction, calculi, and chronic pyelonephritis. Spiral CT can provide definitive information when the diagnosis is not evident on clinical grounds. Voiding cystourethrography and retrograde ureterography occasionally are indicated in the evaluation of recurrent infections, particularly in children.

E Therapy

1. **Antibiotics.** Initial antibacterial therapy is selected on the basis of the urinalysis and an understanding of the epidemiology and bacteriology of the infection. The appropriateness of this therapy must be confirmed by culture and sensitivity testing in refractory, relapsing, and atypical cases.
   a. **Uncomplicated lower tract infection** may be treated with amoxicillin (3.0 g orally over 3 days) or trimethoprim–sulfamethoxazole (320 mg/1.6 g orally over 3 days). Resistance to this therapy has begun to emerge, so clinicians should be aware of local patterns of bacterial susceptibility when choosing therapy. Special recommendations exist for gonorrhea, syphilis, and trichomoniasis.
   b. **Relapsing urinary tract infection and pyelonephritis** should be treated for 14 days. Clinically stable patients may be treated at home with trimethoprim–sulfamethoxazole (80 mg/400 mg orally, twice daily) or a first-generation cephalosporin.
   c. **Prostatitis** must be treated for at least 14 days with antibiotics that penetrate and remain active in prostatic tissue and fluid (e.g., trimethoprim, carbenicillin).
   d. **Recurrent infections** typically require regimens that include trimethoprim–sulfamethoxazole (40 mg/200 mg orally, once daily), methenamine mandelate (500 mg orally, four times daily), and sulfisoxazole (500 mg orally, once daily). Use of agents such as ciprofloxacin (500 mg daily) may result in sterilization of the urine.
   e. **Catheter-associated bacteriuria** in acutely catheterized patients usually resolves following removal of the catheter. Failure to do so or the development of symptoms within 12–24 hours necessitates appropriate antibacterial therapy.
2. **Surgery.** Corrective surgery is indicated for the removal of calculi and for the repair of obstructing anatomic lesions.

F Complications

1. **Abscess formation,** in either the kidney parenchyma or the surrounding retroperitoneal space, often complicates infection proximal to unrelieved obstruction. Persistent systemic symptoms and resistant bacteriuria should prompt diagnostic study using ultrasonography or CT.
2. **Xanthogranulomatous pyelonephritis** is a form of chronic bacterial infection characterized by granuloma formation with lipid-laden macrophages, often in a nonfunctioning kidney. *Proteus mirabilis* is the organism most frequently recovered from renal abscess fluid. Three-fourths of

patients have a history of nephrolithiasis, and in many cases a staghorn calculus is identified at surgery.

3. **Emphysematous pyelonephritis** is a rare, life-threatening complication of bacterial pyelonephritis. Seen most frequently in diabetics, this disease is characterized by gas-forming bacterial infection.
4. **Chronic renal failure** with end-stage renal disease may result from chronic pyelonephritis, particularly if it coexists with renal calculi or obstruction. Most cases of chronic renal failure due to chronic pyelonephritis are not bacterial in origin but represent a broad spectrum of chronic tubulointerstitial disease.

X GLOMERULAR DISEASE

A Hereditary nephritis (Alport's syndrome)

1. **Inheritance and incidence.** Hereditary nephritis is inherited as an X-linked or autosomal dominant trait with variable penetrance. Recent studies have shown that the disease is caused by a defect in one of the genes encoding the subunits of type IV collagen, a basement membrane protein.
2. **Clinical features**
   a. **Hematuria, RBC casts, pyuria, proteinuria,** and **progressive renal failure** occur with variable severity. Renal failure is more common in men.
   b. **High-frequency sensorineural hearing loss,** often without clinically significant deafness, is characteristic.
3. **Therapy and prognosis.** No treatment is successful in slowing or preventing the renal failure, and prognosis is variable. Occasionally, affected patients who undergo renal transplantation develop antiglomerular basement membrane (anti-GBM) antibody disease (Goodpasture's syndrome) if the Alport host recognizes the normal type IV collagen of the transplanted kidney as a "foreign" antigen.

B Minimal change disease (lipoid nephrosis, nil lesion nephrotic syndrome)

1. **Incidence.** Minimal change disease accounts for three-fourths of cases of idiopathic nephrotic syndrome in children but only one-fourth of cases in adults.
2. **Pathology.** Information is scant and nonspecific. Fusion of epithelial foot processes is seen with electron microscopy, but this lesion is common to all proteinuric states.
3. **Clinical features**
   a. **Nephrotic syndrome** is the typical presentation by patients of all ages.
   b. Hypertension occurs in 10% of children and in 35% of adults.
   c. Hematuria is uncommon.
   d. Azotemia develops in 23% of children and in 34% of adults.
4. **Therapy**
   a. **Glucocorticoids.** The remission rate with adequate steroid treatment (i.e., 1–2 mg/kg/day for 4–8 weeks) is 90% for both children and adults. Prolonged remission is seen in 10%–60% of patients; however, relapse is common and is multiple in 25%–50% of patients. Relapses typically are responsive to steroids, with only 5% of initially steroid-responsive patients developing steroid resistance or dependence. Recent studies have demonstrated that adults may have a poorer response to glucocorticoids than previously believed, with 60% of patients having a reduced GFR by 10 years.
   b. **Cytotoxic agents.** Drugs such as cyclophosphamide and chlorambucil have been effective in steroid-resistant and multiple relapsing cases. Occasionally, steroid-resistant patients develop steroid sensitivity following treatment with cytotoxic alkylating agents. The possibility of gonadal (chromosomal) damage caused by these drugs must be carefully considered.

c. **Cyclosporine.** Research has recently shown that this agent is effective in patients with frequent relapsing disease in whom cyclophosphamide has failed or is contraindicated because of gonadal toxicity.

5. **Prognosis.** Minimal change disease is associated with low mortality rates (i.e., 10% among adults and 1.5% among children), with only 10% of deaths caused by renal failure.

C Membranous glomerulonephritis (or glomerulopathy)

1. **Etiology**
   a. **Primary (idiopathic) membranous glomerulonephritis** accounts for 30%–50% of cases of idiopathic nephrotic syndrome in adults but less than 1% of cases in children.
   b. **Secondary membranous glomerulonephritis** may occur with a variety of underlying conditions, including:
      (1) **Infection** [e.g., chronic hepatitis B (HBV) or hepatitis C (HCV), syphilis, malaria, schistosomiasis, filariasis]
      (2) **Rheumatic disease** (e.g., SLE)
      (3) **Neoplasm** (e.g., carcinoma of the lung, colon, stomach, breast, and kidney; non-Hodgkin's lymphoma; leukemia; Wilms' tumor)
      (4) **Drug therapy** (e.g., mercury, gold, D-penicillamine, captopril)
2. **Pathology.** The findings presented in Table 6–5 characterize the stages of membranous glomerulonephritis.
3. **Clinical features.** More than 85% of adults present with proteinuria (> 3 g/day/1.73 m^2 body surface area). The GFR usually is normal at diagnosis and often remains normal for 4–5 years thereafter.
4. **Clinical course.** Membranous glomerulonephritis has a variable course. About 20%–30% of patients achieve a lasting spontaneous remission, 20%–30% develop variable degrees of persistent proteinuria and nonuremic azotemia, and the rest advance to end-stage renal disease, usually over a 5-year period. Male patients, those with heavy proteinuria (> 10 g/day), and those who do not respond with a remission in proteinuria have a worse prognosis.
5. **Therapy.** A combination of steroids and cytotoxic agents has proved effective, but the unpredictable outcome of the disease makes the evaluation of therapy difficult. Recent randomized trials find that steroids alone should not be used as primary therapy. The use of alternating cycles of chlorambucil or cyclophosphamide and prednisone is effective in halting progression to end-stage renal failure in patients with nephrotic syndrome and mild renal insufficiency. Patients treated with cytotoxic drugs are more likely to experience remission of proteinuria.
6. **Complications.** Problematic conditions may intervene, causing an abrupt decrease in renal function.

TABLE 6–5 Stages of Membranous Glomerulonephritis

Stage	Characteristics
I	Normal appearance with light microscopy; subepithelial electron-dense deposits with electron microscopy
II	Spike-like projections of basement membrane material with light microscopy (best visualized with a silver impregnation stain); variable basement membrane thickening
III	Thick glomerular basement membrane (GBM), with a "moth-eaten" or "Swiss-cheese" appearance due to encirclement of immune deposits by spike-like projections of normal GBM
IV	Thickening of the capillary wall, with areas of segmental or global glomerulosclerosis; possible tubulointerstitial fibrosis

a. A **hypercoagulable state** exists in nephrotic patients. Renal vein thrombosis is a recognized problem; pulmonary embolism and arterial thrombosis also have been described.
b. **Intravascular volume depletion** secondary to vigorous diuretic administration leads to decreased renal blood flow.
c. **Hypertension, obstruction,** or **infection** may impair filtration.

D Mesangial proliferative glomerulonephritis

1. **Etiology.** The cause is unknown.
2. **Pathology.** The mesangial proliferative lesion is a global and diffuse increase in the number of mesangial cells and in the mesangial matrix.
3. **Clinical features.** Asymptomatic proteinuria or hematuria may occur. Although 24-hour urinary protein excretion can exceed 3.0 g, the complete nephrotic syndrome is inconsistently seen. One-third of patients are hypertensive at the time of diagnosis. Creatinine clearance is reduced in only 25% of patients at presentation. Serum complement component levels are normal.
4. **Clinical course.** The disease has an extremely variable course.
5. **Therapy.** High-dose (1–2 mg/kg/day) glucocorticoids are reportedly effective in remission induction. Some steroid failures respond to treatment with cyclophosphamide or chlorambucil.

E Membranoproliferative glomerulonephritis

1. **Incidence and etiology**
   a. Collectively, the disorders in this group account for 41% of cases of idiopathic nephrotic syndrome in children and 30% of cases in adults. Males and females are affected equally.
   b. Membranoproliferative glomerulonephritis may be idiopathic or secondary to SLE, cryoglobulinemia, or chronic viral or bacterial infection.
2. **Pathology.** The three pathologic types of membranoproliferative glomerulonephritis, each with distinct features, are described in Table 6–6.
3. **Clinical features.** The presentation is highly variable.
   a. Rapid progression to renal failure with edema and severe hypertension (acute nephritis) has been described.
   b. **Hypocomplementemia** is the most characteristic laboratory finding but is not universally present. The degree of C3 depression may be used as a rough guide to disease activity.
4. **Clinical course.** Chronic glomerulonephritis with end-stage renal disease develops in most cases.
5. **Therapy.** Treatment is not predictably effective, although occasional reports claim some therapeutic benefit. In children with proteinuria or impaired renal function, high-dose steroid therapy

TABLE 6–6 Pathologic Types of Membranoproliferative Glomerulonephritis

Type	Features
I	Intact glomerular basement membrane, subendothelial and mesangial deposits, significant mesangial prominence with matrix interposition Immunofluorescent positivity for immunoglobulin G (IgG), complement compounds (C1q, C4, and C2), and properdin
II (also called dense deposit disease)	Intramembranous and subepithelial deposits ("humps") in 50% of cases, mesangial deposits, moderate mesangial prominence with interposition Immunofluorescent positivity for IgG, C3, and properdin
III	Features of true membranous glomerulonephritis (i.e., with subepithelial deposits) and features of type I membranoproliferative glomerulonephritis

should be tried and maintained for 6–12 months. In adults with heavy proteinuria (> 3 g/day), the **antiplatelet agents** dipyridamole and aspirin may be used. However, evidence does not definitively support the effectiveness of this regimen.

F Focal glomerulosclerosis

1. **Incidence and etiology**
   a. Focal glomerulosclerosis accounts for 30% of cases of idiopathic nephrotic syndrome in adults and is the most common cause of steroid-resistant nephrotic syndrome in children.
   b. This condition is reported to recur in 30%–40% of renal allografts within 3 weeks to 1 year following transplantation.
   c. The etiology is unknown. Focal glomerulosclerosis is seen occasionally in the context of AIDS, heroin and other intravascular drug use, and chronic vesicoureteral reflux, but the causal relationships are uncertain.
2. **Pathology.** The hallmark lesion of focal and segmental glomerulosclerosis evolves through several stages, including mild mesangial prominence, loss of glomerular cellularity, and collapse of capillary loops.
3. **Clinical features and diagnosis**
   a. **Nephrotic syndrome** is the most common clinical presentation. Hypertension and renal failure occur infrequently in childhood but become more prevalent with advancing age.
   b. There are no specific laboratory findings. Proteinuria tends to be heavy (i.e., > 15 g/24 hr), and the biochemical derangements of nephrotic syndrome are accordingly severe.
4. **Therapy**
   a. Recent studies suggest that prolonged glucocorticoid therapy (i.e., ≥ 6 months) may lead to remission of proteinuria, although no randomized trials support this recommendation.
   b. Cyclosporine may be effective in reducing proteinuria.

G Goodpasture's syndrome (see also Chapter 2 XIV B)

1. **Definition.** Goodpasture's syndrome refers to a group of illnesses defined by the following triad of findings: **glomerulonephritis** (usually crescentic), **pulmonary hemorrhage,** and **anti-GBM antibody.** The renal and pulmonary components may be severe or clinically silent. The presence of the anti-GBM antibody, however, has become the essential feature of the diagnosis. Although many systemic illnesses include renal disease and pulmonary hemorrhage [e.g., SLE (see Part I: X M), necrotizing vasculitis (see Part I: X N), Wegener's granulomatosis (see Part I: X N 3), Henoch-Schönlein purpura (see Part I: X K), cryoglobulinemia (see Part I: X O), thrombotic thrombocytopenic purpura (TTP; see Part I: XIV D), legionnaires' disease, and renal disease complicated by pulmonary embolism or CHF], only those illnesses with detectable anti-GBM antibody are considered true Goodpasture's syndrome.
2. **Clinical features and diagnosis**
   a. **Clinical presentation** is highly variable.
      (1) **Generalized, systemic symptoms** may precede organ-specific complaints. Fever and myalgia are common.
      (2) **Renal involvement** usually is in the form of rapidly progressive renal failure. Proteinuria usually is mild, and the urinary sediment contains erythrocytes and RBC casts. This "nephritic" picture may be mild or severe.
      (3) **Pulmonary manifestations** include radiographic infiltrates, hemoptysis, cough, and dyspnea. The lung disease usually precedes kidney disease by a period of days to weeks.
   b. **Laboratory findings**
      (1) The most important finding is evidence of circulating immunoglobulin G (IgG) anti-GBM antibody, which is present in more than 90% of patients.

(2) The pathologic appearance of the kidney is typically that of a crescentic, proliferative glomerulonephritis. Crescents involve 80%–100% of glomeruli and are highly cellular.

3. **Clinical course.** Like the clinical presentation, the course of disease is variable, ranging from a minor recurrent pulmonary hemorrhage that occurs for years—until an abnormal urinary sediment prompts measurement of anti-GBM antibody—to abrupt-onset, fulminant disease, complete renal failure, and asphyxiation by massive pulmonary bleeding over a period of hours to days.

4. **Therapy.** Several treatment methods appear to benefit patients. Poor prognostic indicators include oligoanuria, serum creatinine above 6 mg/mm^3 for many weeks, and advanced histopathologic lesions.
   - **a.** High-dose prednisone should be given as an initial therapy. Cyclophosphamide should also be administered to patients under 55 years of age. A variety of successful but uncontrolled clinical trials have involved combinations of corticosteroids and alkylating immunosuppressive agents.
   - **b.** Intensive, daily plasmapheresis should be administered for 14 days or until anti-GBM antibody disappears.

H **Idiopathic crescentic glomerulonephritis** Individuals with this pathologically defined entity typically present with rapid, progressive deterioration of renal function. It is imperative to recognize that other lesions may induce the clinical syndrome of **rapidly progressive glomerulonephritis (RPGN)** (Table 6–7). This section considers only the idiopathic cases (i.e., those cases not due to other crescentic glomerular diseases). Idiopathic crescentic glomerulonephritis may be classified into three entities: **anti-GBM antibody disease** (see Part I: X G); **immune complex RPGN;** and

TABLE 6–7 Causes of Acute Renal Failure with Crescentic Glomerulonephritis

In primary glomerular diseases
Primary (idiopathic) diffuse crescentic glomerulonephritis
Type I: anti-GBM antibody disease **without** pulmonary hemorrhage
Type II: immune complex disease
Type III: pauci-immune glomerulonephritis (ANCA-associated)
Mesangiocapillary glomerulonephritis (especially type II)
Membranous glomerulonephritis with or without superimposed anti-GBM antibody disease
IgA nephropathy (Berger's disease)
In association with infectious diseases
Poststreptococcal glomerulonephritis
Infective endocarditis
Occult visceral bacterial sepsis
Other infections (e.g., hepatitis B)
In association with multisystem diseases
SLE
Goodpasture's syndrome (anti-GBM antibody disease with pulmonary hemorrhage)
Henoch-Schönlein purpura—disseminated vasculitis
Wegener's granulomatosis
Microscopic polyarteritis (hypersensitivity angiitis)
Other variants
Cryoimmunoglobulinemia (mixed, essential)
Relapsing polychondritis
Lung cancer, lymphoma

Anti-GBM = anti-glomerular basement membrane; IgA = immunoglobulin A; SLE = systemic lupus erythematosus.

pauci-immune RPGN, in which glomerular inflammation and necrosis are present but without immune deposits.

1. **Incidence and etiology.** Idiopathic crescentic glomerulonephritis accounts for about one-third of all cases of crescentic glomerulonephritis. Males are affected twice as often as females.
2. **Clinical features.** Patients present with abrupt-onset renal failure, with rapid loss of renal function (in less than 3 months); frequently normal blood pressure; and normal kidney size. Nonspecific symptoms (e.g., weakness, nausea, cough, weight loss, fever, myalgia, arthralgia) often announce the disease. Extrarenal involvement, with the exception of lung involvement, is rare.
   a. **Renal manifestations.** Approximately 50% of patients are oliguric and azotemic at the time of presentation.
   b. **Pulmonary manifestations.** Transient, mild pulmonary infiltrates or hemoptysis is seen in one half of patients.
3. **Diagnosis.** There are no diagnostic laboratory findings. However, when intrarenal vasculitis (i.e., pauci-immune glomerulonephritis) is the underlying cause, the **antineutrophilic cytoplasmic antibody (ANCA)** test is positive. The diagnosis is based on the discovery of epithelial crescents in a majority of glomeruli in the renal biopsy specimen.
4. **Clinical course and prognosis.** The prognosis may be very bleak, depending on the level of renal function at the time of presentation. Renal failure requiring renal replacement therapy develops in 3–6 months in more than 50% of patients. However, recent data using aggressive immunosuppressive regimens have demonstrated that 50%–75% of patients may enter remission.
5. **Therapy.** In anti-GBM disease, plasmapheresis and immunosuppressives should be used as described for Goodpasture's syndrome (see Part I: X G). In immune complex glomerulonephritis, treatment depends on the individual causative disorder. In pauci-immune deposit disease, treatment involves pulse methylprednisolone and cyclophosphamide.

I **Postinfectious glomerulonephritis** This acute glomerulonephritis occurs with a variety of local or systemic infections. (Glomerulonephritis associated with infective endocarditis and visceral abscess is discussed in Part I: X Q.) Postinfectious glomerulonephritis has been described as a sequela of disease caused by viruses, fungi, protozoa, and helminths. However, the prototypical postinfectious glomerulonephritis is **poststreptococcal glomerulonephritis.**

1. **Incidence and etiology**
   a. The disease primarily affects school-aged children. The disease is rare before 2 years of age but has been reported in adults. Males are affected twice as often as females.
   b. Preceding infection with nephritogenic strains of group A β-hemolytic streptococci (particularly type 12) is the rule, although positive culture of the organism is demonstrated in less than 20% of cases at the time of renal disease. The site of infection (i.e., skin or pharynx) appears to vary with the geographic area of study. The latent period between infection and clinical glomerular disease is 7–15 days; rarely, it is as long as 3 weeks.
2. **Pathology.** Poststreptococcal glomerulonephritis is a diffuse proliferative disease with mesangial and endothelial hypercellularity. Electron-dense deposits (subepithelial "humps") and foot process fusion are seen by electron microscopy. Immunofluorescence often identifies granular deposits of C3 along the capillary basement membrane.
3. **Clinical features and diagnosis**
   a. The typical clinical presentation is a sudden onset of hematuria and edema. Nephrotic syndrome develops in less than 15% of patients.
   b. The characteristic, but not diagnostic, laboratory profile is azotemia, hypocomplementemia (CH_{50} or C3), hematuria, leukocyturia, and proteinuria. Supporting data include elevated titers of antistreptolysin O, antihyaluronidase, and anti-deoxyribonuclease B antibodies, all of which suggest preceding streptococcal infection.

4. **Clinical course and diagnosis**
   a. The typical course of acute disease is recovery, particularly among children. The acute nephritis resolves with amelioration of edema and hypertension 1–3 weeks after onset. Proteinuria may persist for several months, exacerbated by erect posture and exercise. Microscopic hematuria similarly disappears slowly over a period of several months.
   b. Long-term prognosis is controversial. Some patients advance to end-stage renal disease. Factors associated with this poor prognosis are severe oliguria or anuria, crescents in the biopsy specimen, persistent heavy proteinuria, and relatively older age. Persistence of hypocomplementemia and progressive renal failure may, however, indicate an alternative diagnosis (e.g., membranoproliferative glomerulonephritis).
5. **Therapy.** Hypertension must be treated aggressively, particularly in children, who develop florid hypertensive encephalopathy at normal adult blood pressures. Furosemide or bumetanide may likely be required for the underlying edema-inducing disease. Antibiotic use is controversial, although a 10-day course of penicillin in nonallergic patients is safe enough for routine use. Prophylaxis following poststreptococcal glomerulonephritis is not indicated because recurrences are exceedingly rare. Immunosuppressive agents or corticosteroids have no therapeutic role.

J IgA glomerulonephritis (Berger's disease)

1. **Definition and incidence.** The disease is characterized by mesangial deposits of IgA in renal biopsies from patients with recurrent hematuria but normal renal function. The incidence of this disease varies remarkably with geographic location, and men are affected three to four times more often than women.
2. **Pathology.** Findings are characteristic.
   a. Diffuse, sometimes irregularly distributed IgA deposits are seen in the mesangium. IgM or IgG also may be present.
   b. Focal and segmental glomerulonephritis with mesangial proliferation is common. Mesangial prominence may be the only pathologic finding.
3. **Clinical features and diagnosis.** Affected patients, who usually are between 20 and 40 years of age, most commonly present with recurrent, often macroscopic hematuria but a normal GFR and normal tubular function. Biopsy specimens from normal-appearing skin have immunofluorescent positivity for IgA in 50% of cases. Measuring serum IgA levels is not useful.
4. **Clinical course and prognosis.** Course and outcome are variable. The 20-year survival rate is about 50%. A minority of patients progress to renal failure. Factors that predict a poor prognosis include advanced age at disease onset, heavy proteinuria, hypertension, and the presence of crescents or segmental sclerosis on renal biopsy.
5. **Therapy.** Patients with mild histologic changes and proteinuria of more than 3 g/day should receive prednisone for 4–6 months. Recent data suggest that fish oil containing a number of anti-inflammatory fatty acids may be useful in some patients with slowly progressive disease.

K Henoch-Schönlein purpura

1. **Definition.** This systemic disease is characterized by purpura (which may be slight and go unnoticed), arthritis, abdominal pain, bloody diarrhea, and nephritis.
2. **Incidence.** Henoch-Schönlein purpura primarily affects children. Clinical nephritis affects 30% of patients, but almost all patients have an abnormal kidney biopsy.
3. **Pathology.** The histopathology ranges from mild, diffuse mesangial prominence to focal and segmental proliferative glomerulonephritis on a background of diffuse mesangial proliferation. The hallmark of Henoch-Schönlein purpura is the invariable immunofluorescent positivity for IgA in the mesangium.

4. **Clinical features and diagnosis**
   a. The clinical presentation often is preceded by an infection [caused by a virus (e.g., herpes zoster), mycoplasma, or streptococcus], vaccination, insect bite, or drug administration. Rash usually develops early and evolves from morbilliform to purpuric. The legs and buttocks are affected most commonly. Arthritis typically is mild and nondeforming. Gastrointestinal bleeding and pain may dominate the presentation.
   b. Laboratory findings are exceedingly nonspecific, although elevated serum IgA is reported frequently. Serum complement component levels usually are normal.

5. **Clinical course and prognosis**
   a. The clinical course is variable. Patients with recurrent purpura, heavy proteinuria, and clinically severe nephritis at the time of presentation and patients whose biopsies show epithelial crescent formation tend to fare poorly.
   b. Among all children with Henoch-Schönlein purpura, the 15-year survival rate is 90%. By 10 years, however, 15% of these patients have persisting disease and 8% have renal impairment. Among adults, 50% heal completely, 15% progress to renal failure, and approximately 35% have persistent disease.

6. **Therapy.** Several treatment methods have been attempted (e.g., immunosuppression, steroid therapy, anticoagulation) but without proven benefit.

L Diabetic nephropathy

1. **Incidence.** End-stage renal disease develops in 30% of all patients with diabetes. Among patients with juvenile-onset diabetes, 30% develop renal disease within 20 years of the onset of diabetes. Among new patients considered for maintenance renal replacement therapy (largely chronic hemodialysis), at least 40% have chronic renal failure secondary to diabetes. African-American, Hispanic, and Native American individuals have a higher likelihood of developing diabetic nephropathy than Caucasian patients who have diabetes.

2. **Pathogenesis**
   a. The evolution of diabetic nephropathy is symptomatically quiet until late in the disease process. Early in diabetes, the GFR often is above normal. This early hyperfiltration may be most striking in those patients who subsequently develop glomerular damage.
   b. Initially, **microalbuminuria** [the loss of small amounts of protein (range: 30–300 mg/d)] occurs. **Proteinuria** develops after 15–20 years of diabetes. **Nephrotic syndrome** and **azotemia** often develop 3–5 years after the detection of proteinuria. **End-stage renal disease** occurs 1–5 years after the onset of azotemia.

3. **Pathology.** Two major pathologic lesions are associated with diabetes.
   a. **Diffuse glomerulosclerosis** is uniformly present in patients with diabetic nephropathy. It is characterized by an eosinophilic thickening of the mesangium and basement membrane due to accumulation of extracellular matrix proteins.
   b. **Nodular glomerulosclerosis,** also known as **Kimmelstiel-Wilson syndrome,** consists of round nodules that are homogeneous at the center and have circumferential layering of nuclei. These nodules often are multiple within a given glomerulus and may be confluent. Nodular glomerulosclerosis is specific for diabetes, but it is found in only 50% of patients with diabetic nephropathy.

4. **Laboratory findings.** Results are indicative of a slowly declining GFR.

5. **Clinical course.** Factors that accelerate renal deterioration include hypertension, poor glycemic control, urinary obstruction, infection, the administration of nephrotoxic drugs, and the use of intravenous radiocontrast material.

6. Therapy

a. Diabetic nephropathy is treated with supportive measures.

(1) There is emerging evidence linking tight control of blood glucose to moderation of renal disease, especially in those patients with the earliest lesions (microalbuminuria).

(2) Studies have demonstrated that restriction of dietary protein (i.e., to < 0.8 g/kg body weight/day) slows development of renal failure once proteinuria occurs.

(3) Strict control of hypertension is crucial to slowing the progression of renal failure. Recent studies indicate that ACE inhibitors and angiotensin receptor blockers play an important role as primary therapy for diabetic patients with renal dysfunction (including any degree of albuminuria, hypertension, or a reduced GFR).

(4) Avoidance of nephrotoxins and surveillance for urinary infection or obstruction (neurogenic bladder) are prudent conservative measures.

b. End-stage renal disease is treated using established modalities.

(1) Patients who undergo transplantation of a kidney from a living relative have a better 5-year survival rate than those who undergo chronic hemodialysis.

(2) Several dialysis treatment centers have reported good results using continuous ambulatory peritoneal dialysis in patients with diabetes, as long as adequate dialysis is provided. Insulin may be given intraperitoneally, and improved diabetic control may be possible.

M Lupus nephritis Presently, four major lesions and three superimposed (secondary) lesions are recognized as part of this spectrum of renal pathology.

1. Major lesions

a. Focal proliferative lupus nephritis develops during the first year of clinical lupus in 50% of patients.

(1) **Pathology.** The lesion is sharply delineated segmental endothelial and mesangial cell proliferation, which usually affects less than 50% of all glomeruli.

(2) **Clinical features and diagnosis**

(a) Proteinuria is seen in almost all cases; however, nephrotic syndrome is rare. Hematuria is common, and mild renal insufficiency is seen occasionally. Hypertension is not present.

(b) Serologic findings include positive fluorescent antinuclear antibody (ANA) and modest elevations in anti-DNA antibodies. Complement components (C3 and C4) are at normal or decreased levels.

(3) **Clinical course and prognosis**

(a) Remission, as measured by cessation of proteinuria, is seen in about 50% of patients. Relapses commonly occur with extrarenal flares of systemic lupus. Transition to other forms of the disease (e.g., diffuse proliferative or membranous lupus nephritis) occurs in at least 20% of patients.

(b) Renal failure is rare unless the disease progresses to diffuse proliferative lupus nephritis.

(c) The 5-year mortality rate is 10%.

b. Diffuse proliferative lupus nephritis most commonly develops within the first year of clinical lupus.

(1) **Pathology.** Mesangial and endothelial cell proliferation affect most glomeruli with varying severity. Capillary lumina are obliterated, and crescents affect up to 30% of glomeruli. Deposits of IgG, C3, C4, and C1q are diffuse. IgA and IgM deposits also are seen frequently.

(2) **Clinical features and diagnosis**

(a) Proteinuria and hematuria are universal; more than 50% of patients present with nephrotic syndrome. Azotemia, which is common early in the course of the disease, may be severe. Hypertension occurs commonly.

(b) Serologic findings include positive fluorescent ANA, highly elevated anti-DNA antibodies, and depressed levels of C3 and C4. Cryoglobulinemia develops in some cases.

(3) **Clinical course and prognosis**

(a) Remission of the nephrotic syndrome, which is seen in 33% of patients, is sometimes sustained. Transition to mesangial lupus nephritis occurs occasionally in association with clinical remission.

(b) The 5-year mortality rate is 50%. Death results from uremia or active systemic lupus, which frequently is complicated by infection. Hypertension and renal failure may occur as sequelae even after long periods of clinical remission.

c. **Membranous lupus nephritis** develops during the first year of clinical lupus in about 50% of patients.

(1) **Pathology.** The histopathologic pattern of membranous lupus nephritis is very similar to that of idiopathic membranous glomerulonephritis (see Part I: X C 2).

(2) **Clinical features and diagnosis**

(a) Proteinuria is seen in all patients, and hematuria is common as well. Nephrotic syndrome is seen at presentation in 50% of patients and ultimately occurs in 80% of patients. Hypertension and renal insufficiency are rare at the outset of membranous lupus nephritis.

(b) Serologic findings include positive fluorescent ANA, normal or only mildly elevated anti-DNA antibodies, and normal or decreased levels of C3 and C4.

(3) **Clinical course and prognosis**

(a) Remission from nephrotic syndrome is seen in 33% of patients, but relapses are common. Transition to focal or diffuse proliferative lupus nephritis has been reported but is rare.

(b) The 5-year mortality rate is 10% for patients who develop hypertension and renal insufficiency during persistent nephrotic syndrome.

d. **Mesangial lupus nephritis** may occur as the earliest form of lupus nephritis.

(1) **Pathology.** Biopsy shows mesangial prominence with an increase in matrix and in the number of mesangial cells.

(2) **Clinical features and diagnosis**

(a) The complete spectrum of clinical findings is not fully known. Many patients are asymptomatic or present with only mild urinary abnormalities.

(b) Serologic findings include positive fluorescent ANA, mild anti-DNA antibody elevations, and normal or mildly decreased C3 and C4 levels.

(3) **Clinical course and prognosis**

(a) Urinary abnormalities may remit, and transition to diffuse proliferative or membranous lupus nephritis occurs in 15% of patients.

(b) This mesangial lesion is associated with clinical progression only if there is transition to a less favorable histology.

2. **Superimposed lesions**

a. **Glomerulosclerosis** is a secondary lesion that is seen most commonly in diffuse proliferative lupus nephritis with a protracted course. Progressive glomerulosclerosis may be a cause of renal failure in patients whose systemic lupus remits.

b. **Interstitial lupus nephritis** usually coexists with glomerular disease but may develop alone.

(1) Pathologically, this lesion is characterized by intense, mononuclear interstitial infiltration, tubular damage, and interstitial fibrosis.

(2) IgG and C3 are identified in peritubular capillaries and in tubular basement membranes. Parallel electron-dense deposits are seen.

(3) Clinical disorders of tubular function (e.g., disorders of potassium excretion, acid excretion, and urine concentration and dilution) are seen in addition to variable, nonselective proteinuria.

c. **Necrotizing vasculitis** usually complicates diffuse proliferative lupus nephritis and presents as rapidly accelerating hypertension and renal failure. Histopathologically, an acellular necrosis of vessel walls is seen with proteinaceous occlusive thrombi.

3. **Therapy.** Criteria for therapy are not rigidly established. The response of membranous lupus nephritis to therapy varies among reported series. Because of the poor prognosis associated with diffuse proliferative lupus nephritis, this lesion currently is treated—even in cases with few clinical signs or symptoms of renal disease.
   a. **Glucocorticoid therapy** involves various regimens. Induction therapy with oral prednisone (1–2 mg/kg/day) and pulse intravenous methylprednisolone (1–2 g/day) has been described.
   b. **Cytotoxic drugs** (e.g., cyclophosphamide), when added to steroids, often induce remission, preserve or improve renal function, or both.

N Vasculitis

1. **Introduction.** The kidney frequently is involved in systemic vasculitis, although the actual incidence is unknown. The spectrum of renal syndromes associated with vasculitis ranges from modest "microscopic" involvement of arterioles, venules, and capillaries (a syndrome referred to as **hypersensitivity vasculitis**) to extensive "classic" involvement of medium-sized vessels (a syndrome referred to as **polyarteritis nodosa**).
2. **Polyarteritis nodosa**
   a. **Etiology.** This type of vasculitis may be primary (idiopathic) or secondary to drugs, viral infections (e.g., HBV), or rheumatic diseases (e.g., lupus, rheumatoid vasculitis).
   b. **Pathology.** The kidneys show a focal necrotizing arteritis in vessels ranging in size from the renal artery to the interlobular veins.
   c. **Clinical features and diagnosis**
      (1) The clinical presentation often is vague, consisting of low-grade fever, myalgia, arthralgia, and weight loss.
      (2) The laboratory findings are numerous and, although nonspecific, frequently suggest the diagnosis of polyarteritis nodosa when considered collectively (see Table 10–9).
      (3) The diagnosis can be confirmed by renal angiography, which shows multiple small aneurysms with segmental infarctions. Positive serum ANCA titers have become a major diagnostic aid in vasculitis.
   d. **Clinical course and prognosis.** Progression to organ destruction or death is the expected outcome.
   e. **Therapy.** Use of daily high-dose glucocorticoids and daily cyclophosphamide (1–3 mg/kg/day) has increased the 1-year survival rate to greater than 80%.
3. **Wegener's granulomatosis** (see also Chapter 2 XIV C), which affects patients of all ages but is more common in middle-aged men, is a special kind of vasculitis (necrotizing granulomatous vasculitis) with renal involvement.
   a. **Pathology.** The characteristic and diagnostic lesion of necrotizing vasculitis and granulomatous inflammation is most reliably discovered in pulmonary or upper airway biopsy material. Often, a focal and segmental necrotizing vasculitis and glomerulitis are found with few (if any) immune deposits.
   b. **Clinical features and diagnosis**
      (1) The disease affects the kidney and upper respiratory tract, including the nose, throat, and bronchi. Ulcerative vasculitic lesions, including nasal septal perforation, are the most recognizable presenting signs.
      (2) The hematologic and serologic features of Wegener's granulomatosis extensively overlap those of polyarteritis nodosa. ANCAs are present in the serum of most patients and may help in diagnosing the disease and in monitoring response to therapy.

c. **Clinical course.** Wegener's granulomatosis has a variable course. Long-term remissions are seen occasionally with therapy. Death usually results from renal failure, sepsis, hemorrhage, or disseminated intravascular coagulation (DIC).

d. **Therapy.** Treatment with daily high-dose glucocorticoids and daily cyclophosphamide (1–3 mg/kg/day) has increased the 1-year survival rate from less than 20% to greater than 80%.

O Cryoglobulins and cryoglobulinemia

1. **Cryoglobulins** are proteins that precipitate at low temperatures and dissolve on rewarming. Three types of cryoglobulins may be defined (Table 6–8).

2. **Cryoglobulinemia** (i.e., presence of cryoglobulins in the blood) occurs in a variety of clinically dissimilar conditions. Renal disease is associated primarily with types I and II and probably has an immune complex–mediated pathophysiology. Many patients with mixed cryoglobulinemia have an underlying infection with **HCV.**
   a. **Clinical features** (see Table 6–8)
   b. **Diagnosis** involves the detection, characterization, and quantitation of cryoglobulins in serum.
   c. **Therapy** in idiopathic cases is not standardized. Immunosuppressives and steroids are occasionally effective. Encouraging results have been obtained with plasmapheresis, particularly in patients with mixed cryoglobulinemia. Antiretroviral therapy may be effective in patients with HCV-caused mixed cryoglobulinemia.

P Multiple myeloma (see Chapter 4 XIV)

1. **Definition.** Multiple myeloma represents a neoplastic transformation of a monoclonal B lymphocyte into a plasma cell, which produces excessive quantities of immunoglobulin or immunoglobulin fragment (paraprotein). More than 50% of affected patients die of complications of renal failure, and a much higher percentage of patients with multiple myeloma have some form of renal involvement.

2. **Pathology.** The many mechanisms of renal injury in multiple myeloma have different effects on the kidney (Table 6–9).

3. **Clinical features and diagnosis.**
   a. The clinical presentation of renal disease in multiple myeloma often is subtle. Anemia and bone pain in the presence of any form of abnormal urinary finding should prompt evaluation

TABLE 6–8 Cryoglobulins and Cryoglobulinemia

Type	Clinical Features
I: Monoclonal cryoglobulins	Associated with hematologic malignancies Heavy proteinuria, hematuria, and, occasionally, anuria Histologic lesion: usually is a membranoproliferative glomerulonephritis
II: Mixed cryoglobulins that include a monoclonal component with antibody activity against polyclonal IgG	Associated with a syndrome of immune-complex vasculitis; approximately 50% of patients have renal disease Wide spectrum of clinical signs that vary greatly in severity Hypertension, azotemia, and anuria, which are poor prognostic signs Endocapillary proliferation and mesangial prominence (common pathologic features)
III: Mixed cryoglobulins in which both components are polyclonal	May be associated with a variety of other diseases, with or without renal disease, including SLE, hepatitis B or C, and systemic infections

IgG = immunoglobulin G; SLE = systemic lupus erythematosus.

TABLE 6–9 Mechanisms of Renal Injury in Multiple Myeloma

Mechanism of Renal Injury	Effect on the Kidney
Bence-Jones proteinuria	Direct tubular toxicity
	Intratubular obstruction by cast formation
Amyloidosis	Glomerular and tubular amyloid deposits
Hypercalcemia	Renal vasoconstriction
	Calcium–phosphate deposition
Hyperuricemia	Acute urate deposition and tubular obstruction
Hyperviscosity	Vascular occlusion
Light chain nephropathy	Glomerular occlusion

for myeloma. Slowly progressive renal insufficiency is typical; however, acute renal failure may be seen in certain circumstances (e.g., in the presence of hypercalcemia).

b. Many chemical abnormalities commonly occur. Pseudohyponatremia develops secondary to the presence of large quantities of paraprotein, altering the nonaqueous phase of plasma. The anion gap is low and occasionally is negative because of the positive charges on the immunoglobulin molecules. Urine protein concentration is increased, reflecting excretion of the huge paraprotein burden. As mentioned earlier, dipstick measurement for protein is insensitive to immunoglobulin and often gives false-negative results. Thus, acid precipitation with sulfosalicylic acid is required.

4. **Therapy and prognosis.** Although no specific therapy exists for the renal disease, chemotherapy for the malignancy, meticulous regulation of intravascular volume and electrolyte status, and dialysis (when necessary) may prolong life. Plasmapheresis may be useful in improving renal function in patients with acute renal failure and circulating light chains.

Q Glomerulonephritis in infective endocarditis This disease represents the prototypical bacterial illness that may lead to the induction of glomerulonephritis, presumably through an immune-complex mechanism. Glomerulonephritis is thought to occur by similar means in visceral abscess and in infections arising from extracorporeal circulation devices (shunt nephritis). It is possible that any endovascular infection can produce this glomerulonephritis.

1. **Pathology.** The histologic severity ranges from mild mesangial proliferation to severe crescentic glomerulonephritis.
2. **Clinical features.** About 15% of patients develop renal involvement. Nonimmune mechanisms of injury include septic emboli, ischemic ATN with severe CHF, and, indirectly, antibiotic nephrotoxicity. Patients with immune-complex glomerulonephritis present with hematuria, RBC casts in the urine, and azotemia.
3. **Therapy.** There is no specific treatment for the renal disease. Except in fairly advanced cases, successful treatment of the underlying infection usually leads to resolution of the renal disease.

XI RENAL CYSTIC DISEASE

A Adult polycystic kidney disease

1. **Definition, etiology, and incidence.** Adult polycystic kidney disease represents the most common cause of renal failure and death in adults with renal cystic disease. It accounts for approximately 5% of all patients on maintenance dialysis.

a. Inherited as an autosomal dominant trait, adult polycystic kidney disease achieves 100% gene penetrance by the time the patient is 80 years of age. In the majority of cases, the affected gene (polycystin-1) is on chromosome 16 (PKD1); however, in a minority of families, the genetic defect (polycystin-2) resides on chromosome 4 (PKD2).

b. Men and women are affected equally. Family history is positive in more than 75% of cases.

c. Adult polycystic kidney disease must be distinguished from **childhood (autosomal recessive) polycystic kidney disease,** which is universally fatal by the third decade of life, and the **congenital multicystic variant of renal dysplasia.**

2. **Clinical features**

   a. The typical presentation of enlarging flank or abdominal masses, abdominal pain, and slowly progressive renal failure becomes clinically evident by the fourth decade of life, and renal replacement therapy becomes necessary within 10 years of the onset of symptoms. Associated clinical findings may include hypertension, polyuria and nocturia, erythrocytosis, and nephrolithiasis.

   b. The onset of renal failure occurs later in the minority of patients who have the genetic defect on chromosome 4 (about 67 years as opposed to about 54 years) compared with the majority, who have the defect on chromosome 16.

   c. Hepatic cysts occur in 33% of cases. However, liver insufficiency is rare, unlike in the childhood form.

   d. Intracranial (berry) aneurysms occur in 12% of patients. In some series, 6% of all patients with berry aneurysms have adult polycystic kidney disease.

3. **Diagnosis.** Diagnosis is made most easily on the basis of specific ultrasonographic findings. Coincident findings include hematuria, impaired urine concentrating ability, and low-grade proteinuria. Heavy proteinuria, persistent hematuria, and pyuria should be investigated because they rarely occur in uncomplicated adult polycystic kidney disease.

4. **Therapy.** Treatment is restricted to the therapy of end-stage renal disease as it develops. Genetic counseling is important, because 50% of offspring are affected. Women with adult polycystic kidney disease are not at an increased risk for fetal demise or hypertension during pregnancy except as contributed by existing renal insufficiency.

B Nephronophthisis (medullary cystic disease)

1. **Definition and incidence.** Medullary cystic disease is the most common cause of end-stage renal disease in children and adolescents.

2. **Pathology.** The kidney is small in medullary cystic disease, which distinguishes this disease from polycystic and multicystic diseases. Cysts may be located at the corticomedullary junction or in the medulla. Acystic forms have been described. Interstitial fibrosis is prominent, but calcification does not occur.

3. **Clinical features.** Loss of urine concentrating ability and failure to conserve sodium appropriately are almost invariable early signs of disease. The initial presentation often includes polyuria, polydipsia, and enuresis, although an azotemic presentation also is common. Progression to renal failure is a constant clinical feature.

4. **Therapy.** Treatment is aimed at maintaining sodium and water homeostasis during the evolution of disease. Genetic counseling may be appropriate in disease that is clearly familial. The possibility of subclinical disease in siblings must be considered when a donor is being selected for transplantation.

C Medullary sponge kidney

1. **Definition and incidence.** Medullary sponge kidney is not a true cystic disease but rather an ectasia of the renal collecting tubule. This common problem is identified in 1 of every 200 urograms in a large series.

2. **Prognosis.** Outcome is excellent; many patients have no detectable impairment of renal function. Hypercalciuria is common, as are subtle defects in the ability to concentrate and acidify the urine. Nephrocalcinosis and nephrolithiasis, of variable severity, is found in 50% of cases.

D Simple renal cyst

1. **Definition and incidence.** The simple cyst is the most common renal cystic disease; at least half of all individuals older than 50 years of age have one or more macroscopic renal cysts. Renal cysts may be solitary or multiple and unilateral or bilateral. They usually are located in the cortex and bulge through the renal capsule, but they may occur in the medulla. Large renal cysts are more common among adults, and multilocular cysts are rare.
2. **Clinical features.** Symptoms are rare; simple cysts usually are diagnosed during patient evaluation for other problems. Bleeding and infection stimulate the cyst wall to thicken, and calcareous plaques often form within the cyst wall.
3. **Clinical course.** Simple cysts usually are static, although regression may occur from one radiographic assessment to the next. Solitary cysts may undergo malignant degeneration, although this finding is rare. Hemorrhagic cysts are more likely to contain a neoplasm than nonhemorrhagic cysts (i.e., in up to 30% of cases as compared with less than 1% of cases). **Multiple simple cysts** may develop in end-stage renal disease in patients who have undergone hemodialysis for longer than 7 years.
4. **Diagnosis** may be made by CT, ultrasonography, urography, or angiography. Cyst puncture (for fluid aspiration and cytology) and contrast radiology should be performed in patients with large cysts with abnormal ultrasonographic appearance.
5. **Therapy.** In the absence of infection or tumor, no specific therapy is indicated for this benign disease.

XII TUBULOINTERSTITIAL DISEASE

A Acute interstitial nephritis

1. **Definition.** Acute interstitial nephritis appears to be a kidney-based hypersensitivity reaction, usually caused by a drug. Although the true incidence of acute interstitial nephritis is unknown, several hundred cases have been formally reported, and an increasing awareness of this disease has come with increased case recognition.
2. **Etiology.** Drugs implicated in the pathogenesis of acute interstitial nephritis include β-lactam antibiotics (e.g., methicillin, oxacillin, and cephalothin) and other antibiotics (e.g., sulfonamides); nonsteroidal anti-inflammatory drugs (NSAIDs; e.g., ibuprofen, indomethacin, fenoprofen, and tolmetin); diuretics (e.g., thiazides and furosemide); and many other unrelated drugs (e.g., phenytoin, cimetidine, sulfinpyrazone, methyldopa, and phenobarbital).
3. **Clinical features.** The **classic** presentation is development of acute renal failure with fever, rash, and eosinophilia, yet only a minority of patients present with this symptom triad.
4. **Diagnosis**
   a. **Urinalysis** classically shows mild or no proteinuria, microscopic hematuria, pyuria, and eosinophiluria. Urine must be examined microscopically with appropriate staining methods for the presence of eosinophiluria. Some patients with acute interstitial nephritis due to NSAIDs present with nephrotic syndrome characterized by urinary protein excretion exceeding 3.0 g/24 hr.
   b. **Biopsy** shows patchy, irregular interstitial infiltration with inflammatory cells. Monocytes and lymphocytes are constant findings. Eosinophils may be abundant or completely absent. Fibrosis is extremely unusual and should suggest underlying or preexisting renal disease.

Rarely, acute interstitial nephritis may progress to chronic interstitial nephritis, and fibrosis may be prominent. Glomeruli are normal or show only mild mesangial prominence.

5. **Therapy.** Treatment includes discontinuation of the etiologic drug and initiation of supportive measures (e.g., dietary restrictions, blood pressure management, acute dialysis). The value of glucocorticoid therapy is unclear; however, the use of steroids may be justified in patients with severe or rapidly progressive renal insufficiency. In such patients, the addition of immunosuppressive agents such as cyclophosphamide is warranted. When interstitial nephritis is associated with circulating antibodies (a rare occurrence), the addition of plasmapheresis is indicated.
6. **Prognosis.** Outcome is excellent provided that the offending drug is promptly withdrawn. Recovery time varies and may be prolonged in patients with oliguria and in those with extensive interstitial cellular infiltrates. Temporary dialysis may be needed. Rarely, patients progress to end-stage renal disease.

B Chronic interstitial nephritis In general, the clinical features common to these interstitial diseases include a relative preservation of glomerular function until late in the disease but an impairment of tubular functions (e.g., urine concentration, dilution, acidification and potassium excretion) early in the course of the disease.

1. **Drug-related nephropathy**
   a. **Analgesic nephropathy** is the prototypical drug-related chronic interstitial nephritis.
      (1) Analgesic nephropathy occurs more commonly in women than in men. Patients usually are older than 45 years of age and from low socioeconomic classes. Patients often complain of frequent headaches or have coincident psychiatric disease.
      (2) Intravenous urography reveals abnormality in more than 90% of cases, and papillary necrosis is seen in more than 50%. Half of the patients are hypertensive, and anemia is common and often out of proportion to the degree of clinically apparent renal disease.
      (3) Several agents have been implicated (e.g., acetaminophen, phenacetin, aspirin), but none has been specifically proven culpable. The risk for analgesic nephropathy appears to be increased in patients who use more than 3 g/day of such agents.
      (4) Treatment of progressive analgesic nephropathy is supportive. Removal of the inciting agent may arrest the deterioration of renal function.

   b. **Gold nephropathy** is a frequent and important complication of parenteral gold therapy for rheumatoid arthritis. Gold accumulation leads to immune-complex membranous glomerulonephritis and nephrotic syndrome. Cessation of gold therapy at the first sign of proteinuria is recommended and often results in regression of signs of renal disease. It is not yet known whether oral gold preparations are equally nephrotoxic.

   c. **Lithium nephrotoxicity** may be important. Lithium carbonate, used in the treatment of bipolar disorder, is filtered freely and undergoes significant (i.e., 60%–70%) reabsorption in the proximal tubules. Lithium toxicity results in antidiuretic hormone (ADH)–unresponsive nephrogenic diabetes insipidus, incomplete distal renal tubular acidosis, and, rarely, azotemia.

   d. **NSAIDs** have been associated with a variety of clinical renal disorders (see Part II for effects on electrolyte metabolism). Table 6–10 gives the mechanism for NSAID-induced disorders.

2. **Toxin-related nephropathy**
   a. **Cadmium nephropathy** may lead to interstitial disease. Cadmium, a highly toxic byproduct of zinc production, has numerous industrial applications. During long-term exposure, cadmium accumulates in the kidney but blood and urine cadmium concentrations remain normal. Cadmium probably leads to end-stage renal disease, although the true incidence is unknown.

   b. **Lead nephropathy (saturnine gout)** is a well-recognized sequela of chronic lead intoxication.
      (1) The earliest cases of lead intoxication involved miners, paint manufacturers, and distillers of "moonshine" liquor. Lead poisoning also has been reported in children who have

TABLE 6–10 Mechanisms for NSAID-Induced Disorders

NSAID-Induced Disorder	Mechanism
Nephrotic syndrome	Severe interstitial nephritis; histologically normal glomeruli
Decreased GFR	Renal vasoconstriction, especially in patients with preexisting renal disease, congestive heart failure, or cirrhosis; patients treated with triamterene at particular risk
Papillary necrosis	Unknown
Edema	Primary renal sodium retention due to prostaglandin inhibition, especially in patients with underlying congestive heart failure
Hyperkalemia	Hyporeninemic hypoaldosteronism

GFR = glomerular filtration rate; NSAID = nonsteroidal anti-inflammatory drug.

ingested lead-based paint. Individuals who recover from acute lead poisoning occasionally are found later to be victims of chronic lead-related renal disease.

(2) Clinical manifestations of lead nephropathy include a reduced GFR, reduced renal plasma flow (RPF), minimal or no proteinuria, normal urinary sediment, gouty arthritis due to hyperuricemia and low urate clearance, and, occasionally, hypertension, hyperkalemia, and acidemia.

(3) Treatment includes removal of lead exposure and chelation therapy with sodium or calcium **ethylenediaminetetraacetic acid (EDTA)** or **D-penicillamine** (in appropriate cases).

c. **Copper nephrotoxicity** is rare but occasionally is seen in Wilson's disease. Clinically, copper nephropathy may resemble cadmium nephropathy (proximal tubular disease) or ATN. **D-penicillamine** is the treatment of choice.

d. **Mercury nephropathy** may also lead to disease. Mercury is associated with several renal lesions, including membranous and proliferative glomerular disease with nephrotic syndrome, proximal tubular atrophy and Fanconi's syndrome with the development of chronic renal failure, and oliguric ATN. Chelation therapy with **British antilewisite (BAL, dimercaprol)** and hemodialysis may reduce mortality if initiated promptly (i.e., within 48 hours following exposure).

3. **Crystalline nephropathy**

a. **Uric acid** produces renal injury in three ways.

(1) **Uric acid stones** may develop in concentrated acid urine.

(2) **Acute uric acid nephropathy** (acute crystalline obstruction of renal tubules) may accompany sudden or extreme elevations in serum uric acid (i.e., serum levels > 25 mg/dL), as occurs in **tumor lysis syndrome.**

(3) **Gouty nephropathy,** a syndrome of interstitial fibrosis and decreased renal function, may be related to cortical microtophi and a nephrotoxic influence of hyperuricemia in some gouty patients. Lead nephropathy (saturnine gout) may account for a significant percentage of patients with renal insufficiency and gout.

b. **Oxalic acid** also produces tubulointerstitial disease. Elevated urine levels of oxalic acid may lead to the formation of calcium oxalate stones or may mimic the syndrome of acute uric acid nephropathy (acute crystalline obstruction). **Primary hyperoxaluria** is an inherited disease of oxalate overproduction, which terminates in renal failure with extensive deposition of oxalate crystals throughout the body (a condition termed **oxalosis**). **Ethylene glycol poisoning** may lead to renal failure in part by the hyperoxaluria that results from the metabolism of ethylene glycol to oxalate. The use of **methoxyflurane** in anesthesia has been linked to an increased oxalate production with resultant nephrotoxicity. Increased oxalate absorption often is seen following ileojejunal bypass surgery for obesity and may lead to nephrocalcinosis. Mild hyperoxaluria may result from pyridoxine or thiamine deficiency.

c. **Antiviral agents.** High-dose **acyclovir** and **ganciclovir** may lead to intratubular crystal deposition and acute renal failure. **Indinavir,** an antiretroviral agent, may also produce this lesion, because its crystals are highly insoluble. High-dose **methotrexate** may induce intratubular crystal deposition as well, and high-dose **sulfadiazine** may lead to a similar complication when urine is particularly acidic.

4. **Miscellaneous nephropathies**
   a. **Amyloidosis**
      (1) **Definition and classification.** Amyloidosis is a disorder of unknown etiology, which involves the deposition of eosinophilic, amorphous material. The major classifications of amyloidosis are **primary amyloidosis** (occurring without pre- or coexisting illness), **secondary amyloidosis** (occurring in the presence of chronic inflammatory disease), and **heredofamilial amyloidosis.**
      (2) **Clinical features.** Amyloid deposition may be focal and restricted to the kidneys or systemic and generalized. Proteinuria is universal, with nephrotic syndrome developing in 76% of patients. Hypertension occurs in 50% of patients. Kidney size occasionally is increased but decreases with advanced disease.
      (3) **Clinical course.** Progressive deterioration of renal function is the rule.
      (4) **Diagnosis.** Biopsy that demonstrates amyloid protein by green birefringence with Congo red stain unequivocally establishes the diagnosis.
      (5) **Therapy.** There is no effective treatment for primary amyloidosis, although **alkylating agents** and **colchicine** have been advocated. Treatment of secondary amyloidosis is limited to the treatment of the underlying inflammatory disease. Amyloidosis recurs in the transplanted kidney.
   b. **Sarcoidosis** (see also Chapter 2 XIV A)
      (1) **Definition.** Sarcoidosis is a granulomatous disease of unknown etiology. Renal involvement may be secondary to noncaseating granulomatous replacement of the renal interstitium.
      (2) **Clinical features.** Renal size usually is normal, and mild nonselective proteinuria is common. Hypercalcemia, hypercalciuria, or both frequently complicate sarcoidosis as a result of increased synthesis of 1,25-dihydroxycholecalciferol [1,25-$(OH)_2D_3$].
      (3) **Clinical course.** The hypercalcemia may induce acute renal failure, and the hypercalciuria may lead to nephrocalcinosis or calcium nephrolithiasis. Hyperglobulinemia, when present, may be associated with distal renal tubular acidosis. Although glomerulonephritis has been noted among patients with sarcoidosis, the existence of a true sarcoid glomerulopathy is not fully established.
      (4) **Therapy.** Steroids are indicated for the management of hypercalcemia.

C Renal papillary necrosis

1. **Definition.** Renal papillary necrosis results from ischemic necrosis of the renal medulla or renal papillae. There are two forms. The papillary form involves the entire papilla, whereas the medullary form begins with focal areas of infarction in the inner medullary zone.

2. **Etiologic factors.** Conditions associated with renal papillary necrosis include diabetes mellitus, urinary tract obstruction, severe pyelonephritis, analgesic abuse, sickle cell hemoglobinopathy, extreme hypoxia and intravascular volume depletion in infants, and renal allograft rejection.

3. **Clinical features.** The clinical presentation of renal papillary necrosis varies with the stage and extent of disease. Patients with sickle cell trait may have completely asymptomatic renal papillary necrosis, which is discovered incidentally during urography for unrelated complaints. Infection frequently complicates renal papillary necrosis and leads to clinical pyelonephritis. The

necrotic papillae may be sloughed and produce typical ureteral colic or ureteral obstruction. Azotemia is an uncommon presenting sign.

4. **Clinical course.** The course of renal papillary necrosis is a function of the underlying disease. End-stage renal disease may develop, particularly among diabetics.
5. **Diagnosis.** Intravenous urography can establish the diagnosis of both forms of renal papillary necrosis. Radiographically, the affected calyces appear irregular and fuzzy early in the disease process. As the lesion progresses, sequestration of the necrotic tissue leads to sinus formation and the appearance of a sinus tract or arc shadow on the urogram. In advanced renal papillary necrosis, the sequestrum may be sloughed and surrounded by contrast material—the so-called ring sign. Calcification, calicectasis, and medullary cavities may be present in this stage.
6. **Therapy.** Treatment includes relief of obstruction, prevention and prompt eradication of infection, and control of pain (colic). Surgery occasionally is necessary to control hemorrhage or to relieve obstruction.

XIII RENAL TRANSPORT DEFECTS

A Meliturias

Excessive quantities of **sugars** may gain access to the urine because of an increase in filtered load (as in the hyperglycemia of diabetes mellitus) or failure of appropriate reabsorption in the nephron.

1. **Primary renal glycosuria** is an autosomal recessive disorder recognized from birth by constant glycosuria in the absence of abnormal carbohydrate metabolism (i.e., hyperglycemia, ketosis, and other meliturias). Two variants are described. Both are associated with a reduction in either the amount of or affinity for the renal transport protein for glucose.
2. **Other meliturias are recognized.**
   a. **Essential pentosuria (L-xylulosuria),** an autosomal recessive defect in the metabolism of glucuronic acid, affects primarily Jews. L-Xylulosuria occurs secondary to a deficiency of nicotinamide–adenine dinucleotide phosphate (NADP)–linked xylitol dehydrogenase.
   b. **Essential fructosuria** also is an autosomal recessive error of metabolism, which is a result of defective phosphofructokinase activity.

B Aminoacidurias

1. **Cystinuria** is an autosomal recessive defect in the transport of cystine, lysine, ornithine, and arginine. The low solubility of cystine accounts for the symptoms and complications of cystinuria in that it predisposes to the formation of renal cystine stones, which may lead to renal failure. Therapy consists of a lifelong alkaline diuresis to prevent stone formation. D-Penicillamine is required in many cases (see Part I: VII D).
2. **Dibasic aminoaciduria** is a selective defect in lysine, ornithine, and arginine (but not cystine) transport. Autosomal recessive and dominant forms are recognized. Symptoms include amino acid–induced diarrhea, malnutrition, hyperammonemia, and growth and mental retardation. Therapy consists of a low-protein diet.
3. **Iminoglycinuria** is a benign, autosomal recessive disorder of proline, hydroxyproline, and glycine transport.
4. **Hartnup disease** is an autosomal recessive defect in the transport of neutral α-amino acids. Patients with Hartnup disease have a reduced ability to convert tryptophan to niacin, resulting in pellagra—a syndrome characterized by photosensitive erythema, cerebellar ataxia, neuropsychiatric symptoms, and delirium. Therapy is oral nicotinamide.

C Fanconi's syndrome

1. **Definition.** Fanconi's syndrome refers to a collection of proximal tubular defects, which may exist in varying number and degree of severity and may be inherited or acquired.

2. **Etiology**
   a. **Inherited causes** include cystinosis, Lowe's syndrome, Wilson's disease, tyrosinemia, galactosemia, glycogenosis, and fructose intolerance.
   b. **Acquired causes** include transplant dysfunction, myeloma, Sjögren's syndrome, hyperparathyroidism, potassium depletion, amyloidosis, nephrotic syndrome, interstitial nephritis, heavy metal toxicity, and outdated tetracycline. **Ifosfamide,** a cyclophosphamide-related drug, can induce a Fanconi-like syndrome when it is used as an antineoplastic agent. Glycosuria and aminoaciduria have been reported in virtually all children treated with this agent.
   c. An **idiopathic** form of Fanconi's syndrome also exists.
3. **Clinical features and course**
   a. Symptoms and signs include glycosuria, aminoaciduria, phosphaturia, bicarbonaturia, vasopressin-resistant polyuria, rickets or osteoporosis, short stature, and uremia.
   b. The natural history of Fanconi's syndrome depends heavily on the course and prognosis of the underlying disease or diseases.
4. **Therapy.** Treatment is designed to replace lost urinary solutes and to correct the underlying disease or diseases. Phosphate, vitamin D, and bicarbonate should be given when indicated by laboratory and clinical data.

XIV RENAL VASCULAR DISEASE

A Ischemic nephropathy Occlusive disease of the renal arterial system encompasses a broad spectrum of clinical syndromes and pathophysiology. Arterial blood flow may be interrupted by in situ thrombosis or by embolism from distant endovascular sites. Occlusion may be sudden and complete or gradual, with resultant functional renal artery stenosis.

1. **Etiology**
   a. **Renal arterial thrombosis** may develop spontaneously in the context of atherosclerosis, aneurysm, arteritis, hypercoagulable states, sickle cell disease, and thrombotic microangiopathy. Thrombosis also may develop as a complication of external trauma, instrumentation with angiography catheters, arterial surgery, and renal allograft transplantation.
   b. **Renal arterial embolism** may be caused by a clot, tumor fragment, or infectious coagulum.
      (1) **Cardiac conditions** that may lead to renal arterial embolism include a dilated left atrium, artificial heart valves, myocardial infarction, infective endocarditis, marantic endocarditis, and myxoma.
      (2) **Noncardiac conditions** that may cause renal arterial embolism include atheromatous plaques and paradoxical, fat, or tumor embolism.
   c. **Cholesterol emboli** may occur spontaneously or follow vascular surgery or angiography. Acute renal failure may be the only manifestation of disease. Occasionally, skin lesions such as petechiae or livedo reticularis may be seen. Pathology of the skin or kidney reveals cholesterol clefts in small and medium-sized vessels. There is no specific therapy, but the disorder may spontaneously regress, leaving the patient with adequate residual kidney function.
   d. **Progressive renal atherosclerosis** affects a large number (perhaps > 20%) of individuals with end-stage renal failure; they have angiographically significant renal artery stenosis. Studies are underway to determine the optimal strategies for identifying and treating these patients. The risks of contrast-dye–associated acute renal failure, cholesterol embolization, and acute renal artery dissection have prevented many clinicians from suggesting an aggressive approach in most patients. Intervention is indicated in those with severe, uncontrollable hypertension, and in those patients with diffuse vascular disease with clearly progressive renal insufficiency.
2. **Clinical features and diagnosis**
   a. **Acute, complete renal arterial occlusion** usually manifests as flank pain, hematuria, fever, nausea, tissue necrosis [as evidenced by elevated lactate dehydrogenase (LDH) and aspartate

transaminase (AST)], and acute renal failure. The diagnosis is confirmed using radionuclide scanning or angiography. Bilateral occlusion and occlusion of a solitary functioning kidney produce severe anuric acute renal failure.

b. **Chronic or segmental occlusion** produces symptoms and signs commensurate with the degree of ischemic damage including progressive renal failure.

3. **Therapy**

a. Therapy for renal arterial thrombosis is surgical removal of the clot to restore renal blood flow. Best results are obtained when the operation is conducted within 48–72 hours following the onset of disease.

b. Therapy for renal arterial embolism, which usually is diffuse and involves large numbers of smaller arterial branches, is anticoagulation with heparin and resolution of the underlying focus of emboli.

c. Therapy for ischemic nephropathy may involve angioplasty, stent placement, or surgical revascularization. While the role of each of these therapies continues to be explored, there is little evidence that kidney function can be substantially preserved or that acute renal insufficiency due to ischemic nephropathy can be reversed.

B **Renal vein thrombosis** Obstruction of renal venous drainage by a clot may be caused by extension of clots in the vena cava, invasion of the renal vein by tumor, severe dehydration in infants, renal amyloidosis, and certain glomerular diseases associated with nephrotic syndrome, particularly membranous glomerulonephritis.

1. **Clinical features and diagnosis.** Slowly evolving renal vein thrombosis may be completely asymptomatic, whereas acute renal vein thrombosis may produce pain, hematuria, costovertebral angle tenderness, and, ultimately, signs of worsening renal function. The affected kidney appears to be enlarged when visualized with the aid of intravenous urography. Selective venography is diagnostic. New techniques such as Doppler ultrasonography may be particularly useful as a noninvasive approach to diagnosis.

2. **Clinical course.** Renal vein thrombosis generally is not a cause of glomerular disease. Renal vein thrombosis may develop during nephrosis because of loss of anticoagulant proteins and procoagulant deactivators in the urine protein.

3. **Therapy.** Treatment is controversial, as is the belief that renal vein thrombosis predisposes to pulmonary embolism. Current therapy is long-term (3–6 months) anticoagulation with warfarin sodium. Longer treatment is recommended if embolic phenomena occur.

C **Renal artery stenosis** In experimental animals, it has been clearly shown that partial reduction in the luminal size of one or both renal arteries produces renovascular hypertension, which is mediated in most cases by increased renin production with resultant activation of angiotensin and aldosterone. In humans, renal artery stenosis is a recognized cause of renovascular hypertension. However, the coincidence of radiographically demonstrated renal artery stenosis and clinically demonstrated renovascular hypertension does not establish a causal relationship.

1. **Etiology**

a. Among prepubertal children, the primary lesion responsible for renal artery stenosis is **medial fibromuscular dysplasia.**

b. Adults over 50 years of age suffer **renal artery atherosclerosis,** which is twice as common in men as in women.

c. Rare causes include **Takayasu's arteritis, arterial wall disease** (e.g., hematoma, dissecting aneurysm, tumor), and **external arterial compression** due to tumor, fibrosis, or cyst.

2. **Clinical features.** Signs and symptoms include a nearly continuous abdominal or flank bruit, hypokalemia, mild metabolic alkalosis, and asymmetric kidney size. None of these is a constant finding, and often there is no feature to distinguish renal artery stenosis from essential hypertension.

3. **Diagnosis.** Diagnostic strategies vary according to clinical suspicion.
   a. **Rapid-sequence intravenous urography** shows disparity in renal length and a delayed and persistent nephrogram on the affected side.
   b. **Renal angiography** (either standard or magnetic resonance imaging) is appropriate if surgical repair is contemplated or a definitive diagnosis is required. Stenotic segments are reliably identified by this study.
   c. **Duplex ultrasonography,** an emerging technique, may allow noninvasive determination of whether renal blood flow is intact. Unfortunately, because of renal vasculature–related anatomic issues, Doppler ultrasonography may not be technically feasible in many patients. Reports indicate that this procedure is very operator-dependent.
   d. **Renal vein renin studies.** Angiographic proof that renal artery stenosis is etiologically important is difficult to obtain. Finding that the renal vein renin from the affected side is 1.5 times greater than that from the unaffected side is helpful, but patients may respond to treatment without this biochemical finding. Although volume depletion and furosemide administration increase sensitivity, up to 30% of renal vein renin studies may be misleading or nondiagnostic. Ultimately, diagnosis relies on demonstration of normal blood pressure with correction of the renal artery stenosis.
4. **Therapy.** Therapeutic options are antihypertensive drugs, percutaneous transluminal angioplasty (PCTA) with or without stenting, and surgical repair of the affected vessel.

D Microangiopathy: hemolytic–uremic syndrome and thrombotic thrombocytopenic purpura (TTP) As members of the disease group termed microangiopathic hemolytic anemia, hemolytic–uremic syndrome and TTP are similar clinical syndromes that share features with DIC, malignant hypertension, postpartum renal failure, sepsis, and systemic sclerosis.

1. **Clinical features**
   a. **TTP** characteristically manifests as fever, microangiopathic hemolytic anemia, thrombocytopenia, fluctuating neurologic signs, purpura, and renal failure. Gastrointestinal involvement (e.g., mucosal bleeding, jaundice) is common. The course usually is fulminant; more than 50% of patients die within 6 weeks of the onset of TTP. In some cases, the etiologic agent is an autoantibody directed toward a protease, which cleaves von Willebrand's factor.
   b. **Hemolytic–uremic syndrome** is primarily a pediatric disorder characterized by microangiopathic hemolytic anemia, thrombocytopenia, and acute renal failure. The disorder may occur in epidemics and has been reported to follow shigellosis. Hemolytic–uremic syndrome usually has a sudden and dramatic onset, with renal failure the dominant clinical feature. As in TTP, other organ systems may be involved. Renal function returns in most patients who recover from systemic disease, but relapses have been reported.
2. **Diagnosis**
   a. **Laboratory findings** are similar in both disorders.
      (1) Anemia is a constant finding, occurring in association with a variety of structurally damaged RBCs in the peripheral circulation. The reticulocyte count and fibrin split products are elevated, leukocytosis is common, and the serum LDH and indirect bilirubin levels are elevated. Thrombocytopenia is severe (i.e., $< 20{,}000$ platelets/mm^3). The bone marrow shows erythroid hyperplasia with adequate or increased megakaryocytes. Azotemia is common, and the degree of renal failure is characteristically severe. Recently, microangiopathic hemolytic anemia has been found in association with the antiphospholipid antibody syndrome.
      (2) Urinalysis shows hematuria, pyuria, hemoglobinuria, and granular cysts.
      (3) Microbiologic studies may reveal verotoxin-producing *E. coli* as the cause, particularly in epidemics.
   b. **Renal biopsy findings** also are similar. Arterioles and small arteries are occluded by eosinophilic, hyaline thrombi containing fibrin and platelet aggregates, which cause impressive vascular

dilatation. Microinfarcts commonly occur, but without inflammatory infiltrates or signs of vasculitis. Renal lesions are focal and almost completely confined to the arterial side.

3. **Therapy.** Controlled trials comparing individual treatment programs have not been performed. Therapeutic methods currently in use include antiplatelet drugs (e.g., aspirin, sulfinpyrazone, dipyridamole), glucocorticoids, exchange transfusion, plasmapheresis, and, rarely, splenectomy. Most recent trials have suggested that plasma exchange therapy gives the best therapeutic outcome.
4. **Prognosis.** Outcome has improved with modern therapy. Untreated TTP is almost universally fatal within 1 year. However, 1-year survival rates for treated patients range from 40%–80%. Less than 5% of patients with hemolytic–uremic syndrome die within 1 month.

E Systemic sclerosis (scleroderma) This generalized disturbance of connective and vascular tissue leads to fibrosis of the affected tissue. Systemic sclerosis may be a very localized disease (called **morphea**) or a lethal, systemic disease. Renal involvement is a common cause of morbidity and death. The incidence of renal involvement in systemic sclerosis is not solidly established but, based on autopsy series, is estimated to range from 42%–80%. Clinical evidence of renal involvement (i.e., azotemia, hypertension, and active urinary sediment) is seen in about 45% of systemic sclerosis patients. In one study, subtle vascular and hemodynamic abnormalities were seen in 80% of patients.

1. **Clinical features and course**
   a. **Acute renal disease** occurs in the context of rapidly accelerating generalized disease activity, with prominent malignant hypertension. Renal failure can ensue precipitously if the blood pressure is uncontrolled. Pathologically, acute renal disease is quite similar to other microangiopathic diseases. The interlobular arteries show marked intimal thickening and mucoid proliferation, which may lead to cortical necrosis. Glomerular changes usually are mild and nonspecific, often consisting of only mesangial prominence. Interstitial edema with some mononuclear infiltrate is common. Unlike isolated malignant hypertension, systemic sclerosis does not primarily affect arterioles but does produce adventitial fibrosis.
   b. **Chronic renal disease** may be present in patients with systemic sclerosis and little or no clinical signs of renal involvement. Kidney size usually is normal, and the earliest sign of disease is proteinuria, which is noted in 30% of patients. Nephrotic syndrome is rare, and hematuria, urinary casts, and pyuria usually are absent. Hypertension complicates chronic renal disease frequently (i.e., in 25%–50% of patients) and is a harbinger of impending deterioration of renal function. Renal failure occasionally develops in systemic sclerosis patients who have neither proteinuria nor hypertension.
2. **Therapy**
   a. **Treatment of acute renal disease** involves, to a large degree, the control of accelerated hypertension. Captopril, enalapril, minoxidil, and nitroprusside may be required. However, recent data suggest that overly aggressive lowering of diastolic blood pressure to less than 85 mm Hg may actually increase the risk of acute renal failure in patients with scleroderma. Propranolol and furosemide are frequently used adjunctive agents.
   b. **Treatment of chronic renal disease** is less clear-cut. It is not known whether some vasoactive therapy during early, nonazotemic, nonhypertensive stages of the disease is protective. Similarly, the role of treatment for patients with abnormal renal biopsy specimens but no clinical renal disease is unclear.

F Sickle cell nephropathy

1. **Pathology**
   a. Sickle cell trait and sickle cell disease are associated with a variety of renal complications. The renal medulla is relatively anoxic and hyperosmolar—factors that favor erythrocyte sickling. Most damage occurs in the renal papillae.
   b. Medullary infarction resulting from occluded (sickled) vessels produces a spectrum of tubular disorders, including impaired urine concentration. Because the injury is located in the

renal papillae, these patients behave as though they have been papillectomized. Papillary necrosis also is seen. Patients with sickle cell trait are affected less severely than those with sickle cell disease.

2. **Clinical features**
   a. Impaired secretion of potassium and hydrogen ion occurs, and a frequent biochemical finding is hyperkalemia with a hyperchloremic (normal anion gap) metabolic acidosis (see Part II: IV D 2).
   b. Hematuria represents the most dramatic of the renal abnormalities in sickle cell disease. Although it is usually self-limited, life-threatening exsanguination occurs in rare cases.
   c. Glomerular disease, including nephrotic syndrome, has been documented in sickle cell disease. Membranoproliferative-like lesions have been reported, as has typical membranous glomerulonephritis.
3. **Clinical course.** Although frequently the GFR is supranormal early in the course of sickle cell nephropathy, gradual deterioration of renal function is common. Progression to end-stage renal disease occurs in some cases.
4. **Therapy**
   a. Careful fluid management to maintain adequate intravascular volume, both during crises and at other times, clearly is important. Volume depletion is injurious to renal function and is more likely to occur because of the urine concentrating defect.
   b. Patients who are prone to hyperkalemia or acidosis should be advised to reduce their dietary intake of potassium and protein.
   c. Hemodialysis is useful and does not increase the number or severity of crises or alter the transfusion requirement in most patients.
   d. Kidney allografts are susceptible to sickle cell damage.

G Radiation nephritis High doses of ionizing radiation are destructive to the kidney and urinary tract. Delivery of at least 2000 rad (radiation-absorbed dose) over a period of several weeks can induce disease. Radiation-induced nephritis most commonly results from inadvertent exposure during radiotherapy for abdominal or retroperitoneal tumor.

1. **Immediate radiation nephrotoxicity** results in decreased renal blood flow, with tubular function and blood pressure remaining normal.
2. **Acute radiation nephritis** develops 6–12 months after exposure. Clinical signs are edema, hypertension, headache, exertional dyspnea, anemia, cylindruria, proteinuria, and microscopic hematuria. Death occurs in nearly 50% of patients as a result of severe azotemia and hypertension. Patients who recover from the acute phase may have some persistent proteinuria.
3. **Chronic radiation nephritis** may follow acute radiation nephritis or develop anew up to 10 years following exposure. Clinical signs are fairly nonspecific and include fatigue, nocturia, hypertension, hyperuricemia with clinical gout, uremia, anemia, proteinuria, cylindruria, and hyposthenuria.

XV THE KIDNEY IN PREGNANCY

A General physiologic effects

1. Under the hormonal influence of pregnancy, renal size increases by 1 cm or more (radiographically); the renal pelvis, calyces, and ureters dilate, as in hydronephrosis; the GFR and RPF increase 25%–40%; a primary respiratory alkalosis develops; and the osmostat resets downward. Uric acid clearance nearly doubles and renal excretion of glucose increases, whereas blood glucose levels remain normal.
2. Clinically, the enlargement of the collecting system should not be mistaken for obstruction. The serum creatinine and BUN values decrease to less than 0.8 mg/dL and 13 mg/dL respectively. The serum bicarbonate concentration is 4–5 mEq/L lower than in the pregravid state, and the serum

osmolality is 10 mOsm/kg lower, with a corresponding drop of 5 mEq/L in serum sodium concentration. The serum uric acid is reduced to 3–4 mg/dL, and 24-hour urine glucose may exceed 20 g at term in the absence of diabetes.

B **Urinary tract infections** that occur in pregnant women frequently are attributable to the rich nutrient content of the urine and to the urinary stasis resulting from ureteral dilatation. (There is some concern that asymptomatic bacteriuria increases the rate of prematurity, particularly if there is kidney involvement.)

1. **Incidence**
   a. **Symptomatic bacteriuria** represents the most common renal problem seen by obstetricians. Although asymptomatic bacteriuria occurs with equal frequency in pregnant and nonpregnant women (i.e., in 4%–7% of all women), clinical infection (i.e., cystitis or pyelonephritis) develops in 20% of pregnant women.
   b. **Acute bacterial interstitial nephritis** occurs in 1%–2% of pregnant women, with signs and symptoms that are comparable to those seen in nonpregnant women. Lower tract infection also presents with typical symptoms.
2. **Laboratory findings and diagnosis.** Results are the same in both pregnant and nonpregnant women.
3. **Therapy.** Although an overwhelming majority of pregnant women respond well to antibiotic therapy without fetal morbidity, antibiotic therapy must be chosen with respect to possible toxic effects on the fetus.
   a. **Agents of choice. Ampicillin** is the drug of choice when no allergy exists. **Cephalosporins** are also safe. Sulfonamides displace albumin-bound bilirubin and may cause kernicterus, and tetracycline has obvious dental and osseous toxicity.
   b. **Duration of treatment.** Asymptomatic bacteriuria should be treated for 10–14 days. Clinical pyelonephritis should be treated for 6 weeks, owing to the very high rate of relapse.

C **Acute renal failure** complicates 1 in 2000–5000 pregnancies and has a bimodal pattern of occurrence. The first peak occurs in the first trimester and is related to septic abortion. The second peak occurs between 34 and 40 weeks' gestation and is related to preeclampsia, hemorrhage, and intravascular volume depletion.

1. **Clinical conditions**
   a. **Cortical necrosis** is a special cause of acute renal failure complicating pregnancy. Acute cortical necrosis accounts for 5% of cases of acute renal failure in the general population but 10%–30% of cases among pregnant women. Cortical necrosis may complicate any phase of pregnancy, particularly with abruptio placentae. The necrosis can be patchy or extensive. Some women recover variable amounts of renal function; however, most cases ultimately progress to end-stage renal disease.
   b. **Idiopathic postpartum renal failure** is a rare cause of renal failure peculiar to pregnancy. Affected patients present several weeks after an uncomplicated delivery with renal failure and severe hypertension. The exact etiology is unknown; however, the pathologic lesion strikingly resembles the hemolytic–uremic syndrome/TTP complex. It is unknown whether a virus, retained placental tissue, or drugs induce this condition by deranging coagulation or endothelial cell function. Dilatation and curettage (D&C) to remove any placental fragments is worth consideration. Some patients improve with anticoagulation.
2. **Prognosis.** Pregnancy-related acute renal failure has a better outlook for recovery than renal failure that is induced by medical or surgical complications. Nonetheless, maternal mortality is significant, ranging from 10%–25%.

D **Hypertension** Blood pressure declines early in pregnancy, reaching diastolic levels that are 15 mm lower than prepregnancy levels by 22 weeks' gestation. Blood pressure then rises gradually to prepregnancy values by term. This blood pressure drop is accompanied by a constant cardiac output, which suggests decreased peripheral resistance as a mechanism.

1. **Clinical conditions.** Hypertensive disorders of pregnancy are classified for clinical purposes as follows:
   a. **Preeclampsia–eclampsia** (see Part I: XV E)
   b. **Chronic hypertension,** which, in most women, is essential hypertension recognized before pregnancy. A secondary cause rarely is present and may, as in the case of pheochromocytoma, result in disastrously high maternal mortality. A standard evaluation for hypertension should be conducted in women who have high blood pressure and contemplate pregnancy.
   c. **Chronic hypertension with superimposed preeclampsia**
   d. **Late or transient hypertension,** which, in most cases, occurs in the third trimester and resolves within 10 days of delivery but tends to recur in subsequent pregnancies. Many of these women may ultimately develop essential hypertension.
2. **Therapy.** The treatment of hypertension during pregnancy is very difficult. Overly enthusiastic lowering of maternal blood pressure may diminish uteroplacental blood flow, leading to fetal compromise. Diastolic blood pressures above 100 mm Hg in noneclamptic women are best treated with **hydralazine, methyldopa,** or **calcium channel blockers.**
   a. For many reasons, some of which remain controversial, diuretics should not be used routinely.
   b. ACE inhibitors and angiotensin receptor blockers are contraindicated for pregnant women because they reduce placental blood flow and induce acute renal failure in the fetus, renal agenesis, and other deformities.

E Preeclampsia–eclampsia (toxemia of pregnancy) is primarily, but not exclusively, a disease of young primiparas.

1. **Definition.** Preeclampsia is a syndrome of **hypertension** (frequently malignant), **proteinuria, edema,** and, in its extreme, a **microangiopathic hemolytic anemia** with vascular endothelial destruction. The hallmark of this disease is the **labile vasospasm,** reflecting a vascular sensitivity to the pressor effects of endogenous peptides and catecholamines. Blood pressure may fluctuate widely, but sustained 4- to 6-hour periods of hypertension are reliable signs of disease. Preeclampsia that is associated with maternal convulsions and coma is referred to as **eclampsia.**
2. **Pathology.** The renal histopathology is glomerular capillary endotheliosis, with swelling of capillary endothelial cells in the absence of hypercellularity. Vacuolization is common.
3. **Clinical features and diagnosis.** The initial clinical presentation may be mild or severe; however, sustained hypertension newly appearing in the third trimester of a first pregnancy is a suitable criterion for a presumptive diagnosis of preeclampsia. Untreated, fulminant preeclampsia progresses rapidly to maternal convulsions, anuric renal failure, and death.
4. **Therapy** includes hospitalization and bed rest, prompt delivery if the fetus is mature, parenteral magnesium sulfate for impending convulsions, and careful titration of blood pressure to a diastolic range of 95–105 mm Hg. Ganglionic blockers induce meconium ileus in the fetus and are to be avoided. Diuretics are not recommended.

PART II: FLUID AND ELECTROLYTE DISORDERS

I WATER METABOLISM

A Normal physiology

1. **Regulation of water intake.** Increased thirst is the normal response to water loss. The neural center that controls the release of **ADH** is anatomically close to the thirst center and responds to increased body fluid tonicity.

a. **Tonicity** refers to the shift of water through biomembranes produced by osmotically active particles such as glucose and sodium. Urea exerts virtually no tonicity because it easily crosses all membranes and produces no osmotic shift of water.
b. **Osmolality** is a function of the number of molecules in solution independent of effects on water movement.

2. **Regulation of water output**
a. **Proximal tubular reabsorption.** Of the 200 L/day of water that are filtered at the glomerulus, 125 L are reabsorbed in the proximal tubule.
b. **Osmotic gradient formation in the medulla.** Glomerular filtrate not reabsorbed in the proximal tubule enters the loop of Henle, where in the thick ascending limb, active sodium chloride reabsorption without water reabsorption causes dilution of the urine and increases the concentration of solutes in the medullary interstitium.
c. **Collecting tubular transport.** Water that reaches the collecting tubule either is excreted (if ADH is absent, causing the tubule to be impermeable to water) or is reabsorbed (if ADH is present, causing the tubule to be permeable to water). Thus, ADH affects the osmolality of urine, which may range from 1200 mOsm/kg to 50 mOsm/kg.

B Hyponatremia

1. **Definition.** Hyponatremia refers to serum sodium concentration of less than 135 mEq/L. The name, however, is somewhat misleading, because hyponatremia is usually a problem of too much water, not too little sodium. In fact, the sodium content of the body may be increased, decreased, or relatively unchanged. Hypotonicity always implies hyponatremia. The opposite is not always true: hyponatremia can coexist with isotonicity, hypertonicity, or hypotonicity.
a. **Pseudohyponatremia** (isotonic hyponatremia) is a laboratory artifact that occurs in the setting of extreme hyperlipidemia or hyperproteinemia. If the laboratory uses an instrument that reports sodium content per unit volume of total plasma rather than sodium content per volume of the aqueous phase, then significant elevations in plasma lipids or γ-globulins can cause the reported sodium concentration to be artificially low. This artifact can be obviated by using an ion selective electrode that measures sodium ion concentration in the aqueous phase.
b. **Hypertonic hyponatremia** results from the shift of water from the intracellular fluid to the extracellular fluid, which is caused by the presence of osmotically active particles (e.g., glucose) in the extracellular fluid space. Serum sodium concentration is reduced, but the osmolality of the extracellular fluid is above normal.
c. **True hyponatremia** (hypotonic hyponatremia) occurs when there is excess total body water relative to solute content, and is clinically significant when the serum sodium concentration is less than 125 mEq/L and the serum osmolality is less than 250 mOsm/kg.

2. **Etiology**
a. **Decreased renal water excretion**
(1) **Decreased GFR.** A decrease in the filtered load of water to less than 10% of normal results in a clinically significant decrease in the ability of the kidney to excrete water.
(2) **Increased proximal tubular reabsorption.** An increase in proximal tubular reabsorption of filtered fluid from the normal 65% to more than 90% may impair the capacity of the kidney to excrete water. Increased proximal tubular reabsorption occurs when the kidney is hypoperfused (e.g., in states of excessive fluid loss from diarrhea or vomiting). Decreased effective renal perfusion in diseases such as CHF, cirrhosis, or nephrotic syndrome also stimulates proximal tubular reabsorption. This group of disorders is characterized by a low urine sodium concentration, indicating increased renal absorption of sodium, high BUN, and the physical finding of either true volume depletion or one of the edematous conditions.

(3) **Increased collecting tubular reabsorption of water.** Nonosmotically stimulated ADH secretion induces such reabsorption. Characteristics of this condition include relatively normal urine sodium excretion (if intake is normal), a high urine osmolality, and signs of body water expansion resulting from excessive retention of ingested water.

b. **Increased fluid intake.** Fluid intake in excess of 1 L/hr exceeds normal excretory capacity and leads to hyponatremia. This situation is seen in patients who are given excessive hyponatric intravenous fluids and in psychiatric patients who drink excessively.

c. **Syndrome of inappropriate ADH secretion (SIADH)** results from nonosmotically stimulated ADH release associated with the following disorders.

(1) **Tumor.** Several tumors have been reported to produce an ADH-like peptide, most notably small-cell carcinoma of the lung.

(2) **CNS disease.** Excessive ADH release has been documented in postseizure patients as well as in those with cerebral trauma, brain tumors, and psychiatric disturbances. Nausea and vomiting may produce excessive ADH release.

(3) **Pulmonary disease.** SIADH has been described with pulmonary tumors, infections, and bronchospastic disease. The mechanism is believed to be stimulation of the so-called **J receptors** in the pulmonary circulation, leading to pituitary ADH release.

(4) **Hypopituitarism.** Individuals with glucocorticoid deficiency as a result of impaired adrenocorticotropic hormone (ACTH) release may have excessive ADH release, resulting from the loss of glucocorticoid inhibition of ADH release. Primary adrenal insufficiency involving both glucocorticoid and mineralocorticoid production may be associated with a syndrome of renal sodium wasting, which exacerbates the hyponatremia.

(5) **Drug-induced SIADH.** Drugs that may produce SIADH include chlorpropamide and clofibrate, both of which may increase ADH release as well as sensitize the renal tubule to the effects of ADH. Many CNS-active drugs also produce SIADH. Thiazide diuretics, which may directly lead to ADH release, also may cause hyponatremia through excessive renal sodium excretion or through potassium depletion.

(6) **Idiopathic SIADH.** Elderly patients may have no apparent reason for SIADH and yet maintain sustained hyponatremia. This condition may be related to the increase in ADH release that occurs with advancing age.

(7) **Reset osmostat,** a variant of SIADH, occurs in chronically ill and malnourished patients in whom the serum sodium concentration is reset at a low value (approximately 125 mEq/L), thus maintaining an abnormally low serum osmolality. This new set point for osmolality is termed a "reset osmostat." These patients are able to maintain water balance, albeit at constant low serum osmolality. Increased water intake leads to inhibition of ADH release, dilution of the urine, and excretion of the water load; water restriction triggers ADH release but at a lower plasma osmolality than normal individuals and leads to increased urine osmolality and water retention.

3. **Clinical features.** CNS dysfunction may develop as the tonicity of the extracellular fluid falls and water diffuses down an osmotic gradient into the brain cells, leading to cellular edema. Acute hyponatremia with a decrease in serum sodium concentration below 125 mEq/L over a period of hours almost always is associated with acute CNS disturbances such as obtundation, coma, seizures, and death if untreated.

4. **Diagnosis**

a. **Physical findings.** Examination may reveal:

(1) Volume depletion (e.g., in cases related to drugs such as diuretics)

(2) Edema (e.g., in cases related to cirrhosis or CHF)

b. **Laboratory data**

(1) Urine osmolality: $>$ 50–100 mOsm/kg in the presence of plasma hypotonicity

(2) Urine sodium concentration: high when plasma volume is expanded in SIADH but low when effective arterial blood volume is reduced, as in edematous conditions. A urine sodium concentration less than 20 mEq/L strongly argues against SIADH.

c. **Water loading test.** When an intravascularly volume-expanded individual is given 20 mL water/kg orally or intravenously over a period of 20–40 minutes, the normal response is excretion of 80% of this water load within 4 hours and reduction of urine osmolality to below 100 mOsm/kg. Failure to achieve these results suggests an impairment in the kidney's ability to excrete water.

5. **Therapy**
   a. **Fluid restriction.** All patients who are severely hyponatremic should reduce free water intake to approximately 700 mm^3/day.
   b. **Inhibition of water reabsorption**
      (1) **Demeclocycline.** This agent has been shown to alter ADH-induced water flow in the collecting tubule. This drug must be given in doses of 600–1200 mg/day and requires 4–5 days to achieve its peak action. Demeclocycline cannot be administered to patients with liver disease, heart failure, or kidney disease, because it may accumulate to toxic levels in these conditions.
      (2) **Furosemide.** Acute administration of this agent in combination with large amounts of saline may lead to increased water excretion.
   c. **Hypertonic infusions.** The infusion of 3% sodium chloride rapidly raises the tonicity of the extracellular fluid. (Serum sodium concentration should not increase faster than 0.5 mEq/L/hr. Elevation faster than 0.5 mEq/L/hr or to a value greater than 135 mEq/L can result in acute pontine demyelination and severe neurologic damage.) Because extracellular fluid expansion may lead to pulmonary edema, hypertonic saline usually is given in combination with bumetanide or furosemide and should be used only in the treatment of symptomatic patients. Elevation of serum sodium concentration to 125 mEq/L usually alleviates the dangers of brain edema. The amount of hypertonic saline (in mEq) needed to raise the serum sodium concentration ($[Na^+]$) is calculated using the following equation:

$$(\text{Normal serum } [Na^+] - \text{current serum } [Na^+]) \times \text{total body water}$$

6. **Complications**
   a. **Acute hyponatremia.** Acute reduction of serum osmolality can produce intracranial hypertension and brain damage, particularly if the serum sodium concentration falls below 125 mEq/L over a period of hours.
   b. **Chronic hyponatremia.** Brain cells adapt to chronic hyponatremia by loss of net intracellular solute (primarily potassium chloride and organic molecules, termed osmolytes). This adaptation, which can occur over a period of a few days, leads to marked reduction in the degree of cell swelling.

C Hypernatremia

1. **Definition.** Hypernatremia refers to serum sodium concentration that is above normal. Clinically significant effects are produced at serum sodium levels greater than 155 mEq/L. Hypernatremia always implies hypertonicity of all body fluids, because the rise in the extracellular fluid osmolality obligates movement of water from the intracellular space, producing increased intracellular osmotic activity and cell dehydration.
2. **Etiology**
   a. **Extrarenal causes**
      (1) **Decreased fluid intake.** Adequate water intake is required to maintain the tonicity of body fluids in the face of continuous water losses through the skin as well as losses through the urine and gastrointestinal tract. In cool environments, this intake equals approximately 700 mL/day. If intake is less than external losses, body fluid osmolality rises.
      (2) **Increased skin losses.** Profuse sweating may lead to excess water losses through the skin. In addition, burns and other widespread inflammatory lesions of the skin may cause marked fluid losses.

(3) **Increased gastrointestinal losses.** Diarrhea and protracted vomiting also may result in water deficits.

b. Renal causes

(1) **Osmotic diuresis.** The presence of osmotically active, nonreabsorbable solute in the glomerular filtrate prevents water and sodium reabsorption and leads to increased renal water losses. Hyperglycemia with glycosuria is a common cause of osmotic diuresis. Because water losses are relatively greater than sodium losses, the serum sodium concentration rises progressively during osmotic diuresis.

(2) **Decreased ADH effect**

(a) **Central diabetes insipidus** (i.e., failure of ADH synthesis or release) may occur in the following settings:

(i) **Tumor.** ADH deficiency may occur either through direct invasion of the neurohypophysis or through increased intracranial pressure compressing the brain stem.

(ii) **Histiocytosis.** Hand-Schüller-Christian disease, in particular, has a predilection for neurohyophyseal involvement, producing ADH deficiency.

(iii) **Sarcoidosis.** The neurohypophysis may be involved, producing diabetes insipidus.

(iv) **Trauma.** Classically, after resection of the pituitary stalk, a phase of acute ADH release is followed by a prolonged period of central diabetes insipidus.

(b) **Nephrogenic diabetes insipidus** (i.e., failure of renal water conservation despite high levels of plasma ADH) may occur in the following settings.

(i) **Renal disease.** Structural disease impairs the integrity of the renal medulla and, thereby, the urine concentrating ability.

(ii) **Hypercalcemia.** Elevation of serum calcium concentration above 12 mg/dL may impair urine concentrating ability, most likely as a result of inhibition of sodium chloride reabsorption in the thick ascending limb of Henle's loop, increased medullary blood flow, dissipation of medullary hypertonicity, and interference with ADH-mediated water flow in the medullary collecting tubule.

(iii) **Hypokalemia.** Reduction of serum potassium concentration below 3.5 mEq/L leads to a direct stimulation of thirst and a mild impairment of urine concentrating ability.

(iv) **Lithium ingestion.** This action blocks ADH-stimulated osmotic water flow in the collecting tubule.

(v) **Demeclocycline.** This tetracycline antibiotic alters ADH-induced water flow through a direct effect on the cell membrane.

(vi) **Sickle cell anemia.** Reduced medullary blood flow produced by sickling erythrocytes within the vasa recta also may impair urine concentrating ability.

(vii) **Urinary tract obstruction** and the **postobstructive state.** These conditions are associated with nephrogenic diabetes insipidus.

3. Clinical features

a. CNS disorders. Generalized CNS depression, including obtundation, coma, and seizures, develops in young children and elderly patients. Intracerebral and subarachnoid hemorrhage may occur if shrinkage of brain volume leads to tears in the bridging veins.

b. Extracellular volume depletion. Excessive water loss in hypernatremic states may lead to this condition. Although the intracellular fluid accounts for two-thirds of water deficits, the extracellular fluid volume also contracts mildly. If loss of water as well as solute occurs, the contraction is more pronounced. However, if the etiology of the hypernatremia is due to excess salt intake (e.g., hypertonic sodium bicarbonate infusion or sea-water drowning), the extracellular fluid volume increases.

c. **Abnormal urine output.** If the kidneys cause water losses, polyuria (i.e., urine output that is inappropriately high given the level of plasma osmolality or extracellular fluid volume) may be present. If the kidneys are normal and water losses are extrarenal, urine volume typically is reduced.

4. **Diagnosis**
   a. **Dehydration test.** Urine concentrating ability may be tested after overnight dehydration to determine whether a patient has renal water wasting.
      (1) Water deprivation begins at 8:00 P.M. and lasts 14 hours, after which the urine osmolality should exceed 800 mOsm/kg. The patient then is given a subcutaneous dose of ADH (5 U aqueous vasopressin). The urine osmolality should not be further increased by this maneuver.
      (2) If the urine osmolality is less than 800 mOsm/kg after water deprivation or if it increases by greater than 15% after ADH administration, some degree of ADH deficiency is present.
      (3) If the urine osmolality does not exceed 300 mOsm/kg after water deprivation and there is no further increase after ADH administration, some form of nephrogenic diabetes insipidus is present.
   b. **Plasma ADH assay.** In nephrogenic diabetes insipidus, the urine osmolality may not be a true reflection of ADH release, and, thus, plasma ADH levels should be measured.
   c. **Assay of urine osmolality and composition**
      (1) It is useful to measure the solute composition of the urine in the evaluation of polyuria. Urine osmolality less than 200 mOsm/L suggests a primary defect in water conservation. Urine osmolality greater than 200 mOsm/L during polyuria suggests an osmotic diuresis.
      (2) After measuring urine osmolality, the urine should be analyzed for sodium, glucose, and urea to determine the etiology of the diuresis. A urine pH greater than 6 may indicate bicarbonate diuresis.
   d. **Physical examination.** Although examination may be helpful in determining if hypovolemia or hypervolemia is present, it is generally not useful in determining the etiology and pathogenesis of polyuria.

5. **Therapy**
   a. **Free water** may be administered orally, which is the preferred route, or intravenously as a 5% dextrose solution (D_5W). The dextrose is readily metabolized, leaving behind free water. Infusion of a fluid with an osmolality less than 150 mOsm/L is dangerous and may lead to acute hemolysis at the infusion site.
   b. **Vasopressin** may be administered in several different forms. Currently, the agent of choice for treatment of ADH deficiency is **1-deamino-8-D-arginine vasopressin (dDAVP** or **desmopressin)**, which may be administered orally or as a nasal spray every 12 hours.
   c. **Thiazide diuretics** impair dilution in the distal nephron and stimulate proximal tubular reabsorption of sodium and water as a result of volume depletion. The latter action reduces the delivery of fluid to the distal nephron, thereby reducing the degree of polyuria. Thiazides are useful as adjunct therapy in patients with nephrogenic diabetes insipidus.
   d. **Other drugs** such as clofibrate, carbamazepine, and chlorpropamide enhance the renal tubular effects of ADH and possibly contribute to the stimulation of ADH release in certain settings.

6. **Complications.** Diseases of water conservation are dangerous only if patients are not allowed access to water. In such settings, cellular dehydration, CNS depression, and severe volume depletion may occur. The serious manifestations of acute hypernatremia are primarily due to brain cell shrinkage. Brain cells adapt to chronic hypernatremia by net gain of intracellular solute (mainly sodium chloride and organic osmolytes such as *myo*-inositol, taurine, betaine, and other methylamines). This adaptation, occurring over several days, leads to marked reduction in the degree of cell shrinkage.

II SODIUM METABOLISM

A Normal physiology Sodium is the primary osmotic component of the extracellular fluid, which contains approximately 3000 mEq sodium. The sodium content of the extracellular fluid determines the volume of that space and the "fullness," or effective volume, of the systemic circulation. A less than 1% change in renal sodium excretion can produce major changes in extracellular fluid volume.

1. **Renal handling.** Approximately 30,000 mEq/day of sodium are filtered at the glomerulus. If sodium intake is approximately 200–300 mEq/day, the entire glomerular filtrate of sodium must be reabsorbed, less 1% (typical amount of ingested sodium), to maintain sodium homeostasis. Although only 10%–15% of the glomerular filtrate is reabsorbed in the distal tubule and collecting duct, this site is the major regulator for determining final urine sodium composition.
2. **Hormonal regulation.** Aldosterone stimulates sodium reabsorption in the cortical collecting duct. Other hormones may alter renal tubular handling of sodium, but none is as well studied as aldosterone. Aldosterone release from the adrenal gland is governed by the **renin–angiotensin system.**
   a. Renin is an enzyme that catalyzes the conversion of **angiotensinogen** to the decapeptide **angiotensin I** (in plasma). Angiotensin I is converted to the octapeptide **angiotensin II** (in the lung and kidney) by ACE. Angiotensin II is a potent vasoconstrictive agent as well as a potent stimulus for increased aldosterone release from the adrenal gland.
   b. Renin secretion by the kidney is stimulated by renal hypoperfusion, adrenergic stimulation, and circulating catecholamines. Renin is released from the **juxtaglomerular apparatus,** which is located between the afferent and the efferent arterioles of the glomeruli.
   c. Other hormones that regulate sodium handling are listed in Table 6–11.

B Edema

1. **Definition**
   a. Edema generally is defined as an increase in the interstitial compartment of the extracellular fluid.
      (1) Normally, the extracellular fluid volume equals approximately 14 L and accounts for one-third of the total body water. About 25% of the extracellular fluid is represented by plasma volume and is contained within the circulation. The other 75% or 11 L is represented by the interstitial fluid between cells.
      (2) If the interstitial fluid volume increases by approximately 2 L, clinically evident edema may result; edema may be **observable** (as **swelling**) or **palpable** (as **pitting**).
   b. Although edema generally is a function of increased extracellular fluid volume, in some instances increased transcapillary hydrostatic pressure (e.g., as occurs in the portal circulation in cirrhosis) also may contribute to edema.
2. **Pathophysiology.** Edema, or the pathologic increase in extracellular fluid volume, primarily is a function of excessive renal tubular reabsorption of sodium. Decreased renal perfusion (e.g., as occurs in CHF with reduced cardiac output, in cirrhosis with reduced effective arterial blood volume, and in the nephrotic syndrome) is the proximate cause of the increased renal sodium reabsorption, which represents the body's attempt to maintain adequate effective arterial blood volume.

TABLE 6–11 Other Hormones and Their Reactions to Sodium Handling

Hormone	Action on Sodium Transport
Atrial natriuretic peptide	Inhibits renal reabsorption (collecting duct)
Dopamine	Intrarenally generated; inhibits proximal tubule sodium reabsorption
Prostaglandins	Intrarenally generated; inhibit tubular sodium reabsorption and vasodilate the kidney

3. Etiology

a. **CHF.** When cardiac output is reduced, effective arterial blood volume is decreased as well. The decrease in effective arterial blood volume triggers the release of renin and aldosterone, leading to stimulation of distal tubular reabsorption of sodium. Additionally, alterations in renal hemodynamics stimulate an increase in the proximal tubular reabsorption of sodium.

b. **Cirrhosis.** The primary cause of sodium retention in liver disease may be ascites formation as a result of high pressure in the portal circulation. Portal hypertension leads to intravascular fluid volume depletion and secondary renal sodium retention. When hypoalbuminemia occurs, effective arterial blood volume drops, stimulating renal sodium retention. Secondary hyperaldosteronism is common and is caused by intravascular volume contraction as well as impaired hepatic clearance of aldosterone; these factors lead to stimulation of distal tubular reabsorption of sodium. A primary increase in renal sodium reabsorption may occur in cirrhosis.

c. **Nephrotic syndrome.** Hypoalbuminemia leads to reduced effective arterial blood volume, as a result of renal protein losses, which stimulates renal tubular reabsorption of sodium.

d. **Chronic renal failure.** When the GFR falls to less than 10 mL/min, the capacity of the kidney to excrete the typical dietary sodium load is limited, and edema may result.

e. **Excessive mineralocorticoid activity.** Tumors of the adrenal gland and pituitary tumors that secrete large amounts of ACTH may be associated with marked sodium retention.

4. Clinical features

a. **Peripheral edema.** Sodium retention may manifest as swelling in the dependent regions of the body.

b. **Pulmonary edema.** If pulmonary venous pressure acutely rises above 18 mm Hg, pulmonary edema may develop.

5. Diagnosis

a. On **physical examination,** peripheral edema may be identified by the persistence of an indentation following palpation of the soft tissues in the dependent areas. Pulmonary edema is identified by the physical findings of rales or wheezes or by chest radiography.

b. **Urine sodium assay** reveals a urine sodium level that is less than sodium intake and that usually is significantly less than 20 mEq/L.

6. Therapy

a. **Dietary sodium restriction** is essential. A sodium intake of 1 g (23 mEq)/day is the lowest practical intake level that can be achieved.

b. **Diuretics** are useful for increasing sodium excretion.

(1) **Loop diuretics** such as furosemide, torsemide, and bumetanide are particularly effective. Side effects of these drugs include intravascular volume depletion with azotemia, hyperuricemia, hypokalemia, metabolic alkalosis, and hypomagnesemia.

(2) **Thiazide diuretics** such as hydrochlorothiazide inhibit sodium reabsorption in the distal convoluted tubule. They can be used effectively, although they are less potent than loop diuretics. Side effects are similar to those of loop diuretics.

(3) **Potassium-sparing diuretics** such as amiloride and triamterene act primarily to block sodium reabsorption and secondarily to block potassium secretion in the distal tubule. Use of these agents may lead to potassium retention and increased sodium excretion.

(4) **Aldosterone antagonists** such as the competitive agent spironolactone also lead to potassium retention and increased sodium excretion.

III POTASSIUM METABOLISM

A Normal physiology Potassium is the primary cationic component of the intracellular fluid, which contains approximately 4000 mEq potassium. In comparison, the extracellular fluid contains very little potassium—about 65 mEq. The ratio of extracellular to intracellular potassium concentration is an important determinant of electrical activity in excitable membranes (e.g., the cardiac conduction system and somatic nerve endings). The normal dietary potassium intake of 60–90 mEq/day must be excreted by the kidney to preserve potassium homeostasis. Also, dietary potassium intake must be taken up rapidly by cells in preparation for renal excretion; otherwise, the serum potassium rapidly rises to life-threatening levels.

1. **Extrarenal handling.** Cellular uptake of potassium is influenced by the following extrarenal factors:
   a. **Insulin.** High insulin levels stimulate cellular uptake of potassium.
   b. **Epinephrine.** This β_2-active catecholamine directly stimulates cellular uptake of potassium. This action may be particularly important during severe exertion, when serum potassium levels rise because of muscle ischemia.
2. **Renal handling.** Most urine potassium is the result of distal tubular secretion. Several factors are known to alter potassium secretion.
   a. **Aldosterone secretion.** Aldosterone directly stimulates potassium secretion and sodium reabsorption in the collecting tubule of the kidney.
   b. **Sodium reabsorption.** The delivery of fluid and sodium to the collecting tubule also stimulates potassium secretion. This mechanism accounts for the increased potassium secretion caused by diuretics, which act at more proximal sites in the nephron to block sodium reabsorption.

B Hypokalemia

1. **Definition.** Hypokalemia is defined as serum potassium concentration of less than 3.5 mEq/L. Because most of the potassium content of the body is within cells and cellular potassium concentration is about 155 mEq/L, cellular potassium can be severely depleted without causing large changes in serum potassium.
2. **Etiology.** Hypokalemia can result from extrarenal or renal causes.
   a. **Extrarenal causes**
      (1) **Dietary deficiency and gastrointestinal losses**
         (a) **Inadequate dietary intake.** Because potassium conservation in the kidney is limited, a severe reduction of intake to less than 10 mEq/day for many days or weeks can lead to a large negative potassium balance and hypokalemia.
         (b) **Diarrhea.** Because the potassium content of diarrheal fluid may be as high as 100 mEq/L, diarrhea can lead to severe potassium depletion.
         (c) **Vomiting.** Although the potassium content of vomitus is relatively small, the secondary effect of intravascular volume depletion, which produces secondary hyperaldosteronism, stimulates renal potassium excretion.
      (2) **Potassium redistribution**
         (a) **Insulin administration.** A therapeutic or replacement dose of insulin can drive potassium into cells, producing acute hypokalemia.
         (b) **Epinephrine infusions.** Epinephrine also can produce acute hypokalemia by an independent action involving β_2-receptors.
         (c) **Folic acid and vitamin B_{12} therapy.** In patients with megaloblastic anemia, folic acid and vitamin B_{12} stimulate cell proliferation, thus producing acute hypokalemia, because potassium is used in cell synthesis. This effect also may be seen in patients with rapidly growing tumors.
         (d) **Hypokalemic periodic paralysis.** In this rare syndrome, potassium levels fall acutely—without a loss of potassium from the body—prior to episodes of paralysis. This syndrome, which is commonly associated with thyroid disease in Asians, probably represents a defect in catecholamine sensitivity.
   b. **Renal causes.** Any hyperactivity of the normal components of renal potassium excretion can produce a negative potassium balance via increased renal losses.

(1) **Drug-induced renal losses**

(a) **Diuretics.** Agents that act proximal to the site of potassium secretion stimulate urinary excretion of potassium by increasing the delivery of sodium and fluid to the distal tubules.

(b) **Penicillins.** Carbenicillin, ticarcillin, and related drugs act as nonreabsorbable anions in the distal tubule and thereby stimulate potassium secretion. Significant hypokalemia is commonly seen.

(c) **Aminoglycosides.** Tubular defects with magnesium wasting and secondary potassium wasting occasionally may be seen in patients treated with large doses of gentamicin or related compounds.

(d) **Amphotericin B.** This antifungal agent causes damage to the apical membrane of the renal tubular cell, thus increasing potassium loss from the cell.

(2) **Hormone-induced renal losses**

(a) **Primary hyperaldosteronism**

(i) **Primary adrenal adenomas** are associated with hypokalemia, hypertension, and metabolic alkalosis.

(ii) **Diffuse bilateral adrenal hyperplasia** may be associated with a milder hypokalemia than is seen with primary adrenal adenoma.

(iii) In **ectopic ACTH syndrome,** massive mineralocorticoid increase and renal potassium wasting may occur in patients with small-cell lung carcinoma (a tumor that produces and secretes ACTH).

(iv) **Exogenous mineralocorticoid**

Licorice ingestion. Licorice produced in Europe (anise) contains a component, **glycyrrhetinic acid,** which prevents conversion of cortisol to cortisone in the renal distal tubule, thus producing a stimulation of mineralocorticoid receptors and an aldosterone-like action. Ingestion of this agent may lead to the development of hypokalemia with hypertension and metabolic alkalosis.

Tobacco chewing. Certain tobacco compounds also contain **glycyrrhetinic acid** and may cause the development of hypokalemia.

(b) **Secondary hyperaldosteronism**

(i) **Renin-secreting tumor.** This rare entity, diagnosed by arteriography, is characterized by intrarenal tumors of the juxtaglomerular apparatus. Severe hypertension and hypokalemia may occur.

(ii) **Renal artery stenosis** may be associated with hypokalemia and hypertension as a result of secondary hyperaldosteronism produced by hyperreninemia.

(iii) In **malignant hypertension,** severe underperfusion of the kidney may occur and may lead to hyperreninemia, secondary hyperaldosteronism, and hypokalemia.

(iv) **Disorders with reduced effective arterial blood volume** produce only mild hypokalemia despite hyperreninemia and hyperaldosteronism. Reduced tubular flow rate reduces potassium secretion.

In **CHF,** secondary hyperaldosteronism may develop, causing mild hypokalemia even in the absence of diuretic use.

In **cirrhosis,** severe hypokalemia is common because of low intake of potassium and secondary hyperaldosteronism.

(3) **Potassium loss due to primary renal tubular disorders**

(a) **Renal tubular acidosis** is often associated with potassium wasting, which may be secondary to sodium depletion and metabolic acidosis or directly attributable to tubular defects in potassium conservation. Potassium wasting is a feature of distal (type I) as well as proximal (type II) renal tubular acidosis of any etiology.

(b) **Bartter's syndrome** and **Gitelman's syndrome** are characterized by renal potassium wasting, metabolic alkalosis, and polyuria. Blood pressure usually is normal or reduced, but renin and aldosterone levels are very high. In **Bartter's syndrome,** the primary defect lies in one of the epithelial transport proteins involved in the reabsorption of sodium chloride, most commonly the furosemide-sensitive Na^+–K^+–Cl^- cotransporter in the ascending limb of Henle's loop. In **Gitelman's syndrome,** the primary defect involves the thiazide-sensitive Na^+–Cl^- cotransporter in the distal convoluted tubule.

(c) **Chronic magnesium depletion** produces a syndrome of renal tubular potassium wasting without other associated defects in ion transport. The potassium wasting can be severe and is unresponsive to potassium repletion until magnesium deficits have been corrected.

(4) **Potassium loss due to surreptitious diuretic use** is associated with a clinical presentation identical to that of Bartter's or Gitelman's syndrome, including hypokalemia, magnesium wasting, metabolic alkalosis, hyperreninemia, and hyperaldosteronism.

3. Clinical features

a. Neuromuscular disorders. Potassium depletion may cause weakness and paralysis.

b. Cardiac disorders. Arrhythmia, particularly in the presence of digitalis intoxication, is a hallmark of severe hypokalemia.

c. Endocrine disorders. Hypokalemia is associated with abnormalities in pancreatic insulin release. Glucose intolerance has been shown to worsen as a result of diuretic-induced hypokalemia.

d. Polyuria. The polyuria of hypokalemia is a function of polydipsia as well as impaired ADH action.

4. Diagnosis

a. Physical examination. The presence or absence of hypertension is a useful differentiating feature in the approach to the patient with hypokalemia.

(1) If the patient is hypertensive, the hypokalemia may be caused by excessive mineralocorticoid activity. Because many hypertensive patients are treated with diuretics, any hypokalemia could be a side effect of such therapy.

(2) If the patient is normotensive, the hypokalemia represents either a gastrointestinal or a primary renal loss of potassium.

b. Serum electrolyte assay. This test rarely is useful for evaluating the specific cause of hypokalemia. However, the finding of combined acidosis and hypokalemia, which suggests renal tubular acidosis, is an exception.

c. Urine potassium assay. Urine potassium levels below 20 mEq/L suggest extrarenal potassium losses, whereas levels exceeding 30 mEq/L suggest renal losses.

d. Renin–aldosterone axis assay

(1) **Noninvasive tests**

(a) **Renin stimulation test.** This test is used to determine whether excessive mineralocorticoid activity is due to excessive renin production or to a primary adrenal disorder. To evaluate renin production, 40 mg furosemide is administered; then plasma renin is measured in both the supine and upright positions.

(i) In normal individuals, renin levels are increased several-fold following furosemide administration, and the levels increase further when the patient assumes the upright position.

(ii) In individuals with renin suppression due to extracellular fluid volume expansion secondary to excessive mineralocorticoid activity, renin levels are suppressed following furosemide administration and are not stimulated when the patient assumes the upright position.

(b) **Aldosterone suppression test.** To document that aldosterone production is independent of normal inhibitory stimuli, 1–2 L of saline are infused; then plasma aldosterone is measured in both the supine and upright positions. Individuals whose aldosterone levels are not suppressed to below normal values may have primary aldosterone overproduction.

(c) **Plasma aldosterone-to-renin ratio.** A value greater than 15 is highly suggestive of primary hyperaldosteronism in patients following maneuvers such as diuretic administration designed to stimulate renin secretion.

(2) **Invasive tests** include measurement of bilateral renal venous renin as well as adrenal venous aldosterone and cortisol concentrations. This information is necessary to establish a definitive diagnosis of primary aldosteronism and to define the presence of unilateral or bilateral adrenal disease. The hypertension associated with bilateral adrenal hyperplasia does not respond to adrenalectomy, whereas hypertension of aldosteronoma is responsive to tumor removal.

e. **Urine chloride assay.** In cases of mineralocorticoid excess, Bartter's or Gitelman's syndrome, and diuretic abuse, urine chloride levels tend to be elevated in the presence of metabolic alkalosis and hypokalemia. The absence of elevated urine chloride levels is highly suggestive of gastrointestinal potassium losses such as surreptitious vomiting.

f. **Diuretic assay.** If Bartter's or Gitelman's syndrome is suspected, the urine must be analyzed for chloride and diuretics, including loop-active agents and thiazides, before a diagnosis of a primary tubular disorder can be established. Such diuretic assays are commercially available.

5. **Therapy.** In many cases, hypokalemia can be corrected by administration of potassium salts.

a. **Forms of potassium salts.** Potassium may be administered with a variety of anions. Potassium chloride is the preferred form of therapy, because many patients have concurrent chloride deficits. In cases of hypokalemia with coincident renal tubular acidosis, potassium citrate, potassium lactate, or potassium gluconate may be given.

b. **Routes of administration.** Potassium may be given intravenously or orally.

(1) Intravenous potassium solutions should not exceed a concentration of 60 mEq/L, and the rate of administration should not exceed 60 mEq/hr. Normally, potassium deficits are on the order of 300–1000 mEq. These deficits should be replaced slowly, over days, except when digitalis intoxication or life-threatening arrhythmias are present.

(2) Oral potassium is absorbed effectively and should be substituted for intravenous potassium whenever possible. Several potassium salts may be given in wax matrix capsules, which avoid the problem of gastrointestinal ulceration caused by the earlier enteric-coated potassium preparations. A variety of potassium salts also are available as liquid suspensions.

c. **Chronic potassium therapy.** Hypokalemic patients receiving diuretics should be given potassium supplementation to maintain the serum potassium level above 3.5 mEq/L. This level may be accomplished with oral potassium supplementation. Although some foods are high in potassium, it is difficult to overcome these deficits solely by ingesting potassium-rich food.

C Hyperkalemia

1. **Definition.** Hyperkalemia is defined as serum potassium concentration greater than 5.5 mEq/L.

2. **Etiology. Pseudohyperkalemia** may be caused by release of potassium from coagulated cells and platelets after blood is withdrawn for analysis. It can also occur if the platelet or white blood cell (WBC) count is extremely high, as in myeloproliferative disorders. Measurement of plasma potassium is required to eliminate this artifact. **True hyperkalemia** may result from extrarenal or renal causes.

a. **Extrarenal causes**

(1) **Insulin deficiency.** Hyperkalemia in diabetic patients may be due to a lack of insulin and to the presence of associated renal and adrenal abnormalities.

(2) **Cell lysis syndromes.** Acute cell necrosis following either chemotherapy or a massive crushing injury (**rhabdomyolysis**) produces hyperkalemia by rapid cellular release of potassium.

(3) **Succinylcholine therapy.** The muscle relaxant succinylcholine may produce hyperkalemia in susceptible individuals with generalized muscle or neurologic disease.

(4) **Hyperkalemic periodic paralysis.** This rare, familial syndrome that may be associated with an acute shift of extracellular potassium. [The hypokalemic form of this syndrome, which is more common, is discussed in Part II: III B 2 a (2) (e).]

(5) **Hyperosmolality.** Acute increases in extracellular fluid osmotic activity may produce a transcellular shift of potassium and result in hyperkalemia. Diabetic patients who are given intravenous glucose on the suspicion of hypoglycemia may develop this entity if hyperglycemia occurs in the setting of insulin deficiency.

(6) **Acidosis.** Mineral acidosis, not organic acidosis, may be associated with an acute shift of potassium from the intracellular to the extracellular fluid as hydrogen ions enter cells.

b. Renal causes. The renal capacity to excrete potassium is approximately 500–1000 mEq/day, which is 10–20 times the normal intake. An impairment of the normal components of renal potassium excretion may reduce this excretory capacity so that normal intake may produce hyperkalemia.

(1) **Severe renal failure.** When the GFR falls to below 10 mL/min, hyperkalemia may occur, even with normal intake. At a GFR above this level, hyperkalemia is not a result of glomerular insufficiency per se but is the result of a specific disorder in tubular potassium transport or an extrarenal potassium disturbance.

(2) **Aldosterone insufficiency.** Aldosterone is the major hormonal determinant of renal potassium secretion.

(a) **Acquired aldosterone deficiency.** This condition may result from renal disease associated with reduced renin production. (Recall that renin is an enzyme that cleaves precursor molecules to produce the aldosterone secretagogue, angiotensin II.) Primary adrenal disease also may be associated with reduced aldosterone production. Aldosterone deficiency due to impaired renin production or adrenal disease may be produced by:

(i) Interstitial renal disease
(ii) Lead nephropathy
(iii) Diabetic nephropathy*
(iv) Obstructive uropathy
(v) Angiotensin antagonist therapy
(vi) Addison's disease

(b) **Inherited aldosterone deficiency.** Several adrenal enzyme defects associated with deficiency of the 17- or 21-hydroxylase enzymes may be associated with aldosterone deficiency.

(c) **Drug-induced aldosterone deficiency.** NSAIDs act to reduce renin secretion and may produce hyperkalemia through aldosterone deficiency.

(3) **Aldosterone resistance.** The following conditions are characterized by tubular defects associated with elevated aldosterone levels but impaired potassium secretion.

(a) Sickle cell nephropathy
(b) SLE
(c) Amyloidosis
(d) Interstitial renal disease
(e) Obstructive uropathy
(f) Hereditary aldosterone resistance
(g) Use of triamterene, amiloride, or spironolactone

3. Clinical features

a. Neuromuscular disorders. By altering transmembrane electrical potential, severe hyperkalemia may alter muscle function or neuromuscular transmission, leading to severe weakness or paralysis.

*Insulin deficiency in this condition may potentiate hyperkalemia.

b. **Cardiac disorders.** Cardiac arrhythmias may occur at any level above normal but generally are noted only when serum potassium concentration exceeds 6 mEq/L. As serum potassium level rises, a series of electrocardiographic (ECG) changes may be seen, including:
   (1) Prolongation of the P-R interval
   (2) T-wave peaking
   (3) Prolongation of the QRS interval
   (4) Ventricular tachycardias, ventricular fibrillation, and asystole

4. **Diagnosis**
   a. **Elimination of pseudohyperkalemia.** In vitro lysis of erythrocytes, leukocytes, or platelets can produce hyperkalemia as a result of intracellular potassium release (pseudohyperkalemia). All hyperkalemic patients should be checked for pseudohyperkalemia by measuring both plasma and serum potassium concentrations and by inspecting the serum for discoloration suggesting hemolysis. The presence of a myeloproliferative disorder may also produce pseudohyperkalemia.
   b. **Urine potassium assay.** Although only a rough correlation exists between urine and serum potassium levels, hyperkalemia induced by increased intake or increased cell lysis should be associated with urine potassium levels exceeding 50 mEq/L. Values less than 30 mEq/L in the setting of hyperkalemia suggest impaired renal secretion of potassium.
   c. **Renin–aldosterone axis assay.** In certain patients, evaluation of aldosterone and renin levels may help define the etiology of hyperkalemia.

5. **Therapy.** Treatment is divided into acute and chronic phases.
   a. **Acute antagonism and redistribution**
      (1) **Calcium.** The intravenous administration of 1–2 ampules of calcium chloride acutely antagonizes the cardiac effects of hyperkalemia. ECG changes may transiently improve, but serum potassium level remains elevated.
      (2) **Glucose and insulin.** The intravenous infusion of 25 g (1 ampule) of dextrose plus 15 units of insulin lowers serum potassium within 10–15 minutes.
      (3) **β_2-Adrenergic agonists,** given by inhalation or intravenously, rapidly induce potassium uptake into cells, but they are not uniformly effective.
   b. **Acute removal**
      (1) **Diuretics.** Furosemide, bumetanide, and, especially, acetazolamide increase potassium excretion in individuals with adequate renal function.
      (2) **Aldosterone.** The administration of aldosterone as either desoxycorticosterone acetate (15–20 mg/day, intramuscularly) or fludrocortisone acetate (0.2–0.6 mg/day, orally) may increase potassium excretion.
      (3) **Dialysis.** A 4-hour hemodialysis treatment effectively removes potassium and lowers the serum potassium level by approximately 40%–50%. Peritoneal dialysis is less effective, but the acute administration of glucose that accompanies infusion of the dialysate stimulates cellular uptake of potassium.
      (4) **Cation-exchange resins.** The administration of sodium polystyrene sulfonate binds potassium in the gastrointestinal tract. About 2 mEq of sodium are exchanged for every 1 mEq of potassium removed, so that a substantial sodium load may result. Sorbitol is administered orally to prevent severe constipation. Cation-exchange resins can remove 50–100 mEq of potassium over a 6-hour period and may be given orally or rectally.
   c. **Chronic removal.** After the acute removal of potassium, potassium homeostasis may be maintained with any of the following agents.
      (1) **Aldosterone** may be administered in the forms and dosages described in Part II: III C 5 b (2).
      (2) **Diuretics.** Furosemide or acetazolamide may be used in combination with fludrocortisone acetate to increase potassium excretion.

(3) **Cation-exchange resins** may be given on a chronic basis to increase gastrointestinal excretion of metabolism.

IV ACID–BASE METABOLISM

A Normal physiology Acid–base balance refers to the maintenance of the hydrogen ion concentration of body fluids by three control systems: body buffers (e.g., bicarbonate), the lungs, and the kidneys. Because hydrogen ions (protons) are highly reactive particles, even slight changes in hydrogen ion concentration can cause marked alterations in physiologic processes.

1. **Hydrogen ion concentration and pH.** The hydrogen ion concentration of body fluids is low compared with the concentrations of other ions. It is more convenient, therefore, to express the concentration as **pH,** or the **negative logarithm of hydrogen ion concentration.** The pH of the extracellular fluid is maintained at about 7.4. Although it cannot be measured routinely, the pH of the intracellular fluid most likely is between 7.0 and 7.2.
2. **Generation and elimination of hydrogen ion.** Normal metabolic processes generate large amounts of carbonic as well as noncarbonic (nonvolatile) acids, which enter the body fluids and must be buffered and eliminated.
   a. **Carbonic acid.** Hydrogen ions are produced through complete oxidation of glucose and fatty acids to carbonic acid. On dehydration, carbonic acid forms a volatile end product (carbon dioxide), which can be eliminated by the lungs.
   b. **Nonvolatile acid.** Approximately 1 mEq of nonvolatile acid per kg of body weight is produced daily and excreted primarily by the kidneys. This acid is produced through incomplete metabolism of glucose and fatty acids to organic acids (e.g., acetoacetic and β-hydroxybutyric acids) as well as metabolism of proteins such as methionine and phosphoprotein to sulfuric and phosphoric acids, respectively.
3. **Henderson-Hasselbalch equation.** The bicarbonate–carbonic acid (HCO_3^-–CO_2) system is the major buffer component of the extracellular fluid. Acid–base disturbances often are characterized in terms of changes in either the bicarbonate (base) or dissolved carbon dioxide (acid) component of this buffer pair. The classic expression of acid–base state is based on the Henderson-Hasselbalch equation, which relates three variables—pH, carbon dioxide tension (P_{CO_2}), and plasma bicarbonate concentration ($[HCO_3^-]$)—as well as two constants—pK and S—as:

$$pH = pK + \log \frac{[HCO_3^-]}{S \times P_{CO_2}}$$

where: pK = the negative logarithm of the dissociation constant for carbonic acid (6.1) and S = the solubility constant for carbon dioxide in plasma (0.03 mmol/L/mm Hg). Normally, the plasma $[HCO_3^-]$ is 24 mmol/L and the arterial P_{CO_2} is 40 mm Hg. Thus:

$$pH = 6.1 + \log \frac{24}{1.2} = 7.4$$

4. **Respiratory regulation of arterial P_{CO_2}.** By regulating the rate of alveolar ventilation, the lungs may retain or excrete carbon dioxide and in this way regulate the "acid" component of the bicarbonate buffer system.
5. **Renal regulation of plasma bicarbonate content.** There are two important aspects of hydrogen ion metabolism in the kidney: the reabsorption of bicarbonate ion and the secretion of hydrogen ion.
   a. **Reabsorption of bicarbonate ion.** Approximately 4500 mEq of bicarbonate are filtered daily at the glomerulus, virtually all of which are reabsorbed into the proximal tubules. The remain-

ing minute portion of the filtered bicarbonate is reabsorbed into the distal and collecting tubules. Proximal tubular reabsorption of bicarbonate occurs indirectly by the following process.

(1) Filtered bicarbonate ion together with secreted hydrogen ion form carbonic acid within the tubular lumen. Sodium ion reabsorption is linked to this secretion of hydrogen ion to maintain electroneutrality.

(2) Carbonic anhydrase in the brush border of the proximal tubule catalyzes the dehydration of carbonic acid to carbon dioxide and water. Being readily diffusible, carbon dioxide diffuses into the proximal tubular cell, where intracellular carbonic anhydrase catalyzes its rehydration to carbonic acid.

(3) The bicarbonate ion formed by the dissociation of carbonic acid is passively reabsorbed into the peritubular blood along with equimolar amounts of sodium ion, which is actively transported into the peritubular blood. The hydrogen ion formed by the dissociation of carbonic acid within the cell serves as a source of another hydrogen ion to be secreted. This may occur in exchange for sodium ions across the apical epithelial membrane.

b. **Addition of "new" bicarbonate.** In addition to conserving bicarbonate, the kidneys add newly synthesized bicarbonate to the plasma **via secretion of hydrogen ion.** This process replenishes the bicarbonate used to buffer acid produced by incomplete metabolism of neutral foodstuffs and by metabolism of nonvolatile acid precursors in the diet.

(1) The addition of new bicarbonate does not involve the bicarbonate reabsorbed into the proximal tubule but, rather, the bicarbonate generated within the distal tubular cell via the hydration of carbon dioxide and the dissociation of carbonic acid. This process is similar to that for the reabsorption of the filtered bicarbonate; however, the formed bicarbonate in the cell is "new."

(2) The renal contribution of new bicarbonate is accompanied by the excretion of an equivalent amount of acid in the urine in the form of titratable acid, ammonium ion, or both.

(a) **Titratable acid formation and secretion.** The exchange of hydrogen ion for sodium ion converts dibasic sodium phosphate or sulfate in the glomerular filtrate into monobasic sodium phosphate or sulfate, which is excreted in the urine as titratable acid. The hydrogen ion secreted into the distal tubules, therefore, can react with filtered phosphate rather than filtered bicarbonate.

(b) **Ammonia formation and secretion.** Unlike phosphate, ammonia enters the tubular lumen by tubular synthesis and secretion, rather than filtration. Ammonia is synthesized in the proximal tubule as a product of glutamine metabolism, and then it diffuses across the renal parenchyma to be secreted into the lumen of the collecting tubules. Virtually all of the nonpolar ammonia that enters the tubular lumen immediately combines with hydrogen ion to form ammonium ion, which is nondiffusible because it is lipid insoluble. The renal excretion of ammonium ion results in the addition of bicarbonate to the plasma.

6. **Concept of compensation.** Compensation can be defined as the physiologic response to an alteration in either the **respiratory** or **metabolic** (renal) component of acid–base balance to restore the body pH value toward normal. **Physiologic compensation generally is not complete.** In the Henderson-Hasselbalch equation, changes in the "numerator" (metabolic component) are associated with secondary changes in the "denominator" (respiratory component), which restore the log ratio toward 24:1.2 (i.e., 20:1) and, therefore, restore pH **toward** normal, but not back to 7.4. Conversely, changes in the respiratory component are associated with compensatory changes in the metabolic component to restore pH **toward** normal.

7. **Concept of correction of metabolic acidosis.** Compensatory processes do not normalize the low pH and serum bicarbonate concentration in metabolic acidosis (e.g., in diarrhea). However, the normal kidney can restore these parameters toward normal by increasing net acid excretion in

the urine (i.e., excretion of excess hydrogen ions). In large part, the kidney increases renal tubular cell production of ammonia, thus increasing excretion of ammonium ions. The resultant generation of new bicarbonate in the distal tubule restores the serum bicarbonate concentration toward the normal range.

B Respiratory acidosis

1. **Definition. Increased blood $Pa{CO_2}$** (i.e., > 40 mm Hg) and **decreased blood pH** (i.e., acidemia) are characteristic.
2. **Etiology.** Respiratory acidosis is associated with a reduced capacity to excrete **carbon dioxide** via the lungs. Causes include all disorders that reduce pulmonary function and carbon dioxide clearance.
   a. **Primary pulmonary disease** that is associated with alveolar–arterial mismatch may lead to carbon dioxide retention, usually as a late manifestation.
   b. **Neuromuscular disease.** Any weakness of the pulmonary musculature that leads to reduced ventilation (e.g., myasthenia gravis) may produce carbon dioxide retention.
   c. **Primary CNS dysfunction.** Any severe injury to the brain stem may be associated with reduced ventilatory drive and carbon dioxide retention.
   d. **Drug-induced hypoventilation.** Any agent that causes severe depression of CNS or neuromuscular function may be associated with respiratory acidosis.
3. **Clinical features**
   a. **CNS disorders.** Because blood flow to the brain is regulated by blood $Pa{CO_2}$, respiratory acidosis is associated with increased blood flow to the brain and increased cerebrospinal fluid (CSF) pressure. These effects may lead to a variety of symptoms of generalized CNS depression.
   b. **Cardiac disorders.** The acidemia in respiratory acidosis is associated with reduced cardiac output and pulmonary hypertension (effects that may lead to critically reduced blood flow to vital organs).
4. **Diagnosis**
   a. **Acute respiratory acidosis.** Acute carbon dioxide retention leads to an increase in blood $Pa{CO_2}$ with minimal change in plasma bicarbonate content. For each 10 mm Hg rise in $Pa{CO_2}$, the plasma bicarbonate level increases by approximately 1 mEq/L and the blood pH decreases by approximately 0.08. Serum electrolyte levels are close to normal in individuals with acute respiratory acidosis.
   b. **Chronic respiratory acidosis.** After 2–5 days, renal compensation (i.e., increased hydrogen ion secretion and bicarbonate production in the distal nephron) occurs; that is, the plasma bicarbonate level steadily increases. Arterial blood gas analysis shows that in the chronic phase of respiratory acidosis, for each 10 mm Hg rise in $Pa{CO_2}$, the plasma bicarbonate level increases by 3–4 mEq/L and the blood pH decreases by 0.03.
5. **Therapy**
   a. **Correction of the underlying disorder.** Attempts should be made to correct muscular dysfunction or reversible pulmonary disease, if either is the cause of the respiratory acidosis. In the case of drug-induced hypoventilation, vigorous attempts should be made to clear the offending agent from the body.
   b. **Respiratory therapy.** A blood $Pa{CO_2}$ of more than 60 mm Hg may be an indication for assisted ventilation if CNS or pulmonary muscular depression is severe.

C Respiratory alkalosis

1. **Definition. Decreased blood $Pa{CO_2}$** and an **increased blood pH** (alkalemia) are characteristic.
2. **Etiology.** Respiratory alkalosis is associated with excessive elimination of carbon dioxide via the lungs. Causes include any disorder associated with inappropriately increased ventilatory rate and carbon dioxide clearance.

a. **Anxiety** (hysterical hyperventilation). This condition is the most common cause of respiratory alkalosis.
b. **Salicylate toxicity.** Initially, salicylate excess causes overstimulation of the respiratory center, resulting in respiratory alkalosis. Metabolic acidosis may develop from the salicylate load, which enhances the hyperventilation.
c. **Hypoxia.** Any disorder associated with decreased oxygen tension (PaO_2) of blood may lead to an increased respiratory rate and, thus, respiratory alkalosis.
d. **Intrathoracic disorders.** Any inflammatory or space-occupying lesion in the lung may be associated with primary stimulation of ventilatory rate, leading to a low $PaCO_2$. Such conditions include:
   (1) Pulmonary embolism
   (2) Pneumonia
   (3) Asthma
   (4) Pulmonary fibrosis
e. **Primary CNS dysfunction.** CNS disorders that may be associated with inappropriate stimulation of ventilation include:
   (1) Cerebrovascular accident (CVA)
   (2) Tumor
   (3) Infection
   (4) Trauma
f. **Gram-negative septicemia.** An early manifestation of gram-negative septicemia or bacteremia is a primary stimulation of ventilation with respiratory alkalosis. The mechanism is unknown.
g. **Liver failure.** The most common acid–base disorder in liver disease is primary respiratory alkalosis through a direct CNS effect of hyperammonemia.
h. **Pregnancy.** Primary stimulation of ventilation is typically seen throughout pregnancy.

3. **Clinical features.** Acute alkalemia may be associated with several organ system disorders.
   a. **CNS disorders.** A generalized feeling of anxiety may be present and may progress to more severe obtundation and even precoma.
   b. **Neuromuscular disorders.** Acute alkalemia may produce a tetany-like syndrome, which may be indistinguishable from that of acute hypocalcemia.
4. **Diagnosis**
   a. **Acute respiratory alkalosis.** Increased respiratory rate leads to a loss of carbon dioxide via the lungs, which in turn increases the blood pH. For each 10 mm Hg decrease in blood $PaCO_2$ acutely, the plasma bicarbonate level decreases by 2 mEq/L and the blood pH increases by 0.08.
   b. **Chronic respiratory alkalosis.** Within hours after an acute decrease in arterial $PaCO_2$, hydrogen ion secretion in the distal nephron decreases, leading to a decrease in plasma bicarbonate. For each 10 mm Hg decrease in blood $PaCO_2$ chronically, the plasma bicarbonate level decreases by 5–6 mEq/L and the blood pH increases by only about 0.02. Serum chloride level also is elevated.
5. **Therapy.** The primary goal of therapy is to correct the underlying disorder. Use of carbon dioxide–enriched breathing mixtures or controlled ventilation may be required in cases of severe respiratory alkalosis (pH > 7.6).

D Metabolic acidosis

1. **Definition.** Metabolic acidosis is characterized by a decreased blood pH and a decreased plasma bicarbonate concentration. This condition may be caused by one of two basic mechanisms: the loss of bicarbonate or the accumulation of an acid other than carbonic acid (e.g., lactic acid).
2. **Etiology.** The causes of metabolic acidosis may be divided into those associated with a normal anion gap and those associated with an increased anion gap. **The anion gap reflects the concentrations**

of those anions that actually are present in serum but are not routinely assayed, including negatively charged plasma proteins (mainly albumin), phosphates, sulfate, and organic acids (e.g., lactic acid). The anion gap, measured in mEq/L, represents the difference between the concentration of unmeasured anions and cations. It can be calculated as follows:

$$\textbf{Anion gap} = [\mathbf{Na^+}] - ([\mathbf{Cl^-}] + [\mathbf{HCO_3^-}])$$

The normal value of the anion gap is 8 ± 4 mEq/L. An increase represents an increase in one moiety, usually the organic acids. No change with decreases in both plasma bicarbonate concentration and serum pH suggests a primary loss of bicarbonate or the addition of mineral acid.

a. **Metabolic acidosis with an increased anion gap**
   (1) **Ketoacidosis.** This condition refers to a state of increased ketoacid formation, which leads to titration of bicarbonate and consequent metabolic acidosis. Ketoacidosis occurs as a complication of diabetes mellitus, prolonged starvation, and prolonged alcohol abuse.
   (2) **Lactic acidosis.** Decreased oxygen delivery to tissues results in increased lactate production, with accompanying severe metabolic acidosis. Lactic acidosis is a characteristic feature of many conditions associated with low tissue perfusion (e.g., shock and sepsis).
   (3) **Renal failure.** Metabolic acidosis results from the inability of the kidney to excrete the daily hydrogen ion load, derived from food and metabolism, as a result of a decline in ammonium excretion resulting from decreased renal mass. The acidosis of renal failure is characterized by either a normal or elevated anion gap, depending on the severity of the decline in renal filtering function. In either case, the serum bicarbonate is reduced due to the titration by the retained hydrogen ions.
      (a) The anion gap is elevated only when the GFR is severely reduced ($< 25\ mm^3/min$) because the anions (sulfates and phosphates) that accompany the retained hydrogen ions cannot be filtered.
      (b) In mild-to-moderate renal failure (GFR = 25–60 mm^3/min), these anions are freely excreted and do not accumulate, resulting in metabolic acidosis with normal anion gap.
   (4) **Intoxication.** The ingestion of a variety of chemical agents may result in the accumulation of organic acids (e.g., lactic acid). Such intoxicants include:
      (a) Salicylate
      (b) Methanol
      (c) Ethylene glycol

b. **Metabolic acidosis with a normal anion gap (hyperchloremic metabolic acidosis)**
   (1) **Renal loss of bicarbonate** may result from the following conditions.
      (a) **Proximal tubular acidosis.** Characteristics include decreased proximal tubular reabsorption of bicarbonate leading to excessive urinary excretion of bicarbonate. Causes include cystinosis, multiple myeloma, heavy metal poisoning, and Wilson's disease.
      (b) **Distal tubular acidosis.** Characteristics include a decreased distal tubular capacity for hydrogen ion secretion and inability to maintain an acidic urine (urine pH often is > 6.0). This defect leads to an inability to generate "new" bicarbonate through elimination of protons buffered by ammonia. Causes include hereditary disorders, amphotericin B toxicity, SLE, obstructive uropathy, Sjögren's syndrome, and other hyperglobulinemic conditions.
      (c) **Hyperkalemic renal tubular acidosis.** Hyperkalemia, particularly that associated with hyporeninemic hypoaldosteronism, is characterized by reduced ammonia excretion, reduced bicarbonate production, and, thus, the inability to buffer nonvolatile acids derived from the diet. Acidosis (i.e., reduced plasma bicarbonate) is due to reduced ammonia production and, therefore, reduced capacity to excrete hydrogen ion and to generate "new" bicarbonate [see Part II: IV A 5 a (3), b (2)].

(d) **Moderate renal insufficiency.** The decline in ammonium excretion resulting from decreased renal mass causes a decrease in net acid excretion and, therefore, a decrease in serum bicarbonate concentration. Recall that when the GFR is greater than 25 mL/min, anions such as sulfate and phosphate are freely excreted in the urine and do not accumulate, resulting in a normal anion gap.

(e) **Carbonic anhydrase inhibition.** Drugs such as acetazolamide (a diuretic) and mafenide (a topical treatment for burns) inhibit the action of carbonic anhydrase and thereby reduce proximal tubular reabsorption of bicarbonate.

(2) **Gastrointestinal loss of alkali** also produces this syndrome and may occur because of:

(a) Diarrhea

(b) Pancreatic fistulas

(c) Ureterosigmoidostomy

3. **Clinical features.** Signs and symptoms usually are related to the underlying disorder. A blood pH of less than 7.2 may lead to reduced cardiac output. Acidosis also may be associated with resistance to the vasoconstrictive action of catecholamines, resulting in hypotension. Kussmaul's (deep and rhythmic) respiration may be prominent as the ventilatory rate increases in response to the fall in serum pH.

4. **Diagnosis**
   a. Serum electrolyte assay shows a decreased bicarbonate and a variable chloride content, depending on whether the acidosis is associated with a normal or an increased anion gap.
   b. Arterial blood gas analysis also demonstrates a decreased bicarbonate level, with a compensatory decrease in blood $Paco_2$. **Winters' formula** predicts that in pure metabolic acidosis the $Paco_2$ should be 1.5 times the bicarbonate concentration plus 8 ± 2 mm Hg. Variance from this predicted response to pure metabolic acidosis suggests a complicating respiratory dysfunction. (A lower-than-predicted $Paco_2$ suggests primary respiratory alkalosis; a higher-than-predicted $Paco_2$ suggests a disorder of pulmonary function, leading to inappropriate carbon dioxide retention.)

5. **Therapy.** Metabolic acidosis may be treated with alkali when the blood pH is less than 7.2, with intravenous therapy aimed at elevating the pH above this point. Sodium bicarbonate is the preferred alkali.
   a. The required amount of bicarbonate can be calculated on the basis that bicarbonate occupies a space that accounts for approximately 50% of body weight. Thus, the amount of sodium bicarbonate needed to raise the plasma bicarbonate from 13 mEq/L to 20 mEq/L is calculated as: 7 mEq/L $\times$ 0.5 $\times$ kg of body weight. This number is an approximation, and measurements of plasma bicarbonate and blood pH must be repeated in patients so treated. This space is much larger if the metabolic acidosis is more severe.
   b. Underestimation of bicarbonate requirements can occur if bicarbonate losses persist (e.g., diarrhea) or if ongoing acid production is sufficiently rapid to consume administered bicarbonate in a buffering reaction (e.g., lactic acidosis).
   c. In the presence of distal tubular acidosis or renal insufficiency, the chronic bicarbonate requirement is 1 mEq/kg/day, which is equivalent to the nonvolatile acid production daily. However, in proximal tubular acidosis, the bicarbonate requirement is much greater (2–4 mEq/kg/day), because of the ineffective reabsorption of filtered bicarbonate.

E Metabolic alkalosis

1. **Definition. Increased blood pH** and **increased plasma bicarbonate concentration** are characteristic.

2. **Etiology.** Increased plasma bicarbonate levels result from either **increased endogenous production of bicarbonate** (in the stomach or kidney), with reduced renal excretion, or **exogenous administration of bicarbonate or other alkali.** Metabolic alkalosis depends on both the factors that initiate alkalemia (generation phase) and those that maintain it (maintenance phase).

Because the renal capacity for bicarbonate excretion is several thousand mEq/day, it is clear that some impairment in renal bicarbonate excretion is mandatory for the maintenance of metabolic alkalosis and a sustained rise in plasma bicarbonate.

a. **Excessive mineralocorticoid action** on the distal convoluted tubule and collecting tubule stimulates hydrogen ion secretion, thereby raising the plasma bicarbonate level. This occurs in all cases of primary or secondary hyperaldosteronism.
b. **Vomiting.** Loss of gastric hydrochloric acid by any means causes an increase in plasma bicarbonate because the source of hydrogen ion for gastric secretion is the dehydration of carbonic acid within the parietal cells. The concomitant decrease in extracellular fluid volume produced by vomiting, plus the chloride deficits, reduces the GFR and increases the rate of proximal tubular reabsorption of sodium and bicarbonate to maintain the metabolic alkalosis. Potassium deficits also develop because of renal potassium wasting, which may potentiate increased proximal tubular reabsorption of bicarbonate. Secondary hyperaldosteronism due to extracellular volume depletion also contributes to urinary potassium wasting.
c. **Diuretics.** Inhibition of renal sodium chloride reabsorption leads to increased flow rate and, therefore, increased hydrogen ion secretion in the distal convoluted tubule and collecting tubule. Increased hydrogen ion secretion causes increased generation of bicarbonate. The volume depletion produced by the sodium deficits following diuretic use reduces the GFR, stimulates proximal tubular reabsorption of bicarbonate, and maintains metabolic alkalosis. Secondary hyperaldosteronism due to volume depletion causes urinary potassium wasting and also contributes to maintenance of metabolic alkalosis by stimulating hydrogen secretion in the distal segments of the nephron.
d. **Administration of alkali,** either as sodium bicarbonate (e.g., during cardiac resuscitation) or as organic ions (e.g., lactate, citrate, and acetate, which are metabolically converted to bicarbonate by hepatic action), results in an increased plasma bicarbonate level. However, unless renal reabsorption of bicarbonate is stimulated, plasma bicarbonate is not sustained at an elevated level.
e. **Rapid correction of hypercapnia.** Following sustained respiratory acidosis, renal bicarbonate production is elevated as a compensatory event by a stimulation of hydrogen ion secretion. If arterial P_{CO_2} is then acutely reduced by mechanical ventilation, a transient state of hyperbicarbonatemia and elevated blood pH ensues (a condition termed **posthypercapnic metabolic alkalosis**).

3. **Clinical features.** Signs and symptoms generally are dominated by the underlying disease state. However, symptoms of tetany may be the most pronounced clinical features.
4. **Diagnosis**
   a. **Serum electrolyte assay** shows an increased bicarbonate level and a decreased chloride level. Hypokalemia is a frequent finding.
   b. **Arterial blood gas analysis** reveals an elevated bicarbonate level and a compensatory increase in Pa_{CO_2} value. Because a decrease in ventilation is required to elevate Pa_{CO_2}, hypoxia also may result.
   c. **Urinary indices** are useful in the diagnosis of metabolic alkalosis. If extracellular fluid volume contraction is not present (e.g., due to excessive mineralocorticoid activity) or if renal reabsorption of sodium chloride is inhibited (e.g., due to diuretic use), urine chloride levels are elevated. If extracellular fluid volume depletion also is present (e.g., due to vomiting), urine chloride level typically is too low to be measured.
5. **Therapy.** Treatment involves correction of the underlying disease state as well as reduction of renal avidity for bicarbonate. The latter effect is accomplished by extracellular volume expansion with sodium chloride–containing solutions.
   a. The metabolic alkalosis caused by excessive mineralocorticoid activity is highly dependent on potassium depletion. Administration of potassium chloride corrects this disorder.

b. In individuals who have posthypercapnic metabolic alkalosis, judicious administration of acetazolamide or other inhibitors of proximal tubular bicarbonate reabsorption is an adjunct to therapy.

V CALCIUM METABOLISM

A Normal physiology

1. Calcium exists in serum in three forms. About 40% of serum calcium is bound to protein, about 5%–15% is complexed with anions such as citrate and phosphate, and the remaining portion is unbound, ionized calcium. The ionized component of serum calcium is the most important clinically. For example, hypoalbuminemia lowers serum calcium by reducing the protein-bound component. The ionized calcium concentration, however, is unaffected by hypoalbuminemia, and the patient is asymptomatic.
2. Ionized calcium homeostasis is maintained by a balance of calcium input into the blood from the gastrointestinal tract and bone and calcium output from the blood into the urine and lower gastrointestinal tract. Calcium transport across the gastrointestinal tract is influenced strongly by **1,25-dihydroxycholecalciferol [1,25-$(OH)_2D_3$, or calcitriol],** which is the active metabolite of vitamin D. **Parathyroid hormone (PTH)** raises serum calcium by increasing calcium release from bone, by reducing renal excretion of calcium, and by stimulating renal activation of vitamin D to calcitriol. This is the second of two steps in the metabolic activation of dietary vitamin D. The first step takes place in the liver, and the product is **25-hydroxycholecalciferol** [25-$(OH)D_3$, or **calcifediol**]. Serum calcium level is the principal regulator of PTH release.

B Hypocalcemia

is defined as a serum calcium concentration less than 8.5 mg/dL. **Hypoalbuminemia** lowers the total serum calcium by reducing the protein-bound component. Generally, the total serum calcium level is decreased 0.8 mg/dL for each 1 g/L decrement in serum albumin. However, **PTH deficiency** is the primary determinant of hypocalcemia. For a complete discussion of hypocalcemia, see Chapter 9 III B.

C Hypercalcemia

results from disorders that cause either increased gastrointestinal absorption or increased bone resorption of calcium. Normal serum calcium level may reach 10.5 mg/dL in men and 10.2 mg/dL in women. Higher values may indicate true hypercalcemia, but serum protein level also must be monitored to confirm that an increased level of protein does not explain the increased total serum calcium. **Hyperparathyroidism** is the result of oversecretion of PTH, which in turn causes hypercalcemia. A full discussion of hypercalcemia can be found in Chapter 9 III A.

VI PHOSPHATE METABOLISM

A Normal physiology

1. **Phosphate function.** Phosphate may be the single most important dynamic constituent required for cellular activity. Virtually all bodily functions are powered by the high-energy phosphate bonds of adenosine triphosphate (ATP). In addition, phosphate is the major anion and buffer of the intracellular fluid. Its contributory role in the renal excretion of hydrogen ion makes phosphate an important constituent of acid–base metabolism as well.
2. **Phosphate distribution.** About 85% of the total body store of phosphate is in bone. Phosphate also is found in the intracellular and extracellular fluid compartments. Plasma phosphate exists primarily in the form of inorganic phosphate, the majority of which is free (not bound to protein). The inorganic phosphate content of the extracellular fluid is a prime determinant of intracellular inorganic phosphate, which is the source of phosphate for ATP. Intracellular phosphate deficits may result in reduced cell energy production and, therefore, generalized cell dysfunction.

3. **Phosphate homeostasis** involves the balance of phosphate intake and phosphate output ("external" balance) as well as the maintenance of normal phosphate distribution within the body ("internal" balance).
   a. **External phosphate balance.** Normal dietary intake of phosphate is 1200 mg/day, which is provided primarily by dairy products, and normal phosphate excretion is 1200 mg/day (800 mg in the urine and 400 mg in the stool). The gastrointestinal tract is a passive component of external phosphate balance, whereas renal phosphate handling is closely regulated.
      (1) Normally, 90% of filtered phosphate is reabsorbed in the proximal tubule, with only a minute portion reabsorbed distally. The main regulator of renal phosphate handling is PTH. A high PTH level inhibits phosphate reabsorption, and a low PTH level stimulates it.
      (2) PTH-independent control of renal phosphate reabsorption also is exerted by dietary phosphate content and other hormones such as calcitonin, thyroid hormone, and growth hormone (GH). A decrease in phosphate intake stimulates proximal tubular reabsorption of phosphate.
   b. **Internal phosphate balance.** This, too, is regulated, because intracellular phosphate levels are 200–300 mg/dL and extracellular levels are 3–4 mg/dL. Increased insulin or β-adrenergic agonist levels, hydrogen ion shifts, and intracellular metabolic disturbances all alter the phosphate distribution in the body.

B Hypophosphatemia

1. **Etiology.** Hypophosphatemia can result from extrarenal or renal loss of phosphate. One of the most common causes of hypophosphatemia is **chronic severe alcoholism,** which leads to most of the features described below.
   a. **Extrarenal causes**
      (1) **Dietary deficiency and gastrointestinal losses**
         (a) **Inadequate dietary intake.** Most food contains some phosphate. Inadequate dietary intake of phosphate is unusual and only occurs under specific iatrogenic circumstances.
         (b) **Antacid abuse.** Large amounts of calcium salts (e.g., acetate, carbonate) and aluminum- or magnesium-containing antacids bind phosphate in the gastrointestinal tract, increase gastrointestinal phosphate losses, and may produce hypophosphatemia.
         (c) **Starvation.** During prolonged starvation, cell breakdown liberates phosphate into the extracellular fluid. The amount of phosphate in remaining, intact cells, however, is preserved at normal levels. As urinary plus stool loss of liberated, extracellular phosphate exceeds dietary intake, negative phosphate balance occurs. Although hypophosphatemia does not follow immediately, severe phosphate deficits may develop on refeeding as cellular uptake of phosphate is stimulated by new cell growth and macromolecule synthesis.
      (2) **Redistribution of body phosphate**
         (a) **Increased glycolysis.** Any condition associated with increased glycolysis within cells causes organic phosphate compounds to accumulate as the phosphorylated carbon residues in the Embden-Meyerhof pathway, with depletion of intracellular inorganic phosphate. Serum phosphate level falls as phosphate diffuses into cells, causing hypophosphatemia. Reduction of intracellular inorganic phosphate through this mechanism may be drastic and lead to ATP depletion and cell dysfunction, such as rhabdomyolysis.
         (b) **Respiratory alkalosis.** Hyperventilation is associated with reduced serum phosphate because of increased cellular uptake of phosphate due to hypocapnia and alkalemia. Glycolysis within cells is stimulated by acute elevation of cellular pH.
         (c) **Sepsis.** Hypophosphatemia is a known concomitant of gram-negative sepsis and may coexist (although independently) with hypophosphatemia because of respiratory alkalosis.

(d) **Epinephrine.** This agent also stimulates cellular uptake of phosphate. This effect is independent of cellular phosphate uptake due to insulin-mediated glycolysis.

b. **Renal causes**

(1) **Excess PTH.** Any form of hyperparathyroidism results in renal phosphate wasting and hypophosphatemia, provided that GFR is not markedly reduced.

(2) **Primary renal tubular defects.** Conditions such as cystinosis, heavy metal poisoning, multiple myeloma, and Wilson's disease may be associated with generalized proximal tubular defects (Fanconi's syndrome) and renal phosphate wasting.

(3) **Specific transport defects for phosphate.** These defects have been designated as **hypophosphatemic vitamin D–resistant rickets,** which may be familial or sporadic and exist in both child-onset and adult-onset forms. In each of these conditions, decreased phosphate transport in the proximal tubule produces excessive renal phosphate wasting.

(4) **Glycosuria.** Phosphate and glucose compete for transport in the proximal tubule. All glycosuric conditions are associated with excessive renal losses of phosphate.

2. **Clinical features**

a. **Neurologic disorders.** Cellular ATP deficiency may produce an encephalopathy characterized by obtundation, coma, and seizures. Peripheral neuropathy and Guillain-Barré syndrome also have been described.

b. **Hematologic disorders.** Hemolytic anemia, a rare complication of profound hypophosphatemia, is due to cellular ATP depletion and abnormal membrane integrity.

c. **Muscular disorders.** Dysfunction of skeletal muscle has been described and attributed to ATP deficits. Acute rhabdomyolysis may be particularly prevalent in alcoholic patients who are acutely hypophosphatemic. Paralysis of respiratory muscles with respiratory failure also may be seen.

d. **Bone disorders.** Increased bone resorption with abnormal mineralization occurs in chronic hypophosphatemia.

3. **Diagnosis.** Hypophosphatemia, unless due to renal phosphate wasting, causes near-complete elimination of phosphate from the urine. A urine phosphate level of more than 100 mg/L strongly suggests renal **phosphate wasting.** A low urine phosphate level suggests antacid-induced phosphate depletion, gastrointestinal losses, or increased cellular uptake of phosphate. Glucose infusion with secondary insulin release is the cause of hypophosphatemia in most hospitalized patients.

4. **Therapy.** All hypophosphatemic patients should be treated. In general, therapy involves correction of the underlying condition, such as discontinuation of glucose infusions. In individuals with severe hypophosphatemia and preexisting phosphate depletion (e.g., alcoholic patients), symptomatic hypophosphatemia should be treated with phosphate supplementation. Oral phosphate is preferred, and 1500–2000 mg/day may be given in divided doses. If a patient is comatose or is unable to take oral phosphate, intravenous phosphate may be administered twice daily in 250-mg doses, if serum phosphate is less than 1 mg/dL, provided that serum phosphate measurements are taken at 12-hour intervals. Infusion of phosphate must be discontinued if the serum phosphate level rises to 1.5 mg/dL.

5. **Complications.** The greatest danger of hypophosphatemia lies in the injudicious administration of intravenous phosphate. Acute hypocalcemia due to the formation of calcium phosphate may lead to shock, acute renal failure, and death. For this reason, intravenous phosphate should be administered only when specific clinical disturbances are clearly attributable to hypophosphatemia.

C Hyperphosphatemia

1. **Etiology**

a. **Renal failure.** Because the kidney is the main regulator of serum phosphate level, renal failure commonly is associated with hyperphosphatemia. This disorder is not seen until the GFR has decreased to at least 25% of normal. Serum phosphate level generally does not exceed 10 mg/dL in renal failure. Values exceeding 10 mg/dL suggest an additional etiologic factor.

b. Cell lysis syndromes

(1) **Rhabdomyolysis.** Acute muscle breakdown of any etiology is associated with the release of cellular phosphate and, therefore, hyperphosphatemia. Severe hyperphosphatemia (i.e., serum phosphate concentration $>$ 15 mg/dL) may be seen in cases associated with acute renal failure.

(2) **Tumor lysis syndrome.** Malignant disorders associated with a high sensitivity to chemotherapy or radiotherapy result in rapid cell death from such treatments. This syndrome may lead to massive release of phosphate and other intracellular substances into the extracellular fluid. Severe hypocalcemia, cardiovascular collapse, and renal failure due to calcium, urate, and phosphate deposition in the kidney have been described.

c. Exogenous phosphate administration. Any route (i.e., via intravenous infusion, by mouth, or via phosphate enemas) may result in severe and unpredictable hyperphosphatemia, especially if the GFR is reduced.

d. Hypoparathyroidism. Because the level of PTH is a key determinant of the rate of renal phosphate handling, any condition associated with parathyroid insufficiency or a lack of renal response to PTH may be characterized by hyperphosphatemia.

e. Tumoral calcinosis. This rare disorder is characterized by hyperphosphatemia, soft-tissue calcified masses, and normocalcemia. Rather than a disorder of calcium metabolism, this condition is due to a specific increase in the renal reabsorption of phosphate. Tumoral calcinosis may represent a heritable condition.

f. Miscellaneous causes. GH excess, hyperthyroidism, and sickle cell anemia are associated with hyperphosphatemia from excessive renal reabsorption of phosphate. However, this finding is of no clinical significance in these disorders.

2. **Clinical features.** Hypocalcemia, hypotension, and renal failure may be seen in severe hyperphosphatemia. Milder cases, typically seen in chronic renal failure, are associated with secondary hyperparathyroidism and renal osteodystrophy.

3. **Diagnosis.** Hyperphosphatemia in the absence of renal insufficiency is due to hypoparathyroidism, cell lysis, or tumoral calcinosis. The etiologic diagnosis of hyperphosphatemia is made on the basis of the patient history, physical examination, and laboratory data.

4. **Therapy.** Acute hyperphosphatemia may be a medical emergency that requires immediate therapy. In cases of tumor lysis syndrome, acute hemodialysis may be necessary and is an effective treatment. Administration of large amounts of phosphate-binding gels may be useful in the long-term treatment of hyperphosphatemic conditions.

VII MAGNESIUM METABOLISM

A Normal physiology

Magnesium is the second most abundant intracellular cation. (Potassium is the most abundant.)

1. **Magnesium distribution.** More than 50% of the total body store of magnesium is in bone, with most of the remaining portion found in soft tissues, mainly muscle. Less than 1% of body magnesium is in the extracellular fluid, 20%–30% of which is bound to protein and the rest existing as free cation.

2. **Magnesium homeostasis.** Magnesium is absorbed into the small intestine, but this process is primarily unregulated. During dietary deprivation of magnesium, stool magnesium losses result in hypomagnesemia. The kidney efficiently conserves magnesium during dietary deprivation and excretes any excess magnesium due to excessive intake.

B Hypomagnesemia

1. **Definition.** Clinically important hypomagnesemia occurs when serum magnesium concentration falls below 1.0 mg/dL, although it has been proposed that even mild degrees of hypomagnesemia may be associated with a variety of clinical disorders.
2. **Etiology**
   a. **Extrarenal causes**
      (1) **Dietary deficiency and gastrointestinal losses**
         (a) **Inadequate dietary intake.** Nutritional hypomagnesemia may develop after prolonged starvation as well as postoperatively.
         (b) **Malabsorption.** Generalized malabsorption syndrome, chronic diarrhea, diffuse bowel injury, and chronic laxative abuse all are associated with reduced gastrointestinal absorption of magnesium.
      (2) **Redistribution of body magnesium.** Acute cellular uptake of magnesium has been described in individuals who are in alcohol withdrawal. Also, following parathyroidectomy for severe osteitis fibrosa cystica, acute bone formation may cause rapid accumulation of magnesium and calcium in bone and consequent hypomagnesemia.
   b. **Renal causes**
      (1) **Primary tubular disorders.** A number of tubular disorders, including Bartter's syndrome, renal tubular acidosis, and postobstructive diuresis, are characterized by a defect in renal magnesium conservation and hypomagnesemia. Hypomagnesemia also may develop in patients following renal transplantation. In a familial form of renal magnesium wasting, the molecular mechanisms involved have been identified.
      (2) **Drug-induced tubular losses.** Diuretics such as thiazides, furosemide, and ethacrynic acid typically produce varied degrees of hypomagnesemia. Even small doses of the chemotherapeutic agent cisplatin produce marked renal magnesium wasting and clinically severe hypomagnesemia. Gentamicin and amphotericin B also may produce a toxic injury to the renal tubule, with magnesium and potassium wasting occurring in the absence of reduced GFR.
      (3) **Hormone-induced tubular losses.** Hyperaldosteronism or hypoparathyroidism can be associated with renal tubular magnesium wasting and hypomagnesemia.
      (4) **Ion- or nutrient-induced tubular losses.** Because calcium and magnesium compete for transport in the ascending limb of the loop of Henle, hypercalcemia is associated with reduced renal magnesium transport. Phosphate depletion, alcohol consumption, or both are associated with decreased renal reabsorption of magnesium, but the mechanisms are unknown.
3. **Clinical features.** Muscle twitching, tremor, and muscle weakness are commonly seen. These physical signs are due to the direct effect of magnesium on neuromuscular function as well as the hypocalcemic effect of hypomagnesemia. Severe chronic hypomagnesemia leads to decreased glandular secretion of PTH as well as impaired bone response to PTH, and both of these effects lead to hypocalcemia. Also, hypomagnesemia produces a defect in renal potassium reabsorption, which eventually produces potassium depletion. Thus, all of the clinical signs of hypocalcemia and hypokalemia may be seen in hypomagnesemic patients. The clinical presentation of hypokalemia and hypomagnesemia includes cardiac arrhythmias, particularly in patients taking digitalis.
4. **Therapy.** In most patients, a normal diet makes up for magnesium deficits. If ongoing losses occur, magnesium supplementation is necessary. Even in severe magnesium deficiency, however, 50% of an administered dose of magnesium is excreted in the urine. Symptomatic deficits usually amount to 1–2 mmol/kg of body weight.
   a. If **oral magnesium therapy** is required, magnesium oxide generally is tolerated and has 25%–50% absorption. It is given four times daily in doses of 250–500 mg.

b. If **parenteral magnesium therapy** is necessary, 12 mL (25 mmol) of 50% magnesium sulfate in 1 L of D_5W are given over 3 hours, and 40 mmol in 2 L of D_5W are given over the remainder of the 24-hour period. An additional 25 mmol of magnesium sulfate in 1 L of D_5W are given daily for the subsequent 3 days.

C Hypermagnesemia

1. **Etiology.** Because the kidneys can excrete several thousand milligrams of magnesium each day, hypermagnesemia usually is iatrogenic and occurs, in a sustained fashion, only in patients who have impaired renal function and ingest magnesium as either laxatives or antacids. Acute magnesium intoxication may occur in women who are treated for toxemia of pregnancy with intravenous magnesium salts that are administered at an excessive rate. Muscular paralysis can develop at serum magnesium levels of 10 mg/dL.
2. **Therapy.** Calcium ion is a direct antagonist of magnesium and should be given to patients who are seriously ill with magnesium intoxication. Hemodialysis may be required following cessation of magnesium therapy.

PART III: HYPERTENSION

I GENERAL CONSIDERATIONS

A Definition

Hypertension is present when the blood pressure exceeds 140/90 mm Hg at several determinations. The relative importance of systolic versus diastolic hypertension has been recently re-emphasized. Many studies suggest that systolic blood pressure elevation is as, if not more, significant than diastolic blood pressure elevation as a risk factor for a variety of cardiovascular and renal diseases.

1. **Primary (essential) hypertension** is hypertension that has no known cause. Primary hypertension accounts for 90%–95% of cases of hypertension.
2. **Secondary hypertension** is attributable to a diagnosable disease and accounts for the remainder of cases of hypertension.

B Diagnosis

1. Blood pressure should be measured with a **loosely fitting cuff.** The width of the cuff should equal at least 50% of the length of the upper arm. Initially, blood pressure should be **determined in each arm** to be sure that arterial obstruction in the upper extremity is not falsely lowering the distal arm arterial pressure.
2. Blood pressure may be quite elevated at times of stress; in fact, in some patients, merely being in a physician's office may induce transient hypertension. **Multiple determinations over several visits** and some form of **home** or **workplace monitoring** should be conducted prior to initiating pharmacologic therapy in hypertensive patients.

C Consequences of hypertension

In general, the mortality rate over 20 years among patients with a systolic blood pressure of greater than 160 mm Hg or a diastolic blood pressure of greater than 100 mm Hg increases 100% in those who are untreated.

1. **Stroke.** Patients with a systolic blood pressure of greater than 160 mm Hg have a fourfold increased risk of stroke if untreated.
2. **Coronary artery disease.** Patients with a diastolic pressure of greater than 95 mm Hg have a more than twofold increased risk of coronary artery disease as compared with normotensive patients. However, the beneficial response to therapy is not as well defined as it is for stroke.

3. **Congestive heart failure (CHF).** Patients with blood pressure of greater than 160/95 mm Hg have a fourfold increased incidence of CHF. In 75% of patients with CHF, hypertension occurs at some time during the course of their illness. Thickening and hypertrophy of the left ventricle as a result of hypertension may produce CHF as a result of diastolic dysfunction.

II MECHANISMS OF HYPERTENSION

A Primary hypertension

1. **Abnormal cardiac and peripheral hemodynamics.** Blood pressure is the product of cardiac output and total peripheral resistance; thus, for hypertension to occur, there must be an elevation in cardiac output, total peripheral resistance, or both.
   a. An abnormality in peripheral resistance is a contributing factor in most cases of hypertension.
   b. Many patients with hypertension have either persistently elevated cardiac output or elevated total peripheral resistance early in the course of the disease.
2. **Impaired pressure natriuresis**
   a. In normal individuals, an elevation in blood pressure leads to an alteration in intrarenal hemodynamics and physical forces that results in natriuresis. This, in turn, causes a diuresis, a decrease in total extracellular volume, and a fall in blood pressure.
   b. In patients with essential hypertension, the kidney fails to respond normally to elevated arterial pressure and natriuresis is impaired. The homeostatic abnormality may either cause or help sustain the elevated arterial pressure.
   c. The cause of the failure of normal pressure natriuresis is unknown. Hormonal factors, abnormalities in the structure and activity of transport proteins (e.g., the sodium–hydrogen exchanger in the renal tubule), and autonomic nervous system activity have all been implicated experimentally and on a clinical basis.
3. **Baroreceptor resetting.** In hypertensive patients, baroreceptors in the carotid arteries and aorta are "reset" so that higher pressures are required to exert an influence toward lowering blood pressure.
4. **Abnormalities in the renin–angiotensin–aldosterone system.** There is increasing evidence that abnormalities in each component of this complex system may contribute to the pathogenesis of hypertension in many patients with hypertension. For instance, recent experimental studies using gene transfer techniques show that mice with increased gene expression for the angiotensinogen gene are hypertensive.
5. **Abnormalities in other vasoregulatory systems**
   a. **Endothelin,** a peptide produced in many organs and tissues, is a vasoconstrictor with potency several times greater than that of norepinephrine.
   b. **Atrial natriuretic peptide (ANP),** derived from cardiac muscle, may play a role in normal vascular regulation as a vasodilator and may contribute to extracellular volume homeostasis and blood pressure control in states of mineralocorticoid excess by enhancing sodium excretion.
   c. **Endothelium-derived relaxation factor (EDRF)** is thought to be **nitric oxide,** a gas derived from arginine metabolism that is crucial in a number of vasoregulatory phenomena. Defects in this system are thought to contribute to the hypertension associated with pregnancy.

B Secondary hypertension

In 5%–10% of patients with hypertension, this condition is secondary to an identifiable disorder in the endocrine system or the autonomic nervous system.

1. **Renovascular hypertension** (see also Part I: XIV C) is an important cause of secondary hypertension. In this disorder, hypertension is the result of a complex interplay between activation of the renin–angiotensin–aldosterone system and the sympathetic nervous system. The pattern of endocrine stimulation may also depend on whether the vascular lesions are unilateral or bilateral.

a. Initially, high angiotensin II levels lead to vasoconstriction and expanded extracellular fluid volume as aldosterone release is stimulated.

b. With time, volume expansion may lead to suppression of total renal renin production so that circulating renin values may be normal in spite of the elevated blood pressure. This may explain why unstimulated plasma renin levels are not a good index of the presence of renovascular hypertension in all cases and why some patients (e.g., those with unilateral vascular lesions) may not even demonstrate increased renin secretion.

(1) The normal levels of renin, which are inappropriate in the presence of hypertension and an expanded extracellular fluid volume, sustain the hypertension.

(2) In addition, during this chronic phase, increased sympathetic nervous system activity resulting from chronic angiotensin II stimulation contributes to hypertension.

2. **Renal parenchymal diseases.** Hypertension frequently accompanies a variety of renal diseases, highlighting the important contribution of renal endocrine and excretory function in the regulation of blood pressure.

a. **Altered excretory function.** Defects in the renal excretion of salt and water no doubt contribute to the pathogenesis of hypertension in patients with advanced renal failure. In patients maintained on hemodialysis or peritoneal dialysis, modest reductions in extracellular fluid volume can produce a striking reduction in arterial blood pressure.

b. **Altered renin–angiotensin–aldosterone activity.** Ischemic changes resulting from intrarenal scarring may activate the renin-angiotensin system and contribute to hypertension in patients with early or advanced renal failure.

3. **Endocrinologic causes**

a. **Oral contraceptives.** These agents cause hypertension in approximately 5% of patients who use them. Hypertension occurs as a result of estrogen-induced increases in angiotensinogen synthesis in the liver. Reduced estrogen levels or the addition of progesterone may ameliorate this complication.

b. **Mineralocorticoid excess syndromes.** Mineralocorticoid excess leads to hypertension by inducing sodium and water retention, leading to expansion of the extracellular fluid volume. The hypertension is often accompanied by hypokalemia, because mineralocorticoids promote renal potassium excretion in the collecting duct of the nephron. A variety of disorders produce mineralocorticoid excess states.

(1) **Primary hyperaldosteronism.** Tumors of the adrenal gland, which are common on autopsy, are functionally active in 1%–3% of patients, leading to mineralocorticoid excess. Tumors may be unilateral or bilateral, or the excess may result from a diffuse bilateral hyperplasia of the adrenal zona glomerulosa.

(2) **Glucocorticoid-remediable hyperaldosteronism.** In rare patients, a defect in adrenal development leads to the synthesis of aldosterone in the adrenal gland under the influence of ACTH. A gene rearrangement allows expression of ACTH-responsive aldosterone synthase in the zona fasciculata rather than the zona glomerulosa, leading to the production of large amounts of mineralocorticoid hormone. Treatment with dexamethasone suppresses this abnormal pathway. This disorder should be suspected in patients with a family history of hypertension and hypokalemia.

(3) **Exogenous hypermineralocorticoidism.** Some patients may develop striking mineralocorticoid excess hypertension from the ingestion of **glycyrrhetinic acid,** a substance found in European licorice and in some forms of chewing tobacco. Glycyrrhetinic acid blocks the action of 11 beta-hydroxysteroid dehydrogenase (an enzyme that prevents glucocorticoid binding to receptors in the renal distal tubule), resulting in a high mineralocorticoid state. Patients present with hypertension, hypokalemia, and low renin and aldosterone levels.

(4) **Cushing's syndrome.** Glucocorticoid excess resulting from exogenous glucocorticoid therapy, a pituitary tumor, or an adrenal adenoma produces hypertension in approximately 80% of patients with Cushing's syndrome. Hypertension may occur because cortisol has mineralocorticoid-like effects and, therefore, leads to the retention of sodium and water. However, many patients with Cushing's syndrome and hypertension do not manifest a low renin state as would be expected in primary mineralocorticoidism, implying that other mechanisms may contribute to the hypertension as well.

(5) **Liddle's syndrome.** This familial disorder is transmitted as an autosomal dominant form of hypertension. It manifests as hypertension and hypokalemia with low renin and aldosterone levels. The cause is a genetic defect in the beta subunit of the sodium channel in the apical membrane of the distal renal tubule. This defect mimics the action of mineralocorticoid hormones to enhance sodium entry in the distal nephron, thereby enhancing sodium absorption, increasing potassium excretion, and expanding the extracellular fluid volume, leading to an elevated arterial blood pressure.

c. **Pheochromocytoma.** This tumor of the adrenal medulla increases the secretion of catecholamines, leading to hypertension. Approximately 50% of patients have episodic hypertension; the rest have constant hypertension.

d. **Miscellaneous causes. Acromegaly, hyperparathyroidism,** and **hyperthyroidism** also may produce hypertension. **Coarctation of the aorta,** as noted in Chapter 1 VII D, is a correctable cause of hypertension.

III APPROACH TO THE HYPERTENSIVE PATIENT

The majority of patients with hypertension have essential hypertension; therefore, the expense, risk, and inconvenience of screening for secondary causes of hypertension should be reserved for a minority of patients suspected of having one of the following disorders.

A Renovascular hypertension

1. Renovascular hypertension **secondary to atherosclerosis of the renal artery** should be suspected in patients with the following conditions:
   a. Severe hypertension associated with advanced hypertensive retinopathy
   b. Hypertension and severe peripheral vascular disease
   c. Hypertension and sudden deterioration in renal function (with or without the recent introduction of ACE inhibitor therapy)
   d. Known disparity in renal size or function

2. Renovascular hypertension **secondary to fibromuscular dysplasia** should be suspected in young women with severe hypertension, systolic and diastolic abdominal bruits, or a strong family history of hypertension. **Captopril renography** is a useful screening test in those patients with a high prior probability of disease (see Part III: III A 1).

B **Hypermineralocorticoid states** should be suspected in patients with persistent hypokalemia and hypertension. There is no doubt that these disorders are underdiagnosed because many patients with proven mineralocorticoid excess states are normokalemic. Nevertheless, persistent and unexplained hypokalemia remains the most typical sign.

1. **Primary hyperaldosteronism.** The diagnosis rests on finding patients with hypokalemia and hypertension and proving that hyperaldosteronism causes both disorders.
   a. Patients who have unexplained hypokalemia and hypertension should have their **24-hour urinary excretion rate for aldosterone** measured while consuming a 150-mEq sodium diet. If the aldosterone value is elevated and plasma renin is low, an **abdominal CT scan** should be performed to determine whether a surgically correctable (i.e., adenomatous) form of

hyperaldosteronism is present. Recent studies suggest that a plasma aldosterone–to plasma renin–ratio of greater than 50 is highly specific for primary hyperaldosteronism.

(1) Surgery relieves hypertension and hypokalemia in over 70% of patients if adenoma is the cause. Although surgery does not cure hypertension in patients with bilateral hyperplasia, the hypokalemia does remit.

(2) Although hypokalemia may not be found in some patients with primary hyperaldosteronism, patients with hypokalemia are more likely to have a positive response to surgery so the finding of spontaneous hypokalemia remains a reasonable screening tool.

b. Patients with a family history of hypertension should undergo a **trial of glucocorticoid therapy** to determine whether glucocorticoid-remediable hyperaldosteronism is present [see Part II: III B 2 b (2)].

c. **Selective adrenal venography and sampling for lateralizing aldosterone levels** may be performed in some patients.

2. **Pheochromocytoma** should be suspected in hypertensive patients who experience episodes of flushing, diaphoresis, weight loss, and diarrhea.

a. **Measurement of urinary catecholamines and catecholamine metabolites** is useful in making the diagnosis.

b. **CT or MRI** should be used to locate the tumor in the adrenal medulla.

c. An ^{131}I MIBG scan may be performed when the suspicion of diagnosis is high but the CT or MRI is negative.

3. **Coarctation of the aorta** should be suspected in any young patient with hypertension when the blood pressure in the leg is at least 20 mm Hg lower than that in the arm.

IV THERAPY FOR HYPERTENSION

A Goals of therapy Treatment of hypertension is aimed at reducing the diastolic blood pressure to less than 90 mm Hg and the systolic blood pressure to less than 140 mm Hg.

B Indications for therapy It is currently believed that almost all patients with a blood pressure of greater than 140/90 mm Hg should be treated. In patients with borderline hypertension, controversy exists about the risks versus the benefits of therapy, but most clinicians believe that the benefits of therapy predominate and that all patients with an elevated blood pressure should receive treatment to restore the values to < 130/80.

C Types of therapy

1. **Nonpharmacologic measures**

a. **Sodium restriction** alone may be sufficient to lower blood pressure in many hypertensive patients, particularly those with a high sodium intake. Limitation of sodium intake to no more than 2 g/day has been shown to reduce blood pressure significantly in susceptible patients.

b. **Weight reduction** in obese patients also significantly reduces blood pressure.

c. **Limitation of alcohol consumption** may be beneficial. Alcohol potentiates the action of catecholamines and may exacerbate hypertension in susceptible individuals.

2. **Pharmacologic measures.** Patient compliance often is best with therapeutic regimens that are simple to follow. In choosing an antihypertensive regimen, consideration should be given not only to side effects, but also to the number of medications and doses per day that the patient must take.

a. **Diuretics,** which often are the first line of antihypertensive therapy, initially reduce extracellular fluid volume. After several months, a continued reduction cannot be measured, yet blood pressure is maintained at a lower level primarily due to decreased vascular resistance. The exact mechanism whereby diuretics reduce peripheral vascular resistance is unknown.

(1) **Agents**

(a) **Thiazide diuretics** (e.g., **hydrochlorothiazide, chlorthalidone, chlorothiazide, metolazone**) are more effective antihypertensive agents than **loop diuretics** (e.g., furosemide, bumetanide, torsemide, ethacrynic acid).

(b) **Potassium-sparing diuretics** (e.g., **amiloride, triamterene**) act in the distal nephron and collecting tubule and are useful in the treatment of hypermineralocorticoid states.

(c) **Spironolactone** and **eplerenone** are competitive inhibitors of aldosterone.

(2) **Side effects.** Hypokalemia, hyperglycemia, hyperlipidemia, hyperuricemia, hypercalcemia (thiazides only), and prerenal azotemia may occur. Therefore, periodic laboratory determination of potassium and BUN levels is indicated. Uric acid should be monitored periodically in patients with a history of gout. Some studies implicate hypokalemia caused by diuretics as an important risk factor for unexplained sudden death, a catastrophic complication that can be avoided by potassium supplementation or use of potassium-sparing diuretics.

b. **β-Adrenergic blocking agents** reduce cardiac output and renin release. However, it is not clear that these are the primary mechanisms by which β-blockers reduce blood pressure. The combination of a β-blocker and a diuretic agent reduces the diastolic blood pressure to below 90 mm Hg in approximately 80% of patients with mild-to-moderate hypertension.

(1) **Agents. Propranolol, nadolol, metoprolol, atenolol, timolol, betaxolol, carteolol, pindolol, carvedilol, acebutolol,** and **labetalol** are among the β-blockers that are currently approved for the treatment of hypertension. (Labetalol is also an α-adrenergic antagonist.)

(2) **Side effects.** Bronchospasm, bradycardia, a worsening of existing CHF, occasional impotence, fatigue, depression, and nightmares may occur.

c. **Centrally acting adrenergic antagonists** inhibit sympathetic outflow from the CNS by stimulating central α-adrenoreceptors, reducing peripheral resistance and blood pressure.

(1) **Agents. Methyldopa, clonidine, guanabenz,** and **guanfacine** are the commonly used centrally acting drugs.

(2) **Side effects.** Somnolence, orthostatic hypotension, Coombs'-positive hemolytic anemia, impotence, and hepatic injury are side effects of methyldopa. With clonidine, the major but rare side effect is a rebound phenomenon that produces severe hypertension after withdrawal of the drug.

d. **Peripherally acting sympathetic nerve antagonists** cause blood pressure to fall by reducing catecholamine release from peripheral sympathetic nerves.

(1) **Agents.** The most commonly used drugs in this category are reserpine and guanethidine. **Reserpine** depletes nerve storage vesicles of norepinephrine and, thus, limits norepinephrine secretion. **Guanethidine** directly inhibits the release of norepinephrine from adrenergic neurons.

(2) **Side effects.** The major side effect of reserpine is depression; it also may increase the incidence of gastric ulceration. Orthostatic hypotension is the most common side effect with guanethidine therapy.

e. **α-Adrenergic blocking agents** pharmacologically antagonize norepinephrine's stimulation of adrenergic receptors, reducing blood pressure by reducing total peripheral resistance. **Prazosin, doxazosin, terazosin,** and **phenoxybenzamine** are the most commonly used α-blockers.

f. **Calcium channel antagonists** reduce smooth muscle tone, thereby acting to produce vasodilatation, by modulating calcium release in smooth muscle. The subsequent reduction in total peripheral resistance reduces blood pressure. Calcium channel blockers may also reduce cardiac output by decreasing venous return and the inotropic state.

(1) **Agents.** Currently, the dihydropyridines (i.e., **nifedipine, nicardipine, isradipine, felodipine, nimodipine, amlodipine, nitrendipine**), **diltiazem,** and **verapamil** are approved for antihypertensive therapy.

(2) **Side effects.** Dihydropyridines may cause headache, flushing, and peripheral edema. Verapamil, and to a lesser extent, diltiazem, have cardiodepressant actions, unlike the dihydropyridines, making their use problematic in patients with CHF. Recent studies have suggested an increased risk of coronary events in patients receiving calcium channel blockers, but it is premature to stop using these valuable agents, particularly in patients with underlying coronary artery disease and hypertension.

g. **Direct vasodilators** dilate arteries and arterioles, reducing blood pressure by reducing total peripheral resistance. They are particularly effective when used with a β-blocker that inhibits the reflex tachycardia caused by direct vasodilation.

(1) **Agents. Hydralazine** and **minoxidil** are the most commonly used direct vasodilators.

(2) **Side effects.** The major side effects of hydralazine are headache and a lupus-like syndrome; the latter is reversed when the drug is discontinued. The major side effects of minoxidil are orthostatic hypotension and facial hirsutism.

h. **ACE inhibitors** block the conversion of angiotensin I to angiotensin II (a vasoconstrictor), thus reducing total peripheral resistance. In addition, aldosterone production is decreased, reducing the retention of sodium and water.

(1) **Agents. Captopril, enalapril, fosinopril, benazepril, quinapril, ramipril,** and **lisinopril** are useful ACE inhibitors.

(2) **Side effects.** The major side effects of captopril are rashes, leukopenia, and cough, which all typically disappear with discontinuation of the drug. Hyperkalemia may occasionally occur with any of the ACE inhibitors as a result of reduced aldosterone secretion. Because angiotensin II maintains the GFR during states of reduced renal blood flow (by maintaining a high vascular resistance in the postglomerular vessels), the use of ACE inhibitors in patients with compromised renal blood flow may lead to a form of acute renal failure. Reduction in dose or discontinuation of drug is usually sufficient to reverse the fall in GFR.

i. **Angiotensin II–type 1 receptor antagonists** (angiotensin receptor blockers) are a class of drugs that provide the benefits of blockade of the angiotensin system without some of the annoying side effects, particularly cough. These agents appear to offer all of the benefits of ACE inhibitors with fewer side effects.

(1) **Agents. Losartan, valsartan, irbesartan, candesartan, telmisartan, eprosartan, and olmesartan** are available.

(2) **Side effects.** These are similar to those of ACE inhibitors, except that cough has not been seen with receptor blockers.

D Therapeutic strategies

1. **First-line therapy.** Various agents are now considered appropriate for initial antihypertensive therapy. Many physicians still begin therapy with a diuretic, but β-blockers, ACE inhibitors, angiotensin receptor blockers, or calcium channel blockers are also appropriate initial drugs. At the very best, monotherapy produces optimal control of blood pressure in only 75% of patients.
2. **Second-line therapy.** Submaximal doses of two or three antihypertensive agents added in a stepwise fashion have been advocated as a successful approach. The addition of 12.5 or 25 mg hydrochlorothiazide will potentiate the action of a number of antihypertensive agents, particularly the ACE inhibitors and the angiotensin II-receptor antagonists. If the blood pressure is still uncontrolled, the use of multiple drug regimens or the addition of direct vasodilators is indicated.

V HYPERTENSIVE CRISIS

This condition is defined as severe hypertension characterized by a diastolic blood pressure of greater than 140 mm Hg. Blood pressure elevation to this degree can cause vascular damage, pulmonary edema, encephalopathy, retinal hemorrhages, renal damage, and death.

A Diagnosis A diastolic blood pressure of greater than 140 mm Hg, funduscopic findings of papilledema, changes in neurologic and mental status, and an abnormal renal sediment are the hallmarks of hypertensive crisis.

B Therapy Immediate lowering of the blood pressure is indicated.

1. Infusion of **sodium nitroprusside** is effective.
   a. The patient's blood pressure should be monitored constantly so that the dose can be adjusted to maintain the blood pressure within the desired range. An excessive reduction in blood pressure can be reversed rapidly by reducing the dose of the infusion.
   b. Long-term administration of high-dose nitroprusside (7 μg/kg/min) can lead to cyanide intoxication. The likelihood of this complication increases in patients with renal dysfunction.
2. **Labetalol, nicardipine,** and **nitroglycerine** are also effective intravenous therapeutic agents.
3. **The use of sublingual nifedipine has been shown to be dangerous (precipitating coronary ischemia or stroke), and it should not be a part of therapy.**

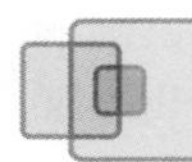

Study Questions

1. A 60-year-old man develops new-onset nephrotic syndrome. A percutaneous renal biopsy is contemplated to determine the nature of the glomerular disease. In which of the following situations is the renal biopsy absolutely contraindicated?

- A The patient has a diastolic blood pressure of 120 mm Hg.
- B The patient has a serum creatinine level of 2.5 mg/dL (normal = 0.8–1.4 mg/dL).
- C The patient has diabetes mellitus.
- D The patient has heavy proteinuria but no other urinary abnormality.
- E The patient has undergone a previous renal biopsy.

2. A 71-year-old man in the surgical intensive care unit is seen for acute renal failure. After an operation for removal of gallstones, he had a persistent drainage from his biliary catheter associated with spiking fevers to 38.9°C. He has been taking gentamicin (70 mg every 8 hours) and cephalothin (2 g four times a day) for the past 10 days. Over the last 4 days, his serum creatinine level has increased at a rate of 1 mg/dL/day, but his urine output of 1.5 L/day has not diminished. At no time has he had any hypotension during this hospitalization.

Physical examination shows normal blood pressure and vital signs. Results of laboratory studies indicate a creatinine level of 7.1 mg/dL, and renal ultrasonography reveals no evidence of obstruction. Which of the following is the most likely cause of the acute renal failure?

- A Sepsis
- B Trauma to the ureter during surgery
- C Gentamicin nephrotoxicity
- D Acute glomerulonephritis
- E Cephalothin-induced acute renal failure

3. A 39-year-old man who is experiencing labored breathing and mental obtundation comes to the emergency department. Physical examination is unremarkable. Laboratory studies show the following: serum sodium = 144 mEq/L, serum potassium = 3.7 mEq/L, serum chloride = 97 mEq/L, plasma bicarbonate concentration $[HCO_3^-]$ = 16 mEq/L, arterial pH = 7.38, and $Pa{CO_2}$ = 21 mEq/L. These findings indicate which of the following acid–base disturbances?

- A Respiratory alkalosis
- B Metabolic acidosis
- C Metabolic acidosis and respiratory alkalosis
- D Metabolic acidosis and metabolic alkalosis
- E No acid–base disturbance

4. A 69-year-old woman has moderately severe renal failure. During her most recent follow-up, laboratory tests showed the following: serum sodium = 142 mEq/L, serum potassium = 5.1 mEq/L, serum chloride = 109 mEq/L, plasma bicarbonate concentration $[HCO_3^-]$ = 15 mEq/L, and creatinine = 4.2 mg/dL. The origin of metabolic acidosis is most likely due to which of the following conditions?

- A Bicarbonaturia
- B Impaired excretion of titratable acids
- C Decreased filtration of hydrogen ions (H^+)
- D Impaired ammonia excretion
- E Hypoaldosteronism

5. A 45-year-old man enters the hospital because of acute flank pain and red urine, which began at night and awakened him. Until this point, the man has been in good health. Physical examination in the emergency department is normal, but he does have hematuria, with essentially normal laboratory studies. Radiography of the abdomen reveals a stone in the right kidney. An intravenous urogram shows the stone to be nonobstructing. Further laboratory studies demonstrate normal serum calcium and phosphate, and a subsequent urine culture is negative. Which of the following types of kidney stone is most likely to have caused this condition?

A. Calcium oxalate stone
B. Uric acid stone
C. Xanthine stone
D. Struvite stone
E. Cystine stone

6. A 70-year-old man with long-standing hypertension has developed more severe hypertension over a 6-month period. In spite of antihypertensive medication, his blood pressure has risen from 140/90 to 175/105 mm Hg. In addition, he had an episode of "flash pulmonary edema" that led to his hospitalization for 1 week. He has continued to take his antihypertensive medication faithfully, but he has developed some intermittent claudication in his left leg. Although he has a long history of smoking, he has had no other medical problems. Which of the following is the most likely cause of this clinical disorder?

A. Renal artery stenosis
B. Pheochromocytoma
C. Hyperaldosteronism
D. Primary worsening of hypertension
E. Coarctation of the aorta

7. A 58-year-old woman is admitted to the hospital for evaluation of polyuria. A water deprivation test is performed for 14 hours under strict medical observation.

Baseline	
Serum sodium	132 mEq/L
Plasma osmolality	275 mOsm/kg
Urine osmolality	145 mOsm/kg

45 Minutes Following Vasopressin	
Serum sodium	130 mEq/L
Plasma osmolality	271 mOsm/kg
Urine osmolality	489 mOsm/kg

Which of the following is the most likely diagnosis?

A. Central diabetes insipidus
B. Nephrogenic diabetes insipidus
C. Electrolyte osmotic diuresis
D. Nonelectrolyte osmotic diuresis
E. Psychogenic polydipsia

8. A 78-year-old man enters the hospital because of abnormalities of urination. Today he is passing large amounts of urine; however, some days he passes no urine at all. He now has a blood pressure of 180/90 mm Hg, and otherwise, his physical examination is normal. Laboratory studies show a blood urea nitrogen (BUN) of 120 mg/dL and a serum creatinine of 4.2 mg/dL. Urinalysis reveals a specific gravity of 1.010; urine that is negative for protein, glucose, ketone bodies, and blood; and an occasional white blood cell (WBC) per high-power field on microscopic examination. Which of the following is the most likely cause of the renal insufficiency?

A Obstructive uropathy
B Acute glomerulonephritis
C Acute interstitial nephritis
D Acute tubular necrosis (ATN)
E Chronic renal failure of unspecified nature

9. A 47-year-old man enters the hospital with nephrotic syndrome. He reports that he initially experienced edema of his feet in the morning, but this condition rapidly progressed until the edema extended to his midcalves and lasted throughout the day. He has been in good health all his life and has not seen a physician in the last 5 years.

On physical examination, blood pressure is 155/100 mm Hg, pulse is 88 bpm, respiratory rate is 15 breaths/min, and temperature is 37.0°C. Examination of the heart and lungs reveals no evidence of congestive heart failure (CHF), examination of the abdomen indicates mild ascites with normal hepatic size, and examination of the extremities reveals 4+ edema to the midcalf. Laboratory studies show a blood urea nitrogen (BUN) of 10 mg/dL and creatinine of 1.0 mg/dL. The rest of the laboratory studies are unrevealing. Urinalysis reveals 4+ protein and one red blood cell (RBC) per high-power field. No RBC casts or other cellular elements are seen on urinalysis. The 24-hour urine contains 9.6 g of protein. Which of the following is most likely to account for this clinical condition?

A Membranous nephropathy
B Poststreptococcal glomerulonephritis
C Lupus nephritis
D Amyloidosis
E Diabetes mellitus

10. A 31-year-old man enters the hospital with acute onset of edema and hematuria. He had been well until 3 weeks earlier, when he had a sore throat and was treated with oral penicillin. Since that time, he has felt generally good but has noted the onset of dark, tea-colored urine and swelling of his legs. He denies any other symptoms, including rash, joint pain, chest pain, and the use of any medication but the penicillin.

On physical examination, blood pressure is 160/110 mm Hg, pulse is 85 bpm, respiratory rate is 15 breaths/min, and temperature is 37.0°C. Other findings include marked peripheral edema extending to midleg. Laboratory studies reveal a blood urea nitrogen (BUN) of 20 mg/dL, creatinine of 1.3 mg/dL, and normal electrolytes. The serum complement level, including CH_{50} and C_4, is reduced by 50%, the anti-deoxyribonuclease B antibody and the antistreptolysin O titer are increased, and the anti-glomerular basement membrane (anti-GBM) antibody assay and antineutrophilic cytoplasmic antibody (ANCA) level are within normal limits. Urinalysis reveals 4+ protein, 4+ blood, and no glucose. Microscopic examination reveals three to four red blood cell (RBC) casts per high-power field as well as many RBCs and white blood cells (WBCs). No bacteria are visible. Which of the following is the most likely cause of this acute renal syndrome?

A Poststreptococcal glomerulonephritis
B Systemic lupus erythematosus (SLE)
C Goodpasture's syndrome
D Immunoglobulin A (IgA) nephropathy
E Allergic reaction to penicillin

11. A 64-year-old man enters the hospital because of renal insufficiency. Until 6 months earlier, when he developed persistent back pain, he was in good health. At that time, he was found to be severely anemic, and his blood urea nitrogen (BUN) and creatinine levels were elevated (42 and 4.6 mg/dL, respectively).

He now undergoes further evaluation. He denies the use of any medications, any past history of renal injury, and any difficulty in voiding. He does complain of persistent weakness and easy fatigability, and his back pain has become more severe over the last 2 weeks.

On physical examination, blood pressure is 120/80 mm Hg, pulse is 70 bpm, respiratory rate is 15 breaths/min, and temperature is 37.0°C. Major physical findings include severe pallor as well as clear evidence of muscle wasting. Urinalysis reveals 1+ protein on dipstick testing and 4+ on sulfosalicylic acid testing. Microscopic examination of the urine reveals an occasional broad and an occasional granular cast. Laboratory studies give the following results: BUN = 61 mg/dL, creatinine = 5.1 mg/dL, serum sodium = 141 mEq/L, serum potassium = 5.6 mEq/L, serum chloride = 101 mEq/L, serum bicarbonate = 14 mEq/L, serum calcium = 11.7 mg/dL, and serum phosphorus = 6.0 mg/dL. Which of the following is the most likely cause of this condition?

- A Renovascular disease
- B Thrombotic renal disease
- C Multiple myeloma
- D Systemic lupus erythematosus (SLE)
- E Analgesic nephropathy

12. A 21-year-old woman enters the hospital because of severe anemia and acute renal failure. Three weeks prior to admission, she had delivered a normal, full-term infant, and had felt extremely weak and fatigued following delivery. Her physician notes that she is extremely pale. A complete blood count (CBC) reveals severe anemia as well as thrombocytopenia. Further laboratory screening reveals elevated blood urea nitrogen (BUN) and creatinine, and she is referred for admission. She denies any medication use postpartum and any previous medical problems similar to this one. Her laboratory studies were normal at the time of discharge from the hospital following delivery.

On physical examination, vital signs are normal, and the only physical findings aside from her pallor are petechiae on the skin and multiple ecchymoses on the lower extremities. Laboratory studies reveal a hemoglobin of 6.3 mg/dL, a hematocrit of 18%, a platelet count of 23,000/mm^3, BUN of 94 mg/dL, and creatinine of 9.1 mg/dL. The serum antinucleophilic cytoplasmic antibody (ANCA) and serum antineutrophilic antibody (ANA) levels are normal. A peripheral blood smear reveals multiple schistocytes. Urinalysis reveals many red blood cell (RBC) casts. Which of the following is the most likely diagnosis?

- A Hemolytic–uremic syndrome
- B Goodpasture's syndrome
- C Systemic lupus erythematosus (SLE)
- D Idiopathic thrombocytopenic purpura
- E A drug reaction

13. A 69-year-old woman complains of easy fatigability, weight loss, and dizziness. Her medical history includes a remote history of tuberculosis. Physical examination reveals a blood pressure of 100/62 mm Hg and increased skin pigmentation. Laboratory studies reveal the following: serum sodium = 129 mEq/L, serum potassium = 6.1 mEq/L, serum chloride = 100 mEq/L, plasma bicarbonate concentration [HCO_3^-] = 21 mEq/L, glucose = 88 mg/dL, and blood urea nitrogen (BUN) = 30 mg/dL. Which of the following diagnoses best fits these findings?

- A Adrenal insufficiency
- B Chronic renal failure
- C Adrenocorticotropic hormone (ACTH)–secreting tumor
- D Distal (type I) renal tubular acidosis
- E Syndrome of inappropriate secretion of antidiuretic hormone (SIADH)

14. A 27-year-old man is referred for evaluation of hematuria. For the past 6 years, he has experienced painless gross hematuria two to three times per year. The condition has always remitted spontaneously within 1–2 days, but on this occasion, bright-red blood has appeared in his urine for the past 8 days. He denies any trauma to his kidneys or any other recent illnesses. Although he has a younger brother with sickle cell anemia, the man has been free from any symptoms of this abnormality. He has no other known family history or evidence of any other renal disease, including kidney stones and infection.

Urinalysis reveals red-to-pink urine, with numerous red blood cells (RBCs) per high-power field, and no proteinuria on orthotoluidine dipstick test. Which of the following is the most likely diagnosis at this point?

- A Nephrolithiasis
- B Carcinoma of the kidney
- C Renal vein thrombosis
- D Prostatitis
- E Sickle cell trait

15. A 28-year-old architect is referred for evaluation of the cause of nephrolithiasis. Over the past 5 years, the man has had six kidney stones, with the most recent one requiring surgical removal. He denies any history of urinary tract infections, but his father and paternal grandfather both had kidney stones.

On physical examination, he is found to be normotensive; all other findings are normal. Laboratory studies reveal normal serum chemistries, including calcium, phosphorus, and magnesium determinations. Urinary determinations of calcium, phosphate, uric acid, and protein also are normal. Urinalysis reveals a urine pH of 5 and occasional hexagonal crystals. Which of the following is the most likely cause of this patient's nephrolithiasis?

- A Calcium oxalate stones
- B Uric acid stones
- C Cystine stones
- D Calcium phosphate stones
- E Magnesium–ammonium–calcium–phosphate (struvite) stones

16. A 21-year-old man enters the hospital complaining that he has been passing dark reddish urine. He has recently recovered from a football-related knee injury incurred 3 months before, and the day before entering the hospital he engaged in vigorous physical activity for the first time since his knee injury. This morning he awoke with sore, painful muscles and the aforementioned change in the character of his urine.

Physical examination is essentially normal except for the painful muscles. Findings on urinalysis include red–brown color; pH of 5.0; specific gravity of 1.02; 3+ dipstick test for blood; and no evidence of glucose, ketones, or bilirubin. Microscopic examination of the urine reveals occasional amorphous debris and three or four granular casts but no red blood cells (RBCs). Which of the following conditions most likely accounts for the urinalysis?

- A Myoglobinuria
- B Hemolyzed blood in the urine
- C Ingestion of foodstuffs containing red dye
- D Urinary tract infection
- E Renal trauma

17. A 37-year-old man enters the hospital with a history of recent onset of hemoptysis and acute renal failure. Until 6 weeks ago, when he noted the onset of a cough which, over the ensuing 3 days, produced streaky, blood-tinged sputum, he had been in good health. His local physician ordered laboratory studies, which revealed a serum creatinine of 1.2 mg/dL. A chest radiograph taken at that time revealed bilateral fluffy infiltrates. The patient was treated with antibiotics and followed over the next 3 weeks; during that time, the lung picture worsened and the serum creatinine rose to 2.5 mg/dL.

Now the man appears ill and in moderate distress. His blood pressure is 120/80 mm Hg, his pulse is 110 bpm, his respiratory rate is 22 breaths/min, and his temperature is 37.2°C. Examination of the chest shows bilateral rales and a few scattered wheezes, and examination of the heart reveals tachycardia but is otherwise normal. A chest radiograph reveals bilateral fluffy alveolar infiltrates. Laboratory examination shows a blood urea nitrogen (BUN) of 65 mg/dL, a creatinine of 4.3 mg/dL, and electrolytes within normal limits. The hemoglobin level is 8.3 mg/dL, and the hematocrit is 28%. Examination of the sputum reveals blood. Urinalysis reveals many red blood cell (RBC) casts. Serum antineutrophilic cytoplasmic antibody (ANCA) levels are negative, as are serum complement levels. The serum antiglomerular basement membrane (anti-GBM) antibody titer is elevated to 1:64. Which of the following represents the most likely cause of this disorder?

- A Wegener's granulomatosis
- B Goodpasture's syndrome
- C Systemic lupus erythematosus (SLE)
- D Microscopic polyarteritis nodosa
- E Idiopathic crescentic glomerulonephritis

18. A 60-year-old man enters the hospital complaining of nausea, weakness, and confusion of 1 week's duration. He has a long-standing history of hypertension and congestive heart failure (CHF) that has been treated with increasing amounts of diuretics and digoxin without apparent benefit.

Physical examination indicates a blood pressure of 145/90 mm Hg (without orthostatic changes), jugular venous distention, bilateral basilar rales, and +2 bilateral ankle edema. Laboratory studies reveal the following: serum sodium = 120 mEq/L, blood urea nitrogen (BUN) = 93 mg/dL, glucose = 135 mg/dL, plasma osmolality = 252 mOsm/kg, and urine osmolality = 690 mOsm/kg. Which of the following is involved in the treatment of hyponatremia in this patient?

- A 3% sodium chloride infusion
- B 0.9% sodium chloride infusion
- C 50 mg hydrochlorothiazide daily
- D Salt and water restriction
- E Demeclocycline

19. A 27-year-old woman presents with a 6-month history of polyarthritis, facial rash, and proteinuria. Urinalysis shows red blood cell casts and white blood cells. Which of the following findings are likely with further testing?

- A Nodular glomerulosclerosis
- B Positive fluorescent antinuclear antibody (ANA)
- C Glomerular capillary endotheliosis
- D Necrotizing granulomatous vasculitis
- E Positive Congo red staining for amyloid

20. A 57-year-old patient with a 13-year history of poorly controlled diabetes mellitus has developed a slow rise in serum creatinine and proteinuria over the past 18 months. Which of the following pathologic or laboratory findings is likely in this setting?

- A Nodular glomerulosclerosis
- B Positive fluorescent antinuclear antibody (ANA)
- C Glomerular capillary endotheliosis
- D Necrotizing granulomatous vasculitis
- E Positive Congo red staining for amyloid

21. A 17-year-old woman in the third trimester of her first pregnancy has a blood pressure of 145/95 mm Hg and 2+ proteinuria. Further testing is most likely to reveal which of the following laboratory or pathologic findings?

A Nodular glomerulosclerosis
B Positive fluorescent antinuclear antibody (ANA)
C Glomerular capillary endotheliosis
D Necrotizing granulomatous vasculitis
E Positive Congo red staining for amyloid

22. A 34-year-old man who is a heavy smoker develops hematuria with red blood cell casts and 2+ proteinuria along with a chest x-ray that shows a nodular, cavitating lesion in the right middle lobe. He also has a necrotic-appearing lesion in his nares. Further testing is most likely to reveal which of the following laboratory or pathologic findings?

A Nodular glomerulosclerosis
B Positive fluorescent antinuclear antibody (ANA)
C Glomerular capillary endotheliosis
D Necrotizing granulomatous vasculitis
E Positive Congo red staining for amyloid

23. A 68-year-old man was diagnosed with multiple myeloma 1 year ago. Over the past 3 months he has developed severe lower extremity edema. Urinalysis shows 4+ proteinuria but no other abnormalities. The serum creatinine is 1.7 mg/dL. Further testing is most likely to reveal which of the following laboratory or pathologic findings?

A Nodular glomerulosclerosis
B Positive fluorescent antinuclear antibody (ANA)
C Glomerular capillary endotheliosis
D Necrotizing granulomatous vasculitis
E Positive Congo red staining for amyloid

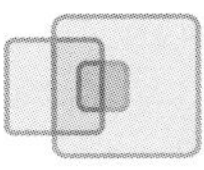

Answers and Explanations

1. The answer is A [Part I: I D 2]. Hypertension is an absolute contraindication to performing a renal biopsy because the incidence of subclinical bleeding at the site is high (75%). In a hypertensive patient, this bleeding may lead to a major, life-threatening hemorrhage. Mild renal insufficiency (as evidenced by a small decrease in creatinine clearance), nephrotic syndrome without urinary casts, and moderately advanced age are not contraindications to performing a renal biopsy. Multiple renal biopsies may be performed in the same patient. A previous renal biopsy is not a contraindication for subsequent biopsies.

2. The answer is C [Table 6–1]. Approximately 5%–10% of patients treated with gentamicin develop a nonoliguric form of acute renal failure. Although the patient has received normal doses of gentamicin, its accumulation in the kidney has produced a late form of acute renal failure. The serum creatinine level then rises while an inappropriately high dosage is maintained. This rise exacerbates the renal insufficiency and prolongs the course of acute renal failure. The nonoliguric nature of this patient's clinical condition also is a typical finding in gentamicin nephrotoxicity. Although the patient could have obstructive uropathy, the negative results of ultrasonography strongly indicate otherwise. Cephalothin can produce an acute interstitial nephritis, but the patient's clinical course is much more compatible with the more common drug-induced disease of gentamicin nephrotoxicity. Acute glomerulonephritis usually is associated with hypertension and an active urinary sediment containing casts, protein, and red blood cells (RBCs).

3. The answer is C [Part II: IV C, D]. Although the arterial pH is within the normal range, the patient is suffering from two separate acid–base disturbances (metabolic acidosis and respiratory alkalosis) which, together, tend to offset their effects on pH. The low Pa_{CO_2} in this case is much lower than would be expected if the patient had only respiratory compensation. Thus, if the patient has a single acid–base disturbance, namely metabolic acidosis, then the expected Pa_{CO_2} is calculated using Winters' formula:

$$\begin{aligned}\text{Expected } Pa_{CO_2} &= 1.5 \times [HCO_3^-] + 8 \pm 2\\ &= 1.5 \times 16 + 8 \pm 2\\ &= 32 \pm 2\end{aligned}$$

The measured Pa_{CO_2} of less than 32 mm Hg indicates that the patient also has a primary respiratory disturbance, namely respiratory alkalosis.

4. The answer is D [Part II: IV D]. The most important factor that leads to metabolic acidosis in renal failure is the impaired synthesis and excretion of ammonia. This combination leads to impaired titration of hydrogen (H^+) ions that are secreted in the distal nephron. The net result is decreased net acid secretion.

5. The answer is A [Part I: VII A; Table 6–4]. The patient most likely has idiopathic calcium oxalate stones. This conclusion is based on the fact that it is the most common form of kidney stone, the stone is radiopaque, and many of the findings suggest that the other answers are wrong. First, uric acid stones are radiolucent, so a stone would not have been seen on the radiographic flat plate prior to the intravenous urogram. Second, xanthine stones are extremely rare and are also radiolucent. Third, struvite stones are found only in the setting of a urinary tract infection. The absence of a positive urine culture strongly suggests that struvite stones are not present. Fourth, while cystine stones could present in this fashion even though the patient is middle-aged, cystine stones typically present much earlier and represent less than 1% of the stones analyzed in large studies. Thus, on a purely statistical basis, the patient is unlikely to have cystine stones. However, all patients with kidney stone formation who have not had their stone crystallography analyzed should have a 24-hour cystine determination to be certain that cystinuria is not present.

6. The answer is A [Part III: III A]. Renal artery stenosis is a common complication in patients with long-standing hypertension and peripheral vascular disease. As many as 80% of patients with this combination of disorders have renal artery stenosis. It is typically atherosclerotic in nature and involves the ostia of the renal arteries. "Flash pulmonary edema" commonly accompanies this condition and probably represents acute changes in hemodynamic status induced by an increased sensitivity to the adrenergic nervous system. Other features of this disorder are worsening of hypertension as well as development of azotemia. This constellation of findings often necessitates intervention, with either percutaneous transluminal angioplasty (PCTA) or surgery.

7. The answer is E [Part II: I C 2 b (1), (2), (a), (b)]. Baseline urine osmolality is quite low, indicating a water diuresis and not an osmotic diuresis. To determine whether the patient has central versus nephrogenic diabetes insipidus (or alternatively, psychogenic polydipsia) requires testing with antidiuretic hormone (ADH). The substantial increase in urine osmolality after administration of vasopressin rules out nephrogenic diabetes insipidus. It is more likely that this patient has psychogenic polydipsia rather than central diabetes insipidus because baseline serum sodium is on the low side. This factor suggests that loss of water in the urine is actually caused by excess water intake, which would tend to decrease serum sodium concentration. In central diabetes insipidus, obligate urinary water losses would tend to raise serum sodium concentration above normal.

8. The answer is A [Part I: VIII A, C]. The incidence of prostatism in elderly men is so great that it must be considered the primary cause of renal insufficiency until proven otherwise. This patient's history is classic in that he had 1 or 2 days on which he seemed to pass no urine followed by days of high urine flow, a pattern that is caused by the gradual accumulation of large amounts of urine in the collecting system under pressure, which eventually may overcome some degree of obstruction. The high pressure is transmitted back to the kidneys and results in renal insufficiency. Acute glomerulonephritis and acute interstitial nephritis are ruled out by the normal results of urinalysis. The possibility of acute tubular necrosis (ATN) should be considered, but no information in the history suggests recent surgery or nephrotoxic drug intake that would have produced ATN. The best way to screen for obstructive uropathy is renal ultrasonography, which would demonstrate dilated upper tract calyces.

9. The answer is A [Part I: X C; XII B 4]. This patient most likely has membranous nephropathy, which is the most common cause of nephrotic syndrome in patients in this age group. It is characterized by an absence of evidence for a high degree of glomerular inflammation. Thus, the urinalysis, which reveals little in the way of cellular elements and heavy proteinuria, supports this diagnosis. Poststreptococcal glomerulonephritis and lupus glomerulonephritis are much more likely to demonstrate active urinary sediments with red blood cells (RBCs) and RBC casts. In addition, these conditions are often associated with systemic manifestations of the underlying disease; none are present in this patient. Amyloidosis could give a clinical picture similar to that described, but the vast majority of patients with systemic amyloidosis have systemic signs such as peripheral neuropathy, autonomic neuropathy, or cardiac disease at the time that they develop nephrotic syndrome. Diabetic nephropathy is unlikely because of the absence of history. Failure to find abnormal retinal findings on ophthalmoscopic examination would also make diabetic nephropathy an unlikely diagnosis.

10. The answer is A [Part I: X I]. The most likely etiology of this patient's acute renal syndrome is poststreptococcal glomerulonephritis. The finding of a reduced serum complement and elevated antistreptolysin O titer in the clinical setting of a streptococcal infection strongly suggests this cause. While systemic lupus erythematosus (SLE) may produce some aspects of the clinical picture, particularly the nephritic renal syndrome, the absence of other systemic signs of SLE makes this condition highly unlikely. However, an antinuclear antibody (ANA) assay should be performed to fully exclude this diagnosis. Goodpasture's syndrome is unlikely in the absence of a history of pulmonary abnormalities or hemoptysis. Immunoglobulin A (IgA) nephropathy can present as a severe, acute nephritic picture but should not produce the other serologic abnormalities seen in this patient. A reaction to penicillin can result in an acute renal injury; however, like IgA nephropathy, it is not associated with the complement and antistreptococcal antibody titers that are seen. Furthermore, nephrotic syndrome would be an uncommon consequence of penicillin reaction, which much more typically presents as an acute interstitial injury to the kidney, with renal insufficiency, eosinophils and other white cell elements in the urine, and minimal proteinuria.

11. The answer is C [Part I: X P]. Multiple myeloma is the most likely etiology. The combination of hypercalcemia and acute renal failure raises the possibility of multiple myeloma as the bone breakdown secondary to tumor involvement releases large amounts of calcium to the extracellular fluid and hypercalcemia ensues. The renal failure in myeloma is primarily related to hypercalcemia combined with proteinaceous cast formation within the renal tubules, producing a form of intratubular obstruction as well as a tubular inflammatory lesion. The major diagnostic clue is the finding of a urinary dipstick that is mildly positive for protein in the urine but a sulfosalicylic acid test that is strongly positive. Dipstick testing does not detect the negatively charged light-chain proteins, only the albumin. The sulfosalicylic acid test detects all forms of proteins. Renovascular lesions and thrombotic renal disease could present with this picture, although they should not be associated with hypercalcemia and severe back pain, and findings on examination of the urine would not include proteins. Systemic lupus erythematosus (SLE) can, of course, be associated with severe anemia and joint manifestations, but hypercalcemia is not part of the picture.

12. The answer is A [Part I: XIV D 1 b]. The most likely cause of this condition is hemolytic–uremic syndrome. This syndrome is associated with platelet consumption as well as acute renal insufficiency. This condition may occur postpartum and can be diagnosed only by examining the entire clinical picture. Patients with systemic lupus erythematosus (SLE) can present with thrombocytopenia and acute renal failure, but the negative antinuclear antibody (ANA) level in the absence of other systemic manifestations makes this answer unlikely. The finding of schistocytes on the peripheral smear also strongly supports the diagnosis of the microangiopathic picture, which explains to a greater extent the anemia seen. The only drug-associated cause of renal insufficiency that manifests as severe thrombocytopenia of this degree as well as severe microangiopathic hemolytic anemia is cyclosporine or penicillamine treatment. Idiopathic thrombocytopenic purpura (ITT) is not associated with concurrent renal disease. The correct therapy for this condition would be to perform plasma exchange, plasma infusions, or both, as the best way of limiting the injury associated with hemolytic–uremic syndrome. The etiology of this syndrome remains unclear, although it can be associated with bacterial infections, particularly when it occurs in epidemic form in children.

13. The answer is A [Part II: I B]. The findings of low blood pressure, increased skin pigmentation, hyperkalemia, and hyponatremia all point to the likely diagnosis of adrenal insufficiency. Adrenocorticotropic hormone (ACTH)–secreting tumors, while they may produce skin pigmentations, are usually associated with hypertension and hypokalemic alkalosis due to excess mineralocorticoid secretion. Hyperkalemia due to renal failure is seen when the glomerular filtration rate (GFR) is below 10–15 mm^3/min. The patient's blood urea nitrogen (BUN) of 30 mg/dL suggests only mildly impaired renal function. Distal (type I) renal tubular acidosis is characterized by hypokalemia (although occasional cases of hyperkalemia have been described).

14. The answer is E [Part I: Table 6–3; XIV F 2 b]. Sickle cell trait, nephrolithiasis, carcinoma of the kidney, renal vein thrombosis, and prostatitis all may be associated with hematuria. The finding of gross hematuria in a young man with a family history of sickle cell anemia, however, strongly suggests that, in the absence of other stigmata of sickle cell disease, he suffers from sickle cell trait. This abnormality commonly is associated with hematuria and is caused by sickling of red blood cells (RBCs) in the vessels on the surface of the renal pelvis and papilla, leading to small areas of infarction and bleeding. Renal tumor can produce bleeding, but it is rarely so persistent in the absence of other symptoms. Renal vein thrombosis can produce hematuria but usually in the setting of severe pain and proteinuria. Nephrolithiasis also may produce relatively silent hematuria if the stone has been present for a long period of time, but pain typically is associated with this condition. Urinary tract infection also can be associated with hematuria, but symptoms of infection (e.g., dysuria, fever) should be present.

15. The answer is C [Part I: Table 6–4]. The patient's clinical presentation is typical of any patient with kidney stone disease. In more than 90% of patients, nephrolithiasis is caused by calcium oxalate stone formation. In 50% of those individuals, hypercalciuria is present. In the absence of hypercalciuria and with the finding of hexagonal crystals in the urine, the physician must be highly suspicious that this patient has cystinuria. A urinalysis revealing cystine crystals is seen in approximately 40%–50% of patients; however, negative urinalysis should not deter the physician from measuring a 24-hour urinary cystine excretion. An initial presentation of cystinuria at age 25 or 30 is not unusual, but in some cases, patients are in their 70s and 80s before they present with cystinuria. The condition is an autosomal dominant trait, but a variety of phenotypic forms may be seen.

Treatment of cystine stones includes maintaining high urine flow rates (i.e., up to 4–5 L/day) and urine alkalinization if a urine pH value over 7.5 can be achieved by sodium bicarbonate administration. Cystine solubility is approximately 100 mg/L; therefore, if an individual excretes between 300 and 400 mg/24 hr, high fluid intake may prevent further stone formation. If, however, excretion is greater than 700 or 800 mg/24 hr, patients often may require D-penicillamine or 2-mercaptopropionylglycine (tiopronine), compounds that form mixed disulfides with cystine and render cystine much more soluble in the urine.

If the patient in question has not had cystine demonstrated in his urine, the next critical test would have been an analysis of the kidney stone.

16. The answer is A [Part I: I A 1 b, 2 a, f; II C 3 a (5).] The finding of dark reddish urine suggests a number of underlying conditions. However, the absence of red blood cells (RBCs) on microscopic examination of the urine combined with the positive dipstick test for blood strongly suggests the possibility of myoglobinuria. Myoglobin is a pigment that is detected by the orthotoluidine reagent on the dipstick. Although hemolyzed blood could be present in the urine, a few RBCs should be noted, whereas none are seen in this patient's urine. Although foodstuffs do contain dyes that may color the urine, these dyes do not produce positive dipstick tests for blood. This clinical picture is most consistent with myoglobinuria caused by sudden, extreme physical exertion by an individual who is not well-conditioned. Such activity leads to muscle cell breakdown and the release of myoglobin into the circulation, with its ultimate filtration by the kidney and appearance in the urine.

17. The answer is B [Part I: X G]. The most likely etiology of this disorder is Goodpasture's syndrome. Wegener's granulomatosis can present with a pulmonary bleeding syndrome associated with acute glomerulonephritis, as seen in this patient and as evidenced by the hemoptysis as well as by the active urinary sediment. However, the negative antineutrophilic cytoplasmic antibody (ANCA) level and the absence of a destructive upper airway lesion on physical examination argue against Wegener's granulomatosis, and the finding of positive anti-glomerular basement membrane (anti-GBM) antibodies strongly points to Goodpasture's syndrome. Systemic lupus erythematosus (SLE) and microscopic vasculitis can present with pulmonary hemorrhage and renal insufficiency but neither is associated with the serologies seen in this patient. Idiopathic crescentic glomerulonephritis describes an entity similar to that seen in this patient, but the finding of positive serum anti-GBM antibody titers eliminates glomerulonephritis as an "idiopathic" entity.

18. The answer is D [Part II: I B 5]. Water restriction should help produce a negative water balance. Salt restriction is also needed because the patient has excess total sodium burden; this change should also optimize the response to diuretics. Hyponatremia in the setting of an expanded extracellular volume [e.g., congestive heart failure (CHF)] develops because of diminished renal ability to excrete water in the face of continuing water ingestion. The renal diluting defect is the result of impaired delivery of tubular fluid to distal diluting nephron segments and is precipitated by enhanced proximal tubular reabsorption. The latter is caused by decreased renal perfusion as a result of impaired cardiac output. A decrease in effective arterial volume also stimulates antidiuretic hormone (ADH) release, which further impairs urinary dilution. Ideally, treatment should be directed at improving cardiac function. Digoxin and diuretics have been administered without significant benefit. The patient certainly cannot tolerate any saline infusions because this treatment would aggravate his congestive symptoms. Hydrochlorothiazide added to his regimen may not be potent enough to improve the refractory congestive symptoms; besides, hydrochlorothiazide itself impairs urinary dilution and may aggravate the hyponatremia. Demeclocycline for the treatment of hyponatremia is reserved for the chronic management of the syndrome of inappropriate antidiuretic hormone (SIADH). Because of its potential nephrotoxicity, demeclocycline is contraindicated in all states of azotemia, as in this case.

19. The answer is B [Part I: X M 1]. The patient has systemic lupus erythematosus (SLE). The glomerular abnormalities of SLE form a disease spectrum, with four associated major lesions: focal proliferative, diffuse proliferative, membranous, and mesangial forms of lupus nephritis. Serologic studies of the four lesions determine differing levels of anti-DNA antibodies and complement components, but common to all four are immunofluorescent findings for antinuclear antibody (ANA). Nodular glomerulosclerosis is a pathologic lesion characteristic of diabetic nephropathy. Glomerular capillary endotheliosis is the pathologic finding in the kidney of patients with preeclampsia. Necrotizing granulomatous vasculitis is characteristic of Wegener's granulomatosis but may be seen in other vasculitic conditions as well. Congo red staining for amyloid is seen in primary and secondary forms of amyloidosis, which can cause the nephrotic syndrome if there is kidney involvement.

20. The answer is A [Part I: X L]. All lesions in the kidneys of individuals with diabetes mellitus are grouped under the term diabetic nephropathy. The foremost clinical feature of diabetic glomerular disease is overt proteinuria, which develops after a prolonged course of diabetes mellitus. Although diffuse glomerulosclerosis is the most common lesion (found in 90% of all diabetic individuals with overt nephropathy) and is correlated with the degree of proteinuria and the renal failure, it is neither specific for nor diagnostic of diabetes. In contrast, the other major renal lesion associated with diabetes, nodular glomerulosclerosis (Kimmelstiel-Wilson syndrome), is both specific for and diagnostic of diabetic glomerulopathy. A positive ANA is a typical feature of systemic lupus erythematosus. Glomerular capillary endotheliosis is the pathologic finding in the kidney of patients with preeclampsia. Necrotizing granulomatous vasculitis is characteristic of Wegener's granulomatosis or other vasculitic conditions. Congo red staining for amyloid is seen in primary and secondary forms of amyloidosis, which can typically cause the nephrotic syndrome.

21. The answer is C [Part I: XV E]. Preeclampsia is the toxemia of pregnancy; this syndrome includes hypertension, edema, and proteinuria. Eclampsia includes the preeclamptic spectrum of symptoms combined with associated maternal convulsions and coma. The primary pathologic renal feature is glomerular capillary endotheliosis. A positive ANA is a typical feature of systemic lupus erythematosus. Necrotizing granulomatous vasculitis is characteristic of Wegener's granulomatosis or other vasculitic conditions. Congo red staining for amyloid is seen in primary and secondary forms of amyloidosis, which can cause the nephrotic syndrome if there is kidney involvement.

22. The answer is D [Part I: X N 3]. Necrotizing granulomatous vasculitis (Wegener's granulomatosis) is characterized by upper or lower respiratory tract symptoms of necrotizing vasculitis and granulomatous inflammation. The kidneys are involved in approximately 50% of patients. Individually, the vasculitis and granulomatous inflammation are not specific for Wegener's granulomatosis; both must be histologically evident for diagnosis. The most recognizable presentation of the condition is the occurrence of necrotizing lesions. A positive ANA is a typical feature of systemic lupus erythematosus. Glomerular capillary endotheliosis is the pathologic finding in the kidney of patients with preeclampsia. Congo red staining for amyloid is seen in primary and secondary forms of amyloidosis, which can cause the nephrotic syndrome if there is kidney involvement.

23. The answer is E [Part I: X P 2]. One of the main associations of multiple myeloma is the development of primary amyloidosis with light-chain restriction. Congo red staining is rather specific for identifying amyloidosis. Primary (AL) or secondary (AA) forms of amyloidosis often affect the kidneys and typically cause the nephrotic syndrome with progressive renal insufficiency. A positive ANA is a typical feature of systemic lupus erythematosus. Glomerular capillary endotheliosis is the pathologic finding in the kidney of patients with preeclampsia. Necrotizing granulomatous vasculitis is characteristic of Wegener's granulomatosis or other vasculitic conditions.

chapter 7

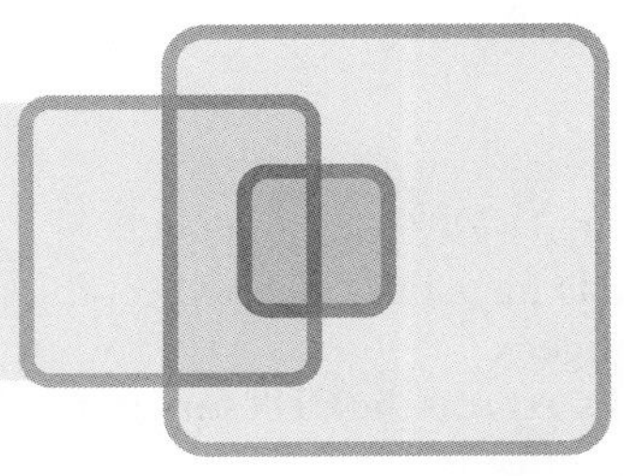

Allergic and Immunologic Disorders

DONALD P. GOLDSMITH, JACK M. BECKER

I OVERVIEW OF THE IMMUNE SYSTEM

Immune responses are generated by natural and adaptive mechanisms that consist of both cellular and humoral components.

A **Natural immunity** is nonspecific; that is, it is not influenced by previous antigen–antibody interactions.

1. **Phagocytic cells, including polymorphonuclear leukocytes (PMNs) [neutrophils and eosinophils], monocytes,** and **macrophages,** form the cellular component of the natural immune response. These cells ingest and destroy pathogenic organisms and other foreign material.
2. **Natural killer (NK) cells** are potent cytotoxic cells whose targets are not antigen-specific.
3. The **complement system,** a complex group of at least 15 serum proteins, mediates inflammatory reactions by attracting granulocytes and macrophages, promoting cell–cell interactions necessary for antigen processing, and stimulating the lysis of enveloped viruses and bacteria.

B **Adaptive immunity** is characterized by direct responses to initial antigen presentation and **memory (anamnestic)** responses on re-exposure.

1. **Humoral immunity** involves the production of **immunoglobulins by mature B lymphocytes.** Antigen binding to membrane-bound immunoglobulin triggers the differentiation of these B cells into mature plasma cells capable of secreting antigen-specific immunoglobulin.
   a. Immunoglobulins are vital to the immune response in three primary ways.
      (1) Immunoglobulins coat invading organisms, thereby impeding their access to the host.
      (2) Immunoglobulin M (IgM) and IgG fix complement (see I A 3).
      (3) Immunoglobulins promote opsonization, which increases the efficiency of phagocytosis.
   b. Immunoglobulins are divided into five classes, or **isotypes.**
      (1) **IgG,** the most prevalent serum immunoglobulin, is normally present at concentrations ranging from 800 to 1500 mg/dL. Four IgG subclasses—IgG1, IgG2, IgG3, and IgG4—have been identified. All subclasses penetrate easily into tissues.
      (2) **IgA** is the principal immunoglobulin in secretory fluids, making it the most important host defense antibody at sites of antigen entry. IgA exists as a dimer linked to an associated secretory component by a J chain. Normal serum levels range from 80 to 350 mg/dL.
      (3) **IgM** exists in serum as a cluster of five monomeric units linked by a J chain and disulfide bonds. It is the initial class of antibody produced as a primary response to antigens. Normal serum levels of IgM range from 40 to 160 mg/dL.
      (4) **IgD** and **IgE** are monomeric proteins present in serum in trace amounts. IgE is the antibody responsible for triggering the allergic reaction. (i.e., approximately 3–5 mg/dL of IgD and 0.05 mg/dL of IgE).

2. **Cellular immunity** is mediated by **T lymphocytes.**
   a. **Subpopulations of T cells** have been defined on the basis of function and the presence of characteristic surface antigens.
      (1) **Cytotoxic T (Tc) cells** express the CD8 surface marker and are responsible for killing cells that express foreign antigens.
      (2) **Helper T (Th) cells** enhance the activity of B cells, macrophages, and other T cells. They express the surface marker CD4.
      (3) **Suppressor T (Ts) cells** are also CD8 positive and inhibit the activity of other cells of the immune system.
   b. Various types of **antigen-presenting cells interact with T cells,** stimulating the release of **lymphokines,** including interleukins, granulocyte–macrophage colony-stimulating factor (GM-CSF), tumor necrosis factor (TNF), interferon-γ (IFN-γ), and other factors. These substances regulate various aspects of the immune response.

II PATHOGENESIS OF THE IgE-MEDIATED ALLERGIC REACTION

Antigen-stimulated release of mediators by cross-linking IgE molecules onto IgE-sensitized mast cells is an **IgE-mediated hypersensitivity reaction.** These reactions are the cause of many allergic disorders, including allergic rhinitis, urticaria, generalized anaphylaxis, insect sting sensitivity, and some drug reactions (see III–VII).

A The allergic response

A hallmark of the allergic diathesis is the tendency to maintain a persistent IgE response after antigen presentation. Initial exposure to antigen stimulates the production of specific IgE molecules, which bind to high-affinity Fc receptors on the surface of mast cells. On re-exposure, antigen cross-linking of these membrane-bound IgE molecules results in the release of vasoactive mediators and the subsequent clinical manifestations of the allergic response, which can include pruritus, sneezing, and bronchospasm.

1. **Fc receptors. Two types of IgE-binding Fc receptors** have been identified.
   a. **High-affinity receptors,** found on mast cells and basophils, bind avidly to IgE. Antigen bridging of IgE bound to these receptors triggers a rapid alteration of calcium and phospholipid metabolism, resulting in release of preformed mediators and the induction of additional, newly synthesized mediators.
   b. **Low-affinity receptors** are found on monocytes/macrophages, lymphocytes, eosinophils, and platelets. Although the function of these receptors is not completely understood, their presence on alveolar macrophages suggests that they play a role in the pathogenesis of allergic asthma.
2. **Mediators**
   a. **Preformed mediators** are synthesized before antigen contact and stored in mast cells and basophils. Examples of such mediators include:
      (1) Histamine
      (2) Heparin
      (3) Serotonin
      (4) Eosinophil chemotactic factor of anaphylaxis (ECF-A)
      (5) Neutrophil chemotactic factor of anaphylaxis (NCF-A)
      (6) Proteases
   b. **Newly synthesized mediators** include:
      (1) Platelet-activating factor (PAF)
      (2) Lipoxin
      (3) Leukotrienes (e.g., leukotrienes B4, C4, D4, and E4)
      (4) Prostaglandin D and thromboxane B_2

B Clinical implications of IgE levels Increased levels of IgE have been implicated in the etiology of allergy.

1. Infants with elevated IgE levels during the first year of life are more likely to develop allergic symptoms later in childhood than are infants with normal levels.
2. Between 60% and 70% of adults with allergic disorders have elevated IgE levels.
3. The presence of antigen-specific IgE in patients with chronic rhinitis and bronchial asthma suggests that these symptoms are associated with allergy.

C Regulation of IgE synthesis

1. **Differentiation of IgE-secreting B cells.** Bone marrow stem cells pass through a series of developmental steps to become mature B cells. **Induction of transcription** occurs during the last of these maturation phases, resulting in plasma cells capable of secreting the IgE isotype.
2. **T-cell involvement in IgE synthesis by B cells**
   a. **Th cells** enhance IgE synthesis, whereas **Ts cells** suppress synthesis. In normal individuals, the population of Ts cells is typically dominant, blunting the IgE-mediated response.
      (1) Primary immunodeficiency disorders (see VIII) are sometimes accompanied by elevated levels of serum IgE.
      (2) In such cases, the number of Th cells is sufficient to induce IgE synthesis, and the number of Ts cells is inadequate to suppress synthesis.
   b. The lymphokines **interleukin-4 (IL-4)** and **IFN-γ,** derived from Th cells, enhance and block IgE synthesis, respectively. An imbalance between IL-4 and IFN-γ may underlie elevated IgE levels in some patients.
3. **Genetic control of IgE modulation**
   a. The **development of IgE antibody to the ragweed antigen Ra5 is associated with a specific human leukocyte antigen (HLA), HLA-Dw2.**
   b. The **development of IgE antibody to rye grass pollen is associated with HLA-B8.**
4. **Anti-idiotypic antibodies** develop as a result of the heterogeneous composition of the variable domain of all immunoglobulins, including IgE. Because IgG anti-idiotypic antibodies inhibit certain antigen-specific IgE responses, a decrease in IgG antibodies leads to elevated IgE levels and an exaggerated IgE expression in some individuals.

D The late-phase reaction The IgE-mediated reaction often has a late-phase component, beginning 3–4 hours after the initial antigen challenge and resolving in 12–48 hours.

1. **Clinical implications.** The late-phase reaction sometimes contributes to the chronicity of allergic rhinitis, atopic dermatitis, and asthma.
2. **Pathogenesis**
   a. Histologically, lesions of the late-phase reaction have greater numbers of mononuclear cells bearing low-affinity IgE receptors. The inflammatory phase is the late response. The bronchoconstrictive phase, is the early response, for example, in an asthmatic patient.
   b. The release of a number of chemical mediators (i.e., chemotactic factors, histamine-releasing factors) is pivotal to the pathogenesis of the late-phase reaction.

III ALLERGIC RHINITIS

A Definition This inflammatory disorder of the nasal mucosa is characterized by nasal blockage, rhinorrhea, sneezing, and pruritus. It is initiated by mast-cell mediators released during the IgE-mediated hypersensitivity reaction. There are two major classifications of allergic rhinitis.

1. **Seasonal allergic rhinitis** has periodic symptoms that occur only during the pollinating season of the antigen to which the patient is sensitive.
2. **Perennial allergic rhinitis** has continuous or intermittent symptoms that occur year round.

B **Incidence** Although accurate estimates are difficult to obtain, it is believed that 10%–30% of adults and up to 40% of children have allergic rhinitis, making this the most common chronic disorder of the respiratory tract. There is no apparent male or female predilection for allergic rhinitis, and no ethnic or racial patterns have been identified. Symptoms may begin at any age but develop in most patients before age 20 years. A history of allergic disorders in the immediate family is common.

C **Etiology** Various aeroallergens (e.g., spores, pollens, organic dusts) trigger the IgE-mediated hypersensitivity reaction that underlies allergic rhinitis.

1. **Common characteristics of aeroallergens**
   a. Aeroallergens usually are smaller than 50 μm.
   b. The allergens are lightweight and therefore easily wind-borne. (Heavier, insect-borne pollens do not cause allergic rhinitis.)
   c. The allergens are released into the environment in large numbers.
   d. The allergenic constituents usually are proteins with molecular weights of 10,000–40,000 daltons.
   e. Seasonal patterns for each pollen are consistent from year to year, but quantities of pollen vary depending on environmental conditions. The type and presence of a pollen is dictated by that specific climate.
2. **Specific seasonal allergens**
   a. **Ragweed pollen** is the most significant cause of allergic rhinitis in the midwestern and eastern United States. Its season usually runs from late summer to early fall (mid-August to early October) in the northeastern United States.
   b. **Tree pollens** elicit symptoms in early spring in the northeastern United States.
   c. **Grass pollens** are the major offenders in late spring and early summer in the northeastern United States. Because roses are fully blooming in late spring, sensitivity to grass pollen often is mistakenly called "rose fever." In the southeastern and southwestern United States, grass pollinates from early spring to late fall and may lead to nearly perennial symptoms.
   d. **Mold spores** initially appear in the early spring, reach peak levels in July and August, and subside after the first frost in the northeastern United States. In the United States, the clinically most important spores are *Alternaria* and *Cladosporium*. The highest mold spore counts occur when a windy period follows a few days of rainy and damp weather.
3. **Specific perennial allergens**
   a. **Dust mites** live primarily in bedding and feed on desquemated skin. They are a significant cause of chronic symptoms.
   b. **Epidermal antigens** are produced primarily by pets such as cats, dogs, and rabbits.
   c. **Indoor molds** (i.e., spores found in homes) include *Aspergillus* and *Penicillium*.
   d. **Nonspecific irritants,** which are not true allergens, include cigarette smoke, air pollution, perfumes, cooking odors, and chemical fumes.
   e. **Occupational allergens** include platinum salts, wood dust, and laundry detergent enzymes, all of which are known to produce both allergic rhinitis and asthma in association with IgE antibodies.
   f. **Other allergens** include cockroach skin casts, which are also considered to be important antigens, particularly in economically depressed areas.

D **Clinical features**

1. **Characteristic symptoms**
   a. **Sneezing**—often with paroxysms of 15–20 sneezes in quick succession—is characteristic and likely to occur in the early morning hours.
   b. **Pruritus** of the nose, palate, and pharynx is common and may lead to the "allergic salute" (repeated pushing up on the end of the nose), which, in turn, often results in a transverse nasal crease.

c. **A thin, watery nasal discharge** usually is present and is associated with varying amounts of nasal obstruction and postnasal drainage. Mouth breathing is common.
d. **Excess lacrimation** and ocular pruritus and soreness are common.
e. **Loss of olfaction and taste** may result from chronic severe nasal congestion.
f. **Otitis media,** resulting from impaired drainage of the eustachian tube, and **sinusitis,** resulting from impaired drainage of the paranasal sinuses, sometimes occur.

2. **Characteristic physical findings** usually are seen at the time of maximal exposure to the offending antigens (e.g., during the height of the pollen season).
   a. **Nasal findings**
      (1) The nasal cavity characteristically contains thin nasal secretions, and the mucosal surface is edematous, boggy, and usually pale or bluish.
      (2) Nasal polyps may be seen but are not common in allergic rhinitis. Their presence usually suggests cystic fibrosis in children and aspirin intolerance in adults.
      (3) Evidence of recent epistaxis in the anterior nasal vault may be seen if a patient's nasal congestion has led to frequent nose-rubbing.
   b. **Conjunctival findings** include injection and swelling, excess lacrimation, granularity, and, occasionally, chemosis. Infraorbital "shiners" (infraorbital venous congestion) may develop.
   c. **Oropharyngeal findings include mucus streaming down the posterior pharynx and cobblestoning of the lymphoid tissue of the same area.**
   c. **Possible findings in children who have severe chronic nasal congestion** include broadened bony dorsum of the nose, narrowed palatal arch, halitosis, retrognathic facies, excess gingival and pharyngeal lymphoid tissue, and dental abnormalities.

E Evaluation

1. **Diagnostic tests**
   a. Accurately applied **skin tests** with potent and specific antigens are the best diagnostic procedures to identify the antigens causing IgE-mediated allergic rhinitis.
   b. The **radioallergosorbent test (RAST)** is an alternative to skin testing and can be ordered by any practitioner. Its sensitivity and specificity have improved dramatically, and for many allergens it is as accurate as skin tests. It is routinely used for patients with extensive eczematoid dermatitis, significant dermatographism, or a complicated history without corroborative skin tests. IgG-blocking antibodies and high total IgE levels may interfere with the RAST.
   c. An **elevated IgE level** is present in only 30%–40% of patients with allergic rhinitis. Clinicians also must consider other possible causes of elevated IgE levels such as immunodeficiency disorders (see VIII). Total serum IgE should not be routinely used in the diagnosis of allergic rhinitis.
   d. **Peripheral eosinophilia** may be seen but is an **inconsistent** finding in patients with allergic rhinitis.
   e. A **stained smear of nasal secretions** at the time of clinically active disease often shows a higher number of eosinophils, but this finding also may be seen in patients with eosinophilic nonallergic rhinitis (see III E 2 d) or hyperplastic sinusitis, as well as in normal infants younger than 6 months of age.
   f. **Fiberoptic rhinoscopy** may be indicated for unilateral nasal blockage, particularly when such blockage is unresponsive to usual medical therapy. This test is routinely performed in office practices.
   g. Selected patients whose skin test and RAST results are negative may benefit from **conjunctival and nasal mucosal challenges** with selected antigens, histamine, or methacholine. Changes in resistance to air flow is measured by the well-standardized technique of rhinomanometry. These types of challenges are not routinely done.
   h. Cytotoxicity testing, provocation–neutralization tests, and measurement of specific or nonspecific IgG4 levels are all unproven and inappropriate tests to use in the diagnosis of allergic rhinitis.

2. **Differential diagnosis**
   a. Nasal congestion with mild rhinorrhea sometimes is seen in **pregnant women** and in patients with **hypothyroidism.**
   b. Abuse of decongestant nasal spray and use of birth control pills, prazosin, thioridazine, perphenazine, propranolol, clonidine, and reserpine are associated with nasal blockage.
   c. **Vasomotor rhinitis** is a syndrome characterized by nasal blockage and rhinorrhea without evidence of immunologic or infectious nasal disease. Increased parasympathetic activity of the nasal mucosa is present. The condition is exacerbated by changes in body or environmental temperature, relatively high humidity, emotional stress, chemical fumes, tobacco smoke, and alteration of body position. Response to medical therapy often is poor.
   d. Symptoms of **eosinophilic nonallergic rhinitis** are similar to those of vasomotor rhinitis; however, in eosinophilic nonallergic rhinitis, nasal eosinophilia is present, nasal polyps are common, and symptoms usually respond to medical management.
   e. **Infectious rhinitis** often occurs in patients with underlying allergic rhinitis and usually is associated with reddened nasal mucosa, thick nasal secretions, sore throat, cervical adenopathy, and low-grade fever. Chronic infectious rhinitis also may occur with bronchiectasis and situs inversus as Kartagener's syndrome [ciliary dysfunction syndrome (CDS)].
   f. A symptom complex known as the **aspirin triad** consists of nasal polyps, chronic sinus disease, and potentially life-threatening asthma, with exacerbation of symptoms after administration of aspirin or other nonsteroidal anti-inflammatory drugs (NSAIDs).
   g. **Anatomic abnormalities,** the most common of which is a partially deviated septum, may cause nasal obstruction. This should be recognizable during routine nasal examination, but sometimes fiberoptic rhinoscopy is needed. When unilateral discharge with a foul odor is present, obstruction by a foreign body should be suspected. Nasal tumors or systemic disorders such as Wegener's granulomatosis and relapsing polychondritis, although rare, may cause nasal blockage.
   h. **Atrophic rhinitis** is seen in older patients and is often secondary to trauma, specific infection, granuloma, or surgery. Mucosal secretions are minimal as a result of unciliated epithelial cells and a decrease in columnar epithelial cells. Anosmia, nasal crusting, and paradoxical symptoms of nasal blockage are characteristic.

F Therapy Management is stepwise and involves avoidance of any offending allergens and provocative substances, administration of selective pharmacologic agents, and, in some instances, initiation of immunotherapy.

1. **Avoidance.** This aspect of management is most successful when a single antigen (e.g., animal dander) is responsible for symptoms. In patients with multiple sensitivities, sensible environmental precautions are recommended and appear to limit severe exacerbation of symptoms.
2. **Environmental measures.** Nonspecific irritants such as cold dry air, paint fumes, and tobacco smoke may contribute to symptoms. Air conditioners reduce indoor mold and pollen counts but must be properly maintained to avoid contamination by molds. Home air purifiers also may be helpful, but the benefits are unproven. Home humidifiers may spew mold into the air if not properly cleaned.
3. **Pharmacologic agents**
   a. **H_1-receptor antagonists** (i.e., **antihistamines**) are useful in controlling rhinorrhea and pruritus but have little clinical effect on nasal congestion. Sedation with impaired school or job performance are undesirable side effects of first-generation H_1-receptor antagonists. Because second-generation antihistamines are not associated with these side effects, they are usually considered first as treatment for allergic rhinitis. Terfenadine, the oldest nonsedating antihistamine, and later astemizole were withdrawn from the market in the United States because prolongation of the Q-T interval may occur, which may lead to the ventricular arrhythmia torsade de pointes.

(1) **First-generation H_1-receptor antagonists**

(a) Ethanolamines (e.g., diphenhydramine) are effective but often produce significant sedation and atropine-like side effects.

(b) Ethylenediamines (e.g., pyrilamine) also are effective, produce less sedation than ethanolamines, and have minimal gastrointestinal side effects.

(c) Alkylamines (e.g., chlorpheniramine) are effective and produce minimal to modest sedation.

(2) **Second-generation H_1-receptor antagonists**

(a) Loratadine, desloratadine, cetirizine, and fexofenadine are administered once daily; they have not been associated with adverse cardiovascular effects.

(b) All second-generation H_1 receptor antagonists lack anticholinergic side effects but may produce mild sedation if given at higher-than-usual doses. Cetirizine will produce sedation in some patients at recommended dosages.

(3) **Intranasal H_1-receptor antagonists.** Azelastine hydrochloride, which is approved for use in the United States, has an efficacy equal to that of oral H_1- and H_2-receptor antagonists. It also may reduce nasal blockage. Twenty percent of patients perceive a bitter taste.

b. **Adrenergic agonists** (also known as **sympathomimetic medications**)

(1) **Oral administration** of α-adrenergic agent (e.g., pseudoephedrine) is effective in reducing nasal congestion but not rhinorrhea. Central nervous system (CNS) stimulation may occur, as well as hypertension and loss of appetite. Short-term use is preferable (<10 days).

(2) **Topical application** of short-acting phenylephrine or long-acting oxymetazoline decreases nasal congestion, but regular administration for more than 3–4 days results in severe rebound nasal congestion (rhinitis medicamentosa).

c. **Cromolyn sodium.** A 4% solution of cromolyn sodium is available for topical nasal use. It must be administered frequently (3–6 times daily) but is effective in treating both seasonal and perennial allergic rhinitis. Because side effects are minimal, cromolyn sodium may at times be preferred to topical nasal steroids, but it is less effective. Pretreatment before allergen exposure may significantly reduce nasal allergic response.

d. **Corticosteroids**

(1) **Systemic agents.** Systemic corticosteroids significantly improve symptoms during the height of a specific pollen season. This treatment is rarely indicated, however, and use of long-term oral corticosteroid therapy for perennial allergic rhinitis is ill-advised because of the deleterious side effects.

(2) **Topical agents.** Highly effective and rapidly metabolized topical steroid preparations (e.g., mometasone furoate monohydrate, budesonide, flunisolide acetate, triamcinolone acetonide, fluticasone propionate) are beneficial in the treatment of seasonal and perennial allergic rhinitis. This class of medications are considered the treatment of choice. In addition, they are useful during withdrawal of topical adrenergic agonists in patients with severe rhinitis medicamentosa. These preparations have minimal systemic side effects; irritation and bleeding rarely occur, and *Candida* overgrowth is very uncommon. No association between these agents and the development of posterior subcapsular cataracts has been demonstrated.

e. **Intranasal anticholinergics.** Ipratropium bromide nasal spray (0.03% and 0.06%) is available for topical use. Rhinorrhea but not other nasal symptoms are effectively reduced. Side effects, although minimal (5%), include dryness and transient epistaxis.

f. **Oral antileukotriene agents.** Data suggest that these medications may be helpful as first-line agents and montelukast sodium has been approved for this indication. Further studies are needed to define the role of these agents in the treatment of allergic rhinitis.

4. **Immunotherapy.** Such treatment may be indicated if patients continue to experience clinically significant symptoms after appropriate environmental avoidance, and pharmacologic measures

have been taken. Although treatment is time consuming and does not provide complete relief for all patients, increased costs of other medications makes immunotherapy relatively cost-effective.

IV URTICARIA AND ANGIOEDEMA

A Definitions

1. **Urticaria** (commonly known as **hives**) is a pruritic and transient skin eruption, with individual lesions presenting as erythematous circumscribed papules, or wheals, often with white edematous centers. Lesions are annular, round, figurate, or confluent. Repeated scratching often results in dermatographism.
2. **Angioedema** may occur alone or jointly with urticaria. Compared with urticarial lesions, angioedema lesions are less pruritic, of longer duration, and found in deeper subcutaneous tissue—particularly in loose areas around the mouth, eyelids, and male genitalia. Angioedema in the submucosa of the upper respiratory tract may lead to laryngeal obstruction, and its occurrence in the gastrointestinal tract may result in abdominal pain with diarrhea.

B Pathophysiology

1. **Histamine** is a primary mediator, causing dilatation of superficial cutaneous and mucosal venules, increased vascular permeability, and stimulation of cutaneous type C sensory neurons that release neuropeptides such as **substance P.** The release of histamine from mast cells and basophils may be stimulated by IgE-related mechanisms, by direct cell activation, or by components of the complement cascade known as **anaphylatoxins** (e.g., C3a, C4a, C5a). C5a also attracts mononuclear cells and neutrophils to the skin.
2. **PAF, prostaglandins,** and leukotrienes evoke histamine-like vascular changes.
3. **Chemotactic factors affecting mononuclear cells, neutrophils, and platelets** are released by activated mast cells and basophils.
4. **GM-CSF** and **IL-3** stimulate basophil histamine release.

C Clinical syndromes according to etiology

1. **Idiopathic urticaria.** In most cases of urticaria lasting several months, no specific cause can be identified, although viral triggers are commonly suspected. This type of urticaria thus is known as **chronic idiopathic urticaria;** it is most common in women 30–50 years of age.
   a. Histologic studies show perivascular infiltrates of the small blood vessels of the skin with no disturbance of vessel integrity. Neither immune complexes nor complement deposition is present, but the infiltrate contains large numbers of both mononuclear cells and hyperreleasable mast cells.
   b. The incidence of chronic idiopathic urticaria is not increased in individuals who have an underlying allergic disorder.
   c. Chronic urticaria also may be attributed to complement disorders, systemic illness, or physical stimuli (see IV C 3–5).
2. **IgE-mediated urticaria.** Many cases of **acute urticaria** can be attributed to an IgE-mediated reaction. The most common antigens eliciting this response are **foods, latex, drugs,** and **venoms.** Inhaled pollen may induce acute urticarial lesions in very sensitive individuals. Pollen exposure on the skin also may induce urticarial-type lesions
   a. Histologic studies of the initial reaction show **partial detachment of the collagen bundles** because of both fluid accumulation and dilatation of small blood vessels. In some individuals, a **late-phase response** characterized by a mixed cellular infiltrate occurs 48 hours after the initial response. This response can occur only if there has been a previous IgE-mediated response (see II A).

b. The incidence of acute urticaria is increased in individuals with an underlying allergic disorder.

c. Acute urticaria also may be brought on by a systemic illness or physical stimuli (see IV C 4–5).

3. **Complement-related disorders,** although rare, are well recognized. **Two major syndromes** exist.

   a. **Disorders associated with complement pathway activation.** Connective tissue disorders such as systemic lupus erythematosus (SLE), hypocomplemententemic vasculitis, and serum sickness caused by drugs or blood products are sometimes associated with **chronic urticaria or angioedema.** In these disorders of the complement system, complement levels are often decreased but they also may be normal.

   b. **A deficiency in the inhibitor of the complement component C1 (C1-INH)** may be hereditary (e.g., in **hereditary angioedema**), idiopathic, or associated with underlying disorders such as SLE or B-cell lymphomas.

      (1) **Genetics.** The inherited form is autosomal dominant, with 85% of patients exhibiting impaired synthesis of C1-INH and the remaining 15% exhibiting functionally inactive C1-INH.

      (2) **Diagnosis.** C1q levels are normal in hereditary C1-INH deficiency and decreased in the acquired forms. In both forms, a depressed C4 level during asymptomatic and symptomatic periods is characteristic, and the diagnosis usually is secured by documenting a quantitative or functional deficiency of C1-INH. Because this disorder is both life-threatening and treatable, recognition is vital.

4. **Systemic diseases.** Urticaria or angioedema sometimes may be the initial sign or a sequela of an underlying systemic illness.

   a. **Acute infectious diseases** in children such as viral upper respiratory infection or streptococcal pharyngitis may be associated with acute urticaria. Rare causes of chronic urticaria in both adults and children are mycobacterial infection, chronic sinusitis, dental abscess, chronic tinea pedis, and helminthic infection.

   b. **Systemic inflammatory disorders** such as SLE, inflammatory bowel disease, hepatitis B (HBV) and hepatitis C (HCV), macroglobulinemia, and the early phase of either hepatitis A (HAV) or infectious mononucleosis may be associated with urticaria. Leukocytoclastic vasculitis of the skin may take the clinical form of urticaria with associated fever and arthralgia. In such cases, C1q-containing circulating immune complexes are present, and, in some cases, even hematologic malignancies.

   c. **Thyroid disorders** (with or without hypothyroidism) are sometimes associated with persistent intractable urticaria. There is a marked female predilection for this condition, and antithyroid antibodies are commonly seen in affected patients.

5. **Physical urticaria and angioedemas** are induced by a physical stimulus such as temperature, sunlight, or physical pressure. Although the pathogenic mechanism for most of these conditions is unknown, some are clearly IgE-dependent. Features of the physical urticarias and angioedemas are described in Table 7–1.

D Therapy

1. **Prevention of further episodes** involves avoidance of known evocative agents (e.g., foods, medications, and physical factors) and identification and management of underlying medical disorders.

2. **Treatment of existing episodes** usually is stepwise, depending on the presumed pathogenic mechanism.

   a. **H_1-receptor blockers** alone often are effective. Cyproheptadine appears to be useful in treating cold-induced urticaria, hydroxyzine in cholinergic urticaria, and diphenhydramine in solar urticaria. Loratadine, desloratadine, cetirizine, and fexofenadine, all second-generation antihistamines, are also effective.

TABLE 7–1 Physical Urticarias and Angioedemas

Type	Stimulus	Clinical Features	Diagnostic Test
Dermatographism	Stroking the skin	Exaggerated triple response of Lewis (wheal, flare, and edema), with occasional passive transfer to normal skin; possible immediate-pressure angioedema; may follow emotional stress or infection	Stroking the skin
Delayed pressure angioedema	Sustained heavy pressure	Deep, erythematous swelling typically affecting the hands or feet; disability secondary to discomfort	Application of pressure using inert weights
Cholinergic urticaria	Increase in core body temperature (e.g., fever, exercise, heat exposure, stress)	Intensely pruritic truncal 1- to 3-mm wheals, sometimes accompanied by excessive sweating, lacrimation, salivation, and abdominal cramping	Methacholine skin test; exercise challenge
Cold urticaria (idiopathic or inherited)	Sudden exposure to cold	Localized pruritus, erythema, and swelling in idiopathic form; papular lesions accompanied by chills, arthralgia, myalgia, and headache in inherited form; possible life-threatening edema of upper or lower respiratory tract	Ice cube challenge
Vibratory angioedema (hereditary or acquired)	Prolonged occupational exposure to vibration	Severe pruritus	Application of laboratory vortex to forearm
Solar urticaria (six types, based on wavelength triggering the reaction)	Exposure to sun or UV light	Progressive excoriation and lichenification of affected areas; possible presence of other metabolic or immunologic disorders (i.e., erythropoietic protoporphyria and SLE)	Exposure to specific UV wavelength
Aquagenic urticaria	Exposure to water	Pruritus sometimes accompanied by small wheals resembling those of cholinergic urticaria	Application of water compresses of varying temperatures

SLE = systemic lupus erythematosus; UV = ultraviolet.

b. **Adding an H_2-receptor blocker** such as cimetidine often has a synergistic effect, because H_2 receptors make up approximately 15% of the histamine receptors in cutaneous blood vessels. H_2-receptor blockers alone are not effective. Doxepin, which blocks both H_1 and H_2 receptors, is sometimes useful in treating refractory urticaria.
c. **Systemic steroids** are reserved for severe cases, with an alternate-day dosing regimen preferred. A skin biopsy is suggested before maintenance steroid therapy is started.
d. **Limited androgens** such as danazol are effective in treating C1-INH deficiency and some cases of steroid-responsive chronic idiopathic urticaria.
e. **Various other medications** such as sulfasalazine, hydroxychloroquine, and dapsone also may be useful, primarily for their corticosteroid-sparing effects.

V GENERALIZED ANAPHYLAXIS

A Definition Anaphylaxis is an acute life-threatening hypersensitivity syndrome. It affects multiple organ systems and results from the precipitous and massive release of mediators from both mast cells and basophils. Symptoms usually begin within minutes of exposure to the causative factor and peak within 1 hour, but can take up to 4 hours for the most severe symptoms.

B Incidence Exact incidence rates are unknown. In Ontario, fatal anaphylaxis from any cause is estimated at 0.4 cases per 1 million population per year. One of every 2700 hospitalized patients in the United States experiences some anaphylactic symptoms. There are approximately 30,000 episodes with 150 deaths in the U.S. each year.

C Etiology A variety of mechanisms, summarized in Table 7–2, can initiate anaphylactic mediator release.

1. **IgE-mediated release.** The binding of IgE antibodies either to complete antigens (e.g., insulin) or to antigenic determinants on hapten–carrier complexes (e.g., the penicilloic acid moiety of penicillin coupled to serum albumin) often precipitates the release of mediators.

TABLE 7–2 Etiologic Mechanisms of Anaphylaxis

Mechanism	Typical Allergens
IgE-mediated mediator release	Drugs
	Sulfonamides
	Tetracyclines
	Penicillins
	Cephalosporins
	Local anesthetics
	Insect venoms
	Allergen extracts
	Chymopapain
	Streptokinase
	Insulin
	Food
	Shellfish
	Nuts
	Eggs
	Milk
	Any food can cause a reaction
Direct mast cell mediator release	Drugs
	Polymyxin B
	Opiates
	Vancomycin
	Radiocontrast media
Anaphylatoxin-induced mediator release (via complement activation)	Human blood products
	Plasma
	Immunoglubulins
	Cryoprecipitates
Other mechanisms	Nonsteroidal anti-inflammatory agents
	Sulfite additives
	Exercise
	Hormones

2. **Non–IgE-mediated release.** Certain substances [e.g., opiate analgesics, radiocontrast media, NSAID (aspirin)] can stimulate degranulation of effector cells directly. This is called an anaphylactoid reaction.

3. **Anaphylatoxin-mediated release.** Significant complement activation generates large amounts of the complement degradation products C3a and C5a. These fragments bind to mast-cell receptors, triggering mediator release.

4. **Other mechanisms.** Other recurrent clinical syndromes have varying etiologies.
   a. **Exercise-induced anaphylaxis:** An anaphylactic reaction that occurs during exercise. This usually occurs after the athlete has ingested some food. The most common foods are carrots, celery, or lettuce, but any food can cause the reaction. The athlete can exercise without having a reaction as well as eat the food without a reaction; only when they are combined does a reaction occur.
   b. **Hormonally related anaphylaxis.** In women of childbearing age, the recurrence of mild-to-severe anaphylactic symptoms that occur during the premenstrual period suggests hormonal triggers. In such women, anaphylaxis also may be provoked by skin tests with progesterone or by infusions of releasing hormones, which induce ovarian secretion.
   c. **Seminal fluid–induced anaphylaxis.** Anaphylaxis caused by coital exposure to seminal fluid is mediated by IgE antibodies to specific seminal proteins. This is an extremely rare reaction.
   d. **Latex-induced anaphylaxis.** This is a reaction that occurs in latex-allergic patients when they are exposed. This exposure can be aerosolized, injected, or through skin contact. The first reactions occurred in patients receiving barium enemas, and later in patients with intravenous tubing sets. Currently, all infusion sets are latex free. Patients with spina bifida as well as health care workers have a higher incidence.

D Clinical features The clinical presentation typically involves multiple organ systems, as summarized in Table 7–3. Physiologic sequelae of mediator release include enhanced permeability of capillaries and postcapillary venules and decreased arteriolar tone. The severity of symptoms is increased in individuals who have a history of asthma.

E Diagnosis Clinical and laboratory findings characteristic of extensive mediator release are the basis for diagnosis.

1. **Essential diagnostic findings** include at least two of the following symptoms:
   a. Bronchial obstruction
   b. Upper airway obstruction
   c. Acute hypotension
   d. Urticaria
   e. Vomiting or diarrhea
2. **Additional findings** that support the diagnosis include:
   a. Characteristic allergic signs and symptoms involving organ systems other than those listed in Table 7–3
   b. Recent exposure to known allergens
   c. Absence of other medical disorders with similar clinical presentations, such as myocardial infarction (MI), vasovagal syncope, arrhythmias, hypovolemic shock, pulmonary embolism, airway obstruction due to a foreign body, and panic disorder
   d. Elevated levels of serum tryptase, as well as urinary histamine and its metabolites. Serum tryptase can be routinely obtained and is used to confirm the diagnosis of anaphylaxis. However, some patients with anaphylaxis will not have detectable levels.
3. **Risk factors** play a role. Individuals with underlying bronchial asthma, ischemic heart disease, or congestive heart failure (CHF) are more likely to suffer severe or fatal anaphylactic reactions.

TABLE 7–3 Signs and Symptoms of Anaphylaxis

Organ or Organ System Affected (% Individuals Involved)	Characteristic Signs and Symptoms
Skin (88%)	Pruritus
	Flushing
	Urticaria
	Angioedema
Eyes (16%)	Ocular pruritus
	Excess lacrimation
	Conjunctival injection
Respiratory system	Nasal congestion
Upper airway edema (56%)	Rhinorrhea
Dyspnea and wheezing (47%)	Cough
	Hoarseness
	Stridor
	Wheezing
	Laryngeal edema
Cardiovascular system (33%)	Weakness
	Palpitations
	Tachycardia
	Hypotension
	Arrhythmias
	Shock
	Cardiac arrest
Gastrointestinal system (30%)	Cramping
	Nausea
	Diarrhea
	Vomiting
	Abdominal distention
	Metallic taste

F Therapy Effective management starts with knowing the duration of the present reaction, the existence of any underlying medical conditions, and the medication currently being taken by the patient.

1. **Specific treatment measures. These should only be performed either after pharmocologic therapy or if pharmocologic therapy is not available.**
   a. Placement in a recumbent position, with legs elevated and neck extended
   b. If possible, elimination of the causative factor or delay of its absorption (e.g., removing an insect stinger or applying a tourniquet between the heart and the site of a precipitating drug injection)
   c. Maintenance of body temperature
   d. Administration of supplemental oxygen
   e. Use of an oropharyngeal airway, tracheal intubation, or cricothyrotomy if necessary to ensure maintenance of a patent airway
2. **Pharmacologic therapy**
   a. **Aqueous epinephrine.** This is the most effective therapy and should given whenever anaphylaxis is considered as a diagnosis. 1:1000 (wt/vol) [0.3–0.5 mL administered subcutaneously] should be repeated every 20–30 minutes as needed. If anaphylaxis is due to an injection, 0.15–0.30 mL placed directly into the injection site limits further absorption of the injected substance. In addition, nebulized epinephrine can be used to assist in airway maintenance.
   b. **Diphenhydramine** (25–50 mg) can be administered orally or by slow intravenous infusion over 5 minutes. Intramuscular injections are no longer recommended. Any antihistamine can

be used. This therapy will not stop an anaphylaxic reaction but is used as adjunctive therapy to epinephrine.

c. **Corticosteroids** (1–2 mg/kg) are administered intravenously. Corticosteroids are used to decrease the later inflammatory response.

d. **Intravenous fluids, volume expanders,** and **pressor agents** are used to maintain blood pressure.

e. Persistent bronchospasm is usually treated with nebulized **β_2-adrenergic agonists.** This can be given continuously by a nebulizer system.

f. Prolonged or biphasic anaphylaxis may be treated by continued cautious administration of **subcutaneous epinephrine** and **intravenous corticosteroids** every 6 hours.

VI INSECT STING SENSITIVITY

Stings by insects of the Hymenoptera order (e.g., **honeybee, yellow jacket, wasp, white-faced and bald-faced hornet**), imported fire ant, and reduvid bug may lead to sensitization and subsequent IgE-mediated hypersensitivity reactions.

A Incidence

Population studies show that up to 25% of people with no history of a systemic reaction after a hymenoptera sting nonetheless may be sensitive, as judged by positive skin tests and the presence of venom-specific IgE antibodies. As many as 20% of these individuals may have a systemic allergic reaction if restung. It is estimated that 75–100 deaths occur in the United States each year from insect sting reactions, with most fatalities occurring in people older than age 40 years.

B Clinical features

A nonallergic reaction to an insect sting consists of transient swelling, pain, and redness surrounding the injection site, all of which usually subside in 1–2 hours but can last up to 48 hours. Allergic reactions vary from scattered patches of urticaria to severe and fatal anaphylaxis.

1. **Large local reactions** extend a significant distance from the sting site (≥ 8 cm), peak in 24 hours, and often take 5–7 days to resolve.
2. **Anaphylactic reactions** may involve the skin (localized or generalized urticaria, angioedema, and generalized pruritus), the respiratory tract (laryngeal edema and bronchospasm), the vascular system (hypotension), and the gastrointestinal system (diarrhea, cramping pain, and nausea). The reaction pattern for repeat stings is often similar. Symptoms usually start within a few minutes of the sting.
3. **Delayed reactions** include serum sickness, vasculitis, Guillain-Barré syndrome, glomerulonephritis, or myocarditis. The etiology of these reactions is unclear.

C Diagnosis

1. An accurate **history** of the symptoms and signs of a systemic allergic reaction after a sting is necessary. Vasovagal reactions often imitate allergic responses; thus physicians must use all available resources to substantiate the clinical findings (e.g., records of the emergency department visit,and or serum tryptase level). Children younger than 16 years of age whose reaction is limited to urticaria are not considered to have had an anaphylactic reaction.
2. **Specific antivenom IgE antibodies** are detected by prick or intradermal tests. Testing should be done for all types of Hymenoptera, for it is extremely difficult for the patient to accurately identify the type of insect that stung them. When skin test results are negative, a specific serum IgE–level RAST is indicated.

D Therapy

1. **Immediate therapeutic measures** are similar to those used in the treatment of anaphylaxis from any cause (see V F).

2. **Prophylactic therapy**
   a. When outside, at-risk individuals should observe **common-sense measures** such as wearing shoes, not wearing heavy perfumes or brightly colored clothes, and staying away from outdoor refuse containers.
   b. All at-risk individuals should own and know how to use an **epinephrine home injection kit.**
   c. Individuals who have had an anaphylatic reaction need to undergo **specific venom immunotherapy. This therapy will allow the patient to decrease their risk down to that of the general population.**
      (1) Immunotherapy often can be stopped after 3–5 years. This has been shown to be the duration needed to effectively desenitize a patient. This therapy will decrease their risk of ananphylaxis down to that of the general population, approximately 1%. Only in those patients in whom anaphylaxis would almost invariably be fatal, i.e., the patient with severe cardiac disease, is immunotherapy continued beyond 5 years.

VII DRUG REACTIONS

A Definitions Adverse drug reactions can be classified as **predictable** or **unpredictable,** with the former accounting for approximately 75% of all untoward effects. Unpredictable responses include **hypersensitivity,** or **allergic,** reactions, which constitute 7%–10% of all adverse reactions.

1. **Type A or predictable responses** most often involve known pharmacologic actions, are dose-dependent, and occur in normal individuals. Examples include overdose, side effects, and secondary effects of a drug, as well as undesirable effects resulting from the interaction of two or more drugs (i.e., cross-reactions, diuretic effect of caffeine, dyspepsia from erythromycin.).
2. **Type B or unpredictable responses** tend to occur in predisposed populations (e.g., on a hereditary basis, as in the association of the HLA-DR2 and DR3 loci with gold-induced nephritis), are not related to the expected pharmacologic action, and are most often independent of dose. Three types of responses have been characterized.
   a. **Intolerance** refers to an adverse reaction that occurs at a subtherapeutic dose (e.g., vomiting at low doses of theophylline).
   b. **Idiosyncrasy** is an unexpected and qualitatively abnormal response to a medication that is unrelated to the drug's known pharmacologic action (e.g., isoniazid-induced neuritis). Idiosyncratic reactions may occur on a hereditary basis [e.g., hemolytic anemia precipitated by quinolines in a patient with glucose-6-phosphate dehydrogenase (G6PD) deficiency].
   c. **Hypersensitivity** results from an immunologic reaction that triggers an abnormal response unrelated to an expected pharmacologic action of the drug (e.g., penicillin-induced urticaria). Drug hypersensitivity reactions usually are categorized according to etiology, using the Gell and Coombs classification system.
      (1) **IgE-mediated reactions** occur when a pharmacologic agent or one of its metabolites binds with drug-specific IgE antibodies on mast cell or basophil membranes. Initial exposure triggers sensitization and the creation of the IgE antibody that then resides on the mast cell. Subsequent exposure to the same drug promotes the cross-linking of the mast cell–bound IgE-specific antibody, which then triggers the mast cell to release mediators, which contribute to the development of urticaria and angioedema, both of which occasionally progress to anaphylaxis.
      (2) **Cytotoxic reactions** result from complement-mediated damage to cell membranes precipitated by the binding of IgM or IgG antibodies to drug antigens on cell surfaces. These reactions usually involve blood cells (e.g., drug-induced thrombocytopenia and hemolytic anemia).
      (3) **Immune complex–mediated reactions** develop when soluble complexes of IgM or IgG antibodies and drug antigen are deposited in tissues. Complement activation occurs in

the soluble phase or when the complex attaches to vessel walls, leading to inflammation and subsequent tissue injury. **Rash** (urticaria or palpable purpura) and **fever** are the most common clinical manifestations of immune complex–mediated reactions, followed by **lymphadenopathy** and **arthralgia** (as can be seen in serum sickness syndrome caused by heterologous serum, sulfonamides, penicillin, hydantoin, any drug, or virus).

(4) **Cell-mediated reactions** require sensitized T lymphocytes that recognize a drug or its metabolite. The antigen–T-cell interaction leads to a lymphokine-induced inflammatory response occurring 24–72 hours after drug administration. **Contact dermatitis** is the most common clinical example of a cell-mediated reaction. Drugs such as topical neomycin penetrate the skin, bind to carrier proteins, and migrate to regional lymph nodes. T cells become sensitized to the bound drug and migrate back to the skin. Subsequent re-exposure to the inciting medication leads to T-cell–mediated inflammation. Another example of cell-mediated hypersensitivity is methicillin-induced interstitial nephritis.

B Clinical features Organ-specific syndromes resulting from drug allergy include the following:

1. **Hepatic syndromes** result primarily in hepatocellular changes, granuloma formation, or cholestasis. Hydantoin and halothane, for example, can cause hepatocellular damage, as can aspirin when administered to children with juvenile rheumatoid arthritis. Allopurinol, methyldopa, or sulfonamides may cause granulomatous changes. Phenothiazines, azathioprine, and erythromycin estolate have been linked to cholestasis and painless jaundice.

2. **Renal involvement** most often takes the form of acute interstitial inflammation. Methicillin, sulfonamides, and cephalosporins have been implicated in this reaction. Fever, eosinophilia, macular rash, pyuria, hematuria, and proteinuria are characteristic. Membranous glomerulonephritis may occur after administration of captopril, gold, penicillamine, or probenecid.

3. **Pulmonary reactions** include pulmonary infiltration and bronchospasm.
   a. **Pulmonary infiltration** has been reported with use of nitrofurantoin, gold compounds, methotrexate, and, rarely, cromolyn sodium.
   b. **Drug-induced bronchospasm** may occur in asthmatic patients after administration of aspirin or other NSAIDs. Excess leukotriene production, resulting from inhibition of the cyclooxygenase pathway, presumably is responsible for this reaction.

4. **Dermatologic reactions** are the most common manifestations of drug sensitivity.
   a. **Urticaria,** occasionally progressing to anaphylaxis, can be precipitated by a variety of medications; the most common offenders are penicillin, sulfonamides, cephalosporins, and allergen extracts. Most urticarial reactions are the result of IgE-mediated or direct histamine release.
   b. **Fixed drug eruptions,** which are most likely attributable to a cell-mediated reaction, may develop after ingestion of tetracycline, sulfonamides, and penicillin. In this reaction, discrete, nonpruritic lesions with a macular to bullous appearance occur at the same place each time the medication is taken.
   c. **Photodermatitis** is characterized by a bright erythematous eruption or eczematoid lesions in areas exposed to ultraviolet light. Two presentations are recognized.
      (1) **Phototoxicity** as a result of ultraviolet light exposure occurs early in drug treatment. Drugs implicated in phototoxic reactions include doxycycline, coal tar derivatives, and psoralens.
      (2) **Photoallergy** occurs 4–21 days after the ingestion of the causative agent. It appears to be a cell-mediated process in which ultraviolet light induces a chemical alteration of the drug, leading to tissue sensitization and subsequent injury. Phenothiazines, griseofulvin, and sulfonamides are common offenders.
   d. **Contact dermatitis** develops 48–72 hours after topical application of the implicated medication and is characterized by a vesicular T-cell–mediated inflammatory reaction. Common preparations causing these skin lesions are *para*-aminobenzoic acid (PABA), neomycin, and antihistamines.

e. **Febrile mucocutaneous reactions** are uncommon but may be severe. Cytotoxic, immune complex, and cell-mediated reactions all contribute to the pathogenesis of these syndromes.
   (1) **Stevens-Johnson syndrome,** a severe form of erythema multiforme, may manifest as papular, urticarial, vesicular, or purpuric lesions involving two or more mucosal surfaces.
   (2) **Toxic epidermal necrolysis** manifests as epithelial bullae with subsequent desquamation. Fever and visceral involvement are common.
   (3) Drugs implicated in both syndromes include rifampin, phenobarbital, phenytoin, trimethoprim–sulfamethoxazole, and penicillins.

C Diagnosis Because so few specific diagnostic laboratory tests are available to confirm drug allergy, obtaining an accurate history is essential. Drug allergy should be considered as the possible cause of almost any clinical symptom or sign because drug allergy reactions may mimic so many other clinical conditions.

1. Clinical features that suggest drug hypersensitivity
   a. Prior exposure to the drug
   b. Onset of symptoms within 48 hours with previous exposure or 7 or more days after initiating drug treatment if there is no prior exposure.
   c. Administration of the drug at the recommended dose
   d. Symptoms and signs commonly associated with known allergic reactions
   e. Prompt disappearance of the symptoms after discontinuation of the implicated drug
2. **Specific diagnostic tests**
   a. **Immediate skin tests** for IgE-mediated reactions (e.g., penicillin, insulin, chymopapain)
   b. **Delayed skin tests** (patch testing; a presumed antigen is placed on the skin, covered, and then reassessed for a reaction at 48 hours after application) for cell-mediated reactions (e.g., PABA, nickel)
   c. **RAST testing** for specific IgE antibodies (e.g., penicillin)
   d. **Coombs' antiglobulin test** for cytotoxic reactions causing hemolytic anemia

D Reactions to selected drugs and biologic agents

1. **Reactions to penicillin** and its semisynthetic derivatives are among the most common adverse drug reactions. From 1% to 10% of patients receiving these drugs experience an allergic response. Monobactams rarely cross-react with penicillin, but carbapenems should be considered equally cross-reactive. Ninety percent of sensitized individuals will outgrow this allergy after 10 years.
   a. **Diagnosis.** When a β-lactam antibiotic is the only drug of choice for patients with a history suggestive of a penicillin allergy, **skin testing** is recommended.
      (1) Serial dilutions of benzylpenicilloyl polylysine (a **major determinant** of penicillin allergy that is associated with immediate or accelerated urticaria and anaphylaxis), aged penicillin G, and fresh penicillin G (both **minor determinants** of penicillin allergy that are associated with severe anaphylaxis) are applied via the prick method and then intradermally.
      (2) If all three tests are negative, the likelihood of a reaction is estimated to be 1%–3%, and penicillin may be administered cautiously. Patients with a positive skin test should not receive penicillin or semisynthetic penicillins. Cephalosporins should be administered to such patients cautiously, because up to 2% of patients who are allergic to penicillin have a cross-reaction to cephalosporins. First-generation cephalosporins appear to carry a greater risk than second- or third-generation cephalosporins.
   b. **Therapy.** Desensitization to penicillin-related IgE-mediated reactions may be accomplished by administering penicillin in increments of increasing strength over 4–6 hours.
      (1) The desensitization procedure should be carried out in a controlled setting with access to appropriate emergency treatment. The oral route, which has been found to be safer than the parenteral route, is preferred. Parenteral administration may be initiated after the completion of oral desensitization.

(2) The refractory, or desensitized, state may be maintained for weeks to months by administering the drug at least every 12 hours. Graded challenges or desensitization to cephalosporins should also be considered. Once the patient has discontinued the medication, protection is lost, and repeating the desensitization would be needed only if the drug needed to be readministered.

2. **Reactions to radiographic contrast dye** occur in 4%–8% of patients studied, with anaphylactoid responses occurring in as many as 1.7% of patients with reactions. This is caused by the high osmolarity of the dye. Repeat anaphylactoid reactions may occur in 16%–44% of patients. Because recently introduced **lower osmolarity contrast dyes** appear to be associated with a decreased risk of anaphylactoid reactions, they are now the agents of choice, particularly for those patients with a history of previous allergic reaction.
   a. **Pathogenesis.** Anaphylactoid responses clinically mimic IgE-mediated anaphylaxis but do not involve IgE or any other immune mechanism.
   b. **Clinical features.** Symptoms of excess vagal stimulation such as bradycardia, hypotension, nausea, or vomiting may occur. These symptoms may be particularly severe, sometimes culminating in shock, particularly in patients taking β-adrenergic blockers and angiotensin-converting enzyme (ACE) inhibitors.
   c. **Therapy.** Treatment of an anaphylactoid reaction is identical to that for anaphylaxis from other causes (see V F). Vagal reactions can be treated with atropine. A pretreatment **prophylactic** regimen of prednisone and diphenhydramine significantly decreases the likelihood of a repeat anaphylactoid reaction. Some experts also recommend the addition of ephedrine and an H_2-specific antihistamine.

3. **Insulin allergy and resistance**
   a. **Allergic reactions.** Because bovine insulin differs from human insulin by three amino acids and porcine insulin differs by only one amino acid, the bovine-based preparation is more allergenic. Bovine insulin is no longer available in the United States. Human insulin, produced by recombinant DNA technology, is much less allergenic than the animal preparations but rarely may still precipitate IgE-mediated hypersensitivity reactions. Certain histocompatibility antigens (HLA-DR2, HLA-DR3, and HLA-B7) may be associated with allergic reactions to insulin, and as many as 50% of people exhibiting insulin allergy also have experienced allergic reactions to other drugs.
      (1) **Local allergic reactions** are characterized by pruritus, swelling, and mild erythema, usually occurring during the first few months of therapy. These reactions often subside completely after a few weeks; if not, antihistamines may be either administered systemically or mixed with the insulin. Dividing the dose among two or more injection sites also may be effective. Prolonged local reactions may result in lipoatrophy.
      (2) **Systemic allergic reactions** are much less common than local reactions (i.e., they occur in <0.1% of patients) and are treated similarly to generalized anaphylaxis (see V F). If insulin therapy is reinstituted less than 24 hours after the systemic reaction, the next dose should be reduced so it is one third to one sixth of the original, with slow incremental increases as needed to obtain metabolic control. A desensitization protocol must be implemented if patients require subcutaneous insulin and more than 24 hours have passed since the systemic reaction occurred.
   b. **Resistance**
      (1) **Nonimmunologic** causes of **insulin resistance** include infection, stress, pregnancy, obesity, Cushing's syndrome, acromegaly, pheochromocytoma, leprechaunism, and **type A insulin resistance syndrome** accompanied by acanthosis nigricans.
      (2) **Immunologic insulin resistance** is mediated by IgG anti-insulin antibodies and is manifested by a need for increasing daily doses (up to 200 U/kg in adults and up to 2 U/kg in

children). The presence of high-titer IgG antibodies to insulin or to the insulin receptor can be confirmed by a competitive binding assay.

4. **Heterologous and homologous sera and vaccines**
   a. **Heterologous sera,** which are used in the management of gas gangrene, botulism, diphtheria, and some snake and spider bites, may evoke serum sickness or anaphylaxis. Antilymphocyte globulin produced in horses or rabbits may cause anaphylaxis and thrombocytopenia. OKT3, a murine monoclonal antibody used to inhibit organ transplant rejection, also can induce various allergic reactions.
   b. **Homologous hyperimmune** sera such as those developed to treat rabies, HBV, tetanus, and cytomegalovirus (CMV) less often cause serum sickness.
   c. **Mumps, measles, rubella, influenza, and yellow fever vaccines** are grown on chick embryos, and anaphylaxis after vaccination in egg-sensitive individuals has been reported but is extremely rare. The current recommendation is that the egg-allergic patient can be given the vaccine without concern. In the extremely sensitive egg-allergic patient who has anaphylactic reactions, testing can be done. This assessment by both prick and intradermal testing should be considered before vaccination. If a patient tests positive, the vaccine should be administered using a desensitization program.
5. **Aspirin reactions** usually manifest as urticaria or wheezing. Chronic rhinitis, sinusitis, and often intractable steroid-dependent asthma develop in a small, well-recognized subgroup of individuals between the ages of 30 and 60 years. In these at-risk individuals, life-threatening severe bronchospasm may occur after aspirin ingestion. However, those in whom chronic asthma develops cannot improve their asthma by abstinence from aspirin or other NSAIDs. Because there are no in vivo or in vitro tests for aspirin allergy, diagnosis can be made only from the medical history and by aspirin challenge. Although oral desensitization has been successful in some individuals, it is rarely indicated.

E Other allergy syndromes

1. **Allergic reactions to latex.** Latex allergy has recently emerged as a significant clinical problem. Natural latex is found in surgical gloves, catheters, balloons, condoms, and dental elastic adhesives.
   a. **Incidence.** Health care workers are particularly susceptible; up to 7.4% of surgeons and 5.6% of operating room nurses are allergic to latex. Children with spina bifida and genitourinary problems have a high incidence of latex allergy.
   b. **Clinical features.** Urticaria on contact, rhinitis, conjunctivitis, and bronchospasm after inhalation are suggestive of latex allergy. Severe anaphylaxis may ensue during surgery, barium enema, or dental procedures.
   c. **Diagnosis.** Latex allergy is IgE-mediated, and the diagnosis is best confirmed by In vitro IgE assays.
   d. **Prevention.** Nonlatex gloves and tubing are available and should be used during surgery in patients with known latex allergy. Premedication, antihistamines, and corticosteroids are also used to prevent severe reactions.
2. **Allergic reactions to streptokinase.** This enzymatic protein is commonly used as a thrombolytic agent.
   a. **Incidence.** The frequency of allergic reaction to streptokinase ranges from 1.7%–18.0%.
   b. **Clinical features.** Although not completely delineated, acute symptoms usually include urticaria, bronchospasm, and hypotension. Re-exposure sensitivity is characterized by a delayed-onset serum sickness–like syndrome.
   c. **Diagnosis.** Allergic reactions to streptokinase are IgE-mediated and corroborated by an immediate reaction to an intradermal test with 100 IU streptokinase. This skin test does not help identify those patients who develop serum sickness.

d. **Prevention.** Substitute forms of thrombolytic therapy should be used in patients who demonstrate intradermal skin sensitivity or in those with known streptokinase allergy.

3. **Protamine sulfate sensitivity.** Protamine sulfate is a low–molecular-weight protein primarily used to neutralize heparin, often during cardiopulmonary bypass procedures, or to act as a complexing agent to prepare neutral protamine Hagedorn (NPH) insulin.
   a. **Clinical features.** Flushing, urticaria, hypotension or hypertension, ventricular fibrillation, wheezing, noncardiac pulmonary edema, transient elevations in pulmonary artery pressure, thrombocytopenia, or neutropenia may develop. Allergic reactions to protamine sulfate have been attributed to IgE-mediated anaphylactic and complement-mediated anaphylactoid mechanisms. Diabetic patients who have used protamine-containing insulins are at increased risk.
   b. **Diagnosis and therapy.** Skin testing is not reliable, but pretreatment with antihistamines and corticosteroids may be helpful for patients suspected of being at high risk for allergic reactions. For high-risk surgical patients, alternative reversal agents should be used.

4. **ACE inhibitors.** These agents exert their effects by pharmacologic blockage of kininase II, which leads to elevated levels of bradykinin and substance P.
   a. **Incidence.** Chronic cough develops in 5%–20% of patients, and angioedema occurs in 0.1%–0.2% of patients taking ACE inhibitors. These medications may also influence the development of anaphylaxis. The occurrence of anaphylaxis during dialysis is known to be more frequent in patients taking ACE inhibitors.
   b. **Clinical features.** A chronic cough starts within 1 week to 6 months after the drug is begun. The cough is most often nocturnal and primarily nonproductive. Angioedema often develops by 24 hours or within 5–7 days after initiation of therapy. Severe laryngeal edema and accompanying stridor may be life-threatening.
   c. **Therapy.** Chronic cough subsides 1–4 weeks after the medication is stopped. Substitution of another ACE inhibitor is not useful. For management of severe angioedema, see IV D. Moderate symptoms resolve gradually when the drug is discontinued.

5. **Sulfonamides and HIV-infected patients.** A maculopapular eruption occurs in up to 3% of sulfonamide recipients, sometimes followed by erythema multiforme or Stevens-Johnson syndrome. In HIV-infected individuals who take sulfonamides, 50% or more develop a maculopapular eruption thought to be related to reduced levels of glutathione reductase. No reliable skin or in vitro tests are available. Oral desensitization protocols have sometimes been used successfully.

6. **Minocycline-induced lupus.** Minocycline is now frequently used in the long-term management of acne vulgaris.
   a. **Clinical features.** Musculoskeletal complaints, fever, weight loss, and pleuropulmonary involvement are characteristic, with symptoms developing an average of 2 years after initiation of drug therapy.
   b. **Diagnosis.** Neurologic, renal, and vasculitic changes are unusual, but hepatic transaminase levels are commonly elevated. A positive antinuclear antibody (ANA) titer is uniformly present, and anti–double-stranded DNA and antineutrophilic cytoplasmic antibody (ANCA) tests are also sometimes positive.
   c. **Therapy.** Symptoms are self-limited once treatment with minocycline is stopped.

F Prevention of drug reactions

1. The concurrent administration of several medications should be avoided.
2. A detailed history of any previous drug reactions should be obtained for all patients to guide selection of a medication that is unlikely to cross-react.
3. Patients with documented allergic drug reactions should be instructed to carry identification (e.g., a medical alert bracelet). Medical records for such patients should be clearly marked.

4. Oral administration, when possible, is preferable to parenteral administration, because the incidence of reactions after oral administration is much lower.
5. Allergic reactions are unlikely to be discovered during premarketing trials, because the number of patients is small when compared with the incidence of reactions, so particular vigilance is indicated when administering any new drug.

VIII IMMUNODEFICIENCY DISORDERS

These disorders, which may be either **hereditary** or **acquired,** represent **four distinct abnormalities** of immune function. The genes that encode for many of the defects that are responsible for these disorders have now been mapped to specific chromosomes.

A **Complement system defects** may affect either the nine complement components or their associated regulatory proteins. The etiology, inheritance pattern, clinical features, and diagnosis of these syndromes are summarized in Table 7–4. This is the rarest of the immunodeficiencies.

B **Phagocyte disorders** (Table 7–5)

1. **Common clinical features.** Recurrent cutaneous and sinopulmonary infections as well as chronic cutaneous and oral inflammation (oral ulcers) may occur. Although the inflammatory response may be delayed, successive infections with *Staphylococcus aureus, Pseudomonas* species, *Haemophilus influenzae,* and *Aspergillus* are common and may be life-threatening.

TABLE 7–4 Complement Deficiency Disorders

Defective Component	Inheritance/ Chromosome Site	Phenotypic Expression	Clinical Features	Diagnosis
C2	Autosomal recessive/6p	Impaired removal of immune complexes	Lupus-like syndrome; severe pyogenic infections with gram-positive bacteria	Assessment of total hemolytic complement (CH_{50})*
C4	Autosomal recessive/19q	Impaired removal of immune complexes	SLE and lupus-like syndrome; Sjögren's syndrome; Henoch-Schönlein syndrome	Assessment of total hemolytic complement (CH_{50})*
C3	Autosomal recessive/19q	Impaired opsonization	Recurrent severe infections due to pyogenic or gram-negative organisms	Assessment of total hemolytic complement (CH_{50})*
C5–C9	Autosomal recessive/C5(9q); C6, C7, C9; C9(5); C8(1p, 9q)	Impaired formation of the membrane attack complex, which mediates bacteriolysis	Recurrent meningococcal and gonococcal infections; increased susceptibility to some viruses; rheumatic disorder	Assessment of total hemolytic complement (CH_{50})*
Properdin (P)	X-linked recessive/ Xp11.23–21.1	Impaired opsonization	Recurrent infections due to pyogenic organisms and fulminant meningococcemia	Alternate pathway hemolytic complement titer (APH_{50}); properdin level

SLE = systemic lupus erythematosus.
*Followed by measurement of specific complement component levels.

TABLE 7–5 Disorders of Phagocyte Function

Disorder	Inheritance/ Chromosome Site	Phenotypic Expression	Clinical Features	Diagnosis
Chronic granulomatous disease	Usually X-linked; may be inherited as autosomal recessive or four chromosomes: 1q25, 7q11.23, 16q24, Xp2H	Abnormal NADPH oxidase function resulting in absence of respiratory burst by stimulated phagocytes	Onset of symptoms by age 1 year; granulomas (e.g., hepatic, pulmonary, lymph nodes)	NBT test, confirmed by chemiluminescence and measurements of superoxide, anion, and H_2O_2. (Prenatal diagnosis is made by sampling fetal blood.)
Chédiak-Higashi syndrome	Autosomal recessive/1q	Impaired chemotaxis, intracellular bacteriolysis, and movement of neutrophils from bone marrow	Frequent viral and enteric bacterial infections; partial ocular and cutaneous albinism; pyoderma; mild neutropenia; bleeding tendency	Presence of giant lysosomal granules in granulocytes, and melanosomes in hair shafts. (Prenatal diagnosis is made by sampling fetal blood.)
Leukocyte adhesion deficiency (surface glycoprotein)	Autosomal recessive/21q22.3	Reduced neutrophil chemotaxis and spreading	Delayed umbilical cord separation, with subsequent omphalitis; cold skin abscesses; necrotizing deep soft tissue abscesses	Sustained granulocytosis; decreased expression of CD 18 on polys by flow cytometry

NADPH = the reduced form of nicotinamide–adenine dinucleotide phosphate; NBT = nitroblue tetrazolium.

2. **Therapy.** Management consists primarily of the diagnosis, treatment, and prevention of pyogenic infections. However, such infections are often refractory to treatment, despite appropriate antibiotic therapy.
   - **a.** A complete diagnostic workup is essential, including taking appropriate cultures and being especially vigilant for the development of superficial or visceral mycosis.
   - **b.** Prompt surgical drainage is essential.
   - **c.** Bone marrow transplantation (BMT) has been used successfully in several children to correct leukocyte adhesion defects. BMT has also been used successfully to effect lasting amelioration of chronic granulomatous disease.
   - **d.** IFN-γ administered subcutaneously three times per week results in a reduced number of infections and is approved for use in chronic granulomatous disease (CGD).
3. **Genetic counseling** should be offered to families of affected individuals.

C **Antibody deficiency syndromes** are characterized by an inability to produce antigen-specific antibodies. These disorders have a variety of causes, including abnormalities of the structural genes for the heavy chain of IgA, congenital infections, and medications. Table 7–6 lists the most common humoral immunodeficiency disorders.

1. **Common clinical features.** Most patients with these disorders present with recurrent infections caused by encapsulated bacteria such as *Streptococcus pyogenes, Streptococcus pneumoniae,* and *H. influenzae.* These patients have primarily sinopulmonary infections.
2. **Diagnosis.** Diagnosis is based on:
   - **a.** Quantitative **determination of serum immunoglobulin levels**—principally IgG, IgA, and IgM
   - **b. Functional immunoglobulin assays**

TABLE 7–6 Humoral Immunodeficiency Disorders

Disorder	Inheritance/ Chromosome Site	Phenotypic Expression	Clinical Features	Diagnosis
X-linked agammaglobulinemia (Bruton's)	X-linked/Xq21.3–22	Dysfunctional gene product: [cytoplasmic tyrosine kinase (Btk)]	Recurrent severe infections due to pyogenic organisms, starting at 9–12 months of age; chronic meningoencephalitis due to echovirus; autoimmune arthritis	Total immunoglobulin < 100 mg/dL; severely reduced IgG, IgM, and IgA levels; marked decrease in mature B cells bearing surface immunoglobulin; marked decrease in surface receptor C19, C20, and C21 cells; absence of plasma cells in lymphoid tissues
Late-onset hypogammaglobulinemia (also known as Common Variable Immunodeficiency)	Unknown pattern; equal sex distribution; high percentage of first-degree relatives with selective IgA deficiency/ likely susceptibility gene in class III region of MHC	Abnormal B-cell terminal differentiation to plasma cells. Half of patients also have abnormal T-cell activation and decreased IFN-γ	Less severe infections due to pyogenic organisms, starting between ages 20 and 40 years; giardiasis; sprue-like syndrome; nodular lymphoid hyperplasia; lymphoreticular malignancy; pernicious anemia; late development of autoimmune disorders	Reduced IgG, IgM, and IgA levels (total immunoglobulin may be < 100 mg/dL); possible slight decrease in B cells bearing surface immunoglobulin; impaired antibody responses
Selective IgA deficiency	Unknown pattern; affects 1 in 400–1000 people (most common immunodeficiency disorder)/ susceptibility gene in the MHC class III region on chromosome 6	Arrested maturation of IgA-bearing cells; terminal block in B-cell differentiation to plasma cells capable of secreting IgA	Recurrent respiratory or gastrointestinal bacterial infections; autoimmune and allergic disorders; no symptoms in 60%–65% of cases; transient deficiency may be seen with certain medications (diphenylhydantoin, D-penicillamine)	Reduced serum IgA and serum IgG; levels (< 5 mg/dL); reduced IgG2 or IgG4 levels in 20% of cases; occasional mild abnormalities of T-cell function

IFN-γ = interferon-γ, MHC = major histocompatibility complex.

(1) Determination of antibodies to **naturally occurring immunogens** (e.g., isohemagglutinins, anti-A, and anti-B IgM antibodies found in individuals with A, B, or O blood types)

(2) Measurement of antibodies to **previously encountered antigens** (e.g., *Streptococcus* species, varicella virus, influenza virus, or Epstein-Barr virus)

(3) Determination of **antibodies to prior immunizations** (e.g., IgG1 antibodies to tetanus and diphtheria toxins or IgG1 antibodies to the carbohydrate capsule of *H. influenzae* and pneumococcus.)

(4) Assessment of **antibody production to newly introduced antigens** (e.g., magnitude of de novo response 3–4 weeks after administration of tetanus toxoid or pneumococcal vaccines)

3. **Therapy**
   a. The treatment of choice for most antibody deficiency syndromes is **replacement therapy** with intravenous immunoglobulin.
   b. Patients with selective IgA deficiency are treated as needed with **appropriate antibiotics** for bacterial infections. Immunoglobulin replacement therapy is limited to those individuals with accompanying IgG subclass deficiency.

D **Cellular immunodeficiencies** include those limited to defects in T-cell function, as well as combined disorders affecting both cellular and humoral immunity (Table 7–7).

1. **Common clinical features.** T-cell deficiencies, whether partial or complete, typically result in recurrent infections of greater severity than those observed in the antibody deficiency syndromes.
2. **Diagnosis.** A demonstrable decrease in the number or function of T cells is the basis of diagnosis. Specific T-cell assays include:
   a. **Quantitative assessment of circulating lymphocytes.** In normal individuals, 80%–85% of the circulating lymphocytes are T cells. Values below 1500 mm^3 are considered abnormal. **Immunofluorescence labeling** with T-cell–specific monoclonal antibodies identifies T-cell subsets (e.g., anti-CD4 labels Th cells, and anti-CD8 labels T-cell populations).
   b. **Delayed hypersensitivity skin tests to previously encountered common antigens** (e.g., *Candida albicans, Trichophyton,* streptokinase–streptodornase, mumps virus). Positive reactions to at least two antigens indicate intact cellular immunity. The *C. albicans* reaction can be blunted or absent in immunologically normal patients with eczema.
   c. **Determination of in vitro responsiveness** of cultured T cells to **specific antigens, mitogens** (e.g., pokeweed, concanavalin A, or hemagglutinin), or **foreign cells**

E **HIV** selectively infects Th cells, leading to progressive deterioration of the immune system and, ultimately, **acquired immunodeficiency syndrome (AIDS).** For a detailed discussion of AIDS, refer to Chapter 8. **Acquired immunodeficiency** may also be secondary to malnutrition, diabetes, nephrotic syndrome, or malignancy/chemotherapy.

TABLE 7–7 T-Lymphocyte–Related Immunodeficiency Disorders

Disorder	Inheritance/ Chromosome Site	Phenotypic Expression	Clinical Features	Diagnosis	Therapy
DiGeorge syndrome	Deletion 22q11; sporadic occurrence	Developmental field defect affecting structures of the third and fourth pharyngeal pouches, leading to thymic, parathyroid, and conotruncal cardiac defects	Anomalies of the cardiac outflow tract; neonatal tetany; hypoplastic mandible; hypertelorism; short philtrum; low-grade or opportunistic infections (occasional or recurrent)	Hypocalcemia; total serum immunoglobulin usually normal; possible failure to make specific antibody after immunization; decreased T cells; mitogen-stimulated proliferation may be normal, decreased, or absent, depending on degree of thymic deficiency	BMT; fetal thymic implantation (short-lived improvement)
Severe combined immunodeficiency syndrome	Classical type: X-linked recessive/ Xq13.1–13.3 Other type: autosomal recessive/20q13, 2q12, 14q13.1	Absence of all adaptive immune mechanisms; vestigial thymus; few thymocytes or Hassall's corpuscles Classical type: Mutation of the γ chain of the IL-2 receptor Other type: ADA (ZAP-70 and PNP deficiency)	Skin infections, sepsis, pneumonia, and diarrhea, starting by age 3 months; marked failure to thrive; severe opportunistic infections (e.g., *Pneumocystis, Candida, varicella*); hypoplastic peripheral lymphoid tissue; chondrodysplasia; possibility of death by age 2 years if untreated	Profound lymphophenia; cutaneous anergy; heterogeneous abnormalities of lymphocyte subpopulations; impaired in vitro lymphocyte proliferative response; serum immunoglobulin levels severely depressed with no response to specific antigens	BMT; intravenous immunoglobulin replacement; experimental gene therapy trial in progress
Wiskott-Aldrich syndrome	X-linked recessive/ Xp11.22–11.3	Disorganization of actin cytoskeleton and lack of membrane-associated glycoproteins; accelerated synthesis and catabolism of all immunoglobulin isotypes; intrinsic platelet abnormality	Eczema; microcytic thrombocytopenia; recurrent pyogenic infections, starting by age 1 year; *Pneumocystis* and herpesvirus infections, starting in late childhood; malignancy (lymphoma) in 15% of cases	Normal IgG levels; elevated IgA levels; slightly reduced IgM levels; impaired humoral response to polysaccharide antigens; mild-to-moderate depression of lymphocyte proliferative response; marked lymphopenia by 6 years of age	Early BMT Splenectomy in patients with bleeding disorders

(*continued*)

TABLE 7–7 Continued

Disorder	Inheritance/ Chromosome Site	Phenotypic Expression	Clinical Features	Diagnosis	Therapy
Ataxia–telangiectasia	Autosomal recessive/ 11q22.23	Hypoplastic thymus; lack of Hassall's corpuscles; intrinsic CD4 and B-cell defects; T-cell chromosomal translocation after x-ray irradiation	Progressive cerebellar ataxia; oculocutaneous telangiectasia; recurrent sinopulmonary infections; increased incidence of malignancy	Absent IgA in 70% of cases; IgG2 subclass deficiency in 35% of cases; low–molecular-weight IgM; mild depression of mitogen-stimulated proliferative response; selective decrease in CD4 cells; persistently elevated serum AFP	Intravenous gamma globulin in IgG2 deficiency; possible gene therapy (future)

ADA = adenosine deaminase; AFP = α-fetoprotein; BMT = bone marrow transplantation; IL-2 = interleukin-2; PNP = purine nucleoside phosphorylase.

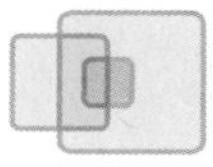

Study Questions

1. A 12-year-old boy is playing in the park near a trash can. He is stung by what he believes is a yellow jacket. He immediately has symptoms of urticaria and wheezing. These symptoms are treated in a local emergency department. He follows up in his primary care provider's office 1 week later. There is a question of the proper diagnosis of insect allergy.

   Which of the following findings provides the best evidence of insect sting hypersensitivity?

   A Positive prick or intradermal skin test
   B Extensive local reaction lasting 5–7 days
   C Documented evidence of a systemic allergic reaction
   D Specific antivenom immunoglobulin E (IgE) antibodies
   E Generalized urticaria in this patient.

2. A 25-year-old man presents to his primary care office with the following symptoms. He has clear rhinorrhea, ocular and nasal puritis, nasal congestion, and sneezing. He knows that it is tree pollen season but has also recently acquired a pet cat for the first time. Which of the following tests is most useful in the diagnosis of the trigger for his allergic rhinitis?

   A Radioallergosorbent test (RAST)
   B Measurement of serum immunoglobulin E (IgE) levels
   C Peripheral blood smear
   D Immediate hypersensitivity skin test
   E Stained nasal smear for eosinophils

3. A 4-year-old boy in your practice has been having many infections. You suspect that he may have an immune dysfunction. Quantitative immunoglobulins were sent and were normal. Which of the following immunodeficiency disorders is associated with normal immunoglobulin G (IgG) levels?

   A X-linked agammaglobulinemia (Bruton's)
   B DiGeorge syndrome
   C Late-onset hypogammaglobulinemia
   D Ataxia-telangiectasia
   E Severe combined immunodeficiency

4. A 35-year-old woman calls for advice. She has a viral syndrome and has developed a rash. You are discussing it with her to help identify whether this is an urticarial rash. Urticarial lesions are best described in which of the following ways?

   A Nonpruritic
   B Linear
   C Evanescent
   D Macular
   E Poorly circumscribed

5. You are attending a lecture about basic immunology. The speaker has just finished discussing the differences between IgE-mediated allergic reactions and IgG-mediated autoantibody reactions. He chooses you out of the audience and asks you the following question. Which one of the following allergic reactions is mediated by immunoglobulin G (IgG) autoantibodies?

   A Insulin resistance
   B Anaphylaxis after ingestion of peanuts

C Latex reaction
D Systemic reaction to an insect sting
E Ragweed-induced rhinitis

6. A 33-year-old man has an acute anaphylactic reaction to an intravenous drug while in the hospital. He is taking a β-adrenergic blockade drug. Which of the following therapeutic choices may be most useful in treating resistant hypotension?

A Subcutaneous aqueous epinephrine
B Intravenous terbutaline
C Intravenous glucagon
D Intravenous aminophylline
E Intravenous diphenhydramine

7. A 28-year-old woman with bronchial asthma is about to start a new job in a health care facility. She hears that health care workers are at a greater risk for developing a latex allergy. She is wondering whether any of her medical conditions make her at a higher risk. Which of the following clinical conditions is most commonly associated with latex allergy?

A Bronchial asthma
B Fibrosing alveolitis
C Diabetes mellitus
D Spina bifida
E Inflammatory bowel disease

QUESTIONS 8–11

Directions: *The response options for Items 8–11 are the same. You will be required to select one answer for each item in the set.*

A Antigen avoidance
B Immunotherapy against known offending antigens
C Antihistamine preparation
D Topical adrenergic agonist

For each of the following patients with allergic rhinitis, select the most appropriate therapeutic intervention.

8. A 34-year-old-woman with severe perennial allergic rhinitis loses 10–15 days of work each year as a result of secondary sinusitis. Immediate skin tests show significant positive reactions to house dustmite, *Cladosporium,* and grass and ragweed pollens. Various medications have been only partially successful in controlling symptoms.

9. A 20-year-old man has mild but persistent year-round symptoms of nasal congestion, rhinorrhea, and watery eyes. He has recurrent epistaxis. Immediate skin tests show positive reactions to house dustmite, *Alternaria,* and grass and ragweed pollens.

10. A 10-year-old girl has rhinorrhea and nasal pruritus after visiting a friend who has a kitten.

11. An 8-year-old boy regularly experiences moderately severe sneezing spells and watery eyes in May and June, September and October, and occasionally during January through March. Immediate skin tests show positive reactions to *Alternaria, Cladosporium,* house dustmite, and grass and ragweed pollens.

QUESTIONS 12–14

Directions: *The response options for Items 12–14 are the same. You will be required to select one answer for each item in the set.*

A. Acute arthritis
B. Acute anaphylaxis
C. Chronic cough
D. Bronchospasm
E. Interstitial nephritis
F. Maculopapular eruption
G. Photoallergic reaction

For each of the following patients exhibiting an adverse drug reaction, select the most likely clinical expression.

12. A 22-year-old man, who is in good health except for recurrent sinusitis, elects to take 81 mg aspirin as antithrombosis therapy.

13. A 54-year-old woman with newly diagnosed hypertension starts enalapril at an appropriate dose.

14. A 34-year-old woman with human immunodeficiency virus (HIV) infection begins to take a prophylactic dose of sulfonamide three times a week.

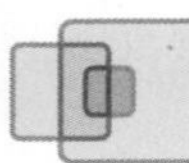

Answers and Explanations

1. **The answer is C** [VI C 1–2]. Clinical documentation of a systemic allergic reaction is essential to the accurate diagnosis of insect sting hypersensitivity. Typically, signs of anaphylaxis develop within minutes after the sting. Subsequent prick or intradermal skin testing, supplemented as necessary by antivenom immunoglobulin E (IgE) levels (determined by radioallergosorbent test [RAST]), provides confirming evidence of hypersensitivity. A large local reaction alone, whether of short or prolonged duration, does not provide sufficient evidence of IgE-mediated hypersensitivity. Generalized urticaria in a child younger than 16 years of age is not considered anaphylaxis and these children do not have a greater risk than the general population of an anaphylactic reaction on their next sting. The only objective test is a serum β tryptase. This test measures tryptase released from mast cells. When elevated, it is useful, but it is not elevated in all anaphylactic reactions.

2. **The answer is D** [III E 1]. An accurately applied skin test is the most valuable tool for identifying the causative antigen in allergic rhinitis, yielding results in approximately 15–20 minutes. The radioallergosorbent test (RAST) has almost equal accuracy but is more expensive and less discriminative than skin testing. Elevated immunoglobulin E (IgE) levels are observed in only 30%–40% of patients with allergic rhinitis and may be secondary to other unrelated disorders. Peripheral eosinophilia seen in a peripheral blood smear is an inconsistent finding. Although eosinophils are usually identified in nasal secretions from patients with allergic rhinitis, they are also detected in eosinophilic nonallergic rhinitis and hyperplastic sinusitis.

3. **The answer is B** [Tables 7–6 and 7–7]. Although reduced levels of immunoglobulin A (IgA) or IgE may be seen in patients with DiGeorge syndrome, a T-cell deficiency disorder, the total serum immunoglobulin level usually is normal, and IgG levels are normal. In X-linked agammaglobulinemia (Bruton's) and late-onset hypogammaglobulinema, IgG, IgM, and IgA levels are all reduced, and the total immunoglobulin level is less than 100 mg/dL. Ataxia-telangiectasia patients have a defect in their DNA repair mechanism. One of the clinical features is low IgA and IgG. Severe combined immunodeficiency results in a decrease in all immunoglobulins.

4. **The answer is C** [IV A 1]. Urticarial lesions are well circumscribed and intensely pruritic; dermatographism may result from prolonged scratching. They are usually bright and described as evanescent. Each lesion is transient, rarely lasting more than a few hours. Bouts of urticaria, however, may persist for several days or even years (as in chronic idiopathic urticaria). Individual lesions that last for longer than 48 hours and that are more painful than pruritic are likely to be due to small vessel vasculitis, not urticaria.

5. **The answer is A** [VII D 3 b (2)]. Insulin resistance is caused by immunoglobulin G (IgG) autoantibodies that bind to insulin receptors, thereby inhibiting their function. This problem usually occurs in women with Sjögren's syndrome, systemic lupus erythematosus (SLE), or a less well-defined clinical syndrome also suggestive of autoimmunity. Food-related anaphylaxis, reactions to latex, systemic reactions to insect stings, and ragweed-induced rhinitis are all IgE-mediated hypersensitivity responses.

6. **The answer is C** [V F 2]. Intravenous glucagon has a positive inotropic and chronotropic effect. In those patients taking β-blocker medications, an even greater increase in blood pressure may occur. Although subcutaneous epinephrine is always the first line of therapy, it may not be effective in patients

using a β-adrenergic blockade drug. The other therapeutic agents are relatively ineffective in the face of β-adrenergic blockade.

7. The answer is D [VII E 1 a]. The highest prevalence of latex allergy occurs in children with spina bifida. This appears to be related to early surgical intervention with constant exposure to the natural latex in catheters and tubing. Surgeons and operating room nurses are at increased risk of developing latex allergy. Bronchial asthma, fibrosing alveolitis, diabetes mellitus, and inflammatory bowel disease are not commonly associated with the occurrence of latex allergy.

8–11. The answers are: 8—B [III F 4], **9—C** [III F 3 a–c], **10—A** [III F 1], **11—C** [III F 3 a–c]. Immunotherapy, which significantly ameliorates symptoms and is used when allergic rhinitis is severe, when medical complications or intolerance to medication occurs, and when various types of medications have been only partially successful, would be recommended for the 34-year-old woman.

Intranasal steroids are the most effective form of therapy, but not an option here. Therefore, antihistamine preparations are the drugs of choice for the treatment of allergic rhinitis. These preparations usually control mild-to-moderate symptoms such as those experienced by the 20-year-old man and the 8-year-old boy; however, some patients experience intolerable side effects such as drowsiness. A second-generation antihistamine such as fexofenadine is less likely to cause such sedation.

If an antihistamine preparation does not relieve symptoms or is not well tolerated, then intranasal therapy with corticosteroids or an H_1 blocker could be considered for the 8-year-old boy. Nasal cromolyn sodium, which in some cases is as effective as a decongestant in treating seasonal allergic rhinitis, could have been recommended for the 8-year-old boy with seasonal symptoms.

Topical adrenergic preparations are used for no longer than 2–3 days to treat acute nasal congestion that could lead to sinusitis. They are used sometimes before air travel by individuals who are susceptible to barotitis media.

Antigen avoidance is most successful when a single antigen can be identified as the causative agent. Because the 10-year-old girl developed symptoms only after being exposed to her friend's kitten, it is likely that avoiding cats will alleviate her symptoms. Antigen avoidance is not feasible for all patients, however. For example, although a patient may be able to avoid animal dander indoors, the avoidance of multiple outdoor antigens is likely to prove difficult, if not impossible. Nonetheless, sensible environmental precautions help limit exacerbation of symptoms.

12. The answer is D [III E 2 f]. This man, an individual with recurrent sinusitis, also may have underlying chronic rhinitis and perhaps undiagnosed nasal polyposis. Bronchospasm, which may be prolonged and severe, typically begins within 30 minutes after aspirin ingestion. The combination of asthma, nasal polyposis, and sinusitis is known as the aspirin triad. However, aspirin-induced anaphylaxis does not occur in patients with underlying sinusitis or polyposis and starts after two or more exposures to aspirin.

13. The answer is C [VII E 4]. Chronic cough has been reported in 5%–20% of patients who take angiotensin-converting enzyme (ACE) inhibitors. The cough is usually nonproductive and nocturnal. Symptoms may begin as early as 1 week or as late as 6 months after drug use. ACE inhibitors also lead to development of angioedema in 0.1%–0.2% of patients, and in certain clinical situations, this group of medications is known to exacerbate anaphylaxis.

14. The answer is F [VII E 5]. A maculopapular eruption is seen in approximately 3% of all recipients of sulfonamide and in more than 50% of those individuals with human immunodeficiency virus (HIV) infection. The combination of trimethoprim–sulfamethoxazole is used for prophylaxis and treatment of *Pneumocystis carinii* infection in immunocompromised individuals. There are no reliable in vitro or in vivo tests to predict sensitivity, so an oral dose challenge and desensitization protocol are sometimes performed in patients who are believed to be particularly vulnerable.

chapter **8**

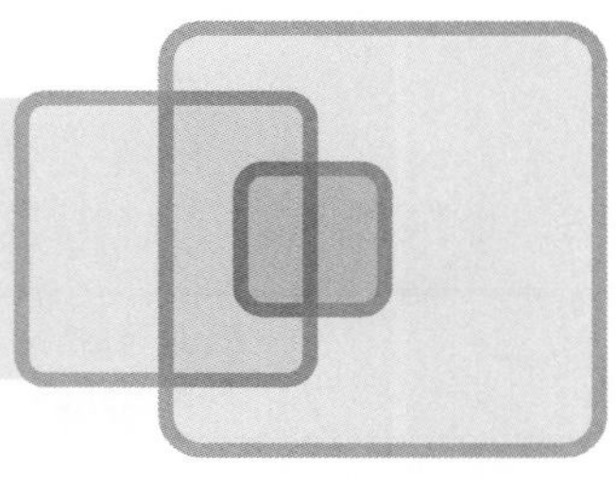

Infectious Diseases

THOMAS FEKETE

I GENERAL PRINCIPLES OF HUMAN–MICROBE INTERACTION

The normal human body harbors a complex microbial ecosystem. Generally, these **commensal** organisms (referred to as the **indigenous flora**) are considered to be nonpathogenic. Infection and disease may result, however, when the body is challenged by a known pathogen or when the body's defense system is disturbed, allowing uncontrolled growth or invasion by the indigenous flora.

A Normal human–microbe ecology

Microorganisms can interact with humans in the following ways:

1. **Most indigenous organisms seldom cause disease.** Many of the organisms normally found on the skin and mucous membranes (e.g., *Staphylococcus epidermidis, Corynebacterium* species) are ubiquitous but may cause disease in unusual settings (e.g., when host defenses are significantly impaired or when artificial material such as a catheter or a prosthetic joint is present).
2. **Some indigenous organisms may cause disease in other body sites.** Many bacteria that normally exist in one body site may cause morbidity elsewhere. For example, α-hemolytic (viridans) streptococci are commensals in the oropharynx but can cause endocarditis if they are inoculated into the blood and settle on a previously damaged heart valve. In addition, enteric aerobes and anaerobes, which normally exist in high density in the colon, can cause peritonitis and abscess formation if the colon is perforated and these bacteria spill into the abdominal cavity.
3. **Transient organisms may cause disease.** The body's normal flora may allow the temporary growth of certain microbes, which disappear spontaneously but may cause disease while present. For example, patients with invasive meningococcal disease first have pharyngeal carriage of *Neisseria meningitidis,* but only a tiny fraction of individuals with meningococci in the pharynx ever develop systemic disease.
4. **Pathogenic organisms usually cause disease.** Most viruses, as well as *Chlamydia* and *Rickettsia,* rarely are isolated from humans except during or following an acute illness. Some pathogenic bacteria include *Brucella* and *Salmonella* species, *Neisseria gonorrhoeae,* and *Mycobacterium tuberculosis.*

B Host defense mechanisms

The human body has many ways of defending itself from potentially pathogenic microorganisms.

1. **Anatomic barriers** are integral in preventing infection. These include physical barriers such as intact skin and mucous membranes, as well as functional barriers such as the muscular protection of the glottis and bladder neck.
   a. **Herpetic whitlow** occurs when broken skin comes into contact with herpes simplex virus. Similarly, nonsterile intravenous injection of drugs may allow skin flora to enter the bloodstream and lead to the development of **endocarditis.**
   b. Mechanical devices such as indwelling bladder catheters and endotracheal tubes allow **bacterial colonization** of normally sterile sites; this colonization may lead to infection.
2. **Cellular immunity** (Table 8–1)

TABLE 8–1 The Human Immune System

Component	Source	Function	Causes of Diminished Function	Opportunistic Organisms
Cellular immunity				
Neutrophil	Bone marrow	Phagocytosis; acute inflammation	Genetic disorders Chronic granulomatous disease Myeloperoxidase deficiency Acquired causes Cytotoxic therapy Leukemia Aplastic anemia Drug reaction	Endogenous flora; enteric bacilli; *Pseudomonas aeruginosa; Candida* species; *Aspergillus* species
Eosinophil	Bone marrow	Modulate hypersensitivity reactions to multicellular parasites	Idiopathic; corticosteroid therapy	None known
Monocyte/macrophage	Bone marrow	Release cytokines; interact with lymphocytes; phagocytosis	Cytotoxic therapy; lymphoreticular malignancy	
T lymphocyte	Thymus; bone marrow	Modulate activity of B lymphocytes, macrophages, and T lymphocytes	Genetic disorders; autoimmune disease; lymphoreticular malignancy; AIDS; organ transplantation; corticosteroid therapy	*Mycobacterium* species; fungi; *Listeria* species; *Nocardia* species
Humoral immunity				
Antibody	Plasma cells	Facilitate phagocytosis; inactivate toxins	Genetic disorders; multiple myeloma; splenectomy	Viruses; pyogenic bacteria
Complement	Liver	Enhance phagocytosis; direct cell destruction	Genetic disorders; severe liver disease	*Neisseria* species (especially with deficiency of complement components (C5–C9)

AIDS = acquired immunodeficiency syndrome.

a. **Neutrophils** (polymorphonuclear leukocytes) [PMNs] are phagocytic cells that are important for ingesting and killing microorganisms that breach normal body defenses.
   (1) When neutrophils are reduced substantially in number (a condition termed **neutropenia**), pyogenic bacteria and fungi that are commensals of the skin or gut such as *Escherichia coli* and *Candida albicans* can cause serious infections.
   (2) Functional abnormalities of neutrophils may result in syndromes of varying type and severity.
      (a) For example, patients with **chronic granulomatous disease,** which is caused by a deficiency of nicotinamide adenine dinucleotide phosphate (NADPH) oxidase, are prone to infections by catalase-producing organisms such as *Staphylococcus aureus,*

many gram-negative bacilli, and fungi. These infections start early in life and tend to be severe and recurrent.

(b) Conversely, patients with **lazy leukocyte syndrome** tend to have mild, easily treatable infections associated with the upper respiratory tract.

b. **Monocytes** and their tissue forms, **macrophages,** also are important for the ingestion of pathogenic microbes as well as for the production of cytokines, interleukins, and other modulators of the immune system. Some microorganisms are resistant to macrophage killing. After phagocytosis, these bacteria may be protected from those antibiotics that do not penetrate macrophages. Examples of these bacteria are *Salmonella, Legionella,* and *Mycobacterium* species.

c. **Lymphocytes** are the third component of the cellular immune system. **T lymphocytes,** or **T cells,** have many roles in modulating the activities of other T cells, monocytes, and **B lymphocytes,** or **B cells** (see Chapter 7 I B).

(1) Antigen-specific T cells are responsible for delayed hypersensitivity and for controlling infections caused by a variety of agents, including species of *Mycobacterium, Pneumocystis,* and *Cryptococcus.*

(2) T cells are broadly divided into **helper T (Th) cells** and **suppressor T (Ts) cells** based on their effect on the immune system in terms of augmenting or diminishing the immune response. Th cells (e.g., CD4 cells) tend to up-regulate the immune response, and Ts cells (e.g., CD8 cells) tend to down-regulate the immune response.

(3) T cells also play a pivotal role in the manifestations of autoimmune diseases.

3. **Humoral immunity** (see Table 8–1)

a. **Antibody-mediated immunity** involves the production of antibody by activated B cells, which are stimulated by exposure to the proper antigen and to Th cells to differentiate into **plasma cells.** Plasma cells essentially are factories for the production of immunoglobulins, which they excrete into their environment. Immunoglobulins facilitate phagocytosis and activate complement, thus resulting in a more rapid clearance of the antigen. The absence or profound deficiency of immunoglobulins leads to recurrent infections caused primarily by encapsulated bacteria (e.g., *Haemophilus influenzae, Streptococcus pneumoniae*).

b. The **complement system,** a cascading series of glycoproteins, tags foreign material to promote phagocytosis or directly damages or destroys infective organisms. Severe complement deficiencies may predispose individuals to infections. For example, the reduced production of one or more of the late complement components (i.e., C5–C9) predisposes to overwhelming neisserial infections.

C Thermal regulation One of the most recognized features of infectious diseases, regardless of the site of infection, is the elevation of body temperature.

1. **Normal regulation of body temperature.** The normal core body temperature is approximately 37°C (±1°). Monocytes secrete a polypeptide called **interleukin-1** (IL-1), which stimulates the hypothalamus to increase the body's temperature **set point.** The rise in set point causes alterations in circulation, metabolism, and perspiration, which ultimately lead to a rise in body temperature. Body temperature usually is measured by placing a thermometer in the mouth or the rectum. It also may be measured directly from the tympanic membrane or the superior vena cava. (Mouth breathing or the recent ingestion of very hot or cold beverages may reduce the accuracy of orally measured temperature readings, which tend to be 0.5°C–1.0°C lower than rectal temperatures.) Temperature readings above 38.3°C are considered abnormal. **Hypothermia** (body temperature < 36°C) is sometimes a response to overwhelming infection, especially in neonates and the elderly.

2. **Conditions associated with fever.** Almost any infectious process may be accompanied by fever, although the absence of fever should not exclude the consideration of an infection. Fever also may occur with myocardial infarction (MI), pulmonary embolism, drug reactions, autoimmune disease, cancer (e.g., lymphoma, renal cell carcinoma), or one of a variety of miscellaneous illnesses

(e.g., inflammatory bowel disease, sarcoid). The actual temperature pattern rarely helps narrow the range of etiologic factors that may be causing the fever.

3. **Fever management. Antipyretic drugs** [e.g., aspirin, acetaminophen, nonsteroidal anti-inflammatory agents (NSAIDs)] can modify a fever, but they seldom completely suppress a fever caused by infection. When fever is extreme (i.e., >42°C) or when the accompanying tachycardia and circulatory changes are poorly tolerated, it is wise to try to reduce body temperature. However, in most settings, fever is merely uncomfortable, and attempts to eliminate it may be comparatively more unpleasant because of the shaking and sweating that are sometimes associated with fever lysis. Cooling blankets are especially unpleasant for many patients and may actually increase the metabolic load by defeating the efforts of the hypothalamus to reset the core body temperature.
4. **Beneficial effects of fever.** Fever does play a role in host defense, because many infective microbes may prefer normal body temperature or lower. However, the clinical significance of this protection is unknown. In addition, some elements of the immune system are more efficient at higher temperatures, whereas others are less efficient. The net effect on recovery from infection is not known.

D **Microbial virulence factors** are important in determining the likelihood of infection. To infect a host, microorganisms or their products must adhere to host tissue.

1. **Some microbes invade host cells or breach barriers** to reach susceptible body sites and, along the way, avoid or overcome host defenses. In some situations (e.g., chickenpox or measles), microbes can easily infect otherwise healthy individuals who have normal host defenses but no prior exposure to the microbe.
2. **Some microbes cause disease at the contact site with the host.** An example is *Giardia intestinalis,* which is confined to the lumen of the small bowel and causes abdominal cramping and diarrhea.
3. **Some microbes have a special ability to produce a toxin or virulence factor** to cause disease. For example, a toxin elaborated by some strains of *S. aureus* [toxic shock syndrome toxin-1 (TSST-1)] is responsible for **toxic shock syndrome** (TSS; see VII D 1 a).
4. **In some situations, microbes work in groups to cause disease** when an individual organism lacks an essential virulence or survival quality to act alone. An example is **delta hepatitis (HDV),** which can occur only in the presence of ongoing hepatitis B (HBV) infection.
5. Because of the selective pressures induced by using antimicrobial agents to treat or prevent infections in humans and animals, **microorganisms that are resistant to antibiotics may have a propensity for causing infections.** This is especially true where antibiotic use is widespread, such as in hospitals and nursing homes. Similar problems have appeared in ambulatory settings, where antibiotic use is widespread. This is most notable in children who receive repeated courses of antibiotics (e.g., for recurrent otitis media) and harbor a more resistant microbial flora as a result.

E **Epidemiologic considerations** In addition to host and microbial characteristics, environmental circumstances also help determine the nature and severity of an infection.

1. **Contagious diseases.** Such diseases are spread from person to person through direct physical contact (e.g., syphilis) or by infectious aerosols (e.g., tuberculosis). Smallpox was eradicated successfully in part because preventive measures could be directed to potential contacts of documented cases.
2. **Vectors and fomites**
   a. Vectors are animals that act as hosts or carriers of a disease without becoming ill themselves. Most vectors are insects or arthropods. In general, infections that are related to animals or their products (e.g., meat, milk, or eggs) are called **zoonoses.**
   b. **Fomites** are inanimate objects capable of spreading infection. Fomites are most commonly identified in hospitals, where enhanced patient susceptibility and a high concentration of virulent organisms coexist.

3. **Geography.** Some diseases occur exclusively or at substantially greater frequency in certain areas. For example, mosquito bites almost never result in the transmission of malaria in the United States. When considering such a disease in a diagnosis, a history of travel to or residence in an appropriate area is important. Duration of exposure can also be important. For example, filariasis leads to elephantiasis only after repeated exposure to the mosquito vector over a period of months to years.
4. **Season.** Many infections occur more commonly during a particular time of the year. This may be because of certain activities that might expose an individual to risk and that are seasonal in nature (e.g., hunting, fishing) or to environmental factors that favor the growth of the microbe or its insect vector.
5. **Institutions.** Certain settings that bring together susceptible individuals may alter the risk of infection. Hospitals and nursing homes can amplify and alter the nature of infections among the sick and the elderly, whereas day-care centers can have a similar effect on the young.

II USE OF ANTI-INFECTIVE THERAPY

A General principles Because the use of antibiotics can be lifesaving, it is important to recognize when to initiate treatment. However, any type of medical intervention presents potential hazards, and the indiscriminate use of antibiotics is no exception. In general, four circumstances prompt antimicrobial therapy.

1. **Organism-based treatment**
   a. When cultures or stains from a patient demonstrate a credible microorganism, appropriate antibiotic treatment is initiated. Note the following examples:
      (1) A wet mount of vaginal secretions showing *Trichomonas vaginalis*
      (2) Blood cultures that are positive for *Streptococcus sanguis* in a patient with a history of mitral valve disease and a fever
   b. Techniques for recognizing specific antigens of microorganisms also may be used to help initiate therapy. An example is the finding of cryptococcal antigens in the cerebrospinal fluid (CSF) in a patient with chronic meningitis.
   c. Isolation of an organism allows in vitro testing of antibiotic susceptibility. However, for many microbes, resistance patterns are predictable enough to permit treatment without these further tests.
2. **Syndrome-based treatment** is initiated when all three of the following conditions apply:
   a. The clinical picture strongly suggests specific organ disease.
   b. The tests needed to make a microbiologic diagnosis are not available or practical.
   c. The most likely causative organisms all respond to the same treatment.
      (1) For example, if an otherwise healthy young woman has painful urination and a positive test for white blood cells (WBCs) in the urine, treatment can be initiated for a urinary tract infection without even submitting a urine specimen for culture.
      (2) However, patients with a poor response to initial treatment, relapse, or complicating concomitant medical illness cannot be optimally managed without further diagnostic evaluation.
3. **Empiric therapy** is given when the diagnosis is uncertain but clinical experience suggests that the patient outcome in a particular setting is improved with antimicrobial therapy.
   a. Generally, empiric therapy is initiated while awaiting the results of diagnostic tests to identify a specific causative organism.
   b. Fever often develops as the first sign of infection in patients with severe neutropenia from cancer therapy. These patients may succumb to their infection before final reports are received from the laboratory. Thus, antimicrobial therapy should begin at the first sign of fever.
4. **Prophylaxis** is used when a specific infection or complication is to be avoided. Generally, this form of empiric therapy is restricted to a fixed and brief period during which there is a risk of

infection. Examples include the use of penicillin before dental procedures in patients with heart valve disease and the use of perioperative antibiotics in surgery. The longer the duration of the prophylaxis, the more likely to have consequences related to antimicrobial toxicity or to the acquisition of resistant flora.

B Dosage and route When considering the use of antibiotics, the appropriate dosage and route of administration must be established.

1. **Dosage**
   a. Dosing usually is based on pharmacologic and clinical data related to the size and age of the patient, the desired level of the drug in the target tissue, the drug's rate of elimination (often estimated by examining kidney and liver function), and the expected penetration of the drug into the infected tissue.
   b. Guidelines for proper dosing usually are provided with the drug itself and are widely available. Occasionally, dosage can be adjusted through the use of blood or tissue levels of the drug. This is commonly done, for example, to provide a safe and effective course of vancomycin therapy in a person with reduced or absent kidney function.
2. **Route.** In terms of comfort and convenience, oral therapy is usually preferred. But parenterally administered (i.e., intravenous or intramuscular) drugs are usually more reliably absorbed than orally administered drugs. They are used in the following situations:
   a. In patients who cannot tolerate orally administered drugs because of vomiting, decreased peristalsis, swallowing difficulty, or depressed mental state
   b. In patients in whom institution of therapy is urgent
   c. When no oral form of the drug exists or when adequate amounts of the oral forms cannot be administered

C Cost This issue has become more important with increased attention to cost containment. When all other factors are equal, cost may influence which drug is prescribed. With intravenously administered drugs, the cost of diluents and of labor involved in preparing and infusing the drugs must be considered. The cost of administration is lower with intramuscularly given drugs and is lowest with oral agents.

D Specific antibiotic spectrum The range or **spectrum** of microorganisms inhibited or killed by an antibiotic is an important consideration in deciding which drug to use. The results of in vitro testing are helpful in selecting an antibiotic that is most likely to be effective against an infective organism. The two most common ways to present the results of in vitro susceptibility testing are to note whether the organism being tested is susceptible, intermediate, or resistant to the drug or to note the concentration of the drug needed to inhibit the organism (this latter number is called the minimum inhibitory concentration or MIC). Even when the particular organism has not been tested, it may be assumed—on the basis of either local patterns of antibiotic susceptibility or general experience in treating certain syndromes—that a given drug is likely to be effective. However, susceptibility patterns merit close scrutiny because they change over time.

E Concentration- or time-dependent effect Some antimicrobials have no greater effect on bacterial inhibition or killing when the tissue levels are raised above a threshold (such as the MIC) needed to see an effect. This is **time-dependent** action since the benefit of the drug is related to the amount of time that it is present at or above this threshold level. Beta-lactams are, in general, time-dependent antibiotics. Other drugs are most effective when they can reach high peak levels or spend prolonged periods at multiples of the threshold needed to inhibit or kill microbes even if their concentration falls below that threshold for a considerable period. This is called **concentration-dependent** activity and is typical of aminoglycosides.

F **Toxicity and side effects** Although life-threatening toxicity rarely occurs with antibiotic treatment, physicians should be familiar with the specific risks of each drug administered so that side effects can be anticipated and minimized.

1. **Allergic reactions,** which are sometimes fatal, can occur with almost any pharmaceutical agent but are more common with the **β-lactam antibiotics** and sulfonamides than with other antimicrobials.
2. **Chloramphenicol,** which is seldom used, is associated with **bone marrow suppression,** including irreversible aplastic anemia.
3. Many drugs can cause **renal dysfunction,** the most prominent being the **aminoglycosides.** This toxicity is reversible and usually of minor clinical significance, but full recovery may take weeks or months. In rare instances, dialysis may be needed. In addition, various forms of **amphotericin B** are used in the treatment of fungal infections. Careful attention to the patient's fluid status may mitigate the reversible nephrotoxicity that is often associated with this agent.
4. **Abnormalities in blood coagulation** (e.g., changes in the levels of clotting factors or in the number or function of platelets) have been associated with several **β-lactam antibiotics** and sometimes result in clinically significant bleeding.
5. **Ototoxicity** is an infrequent but potentially debilitating side effect of **aminoglycosides.** Either auditory or vestibular impairment can occur; often, it is irreversible.
6. **Phototoxicity** is an exaggerated response of the skin to sun exposure. This can result in severe "sunburn" and is associated with some fluoroquinolones.
7. **Toxicity to cardiac conduction** can arise from any number of drugs (including non-antibiotic compounds). The most common arrhythmia is associated with QT prolongation. At the extreme end of QT prolongation is a self-sustaining arrhythmia called torsade de pointes, which can be life-threatening. A number of antibiotics (macrolides and fluoroquinolones) have been associated with QT prolongation, and their actions are more likely to be serious if other medications also prolong the QT interval or if the patient has a predisposition to a long QT to begin with.

G **Adult immunization**

1. It is important for adults to have immunity to **all of the childhood diseases except pertussis.** (Although pertussis may occur in adults, it usually is mild, and the available vaccines are not well tolerated when administered to adults.)
   - **a.** If individuals have not been previously vaccinated against tetanus and diphtheria, a series of such vaccines should be administered. Booster doses of tetanus should be given every 10 years to all adults but may be given earlier if an individual has a tetanus-prone wound and the previous dose of toxoid was given more than 5 years earlier. Passive immunization with tetanus immunoglobulin is indicated if a wound has been extensively contaminated with dirt. Diphtheria toxoid is usually coadministered with tetanus.
   - **b.** Killed poliovirus vaccine should be given to adults who are not already immune, especially those with children who are due to receive live poliovirus vaccine. Although polio may be eradicated worldwide in the early years of the twenty-first century, cessation of standard childhood polio vaccination may not follow until several years of eradication have elapsed.
   - **c.** Because rubella in a pregnant woman can result in a devastating infection of the fetus, all women of childbearing age should be immune to rubella. Serum tests for antibody to rubella are widely available to help identify adults who need vaccination. Rubella is a part of the standard panel of childhood vaccines.
   - **d.** If there is no history of mumps or measles illness or vaccination, the appropriate live virus vaccines for these illnesses should be given. Although measles may rarely occur in vaccinated individuals, this is a rare event when two doses of vaccine have been appropriately administered.

2. Special vaccination issues concern the **elderly** (aged 65 years and older) and **chronically ill** patients, especially those with cardiac or pulmonary disease. All such patients should receive **pneumococcal vaccination** once and, in the appropriate season, should have annual **influenza vaccination.** Reimmunization with pneumococcal vaccine may be considered for those individuals who had their first dose before the age of 65 if more than 5 years has elapsed since that dose. A new conjugate vaccine to prevent pneumococcal infections has been developed for children, and it has reduced the burden of pneumococcal disease. This vaccine is not currently recommended for adults.
3. **Travelers** to countries where **yellow fever** is endemic (most of tropical Africa and South America) should receive this vaccine. **Typhoid** immunizations may be recommended for certain travelers. **Hepatitis A** (HAV) vaccine is recommended for travelers who expect to encounter poor sanitary facilities, especially those resulting in human fecal contamination of food or water. Hepatitis A vaccine has largely supplanted the use of immune serum globulin (ISG), which has been in short supply. Direct intramuscular injection of ISG is still suggested if there is not a window of at least 2 weeks before a high-risk exposure to hepatitis A.
4. Universal immunity to **HBV** and **varicella** are current public health goals. Although individuals who are already immune by virtue of prior infection or vaccination do not usually benefit from vaccination, both vaccines can be given safely to persons whose exposure history is unknown. Both vaccines are less effective in individuals with impaired immune status. Because varicella vaccine is a live virus vaccine, it should be used cautiously or not at all in patients with known advanced immunodeficiency.
   a. Adults who have durable immunity to varicella-zoster virus from a clinical bout of chickenpox in childhood do not need vaccination.
   b. Adults with no history of chickenpox or no serologic evidence of immunity should receive two doses of vaccine.
   c. Adults with no history of HBV or vaccination for it should receive three doses of vaccine in an appropriate schedule. Although universal administration of hepatitis A vaccine is not yet recommended, there is a formulation of hepatitis A and hepatitis B vaccine combined that would reduce the total number of injections.
5. **Asplenic individuals** should have **pneumococcal** and **meningococcal vaccinations,** even though protection from these infections is incomplete. In preparation for elective splenectomy, immunizations should be performed before surgery.
6. **Hepatitis A** (HAV) vaccine is highly immunogenic and safe. It is recommended in areas with unusually high rates of HAV, for travelers to parts of the world where HAV is more common than it is in the United States, and for people with hepatitis C (HCV).
7. **Meningococcal vaccine** has been recommended for college-age students—especially those living in dormitories. There have been outbreaks of serious meningococcal infections on college campuses, although the number of cases per year is small. The vaccine is well tolerated but has a limited duration of effectiveness (a few years) and does not protect against type b meningococcal infections.

III EFFECTIVE USE OF THE MICROBIOLOGY LABORATORY

To maximize the usefulness of any microbiology laboratory, it is necessary to be familiar with its specific capabilities and procedures. The following are general guidelines.

A Obtaining and handling specimens

1. **Fresh specimens are superior to old ones.** This is especially true when quantitative results are important (e.g., colony counts of urine cultures) or when the target organism is fragile (e.g., pro-

tozoal trophozoites in stools). If immediate delivery of a specimen is not possible, proper maintenance of the specimen should be ensured until it can be processed.

a. Some bacteria (e.g., *N. gonorrhoeae*) are sensitive to cold and should not be refrigerated.
b. Specimens to be cultured for anaerobes should be maintained in a prereduced, oxygen-free environment or in a syringe without any air and without a needle. They should be transported to the laboratory for immediate plating.

2. **Large specimens are better than small ones.** In most cases it is preferable to have adequate material to culture than to have only a swab; the laboratory technologist should have the final choice as to which portion to use. Sometimes, multiple specimens are needed to identify microorganisms (e.g., *M. tuberculosis*) that are shed infrequently or in small numbers.
3. **Biological hazards should be labeled and handled properly.** Laboratories have instituted **universal precautions** and treat all specimens as potentially infectious. Some bacteria and fungi may be especially hazardous in pure culture (e.g., *Brucella, Francisella, Coccidioides*), and the laboratory should be notified if these organisms are suspected clinically so that appropriate care can be taken.
4. **Newer techniques may bypass or accelerate culture results.** Tests for gonorrhea and chlamydia can now be done without concern for maintaining bacterial viability and with results that are much faster than before. Similarly, culture testing for mycobacteria is now faster than before (positive results back in 10 days vs. 30 days), and DNA probes can identify mycobacteria in less than a day once cultures are positive.

B **Interpreting negative and positive cultures** When a diagnosis rests on identifying an organism obtained from a clinical specimen, it is crucial to recognize what represents simple contamination by other body flora or inanimate sources. Laboratory results are more credible when a specimen has been stained and shown to contain the appropriate cell type (e.g., neutrophil or alveolar macrophage in sputum) and lacks evidence of contamination (e.g., squamous epithelial cells in sputum or urine). When care and attention have been lavished on a good specimen, almost any positive result is significant.

1. If antibiotics have been administered, the potential for positive cultures is reduced, and the predictive value of negative cultures also is diminished.
2. When cultures are truly negative, the use of special media and growth conditions should be considered. Supplementary nutrients or suppression of other organisms may be necessary to permit growth and identification.
3. Cultures that are repeatedly positive for a given organism may be more convincing than a single positive specimen. This is especially true for blood cultures. Specimens taken from normally sterile sites such as CSF and joint and pleural fluids usually are reliable when obtained aseptically. However, if they are culture-positive for skin or mucous membrane commensals, repeat cultures can be helpful.
4. Corroborative tests such as antigen detection, specific nucleic acid probes, and seroconversion (i.e., the development of antibodies to a pathogen) can establish the significance of a single culture-positive specimen or establish a diagnosis when cultures have not been obtained or are negative.
5. Quantitative tests such as viral load for human immunodeficiency virus (HIV) and quantitative bronchoalveolar lavage (BAL) fluid cultures may be useful in assessing the severity of disease or the probability that a positive culture represents true infection.

C **Interpreting antimicrobial susceptibility tests** In vitro testing of antimicrobial susceptibility can provide useful information about the specific microbe causing an infection. For many bacteria, these tests can be accomplished rapidly, with results sometimes available in hours. However, **the conditions used in susceptibility testing do not necessarily simulate conditions in the patient.**

1. The results of susceptibility testing may show the microorganism to be susceptible, intermediately susceptible, or resistant to the drug being tested. This information presupposes that the drug

concentration at the site of infection will be similar to what usually is found in serum. It also assumes that the organism will be inhibited or killed at the infection site if it is exposed to such a drug concentration.

2. Another way to assess susceptibility is to determine the actual concentration of antibiotic needed to inhibit the microorganism. This usually is done by exposing the microbe to varying concentrations of the drug and observing which is the lowest one to inhibit growth [**minimum inhibitory concentration (MIC)**]. The lower the MIC, the more susceptible the organism. The epsilometer test (E-test) is usually a reliable way to obtain an MIC without the inconvenience of preparing serial dilutions of drug. In some instances, clinical experience shows that a drug is ineffective despite in vitro data that suggest it would work. For example, cephalosporins are not useful in treating infections caused by methicillin-resistant *S. aureus,* although blood and tissue levels in excess of the MIC are easily achievable.
3. Direct measurement of serum or tissue levels of the drug being used may be desirable so that the dosage can be adjusted to avoid toxicity and to maximize therapeutic benefit. This is especially true for patients who may have less predictable blood or tissue levels of antibiotic because of altered drug metabolism or excretion secondary to renal or hepatic dysfunction. For example, vancomycin is a time-dependent antibiotic, and levels should be >8 μg/mL at all times. For most patients, standard dosing regimens can achieve this goal, but patients with fluctuations of renal function or certain forms of continuous dialysis can have unpredictably low levels and may need to be redosed. High levels of vancomycin have not been clearly associated with toxicity, but peak levels higher than 40 μg/mL are unnecessary.

IV RISK FACTORS FOR INFECTION

Sometimes it is possible to identify patient characteristics that modify the likelihood or severity of an infection. In general, the intensity or frequency of exposure and the degree of susceptibility correlate with potential hazard of infection.

A Diabetes In general, patients with diabetes are not known to have infections more frequently than individuals without glucose intolerance. However, there are a few significant differences.

1. **Foot and lower leg ulcers,** which may become infected, are more likely to occur in patients with diabetes. Such soft tissue infections are more likely to involve gram-negative rods, and they are more difficult to cure than those occurring in nondiabetic individuals. These infections tend to occur in patients with neuropathy or severe vascular disease.
2. **Genital infections** with *Candida* species, especially vulvovaginal candidiasis, are more likely to occur in patients with diabetes. Urinary tract infections may be more common and more severe in these patients, and the increased morbidity probably is related to bladder dysfunction in those patients with diabetic neuropathy. It is often recommended that urinary tract infections be more vigorously treated in patients with diabetes.
3. Some **rare diseases** occur almost exclusively in diabetic patients.
   a. **Malignant otitis externa** is a painful, rapidly progressive, and locally destructive disease of the external auditory canal that may extend to the temporal bone and the brain. *Pseudomonas aeruginosa* is the causative agent (see V B 1 a).
   b. **Rhinocerebral mucormycosis,** a fungal infection that starts in the nose or paranasal sinuses, is locally destructive. It is found in patients with severe metabolic acidosis (e.g., in patients with diabetes and ketoacidosis).
   c. **Synergistic gangrene** is a soft tissue infection that often is attributable to streptococci and obligate anaerobes. It may involve the skin or the underlying fascial structures and tends to progress relentlessly unless treated with extensive surgical débridement.

d. **Emphysematous cholecystitis** is a rare but severe infection of the gallbladder. Unlike ordinary cholecystitis, it requires urgent antibiotic administration and consideration of surgery. The clinical clues are similar to that of cholecystitis but there is often high fever, tachycardia, hypotension, and other evidence of sepsis. X-rays, computed tomography (CT) scan, and other imaging studies show gas in the gallbladder wall.

B Alcoholism Acute and chronic alcohol use can impair neurologic function and decrease the efficacy of neutrophils. In addition, chronic alcohol use can result in severe organ damage, especially to the liver.

1. The incidence of pneumococcal, aspiration, and gram-negative bacillary **pneumonias** is greater in alcoholics than it is in the general population. Tuberculosis, anaerobic lung abscess, and empyema also are more common.
2. When ascites is present, alcoholics may develop **spontaneous bacterial peritonitis,** a bacterial infection of ascitic fluid that occurs in the absence of bowel perforation. This infection, usually caused by gram-negative aerobic bacilli or enterococci, also occurs in nonalcoholic patients with ascites (e.g., nephrotic syndrome).

C Injection drug use Several infections are more common in injection drug users than in comparable individuals who do not use such substances. **Fever** in such drug users must be evaluated carefully because pyogenic bacterial infections can progress rapidly if treatment is delayed.

1. **Infections related to unsterile techniques.** Injection drug users are prone to a variety of suppurative complications because, in most cases, the preparation of the drug is not aseptic, equipment is not sterile, and skin cleansing is inadequate.
   a. **Bacterial endocarditis,** which often occurs on the tricuspid valve (a valve rarely infected in other populations), is the most serious infection. Usually, the bacterium responsible is *S. aureus.*
   b. **Superficial skin infections** are common, and infectious arthritis, usually caused by *P. aeruginosa* or *S. aureus,* is seen frequently.
   c. **Tetanus,** although rare, occurs more frequently, because injection drug users are more likely to have improperly cleaned wounds and low levels of immunity.
2. **Infections related to needle sharing.** Some contagious diseases can be transmitted efficiently via the small amount of blood in used needles and syringes. For example, the incidence of HBV, HCV, and HIV infection is increased in injection drug users.

D Homosexuality

1. **Homosexual men.** Infectious agents include *Shigella* species, *N. gonorrhoeae, G. intestinalis, Chlamydia trachomatis, Entamoeba histolytica, Treponema pallidum,* HAV, and human papillomavirus (HPV). HIV, HBV, and non-A, non-B hepatitis virus have been recognized as being hyperendemic among American homosexual men, especially those living in urban communities. The incidence of many of these infections has declined as sexual practices have changed in response to the HIV epidemic.
2. **Homosexual women.** The incidence of infectious diseases is not known to be increased in homosexual women.

E Occupational exposure

1. The risk of occupation-related infection may be **unpredictable,** as in the outbreaks of **Pontiac fever,** which were related to the aerosolization of *Legionella pneumophila*–contaminated water via air-conditioning ducts throughout an office building.
2. The risk of infection also may be influenced by factors outside the immediate work environment. For example, the risk of brucellosis among slaughterhouse workers is determined largely by the

number of livestock infected and to a lesser extent by the degree of the worker's exposure to the blood of infected livestock.

3. When an increased risk is **predictable,** certain preventive measures can be instituted (e.g., immunization of veterinarians against rabies).

F **Internal prostheses** When a prosthesis (or any foreign material such as heart valves) is inserted into the body, there is a possibility that an infection will develop at the site of insertion. Because of the human body's reaction to foreign material, a prosthetic organ is susceptible to infection by a greater number and variety of organisms than is the native, damaged organ. In addition, the clinical presentation of these infections may be atypical, and the interval between surgery and any manifestation of sepsis may be long (e.g., many years). *S. epidermidis* is involved in many of these infections. In most cases, bacteria are inoculated at the time of surgery, although secondary hematogenous or percutaneous spread is possible.

1. **Diagnosis.** The diagnosis of these infections depends on recognition of the characteristic clinical presentation. Infected joints almost always cause local pain and may be accompanied by erythema, loosening of the prosthesis, tenderness, and fever. Infected heart valves are almost always associated with fever and may be accompanied by valve dysfunction. These infections resemble native valve endocarditis.
2. **Therapy.** Treatment is most successful when it includes the removal or replacement of the prosthetic device as well as systemic antibiotic treatment.

G **Indwelling catheters** Despite the high risk of infection with the use of catheters, there is no indication for systemic antibiotic prophylaxis before or during catheterization.

1. Like internal prostheses, catheters such as intravenous or intra-arterial lines, bladder catheters, and endotracheal tubes offer sites of diminished host responsiveness. Furthermore, they provide communication between the external environment and the ordinarily sterile internal environment of the body.
2. In addition to intrinsic host factors, **two important factors determine the likelihood of catheter-related infection:** the **duration of catheterization** and the **degree of asepsis maintained during catheterization.** Duration is the most important factor in tracheal and urethral catheterization. Both factors are important in vascular catheterization.
   a. For long-term intravenous access with a surgically implanted catheter such as a Hickman silastic catheter, the risk of infection can be reduced, although not eliminated, by meticulous attention to sterile technique during insertion and by avoiding sites such as the groin that are prone to microbial contamination.
   b. For the patient who needs intravenous access for a short or intermediate period and has catheters placed in the arms, the sites should be changed every 48–72 hours. When a catheter is placed in a central vein for temporary intravenous access, the maximal duration of the catheterization at a given site is not absolute; however, there is a substantial risk of infection after a few days, and catheters should be removed as soon as possible or at the first sign of sepsis. Long catheters can be inserted in the arm but have their tip in the vena cava. These peripherally inserted central catheters (PICC) are used to deliver medications that can irritate peripheral veins or cause problems if the catheter gets dislodged.
   c. Vascular catheters generally are maintained with a high degree of care to avoid infection (e.g., aseptic dressing changes and the application of antibiotic-containing ointments to the insertion site); however, the importance of these measures in preventing infection is unknown. Most catheter-related infections show little or no evidence of disease at the catheter insertion site, although pus or significant redness at the insertion site are usually associated with infection of the catheter.

d. Some catheters are impregnated with silver or with antibiotics, and these are associated with fewer infections. However, whether the rate of serious infection such as bacteremia is significantly lower with these catheters is not certain.

H **Granulocytopenia** A specific risk that has been identified and carefully studied is related to **granulocytopenia,** the absence of adequate numbers of circulating neutrophils. The risk of infection is inversely related to the duration and degree of granulocytopenia. Neutrophil counts greater than 500/mm^3 are adequate protection against most opportunistic infection.

1. In most patients with granulocytopenia, the underlying disease is a hematologic malignancy, although reduced neutrophil levels can be seen in association with aplastic anemia, drug-induced agranulocytosis, and cytotoxic chemotherapy. Patients with hematologic malignancy have an additional infection risk when they get chemotherapy, which also disrupts the lining of the gastrointestinal tract and permits bacterial and fungal invasion.
2. The indigenous flora of patients with granulocytopenia is likely to be altered during hospitalization and with the administration of antibiotics. The microflora most commonly associated with infections in affected patients is derived from their indigenous flora. Bacteria such as *E. coli* and *P. aeruginosa,* as well as fungi such as *C. albicans,* are most often found.
3. Molds such as *Aspergillus* species may cause serious, often fatal, infections in patients with granulocytopenia. Spores are inhaled from the environment.
4. Persistent **fever** is the hallmark of infection in patients with neutropenia. Because uncontrolled infection can result in rapid clinical deterioration, antimicrobials are given immediately after appropriate culture specimens are obtained.
5. Granulocytes released into the circulation after the use of colony-stimulating factors such as filgrastim are fully functional. Thus, granulocytopenia after chemotherapy of solid tumors is often brief and unaccompanied by serious infection.

I **Corticosteroids** These agents are used to treat a variety of medical problems. Although steroids typically cause an increase in the number of circulating WBCs, they have an immunosuppressive effect that is strongly dose related.

1. The expression of this immunodeficiency is seen mostly in the increased incidence of infection usually controlled by cellular immunity (e.g., mycobacterial, fungal, nocardial, cytomegaloviral infections). Steroids also alter some diagnostic tests, most notably the expression of delayed hypersensitivity.
2. Steroids are used widely in transplantation procedures involving the kidney, heart, lung, liver, and bone marrow. In part, the infections experienced by these patients are related to corticosteroids and the other drugs (i.e., cyclosporine, tacrolimus, azathioprine, mycophenylate mofetil) used to prevent organ rejection. These latter drugs are sometimes referred to as "steroid sparing," but this refers to their use in reducing risk for nonimmune steroid-associated effects.
3. Injectable tumor necrosis factor (TNF)–inhibiting drugs are useful in the treatment of rheumatoid arthritis and inflammatory bowel disease. However, these drugs (especially infliximab) have been associated with an excess of cases of tuberculosis (TB; including extrapulmonary TB).

J **Neurologic deficits** Neurologic dysfunction may predispose patients to infection if such deficits cause body defenses to be more easily breached. The following are examples.

1. Elimination of the gag reflex, whether by stroke or coma. This may predispose patients to aspiration of oral or gastric contents.
2. Secondary infection of a hypoesthetic limb. Diabetic neuropathy can result in skin ulceration and infection.

3. Loss of neuromuscular control of the bladder. Long-term catheterization (with its attendant complications) may be necessary.

K Age The likelihood of acquiring certain infections varies considerably with age. In general, the maturation of the immune system is responsible for the changing pattern of infections in early childhood, and the presence of other medical illnesses accounts for most of the changes in late adulthood. Diminished immune response in the elderly may predispose them slightly to infection. For example, lower titers of antibody to influenza virus are found after immunization in the elderly than in younger adults.

L Nosocomial infection Although nosocomial infections (i.e., infections acquired after 2 or more days in the hospital) can involve any body site, they have some important common characteristics.

1. **Etiology and pathogenesis**
   a. **Residence in the hospital** predisposes patients to skin and mucosal colonization by microbial flora different from that found in ambulatory patients. Specifically, enteric gram-negative rods (e.g., *E. coli, Klebsiella*) or *P. aeruginosa* in the alimentary tract may spill over onto the skin or into the respiratory tree. The degree of illness influences the likelihood and rapidity of acquiring hospital flora.
   b. **Antimicrobials** given to prevent or treat infection may predispose patients to colonization and subsequent infection by hospital flora.
   c. **Instrumentation** (e.g., endotracheal tubes, intravenous catheters) may bypass some of the natural host defenses.
   d. **Failure to observe appropriate infection control measures** may permit the dissemination of hospital flora. The most important route for such dissemination is on the hands of health care workers.
   e. **Environmental factors,** such as those that permit colonization of water by legionella or imperfect air filtration that allows for fungal spores, may permit infection to occur at excess rates because of the inherently decreased resistance to infection by some patients.
2. **Therapy.** The duration of hospitalization and the likelihood that the infection was acquired nosocomially influence the use of empiric antibiotics to treat suspected infections. Knowledge of the antimicrobial susceptibility patterns of nosocomial microbes can be especially helpful.
3. **Prevention**
   a. **Proper technique on insertion** of devices such as endotracheal tubes and intravenous catheters is essential. Prompt discontinuation when they are no longer needed may reduce the burden of nosocomial infections.
   b. **Hands must be washed** or gloves changed between patient contacts. Alcohol-based gels or creams are effective and easier to use regularly than is thorough handwashing before and after each patient encounter.
   c. **Universal precautions** have been instituted in health care facilities to reduce the risk of transmission of many potentially hazardous microbes, including blood-borne viruses such as HIV type 1 (HIV-1) and HBV. It is extremely important to be familiar with the institutional policy of the health care facility in which one works. The essential principles of universal precautions are to treat each clinical specimen as potentially infective, to reduce sharp (e.g., needlestick) exposures, to avoid splashes of body fluids onto mucous membranes, and to dispose of potentially hazardous substances safely.
   d. For some diseases, especially tuberculosis, **reduction of exposure of health care workers** and **other patients** to aerosol droplets exhaled by an infected patient is important. In the setting of documented or suspected infection by such organisms, a private room with appropriate ventilation is required. Reduction of time spent in the room and fastidious use of masks by patients and health care workers can reduce risk of transmission.

e. **Protective isolation** is intended to protect patients from exogenous sources of colonization or infection. This measure is usually applied to patients with extensive burns or with extreme neutropenia. There are many different practices of protective isolation, but careful handwashing and use of gloves are probably most important.

V SPECIFIC INFECTIONS ACCORDING TO BODY SITE

A Central nervous system (CNS) infections

1. **Meningitis**
   a. **Acute meningitis** is an inflammatory disease involving the arachnoid layer of the meninges and the fluid that circulates in the ventricles and the subarachnoid space—the **CSF.**
      (1) **Classification.** There are two major classifications of meningitis: **bacterial** and **aseptic.** In both forms, fever, headache, and stiff neck occur.
         (a) In bacterial meningitis, the CSF has a pyogenic nature, with an elevated WBC count, an increased fraction of neutrophils, an elevated protein level, and a normal or lowered glucose level.
         (b) In aseptic meningitis, the CSF is characterized by a mildly elevated WBC count with a preponderance of lymphocytes, a normal or mildly elevated protein level, and a normal glucose level (i.e., more than two thirds of the serum level).
      (2) **Etiology.** The etiologic agents of meningitis can be divided into those causing bacterial meningitis and those causing aseptic meningitis.
         (a) **Bacterial meningitis.** The **causes vary with the age of the patient.** *E. coli* and *Streptococcus agalactiae* occur most frequently in infants; *H. influenzae,* which used to predominate in young children (2 months–6 years), has been practically eradicated by universal vaccination; *N. meningitidis* is most common in adolescents and young adults; and *S. pneumoniae* is most common in adults older than 25 years. *Listeria monocytogenes,* which enters the body through the gastrointestinal tract, is found most commonly in cancer patients and immunosuppressed individuals.
         (b) **Aseptic meningitis.** Usually a **viral disease,** aseptic meningitis may also reflect an **inflammatory process adjacent to the meninges** (e.g., cerebritis, brain abscess, sinusitis, or otitis). In partially treated bacterial meningitis, the CSF usually has a pyogenic nature, although antibiotics may modify the disease in such a way as to create an aseptic pattern. Drug hypersensitivity also may cause an aseptic meningitis (usually with a predominance of neutrophils in the WBCs) and may occur rarely with ibuprofen or a variety of other agents.
      (3) **Clinical features.** When bacteria cause meningitis, this manifestation usually is part of a **systemic, bacteremic infection.** An exception occurs when bacteria gain access to the meninges after trauma or surgery or via a bony defect (usually in the temporal area or the cribriform plate).
         (a) With disease due to *H. influenzae* or *S. pneumoniae,* focal infection such as **pneumonia** or **otitis** also may be apparent.
         (b) With disease due to *N. meningitidis,* there may be a characteristic systemic infection consisting of a **petechial** or **purpuric skin rash and hypotension,** which can develop rapidly.
         (c) With aseptic meningitis due to echoviruses or coxsackieviruses, there may be a characteristic **rash resembling rubella** or a **vesicular** or **petechial rash.**
      (4) **Therapy**
         (a) **Bacterial meningitis. Antibiotics** have a significant impact on the outcome of this disease. Without treatment, death is almost certain; with treatment, however, the mortality rate is reduced to approximately 20% of those patients who are not moribund at

the time of diagnosis. Bactericidal antibiotics should be given in dosages that permit the drug to achieve killing levels in the CSF. Because the blood-brain barrier blocks virtually all drugs and reduces drug penetration from the blood into the CSF, maximum tolerated systemic dosages should be given even at the end of the treatment course (usually a total of 2 weeks).

(i) In adults, initial therapy with a combination of a broad-spectrum cephalosporin and vancomycin is used initially. Frequently, this can be simplified once the results of cultures and sensitivities have been obtained. Ampicillin is still usually effective against *S. pneumoniae* and virtually always effective against *N. meningitidis* and *Listeria.*

(ii) If resistant organisms are found, the appropriate drug (e.g., cefotaxime or vancomycin) is begun or continued, and other agents are stopped. *S. pneumoniae* resistant to penicillin (and sometimes cephalosporins) is being isolated more frequently. In critically ill patients with suspected or established pneumococcal meningitis, vancomycin should be added to the regimen until susceptibility information is available.

(iii) If pyogenic meningitis is present, a short course of corticosteroids such as dexamethasone starting **before or with** the antibiotics can prevent death and substantial morbidity in adults or children.

(b) **Aseptic meningitis.** There is **no specific chemotherapy** for this condition. Any underlying disease should be treated. If drug hypersensitivity is suspected, the offending agent should be stopped.

b. Chronic meningitis

(1) **Etiology.** The most common causes of chronic meningitis are tuberculosis, cryptococcal disease, malignancy, and sarcoidosis.

(2) **Clinical features.** Chronic meningitis may have an indolent presentation, with symptoms similar to those of acute meningitis or with altered mentation with or without fever. CSF abnormalities may progress if the underlying disease is untreated. In many of these diseases, the CSF glucose level is low. Chronic meningitis should be considered when a low CSF glucose level is noted in patients who are found not to have acute bacterial meningitis.

(3) **Therapy.** Treatment is directed at the underlying disease.

(a) **Tuberculosis** is treatable if there is not already extensive neurologic deterioration. Almost all **antituberculous drugs** (e.g., isoniazid, rifampin) achieve good levels in the CSF and are useful in the treatment of tuberculous meningitis (see VII C).

(b) **Cryptococcal meningitis** may be difficult to treat and has a high relapse rate, especially when it occurs as a complication of HIV infection [see VIII G 1 c (1)]. Treatment usually begins with **amphotericin B alone or in combination with flucytosine,** but there is a high rate of failure and relapse. **Triazole drugs** such as fluconazole are useful in the prevention of relapse; they also may be appropriate as first-line therapy in mild cases.

(c) **Malignancy** involving the meninges is difficult to treat and may require **neural radiation therapy** or **intrathecal chemotherapy.**

(d) **Sarcoidosis** usually is treated with **corticosteroids.**

2. Encephalitis

a. Etiology. Most encephalitides are caused by viruses, several of which are transmitted by the bites of infective mosquitoes.

b. Clinical features. Patients with encephalitis usually present with altered mentation, seizures, or both. The CSF may be normal or have an aseptic pattern.

c. Diagnosis. Diagnosis involves measuring rising titers of antibody to one of the encephalitis viruses in patients with a compatible clinical syndrome. When **herpes simplex encephalitis** is suspected, early antiviral treatment is recommended. Measurement of herpes simplex virus–specific nucleic acid in CSF has largely supplanted brain biopsy for diagnosis. Successful treatment of herpes encephalitis depends on initiation of medications before neurologic deterioration becomes extensive. West Nile virus was first described as a cause of encephalitis in New York in 1999, but since then this mosquito-borne infection has been found through much of North America. Patients with West Nile encephalitis can have a complete recovery of function, but many patients have severe weakness during the infection and may recover only partially if at all.

d. Differential diagnosis

(1) *Toxoplasma gondii* can cause encephalitis in patients with diminished T-cell function [e.g., due to acquired immunodeficiency syndrome (AIDS) or post-transplantation immunosuppressive therapy].

(2) Some intoxications and immune diseases [e.g., systemic lupus erythematosus (SLE)] may have a presentation indistinguishable from encephalitis.

(3) Endocarditis also should be considered.

e. Therapy. Treatment of viral encephalitis is **supportive,** with the exception of acyclovir for herpes simplex encephalitis. Toxoplasmosis, drug intoxication, endocarditis, and immune diseases are treatable, and patients with associated encephalitis usually respond.

3. Intracranial abscess. Suppurative infections can involve the contents of the calvarium, usually by direct spread from an infected sinus or ear.

a. Etiology. The bacteriology of intracranial infections reflects the types of organisms that cause disease in more superficial contiguous structures such as streptococci and anaerobic bacteria. Abscesses can be localized to the extradural (also called epidural) or subdural spaces or in the brain parenchyma. Rarely, hematogenous spread of bacteria can give rise to intracranial abscesses. Less common agents are *Toxoplasma, Nocardia,* and *Cryptococcus* species, which usually are seen in immunocompromised patients with reduced helper T cell numbers or function.

b. Diagnosis. Magnetic resonance imaging (MRI) [more sensitive] or **computed tomography (CT)** [more widely available and less expensive] of the brain is helpful in making the diagnosis. Early scans may be equivocal, but studies repeated within a few days are almost always positive, especially with the use of contrast. Definitive diagnosis requires aspiration for stain and culture.

c. Therapy. Bacterial abscesses are treated with appropriate **antibiotics** that penetrate brain tissue well. These may include penicillin, chloramphenicol, and metronidazole. The usual treatment is given for infection by *Toxoplasma* (e.g., pyrimethamine, sulfadiazine), *Cryptococcus* (e.g., amphotericin B, flucytosine), or *Nocardia* (e.g., a sulfa drug with or without trimethoprim). Surgical excision or decompression is not always needed, but some patients, especially those with large lesions or slow response to treatment, require **serial aspirations** or more aggressive surgical débridement.

B Head and neck infections

1. Otitis. Infections of the ear can involve any of the ear's three major anatomic areas—the outer, middle, or inner ear.

a. Outer ear infections tend to be minor irritations of the external auditory canal. Topical antibiotic treatment is used for external otitis. An exception is **malignant otitis externa,** a destructive process most commonly found in diabetic patients (see IV A 3 a). Malignant otitis externa requires antibiotics that are effective against *P. aeruginosa* infection plus surgical débridement and drainage.

b. Middle ear infection, or **otitis media,** typically is a disease of children and manifests as ear pain and reduced auditory acuity. Otoscopy shows a dull, poorly mobile tympanic membrane with or without pus behind it. The most common causes are pneumococci, *Streptococcus pyogenes, Moraxella catarrhalis,* and *H. influenzae.* In chronic cases, especially if multiple courses of antibiotics have been given, enteric gram-negative rods and anaerobes may be involved. Therapy for acute otitis media is amoxicillin, amoxicillin with clavulanic acid, trimethoprim with sulfamethoxazole, a macrolide such as azithromycin or clarithromycin, or an oral cephalosporin. Cultures and appropriate therapy are suggested for chronic otitis media.

c. **Inner ear infections** rarely are caused by bacteria. However, several viruses may be associated with a syndrome of **vertigo** with or without **tinnitus.** No treatment is helpful.

2. **Sinusitis.** The paranasal sinuses have continuous exposure to the external environment via the ostia in the nose. Under normal conditions, host defenses maintain the sterile environment of the sinuses. However, when mucociliary clearance is interrupted because of structural or functional abnormalities, infection can supervene. In addition, patients with mid- to late-stage HIV infection are prone to recurrent or chronic sinusitis.

   a. **Etiology.** As in middle ear infections, **virulent bacteria** such as pneumococci and *H. influenzae* are most likely to cause acute disease, and anaerobic or enteric organisms are associated with more chronic infections. Bacterial sinusitis may follow and mimic viral upper respiratory infections; however, only the bacterial infections go on to develop suppurative complications of the CNS.

   b. **Diagnosis. Sinus radiography** shows mucosal thickening or opacification or air–fluid levels in sinusitis. Tenderness and edema help localize disease to the sinuses but are not present in all patients. **CT scanning** is more sensitive than sinus radiography, but it should not be performed in the early stages of "colds," because minor sinus abnormalities are commonly seen on CT scan in patients without significant ongoing sinusitis. Most cases of sinusitis are diagnosed clinically, and imaging is reserved for patients with refractory or recurrent disease.

   c. **Therapy**

      (1) In mild cases, **antibiotics** (e.g., penicillin, cephalosporins, macrolides, or sulfa drugs) alone or in combination with decongestants are adequate.

      (2) Functional **endoscopic sinus surgery** can be useful in patients with repeated or persistent infection.

3. **Odontogenic infections,** the most common infections occurring in the oral cavity, usually are local and respond to simple measures such as draining abscesses, restoring carious teeth, and maintaining good oral hygiene. Sometimes, however, soft tissue infections in the mouth can dissect through tissue planes and involve deeper structures of the face or neck. Examples are **Ludwig's angina,** which is an infection extending to the floor of the mouth, and **retropharyngeal abscess,** which can track down to the mediastinum. The involved bacteria are streptococci and indigenous oral anaerobes.

4. **Eye infections.** Normally, the eyes are resistant to infections.

   a. **Conjunctivitis.** Superficial infections of the conjunctiva usually are bacterial or viral and resolve spontaneously. An exception is **gonorrheal conjunctivitis,** a rare adult disease that must be treated vigorously.

   b. **Keratitis.** Because the transparency of the cornea is crucial for vision, diagnostic tests such as bacterial and viral smears and cultures are warranted. Initial therapy is guided by the clinical picture, because a variety of organisms can cause keratitis, including *S. aureus, P. aeruginosa,* streptococci, numerous fungi, and herpes simplex and varicella-zoster viruses. It is important to recognize keratitis caused by herpes simplex virus so that appropriate antiviral therapy to prevent blindness can be instituted.

   c. **Endophthalmitis.** Bacteria most commonly cause this infection of the internal structures of the eye, which may follow eye surgery or infection elsewhere in the body. Systemic and topical antibiotics, selected on the basis of clinical findings and Gram stain of ocular material, are administered to prevent irreversible destruction of the eye. However, the prognosis for normal visual acuity after endophthalmitis is poor.

C Respiratory tract infections

1. **Upper respiratory infections.** Infections involving the nose, throat, larynx, airways, and adjacent structures are the most common causes of morbidity in the United States.

a. **Etiology.** Upper respiratory infections almost invariably are viral. Rarely is a specific cause sought or found.
b. **Clinical features.** These "colds" and "flus" involve rhinorrhea, coryza, cough, a slight fever, and, sometimes, sore throat. During seasons when influenza is epidemic in a community, headache, cough, myalgia, and a more marked temperature elevation may suggest the diagnosis.
c. **Therapy.** Treatment for "colds" is symptomatic, although influenza A virus infections may resolve more quickly when an antiviral such as amantadine, rimantidine, oseltamivir, or zanamivir is administered. These medications can be useful in preventing influenza in high-risk patients when immunization is not feasible or is performed too late to offer meaningful protection.
d. **Prevention.** Because of the ubiquity and extreme infectivity of most epidemic viruses, prevention of most upper respiratory disease is difficult. Careful handwashing is a simple measure to prevent the spread of upper respiratory infections. In many cases, timely administration of vaccine developed against the epidemic strains that exist during a particular season also may prevent influenza. Immunization should be directed at individuals who are at greatest risk for complications of upper respiratory infection such as elderly or chronically ill individuals. Yearly immunization has a favorable impact on influenza morbidity and mortality. In addition, immunization of healthy adults may reduce absenteeism at work, and vaccination of health care providers may prevent or slow epidemics of influenza in nursing homes and hospitals.

2. **Pharyngitis**
   a. **Etiology.** The major etiologic agents of pharyngitis, a common illness, are viruses, *Mycoplasma pneumoniae, Chlamydia pneumoniae,* and *S. pyogenes* (group A streptococci).
   b. **Clinical features. Sore throat** that occurs with or without objective findings of erythema or exudate on the oropharynx or tonsils is characteristic.
   c. **Therapy**
      (1) Treatment for group A streptococcal pharyngitis may accelerate healing and reduce symptoms, but the major purpose of treating this disorder is **prevention of subsequent rheumatic fever,** a rare sequela.
      (2) Viral pharyngitis does not improve with any known chemotherapy.
      (3) Whether treatment of mycoplasmal or chlamydial pharyngitis is beneficial is not known.

3. **Tracheobronchitis** is an infection of the airways.
   a. **Etiology.** Most cases of tracheobronchitis are associated with infection by mycoplasma or by **viruses,** such as influenza or parainfluenza virus (in adults) or respiratory syncytial virus (in young children). However, bacteria may play a role in patients with chronic obstructive pulmonary disease (COPD) and cystic fibrosis. *H. influenzae, S. aureus,* and *P. aeruginosa* are believed to be pathogenic in those with cystic fibrosis (see Chapter 2 IV B).
   b. **Clinical features and laboratory findings.** Cough with abundant, thick sputum is characteristic of tracheobronchitis. Fever, chest pain, and wheezing also may occur. If rales or consolidation is found, pneumonia is suggested. The WBC count and chest radiograph are unchanged from baseline in uncomplicated tracheobronchitis.
   c. **Therapy.** Simple supportive measures usually suffice. Antibiotics usually are given to patients with COPD exacerbation, although the benefit of such therapy is modest and most pronounced when all three elements of exacerbation are present: dyspnea, increased volume of sputum, and increased purulence of sputum. Cystic fibrosis patients undergo chest physical therapy and receive antimicrobial agents according to sputum bacteriology (see Chapter 2 IV B 6 b).

4. **Pneumonia**
   a. **Etiology.** The causes are innumerable and include bacteria, viruses, fungi, and parasites. Although identification of the specific cause of pneumonia is ideal, many patients can be treated initially on the basis of clinical and demographic features.

b. Clinical features and diagnosis

(1) **Patient history** may indicate an underlying condition. For example, the incidence of bacterial pneumonia is increased in association with COPD or alcoholism. Fever is usually, but not invariably, present. Evidence of extra fluid in the lungs is noted as rales or consolidation on physical examination and infiltrate on chest radiograph. In addition, the appearance of the sputum can be useful for making the appropriate diagnosis.

(2) Because of the **vast differential diagnosis,** it is helpful to consider pneumonia in two ways (recognizing that a considerable overlap is possible):

(a) Whether it developed at home **(community-acquired)** or in a hospital or institution **(hospital-acquired** or **nosocomial)**

(b) Whether it had a rapid onset with chills, fever, and cough **(classical)** or a more indolent onset **(atypical)**

c. Pneumonia syndromes

(1) **Classical community-acquired pneumonia**

(a) **Etiology.** This syndrome most frequently is caused by *S. pneumoniae.* However, *H. influenzae, M. catarrhalis,* and enteric gram-negative bacilli also can cause this clinical picture.

(b) **Diagnosis.** Gram staining of expectorated sputum shows large numbers of neutrophils (i.e., > 25 per low-power field) and few squamous cells (< 10 per low-power field). The bacterial flora may be mixed, but often there is a predominance of one morphologic type such as the lancet-shaped gram-positive cocci, which appear in pairs in pneumococcal pneumonia.

(c) **Therapy.** When the presentation is truly classic, with a single shaking chill, rust-colored sputum, and a moderate fever accompanied by a Gram stain suggesting pneumococci, penicillin used to be the drug of choice. Because so many areas have a high incidence of pneumococcal penicillin resistance, an alternative agent such as a macrolide or fluoroquinolone active against gram-positive bacteria (e.g., gatifloxacin, moxifloxacin, or levofloxacin) is preferred as initial treatment.

(i) A macrolide or fluoroquinolone is used in penicillin-allergic patients when symptoms blend into those seen in the atypical form or when the Gram stain is inconclusive.

(ii) If the Gram stain shows gram-negative rods, therapy appropriate for *Haemophilus* or enteric gram-negative bacilli is given, usually in the hospital.

(iii) If gram-negative cocci appear singly or in pairs, treatment should be directed toward *M. catarrhalis.*

(2) **Atypical community-acquired pneumonia**

(a) **Etiology.** This syndrome usually is caused by *M. pneumoniae* or *C. pneumoniae,* although a variety of viruses may be responsible, including adenovirus, parainfluenza virus, and respiratory syncytial virus.

(b) **Diagnosis.** Atypical community-acquired pneumonia is less severe than the classical form, with a less diagnostic sputum. Systemic symptoms (e.g., myalgia, arthralgia, skin rash) are more prominent, and chest complaints (e.g., pleuritic pain, productive cough) are less marked in atypical pneumonia than in classical pneumonia. Gram stain shows some neutrophils and a variety of bacterial forms. Cultures seldom are diagnostic. Chest radiographs usually show patchy, bilateral infiltrates and little or no pleural effusion.

(c) **Differential diagnosis**

(i) **Aspiration pneumonia** may result from pulmonary aspiration of oral secretions, especially with diminished protection of the airways (e.g., after unconsciousness, a seizure, or vocal cord paralysis).

(ii) **Tuberculosis** is also a consideration in a case of a slowly evolving pulmonary infection. However, there usually is other evidence of tuberculosis (e.g., radiographic findings, an exposure history, or a positive acid-fast smear of the sputum) [see VII C].

(iii) **Legionnaires' disease** also may occur in this way (see VII E).

(d) **Therapy.** Patients with atypical pneumonia often present after they have had many days or over a week of symptoms. Effective treatment may not bring immediate relief but may further shorten the course of the illness. Any of the macrolides or fluoroquinolones is appropriate, and the oral route is adequate. Therapy for other nonclassical pneumonias involves the following measures:

(i) When **aspiration pneumonia** is suspected, an antibiotic with consistent activity against oral anaerobes and streptococci (e.g., penicillin or clindamycin) is suggested.

(ii) **Tuberculosis** always is treated with combinations of antibiotics (see VII C 2).

(iii) **Legionnaires' disease** usually responds to macrolides or fluoroquinolones, although some severely ill patients may require hospitalization (see VII E 5).

(3) **Classical (acute) hospital-acquired pneumonia**

(a) **Etiology.** This syndrome can be caused by a variety of bacteria. Patients often are granulocytopenic, postoperative, or intubated. Because these patients usually have pharyngeal colonization by enteric gram-negative aerobes, the pneumonia is likely to involve these organisms. All risk factors should be taken into consideration when assessing these patients.

(b) **Diagnosis.** Gram stain and culture of sputum are important in determining the organisms involved in this infection. Even though good respiratory specimens can be hard to obtain, it is worth the effort to make a microbial diagnosis for pneumonia patients either in or recently discharged from the hospital. More invasive tests such as bronchoscopy and lung biopsy may be needed to confirm the diagnosis.

(c) **Therapy.** When the Gram stain suggests inflammation and shows abundant gram-negative rods, recommended treatment is a β-lactam antibiotic with activity against a wide variety of enteric gram-negative organisms, with or without an aminoglycoside. Knowledge of susceptibility patterns in the hospital can help in choosing empiric therapy. When culture results are available, more specific therapy can be given. In patients with neutropenia, broad coverage (including activity against *P. aeruginosa*) is used. If *Legionella* is seriously considered, a macrolide or fluoroquinolone should be added. Hospitals with significant rates of infection caused by methicillin-resistant *Staphylococcus aureus* are settings where the use of vancomycin is prudent when the Gram stain suggests a staphylococcal infection or where the specimen could not be obtained.

5. **Lung abscess**

a. **Etiology.** This infection may be the result of a pyogenic pneumonia caused by pathogens such as *S. aureus* or *S. pyogenes.* More commonly, however, lung abscess occurs as a late stage in the evolution of an untreated anaerobic or mixed flora pneumonia, such as when oral or gastric contents enter the airway. Neurologic impairment of normal glottal reflexes predisposes patients to aspiration and lung abscess.

b. **Clinical features.** Approximately half of patients are afebrile, and some have long-standing constitutional complaints such as weight loss. A foul-smelling sputum is highly suggestive of anaerobic infection.

c. **Therapy.** Most lung abscesses drain into the tracheobronchial tree and can be cured with appropriate antimicrobial therapy, although the duration of therapy often is long.

6. **Thoracic empyema**

a. **Etiology.** This infection also is related to underlying pneumonia. Any pyogenic pneumonia may give rise to a pleural effusion, which may become infected. Rarely, anaerobic empyema is the only manifestation of thoracic infection; presumably, this occurs as a sequela to an anaerobic pneumonia or lung abscess, which may not be apparent at the time of the empyema.

b. Therapy

(1) Noninfected parapneumonic effusions with a relatively low WBC count and a pH above 7.2 usually resolve with systemic antimicrobial therapy.

(2) Infected effusions, or those with a very low pH or a high WBC count, usually require thoracostomy drainage.

D Gastrointestinal infections

1. **Food poisoning.** These syndromes represent a diverse collection of intoxications or infections associated with ingestion of food or beverage that has been contaminated with pathogenic organisms, toxins, or chemicals. Disregarding the purely chemical entities such as heavy metal poisoning, mushroom poisoning (see Chapter 5 IV D 5 b), and polychlorinated biphenyl (PCB) poisoning, food poisoning syndromes can be divided into those causing **gastrointestinal symptoms** and those causing **neurologic symptoms.** In all cases of suspected food poisoning, some epidemiologic assessment should be done to identify other infected individuals and to report outbreaks to public health authorities.

a. Gastrointestinal food poisoning is the most familiar type of food poisoning (see Chapter 5 IV D 4 and Table 5–1). Diarrhea, nausea, vomiting, and abdominal pain are the most common manifestations.

(1) **Clinical categories** usually are based on the incubation period, the food vehicle, and the nature of the gastrointestinal complaint.

(a) Preformed toxins give rise to the shortest-onset syndromes. For example, the enterotoxin-mediated syndromes caused by staphylococci, *Bacillus cereus,* and *Clostridium perfringens* manifest within a few hours after ingestion of the contaminated food.

(b) Diseases that depend on the growth of bacteria require a period of hours to days to manifest, and it may be difficult to relate the illness to a specific exposure. Sometimes cultures of various leftover foods are helpful; in other cases, careful recall of foods consumed is diagnostic.

(2) **Therapy.** Almost all forms of gastrointestinal food poisoning are self-limited and remit spontaneously within 1 or 2 days. Careful replacement of fluid and electrolytes may be needed for young children or those adults with significant underlying medical disease, but watchful waiting is usually sufficient.

b. Neurologic food poisoning is rare. However, it is important to establish the diagnosis so that appropriate therapy can be instituted immediately.

(1) **Botulism.** This syndrome is an intoxication caused by a preformed toxin of *Clostridium botulinum.* Although the toxin is destroyed by heating, the duration or degree of heating may be inadequate. Often, a gastrointestinal prodrome occurs before the classic flaccid paralysis sets in. Infants have the highest rate of botulism, and it is characterized by the germination *of C. botulinum* spores inside the baby and elaboration of the toxin directly into the gastrointestinal tract. When adults develop botulism from this mechanism of endogenous production of toxin, it is called **hidden botulism.**

(2) **Fish poisoning** (see Chapter 5 IV D 5 a)

(a) **Consumption of contaminated shellfish** can result in two types of poisoning: paralytic and neurotoxic.

(i) **Paralytic shellfish poisoning** results from contamination by neurotoxin-producing dinoflagellates of the genus *Gonyaulax.* This syndrome includes paresthesias followed by muscle weakness.

(ii) **Neurotoxic shellfish poisoning** results from shellfish contamination by dinoflagellates of the genus *Gymnodinium.* This syndrome is characterized by paresthesias without muscle weakness. Consumption of fleshy fish can give rise to a similar neurologic syndrome called **ciguatera** [see Chapter 5 IV D 5 a (1)].

(b) **Consumption of certain contaminated fish** such as tuna and bonito can result in an illness resembling a histamine reaction. This syndrome is called **scombroid.**

(3) **Monosodium glutamate intoxication** (sometimes called **Chinese restaurant syndrome**). This condition is characterized by a burning and tightness in the upper body accompanied by systemic symptoms such as flushing, diaphoresis, cramps, and nausea.

(4) **Therapy.** Neurologic food poisoning syndromes usually resolve completely but require patient reassurance and supportive medical care. Supportive measures may include tracheal intubation for patients with botulism or paralytic shellfish poisoning. Identifying the vehicle is crucial to prevent further occurrences. Specific antitoxin therapy is available for botulism and should be administered as soon as possible after the diagnosis is established.

2. **Infectious diarrhea.** Acute diarrhea often can be attributed to microorganisms. The occurrence of any infectious diarrhea suggests a break in optimal hygienic measures. The disease is transmitted either through fecal contamination of food or water or from human to human via fomites or by sexual contact (see Chapter 5 IV D 4).

a. **Etiology and pathogenesis.** Determining the specific etiologic agent of infectious diarrhea can be laborious and is often unsuccessful. It may be useful to distinguish invasive from non-invasive processes.

(1) **Invasive processes.** Certain agents of acute diarrhea (e.g., *Shigella, Salmonella, Entamoeba, Campylobacter*) invade the terminal ileum and colon, where they destroy mucosal cells and cause inflammation. A bloody diarrhea has been associated with some strains of *E. coli* that bear a toxin. Most of these strains belong to the O157:H7 serotype of *E. coli* and can be cultured by a clinical laboratory if they are alerted to the suspicion of this organism.

(2) **Noninvasive processes.** Other agents of acute diarrhea [e.g., enterotoxigenic *E. coli, Vibrio cholerae* (rarely found in the United States), *Cryptosporidium, G. intestinalis,* rotavirus] are enterotoxigenic and adhere to mucosal cells in the small intestine, where they produce diarrheal toxins.

b. **Clinical features.** Manifestations vary with respect to the presence of abdominal pain, cramps, and blood or mucus in the stool, as well as to the frequency and nature of the bowel movements.

(1) **Diarrhea due to invasive agents** generally is associated with rectal bleeding, fever, and systemic symptoms such as headache.

(2) **Diarrhea due to noninvasive agents** usually occurs without fever and is associated with fewer systemic complaints. However, substantial fluid loss from watery diarrhea in these patients may occur.

(3) **Diarrhea due to enterohemorrhagic *E. coli* (O157:H7)** is usually self-limited, but it can lead to hemolytic-uremic syndrome (HUS). This is a serious illness that tends to occur mostly in children and has a substantial mortality rate.

c. **Diagnosis.** It is important to distinguish among the various infectious diarrheal diseases because their therapies are different.

(1) **Microscopic examination**

(a) **Fecal leukocytes.** A useful test is to examine the stool for WBCs using Gram stain or preparations stained with methylene blue.

(i) **Invasive agents** may secrete cytotoxin or penetrate the mucosal wall of the bowel. Either mechanism may lead to the presence of leukocytes in the stool. [The diarrhea associated with *Clostridium difficile,* sometimes called **pseudomembranous colitis** (see Chapter 5 V I), also is associated with pus in the stool, as are several of the sexually transmitted proctitides and **inflammatory bowel diseases** (i.e., ulcerative colitis and regional enteritis or Crohn's disease).]

(ii) **Noninvasive agents** do not cause the migration of leukocytes into the bowel wall and the stool. However, special techniques are needed to identify *Microsporidium* or *Cryptosporidium* in the stool, and the laboratory may not perform these tests routinely.

(b) **Trophozoites or cysts** in the stool suggest the presence of protozoa such as *E. histolytica* or *G. intestinalis.*

(2) **Stool culture**

(a) The presence of fever or the identification of fecal leukocytes suggests an invasive pathogen. When the clinical severity or the epidemiologic setting makes the precise diagnosis important, the stool can be cultured for the most common of these pathogens (i.e., *Shigella, Salmonella,* and *Campylobacter*). Stool cultures take at least 2 days to process, so therapeutic decisions are often made clinically.

(b) Evaluation of the stool for protozoa (i.e., the **ova and parasite test**) also is recommended.

(c) *C. difficile* produces an enterotoxin leading to diarrhea, fever, and stool leukocytosis. (In severe cases, a pseudomembrane may be present in the rectum or colon.) Disease occurs during or shortly after the administration of antibacterial agents and is especially common in **nosocomial diarrhea.** Culture and toxin assays are available to diagnose *C. difficile* infection.

(3) **Proctosigmoidoscopy or colonoscopy.** These techniques may aid in the diagnosis of inflammation-related diarrhea, especially by allowing differentiation of infectious from noninfectious causes.

(4) **Biopsy.** In cases of persistent diarrhea in which less invasive techniques have failed to provide a diagnosis, **biopsy** of the large bowel (for *E. histolytica*) or the small bowel (for *G. intestinalis or Cryptosporidium*) may be diagnostic.

d. Therapy

(1) **Fluid and electrolyte replacement** is paramount, regardless of the causal agent, and should be adjusted according to the patient's degree of depletion.

(2) Specific **antimicrobial therapy** may be necessary.

(a) Among the bacterial causes of acute diarrhea, only *Shigella* infections are routinely treated. The inherent delay in diagnosis makes it unnecessary to treat most *Campylobacter, Salmonella,* and *E. coli* infections except in severely ill patients or those with impaired immunity. Most cases in previously healthy people resolve without incident within a few days to 1 week. When treatment is indicated, fluoroquinolones are usually effective, although increasing resistance to fluoroquinolones has been noted. Treatment of enterohemorrhagic *E. coli* (O157:H7) is not indicated, and, under some conditions, it may exacerbate the disease and lead to an increased risk of HUS.

(b) Antiprotozoal agents usually are indicated for giardiasis and amebiasis.

(c) Disease associated with *C. difficile* is treated with cessation of the causative antibiotic (when possible) and oral metronidazole. If this therapy fails, oral vancomycin may be used. Approximately 20% of patients will have recurrence after apparently successful treatment, and they can be retreated with the same regimen. A small number of patients have frequent recurrences despite good therapy.

e. Prognosis. The prospect for complete recovery from infectious diarrhea is excellent for all patients except those who are severely immunocompromised. In most cases, a cause is not established or even investigated. Diarrhea associated with *C. difficile* is normally easy to manage, but some patients can have poor outcomes, including death. This is almost always associated with significant underlying disease including prior organ transplantation and immune suppression.

E Intra-abdominal infections

1. **Peritonitis.** An inflammation of the lining of the abdominal cavity, peritonitis may result from bacterial infection or chemical irritation. It is characterized by sharp abdominal pain often with tenderness and rebound tenderness. Bowel sounds are often diminished or absent because of the

secondary ileus associated with peritonitis. There are two types of bacterial peritonitis. **Primary** (spontaneous) **peritonitis** occurs without other abdominal disease, and **secondary peritonitis** occurs after rupture or perforation of a hollow organ. It is crucial to distinguish between primary and secondary peritonitis, because a ruptured viscus requires surgical repair.

a. Primary peritonitis

(1) **Etiology.** Primary peritonitis is almost always preceded by ascites, usually secondary to hepatic cirrhosis. The causative organism most often is an enteric pathogen, usually *E. coli.* Other gram-negative rods, enterococci, and pneumococci are also seen.

(a) **In children,** primary peritonitis historically has been seen most often in association with **nephrotic syndrome** and ascites. Causative organisms usually are streptococci, pneumococci, and enteric gram-negative bacteria.

(b) **In adults,** primary peritonitis usually develops in the setting of **hepatic cirrhosis** and ascites. Most often, the causative organism is an enteric pathogen, usually *E. coli,* another enteric gram-negative rod, or an enterococcus.

(2) **Clinical features.** Anorexia, abdominal pain and distention, rebound tenderness, nausea, vomiting, fever, and hypotension may occur.

(3) **Diagnosis.** Paracentesis of peritoneal fluid, with smear and culture for appropriate bacteria, is necessary. Cultures may be somewhat insensitive and may need to be repeated. WBC counts greater than 250/mm^3 in peritoneal fluid suggest bacterial infection. Abdominal free air is not seen on abdominal radiograph. In some cases, exploratory laparotomy is required to rule out secondary peritonitis.

(4) **Therapy. Systemic antibiotics** are necessary for the treatment of primary peritonitis. If the Gram stain does not show a characteristic organism, empiric therapy for *E. coli, Klebsiella pneumoniae,* and pneumococci should be started. Because patients with advanced liver disease are already very sick, the mortality rate, even in appropriately treated patients, may be 20%.

(5) **Prevention.** After the first episode of primary peritonitis, a patient with liver disease should be offered antibiotic prophylaxis (e.g., with a fluoroquinolone) to prevent further bouts. Treatment of the liver disease is also important.

b. Secondary peritonitis

(1) **Etiology.** The causes of secondary peritonitis are many, but the process is the same in most cases. Usually, enteric pathogens gain access to the abdominal cavity through a tear or necrotic defect of an abdominal organ. Common examples include ruptured appendix and perforated peptic ulcer. In most cases, the infection is polymicrobial, and the causative organisms are endogenous.

(2) **Clinical features.** The early symptoms of secondary peritonitis are similar to those of spontaneous peritonitis. Abdominal pain, nausea, vomiting, and fever are common complaints. Tachycardia and shock may develop.

(3) **Diagnosis.** Diagnosis may be difficult in patients without the usual clinical features. For example, corticosteroid therapy may mask the pain and tenderness that usually characterize peritonitis, but septic complications continue to develop.

(a) The most important laboratory finding in secondary peritonitis is the presence of **free air in the abdomen,** as determined by chest or abdominal radiograph.

(b) Careful and repeated observation and consultation with a general surgeon help distinguish surgically remediable disease from mimicking conditions.

(4) **Therapy.** In most cases, **surgical repair** of the damaged viscus and **drainage of abdominal pus** are the cornerstones of therapy. Antibiotics with activity against enteric gram-negative bacilli and anaerobes (especially *Bacteroides fragilis*) also are important. The need for coverage for enterococci is controversial.

c. Peritonitis and peritoneal dialysis. Peritonitis is a frequent complication of peritoneal dialysis, whether it is performed acutely or on a continuous basis. Ordinarily, the dialysis need not be interrupted, and systemic or peritoneally administered antibiotics can be used for treatment. Skin flora are often implicated, but gram-negative rods and fungi are sometimes seen.

2. **Postoperative intra-abdominal abscesses.** Diagnosis of these infections is often difficult.
   a. **Etiology and pathogenesis**
      (1) Postoperative abscesses develop most frequently when the bowel has been breached in an operative procedure. However, they may occur when nonviable tissue or accumulations of blood, serum, urine, or bile are present in the abdominal cavity.
      (2) Although these infections usually occur within several days of the operative procedure, they may be delayed by weeks or months. They tend to develop near the anatomic site of the surgery, although the contour of the abdomen may allow infected fluid to move to other locations.
   b. **Diagnosis.** CT and ultrasonography are the most commonly used techniques for locating these abscesses. Most importantly, there must be a high index of suspicion for patients who have prolonged fever, abdominal pain, or both after surgery.
   c. **Therapy.** Once intra-abdominal abscesses have been identified, **they should be evacuated,** either by repeat surgery or through a temporary flexible drainage catheter. **Antimicrobial therapy** should be administered based on the results of Gram stain and cultures. Anaerobes play a major role in intra-abdominal abscesses and should be suspected when the fluid is foul-smelling or shows polymicrobial morphology on Gram stain. In selecting antimicrobial treatment, the onus is to prove that anaerobes are *not* present.
3. **Hepatic and splenic abscesses**
   a. **Etiology and pathogenesis.** Bacterial (pyogenic) abscesses may develop in the liver and spleen, although these sites are relatively protected from infection. They may be single or multiple and often are multibacterial. Hepatic abscesses usually are associated with biliary disease or portal vein bacteremia. Splenic abscesses are associated with systemic bacteremia, hemoglobinopathy, trauma, endocarditis, or intravenous drug use.
   b. **Clinical features.** Fever, chills, and pain near the affected organ are common. However, clinical findings may be subtle, making localization and diagnosis difficult.
   c. **Diagnosis.** Cross-sectional anatomic imaging such as CT scanning, MRI, or ultrasonography are usually used to make the diagnosis. Blood cultures should always be obtained. In travelers to areas endemic for ameobiasis or for immigrants from those areas, an evaluation for amoebic abscess using serologic tests or a cytologic analysis of the abscess fluid can be very helpful.
   d. **Therapy. Treatment is primarily surgical,** with excision of abscesses from the liver or splenectomy. Catheter drainage is another option for selected patients. **Systemic antimicrobial therapy is mandatory.** Sometimes small liver abscesses can be treated with antibiotics alone and have a good outcome.
4. **Cholecystitis and cholangitis**
   a. **Cholecystitis** is a common medical problem (see Chapter 5 VIII B, C).
      (1) **Etiology and pathogenesis.** Infection need not be present or prominent. In most cases, obstruction of the gallbladder is found, and the bile, which is normally sterile, may be colonized by bacteria such as *E. coli, K. pneumoniae,* or enterococci.
      (2) **Clinical features.** Right upper quadrant abdominal pain, anorexia, nausea, vomiting, and low-grade fever with chills may be present.
      (3) **Diagnosis.** The diagnosis is made on the basis of the clinical presentation and evidence of gallstones or gallbladder dysfunction as demonstrated by ultrasonography or radionuclide cholecystography.
      (4) **Therapy.** Cholecystitis usually is treated adequately with **conservative measures.** Cholecystectomy is recommended for recurrent disease, rupture, or empyema of the gallbladder. Chemical dissolution of gallstones with bile acids or lithotripsy may be useful, but only in selected patients. Antibiotics are seldom needed in patients who do not require surgery.

b. Cholangitis is a more serious problem than cholecystitis (see also Chapter 5 VIII G).

(1) **Etiology and pathogenesis.** Cholangitis tends to occur with obstruction of the intrahepatic or common bile duct (usually by gallstones or malignancy). Bacterial colonization (most often with *E. coli*) in this setting usually leads to infection.

(2) **Clinical features.** Clinical manifestations are similar to but more severe than those for cholecystitis. Right upper quadrant abdominal pain, high fever with shaking chills, and jaundice **(Charcot's triad),** often in the setting of gallbladder disease, may occur.

(3) **Diagnosis.** The characteristic presentation of **Charcot's triad** and the finding of **moderate to severe leukocytosis** with elevated serum bilirubin and alkaline phosphatase form the basis of diagnosis. Bacteremia also is commonly found. Patients with recent biliary surgery or cancer in the liver or pancreas have an especially high risk for developing cholangitis.

(4) **Therapy.** Treatment usually consists of **antimicrobial agents** that are active against enteric organisms, accompanied by **decompressive surgery. Endoscopic sphincterotomy** or **percutaneous transhepatic drainage** may be used in lieu of or in preparation for open surgical drainage. In patients with percutaneous drainage for malignancy, recurrent disease is especially common.

F Urinary tract infections (see Chapter 6, Part I: IX)

1. **Incidence.** These are the most common bacterial infections encountered in clinical practice and occur much more frequently in women than in men.
2. **Etiology.** Most urinary tract infections are caused by gram-negative bacteria, including *E. coli* (most commonly), *Klebsiella* species, and *Proteus* species. Less common causes include gram-positive cocci such as *Staphylococcus* species (especially *Staphylococcus saprophyticus*) and enterococci.
3. **Clinical features**

a. In general, symptomatic urinary tract infections are characterized by the irritative symptoms of urinary frequency, urgency, and pain. Flank pain and fever suggest upper tract involvement.

b. The composition of the urinary sediment in urinary infections is characterized by a large number of neutrophils and a variable number of red cells. WBC casts may be observed in kidney infections.

c. Quantitative urine cultures do not distinguish between upper (kidney or ureter) and lower tract (bladder and urethra) infections.

4. **Clinical syndromes**

a. There is standard agreement that a bacterial count exceeding 10^5 organisms per milliliter of urine combined with irritative voiding symptoms and pyuria indicate significant disease, not simple contamination. However, two clinically important situations are not covered by this definition of urinary tract infections.

(1) Patients with symptoms of true urinary tract infection but with fewer than 10^5 bacteria per milliliter of urine

(2) Patients with no symptoms of urinary tract infection but a urine bacterial count exceeding 10^5/mL. This condition, which is termed **asymptomatic bacteriuria,** is not rare and occurs most often in women and in older patients.

b. **Catheter-related bacteriuria** is an inevitable concomitant complication of prolonged bladder catheterization. It can be delayed by careful aseptic insertion, silver-impregnated catheters, and strict closed drainage. However, after 1 or 2 weeks, some degree of colonization is common, and eventually, bacterial counts exceeding 10^5/mL of urine are reached.

c. **Prostatitis** is a complication of many urinary tract infections in men. Acute prostatitis is characterized by perineal pain and irritative voiding symptoms.

d. **Urethritis** is often a symptom of a sexually transmitted disease (e.g., gonorrheal or chlamydial infection). Copious urethral discharge is diagnostic, but mildly symptomatic urethritis can mimic a urinary tract infection.

5. **Diagnosis.** Diagnostic tests seldom are needed to make a decision to treat patients with symptoms of urinary infection, dipstick evidence of bacteriuria, or pyuria. In patients with previous infections or other risk factors, urine culture helps ascertain the exact microbiology of the infection.
   a. The issue of when to examine patients for anatomic abnormalities as an explanation for urinary tract infections is controversial. Most evidence suggests that cystoscopy and urography seldom show treatable causes of infection and should be reserved for patients with frequent recurrences and jeopardized kidney function. Men have a higher rate of anatomic complications (usually prostate-related) than women.
   b. When blood cultures are positive in the context of a urinary tract infection, involvement of the kidneys or prostate gland is implied. Fever also suggests renal involvement.
   c. Rectal examination may indicate enlargement or tenderness of the prostate, and purulent discharge may be expressed from the urethra after prostatic examination.
6. **Therapy.** Treatment is usually directed at the agent most likely to be responsible for the infection.
   a. ***E. coli*–caused infections.** Because *E. coli* has a propensity for causing infections in otherwise healthy individuals, antibiotics effective against *E. coli* should be given in the absence of cultures. Many oral agents can be used, including trimethoprim and sulfamethoxazole used alone or together, quinolones, tetracyclines, and some penicillin preparations such as amoxicillin with clavulanic acid. Used alone, ampicillin is likely to be ineffective because of the large number of ampicillin-resistant *E. coli.* Cephalosporins are widely used to treat uncomplicated urinary tract infections, but they possess no special qualities for this indication and are often expensive.
      (1) A 3-day course of therapy is adequate to cure most infections (especially cystitis) where urine drug levels seem to be the most important determinant of effectiveness.
      (2) Failure to cure infections rapidly does not alter the efficacy of future therapy. In rare instances, refractory infection may require a long course of therapy—sometimes up to several months—although briefer courses (i.e., 2 weeks) often are successful.
   b. **Asymptomatic bacteriuria.** The therapeutic approach is a matter of debate. However, treatment is indicated for patients with a known structural or functional abnormality of the kidneys (including renal transplant) and those who are pregnant.
   c. **Catheter-related bacteriuria.** Frequent bladder catheterizations (several times daily) rather than use of an indwelling catheter may lessen the risk of this infection. This approach has been most effective in paraplegic patients who otherwise would require prolonged bladder drainage through an indwelling catheter.
   d. **Prostate infections.** These conditions are difficult to treat. Fluoroquinolones, which enter the prostate gland, are the best therapeutic agents for prostatitis; the duration of treatment should be at least 2 weeks, although it may extend considerably longer.

G Skin and soft tissue infections Bacterial, fungal, and viral infections of the skin and related structures (e.g., hair follicles, sweat glands) are common.

1. **Bacterial skin infections** usually start in areas of trauma or previous disease.
   a. **Etiology.** In otherwise healthy individuals, gram-positive cocci such as *S. pyogenes* and *S. aureus* cause most skin infections. Immunocompromised individuals are subject to the usual gram-positive flora as well as a wider variety of pathogens, including enteric gram-negative bacilli and *P. aeruginosa.*
   b. **Clinical features.** The three major forms of bacterial skin infection are **cellulitis, abscess,** and **ulcer.**
      (1) **Cellulitis** is characterized by redness, warmth, and tenderness of the skin. It may involve a limited area or may spread widely and rapidly. Any part of the body may be affected. Fever and leukocytosis are common. [In some patients, a rapidly progressive cutaneous infection (streptococcal TSS) caused by group A streptococci and characterized by significant systemic features can cause severe skin damage and even death.]

(2) **Abscesses** represent deeper, circumscribed infections, which often start in accessory structures such as hair follicles. They may be warm or of normal skin temperature and frequently contain pus. Fever is most likely to be present in individuals with large, multiple, or deep abscesses.

(3) **Ulcers** are not usually the result of bacterial infection alone but reflect tissue damage from ischemia or trauma. Invariably, ulcers are colonized by bacteria and may lead to deep soft tissue or bone infection. They usually occur in dependent areas (e.g., the sacrum) or in areas of poor blood flow or decreased sensation (e.g., in the feet of a patient with diabetes).

c. **Therapy**

(1) **Cellulitis requires antibiotic management.** Agents active against streptococci and staphylococci usually are effective, including semisynthetic penicillins (e.g., nafcillin), cephalosporins, vancomycin, clindamycin, and linezolid.

(2) **Abscesses should be drained,** although some rupture spontaneously. Antibiotics are seldom needed unless there is accompanying cellulitis.

(3) **Skin ulcers** usually are managed by **débridement and antibiotic therapy** with broad-spectrum agents active against enteric gram-negative rods, gram-positive cocci, and anaerobes. Skin grafting may be beneficial.

2. **Fungal skin infections** usually are acquired by exposure of the skin to pathogenic fungi. Exceptions are cutaneous manifestations of blastomycosis or candidal fungemia.

a. **Clinical features.** Fungal infections that start in the skin fall into three groups.

(1) **Dermatophytosis** is a superficial infection of the epidermis due to dermatophytic fungi (e.g., *Trichophyton, Microsporum,* and *Epidermophyton* species). Athlete's foot and ringworm are examples. The skin usually is flaky and may be slightly discolored but is not frankly painful.

(2) **Candidiasis** is a red, tender edematous rash occurring in moist body parts and caused by *C. albicans.* Intertrigo in the axillary or inframammary area is an example.

(3) **Mixed bacterial flora and fungi** (usually *Candida* species) can be involved in superficial infection. This may be evident during or after administration of antibacterial therapy.

b. **Diagnosis.** Potassium hydroxide preparations (or Gram stains) and fungal cultures are the foundation of diagnosis.

c. **Therapy**

(1) Dermatophytosis is treated with topical therapy for limited disease or with oral therapy for extensive infection. **Azoles** (e.g., ketoconazole, fluconazole) are most commonly used.

(2) Candidiasis is treated topically, but special attention should be given to keeping the affected area clean and dry. Rarely, systemic azole therapy is required.

(3) Mixed bacterial and fungal infections usually do not require specific antifungal therapy.

3. **Viral skin infections** may be cutaneously inoculated, as in the case of herpes simplex, but more commonly are a manifestation of systemic viral infection or an immune response to infection. An example of this is **varicella (chickenpox),** in which the virus is acquired via the respiratory tract and spreads to the skin after a viremia.

4. **Deep soft tissue infections** are rare but serious infections usually caused by streptococci, anaerobes, and gram-negative rods. There may be comparatively little abnormality of the skin in some of these infections (e.g., **fasciitis**). Combinations of medical and surgical therapy usually are used, but even so, many patients succumb to these infections.

a. **Gangrene** is an infection of the skin and soft tissues caused by a mixed anaerobic and aerobic bacterial flora that usually includes *C. perfringens.* It is characterized by cellulitis and gas in the soft tissues. Therapy involves surgical débridement and antibiotic therapy (e.g., with penicillin).

b. **Fasciitis** is a rare infection between tissue planes. It usually occurs postoperatively, after rupture of an abdominal viscus, or in diabetic patients. Pathogenic bacteria include mixed anaerobes, streptococci, and, occasionally, gram-negative bacilli.

H Osteomyelitis Bone infections can be classified according to their pathogenesis. In general, bone infections develop in three ways: by extension from a contiguous infection, by direct inoculation during surgery or as a result of trauma, and by hematogenous spread.

1. **Osteomyelitis due to contiguous infection or inoculation.** Bone infection should be suspected in patients with a history of **trauma** or **surgery** or with obvious **soft tissue infection** overlying bone, although the bone involvement may be difficult to prove.
   a. **Etiology.** Almost any bacterium can be responsible including *S. aureus, P. aeruginosa,* or anaerobes.
   b. **Clinical features.** Symptoms and signs may simply be those of the adjacent infection. Pain is common, and fever is variable.
   c. **Diagnosis.** This process may be difficult. Radiographic evidence of osteomyelitis lags behind the symptoms and pathologic changes by approximately 7–10 days. Although bone scanning is sensitive for osteomyelitis, it may not distinguish bone infection from more superficial soft tissue infection. The definitive diagnosis rests on bone biopsy and bacterial culture. An expensive but useful test is the MRI scan, which shows changes in the bone marrow that can be detected well before change in plain X-rays.
   d. **Clinical course and therapy.** The clinical course guides the length of treatment, but, generally, **long courses of antibiotics** are necessary. Devitalized bone, poor blood supply, and adjacent infection may be reasons for extended (months) therapy.
2. **Hematogenous osteomyelitis.** This type of disease should be suspected in febrile patients who experience pain and swelling over a bone but have no obvious source of infection.
   a. **Etiology.** The bacteriology involves largely *S. aureus.* However, *Salmonella* species seem to be more important in patients with sickle cell disease. Vertebral osteomyelitis also is somewhat different in that gram-negative bacilli may be introduced from the urinary tract through venous channels.
   b. **Diagnosis.** Radiography and bone scanning are helpful. The erythrocyte sedimentation rate usually is elevated but this is quite a nonspecific finding. Bone aspiration and culture are recommended for microbiologic diagnosis. Blood cultures also should be obtained.
   c. **Therapy.** Treatment is a prolonged course of **antibiotics.** Nonviable bone may need to be removed surgically because it provides a site for potential relapse.

I Intravascular infections and endocarditis Intravascular infections manifest as **viremia, bacteremia, fungemia,** or **parasitemia,** depending on the type of infective organism demonstrated in the blood. Such infections may reflect **invasion or failure of containment at a localized site** (e.g., bowel or lung) or a **primary infection of the blood vessels or the heart** (e.g., endocarditis).

1. **Local infections** lead to positive blood cultures, with a frequency dependent on the site and severity of the infection and on the organism or organisms responsible for the infection.
   a. For example, among hospitalized patients with pneumococcal pneumonia, 10%–25% have bacteremia. The prognosis for these patients is worse than for those without bacteremia because those with bacteremia tend to have more diffuse lung involvement and more virulent organisms.
   b. Even when blood cultures do not demonstrate a particular organism, metastatic infection or dissemination (e.g., cryptococcal meningitis or miliary tuberculosis) strongly suggests blood-borne spread.
2. **Septic shock** is a commonly recognized clinical entity defined as a systemic infection accompanied by hypotension that is not attributed to hypovolemia or intrinsic cardiac disease. In most cases, blood cultures are positive during these episodes.
   a. **Etiology.** Septic shock sometimes is called **gram-negative sepsis** based on the observation that the bacteria most frequently responsible are gram-negative enteric bacilli. **Endotoxin** (the lipopolysaccharide coat of gram-negative organisms) is the cause. However, an indistinguishable clinical disease can be caused by gram-positive bacteria, viruses, and yeast.

b. **Therapy. Antibiotic treatment** is critical for patient recovery. High-dose corticosteroid therapy to supplement usual supportive measures is not thought to improve survival. Various immunomodulators such as tumor necrosis factor (TNF) inhibitors and antibody to endotoxin have failed to improve the prognosis of septic shock. Activated protein C (drotrecogin) has anti-coagulant properties but also seems to block some of the destructive positive feedback loops that promote organ damage in shock. It is useful in the most severely ill patients.

3. **Catheter-related infections** are serious problems associated with hospitalization. Infection seldom is caused by the infusion of contaminated fluid. Rather, these infections most commonly occur at the **site of cannulation.**
   a. **Diagnosis.** Diagnosis involves demonstration of either local skin infection at the cannulation site or positive blood cultures and the presence of the same bacteria in significant numbers on a semiquantitative culture of the catheter. Sometimes a vein infection may not be apparent until after the catheter has been removed. Infected veins are almost always clotted at the site of the infection.
   b. **Therapy.** Removal of the catheter when local infection is present is necessary. When vascular access is crucial and the catheter has been aseptically inserted into the vena cava (e.g., a **Hickman catheter**—a wide-bore silastic catheter used for chemotherapy, hyperalimentation, or drawing blood), conservative therapy with antibiotics alone may cure the infection. Fungal infections or those caused by highly resistant bacteria usually cannot be cured without removal of the catheter. Tunneled catheters that exhibit erythema and other signs of inflammation along the catheter tract also need to be removed. Rarely, an infected peripheral vein will require surgical management because pus needs to be drained.

4. **Vascular graft infection** is one of the most serious consequences of vascular surgery. Although native blood vessels may become infected in atherosclerotic processes or in pyogenic processes involving the arterial wall itself **(mycotic aneurysm),** these events are rare. When arteries are bypassed because of arterial insufficiency or for hemodialysis vascular access, the surgical site can become infected.
   a. **Diagnosis.** This rests on finding consistently positive blood cultures in a patient with such a graft. Nuclear studies such as a tagged WBC scan may be useful diagnostically.
   b. **Therapy.** The best chance of cure involves removal of the entire prosthetic device. When this is not possible, revascularization (i.e., circumventing the site of infection) can be tried. Antibiotic therapy alone cannot ensure a positive outcome and must be carried out for usually 6 weeks or more.

5. **Endocarditis** usually results from infection of the cusp of a heart valve, although any part of the endocardium or any prosthetic material inserted into the heart may be involved.
   a. **Etiology.** A variety of organisms may cause endocarditis, although bacteria account for almost all cases. The specific agent of endocarditis depends on which cardiac structures are affected.
      (1) **Infection of normal valves,** which is rare, is usually associated with intravenous drug use. *S. aureus* is the most common pathogen.
      (2) **Infection of previously damaged valves** usually is attributable to viridans streptococci. Other agents of endocarditis in this setting are enterococci, *S. aureus,* and various small gram-negative rods constituting part of the normal oral flora.
      (3) **Infection of prosthetic valves** involves staphylococci (both coagulase positive and coagulase negative) as the most common agents of early-onset disease (occurring < 2 months postoperatively). Streptococci are the most common agents of late-onset disease (occurring > 2 months postoperatively).
   b. **Clinical features.** Signs and symptoms vary widely.
      (1) Common findings include **fever,** which is almost universal, and a **heart murmur.** Endocarditis is one of the most common causes of fever of unknown origin.
      (2) Less commonly, **embolic disease** such as stroke or splenic artery embolism and infarction is evident. Most emboli are small and may give rise to uncommon but diagnostically

helpful physical findings including **Roth's spots, Osler's nodes, Janeway lesions,** and **conjunctival hemorrhage.**

(3) A variety of constitutional symptoms such as myalgia, back pain, confusion, or fatigue may occur.

c. **Laboratory diagnosis**

(1) **Blood cultures** are critical and are positive in more than 90% of cases of endocarditis. (Previous use of antibiotics may lower this figure.) Because of the continuous bacteremia of endocarditis, virtually all cultures are positive, and it is rarely necessary to obtain more than three or four cultures.

(2) For patients with culture-negative endocarditis, there is little incremental value in collecting several additional blood samples for culture. Sometimes, the microbiology laboratory can enhance isolation by using **special culture techniques.**

(3) Immune complexes may cause a **glomerulonephritis,** which is characterized by elevated serum creatinine, hematuria, and casts in the urine, or rheumatologic manifestations such as sterile arthritis. The role of immune complexes in other aspects of endocarditis is not well understood.

(4) **Moderate anemia** is associated with endocarditis that has been present for more than 2 weeks.

d. **Therapy.** Treatment has been carefully studied. When endocarditis is untreated, it is almost uniformly fatal. In general, prosthetic valve disease is more difficult to treat medically or surgically.

(1) **Antibiotic therapy** alone provides an excellent chance of cure for streptococcal disease on a native valve and for staphylococcal disease on the tricuspid valve. The key is to provide an adequate dosage for a long enough period, usually 2–6 weeks, depending on the organism.

(2) In medical failures, **valve replacement** may be a necessary adjunct to antibiotic therapy. Other indications for valve surgery include:

(a) Fungal endocarditis (an absolute indication)

(b) Congestive heart failure (CHF)

(c) Recurrent major emboli

(d) Inability to provide a full course of antibiotic therapy

(e) Inability to sterilize the blood after 10–14 days

VI SEXUALLY TRANSMITTED DISEASES (STDs)

A Modes of transmission STDs usually affect healthy adults. Multiple STDs can be present at once. Microorganisms may be transmitted during intimate sexual relations in three ways.

1. **Cutaneous inoculation** is the most common route for the five "classical" STDs (i.e., syphilis, gonorrhea, chancroid, lymphogranuloma venereum, and granuloma inguinale) as well as for herpes simplex. Apposition of an infected site to a susceptible site in a partner results in a physical transfer of microorganisms. Abrasion or trauma may facilitate the infection of skin.

2. **Blood-borne infection** can be transmitted by sexual activity. HBV, HCV, cytomegalovirus (CMV), and HIV are all transmitted by inoculation of microscopic amounts of blood or serum.

3. **Enterically acquired infection** may occur with sexual activity because the anal area is close to the genitals or is also used for sexual interaction. *Shigella, Entamoeba,* and HAV are examples of sexually transmissible enteric diseases.

B Urethritis

1. **Etiology.** Urethritis is classified as **gonococcal** or **nongonococcal.**

a. **Gonococcal urethritis** is caused by *N. gonorrhoeae.* In almost all cases of gonococcal urethritis, Gram stain of the urethral discharge shows gram-negative intracellular diplococci.

b. **Nongonococcal urethritis** is caused by *C. trachomatis, Ureaplasma urealyticum,* or some other, yet unidentified, agent. (In 25% of cases of gonococcal urethritis, one of these organisms also is present, and patients may have recurrent symptoms after therapy for gonorrhea.)

2. **Clinical features**
   a. **Dysuria** is observed in most cases of urethritis, whether gonococcal or nongonococcal.
   b. **Urethral discharge** is observed more frequently in men than women and may be purulent (usually in gonococcal disease) or cloudy and mucoid (usually in nongonococcal disease).

3. **Therapy**
   a. A variety of **antibiotic regimens** can be used to treat gonorrhea. However, resistance patterns change, and up-to-date recommendations should be sought.
   b. Many clinicians recommend that treatment with a tetracycline or macrolide follow gonococcal therapy to eliminate possible simultaneous nongonococcal urethritis. A 7-day course of a tetracycline or erythromycin or a single dose of azithromycin is usually sufficient, although some patients experience a relapse within a few weeks. These patients usually respond to another course of antibiotics.

C Pelvic inflammatory disease (PID)

PID refers to a complex of infections involving the uterus, fallopian tubes, or ligaments of the uterus.

1. **Etiology**
   a. *N. gonorrhoeae, C. trachomatis,* or a mixture of pelvic anaerobes may be involved, although it is difficult to determine which of these is responsible when instituting therapy.
   b. The presence of an intrauterine device (IUD) may predispose patients to PID.

2. **Clinical features and laboratory findings.** The symptoms may be contemporaneous with menstruation and usually consist of lower abdominal or pelvic pain and tenderness on palpation of the cervix, uterus, or adnexa. Fever is not necessarily a significant feature. A cervical discharge or pelvic mass may be present, and the WBC count may be normal or elevated.

3. **Diagnosis**
   a. It is important to obtain cultures or other diagnostic tests for *N. gonorrhoeae.* If there is fluid in the retro uterine cul-de-sac, culdocentesis can be performed and may help differentiate the possible causes.
   b. Ultrasonography of the pelvis may demonstrate an adnexal mass or abscess, which should be followed carefully.

4. **Therapy.** No simple therapy is effective in all cases of PID. Hospitalization is suggested when pain is incapacitating or when parenteral therapy is given. Combinations of antibiotics are usually needed to cover the three major categories of possible pathogens.

5. **Complications.** The most serious long-term complications of PID are infertility, ectopic pregnancy, and the need for hysterectomy.

D Infectious proctitis

1. **Etiology.** Infectious proctitis can be caused by a variety of microorganisms. When anal sex is practiced, gonorrhea, syphilis, chlamydial infection, and herpes should be considered. When there is no history of anal sex, shigellosis and amebiasis are more likely causes.

2. **Clinical features and diagnosis.** Proctalgia (rectal pain), a change in bowel habits, and a mucoid or bloody anal discharge between bowel movements suggest infectious proctitis. A sexual history should be obtained to aid in the diagnosis, and appropriate diagnostic studies (e.g., sigmoidoscopy, culture and Gram stain of the discharge, biopsy) should be performed.

3. **Therapy.** When specific agents of infectious proctitis can be identified, appropriate antibiotic treatment should be administered. In general, the same regimens used to treat these pathogens

in other body sites are effective in proctitis. However, for gonorrheal proctitis, cure rates are lower than for gonorrheal urethritis, and post-therapy cultures should be obtained.

E Syndromes of genital ulcers and lymphadenopathy

1. **Incidence.** Ulcerative lesions of the genitalia are common outpatient problems.
2. **Etiology.** There are many causes, which vary in different parts of the world. In the United States, **genital herpes** is the most common cause of genital ulcers, followed by **syphilis.** Other causes include **lymphogranuloma venereum, chancroid,** and **granuloma inguinale (donovanosis),** all of which are uncommon in the United States. (Gonorrhea is an STD that does not cause genital ulcer syndromes.)
3. **Clinical features** (Table 8–2 [Color figures of these conditions are shown on the accompanying CD.])
   a. **Genital herpes** initially manifests as itching and soreness followed by the appearance of erythema and, eventually, the development of herpetic vesicles. In immunocompromised patients (e.g., transplant recipients, patients with HIV), vesicles may be confluent and lead to large ulcers.
   b. **Syphilis,** in its primary form, manifests as a painless, often solitary, chancre (ulcer) with a hard, indurated base. Oral and vulvar lesions may be subtle, and oral lesions may be painful.
   c. **Lymphogranuloma venereum** manifests as nodes that are disproportionately large compared with the ulcers. There often is a depression between the inguinal and femoral nodes **(groove sign).**

TABLE 8–2 Syndromes of Genital Ulcers and Lymphadenopathy

Disease	Causative Organism	Diagnostic Tests	Clinical Findings	Therapy
Genital herpes (see Color Figure on CD)	Herpes simplex virus	Direct immunofluorescence; culture	Lesion—multiple, vesiculopustular; painful	None; acyclovir
Syphilis (see Color Figures on CD)	*Treponema pallidum*	Darkfield microscopy; RPR test	Lesion—usually solitary; indurated; painless Nodes—rubbery; not fluctuant	Penicillin; tetracycline
Lymphogranuloma venereum (see Color Figure on CD)	*Chlamydia trachomatis*	Culture; serologic examination	Lesions—small papule or vesicle Nodes—large; suppurative; both sides of inguinal ligament affected (groove sign)	Tetracycline; erythromycin
Chancroid (see Color Figure on CD)	*Haemophilus ducreyi*	Gram stain; culture (special media needed)	Lesion—ragged; soft; dirty looking Nodes—tender; suppurative	Erythromycin; ceftriaxone; trimethoprim–sulfamethoxazole; fluoroquinolone
Granuloma inguinale (see Color Figure on CD)	*Calymmatobacterium granulomatis*	Biopsy with Giemsa or Wright's stain	Lesion—large; slowly advancing; rolled edges; not indurated Nodes—not prominent	Tetracycline; trimethoprim–sulfamethoxazole

RPR = rapid plasma reagin.

   d. **Chancroid** is characterized by multiple, painful ulcers with ragged, undermined edges and suppurative inguinal nodes.
   e. **Granuloma inguinale** is a more indolent infection characterized by a painless, beefy-red lesion with ragged edges and less prominent adenopathy. It is rare in the United States. The clinical characteristics and course of illness are more like genital cancer than other STDs.

4. **Diagnosis**
   a. When a **genital ulcer** is noted, a **Tzanck smear** for herpes and a **dark-field examination** for spirochetes can help make a quick diagnosis. However, dark-field examinations can be technically difficult. In all cases, serologic testing for syphilis should be performed. Viral cultures for herpes simplex are reliable, rapid, and reasonably inexpensive.
   b. Diagnosis of **lymphogranuloma venereum** is difficult. The culturing *C. trachomatis* from a lesion or a node or by showing a serologic reaction to this organism may confirm the diagnosis.
   c. Diagnosis of **chancroid** involves eliminating other causes of genital ulcers and isolating *Haemophilus ducreyi* from the ulcers or suppurative nodes. However, *H. ducreyi* can be difficult to grow in culture, even under optimal conditions. In most patients, a clinical suspicion of chancroid and negative tests for syphilis and herpes simplex are sufficient to initiate treatment.
   d. Diagnosis of **granuloma inguinale** is confirmed by demonstration of Donovan bodies in edge scrapings prepared with Giemsa or Wright's stain. An experienced cytopathologist may be needed to make the identification.

5. **Therapy.** Identification and treatment of sexual contacts is always desirable.
   a. **Herpes infections** are self-limited but recurrent. Acyclovir, famciclovir, or valacyclovir may shorten the course and reduce symptoms but not affect the natural history of these infections. Patients with frequent recurrences can use lower doses of these same medicines as prophylaxis.
   b. **Syphilis** is treated with varying schedules of penicillin, depending on the stage. Tetracycline may be useful for patients with penicillin intolerance or other special requirements, but penicillin is clearly preferred even if it requires desensitization.
   c. **Lymphogranuloma venereum** is treated with a tetracycline or a macrolide.
   d. **Chancroid** is treated with azithromycin, ceftriaxone, fluoroquinolones, or erythromycin. However, resistance patterns of *H. ducreyi* are variable, and up-to-date recommendations should be acquired.
   e. **Granuloma inguinale** is treated with a tetracycline or trimethoprim–sulfamethoxazole.

6. **Late complications**
   a. **Herpes simplex recurrences** tend to be most common early after acquisition but may continue to occur for many years and may become severe in immunocompromised patients. Herpes also can complicate parturition and cause devastating infection of neonates.
   b. **Syphilitic chancres** heal spontaneously after 1–2 weeks. However, in the secondary phase, syphilis can manifest as a multisystem disease including, but not limited to, lymphadenopathy, rash (especially on the palms and soles), fever, pharyngitis, and meningitis. The multisystem disease resolves spontaneously, and a latent, noninfective phase ensues. Most patients remain seropositive. In tertiary syphilis, approximately 10% of patients develop serious late complications of the aorta or the CNS. The neurologic lesions are varied but include pupillary disturbances, posterior spinal column problems, and major cognitive impairment. Treatment may halt progression but is unlikely to reverse damage.
   c. **Lymphogranuloma venereum** may rarely lead to genital or rectal scarring.
   d. **Chancroid and granuloma inguinale** tend to cause only local problems.

VII OTHER INFECTIOUS DISEASES AND SYNDROMES

A Infections associated with adenopathy and splenomegaly Syndromes of adenopathy (both local and general), splenomegaly, and fever are common medical problems. The differential diagnosis should include tumors, rheumatic diseases, and vasculitis as well as specific infectious processes.

1. **Generalized lymphadenopathy and fatigue** are the classic signs of **infectious mononucleosis.**
   a. Mononucleosis most commonly is caused by the **Epstein-Barr virus** and is associated with splenomegaly, pharyngitis, and an atypical lymphocytosis.
   b. **CMV** causes a mononucleosis syndrome that is virtually indistinguishable from Epstein-Barr virus–induced mononucleosis.
   c. Both infections tend to occur in adolescents and young adults and may be subclinical.
      (1) They are distinguished by serologic tests such as the **Monospot test,** which usually demonstrates the presence of heterophile antibody in Epstein-Barr virus infection and the absence of heterophile antibody in CMV infection.
      (2) Specific antibody testing for the two viruses can confirm the diagnosis in equivocal cases.
      (3) Both viruses can be transmitted by intimate contact including, but not limited to, sexual intercourse.
   d. Some cases of mononucleosis are caused by *T. gondii,* but this infection usually is subclinical or presents as a mild "viral-type syndrome" in healthy adults.
   e. **Early HIV infection** may manifest as fever, lymphadenopathy, and fatigue, as well as rash, neck stiffness, or other features of a "viral infection." This set of symptoms occurs in 30%–60% of patients who experience acute HIV infection. (This is sometimes called seroconversion illness, because antibodies to HIV become apparent at the end of this period.)
2. Fever, adenopathy, and fatigue also may be **manifestations of secondary syphilis.**
3. **Splenomegaly out of proportion to adenopathy**
   a. This clinical presentation is characteristic of only a few infections such as malaria, schistosomiasis, and kala-azar (visceral leishmaniasis).
   b. This syndrome also should suggest a **malignancy** such as lymphoma or Hodgkin's disease, an **infiltrative disease** such as Gaucher's disease, a **congestive disease** such as hepatic cirrhosis, or a **connective tissue disease** such as SLE.
   c. **Local infections** such as splenic abscess and left-sided subphrenic abscess may manifest as a palpable spleen.
4. **Localized adenopathy** helps pinpoint a potential **infection** or **tumor.**
   a. A few small (< 8 mm) lymph nodes in the inguinal, axillary, or cervical region may be present in most healthy adults. If the nodes are nontender and firm but not rock hard and do not change over a period of weeks to months, they usually do not warrant attention.
   b. Lymphadenopathy in other areas is unusual without an obvious infection in the region drained by those nodes.
   c. Cutaneous inoculation with an infective agent may result in a local lesion and regional adenopathy. Examples are sporotrichosis (from exposure to *Sporothrix schenckii,* a plant-associated fungus) and cat-scratch disease (*Bartonella henselae* infection following cat bite or scratch).
   d. Lymphadenopathy alone or with a variety of constitutional problems occurs in mid to late stages of HIV infection.

B Infections associated with eosinophilia Eosinophils are granulocytes that have limited ability to phagocytose bacteria but are prominent in hypersensitivity reactions and in infections by multicellular parasites that have an invasive phase.

1. The finding of eosinophilia (i.e., an increase in the number of circulating eosinophils > 500/mm^3) should stimulate the search for an infection.
   a. Eosinophilia is seen most often with infection by helminths that are not limited to the lumen of the bowel such as the **schistosome** (blood fluke), which belongs to the **trematode** group. The pinworm (from the **nematode** group) does not tend to stimulate eosinophilia because it has no tissue phase.
   b. *Strongyloides stercoralis* is the most important helminth associated with eosinophilia in the United States. Strongyloidiasis should be suspected in persons who live or have lived in trop-

ical areas (or in the southeastern United States) and who have persistent eosinophilia with or without cutaneous or gastrointestinal complaints. Because the *Strongyloides* larvae can cross the bowel wall, they may be associated with episodes of polymicrobial bacteremia involving typical bowel flora. Untreated disease can last for decades and worsen during periods of immunosuppression.

c. Protozoa (e.g., *Entamoeba, Giardia*) seldom elicit eosinophilia.

d. Most bacterial infections cause eosinopenia because of the effect of endogenous steroid production. Medically prescribed corticosteroids or endogenous excess steroid production (e.g., Cushing's disease) reduce eosinophilia of any origin.

2. Many noninfectious diseases may stimulate eosinophil production, release, or both. The most frequently encountered are **atopic** or **allergic diseases.**

3. When a drug such as an antibiotic is the allergen or hapten, eosinophilia acts as a marker for an allergic reaction to the drug. The eosinophilia tends to resolve quickly after the offending drug has been withdrawn.

C Tuberculosis This illness remains a major medical problem in certain immigrant and underprivileged groups in the United States as well as a widespread disease throughout the world. The diagnosis is based on identification of acid-fast bacilli—specifically, *M. tuberculosis*—on special stain or culture. However, the diagnosis may be difficult to establish, because many patients have too few bacteria to be seen on direct stain, and it takes several weeks of incubation for specimens to grow.

1. **Clinical syndromes**

   a. **Pulmonary tuberculosis** is the most common form. In most adults, this condition is characterized by an increased cough (possibly with altered sputum), weight loss, hemoptysis, and fatigue. The chest radiograph usually is abnormal and shows signs of a prior exposure to *M. tuberculosis* (e.g., calcified or enlarged intrathoracic lymph nodes and infiltrates in the posterior segment of the upper lobes). Most cases of pulmonary tuberculosis are believed to be a reactivation of *M. tuberculosis* acquired months to years earlier rather than reinfection or initial infection by this bacterium. However, reinfection has been confirmed in patients both with and without HIV infection. Primary disease may resemble bacterial pneumonia and should be especially suspected when a close contact has recently been discovered to have active tuberculosis.

   b. **Extrapulmonary tuberculosis** can develop in any organ, but the most seriously affected are the kidneys, bones, and meninges. Again, the diagnosis rests on finding *M. tuberculosis* in body fluid or tissue. Only approximately 40% of patients with extrapulmonary tuberculosis have clinical or radiographic evidence of lung involvement at the time of diagnosis of the extrapulmonary disease.

2. **Therapy.** Treatment is aimed at curing the patient who has a definite diagnosis of tuberculosis. To be effective, the therapy must include **at least two antimicrobial agents.** Single-agent treatment has a high risk of failure because of the selection of drug-resistant strains of the infecting tubercle bacillus.

   a. Because of their potency and reliability, **isoniazid** and **rifampin** are the drugs of choice for tuberculosis. Other first-line drugs include ethambutol, pyrazinamide, and streptomycin. Most authorities recommend starting four drugs initially to provide adequate coverage, in view of possible isoniazid or rifampin resistance.

   b. Second-line drugs are used primarily for patients who are intolerant of the first-line agents or who have drug-resistant disease. These drugs include ethionamide, kanamycin, and cycloserine. Fluoroquinolones have activity against *M. tuberculosis,* which would make them seem to be reasonable first-line drugs, but the need for long courses and the concern about selecting a resistant bacterial flora pushes them to second-line status.

c. The usual duration of treatment is 6–12 months, depending on the patient and the regimen. Shorter courses have an unacceptably high rate of failure.

3. **Prevention**

a. **Skin testing.** The **tuberculin skin test** is used widely to screen certain high-risk populations, particularly those who have been exposed to an infectious individual. The test involves an intradermal injection of the **purified protein derivative (PPD)** of tuberculin. After 48–72 hours, the injection site is examined for visible and palpable induration. Because of a possible cross-reaction after exposure to other mycobacteria, a single tuberculin skin test to determine sensitization to *M. tuberculosis* is considered positive only if the induration at the skin test site measures at least 15 mm in diameter in immunocompetent individuals, 10 mm in sick persons without primary depression of their immune system, and 5 mm in immunosuppressed individuals (e.g., organ transplant recipients or patients with advanced HIV infection). Newer tests looking for direct immune responsiveness of lymphocytes to mycobacterial components can be done in vitro and may yield less equivocal and more rapid results than skin tests.

b. **Chemoprophylaxis.** Certain individuals are at extremely high risk for the development of significant symptomatic tuberculosis. In many cases, disease can be prevented by administering isoniazid alone for 6–12 months, at a dosage of 300 mg/day. Pyridoxine is coadministered with isoniazid to prevent peripheral neuropathy. The high-risk groups include:

(1) Individuals younger than 30 years of age who have positive skin tests for tuberculosis

(2) Individuals of any age who previously had negative skin tests but recently (within the past year) developed positive skin tests for tuberculosis

(3) Individuals with positive skin tests who receive chronic corticosteroid therapy

(4) Individuals who live in the same house or come in close contact with an infected and contagious individual

(5) Prior BCG vaccination does not alter the decision to use chemoprophylaxis

c. **Immunization.** Vaccination of children and adults with bacille Calmette-Guérin (BCG) has been reported to reduce the risk of acquiring tuberculosis. BCG, a live bacterial vaccine, should not be used when there is known immunodeficiency. The PPD skin test can become positive after BCG administration. The BCG vaccine is seldom used in the United States, but it is widely used in other countries.

d. **Isolation.** Because of the **potential hazard of transmission** of tuberculosis in the hospital, it is important to identify potentially infective patients and to ensure adequate containment of their infectious aerosols.

(1) Waiting for a positive acid-fast bacillus smear may introduce an excessive delay, so any patient suspected of having highly contagious tuberculosis should be housed in a private room with air pressure less than that in the hallway. Visitors and staff should wear masks.

(2) Smears are useful in confirming the diagnosis. Finding three consecutive negative smears may be enough to discontinue isolation, but in some clinical settings, it may still be appropriate to continue treatment until the final cultures are available weeks later.

D Infections associated with diffuse rash and fever

1. **Toxin-associated diseases**

a. **Toxic shock syndrome** (TSS) occurs when a susceptible individual is colonized or infected by a strain of *S. aureus* that produces a toxin (TSST-1). This toxin is a superantigen that can stimulate the immune system in a way that leads to severe hypotension and organ damage. Most adults have antibody to this toxin and are thus immune. Many cases have been associated with tampon use in young women, but current tampons seem to be safer, and menstrual TSS is considerably less common than it was in the early 1980s. Toxin-producing *S. pyogenes* (group A streptococci) can cause a very similar illness.

(1) **Clinical features**

(a) TSS is characterized by fever, hypotension, diarrhea, mucous membrane changes, and a diffuse erythematous rash with desquamation on the hands and feet. Multisystem involvement is the rule, with involvement of gastrointestinal, renal, hepatic, hematopoietic, and musculoskeletal organs.

(b) TSS varies from a mild illness to a life-threatening disease. Hypotension from fluid loss and lack of vascular tone is the most ominous prognostic sign. There may be recurrences until protective antibody is formed.

(2) **Therapy.** The treatment for acute illness is **supportive,** consisting of fluids and pressors. Antibacterial therapy is given to prevent recurrence.

b. **Scarlet fever** is an illness caused by infection with toxigenic *S. pyogenes* (group A streptococcus). It is characterized by fever, rough erythematous diffuse rash, mucous membrane erythema (including strawberry tongue), and local streptococcal infection (usually involving the skin). Less severe than TSS, scarlet fever usually responds to supportive measures and antistreptococcal therapy.

2. **Non–toxin-mediated illness with fever and rash**

a. **Kawasaki disease** usually affects young children. It is characterized by prolonged fever, digital swelling, conjunctivitis, mucous membrane erythema, lymphadenopathy, and thrombocytosis. The major late sequela is vasculitis, especially coronary artery aneurysm. Treatment involves aspirin and gamma globulin.

b. **Adverse reactions to medications** include combinations of fever, rash, and eosinophilia. Reaction severity ranges from trivial to life-threatening.

(1) The most common offending agents include anticonvulsants, oral hypoglycemics, abacavir for HIV disease, and antibiotics (especially β-lactams and sulfa drugs). Unlike acute hypersensitivity reactions, which occur within minutes to hours of administration, the rash or fever of drug-induced reactions usually appears after a variable interval of uneventful therapy.

(2) The most serious reaction, toxic epidermal necrolysis **(Stevens-Johnson syndrome),** is characterized by diffuse macular eruption and extensive involvement of the mucous membranes. If the affected skin sloughs, fatality may occur because of fluid derangement and sepsis.

c. A number of **viral exanthems** (skin rashes) and **enanthems** (mucous membrane rashes) are well described. Most usually affect children and unvaccinated individuals and are mild, each having a characteristic appearance and course. Measles (rubeola), erythema infectiosum, and coxsackievirus are among the best known.

d. **Spotted fevers** are caused by *Rickettsia* species. In the United States, the most well known is **Rocky Mountain spotted fever (RMSF),** caused by *Rickettsia rickettsii.* RMSF, which is transmitted by the bite of the dog tick (*Dermacentor* species), most often occurs in the southeastern part of the country. After a delay of several days, there is headache, fever, and a rash, which starts peripherally and moves centrally. Infection involves the vascular endothelium and may be fatal in 15%–20% of untreated patients. Usually, tetracycline or chloramphenicol is effective if given early enough. A similar syndrome, usually without rash, can be caused by *Ehrlichia chaffeensis,* another tick-borne rickettsial pathogen.

E Legionnaires' disease

1. **Etiology.** Legionnaires' disease is a pneumonia caused by *L. pneumophila,* a gram-negative bacterium that dwells in warm aquatic environments. Several legionella-like organisms have been discovered, which produce similar but distinct disease patterns.

2. **Epidemiology**

a. Infection occurs when contaminated water is aerosolized and then inhaled (e.g., during nebulizer treatments). Some outbreaks of legionnaires' disease have been connected to the airborne spread of contaminated fluid from air-conditioning cooling towers or from potable water.

b. Individuals who are particularly vulnerable to infection include cigarette smokers, people with underlying lung disease, and immunosuppressed individuals (e.g., those receiving steroid therapy).

3. **Clinical features**
   a. Fever occurs in almost all cases, is abrupt, and usually is associated with shaking chills. A sudden headache may precede the rapid increase in temperature.
   b. Cough is a common symptom, which initially is nonproductive but progresses to a productive cough that may be associated with slight hemoptysis.
   c. Less common symptoms include diarrhea, nausea, vomiting, and pleuritic pain.
4. **Diagnosis.** The diagnosis is made by **culturing the bacterium** from infected body sites (e.g., lung tissue, pleural fluid, or sputum) or by demonstrating the bacterium by immunofluorescent, nucleic acid hybridization, or antigen detection techniques. When *L. pneumophila* infection cannot be confirmed by these methods, increasing titers of antibodies from the acute phase to convalescence can be diagnostic.
5. **Therapy.** The preferred therapy for all *Legionella* infections is a **macrolide** (e.g., azithromycin) or a **fluoroquinolone** (e.g., levofloxacin).

F Lyme disease

1. **Etiology.** Lyme disease is a multisystem infection caused by a spirochete, *Borrelia burgdorferi,* which is transmitted by tick bite.
2. **Epidemiology.** The incidence of Lyme disease is related to the presence of its vector (usually *Ixodes* ticks) and infected wild mammals such as deer and mice. In the United States, endemic foci have expanded from initial small areas in New England to include areas as far south as Georgia as well as areas in the Midwest and the Pacific states. Lyme disease is the most common tick-borne illness in the United States.
3. **Clinical features.** Lyme disease is divided into three phases. The phases may follow each other closely or be separated by periods without symptoms.
   a. The **first phase** is characterized by an enlarging erythematous rash **(erythema migrans)** at the site of the original tick bite. There may be central clearing or a few satellite lesions. Patients are often constitutionally ill with malaise, headache, and mild fever.
   b. The **second phase** involves the heart (conduction abnormalities, arrhythmias) or the nervous system (cranial or peripheral neuropathies or aseptic meningitis). **New onset of Bell's palsy** (paralysis of cranial nerve VII) should suggest the possibility of Lyme disease.
   c. The **third phase,** which affects only a few patients, consists of an oligoarticular arthritis or some persistent, mild neuropsychiatric disturbances.
4. **Diagnosis.** The diagnosis is difficult. In early illness, the production of antibody to *B. burgdorferi* may not be detectable. Conversely, people living in endemic areas may have antibody without any clinical illness. The organism may be demonstrated rarely in skin biopsies and can sometimes be cultured. High levels of immunoglobulin M (IgM) antibody and increasing levels of IgG antibody to one or more *B. burgdorferi* antigens corroborate clinical suspicions of Lyme borreliosis.
5. **Therapy.** Early **antibiotic therapy** seems to prevent disease progression for most patients. Tetracyclines are preferred for adolescents and adults; penicillin is an alternative. For later-stage disease, high dosages of penicillin, tetracycline (especially doxycycline), and ceftriaxone have been shown to relieve symptoms. Some oral cephalosporins and azithromycin have also been shown to be useful. A vaccine that had been marketed to prevent Lyme disease is no longer available.

VIII RETROVIRUS INFECTION OF HUMANS

A Introduction Retroviruses are single-stranded RNA viruses characterized by the presence of **reverse transcriptase,** an enzyme that uses the viral RNA as a template to make a copy of complementary DNA for integration into the host cell. Many animals can be infected with species-specific retroviruses.

1. Retroviruses known to cause disease in humans are the **human T-cell lymphotropic viruses types I and II** (HTLV-I and HTLV-II) and HIV.
2. HIV comprises two types: type 1 (HIV-1) and type 2 (HIV-2).

B **Epidemiology** All of these agents can be transmitted from person to person via sexual activity or mingling of blood (as occurs via blood transfusion or sharing of blood-contaminated needles) and from mother to child in utero.

1. **HTLV-I** is found most commonly in the Caribbean basin and in southern Japan. Up to 10% of the population in certain villages may be infected.
2. **HTLV-II** is not known to have such marked geographic clusters, and incidence seems to be low worldwide.
3. **HIV**
   a. **HIV-1** is found worldwide. Because of a long latent period and the possibility of one person infecting many others via sexual activity or needle sharing, an explosive spread of this virus has led to a striking change in its distribution since 1981, when it was first identified. Male homosexual activity was the predominant mode of transmission in North America and Europe during the 1980s. Intravenous drug use and heterosexual transmission account for an increasing share of new infections, especially among women, who constitute one of the fastest growing groups to be infected. In Africa, heterosexual activity is the predominant mode of transmission.
   b. **HIV-2** is found primarily in west Africa.

C **Clinical features**

1. **HTLV-1** is the causative agent of adult T-cell leukemia–lymphoma. This unusual malignancy, which is associated with skin involvement and hypercalcemia, is difficult to treat. However, **most people** infected with HTLV-I **have no clinical illness** even after years or decades of infection.
2. **HTLV-II** has not been categorically associated with any illness.
3. **HIV**
   a. **HIV-1** infection has traditionally been divided into three overlapping stages.
      (1) In **early illness** (seroconversion stage), within a few weeks or months after exposure to HIV, whole virus and viral antigens and nucleic acid can be found in the blood and body fluids. Although many patients are asymptomatic, approximately 40% of patients have a brief illness marked by headache, fever, skin rash, or lymphadenopathy, which resolves spontaneously within a few weeks. Most people who become infected with HIV-1 develop antibody within 1–6 months of exposure.
      (2) Almost all HIV-1–infected patients have a clinical **latent period,** during which there is no clinical illness but virus can be detected and is replicating. Depending on both host and viral factors, the intensity of viral infection varies across a wide range. It is usually measured in copies/mL of blood and can be as low as <50 to as high as several million. With time, the virus alters the host immune response, the earliest indications of which may be declining numbers of Th cells (CD4), normal to increased numbers of Ts cells (CD8), and a dramatic change in the ratio of Th to Ts cells from the normal ratio of 2:1. Some patients have minor viral infections or other symptoms (e.g., more-frequent-than-usual recurrences of oral or genital herpes simplex, herpes zoster, oral hairy leukoplakia, mild fever, sweats, weight loss, and diarrhea). Common bacterial infections (e.g., pneumonia, tuberculosis) may occur with increased frequency at any point in HIV-1 infection, including the early stage of disease. These complications tend to become more common as the duration of HIV-1 infection increases.
      (3) **Advanced symptomatic HIV-1 infection** is manifested as AIDS. HIV infection is best thought of as a continuum, with evidence of progressive immune depletion correlating

with increased probability of specific infection or malignancy; nonspecific localized or generalized complaints such as fever, fatigue, or night sweats; or organ dysfunction such as renal failure or dementia. Older definitions of AIDS are mostly used to determine eligibility for disability insurance rather than to guide therapy.

b. **Monitoring HIV-1** disease is very helpful in establishing prognosis and adjusting treatment. Various quantitative assays of viral nucleic acid predict the rate of progression of disease; those patients with the lowest viral loads tend to remain symptom free and live longer than those with high viral loads. When treatment is effective, these assays show a drop to low or undetectable **viral load.** If viral load has been very low and is now increasing, treatment may be failing.

c. **HIV-2** infection follows the same general pattern as HIV-1, but much less is known. The clinical course is usually milder or slower. Several well-described cases of AIDS have been associated with HIV-2 in the absence of HIV-1. It will probably be shown that determinants of immunosuppression are the most significant predictors of whether opportunistic infection or malignancy will occur.

D Therapy

1. **HTLV-I.** Treatment of HTLV-I–related malignancies with conventional cancer chemotherapy has been disappointing. However, the use of anti-retrovirals directed against HIV-1 has resulted in some durable remissions. No treatment of asymptomatic HTLV-I infections is necessary.
2. **HTLV-II.** There is no need to treat HTLV-II infection at any stage.
3. **HIV**

   a. **HIV-1. At all stages of illness, the goal of therapy is to suppress viral replication as measured by viral load.** Improvement in clinical and immune parameters may be delayed but usually follows in a matter of weeks to months. Chemotherapy may influence the progression of HIV-1 infection. Careful evaluation and timely antiretroviral therapy may delay or prevent the development of significant complications. When to start therapy is a complex question that depends on a number of factors. For patients with **symptomatic** infection, therapy should be started as soon as possible. For patients with rapidly progressive infection (as determined by high viral loads and dropping CD4 counts), early therapy is also appropriate. What is most unclear is when to initiate therapy in a person with good immune function. Early intervention will preserve immune function but can be taxing vis-à-vis side effects and cost. Interruptions of therapy are controversial but there does seem to be a risk that getting back control of viral replication might be challenging.

   (1) A variety of drugs have been shown to be effective in reducing the viral load and improving immune function. Because recommendations change quickly, the decision about which therapy to use should be based on current studies. As of 2004, five classes of drugs for the treatment of HIV-1 are available: **nucleoside reverse transcriptase inhibitors (NRTIs), nucleotide reverse transcriptase inhibitors, non-nucleoside reverse transcriptase inhibitors (NNRTIs), fusion inhibitors,** and **protease inhibitors.**

   (2) Evidence indicating that **combinations** of agents are much more effective is very strong. Although single agents can be shown to have activity (as measured by reducing viral load and increasing CD4 counts), there is no occasion to use them alone.

   (3) **Failure to adequately suppress viral replication** or rebound viral replication is a **poor prognostic sign.** A reevaluation of treatment is warranted at this time.

   (4) **Resistance** to antiretroviral drugs occurs by mutational change in the viral genome. Exposure to any of the agents is predictably followed by resistance within weeks to months unless viral replication is successfully suppressed. Once resistance occurs, it is very stable and does not disappear even with drug cessation. Resistance to various antiretroviral drugs can be measured by genotypic analysis (looking for known mutations that confer specific resistance) or phenotypic analysis (akin to the tests to look for bacte-

rial drug resistance). Both of these methods are expensive and somewhat inconclusive although they can be helpful in guiding therapy.

(5) **Drug–drug interactions** are common and potentially severe. Some antiretrovirals such as the protease inhibitors can have powerful effects on hepatic cytochrome enzymes. This may result in unexpectedly high or low levels of other drugs that depend on liver metabolism.

(6) **Direct drug toxicity** is common although usually manageable. Akin to cancer chemotherapy, different agents tend to have different side effects and toxicities. Therefore assembling a combination of HIV-1 medications needs to take into account various toxicities. Some of the most severe toxicities include pancreatitis, peripheral neuropathy, severe hypersensitivity reactions, lactic acidosis, and dyslipidemia.

(7) **Drug costs** are high, and the cost of monitoring is also considerable. Whereas effective HIV-1 care is money saving in the long run (as compared with the cost of hospitalizations, decreased productivity, and early mortality), it can be difficult to afford good HIV-1 care.

b. HIV-2. Treatment for HIV-2 infection tends to mirror that of HIV-1 and is much less extensively studied.

E **Prognosis** The prognosis of HIV-1 infection has changed radically with the awareness that suppressing viral replication can allow for immune reconstitution. Individuals who contracted HIV-1 infection in the past could live in good health for many years, even without medical intervention, and then experience declining health for several years. Now, with careful medical management, HIV-1 can be controlled in many individuals, although the duration of this response is not yet known. This has considerably influenced the mortality rates of AIDS. Even for those patients who are unwilling or unable to follow the complex drug regimens needed to restore immune function, intermittent antiviral therapy may provide some benefit, although the long-term prognosis may not be good. With the many new treatment modalities in development for HIV-1–infected individuals, further prognostic changes may occur in the foreseeable future.

F Prevention

1. **Screening.** There is **no systematic screening program** for retroviral infections. Applicants to the military are screened for HIV-1 infection, and blood donors are screened for HTLV-I and HIV-1. Most testing is done on a voluntary basis, and many states require an informed consent or some equivalent document for HIV-1 testing. Because most HTLV-I–and HTLV-II–infected patients never develop clinical disease, there is little call for screening for these agents. HIV-1 screening tests are very sensitive, specific, and widely available for HIV-1 infection, but they may not detect the antibody response to HIV-2. Home testing and point-of-use testing for HIV-1 are available and accurate, but standard tests should always be done to corroborate positive results.
2. **Controlling spread of infection.** Preventive measures for controlling the spread of HIV include **education** about risk factors, **sexual abstinence,** use of **barrier precautions** (condoms), **avoidance of childbirth** in women known to be HIV-1 infected, **needle exchange programs,** and **universal testing blood products.** Treatment of HIV-1–infected pregnant women with antiretrovirals substantially decreases prenatal and peripartum transmission of HIV, as does delivery by cesarean section. Breast feeding should be avoided by women infected with HIV-I. Suppression of HIV-1 in the blood is accompanied by reduction of viral loads on mucosal surfaces so it should also decrease infectivity. This in no way should be construed as a reason to reduce cautiousness with regard to safer sex practices and needle sharing.
3. **Public health.** HIV-1 infection is a disease that must be reported to the Department of Health irrespective of the clinical status of the patient. Partner notification requirements vary considerably among legal jurisdictions.

G **Complications** Effects of HIV-1 infection can result from direct damage caused by the virus or from the opportunistic infections or malignancies that accompany the decline of the immune system in late-stage HIV-1 infection. In general, direct effects of HIV-1 include fevers, night sweats, weight loss, decreased libido, cognitive deficits, and muscle wasting.

1. **Types of complications**
   a. **Skin lesions**
      (1) Some lesions are rare in individuals without HIV infection but are relatively common in those with HIV-1 infection.
         (a) Kaposi's sarcoma, which is caused by a herpesvirus (HHV-8)
         (b) Eosinophilic folliculitis
         (c) Disseminated molluscum contagiosum
         (d) Bacillary angiomatosis (Bartonella)
         (e) Thrush (Candida)
      (2) The following common disorders are more severe in individuals with HIV-1 infection.
         (a) Psoriasis (including psoriatic arthritis)
         (b) Seborrheic dermatitis
         (c) Alopecia
         (d) Onychomycosis (fungal infections of the nail beds)
         (e) Severe or recurrent genital candidal infection
   b. **Lymphatic system.** Lymph nodes are often enlarged, although usually this is not reflective of a specific infection or tumor. The enlarged nodes are characterized on biopsy as having reactive hyperplasia.
      (1) **Lymphomas** often occur as extranodal disease but may cause nodal enlargement later.
      (2) Several **infectious agents** can cause lymph node enlargement, including *T. pallidum, M. tuberculosis,* and *Histoplasma capsulatum.* Node aspirate or biopsy is useful in distinguishing among these organisms.
      (3) **Kaposi's sarcoma** may be found in lymph nodes.
   c. **Nervous system.** Such involvement may be diffuse or focal. Some cognitive or motor dysfunction is common and tends to become more severe. Usually, there is evidence of cerebral atrophy, and no opportunistic agent can be found to explain the dementia.
      (1) **Meningitis** is caused most frequently by *Cryptococcus neoformans,* a ubiquitous yeast. Headache and neck stiffness range from mild or transient to severe, and the CSF is often normal or near normal with regard to cell count, protein level, glucose concentration, and general appearance. Cryptococci are seen on India ink preparations, and cryptococcal antigen can be demonstrated in serum and CSF. *Cryptococcus* is easily cultured from CSF and less commonly from blood.
         (a) Aseptic meningitis with headache, nuchal rigidity, and lymphocytic pleocytosis often occurs in the early stage of HIV-1 infection and occasionally in later stages.
         (b) Other forms of meningitis, although relatively uncommon, occur more often than in the general population.
      (2) **Neuropathy** may be a part of HIV-1 infection, an opportunistic infection, or a side effect of treatment. For example, vincristine, which may be used for some AIDS-related malignancies, induces dose-related peripheral neuropathy, as do certain NRTIs such as zalcitabine (ddC) and didanosine (ddI).
      (3) **Space-occupying lesions of the CNS** are found with some frequency in HIV-1 infection. The presentation is usually one of focal neurologic abnormality (often accompanied by seizures) and an abnormal CT or MRI scan.
         (a) *T. gondii,* a protozoan parasite found worldwide, is the most common cause of **brain abscess** in AIDS patients.
         (b) **Lymphomas** located in deep brain structures and **progressive multifocal leukoencephalopathy** (caused by the JC virus) are also disproportionately common.
   d. **Eye.** HIV-1 may be associated with some direct toxicity to the eye and optic nerve, but **CMV retinitis** is the most common and serious ocular complication of AIDS. The lesions are pre-

dominantly retinal and spare the choroid. They usually progress over weeks and can lead to blindness. Involvement of both eyes is the rule, and CMV retinitis is often part of a systemic illness including predominantly the gastrointestinal tract. Serious CMV ocular disease occurs in late-stage HIV infection when the CD4 count is very depressed. Treatment of HIV that results in CD4 increases will often stop progression of disease.

e. Upper alimentary tract

(1) The upper gastrointestinal tract is most frequently affected by **local candidal or herpes simplex infections,** which can extend into the esophagus, or by **Kaposi's sarcoma,** which can be found throughout the intestine. Endoscopic esophageal brushes or biopsy can distinguish between the two most common opportunists.

(2) Visual examination of the oral cavity is sufficient for identifying **oral hairy leukoplakia,** an Epstein-Barr virus–related infection that predominantly involves the lateral tongue but may extend to other parts of the oral cavity.

(3) **Aphthous ulcers** of the mouth and esophagus are common, and esophageal ulcers can be large and painful.

f. Liver

(1) In the late stage of HIV-1 infection, the liver often is the site of **opportunistic infections** such as histoplasmosis, mycobacteriosis [due to *M. tuberculosis* and *Mycobacterium avium-intracellulare* (MAI)], cryptococcosis, and CMV. Hepatic candidiasis, which is sometimes seen in leukemia as part of systemic fungal disease, is not seen in AIDS.

(2) The same populations who are at risk for HIV-1 infection are also at risk for blood-borne hepatitis: **HBV; HCV; HDV;** and **non-A, non-B hepatitis.** Peliosis hepatis is a treatable liver infection caused by *B. henselae,* the agent of cat-scratch disease.

g. Gastrointestinal tract distal to the esophagus

(1) **HIV-1** can cause an **enteropathy** distinct from the infectious diarrheas.

(2) In addition, ***Cryptosporidium*** species, ***Microsporidium, Cyclospora, Isospora,*** and ***G. intestinalis*** are potentially causes of **watery diarrhea** and **diffuse abdominal pain** in HIV-1–infected patients.

(3) The stomach and small bowel also may be sites of origin of **extranodal lymphoma.**

(4) **CMV colitis** can be the cause of severe abdominal pain, diarrhea, and fever, and it occasionally can lead to perforation or megacolon.

h. Lungs. In AIDS, the lungs are the most common target organ for symptomatic disease.

(1) ***Pneumocystis carinii*** **pneumonia (PCP)** develops in most patients who do not receive prophylaxis and whose CD4 cell count drops below 200/mm^3. In HIV-1–infected individuals, PCP has a subacute presentation that delays diagnosis, often for weeks. By the time patients come to medical attention, they have fever, dry cough, and hypoxemia. Chest radiographs may be normal or have interstitial markings or fluffy infiltrates. Usually, diagnosis is made by examining sputum, BAL fluid, bronchial washings or brushings, or lung biopsy specimens. Even after initiation of treatment, the disease may progress temporarily but ultimately yields to effective therapy in 90% of patients. Short courses of steroids are often given to abort an early worsening with the initiation of therapy.

(2) **Bacterial pneumonias** also occur more commonly in HIV-1–infected patients than in otherwise healthy individuals. Although these pneumonias may be more severe than in immunocompetent patients, they usually respond to routine antimicrobial therapy. Pneumococcus is the most common cause of bacterial pneumonia in adult HIV-1–infected patients. Bacterial pneumonia can occur simultaneously with PCP.

(3) **Fungal pneumonia** is less common and is usually a part of systemic cryptococcal, *Coccidioides,* or *Histoplasma* infection. Awareness of exposure to the agents of endemic mycoses (e.g., *Coccidioides* or *Histoplasma*) is crucial to make the diagnosis and to initiate appropriate therapy.

(4) **Viral pneumonia** can be severe in HIV-1–infected patients. CMV, a herpesvirus known to cause severe lung disease in other patients with Th-cell deficiencies (especially bone marrow transplant recipients), may cause a fatal pneumonia alone or with PCP in HIV-1–infected patients.

(5) **Mycobacterial disease** is common.

(a) Infection with ***M. tuberculosis*** may appear relatively early in HIV-1 infection. Although it has a higher propensity to disseminate in patients who have Th-cell (CD4) depletion, it usually responds to antimycobacterial therapy. Multiply resistant (to isoniazid and rifampin) *M. tuberculosis* is still uncommon, but these strains are difficult to treat. In immunologically competent individuals, the clinical response may only be 60%, whereas it is considerably lower in HIV-infected patients.

(b) **Nontuberculous mycobacteria,** usually MAI, may be found in sputum. In HIV-1–infected patients, the lungs are a fairly minor target organ for this pathogen, which usually infects the liver, spleen, blood, and bone marrow.

(6) A **noninfectious pneumonitis** characterized by lymphocytic infiltration of the lungs has been seen frequently in children with HIV-1 infection and is being recognized more commonly in adults.

i. Cardiovascular system. Cardiomyopathy may be found in HIV-1–infected patients, presumably as a direct consequence of the virus.

j. Musculoskeletal system. This system is frequently involved in all stages of HIV-1 infection. Manifestations are seldom life-threatening but do cause substantial morbidity. Except for AIDS-associated arthritis, most of these manifestations are clinically similar to entities in individuals without HIV-1 infection. However, the incidence and severity of these manifestations are greater in HIV-1–infected patients and tend to be worse in the late stage of HIV-1 infection.

(1) **Articular manifestations**

(a) **Arthralgias** occur in up to one third of HIV-1–infected individuals. The pain is intermittent and usually affects the large joints.

(b) **Reiter's syndrome** has been reported to affect approximately 5% of HIV-1–infected homosexual men, although it seems to be rarer in individuals who acquire HIV-1 through needle sharing or heterosexual activity.

(c) In patients with psoriasis, HIV-1 infection increases the risk of developing **psoriatic arthritis.**

(d) **AIDS-associated arthritis** is severe and debilitating. It affects the large joints and produces only a mild synovitis. Intra-articular steroids may give considerable relief.

(2) **Muscular diseases**

(a) **Myalgias** are common in HIV-1 infection, especially in the early mononucleosis-like illness associated with seroconversion.

(b) **Polymyositis** with proximal muscle weakness and elevated serum levels of muscle enzymes [e.g., creatine kinase (CK)] occurs in approximately 2% of HIV-1–infected individuals. It also may occur as a side effect of zidovudine therapy.

(3) **Bone and joint infections** are fairly uncommon in HIV-1 infection, except among injection drug users. The causative agents are a mixture of common organisms (see V H) and opportunistic agents such as mycobacteria and fungi.

(4) Various forms of **vasculitis and connective tissue disease** (e.g., Sjögren's syndrome) seem to occur with higher-than-expected frequency.

k. Hematopoietic abnormalities. These conditions are common in HIV-1 infection.

(1) **Immune thrombocytopenia** may occur in mid- to late-stage HIV-1 infection and resembles idiopathic thrombocytopenic purpura (ITP) or thrombotic thrombocytopenic purpura (TTP).

(2) **Anemia** is common in late HIV-1 infection. The pattern is usually one of chronic disease with normochromic, normocytic indices. Some antiretroviral therapies and antimetabo-

lites used to prevent infections may induce macrocytic anemia. Serum levels of vitamin B_{12} are often low, but vitamin B_{12} therapy does not improve hematologic parameters. Many patients with low levels of erythropoietin respond to erythropoietin replacement therapy.

(3) **Neutropenia,** along with the expected depletion of lymphocytes, may accompany HIV-1 infection. This may be a sign of disseminated bacterial or opportunistic infection, and blood and bone marrow culture (including mycobacterial cultures) can be helpful. Antiretroviral and antimetabolite therapies may contribute to neutropenia.

(4) **Immunoglobulin disorders** are common. The most frequently described is a polyclonal increase in gamma globulin with an inability to produce novel immunoglobulins. Thus, patients with advanced HIV-1 infection may respond poorly to vaccination and may not demonstrate good serologic responses to acute infections, especially when challenged during the late stages of HIV infection.

l. **Endocrine system.** A variety of endocrine abnormalities, including thyroid and adrenal insufficiencies, have been reported in HIV-1 infection.

m. **Reproductive system**

(1) Carcinoma of the uterine cervix and dysplastic changes occur more commonly in HIV-1–infected women.

(2) Fungal (candidal) vulvovaginitis is more frequent and may be caused by antifungal drug-resistant strains.

(3) Herpes simplex infections can become very severe with the advanced immune depression associated with HIV-1. Patients with herpes genital infections can have large, confluent painful areas of involvement.

2. **Treatment of infections associated with HIV infection.** Therapeutic regimens may be the same or more intensive than those for the same infection in immunocompetent individuals or patients with other causes of immune depression. Many of the infections associated with HIV are potentially chronic; lifelong secondary prophylaxis and close vigilance are necessary to control recurrences. Recommendations concerning the treatment of these conditions are revised constantly, and current information should always be sought.

3. **Prevention of complications**

a. **Tuberculosis**

(1) **Screening.** Early skin testing is most useful for identifying individuals at risk for recrudescence of previously acquired infection, because many patients become anergic in the later stages of HIV infection. Only 5 mm of induration is needed to qualify as a positive skin test in a person with HIV infection. Aggressive contact tracing of persons who are known to be infectious with tuberculosis also can identify individuals at risk before they become ill with recently acquired tuberculosis.

(2) **Prophylactic isoniazid** reduces the risk of recurrent tuberculosis when administered for 6–12 months to patients who have had positive PPD skin tests.

b. **MAI infection. Macrolides** or **rifabutin** can be given when the CD4 count drops to less than 75 cells/mm^3.

c. **PCP.** Every individual who has already had PCP should receive secondary prophylaxis. Because PCP is a common complication of mid- to late-stage HIV infection, and because preventive therapy is safe and effective, it has become general practice to offer PCP prevention to every HIV-infected person when the CD4 count falls to below 300 cells/mm^3. First-line prophylaxis for PCP is trimethoprim–sulfamethoxazole. For patients intolerant of this medication, dapsone, clindamycin/primaquine, or atovaquone should be considered. Therapy is lifelong unless immune function is improved by HIV-1 suppression.

d. **Syphilis** can recrudesce in HIV-infected persons. **Standard treatments** are usually effective, but careful follow-up is indicated. When there is a question of whether a cure has been achieved, a more intensive regimen (e.g., that for the treatment of neurosyphilis) is recommended.

e. **Cryptococcal disease** can be prevented or delayed by the use of **fluconazole** in patients with late-stage HIV infection. Although fluconazole is safe and prevents or delays the occurrence of thrush, controlled studies show no survival benefit to this regimen as compared with treating fungal infections as they occur. Patients with cryptococcal meningitis should continue to receive antifungal therapy until their CD4 counts exceed 200/mm^3.

f. **Toxoplasmosis.** Many prophylactic regimens for PCP also can prevent clinical toxoplasmosis from occurring. However, it is not usually advisable to add anti-*Toxoplasma* medications to the preventive regimen of an individual who is intolerant to the kind of PCP prophylaxis that also prevents toxoplasmosis.

g. **Bacterial pneumonia.** Early administration of **pneumococcal vaccine** is recommended for every HIV-infected person. A single dose should be adequate for a lifetime.

h. **Hepatitis. HBV vaccine** is recommended for universal use. Because the vaccine is safe and the route of transmission of HBV is similar to that of HIV, vaccination of HIV-infected persons is logical.

i. **Enteritis.** Because many meats and animal products such as milk and eggs can be contaminated with bacteria that cause enteric infection, HIV-infected persons should be advised to consume only pasteurized milk and to eat well-cooked eggs and meats.

j. **Cryptosporidial infection.** The discovery of *Cryptosporidium* in municipal water supplies is worrisome for patients with advanced HIV infection. It is not clear whether the use of water filters and bottled water can substantially reduce the risk of this infection.

k. **Immune reconstitution.** Prophylaxis can be stopped when immune function is restored. Some individuals experience transient worsening of infections as immune function improves. This can be a fairly severe reaction that might require reinstitution of therapy for the previously quiescent infection. Most of the time it is most helpful to continue anti-retroviral therapy despite the clinical worsening because immune reconstitution eventually goes away.

l. In general, prophylaxis against the common HIV-1–associated infections can be stopped when the CD4 count passes the level at which the risk of that infection begins to increase significantly. Usually this is done after at least two CD4 measurements have been high enough and when the patient is clinically stable. If the CD4 drops, it may be necessary to restart prophylaxis.

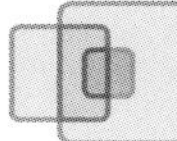

Study Questions

1. A 70-year-old man is admitted to the hospital for an elective hernia repair. The night before surgery, a nurse reports a rectal temperature of 38.1°C. After a careful examination shows no obvious source of infection, a single blood sample is sent for culture. The surgery is uneventful, but 3 days later, *Corynebacterium* is identified on blood culture. Which of the following best explains this finding?

- A The patient has bacterial endocarditis caused by *Corynebacterium.*
- B While taking the rectal temperature, the nurse inadvertently caused *Corynebacterium* bacteremia.
- C Tooth brushing just before the blood collection resulted in transient *Corynebacterium* bacteremia.
- D Inadequate skin preparation or careless handling resulted in contamination of the blood culture.
- E The laboratory mistook *Escherichia coli* for *Corynebacterium.*

2. A 19-year-old man with acute nonlymphocytic leukemia is admitted to the hospital 2 weeks after his first round of chemotherapy. His temperature is 39.2°C, and physical examination shows no localized abnormalities. Chest radiograph shows a Hickman catheter with its tip in the right atrium. The white blood cell (WBC) count is 300/mm^3 with no polymorphonuclear or band cells in the differential count. Blood cultures are obtained. Which of the following is the next step?

- A Initiate antistaphylococcal treatment for the possibility of Hickman catheter–related bacteremia.
- B Administer broad-spectrum antibiotics with excellent activity for enteric gram-negative rods and *Pseudomonas aeruginosa.*
- C Await results of blood cultures and other diagnostic tests because infection could be caused by almost any microorganism.
- D Initiate oral prophylaxis to prevent bacterial and fungal infections.
- E Administer parenteral antifungal therapy.

3. A 20-year-old woman with a history of seizures for which she has taken phenytoin for 4 months has a fever of 38.7°C; she has felt febrile for 2 weeks. She has no respiratory or urinary symptoms. Physical examination findings are normal except for elevated body temperature. Chest radiograph, urinalysis, and complete blood count (CBC) findings are normal. Which of the following would be the best next step?

- A Admit the patient for toxic shock syndrome (TSS).
- B Administer acetaminophen.
- C Treat occult urinary tract infection with antibiotics.
- D Discontinue phenytoin and prescribe another anticonvulsant.
- E Cool the patient with a cooling blanket.

4. A sexually active 24-year-old woman known to be HIV-1–infected has had a fever for 2 days and has a productive cough. Chest radiographs show an infiltrate in the right lung. Two weeks earlier, her helper T (Th) cell (CD4) count was 510/mm^3. Gram stain of sputum shows many white blood cells (WBCs) and squamous epithelial cells with a mixed bacterial flora. Testing for nontreponemal antigen (rapid plasma reagin) is positive at two dilutions, and treponemal antigen testing is also positive. Which of the following is the most likely cause of the pneumonia?

- A *Streptococcus pneumoniae*
- B *Pneumocystis carinii*

C Cytomegalovirus (CMV)
D *Mycobacterium avium-intracellulare* (MAI)
E Syphilis

5. A 62-year-old man has right upper quadrant abdominal pain, nausea, and vomiting. Physical examination shows only guarding over the liver. Ultrasound examination confirms the diagnosis of gallstones without dilated bile ducts. The man is allergic to penicillin (a rash developed after penicillin therapy for a sore throat). In addition to dietary changes, which of the following treatments would be best?

A No antibiotics
B Erythromycin
C Oral quinolone
D Trimethoprim–sulfamethoxazole
E Amoxicillin

6. Two weeks after emergency surgery for a perforated duodenal ulcer, a 39-year-old woman complains of fever and vague abdominal pain. Her only medication is ranitidine. On physical examination, she appears a little pale, has a temperature of 38°C, and has a slight fullness in the epigastrium. Computed tomography (CT) scan of the abdomen shows an area of fluid collection measuring 3 × 3 × 8 cm in the left paracolic gutter. Which of the following would be the most effective next step?

A Administer antibiotic therapy with an agent highly effective against aerobic gram-negative rods (e.g., aztreonam).
B Administer antibiotic therapy effective against abdominal anaerobes (e.g., clindamycin).
C Provide catheter drainage of the fluid collection and antibiotics appropriate for culture results.
D Administer no therapy unless blood cultures are positive or the collection changes in size.
E Order a magnetic resonance imaging (MRI) scan to confirm the CT findings.

7. A 64-year-old woman presents to the emergency department with abdominal pain and fever. She has had a long history of mild, intermittent dyspepsia that frequently has followed meals. She has had diabetes for 12 years, and although her response to oral hypoglycemic agents has been poor, she has refused to use insulin. At the time of presentation, she has been ill for 36 hours with vomiting, fever, and abdominal pain. On examination, she is febrile with a temperature of 38.9°C and has tachycardia of 124 beats/min. She is mildly jaundiced. Bowel sounds are diminished, and tenderness and guarding are most marked in the right upper quadrant. Toward the end of the examination, rigor is evident, and she has broken into a sweat. Which of the following is most likely to be her problem?

A Pancreatitis with abscess
B Cholangitis
C Perforated peptic ulcer
D Splenic abscess
E Esophageal reflux

8. A 24-year-old man takes an exotic "around the world" vacation to Europe, Africa, India, and China. On his holiday, he has frequent sexual encounters and does not use condoms. In addition, he is bitten by mosquitoes many times. On his return, he notes fever, and his physician finds generalized lymphadenopathy. Which of the following is least likely to account for both these symptoms?

A Human immunodeficiency virus type 1 (HIV-1)
B Infectious mononucleosis
C Malaria
D Syphilis
E Cat-scratch disease

9. A 14-year-old girl from Pennsylvania goes to Wisconsin for a 2-week camping trip. Two weeks after she returns, she notices a solitary circular rash on her left calf just above the area normally covered by her socks. Overall, she feels well, and there is gradual progression of the rash over the next week. Which of the following diseases endemic in Wisconsin or Pennsylvania did she most likely acquire?

- A Blastomycosis
- B Lyme disease
- C California encephalitis
- D Rocky Mountain spotted fever (RMSF)
- E Syphilis

10. Which of the following is the strongest indication to consider valve replacement surgery in a patient with infective endocarditis?

- A Hematuria
- B Positive cultures for *Staphylococcus aureus* on the second day of therapy
- C Splinter hemorrhages and Osler's nodes
- D Progressive congestive heart failure (CHF)
- E Splenomegaly

11. An 18-year-old woman takes a summer job working in a day-care center. A month after starting, she develops a rash over her whole body. The lesions are small vesicles on a slightly erythematous base. Except for a slight cough and fever of 38°C, she feels well. She has proof of having received her childhood immunizations before she started school. Which of the following statements is most correct?

- A The patient probably has an elevated total white blood cell (WBC) count and a differential with an abundance of neutrophils and band forms.
- B Within 1 week, the patient will recover totally with lifelong immunity and no further sequelae.
- C The patient probably developed an allergy to some of the fabric in the toys at the daycare center.
- D The patient may be infectious to other family members.
- E If the patient becomes pregnant 1 year or more later, she will require close obstetric observation.

12. After a recent bad cold, an 18-year-old man has symptoms of sinusitis with nasal drainage and stuffiness. On examination, papilledema is evident. The physician is convinced that the patient has a brain abscess. Which of the following statements is correct?

- A Magnetic resonance imaging (MRI) scans are usually not helpful.
- B The source of infection is usually cardiac.
- C Antimicrobials active against *Pseudomonas aeruginosa* are usually a part of the treatment.
- D Complete surgical excision is usually not needed.
- E The patient is likely to develop bacterial meningitis in the next 5 years.

13. A 12-year-old boy has had fever and bloody diarrhea for 2 weeks and has lost 4 pounds of body weight. Three stool specimens have yielded no enteric pathogens on culture, and no ova or mature parasites are observed on direct examination. Which of the following is the best reason for his illness?

- A Regional enteritis
- B Giardiasis
- C Travelers' diarrhea caused by enterotoxigenic *Escherichia coli*
- D Cryptosporidiosis
- E Jejunal infarction

14. Which of the following features of the cerebrospinal fluid (CSF) is typical of bacterial meningitis but rare in viral meningitis?

A Headache and stiff neck
B Leukocyte pleocytosis
C Increased cerebrospinal fluid (CSF) protein
D Decreased CSF glucose (i.e., to less than half of the serum level)
E Fever

15. A 70-year-old man has chronic lung disease. Which of the following immunizations should he receive annually?

A Influenza
B Tetanus
C Pneumococcal pneumonia
D Pertussis
E Hepatitis B (HBV)

16. A 49-year-old man reports recent sexual contact with a commercial sex worker. About 9 days later, he experiences dysuria and has a very modest urethral discharge. Which of the following infectious agents most likely accounts for his symptoms?

A *Chlamydia trachomatis* infection
B Syphilis
C Trichomoniasis
D Granuloma inguinale
E *Escherichia coli*

17. A 41-year-old man with a history of weight loss and hairy leukoplakia reports that a recent HIV-1 blood test came back positive. His CD4 count is 204/mm^3, and his viral load is 58,000 copies/mL by reverse transcriptase polymerase chain reaction (moderately high). A purified protein derivative (PPD) skin test is negative for tuberculosis, and you find that he has already had a pneumococcal vaccination. Which of the following would be the next step?

A Wait until he develops a more significant opportunistic infection before beginning antiretroviral therapy.
B Begin zidovudine at standard doses and take the patient's CD4 count and a viral load in 6 weeks.
C Begin a combination regimen with three active agents such as zidovudine, lamivudine, and efavirenz.
D Begin a course of fluconazole to prevent thrush and rifabutin to prevent *Mycobacterium avium-intracellulare* (MAI) infection.
E Refer the patient to a dentist for management of the hairy leukoplakia.

18. When a patient needs a peripheral intravenous catheter for approximately 1 week, which of the following methods is the most important way of preventing catheter-related infections?

A Using a powerful antimicrobial ointment at the junction of the hub and the skin
B Changing the catheter site every 48–72 hours
C Giving systemic antibiotics for the entire duration of catheter placement
D Shaving the skin before cleansing it
E Using the leg rather than the arm

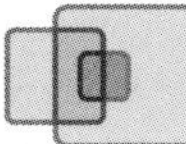

Answers and Explanations

1. The answer is D [I A; III B]. Inadequate skin preparation or careless handling results in contamination of the blood culture. Even though all of the answers are possible, the most likely one is simple contamination; 2%–5% of blood cultures are contaminated by skin flora from the patient or the phlebotomist. *Corynebacterium* makes up a small fraction of oral and rectal flora and is less likely to enter the blood from these sites. Endocarditis caused by *Corynebacterium* is rare and almost never involves native valves. *Escherichia coli* and *Corynebacterium* are essentially impossible to confuse in the laboratory.

2. The answer is B [II A 3]. The next step is to administer broad-spectrum antibiotics with activity against enteric gram-negative rods and *Pseudomonas aeruginosa.* The heightened susceptibility of neutropenic patients to die quickly of overwhelming sepsis makes early intervention obligatory. Even though many clinicians include antibiotic coverage for staphylococci, the most common bacteria encountered are gram-negative rods. Antifungal treatment is used if antibacterial therapy fails to control the fever or if a specific fungal infection is found. Prophylaxis is started before having evidence of active infection.

3. The answer is D [VII D 2 b]. The next best step is to discontinue the phenytoin and prescribe another anticonvulsant. Of the many drugs that cause fever as an unwanted side effect, anticonvulsant agents lead the list. Prolonged fever can have many causes other than medication reactions and may be difficult to diagnose. In ambulatory patients, common bacterial infections are fairly well excluded by normal findings on chest radiograph, urine, and blood tests. Toxic shock syndrome (TSS) is a multisystem illness in which fever is only one component. Although juvenile rheumatoid arthritis affects patients in this age group, aspirin would be more appropriate than acetaminophen. Cooling blankets are used only in severely ill patients.

4. The answer is A [V C 4 b, c (1); VIII G 1 h (1)]. The most likely cause of the pneumonia is *Streptococcus pneumoniae.* Although *P. carinii* is the most common serious opportunistic infection in patients with HIV-1 infection, the productive cough, localized infiltrate, and brief duration argue against *P. carinii* pneumonia (PCP). In addition, the Th cell (CD4) count of more than 500 cells/mm^3 suggests that serious opportunistic infections such as PCP, cytomegalovirus (CMV), or *Mycobacterium avium-intracellulare* (MAI) are unlikely for some time. Syphilis, which may have been present, almost never involves the lungs.

5. The answer is A [V E 4 a]. Uncomplicated cholecystitis without obstruction of the biliary ducts or empyema of the gallbladder is best managed conservatively. Although some bacteria may be found in the bile at the time of cholecystectomy, there is rarely progression to infection. Erythromycin essentially has no activity for any of the agents associated with cholecystitis or cholangitis. Amoxicillin is contraindicated for patients who are allergic to penicillin. Severely ill patients should be hospitalized to manage the possibility of serious complications.

6. The answer is C [V E 2]. Catheter drainage of the fluid collection and antibiotics appropriate for culture results would be the most effective step to take next. The most likely explanation for the clinical findings and the computed tomography (CT) abnormality is a postoperative intra-abdominal abscess. These rarely heal without drainage. Surgical drainage is effective, but a lesion that can be reached safely with a catheter may be drained equally effectively and more safely. Antibiotics are usually used as adjunctive therapy. The flora of these abscesses is usually mixed with enteric aerobes and anaerobes. Good cultures can be useful in refining the exact therapeutic regimen. Magnetic resonance imaging (MRI) is a fine test, but the CT scan has already led to a diagnosis.

7. The answer is B [V E 4]. According to the patient, she has certainly had cholecystitis in the past. With gallstones in the gallbladder, there is always some risk of migration to the common bile duct and subsequent obstruction of the duct. The infection that may follow obstruction of the common bile duct may be very serious, with bacteremia and sepsis as common sequelae. Pancreatic abscess can manifest as abdominal pain, but it does not have the associated localized right upper quadrant findings as often as cholangitis. Perforated ulcers lead to peritonitis. Splenic abscesses are almost always the sequelae of bacteremia (e.g., with endocarditis). Reflux esophagitis can cause severe heartburn but does not result in sepsis.

8. The answer is C [VII A 1, 2]. Malaria is characterized by lack of lymphadenopathy, although splenomegaly and fever are characteristic. Although generalized enlargement of lymph nodes is a nonspecific finding, it often can lead to the diagnosis of a clinical entity. When the lymphadenopathy is coupled with fatigue and an atypical lymphocytosis, infectious mononucleosis is suggested. This syndrome most often is caused by Epstein-Barr virus, but a similar clinical picture is produced by cytomegalovirus (CMV) infection. The infections can be distinguished by using serologic tests (e.g., Monospot test) or specific antibodies. Secondary syphilis also should be considered in patients with adenopathy of short duration; this can be confirmed on the basis of serologic tests and the finding of an appropriate rash. Reactive, hyperplastic lymph nodes are common in HIV-1 infection. For this patient, all of these are possibilities, but the malaria would not account for the enlarged lymph nodes. Cat-scratch disease usually causes enlarged lymph glands, with stellate microabscesses apparent histologically.

9. The answer is B [VII F]. Only Lyme disease and Rocky Mountain spotted fever (RMSF) occur with a rash as a common feature. California encephalitis (which is spread by mosquito) has few, if any, skin manifestations but does cause a syndrome of progressive neurologic deterioration that resolves spontaneously in most cases. Blastomycosis, a disease that enters the body through the respiratory tract and may metastasize to other organs, almost never generates a circular rash. RMSF has a rash that usually begins peripherally but is rarely solitary. The course of disease is usually fairly rapid, in contrast to the indolent but progressive lesion that is typical of erythema migrans. Syphilis causes a rash but almost never involves only one spot on the leg.

10. The answer is D [V I 5 d]. Although all of the answers reflect aspects of endocarditis, the only absolute indications for valve replacement are fungal endocarditis, congestive heart failure (CHF), valve ring abscess, and failure to clear infection after a long course of antimicrobial therapy. Some authorities recommend valve replacement after multiple significant emboli. Minor emboli, an enlarged spleen, and immunologic phenomena are not cause for valve replacement.

11. The answer is D [II G 4]. Although a varicella vaccine does exist, its implementation has not been universal among older children or adults. Thus, many children and adults are still susceptible to varicella. Sequelae of varicella infection are rare and include pneumonia, meningitis, and hepatitis as well as herpes zoster (shingles). The white blood cell (WBC) count is normal or slightly depressed in most of the childhood exanthems. Varicella in pregnancy can be severe, but this patient will be safe once her rash disappears.

12. The answer is D [V A 3]. Cross-sectional imaging studies [e.g., computed tomography (CT) and magnetic resonance imaging (MRI)] are critical to the diagnosis and management of intracranial abscess. Surgery is often undertaken to obtain a specimen for culture or to decompress the abscess. Total surgical excision is rarely required in the patient who is responding well to medical therapy. Although occasional patients do have cardiopulmonary sources for infection, most patients have contiguous infection of the middle ear or, as in this case, the sinus. Meningitis can follow trauma to the cribriform plate but rarely follows a brain abscess.

13. The answer is A [V D]. Regional enteritis, ulcerative colitis, and a variety of invasive infectious pathogens can cause bloody diarrhea. A single stool specimen may miss any of these agents. *Giardia lam-*

blia and *Cryptosporidium* usually cause an upper small bowel lesion that leads to watery diarrhea without fever. Travelers' diarrhea is a toxin-mediated infection that also leads to minimal inflammatory changes in the bowel. Bowel infarcts are extremely rare in children.

14. The answer is D [V A 1 a (1)]. Acute meningitis is an inflammatory process involving the arachnoid layer of the meninges and the cerebrospinal fluid (CSF). Two major forms of acute meningitis are recognized—bacterial and aseptic. Because the two forms have a similar clinical presentation of fever, headache, and stiff neck, the interpretation of CSF findings is important in the management of acute meningitis. Aside from a diagnostic Gram stain, lowered CSF glucose (i.e., to less than half of the simultaneous serum level) and the presence of a neutrophil pleocytosis are the most characteristic findings in bacterial meningitis. An increased CSF protein level also is a consistent finding in bacterial meningitis; however, CSF protein may be mildly elevated in the aseptic form as well. The pleocytosis in aseptic meningitis is modest (usually < 100 cells/mm^3) and is characterized by a preponderance of lymphocytes.

15. The answer is A [II G 2]. Immunity to pertussis is not essential for adults of any age, and a periodic booster for tetanus is all that is required. A single vaccination for pneumococcal infection should be given to all persons with chronic cardiopulmonary disease and to all adults older than age 60 years. Reimmunizations may not be needed at all, and certainly no more than once every 5–7 years. However, the immunity conferred by influenza vaccine is short-lived and strain specific. Yearly immunizations for influenza are strongly recommended for the elderly and those with chronic cardiopulmonary diseases. Hepatitis B (HBV) vaccine is not routinely indicated in the elderly, and vaccination is not needed for at least 5 years.

16. The answer is A [VI B 1,2]. Chlamydial infection is one of the most common causes of urethritis and frequently manifests with dysuria. Syphilis and granuloma inguinale do affect the external genitals but tend to spare the urethral mucosa. Trichomonas is sometimes found in the male genitals, but it is almost always without symptoms. *Escherichia coli* can cause a urinary tract infection but not a sexually transmitted disease (STD).

17. The answer is C [VIII D 3]. Symptomatic HIV-1 infection can be treated using combination therapy with exceedingly good results. With luck, the correct antiretroviral drug combination will lead to an improvement in this patient's immune function, and he might be able to avoid all chemoprophylaxis indefinitely. Delay in treatment now might spare him some drug side effects, but he is almost to the point of developing severe complications from HIV-1 itself. Treatment with a single drug such as zidovudine is not useful because of its limited impact on viral burden and the early emergence of resistance. Although prophylaxis for *Mycobacterium avium-intracellulare* (MAI) and fungal infections may reduce the number of such infections, it need not be started until immune dysfunction has progressed considerably. Hairy leukoplakia is not serious and will subside with improved immune function.

18. The answer is B [IV G]. Assuming that all catheters are placed under the best possible conditions, keeping them clean and dry is all the daily care they need. Short plastic catheters are prone to infection over time, so routine replacement is recommended. This rule does not apply to central catheters (placed directly into a central vein or threaded up along the arm). There is no benefit to shaving the skin except to provide a better surface for the adhesive tape used to secure the catheter. Intravenous lines in the leg, which are trickier to maintain and have a higher rate of infection, should be avoided whenever possible.

chapter **9**

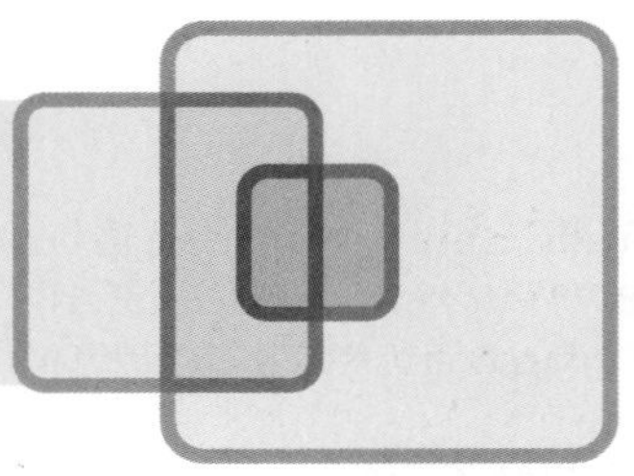

Endocrine and Metabolic Diseases

E. VICTOR ADLIN

I DISORDERS OF THE PITUITARY GLAND

A **Anterior pituitary disease** results from insufficient production of pituitary hormones (hypopituitarism), excessive production of pituitary hormones (acromegaly, Cushing's disease, or hyperprolactinemia), or the local effects of pituitary tumors.

1. **Pituitary tumors** make up 10% of intracranial tumors. Most are benign, but their continued slow growth in the confined sellar and suprasellar areas may cause serious neurologic damage.
   a. **Types**
      (1) **Pituitary adenomas** are classified by cell type, based on electron microscopy and immunohistochemical staining.
         (a) **Somatotroph tumors** produce growth hormone (GH), **corticotroph tumors** produce adrenocorticotropic hormone (ACTH), and **lactotroph tumors** produce prolactin.
      (2) **Craniopharyngiomas,** the most common tumors of the hypothalamic–pituitary area in children, arise from remnants of cells from Rathke's pouch.
         (a) These tumors usually are located above the sella turcica, but they may produce changes within the sella itself.
         (b) They may be solid or cystic, may contain cholesterol-rich fluid, and often contain areas of calcification.
      (3) **Meningiomas** and **metastatic tumors** may involve the hypothalamic–pituitary area.
   b. **Clinical features**
      (1) **Excess hormone production** by pituitary adenomas may lead to **acromegaly** (see I A 3), **Cushing's disease** (see V B 1 a), or **hyperprolactinemia** (see I A 4).
         (a) In rare cases, these tumors may produce excess thyroid-stimulating hormone (TSH), causing hyperthyroidism.
         (b) Follicle-stimulating hormone (FSH) and luteinizing hormone (LH) are frequently produced in excess by pituitary tumors, but this usually does not result in a clear-cut clinical syndrome.
      (2) **Insufficient hormone production,** due to compression or destruction of pituitary and hypothalamic cells, produces the syndrome of **hypopituitarism** (see I A 2).
      (3) **Neurologic effects**
         (a) **Optic nerve compression** may occur. Pituitary tumors may press upward on the inferior surface of the optic chiasm. Vision loss tends to occur first in the superior temporal quadrants, with bitemporal hemianopia in more advanced cases.
         (b) **Headache** is common.
         (c) Other neurologic manifestations such as mental status changes, cranial nerve abnormalities, vomiting, and papilledema are less common.

(4) Sensitive imaging techniques [e.g., magnetic resonance imaging (MRI)] can show pituitary **microadenomas** (tumors < 10 mm in diameter) in 10% of normal individuals. If hyperprolactinemia or other hormone abnormalities are not present and if follow-up study shows no progressive enlargement, these tumors should be regarded as incidental findings of no clinical significance.

(5) **Multiple endocrine neoplasia, type I** (**MEN I, Wermer syndrome**) is a syndrome consisting of tumors, often functioning, of the pituitary, parathyroids, and pancreatic islets.

c. Diagnosis

(1) **Diagnostic imaging**

(a) **Skull radiographs** may show enlargement or distortion of the sella when tumors are 10 mm or more in diameter (**macroadenomas**). Suprasellar calcification suggests the presence of a craniopharyngioma.

(b) **Microadenomas** may be visualized with more sensitive procedures such as **MRI with gadolinium enhancement** or **computed tomography** (**CT**).

(2) **Hormone studies.** Pituitary adenomas that secrete excess GH, ACTH, or prolactin can be diagnosed by measuring the pituitary hormones, or in some cases the hormones produced by target organs, even if the adenoma is too small to be visualized by diagnostic imaging.

d. Therapy

(1) **Surgery** is indicated for pituitary adenomas that produce neurologic symptoms and for some tumors that cause syndromes associated with hormone overproduction.

(a) **Transsphenoidal pituitary microsurgery** is used for intrasellar tumors that have minimal or no suprasellar extension. Small adenomas often can be removed without damage to normal pituitary tissue.

(b) **Transfrontal resection** may be necessary for large tumors that extend far outside the sella turcica or compress the optic chiasm.

(2) **Radiation therapy,** used alone or in conjunction with surgery, may decrease the size of pituitary tumors and decrease hormone production.

(3) **Medical therapy**

(a) **Hormone replacement** is required if hypopituitarism is present.

(b) Dopamine agonists such as **bromocriptine** and **cabergoline** as well as somatostatin analogs such as **octreotide** may decrease the size and hormone production of certain pituitary tumors [see I A 3 d (3) and I A 4 d (2)].

2. Hypopituitarism

a. Etiology

(1) **Pituitary tumors,** most commonly pituitary macroadenomas and craniopharyngiomas, may destroy normal hypothalamic–pituitary tissue.

(2) **Sheehan's syndrome** is hypopituitarism caused by infarction of the anterior pituitary gland during childbirth. The pituitary gland doubles in size during pregnancy, largely because of hyperplasia of the lactotrophs. The blood supply does not keep pace with the enlargement, however, and hypotensive episodes during a complicated delivery may lead to infarction.

(3) **Surgery** for the removal of pituitary or other brain tumors may damage the hypothalamus, the pituitary gland, or both.

(4) **Less common causes** of pituitary or hypothalamic destruction include **sarcoidosis, hemochromatosis, Hand-Schüller-Christian disease, tuberculosis, syphilis,** and **fungal infections.**

b. Clinical features

(1) **GH deficiency** has different effects in children and adults.

(a) In children, **growth failure** occurs, leading to short stature in adulthood (**pituitary dwarfism**).

(b) In adults, GH deficiency was once thought to have no important clinical effects. It is now recognized that GH deficiency causes undesired changes in body composition, with an **increase in body fat** and a **decrease in lean body mass.** These changes may be accompanied by decreased strength and exercise capacity.

(c) Other adverse effects of GH deficiency may include an increase in cardiovascular risk factors such as insulin resistance and hyperlipidemia, atherosclerosis, impaired quality of life, and perhaps shortened life expectancy.

(2) **Gonadotropin (LH and FSH) deficiency** causes **amenorrhea and genital atrophy in women** and **loss of potency and libido in men.** If adrenal androgens are deficient as well, because of concomitant ACTH deficiency, pubic and axillary hair may be lost, especially in women.

(3) **TSH deficiency** results in the symptoms and physical changes of **hypothyroidism** (see II B 2 a–b).

(4) **ACTH deficiency** leads to **adrenal insufficiency** (see V C). Secondary adrenal insufficiency (caused by pituitary disease) differs in several clinical manifestations from primary adrenal insufficiency (caused by adrenal disease).

(a) **Hyperpigmentation** of the skin and mucous membranes is characteristic of primary adrenal disease.

(i) It is caused, indirectly, by the negative-feedback stimulation of ACTH by low plasma cortisol levels. [ACTH and melanocyte-stimulating hormone (MSH) are derived from the same large precursor molecule (pro-opiomelanocortin), so when ACTH is increased, MSH is increased as well. MSH stimulates melanocytes and causes pigmentation.]

(ii) ACTH (and therefore, MSH) levels are low in secondary adrenal insufficiency; consequently, hyperpigmentation is not characteristic of this condition.

(b) **Electrolyte changes** (i.e., decreased serum sodium and increased serum potassium levels) are minimal in secondary adrenal insufficiency, because aldosterone production by the adrenal cortex (which promotes sodium retention) depends primarily on renin and angiotensin (which are undisturbed) rather than on ACTH.

(5) **Prolactin deficiency** may be responsible for the postpartum failure of lactation in Sheehan's syndrome but otherwise produces no clinical manifestations.

(6) With slow, progressive destruction of pituitary tissue, **failure of GH and gonadotropin secretion** occurs early. With continuing loss of tissue, TSH and finally ACTH and prolactin fall below normal levels.

(7) **Deficiency of individual pituitary hormones** may occur. Isolated GH deficiency and isolated gonadotropin deficiency are not uncommon, especially in children. Isolated deficiencies of TSH and ACTH are very uncommon.

c. Diagnosis

(1) **Evaluation of target organ function** is often the first step in the diagnosis of hypopituitarism; this condition is often suspected because of failure of more than one target organ (i.e., thyroid, adrenal glands, gonads). Tests of thyroid, adrenal, ovarian, and testicular function are described in sections II, V, VI, and VII, respectively.

(2) **Measurement of pituitary hormones**

(a) **GH levels** may be undetectable under basal conditions in normal individuals; therefore, provocative maneuvers may be needed to prove inadequacy of hormone production.

(i) **Insulin-induced hypoglycemia** (the insulin tolerance test) is the most consistently effective test stimulus for GH. Regular insulin, in a dose of 0.1–0.15 U/kg, is given as an intravenous bolus, and GH levels are measured after 30, 60, and 90 minutes have passed. The fall in the serum glucose level, usually maximal at 30 minutes, is followed by a rise in GH to a level greater than 8–10 μg/L in normal individuals. A peak GH level less than 2.5–5 μg/L after insulin infusion indicates GH deficiency.

(ii) The patient must be observed closely during the test; central nervous system (CNS) symptoms of hypoglycemia require immediate intravenous administration of glucose. This test should not be performed in persons older than 65 years, or persons with coronary disease or a seizure disorder.

(iii) Because the insulin tolerance test is uncomfortable, inconvenient, and unsafe in some patients, other provocative tests are sometimes used. The next most effective stimulus for GH, after insulin-induced hypoglycemia, is **the IV infusion of arginine and GH-releasing hormone.**

(iv) In patients with panhypopituitarism, provocative tests may not be necessary to diagnose GH deficiency. If three or more other pituitary hormone deficiencies exist (i.e., TSH, ACTH, LH or FSH, or vasopressin) the probability that GH is also deficient exceeds 95%. This probability is even higher if IGF-1 levels are low (although a third of GH-deficient patients may have normal levels of IGF-1.)

(b) **Levels of other pituitary hormones** can be measured by radioimmunoassay, but because low values cannot be distinguished reliably from normal values, the evaluation is useful only in special situations.

(i) If thyroid function is decreased [i.e., low free thyroxine (T_4) or free T_4 index], the TSH level should be elevated if the disorder originates in the thyroid; a low (or normal) TSH value strongly suggests hypopituitarism.

(ii) If adrenal insufficiency is present (e.g., if levels of serum cortisol are low), the ACTH level should be elevated if the disorder originates in the adrenal glands; a low (or normal) ACTH level strongly suggests hypopituitarism.

(iii) In postmenopausal women, or in men with inadequate testicular function (i.e., a low testosterone level), LH and FSH levels should be high; low (or normal) values suggest hypopituitarism.

(3) **Other provocative tests**

(a) **Insulin-induced hypoglycemia** stimulates cortisol production as well as GH production. Cortisol levels can be measured in the same blood samples in which GH is measured. An increase in serum cortisol of at least 10 μg/dL to a level of 20 μg/dL or higher indicates normal function of the entire hypothalamic–pituitary–adrenal axis.

(b) The **metyrapone test** evaluates ACTH reserve function.

(i) Metyrapone inhibits 11β-hydroxylation, the enzymatic step that produces cortisol from its precursor, 11-deoxycortisol. Oral metyrapone administration causes a decrease in cortisol production, which stimulates ACTH output by the pituitary gland. The increased ACTH stimulates production of 11-deoxycortisol.

(ii) If the serum level of 11-deoxycortisol increases as expected after metyrapone administration, it indicates that both pituitary ACTH reserve and adrenal response to ACTH are normal.

d. Therapy

(1) The **underlying cause** of the pituitary insufficiency (e.g., enlarging pituitary tumors, granulomatous diseases) should be sought and treated, if possible.

(2) **Hormone replacement**

(a) **GH administration** can stimulate growth and increase the ultimate height in children with isolated GH deficiency or panhypopituitarism. Synthetic human growth hormone of recombinant DNA origin is available but must be given by injection and is expensive. GH replacement is given to some adults with GH deficiency; however, the inconvenience and expense of this treatment must be weighed against its possible benefits on a case-by-case basis.

(b) **Thyroid hormone** is given in usual replacement doses (see II B 4).

(c) **Cortisol** (hydrocortisone) is given in usual replacement doses (see V C 4).

(d) **Estrogen–progesterone combinations** may be given to women, and testosterone to men, to prevent or treat the manifestations of hypogonadism (see VI A, VI B, and VII A).

(e) Fertility is considerably more difficult to achieve because it depends on the precisely controlled administration of **gonadotropins** or **gonadotropin-releasing hormone (GnRH).**

(i) GnRH has been successful in restoring ovulation in women and sperm production in men, but only in cases in which hypothalamic production of GnRH is impaired but the pituitary retains its ability to secrete LH and FSH in response to GnRH.

(ii) **GnRH** stimulates LH and FSH production only if it is administered in a way that mimics normal physiologic secretion; that is, it must be given by regular pulsatile injection every 90–120 minutes. (Constant, rather than pulsatile, administration of GnRH has the opposite effect. It decreases pituitary LH and FSH production).

3. Acromegaly

a. Etiology. Acromegaly is caused by a pituitary adenoma that produces GH.

(1) In many cases, the adenoma is large enough to distort the sella turcica and can be seen on lateral skull radiographs; in other cases, CT scan or MRI is needed to visualize the tumor, and in a few cases, no tumor can be visualized.

(2) Immunohistochemical staining shows that these adenomas are composed of somatotroph cells.

b. Clinical features. Excess GH secretion may cause changes in bone, soft tissues, and metabolic processes.

(1) **Bone and soft tissue changes**

(a) In children, excess GH secretion may cause increased linear growth of long bones, resulting in **gigantism.** After closure of the epiphyses at puberty, these changes cannot occur.

(b) In adults, soft tissue growth and bone enlargement, especially in the acral areas of the skeleton, lead to **diverse manifestations,** many of **which affect the patient's appearance** (Table 9–1). These changes are gradual and may not be obvious to the patient or the patient's family until the present appearance is compared with that on old photographs.

(2) **Metabolic changes**

(a) **Decreased glucose tolerance,** a result of the anti-insulin actions of GH, is common, although overt diabetes occurs in only 10% of patients with acromegaly.

(b) A tendency to develop **hyperphosphatemia** is caused by the increased tubular reabsorption of phosphate that is induced by GH.

c. Diagnosis. Clinical manifestations raise the suspicion of acromegaly. Abnormalities in the blood levels of GH, insulin-like growth factor I (IGF-I, formerly called somatomedin C), or both, confirm the diagnosis.

(1) Because glucose suppresses GH in normal subjects but not in acromegaly, **GH measurement after a glucose load** may best distinguish between normal and acromegalic subjects.

(2) **IGF-1** is a growth factor produced by the liver under the stimulation of GH. IGF-1 levels may be elevated in patients with acromegaly whose GH level is normal or equivocal. Elevated levels of IGF-1 provide an additional index of GH activity and further evidence of the diagnosis.

(3) Initially, fasting levels of GH and IGF-1 should be measured. If the GH level is less than 0.4 μg/L, and IGF-1 is normal, acromegaly is excluded.

(4) If either the GH or IGF-1 level is not low enough to exclude acromegaly, a 75-g oral glucose tolerance test should be performed, with GH measurements every 30 minutes for

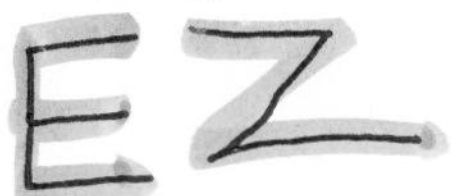

TABLE 9–1 Skeletal and Soft Tissue Manifestations of Acromegaly

Enlargement of hands (especially fingertips) and feet
Increased ring, glove, and shoe sizes
Coarsening of facial features
Thick skin folds
Brows and nasolabial creases
Enlargement of nose
Enlargement of mandible
Prognathism
Spreading of teeth
Enlargement of internal organs
Heart, lungs, liver, spleen, and kidneys
Skin thickening and interstitial edema, with swelling and firmness of soft tissues
Osteoarthritis
Entrapment neuropathies (especially carpal tunnel syndrome)
Radiographic changes
Enlargement of sinuses
Tufting of distal phalanges, cortical thickening

2 hours. If the GH level does not fall below 1.0 μg/L, a diagnosis of acromegaly is suggested; an elevated IGF-1 level increases the liklihood of this diagnosis.

(5) False-positive GH responses (i.e., failure of suppression) may occur after surgery and in patients with diabetes mellitus, liver disease, kidney disease, and malnutrition.

d. Therapy

(1) **Transsphenoidal pituitary adenomectomy** causes prompt normalization of GH levels in most patients. Permanent cure is common when the adenoma is small but uncommon when the tumor is large and extends beyond the sella turcica.

(2) **Conventional radiation therapy** lowers GH levels slowly; normal levels may not be reached until 3–10 years after treatment, if at all.

(3) **Octreotide,** an analog of somatostatin, can be given by subcutaneous injection. It lowers GH levels in many patients with acromegaly and may be useful in patients in whom surgery and radiation therapy have been unsuccessful.

(4) **Pegvisomant**

(a) **Pegvisomant** is an analog of GH that binds to GH receptors, blocking the binding of GH and thus inhibiting its actions. The result is a decrease in IGF-1, and lessening of the effects of excessive GH in acromegaly.

(b) Pegvisomant is given by injection once daily. It may be indicated in patients who have not responded adequately to other treatments.

4. Hyperprolactinemia. As many as 50% of all pituitary adenomas have been found to secrete prolactin.

a. Etiology

(1) **Prolactin-secreting pituitary adenomas (prolactinomas)** are more common in women than in men, usually appearing during the reproductive years and causing menstrual abnormalities and galactorrhea (**the galactorrhea-amenorrhea syndrome**). Men tend to have larger tumors at the time of diagnosis, which usually are suspected because of neurologic impairment and hypogonadism.

(2) **Damage to the hypothalamus or pituitary stalk** by tumors, granulomas, and other processes may prevent the normal regulatory effect of hypothalamic dopamine on lactotrope activity, resulting in hypersecretion of prolactin.

(3) **Drugs** that can inhibit dopamine activity and, thus, interfere with its regulation of prolactin secretion include psychotropic agents (e.g., phenothiazines, butyrophenones,

tricyclic antidepressants), antihypertensives (e.g., methyldopa, reserpine), metoclopramide, cimetidine, and others.

b. Clinical features

(1) **Amenorrhea** or menstrual irregularity is due to the inhibition of hypothalamic GnRH production by prolactin as well as the direct effects of the prolactin on the ovaries.

(2) **Galactorrhea** is a direct result of prolactin excess.

(3) **Loss of potency and libido,** with low testosterone levels, is the common endocrine manifestation in men.

c. Diagnosis

(1) **Prolactin levels** are elevated. A serum prolactin level greater than 300 ng/mL strongly suggests the presence of a prolactinoma. Functional causes of hyperprolactinemia such as drugs seldom elevate the level above 100–200 ng/mL.

(2) **CT scanning** and **MRI** are used to visualize an adenoma.

d. Therapy. Treatment of prolactinoma depends on the size of the tumor and its manifestations. A small, nonenlarging tumor in a woman with insignificant galactorrhea who does not desire pregnancy may not require treatment. If pregnancy is desired, if the galactorrhea or amenorrhea is unacceptable, or if the tumor is enlarging or causing local symptoms, therapeutic options include **surgery, administration of bromocriptine or another dopamine agonist,** and **radiation therapy.**

(1) **Transsphenoidal surgery** cures most patients with small prolactinomas. Large tumors with suprasellar extension, however, usually are not cured by surgery.

(2) **Dopamine agonists** (bromocriptine, cabergoline, pergolide) are remarkably effective in decreasing prolactin levels, usually to normal, which promptly relieves the galactorrhea and restores normal menses and fertility; it frequently reduces tumor size as well.

(a) Many patients may not tolerate bromocriptine; its side effects include nausea, headache, dizziness, and fatigue. Initial dosages of 1.25 mg once or twice daily may need to be increased to 10–20 mg daily for full effect.

(b) Cabergoline may be better tolerated and needs to be given only twice weekly.

(c) Because of the poor surgical results in patients with large tumors, initial treatment with bromocriptine is given. If the tumor shrinks, there is a greater chance for successful surgery, or medical treatment alone may be continued indefinitely.

(3) **Radiation therapy** may be used in conjunction with surgery and dopamine agonists to further reduce tumor size and function.

B Posterior pituitary disease **Arginine vasopressin** [**antidiuretic hormone** (**ADH**)] is produced by cells in the supraoptic and paraventricular nuclei of the hypothalamus, travels down the pituitary stalk in the axons of these cells, and is stored in the nerve endings in the posterior lobe of the pituitary gland (i.e., in the neurohypophysis). Inadequate ADH production may follow damage to the hypothalamus, the pituitary stalk, and, less commonly, the posterior pituitary gland, and it results in **diabetes insipidus.** Excessive ADH production produces the **syndrome of inappropriate secretion of ADH (SIADH).**

1. Diabetes insipidus. The term **central diabetes insipidus** is used to describe disease due to ADH insufficiency, and the term **nephrogenic diabetes insipidus** is used to describe disease due to renal unresponsiveness to ADH.

a. Etiology

(1) Approximately 50% of cases are **idiopathic.**

(2) **Injury to the hypothalamic–pituitary area** may result from head trauma, brain tumors, and neurosurgical procedures.

(3) **Less common causes** include **sarcoidosis, syphilis, Hand-Schüller-Christian disease,** and **encephalitis.**

b. Clinical features

(1) **Polyuria,** with urine volumes of 3–15 L daily, results from the inability to reabsorb free water and to concentrate urine in the absence of adequate ADH.

(2) **Thirst** results, which leads to **increased fluid intake.** A conscious patient with a normal thirst mechanism and free access to water will maintain hydration; the disease in such a patient is an inconvenience rather than a threat to life. However, rapid and life-threatening dehydration may occur in an infant or in an unconscious patient.

(3) Laboratory abnormalities include a **dilute urine** (osmolality < 200 mOsm/kg and specific gravity < 1.005) and a high-normal or slightly **elevated plasma osmolality.**

c. Diagnosis

(1) **Measurement of plasma osmolality.** In untreated patients, this determination helps distinguish the causes of polyuria. In diabetes insipidus, the loss of free water is primary, and plasma osmolality tends to be high (280–310 mOsm/kg). In psychogenic polydipsia, excessive fluid intake is primary, and plasma osmolality tends to be low (255–280 mOsm/kg).

(2) **Water deprivation test**

(a) **Method.** Fluid intake is withheld until urine osmolality reaches a plateau (i.e., an hourly increase of < 30 mOsm/kg for 3 consecutive hours). When urine osmolality is stable, plasma osmolality is measured. Two μg desmopressin (dDAVP) is then injected subcutaneously, and urine osmolality is measured again 1 hour later.

(b) **Response.** The responses typical of normal individuals and of patients with partial, complete, and nephrogenic diabetes insipidus are shown in Table 9–2. Patients with partial diabetes insipidus show an increase in urine osmolality with dehydration, but the incompleteness of their response is demonstrated by a further increase after ADH is injected.

(3) **Administration of hypertonic saline.** Infusion of a solution (2.5% sodium chloride given intravenously for 45 minutes at 0.25 mL/kg/min) after a water load (20 mL/kg in 30–60 minutes) causes a sharp decrease in urine flow in normal subjects because of stimulation of ADH secretion. Patients with diabetes insipidus cannot respond to this stimulus.

(4) **Differential diagnosis.** In patients with polyuria and dilute urine, central diabetes insipidus must be differentiated from nephrogenic diabetes insipidus and compulsive water drinking.

(a) **Nephrogenic diabetes insipidus** is a condition in which the renal tubules fail to respond to normal circulating levels of ADH.

(i) The condition may be primary and familial, starting in infancy, or it may occur later in life as a secondary condition in association with hypokalemia, hypercalcemia, chronic renal disease, sickle cell anemia, amyloidosis, or the use of certain drugs (e.g., lithium, demeclocycline, methoxyflurane).

TABLE 9–2 Response to Water Deprivation Test

Diagnosis	Increase in Urine Osmolality above 280 mOsm/kg with Dehydration	Further Increase in Urine Osmolality in Response to ADH
Normal	+	–
Complete central diabetes insipidus	–	+
Partial central diabetes insipidus	+	+
Nephrogenic diabetes insipidus	–	–

ADH = antidiuretic hormone.

(ii) The clinical features are the same as those caused by ADH deficiency. The difference is seen in the failure of nephrogenic diabetes insipidus to respond to administration of ADH.

(b) **Compulsive water drinking (psychogenic polydipsia)** is a primary psychiatric abnormality that leads to polyuria and dilute urine. Differentiation from diabetes insipidus may be difficult. It is most common in young or middle-aged women who often have a history of psychiatric disorders.

d. Therapy

(1) **Desmopressin (dDAVP),** a synthetic analog of vasopressin, can be administered orally, 0.1–1.2 mg daily in 2 or 3 doses. It also can be given as a nasal spray, and a parenteral preparation is available for use in acutely ill or postoperative patients.

(2) **Chlorpropamide,** an oral hypoglycemic agent, has the additional effect of potentiating the action, the secretion, or both, of endogenous ADH. This effect may be used in the treatment of diabetes insipidus.

(a) Patients who have at least partial ADH production often become asymptomatic when 250–500 mg of chlorpropamide is taken daily.

(b) Physicians and patients must watch for hypoglycemia, a possible side effect.

(3) **Thiazide diuretics** have the paradoxical effect of decreasing urine output in patients with diabetes insipidus.

(a) The volume depletion induced by diuretics increases sodium and water reabsorption in the proximal tubule, thus blunting the effect of the defective water absorption in the distal and collecting tubules.

(b) Thiazides are only partially effective, decreasing urine volume by 30%–50%. However, unlike dDAVP, they are useful for treating nephrogenic diabetes insipidus, because their action does not depend on distal tubular response to ADH.

2. Syndrome of inappropriate secretion of ADH (SIADH)

a. Etiology

(1) ADH production by **malignant tumors,** particularly oat cell carcinoma of the lung and carcinoma of the pancreas, was the originally recognized cause of SIADH.

(2) More commonly, excess ADH production by the neurohypophysial axis or by diseased tissue is caused by other disease processes through unknown mechanisms. These disease processes include **pulmonary diseases** (e.g., pneumonia, tuberculosis) and **CNS disorders** (e.g., stroke, head injury, encephalitis).

(3) **Drugs** (e.g., chlorpropamide, carbamazepine, vincristine, clofibrate) may stimulate hypothalamic–neurohypophyseal ADH production.

b. Pathophysiology. ADH excess causes water retention and extracellular fluid volume expansion, which is then compensated for by increased urinary sodium excretion. Clinically, significant volume expansion (i.e., edema or hypertension) is not present, because of the natriuresis. However, the water retention and the sodium loss both contribute to **hyponatremia,** which is **the hallmark of SIADH.** If water intake is minimized, this sequence of events does not occur, and serum sodium levels do not fall.

c. Clinical features. Hyponatremia refers to a serum sodium level less than 135 mEq/L.

(1) Symptoms of lethargy, confusion, agitation, headache, nausea and vomiting, and focal neurologic abnormalities are common when the sodium level declines rapidly or when it reaches a level less than approximately 125 mEq/L.

(2) Seizures and coma may occur with more severe hyponatremia.

d. Diagnosis. The following conditions are the basis of diagnosis.

(1) **Hyponatremia** is present, with low serum osmolality.

(2) **Daily urinary sodium excretion exceeds 20 mEq/L,** despite the low serum sodium levels, and urine osmolality is higher than serum osmolality. (Other causes of hyponatremia such as sodium depletion cause renal retention of sodium, with < 20 mEq/L excreted daily.)

(3) Conditions that might *appropriately* stimulate ADH secretion because of volume depletion must be excluded. These include adrenal insufficiency, fluid loss, edematous states (e.g., heart failure, nephrosis, cirrhosis), and renal failure.

e. **Therapy.** The cause of SIADH should be treated when possible.

(1) **Fluid restriction** to 500–1000 mL daily is effective in increasing the serum sodium level and is the mainstay of treatment. The limiting factor is patient adherence.

(2) If hyponatremia is severe, **hypertonic (3%) saline** should be administered to elevate the serum sodium level above 120 mEq/L.

(a) Serum sodium must not be increased rapidly to a level exceeding 125 mEq/L, or CNS damage may result (see Chapter 11 XI B 1).

(b) Salt loading is of only temporary value because the additional sodium is soon excreted in the urine.

(3) If fluid restriction cannot be enforced, 300 mg **demeclocycline** can be administered three or four times daily. Demeclocycline is an antibiotic with the useful side effect of inhibiting renal tubular response to ADH.

II DISORDERS OF THE THYROID GLAND

The thyroid may produce too little or too much hormone; it may undergo chronic enlargement and inflammation (**chronic thyroiditis**); and it is a common site for benign and malignant tumors. Thyroid disease is suggested by symptoms of **hypothyroidism** (i.e., insufficient thyroid hormone effect) or **hyperthyroidism** (i.e., excess thyroid hormone effect), as well as by localized or diffuse thyroid enlargement (**goiter**). Initially, thyroid disease usually is evaluated by thyroid function tests, which measure blood hormone levels. Information on the physical characteristics and function of separate areas of the thyroid may then be obtained, if necessary, by isotope scans and other imaging techniques.

A Thyroid function studies

1. **Serum total T_4 determination** measures the total bound (99.95%) and free (0.05%) T_4 in the circulation. The serum T_4 concentration is elevated in hyperthyroidism and decreased in hypothyroidism.

a. The proteins that bind T_4, mainly **thyroxine-binding globulin (TBG)**, are elevated by estrogen treatment, pregnancy, liver disease, and congenital TBG excess.

(1) If the binding proteins are elevated, the total T_4 concentration in the blood is high, but the concentration of free T_4 (the active form of the hormone at the tissue level) remains normal. It is regulated by the normally functioning thyroid hormone–TSH feedback mechanism.

(2) If the concentration of free T_4 is normal, the patient is euthyroid, and the elevated level of total T_4 is misleading.

b. The converse is also true. TBG levels may be lowered by androgen treatment, cirrhosis, the nephrotic syndrome, or congenital TBG deficiency. In this case, the concentration of total T_4 is low, but the patient maintains a normal level of free T_4 and is euthyroid.

c. Therefore, the total T_4 concentration alone is not an adequate test to evaluate thyroid function. Either the T_4 concentration must be measured in conjunction with a test that evaluates protein binding [e.g., the triiodothyronine (T_3) uptake test] or free T_4 itself must be measured.

2. **Serum total T_3 determination** measures the concentration of the total bound and free T_3 in the circulation. The total T_3 measurement may give the same misleading results as the total T_4 measurement if there is an abnormality in binding proteins.

3. **T_3 uptake test**

a. **Method.** This test is performed by combining in a tube the patient's serum, a known amount of radiolabeled T_3, and an insoluble binder of T_3 such as a small piece of resin. The binding proteins from the patient's serum and the resin compete for the labeled T_3.

(1) If the binding proteins are increased, less T_3 binds to the resin, and if the proteins are decreased, more T_3 binds to the resin.

(2) The result, which is expressed as a percent of labeled T_3 bound to the resin, is a measure of the unoccupied binding sites on the patient's thyroid hormone–binding proteins.

b. Interpretation

(1) The T_3 resin uptake is elevated in hyperthyroidism. Thyroid hormone is increased in the blood; therefore, the hormone bound to protein is also increased, leaving fewer unoccupied binding sites. Consequently, there is increased labeled T_3 binding to resin. Conversely, the T_3 resin uptake is decreased in hypothyroidism.

(2) In both instances, the T_3 resin uptake varies directly with changes in the total T_4 and total T_3 concentrations and confirms the diagnosis suggested by the total T_4 and total T_3 levels.

(3) However, if the levels of total T_4, total T_3, or both are increased or decreased because of abnormalities of the binding proteins, rather than hypothyroidism or hyperthyroidism, the T_3 resin uptake changes in the opposite direction. For example, when binding protein is increased, there is an increase in total T_4, as well as an increase in unoccupied binding sites that causes a decrease in the T_3 resin uptake.

4. Free T_4 index

a. If the total T_4 level and T_3 resin uptake are known, an index can be calculated that estimates the free T_4 level.

(1) The patient's T_3 resin uptake is divided by the average normal T_3 resin uptake, and the total T_4 is multiplied by this fraction.

(2) The result, which is called the free T_4 index, has approximately the same normal range as the total concentration of T_4. This process considers the effects of abnormalities of thyroid hormone–binding proteins on the total T_4 measurement.

b. Example. A patient has a total T_4 of 15.0 μg/dL (normal = 4.5–12.5 μg/dL). If the T_3 resin uptake is 45%, the free T_4 index equals 45% divided by 30% (which is the average normal uptake) multiplied by 15.0, or 22.5. This result suggests a diagnosis of hyperthyroidism. If the T_3 resin uptake is 15%, the free T_4 index is 7.5 ($15/30 \times 15.0$), suggesting that the patient is euthyroid but has an increased level of T_4-binding proteins.

5. Serum TSH measurement

a. In primary **hypothyroidism,** measuring the serum TSH concentration is a very sensitive test, because it usually becomes elevated even before thyroid hormone levels decline below normal. TSH elevation is caused by the negative feedback effects of low thyroid hormone levels.

b. In **hyperthyroidism,** the elevated thyroid hormone concentrations lead to suppression of serum TSH to levels below normal. This finding is a very sensitive indication of hyperthyroidism, because TSH may be suppressed even when thyroid hormone levels are not elevated above the normal range.

6. Radioactive iodine uptake by the thyroid gland 24 hours after administration of the isotope is increased in hyperthyroidism and decreased in hypothyroidism. This test is especially useful in detecting forms of hyperthyroidism in which the thyroid gland itself is not synthesizing excess hormone; that is, the hyperthyroidism associated with exogenous thyroid hormone administration, subacute thyroiditis, and ectopic hormone production (e.g., caused by struma ovarii). In these situations, blood hormone levels are high, but the radioactive iodine uptake is low.

B Hypothyroidism

1. Etiology

a. Chronic autoimmune thyroiditis (see II D 2) is the most common cause of spontaneous hypothyroidism in the United States. This condition has a goitrous form (Hashimoto's disease) and an atrophic form; in both forms antithyroid antibodies are typically present in the serum.

b. **Hypothyroidism frequently develops after the treatment of Graves' disease,** and the prevalence exceeds 50% in patients treated with radioactive iodine. However, hypothyroidism also may occur after Graves' disease is treated by subtotal thyroidectomy or antithyroid drugs.

c. **Secondary hypothyroidism** is caused by any of the conditions that may affect the hypothalamic–pituitary axis and cause hypopituitarism (see I A 2 a).

d. **Less common causes** of hypothyroidism include congenital athyreosis, congenital biochemical defects that prevent thyroid hormone production, and insensitivity of the tissues to thyroid hormone. Iodine deficiency is an uncommon cause of hypothyroidism in most highly developed countries, but it is common in some areas of the world.

2. **Clinical features**

a. **Symptoms** (Table 9–3)

(1) As metabolism slows because of the lessened effects of thyroid hormone on tissues, patients may experience **weakness, lethargy, sleepiness and fatigue, and slowness of speech and thought.**

(2) A **puffy appearance, constipation,** and a **constant feeling of cold** may be present. **Muscle cramps** are common.

(3) Slight-to-moderate **weight gain** reflects the decreased metabolism, but massive weight gain does not occur because appetite tends to be diminished.

(4) Edema of the larynx and middle ear may cause **voice changes and hearing loss** in severe cases.

(5) Excess and **irregular menstrual bleeding** may be associated with anovulatory cycles.

b. **Physical findings** (Table 9–4)

(1) **Puffiness** and **nonpitting edema** are caused by the accumulation of mucinous mucopolysaccharide-rich material in the tissues. The term **myxedema** describes this phenomenon and is sometimes used synonymously with severe hypothyroidism.

(2) The characteristic puffy, dull appearance and the **slow return phase** of the Achilles and other **deep tendon reflexes** are perhaps the most helpful physical findings in suggesting hypothyroidism.

c. **Effects on organ systems.** All organ systems are affected; some of the most important changes are listed in Table 9–5.

d. **Cretinism** is severe **hypothyroidism beginning in infancy.** Cretinism is marked by mental retardation and impairment of physical growth and development.

(1) Short limbs and a large head, with a broad, flat nose, widely set eyes, and a large tongue characterize this form of dwarfism. Epiphyseal dysgenesis, with abnormalities of the ossification centers, affects the femoral and humeral heads and other parts of the skeleton.

(2) Early recognition and treatment prevent the otherwise irreversible mental and physical impairment.

e. **Myxedema coma** may result if severe hypothyroidism goes untreated. This serious condition may occur gradually (over years) or more acutely in response to precipitating factors (e.g., infection, exposure to cold). The mortality rate is 50%–75%. Hypothermia, hypoglycemia, shock, hypoventilation, and ileus may be present in addition to the severely depressed state of consciousness.

TABLE 9–3 Symptoms of Hypothyroidism

Weakness, lethargy, and fatigue ("slowing down")	Muscle cramps
Dry skin and coarse hair	Weight gain
Puffy eyelids, face, and hands; swollen legs	Hoarseness
Cold intolerance	Menorrhagia
Constipation	Hearing loss

TABLE 9–4 Physical Findings in Hypothyroidism

Thickened, puffy features	Bradycardia
Yellowish, dry skin	Slow return of deep tendon reflexes
Nonpitting edema	Loss of lateral portion of eyebrows
Hypothermia	

3. **Diagnosis**
   a. **Overt hypothyroidism** is suggested in severe cases by the characteristic symptoms and physical findings; however, mild cases may escape detection unless laboratory tests are performed. Routine laboratory screening is especially recommended for newborns and women older than 50 years of age. TSH levels should also be measured in elderly persons with nonspecific complaints, because many hypothyroid symptoms such as fatigue and constipation may be mistaken for the changes of aging.
      (1) Serum T_4 and T_3 levels, as well as T_3 uptake, are decreased.
      (2) An increased serum concentration of TSH is the earliest and most sensitive indicator of primary hypothyroidism, and a sensitive TSH assay should be used for screening. If the TSH level is elevated, the diagnosis may be confirmed by the finding of a decreased serum free T_4 or free T_4 index.
   b. **Subclinical hypothyroidism** is a common condition in which serum TSH is elevated but serum free T_4 or the free T_4 index is normal rather than decreased. Many affected patients progress to overt hypothyroidism. The decision to treat patients with subclinical hypothyroidism must be made on a case-by-case basis. A greater degree of TSH elevation, the presence of symptoms that might be caused by hypothyroidism, and the presence of antithyroid antibodies are factors favoring a decision to treat.
4. **Therapy**
   a. **Thyroid hormone preparations.** Thyroid extract derived from animal sources and synthetic preparations containing both T_4 and T_3 have been used in the past and are still available. However, synthetic L-thyroxine sodium is the agent of choice.
      (1) The administered T_4 is slowly converted to T_3, and the proportions of circulating T_4 and T_3 approximate those of euthyroid individuals.
      (2) The peaks and valleys of blood T_3 levels, which are seen when exogenous T_3 is given, are avoided.
   b. **Initiation of treatment**
      (1) Patients with severe hypothyroidism, older patients, and patients with cardiovascular disease may have an increased sensitivity to thyroid hormone and are at risk for acute cardiovascular and other complications if the hypothyroidism is corrected too quickly. Therefore,

TABLE 9–5 Effects of Hypothyroidism on Organ Systems

Cardiovascular system	Nervous system
Decrease in cardiac output	Decreased mental function
Pericardial effusion	Psychiatric changes (e.g., psychosis, depression)
Respiratory system	Blood
Hypoventilation	Normochromic normocytic anemia
Pleural effusion	
Gastrointestinal tract	
Constipation	

these patients should be given a very small dose of thyroid hormone initially (e.g., 25 μg of L-thyroxine), which is increased to a full maintenance dose during a 6- to 12-week period.

(2) Younger patients and patients with less severe hypothyroidism may be started on a slightly higher dose (50 μg of L-thyroxine) and advanced to a full replacement dose more quickly (e.g., the dose may be raised to 100 μg in 2 weeks and to 125 μg or 150 μg in another 2 weeks).

c. **Maintenance therapy.** Most patients require approximately 0.7 to 0.8 μg L-thyroxine per pound of ideal body weight for physiologic replacement of thyroid hormone. When this dose is tolerated and symptoms of hypothyroidism have resolved, the dose should be further adjusted so that serum TSH is maintained in the normal range.

d. **Myxedema coma** has a high mortality rate **and must be treated rapidly,** despite the risk associated with sudden hormone replacement.

(1) L-thyroxine is given intravenously as a 500-μg bolus injection, followed by daily maintenance doses.

(2) Ancillary treatment includes the temporary use of adrenal corticosteroids and respiratory support.

C Hyperthyroidism

1. **Etiology**

a. **Graves' disease (diffuse toxic goiter) is the most common cause of hyperthyroidism.** It is a form of autoimmune thyroid disease in which an abnormal immunoglobulin G (IgG) [thyroid-stimulating immunoglobulin] binds to TSH receptors on the thyroid follicular cells, causing diffuse enlargement of the gland and stimulation of thyroid hormone production. Graves' disease is most common in women between the ages of 20 and 50 years, although others may be affected.

b. **Toxic nodular goiter (Plummer's disease)** and **toxic thyroid adenoma** are less common than Graves' disease and usually affect older individuals.

(1) Discrete areas of the thyroid function autonomously, secreting excessive amounts of thyroid hormone. The cause is unknown, but activating mutations in the TSH receptor gene or in the stimulatory G protein that couple the TSH receptor to cyclic adenosine monophosphate (cAMP) formation have been found in many cases.

(2) The presence of both normal thyroid tissue and autonomously functioning abnormal tissue is the pathognomonic feature. Radionuclide scanning shows that the normal tissue is hypofunctioning; this occurs because TSH is suppressed by the excessive levels of thyroid hormone produced by the abnormal tissue. Cure of the hyperthyroidism restores function to the suppressed normal tissue.

c. **Subacute thyroiditis** (see II D 1) may cause transient hyperthyroidism.

d. **Factitious hyperthyroidism** may be caused by surreptitious ingestion of thyroid hormone by patients. Inadvertent administration of excessive doses of the hormone by physicians may have the same result.

e. **Rare causes** of hyperthyroidism include excess TSH production by **pituitary tumors, teratomas of the ovary** that produce thyroid hormone **(struma ovarii),** and overproduction of hormone by the thyroid gland following iodine ingestion, which is called jodbasedow.

2. **Clinical features.** Thyroid hormone increases oxygen consumption by tissues, raising heat production and energy metabolism. It interacts with the sympathetic nervous system in a way that seems to increase tissue sensitivity to catecholamines and adrenergic stimuli. In addition, it affects protein, fat, carbohydrate, and vitamin metabolism. These and other actions lead to profound changes in many organ systems when thyroid hormone is in excess.

a. **Metabolic changes** include an **elevated basal metabolic rate** and **weight loss** despite increased appetite and food intake. **Sweating** and **heat intolerance** reflect the increased heat production.

b. **Cardiovascular effects**
   (1) The heart rate is increased; **sinus tachycardia** is common, with rates of 120 beats/min or higher in severe cases.
   (2) Systolic blood pressure tends to be elevated and diastolic blood pressure decreased, with a **wide pulse pressure.**
   (3) Myocardial excitability is increased, and arrhythmias [e.g., **atrial fibrillation, premature ventricular contractions (PVCs)**] may occur.

c. **Gastrointestinal symptoms** of loose stools or **diarrhea** are common.

d. **Skin and hair changes.** The **skin is warm and moist** because of peripheral vasodilation and increased sweating. **Fine, silky hair** is characteristic.

e. **CNS effects** include **emotional lability, restlessness,** and **fine tremor.**

f. **Muscle weakness** and **fatigue** are common.

g. **Ophthalmopathy**
   (1) **Stare** and **lid lag** (i.e., slow closing of the upper lid when the eye moves downward, revealing sclera between the lid and cornea) may occur in any form of hyperthyroidism.
   (2) True **thyroid exophthalmos,** however, is seen only in Graves' disease, occurring in approximately 50% of cases. The eye is pushed forward because of mucinous and cellular **infiltration of the orbit and extraocular muscles.** There is **inflammation of the conjunctiva** and surrounding tissues. Patients may complain of **tearing, eye irritation, pain,** and **double vision.** In severe cases, vision may be threatened.

h. **Thyroid storm** is a sudden exacerbation of the signs and symptoms of hyperthyroidism.
   (1) Precipitating events may include intercurrent illness, trauma, surgery, or childbirth.
   (2) The exacerbation of hyperthyroidism may be caused by an increase in the unbound fraction of thyroid hormone, which may occur with severe nonthyroidal illness.
   (3) Marked fever, tachycardia, and agitation are present and may progress to stupor and coma, with vascular collapse.
   (4) The mortality rate is 50%–75%.

3. **Diagnosis**

a. **Presenting symptoms** of weight loss, nervousness, palpitations, muscle weakness, and diarrhea are characteristic.

b. **Family history** of thyroid disease is common.

c. **Physical examination** often reveals a fidgety, hyperkinetic patient with warm, moist skin; fine, silky hair; and a fine tremor of the hands.
   (1) The eyes may be prominent, with retraction of the upper lid and a staring appearance.
   (2) The thyroid is enlarged in most cases. In Graves' disease, the enlargement is uniform, and a bruit may be heard over the gland; in toxic nodular goiter one or more nodular areas are usually felt.
   (3) The heart rate often exceeds 100 beats/min.
   (4) The return phase of the deep tendon reflexes is brisk.

d. **Laboratory studies** show an increase in the serum concentration of total T_4 and free T_4, serum concentration of total T_3 and free T_3, and T_3 resin uptake. The radioactive iodine uptake is high. Serum TSH levels are low.

4. **Therapy.** The **adrenergic manifestations of hyperthyroidism** (e.g., sweating, tachycardia, tremor) may be diminished by **β-blockers.** These drugs do not affect thyroid function but provide symptomatic relief until thyroid hormone levels can be lowered to normal.

a. **Treatment of Graves' disease.** The most common methods for treatment of Graves' disease are **antithyroid drugs, subtotal thyroidectomy,** and **radioactive iodine.**
   (1) **Antithyroid drugs**
      (a) **Mechanism of action. Methimazole** and **propylthiouracil (PTU)** inhibit the oxidation of iodide and the coupling of iodotyrosines, thus decreasing the synthesis of thyroid hormone. In addition, PTU decreases the conversion of T_4 to T_3 in peripheral tissues.

(b) **Medical treatment of Graves' disease.** Full doses (i.e., 30–40 mg methimazole or 300–400 mg PTU) are given daily until the patient is euthyroid.

(i) Although blockade of hormone synthesis is rapid, clinical improvement occurs only after a few weeks or months, because a large pool of stored hormone continues to be released from the thyroid.

(ii) After clinical improvement, the dose is tapered to the lowest dose that maintains euthyroidism, and the drug is continued for 1–1½ years. Treatment is then discontinued in the hope that a lasting or permanent remission has occurred.

(c) **Drug toxicity**

(i) **Skin rash or joint pain** occurs in 3%–5% of patients, necessitating a switch to the alternative drug.

(ii) **Agranulocytosis** occurs in fewer than 0.5% of patients but is life threatening. For early detection of agranulocytosis, patients should be instructed to stop the drug immediately if fever, sore throat, mouth ulcers, or other unexplained symptoms occur. Treatment should be resumed only after examination shows a normal white blood cell (WBC) count.

(d) **Advantages of medical treatment with antithyroid drugs**

(i) Hospitalization, surgery, and anesthesia are avoided.

(ii) There is less likelihood of the occurrence of post-treatment hypothyroidism than in patients treated with radioactive iodine.

(e) **Disadvantages of antithyroid drugs**

(i) Permanent remission occurs in fewer than 50% of patients treated.

(ii) Successful treatment depends on patient adherence, which is less of a problem when treatment is by surgery or radioactive iodine.

(2) **Subtotal thyroidectomy**

(a) **Preparation for surgery.** Operation on thyrotoxic patients involves the risk of thyroid storm; therefore, treatment should be initiated with antithyroid drugs long enough in advance for patients to return to a euthyroid state before surgery.

(b) **Advantages of surgery**

(i) Cure of hyperthyroidism is rapid (once a euthyroid state has been produced by antithyroid drugs).

(ii) The success rate is high; most patients are cured, and fewer become hypothyroid after surgery than after treatment with radioactive iodine.

(iii) Patient adherence is required for a shorter period than it is in prolonged antithyroid drug treatment.

(c) **Disadvantages of surgery**

(i) Patients usually must be hospitalized, and surgical and anesthetic risks are incurred.

(ii) Surgical complications include hypoparathyroidism and recurrent laryngeal nerve paralysis.

(3) **Radioactive iodine**

(a) **Method of treatment.** A single dose of iodine 131 (^{131}I) causes a decrease in function and size of the thyroid gland in 6–12 weeks. Approximately 75% of patients with Graves' disease are made euthyroid by a single dose; those who are still thyrotoxic after 12 weeks are given a second dose. Additional doses can be given if needed. Eventually, almost all patients are cured in this way.

(b) **Advantages of radioactive iodine**

(i) Hospitalization, surgery, and anesthesia are avoided.

(ii) The rate of cure approaches 100%.

(iii) Little patient adherence is required.

(c) **Disadvantages of radioactive iodine**

(i) Multiple treatments may be needed.

(ii) Hypothyroidism, the treatment of which requires long-term patient adherence, occurs in approximately 10% of patients after 1 year and continues to develop at a rate of 2%–3% each year. After 10–15 years, more than 50% of patients are hypothyroid. This complication is easily treated, however, with a single daily dose of L-thyroxine sodium.

(iii) There is a slight risk of genetic effects (comparable in magnitude to the effects of a barium enema or intravenous urogram) in future offspring. However, no increase in the risk for leukemia, thyroid cancer, or other malignancies has been found in patients treated with radioactive iodine.

(4) **Choice of therapy**

(a) Radioactive iodine is the treatment of choice for most patients older than 30–40 years and is frequently used in younger individuals.

(b) In younger patients, the choice is more difficult. In patients with mild clinical manifestations, slightly to moderately elevated thyroid hormone levels, and an only moderately enlarged thyroid, a trial of antithyroid drugs is reasonable, because patients with mild disease have a better chance for a lasting remission.

(c) Surgery may be a better choice for patients with large goiters and severe disease and for patients who are unwilling to take antithyroid drugs for a prolonged period.

b. **Treatment of toxic nodular goiter and toxic adenoma.** Because antithyroid drug therapy does not lead to permanent remission in affected patients, the options for treatment are surgery and radioactive iodine.

(1) **Thyroidectomy** or removal of a hyperfunctioning nodule rapidly cures the hyperthyroidism and relieves symptoms of pressure or tracheal or esophageal obstruction that may be caused by a large goiter.

(2) **Radioactive iodine** treatment requires much larger doses in patients with toxic nodular goiter than in patients with Graves' disease because the affected thyroid cells are relatively radioresistant. However, because the unaffected thyroid cells are functionally suppressed, they do not trap ^{131}I and are spared the effects of radiation; therefore, hypothyroidism after radioactive iodine treatment is less common in these patients.

c. **Treatment of thyroid storm**

(1) The mainstay of treatment is iodine, which acts within 24 hours by inhibiting the release of thyroid hormone. Sodium iodide is given in an intravenous dose of 1–2 g over 24 hours, or potassium iodide may be given orally.

(2) Antithyroid drugs are administered, but because they block hormone synthesis without inhibiting the release of preformed hormone, their effect is less rapid.

(3) β-Blockers and adrenal corticosteroids also are used.

D Thyroiditis

1. **Subacute thyroiditis** (also called granulomatous thyroiditis or de Quervain's thyroiditis)

a. **Etiology.** The cause of subacute thyroiditis generally is considered to be viral. Mumps and coxsackievirus, among others, have been suspected.

b. **Clinical features**

(1) **Early symptoms.** A prodrome of malaise, upper respiratory symptoms, and fever that lasts 1 or 2 weeks may occur. Then, the thyroid gland becomes enlarged, firm, and tender, with pain radiating to the ears, neck, or arms.

(2) **Hyperthyroidism.** Leaking of thyroid hormone from damaged follicles into the circulation may lead to hyperthyroidism.

(3) **Disease course.** The thyroid pain and hyperthyroidism subside in a few weeks or months. The gland usually returns to normal size; if enlargement persists, chronic autoimmune thy-

roiditis should be suspected. A self-limited period of **hypothyroidism** may occur after the released hormone has been metabolized but before new hormone production has resumed.

c. **Diagnosis.** When the thyroid becomes acutely swollen, tender, and painful, especially if symptoms of hyperthyroidism are present, subacute thyroiditis is suspected. The diagnosis is confirmed by a **very low radioactive iodine uptake in the face of high serum T_4 and T_3 levels.** The radioactive iodine uptake is low because the follicular cells are injured and unable to trap iodine and because the high levels of circulating thyroid hormone suppress TSH.

d. **Therapy.** Treatment is **symptomatic,** because the disease is self-limited.
   (1) Aspirin, nonsteroidal anti-inflammatory drugs (NSAIDs), and adrenal corticosteroids (in severe cases) relieve the pain and tenderness.
   (2) β-Blocking drugs can be used to relieve symptoms of hyperthyroidism.

2. **Chronic autoimmune thyroiditis (Hashimoto's thyroiditis)**
   a. **Etiology.** Chronic thyroiditis is a common autoimmune disorder that primarily affects women. Antithyroid antibodies are present in most patients.
   b. **Clinical features**
      (1) **Thyroid gland enlargement,** the main clinical manifestation, is the result of autoimmune damage that leads to lymphocytic infiltration, fibrosis, and a weakened ability of the thyroid to produce hormone (Figure 9–1).
      (2) **Hypothyroidism** is present in many patients when the disease is first diagnosed and may affect additional patients as the disease progresses.
      (3) **Pain and tenderness of the gland** sometimes occur, as in subacute thyroiditis.
   c. **Diagnosis.** Chronic thyroiditis is suspected in any patient with a firm, nontoxic goiter; a high titer of antithyroid peroxidase antibodies or antithyroglobulin antibodies, or both, is confirmatory. Thyroid function tests usually are normal unless the patient has hypothyroidism.
   d. **Therapy.** Treatment with L-thyroxine sodium often decreases the size of the goiter and, therefore, is useful even in patients with normal thyroid function. If hypothyroidism is present, this treatment is, of course, essential.

3. **Painless thyroiditis** (also called silent thyroiditis or postpartum thyroiditis). This syndrome resembles subacute thyroiditis in some ways and chronic thyroiditis in others.
   a. Like subacute thyroiditis, painless thyroiditis is associated with transient, self-limited hyperthyroidism, often with thyroid gland enlargement, and a low radioactive iodine uptake. Thyroid pain and tenderness are absent, however.
      (1) Recognition of this cause of self-limited hyperthyroidism is important, because, in the absence of thyroid pain to suggest thyroiditis, the syndrome could easily be mistaken for Graves' disease and be treated inappropriately.
      (2) The low radioactive iodine uptake is the most useful finding for distinguishing painless thyroiditis from Graves' disease.

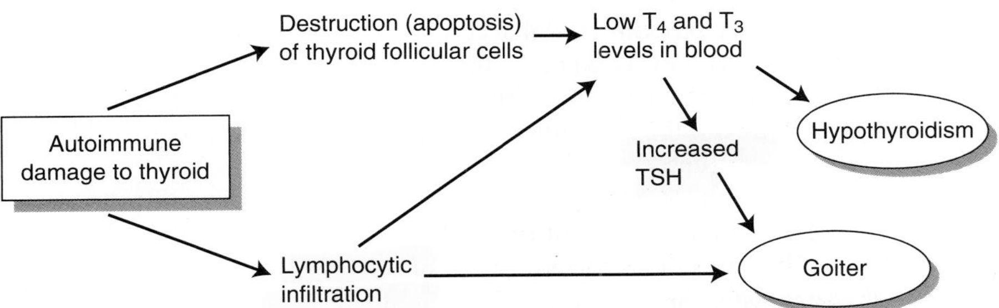

FIGURE 9–1 Pathogenesis of chronic autoimmune thyroiditis. (Adapted from Adlin EV: *Endocrinology Science and Medicine.* Philadelphia, Lippincott Williams & Wilkins, 2001, p 32.)

b. Like chronic thyroiditis, painless thyroiditis is characterized by lymphocytic infiltration of the thyroid and is considered to be an autoimmune disease. However, although antithyroid antibodies may be present, the titers are lower than in chronic thyroiditis.

c. Painless thyroiditis is common after delivery; **postpartum thyroiditis** occurs after 5%–10% of pregnancies.

4. **Rare forms of thyroiditis**

a. **Suppurative thyroiditis** is caused by pyogenic bacterial infection. This thyroid condition is treated with antibiotics and surgical drainage, if necessary.

b. In **Riedel's struma** (fibrous thyroiditis), fibrous connective tissue replaces normal thyroid tissue and infiltrates surrounding structures. Surgery is indicated to exclude cancer and to relieve tracheal compression.

E Thyroid cancer

1. **Epidemiology**

a. Thyroid cancer is common; it is found at autopsy in approximately 5% of patients with no known thyroid disease. However, death due to thyroid cancer is uncommon—approximately 1200 individuals die of this condition each year in the United States.

b. These contradictory observations are explained best by the behavior of thyroid cancer. It is usually indolent and tends to remain localized to the thyroid for many years, which is the reason for the low mortality rate.

2. **Etiology**

a. **Radiation exposure.** Incidence of thyroid cancer is increased in atomic bomb survivors and in individuals who received radiation therapy to the neck (e.g., for enlarged thymus or enlarged tonsils) in childhood.

b. **Genetic factors.** One form of thyroid cancer, medullary carcinoma, may be familial.

c. **TSH** can induce thyroid cancer in animals and may stimulate the growth of many human thyroid cancers.

3. **Types.** Thyroid cancer may manifest as a solitary thyroid nodule or, less commonly, as multiple nodules or a mass in the neck. These tumors occasionally cause hoarseness, symptoms of tracheal or esophageal compression (e.g., dyspnea, dysphagia), or pain.

a. **Papillary carcinoma,** which accounts for 80% of all thyroid cancer, affects the youngest age group—50% of patients are younger than 40 years of age.

(1) The neoplasm consists of columnar cells in folds (the papillae). It tends to grow slowly, often remaining localized to the thyroid for years, and eventually spreads via the lymphatic system to other parts of the thyroid and to regional nodes.

(2) There are few recurrences after treatment, especially in young patients with small primary tumors.

b. **Follicular carcinoma,** which constitutes 10% of all thyroid cancers, histologically may resemble normal thyroid tissue. Follicular carcinoma is more malignant than papillary cancer and often spreads to bone, the lungs, and the liver. The 10-year survival rate is 50%.

c. **Medullary carcinoma,** which accounts for 5% of all thyroid cancers, arises from the parafollicular cells (or C cells) of the thyroid. It has a hyaline stroma, which may stain for amyloid.

(1) Approximately 20% of these carcinomas are familial and may be a component of **MEN type II** (Sipple's syndrome), a syndrome of medullary thyroid carcinoma and pheochromocytoma.

(2) This tumor often produces calcitonin and occasionally produces other hormones.

(3) It is more malignant than follicular carcinoma, with both local lymphatic and distant hematogenous spread.

d. **Anaplastic carcinoma,** which accounts for 5% of thyroid cancers, usually affects patients older than 50 years of age and is highly malignant. It invades rapidly, metastasizes widely, and usually causes death within a few months.

4. **Therapy.** Papillary, follicular, and medullary carcinoma usually are treated with a combination of surgery, suppression with thyroid hormone, and radioactive iodine. Anaplastic carcinoma generally is treated palliatively. It may require surgery to relieve obstruction; chemotherapy may delay death.

   a. **Surgery**

      (1) Papillary carcinoma, when small and limited to a single area of the thyroid, often is treated by removal of the involved lobe and the isthmus.

      (2) Follicular carcinoma and more extensive papillary tumors usually are treated by near-total thyroidectomy; just enough tissue is left in association with the posterior capsule to spare the parathyroid glands. This more extensive procedure is more likely to be complicated by hypoparathyroidism, but it is followed by less tumor recurrence.

   b. **Radioactive iodine therapy.** Differentiated thyroid cancer (papillary and follicular) often accumulates radioactive iodine.

      (1) Radioiodine can be used to ablate any normal thyroid tissue that remains after near-total thyroidectomy; normal thyroid tissue has greater affinity for radioiodine than tumor tissue, and therefore limits the amount of radioiodine that would be taken up by tumor.

      (2) After all normal thyroid tissue has been ablated, whole-body scans with radioiodine will be more likely to reveal functioning metastatic tumor, which can be treated with subsequent large doses of radioiodine.

   c. **Suppression therapy.** Because many thyroid cancers grow more rapidly with TSH stimulation, TSH should be suppressed by treatment with L-thyroxine.

      (1) Because suppression of TSH produces a state of subclinical hyperthyroidism, which may decrease bone density, increase cardiac irritability, and have other deleterious effects, to what extent TSH should be suppressed is not clear.

      (2) A reasonable approach may be to aim for full suppression (undetectable TSH) in patients with high-risk thyroid cancer (large tumor, known metastases, etc.) and to aim for TSH in the low-normal range in patients with low-risk cancer.

F **Thyroid nodules** are present in 1% of individuals in their 20s and in 5% of individuals in their 60s; cancer is found in approximately 5% of these nodules.

1. **Pathology.** Thyroid nodules may be true adenomas, cysts, localized areas of chronic thyroiditis, colloid nodules, hemorrhagic necrotic tissue, or carcinoma.

2. **Diagnosis**

   a. **Risk assessment**

      (1) **Radiation treatment** of the head or neck in childhood is associated with an increased prevalence of thyroid nodules and thyroid cancer in adult life.

      (2) **Sex.** A higher percentage of nodules are malignant in men than in women (although nodules are much more common in women).

      (3) **Age.** A higher percentage of nodules are malignant in younger individuals (although nodules are much more common in older individuals). In children, 50% of nodules are malignant.

      (4) **Disease course.** Malignancy is suggested by recent growth of the nodule or by continuing growth despite suppressive therapy with L-thyroxine. Malignancy is less likely if the nodule disappears after aspiration of cyst fluid, if the nodule is visible as a "warm" or "hot" spot on scintiscan (i.e., as demonstrated by its uptake of radioactive iodine), or if the nodule shrinks with suppressive therapy.

      (5) **Physical examination**

         (a) Malignancy is suggested when the nodule is fixed in place and no movement occurs on swallowing.

         (b) Unusually firm consistency, irregularity of the nodule, or regional lymph node enlargement also suggest malignancy.

(c) Malignancy is less likely if there are multiple nodules or if the nodule is less than 1 cm in diameter.

b. Laboratory evaluation

(1) **Radionuclide thyroid scintiscanning** identifies the nodule as "hot," "warm," or "cold."

(a) Because most cancers appear on scan as cold areas, only cold nodules are considered to have a significant risk of malignancy.

(b) Of all nodules, 70%–90% are cold, and most of these are benign. Therefore, scanning may indicate a greatly reduced risk of malignancy in a nodule that is warm or hot, but it does not yield much additional information on the risk of malignancy in a nodule that is cold.

(2) **Fine-needle aspiration biopsy** is safe and easily performed in an office setting. Cells, not sections of tissue, are obtained and must be evaluated by a skilled cytopathologist. The overall results and predictive values are shown in Table 9–6.

3. **Management.** The goal of management is surgical removal of the nodules with a high probability of malignancy and careful observation of the others, sometimes with attempted suppression by L-thyroxine. An algorithm for the management of thyroid nodules is shown in Figure 9–2.

III DISORDERS OF THE PARATHYROID GLANDS

A Primary hyperparathyroidism and hypercalcemia Primary hyperparathyroidism is the result of oversecretion of parathyroid hormone (PTH), which in turn causes hypercalcemia. When primary hyperparathyroidism was first recognized in the early 1920s, patients exhibited severe bone disease, recurrent urinary calculi, and systemic illness caused by marked hypercalcemia. Now the disease is diagnosed much earlier, and, as a result, most cases are less severe.

1. **Epidemiology.** Primary hyperparathyroidism is common, affecting approximately one individual in every 1000 who are screened. The disease is especially common in middle-aged and elderly women.

2. **Etiology**

a. A single **parathyroid adenoma** causes 80%–90% of cases, and **hyperplasia** of all four glands causes 10%–20% of cases of primary hyperparathyroidism. Parathyroid carcinoma is a rare cause.

b. **Predisposing factors**

(1) Although most cases seem to arise without a known cause, a history of **radiation to the neck** is present in 10% or more of patients.

(2) Familial occurrence of parathyroid hyperplasia and of the MEN syndrome, which often involves parathyroid adenomas or hyperplasia, indicates that **genetic factors** may be important.

3. **Pathophysiology.** PTH is important in maintaining normal calcium homeostasis (Figure 9–3).

a. PTH raises the serum calcium level by stimulating vitamin D production (which is important for gastrointestinal absorption of calcium), by increasing renal tubular reabsorption of cal-

TABLE 9–6 Results of Fine-Needle Aspiration Biopsy of Thyroid Nodules

Cytologic Findings	% of Nodules	% Positive for Cancer
Benign	75	1–5
Suspicious or indeterminant	20	20
Malignant	5	97

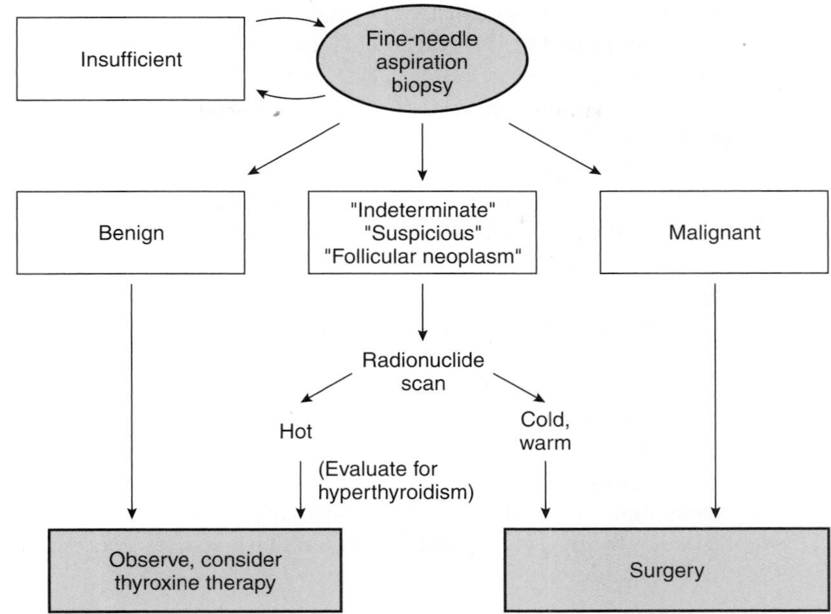

FIGURE 9–2 Algorithm for evaluation and management of patients with a thyroid nodule. (From Adlin EV: *Endocrinology Science and Medicine.* Philadelphia, Lippincott Williams & Wilkins, 2001, p 48.)
(Adapted from Mazzaferri EL: Management of a solitary thyroid nodule. *N Engl J Med* 1993;328:553–559; and Singer PA, Cooper DS, Daniels GH, et al: Treatment guidelines for patients with thyroid nodules and well-differentiated thyroid cancer. *Arch Intern Med* 1996;156:2165–2172.)

cium, by decreasing renal tubular reabsorption of phosphate, and by promoting movement of calcium from the bone.

b. Decreased circulating levels of ionized calcium stimulate PTH production, tending to raise calcium levels back to normal; conversely, increased circulating levels of ionized calcium inhibit PTH production. However, a parathyroid adenoma may function autonomously, producing excessive PTH despite high serum calcium levels and causing the abnormalities of primary hyperparathyroidism.

4. Clinical features. The routine measurement of serum calcium levels in multichannel screening tests has led to early diagnosis of primary hyperparathyroidism. The disease commonly manifests as mild asymptomatic hypercalcemia, although occasionally patients are seen with the classic findings of advanced kidney and bone disease. Patients with serum calcium levels greater than 11 or 12 mg/dL often have gastrointestinal symptoms, neurologic symptoms, or both.

a. Renal manifestations

(1) Although PTH increases renal calcium reabsorption, the hypercalcemia and resulting increased glomerular filtration of calcium commonly lead to **hypercalciuria,** which may cause the formation of **urinary calculi.**

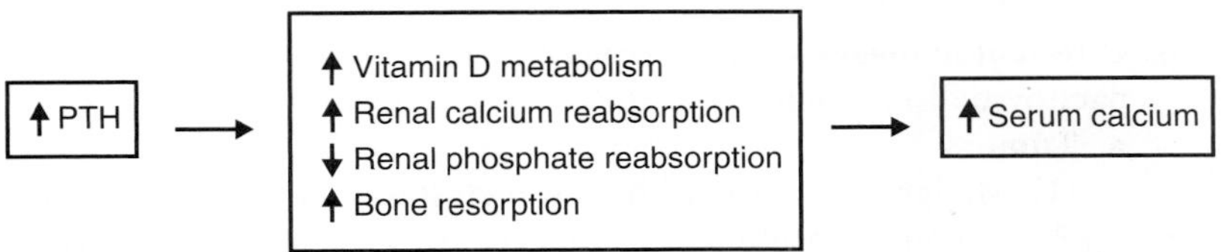

FIGURE 9–3 Actions of parathyroid hormone (PTH) in maintaining normal calcium homeostasis.

(2) Chronic hypercalcemia may cause deposition of calcium within the renal parenchyma (nephrocalcinosis) and eventual **renal failure.**

b. **Skeletal manifestations.** PTH excess increases the rate of osteoclastic bone resorption and can lead to the disorder of bone metabolism called **osteitis fibrosa cystica.**

(1) **Symptoms** include bone pain, fractures, and areas of swelling and deformity localized to involved bones.

(2) There are areas of **demineralization** in the skeleton. In severe cases, there may be **bone cysts** and "**brown tumors,**" which are localized lesions consisting of proliferating osteoclasts, osteoblasts, and fibrous tissue.

(3) Radiographs may show **generalized osteopenia,** with demineralization of the skull and other areas. **Subperiosteal resorption** of bone occurs in the phalanges and distal portions of the clavicles. Loss of the lamina dura around the teeth is characteristic.

c. **Gastrointestinal manifestations.** Symptoms related to the hypercalcemia of hyperparathyroidism include anorexia, weight loss, constipation, nausea and vomiting, and abdominal pain. Patients with hyperparathyroidism may have an increased incidence of peptic ulcer disease and pancreatitis.

d. **Neurologic manifestations.** Emotional changes and abnormal mentation, which also are related to the hypercalcemia of hyperparathyroidism, may occur. Fatigue and muscle weakness are common.

5. **Diagnosis**

a. **Laboratory findings**

(1) **Blood chemistry**

(a) **Elevation of the serum calcium level is the hallmark of primary hyperparathyroidism.**

(b) The serum phosphate level is lowered in many, but not all, cases.

(c) Because the serum chloride level tends to be increased (because of PTH–induced bicarbonaturia), the serum chloride-to-phosphate ratio usually is elevated (>33); this finding is more consistent than that of hypophosphatemia.

(d) The serum alkaline phosphatase level is elevated only in patients with significant bone disease.

(2) **Urine chemistry. Hypercalciuria** is common but, because of the calcium-reabsorbing action of PTH, approximately one third of patients have normal urine calcium levels.

b. **PTH assay.** An elevated blood PTH level in the presence of hypercalcemia is strong evidence for primary hyperparathyroidism because other causes of calcium elevation tend to suppress PTH levels. The **immunoradiometric assay for intact PTH** is more sensitive and specific than previously used assays.

c. **Diagnostic imaging**

(1) Noninvasive techniques such as **ultrasonography, CT scanning, MRI,** and **isotope scans** may demonstrate parathyroid adenomas in 60%–80% of cases.

(2) **Selective venous catheterization,** in which blood samples are taken from veins draining various areas of the neck and mediastinum, is a much more difficult procedure. A marked increase in PTH concentration suggests the location of the adenoma. This procedure is seldom performed except in patients facing a second operation after an unsuccessful neck exploration.

6. **Differential diagnosis.** Hypercalcemia may be caused by entities other than primary hyperparathyroidism (Table 9–7)

a. **Tumors**

(1) **Malignant tumors with bone metastases** may cause hypercalcemia through an increase in bone resorption due to local effects and sometimes through locally acting humoral substances (e.g., osteoclast activating factor) produced by the metastatic tumor.

TABLE 9–7 Causes of Hypercalcemia

Primary hyperparathyroidism	Sarcoidosis
Malignancy	Benign familial hypercalcemia
With bone metastases (e.g., breast cancer, myeloma, lymphoma)	Hypervitaminosis D
Without bone metastases (e.g., hypernephroma; pancreatic cancer; squamous cell carcinoma of the lung, cervix, and esophagus; head and neck tumors)	Milk–alkali syndrome
	Hyperthyroidism
	Thiazide therapy
	Immobilization

(2) **Tumors that cause hypercalcemia in the absence of bone metastases** do so by producing **PTH-related peptide (PTHrP),** a humoral factor that acts like PTH and binds to PTH receptors but is not measured by the PTH radioimmunoassay. PTHrP may produce biochemical effects like those of PTH, including hypophosphatemia and increased urinary nephrogenous cyclic adenosine 3′,5′-monophosphate (cAMP). Humoral hypercalcemia of malignancy may be differentiated from primary hyperparathyroidism by finding an elevated level of PTHrP and a normal or low level of PTH.

b. Sarcoidosis may cause hypercalcemia because of production of 1,25-dihydroxyvitamin D_3 by granulomatous tissue. If no other findings indicate the presence of sarcoidosis and the PTH concentration is not elevated, a therapeutic trial may be helpful. Serum calcium levels decline within 1 week of the start of glucocorticoid administration (e.g., 40 mg prednisone daily) in most cases of sarcoidosis but are unaffected in most cases of primary hyperparathyroidism.

c. Benign familial hypercalcemia (familial hypocalciuric hypercalcemia) is an autosomal dominant disorder caused by an inactivating mutation of the gene encoding the calcium-sensing receptor. The parathyroid glands and the renal tubules fail to recognize the true concentration of extracellular calcium, leading to overproduction of PTH and increased renal reabsorption of calcium.

(1) The resulting syndrome consists of mild-to-moderate hypercalcemia with normal or slightly elevated serum PTH levels and hypocalciuria. Patients remain asymptomatic, without renal calculi, renal parenchymal damage, or bone disease.

(2) Diagnostic clues are the familial occurrence and the low (rather than high) urinary calcium excretion.

(3) Because surgical treatment is not beneficial and is not recommended, this condition should be ruled out in patients with apparent primary hyperparathyroidism.

d. Vitamin D intoxication, which is usually seen in patients receiving pharmacologic doses of the vitamin for the treatment of hypoparathyroidism, results in hypercalcemia.

(1) The diagnosis should be apparent from the patient's history.

(2) If a sufficiently rapid fall in serum calcium levels does not result when vitamin D ingestion is stopped, glucocorticoids should be given. Glucocorticoids inhibit the action of vitamin D on intestinal calcium absorption and rapidly lower serum calcium levels.

e. Milk–alkali syndrome is caused by the ingestion of large quantities of calcium and absorbable alkali. It is characterized by hypercalcemia, systemic alkalosis, and renal damage due to nephrocalcinosis. This syndrome is unlikely to develop unless calcium intake exceeds 5 g calcium carbonate (2 g elemental calcium) daily, which is approximately double the dose usually recommended for the prevention or treatment of osteoporosis.

f. Other causes of hypercalcemia

(1) **Hyperthyroidism.** This condition may cause hypercalcemia because of increased bone turnover. The diagnosis is usually evident because the hyperthyroidism, not the hypercalcemia, is the presenting syndrome.

(2) **Thiazide diuretics.** These agents decrease urinary calcium excretion but rarely cause hypercalcemia; they should be avoided, however, in patients with hyperparathyroidism.

(3) **Prolonged immobilization.** Because of continuing bone resorption in the absence of normal postural stimuli for bone formation, hypercalcemia may occur. This problem is particularly common in children who are confined to bed for long periods (e.g., in a total body cast for treatment of multiple traumatic fractures).

(4) **Paget's disease.** Increased bone turnover and localized bone tumors due to defective regulation of bone metabolism may produce hypercalcemia, especially during periods of immobilization.

(5) **Recovery from acute renal failure.** A syndrome of hypercalcemia may develop during the recovery period after rhabdomyolysis and acute renal failure. During the first 2–3 days after muscle injury, the initial muscle damage leads to local calcium and phosphate deposition. When renal function returns to normal, calcium and phosphate exit from sites of muscle damage and enter the circulation to produce hypercalcemia. This defect typically occurs 2–3 weeks after the acute muscle injury.

7. Therapy of primary hyperparathyroidism

a. Surgery

(1) **Indications.** Asymptomatic patients with minimal elevation in serum calcium and no complications often have no progression of the disease for 10 years or longer. Such patients may be followed closely and considered for surgery only if they develop specific indications (Table 9–8).

(2) **Initial surgical exploration.** In most cases, a **single adenoma** is found and removed. If **parathyroid hyperplasia** is found, the surgeon may remove three glands and part of the fourth, or all parathyroid tissue and transplant a portion to the muscles of the forearm or neck. The removal of additional parathyroid tissue from the transplanted portion may be accomplished easily if necessary.

(3) **Repeat surgical exploration.** Approximately 10% of initial neck explorations fail to indicate abnormal parathyroid tissue or cure the disease. After the patient is reevaluated, additional invasive and noninvasive localizing procedures are considered before a second operation is performed.

(4) **Postoperative course.** Transient hypocalcemia is common after the removal of a parathyroid adenoma because the remaining normal glands are likely to have been suppressed by long-standing hypercalcemia.

(a) Patients usually recover within a few weeks.

(b) In the occasional patient with severe bone disease, marked intractable hypocalcemia may persist for several months, because, when the excess PTH stimulus is suddenly

TABLE 9–8 Indications for Surgery in Primary Hyperparathyroidism

Indication
Symptoms related to hypercalcemia
Serum calcium levels > 1 mg/dL above normal range
Age < 50 years
Renal manifestations
Renal calculi
Reduced creatinine clearance
24-Hour urine calcium excretion > 400 mg/dL
Bone mineral density > 2.5 SDs below peak bone mass (t-score)
Patient preference for surgery or unwillingness/inability to undergo prolonged follow-up

SD = standard deviation.

removed, the demineralized bone becomes avid for calcium (the "hungry bones" syndrome).

b. **Medical therapy** may be used if no indications for surgery are present (see Table 9–8), if other illness contraindicates surgery, or if the patient refuses surgery.
   (1) **Increased fluid intake** and activity help to minimize hypercalcemia.
   (2) **Oral phosphate** in doses of 1–2 g daily often lowers the serum calcium level. The main complication, extraskeletal calcification, is uncommon if this dose is not exceeded.
   (3) **Estrogen** may lower mildly elevated serum calcium levels to normal, apparently by decreasing bone resorption. This treatment may be considered in postmenopausal women, who make up two-thirds of the cases of primary hyperparathyroidism.

c. **Emergency treatment** is necessary if the calcium level increases above 13–15 mg/dL before the adenoma can be removed or if surgical treatment is refused or is unsuccessful. Hypercalcemia caused by diseases other than hyperparathyroidism (e.g., hypercalcemia due to malignancy) also may be treated by the following methods.
   (1) **Hydration with sodium diuresis.** Four to six liters or more of intravenous saline daily, with large doses of furosemide, increase renal calcium excretion and reduce serum calcium levels.
   (2) **Bisphosphonates** such as **pamidronate** bind to hydroxyapatite in bone and block dissolution of this mineral; they also inhibit osteoclast activity. The resulting inhibition of bone resorption produces a decline in serum calcium levels over 1–7 days. Pamidronate (60–90 mg) is given intravenously in a single dose over 24 hours; this can be repeated in 7 days if necessary.
   (3) **Plicamycin** (formerly called mithramycin) is an antineoplastic agent that lowers serum calcium levels by inhibiting osteoclastic bone resorption. A single intravenous dose of 25 μg/kg administered over 4–6 hours may lower the serum calcium levels for several days. This drug is commonly used in treating hypercalcemia due to malignancy.
   (4) **Gallium nitrate** is a potent inhibitor of bone resorption. It is given in a dose of 200 mg/m^2/day by continuous infusion for 5 days. Potential nephrotoxicity limits its use to patients without renal failure.
   (5) **Calcitonin** lowers serum calcium levels by inhibiting osteoclastic bone resorption. It is the fastest acting hypocalcemic agent and is very safe, but it is less potent than plicamycin, gallium nitrate, or pamidronate, and its effect tends to decrease after several days. Salmon calcitonin, 4 U/kg, is given intramuscularly or subcutaneously every 12 hours.
   (6) **Glucocorticoids** lower serum calcium levels in patients with sarcoidosis and vitamin D intoxication, and sometimes in those patients with myeloma and hematologic malignancy. However, glucocorticoids do not lower serum calcium levels in patients with hyperparathyroidism.

B Hypoparathyroidism and hypocalcemia

1. **Etiology**
   a. **Surgical removal of the parathyroid glands** is the most common cause of hypoparathyroidism.
      (1) This may be an unavoidable result of radical neck dissection for cancer or a rare complication of subtotal thyroidectomy.
      (2) **Temporary hypoparathyroidism** after neck surgery is not uncommon and may be due to ischemic injury to the glands. Recovery usually occurs in a few weeks or months.
   b. **Idiopathic hypoparathyroidism** of autoimmune etiology is much less common. It usually is diagnosed in childhood, may be familial, and sometimes is associated with adrenal insufficiency and mucocutaneous candidiasis.

2. **Pathophysiology. PTH deficiency leads to hypocalcemia, the hallmark of hypoparathyroidism,** through the same mechanisms by which increased secretion of PTH causes hypercalcemia (see

III A 3). In addition, the decreased renal phosphate clearance leads to **hyperphosphatemia,** which is present in most cases of hypoparathyroidism.

3. **Clinical features and diagnosis.** Hypocalcemia produces acute symptoms related to increased neuromuscular irritability. In addition, long-term changes may occur as a result of effects on ectodermal tissues and ectopic calcium deposition.
   a. **Symptoms and signs**
      (1) **Latent tetany**
         (a) Mild hypocalcemia may cause **muscular fatigue and weakness** as well as **numbness** and tingling around the mouth and in the hands and feet.
         (b) **Chvostek's sign** may be positive (i.e., a tap over the facial nerve in front of the ear elicits a contraction of the facial muscles and upper lip). However, Chvostek's sign may be positive in 10% of normal individuals.
         (c) **Trousseau's sign** may be positive; that is, inflation of a blood pressure cuff on the arm to a pressure higher than the patient's systolic pressure for 3 minutes elicits carpal spasm [flexion of the metacarpophalangeal (MCP) joints and extension of the interphalangeal joints, with drawing together of the fingers and adduction of the thumb].
      (2) **Overt tetany.** Severe hypocalcemia causes **twitching and cramps of the muscles with carpopedal spasm. Laryngeal stridor** and **seizures** may occur in severe cases.
      (3) **Long-term effects of hypocalcemia**
         (a) **Ectodermal changes** include atrophy, brittleness, and ridging of the nails; dryness and scaling of the skin; and enamel defects and hypoplasia of the teeth.
         (b) **Calcification of the basal ganglia** may occur and is occasionally associated with parkinsonian signs and symptoms.
         (c) **Calcification of the optic lens may lead to cataract formation.**
   b. **Laboratory abnormalities. Hypocalcemia** and **hyperphosphatemia** are consistently present in hypoparathyroidism. PTH levels, of course, are low, but clinical assays may not be sufficiently sensitive to distinguish between low and normal levels.

4. **Differential diagnosis**
   a. **Pseudohypoparathyroidism**
      (1) Pseudohypoparathyroidism is a hereditary disease with two distinct areas of clinical expression.
         (a) **Calcium metabolism is abnormal** because of end-organ resistance to the action of PTH; that is, the kidney and bone cannot respond to PTH, even though its concentration in the serum is normal or increased. The result is hypocalcemia and hyperphosphatemia, as are seen in true hypoparathyroidism.
         (b) **Developmental and skeletal abnormalities** (**Albright's hereditary osteodystrophy**) are present.
            (i) The most common abnormalities are short stature, shortening of the metacarpal and metatarsal bones, and mental deficiency.
            (ii) The skeletal abnormalities sometimes occur in the absence of any disorder of calcium metabolism; this has been called "pseudopseudohypoparathyroidism."
      (2) If Albright's hereditary osteodystrophy is not present and if hypocalcemia is not clearly postsurgical in its onset, the differentiation between true hypoparathyroidism and pseudohypoparathyroidism may depend on laboratory tests.
         (a) PTH levels may be sufficiently elevated in pseudohypoparathyroidism to distinguish the syndrome clearly from hypoparathyroidism.
         (b) Injection of PTH is followed promptly by increased urine concentrations of phosphate and cAMP and, within 1 or 2 days, by an increase in serum calcium in patients with hypoparathyroidism. No response occurs in patients with pseudohypoparathyroidism.

b. **Hypoalbuminemia** causes a decrease in the fraction of serum calcium that is bound to protein and, therefore, a decrease in total serum calcium; because the ionized fraction of serum calcium remains normal, however, there are no clinical manifestations of calcium deficiency. This should not be considered a form of true hypocalcemia. For each decrement in serum albumin of 1 g/L, the serum calcium is expected to decline by approximately 0.8 mg/dL.

c. Hypocalcemia in **renal failure** is caused by many factors. These include renal phosphate retention (with resultant hyperphosphatemia), reduced production of 1,25-dihydroxyvitamin D_3 by the diseased kidneys, and bone resistance to the calcemic action of PTH.

d. **Malabsorption** associated with gastrointestinal disease may lead to inadequate calcium or vitamin D absorption and consequent hypocalcemia.

e. **Vitamin D deficiency** or resistance to the actions of vitamin D may cause hypocalcemia through decreased gastrointestinal absorption of calcium.

f. **Acute pancreatitis** may lead to intra-abdominal precipitation of calcium soaps in areas of fat necrosis. Whether this explains why hypocalcemia is sometimes seen in patients with acute pancreatitis is uncertain.

g. **Osteoblastic metastasis** of prostate, breast, or lung cancer may produce hypocalcemia, presumably because of rapid bone uptake of calcium.

h. **Hypomagnesemia** decreases production of PTH and inhibits the actions of PTH and vitamin D on bone, leading to hypocalcemia.

5. **Therapy**

a. **Hypoparathyroidism.** PTH, which must be injected twice daily, is not commonly used for long-term therapy. Instead, treatment with **supplemental calcium,** combined with **vitamin D** to enhance its absorption, is effective in correcting the hypocalcemia and hyperphosphatemia of hypoparathyroidism, even in cases caused by end-organ unresponsiveness to PTH (e.g., pseudohypoparathyroidism).

(1) **Calcium supplementation.** Usually 1–2 g elemental calcium is given daily.

(a) Commonly used preparations include calcium gluconate (each 1-g tablet contains 90 mg elemental calcium), calcium carbonate (each tablet of Os-Cal 500 contains 500 mg calcium), and calcium glubionate (each tablespoon of Neo-Calglucon contains 345 mg calcium).

(b) The calcium is given in three or four divided doses. The dose can easily be raised or lowered to regulate serum calcium levels.

(2) **Vitamin D. Vitamin D_2 (ergocalciferol)** has been used for years in the treatment of hypoparathyroidism, but **calcitriol** has largely replaced it.

(a) **Calciferol**

(i) Because vitamin D_2 must be converted to 1,25-dihydroxyvitamin D_3 to be fully effective (a conversion that is greatly inhibited in the absence of PTH), large doses are necessary. The average daily dose is 50,000 U, with a range of 25,000–150,000 U, although the recommended dietary allowance in normal persons is only 400 U.

(ii) The onset of action is slow (1–2 weeks), but the effect may persist for months after administration is stopped.

(b) **Calcitriol (1,25-dihydroxyvitamin D_3).** The main advantage of calcitriol over vitamin D_2 is the faster onset and cessation of action, which may lead to more precise control of blood calcium levels. Calcitriol is given in doses of 0.25–2.0 μg/day.

b. **Acute hypocalcemia.** Treatment of this condition, which may occur shortly after parathyroid resection and may cause severe tetanic symptoms, consists of intravenous administration of calcium. Calcium gluconate (10%) in a dose of 1–2 g is given intravenously in approximately 10 minutes followed by slow infusion of 1 g calcium gluconate over the next 6–8 hours.

IV DISORDERS OF GLUCOSE HOMEOSTASIS

A Diabetes mellitus This condition is **characterized by hyperglycemia** and other metabolic derangements that are **caused by inadequate action of insulin** on body tissues, because of either reduced circulating levels of insulin or resistance of target tissues to its actions. Because of the prevalence and importance of certain complications, diabetes may be considered to be a syndrome consisting of metabolic abnormalities, microvascular disease (i.e., retinopathy and nephropathy), large-vessel disease (i.e., accelerated atherosclerosis), and peripheral and autonomic neuropathy.

1. **Classification** (Table 9–9). Diabetes mellitus is divided into two categories—**type 1 diabetes** (formerly called insulin-dependent diabetes) and **type 2 diabetes** (formerly called noninsulin-dependent diabetes). Syndromes with features from either of these categories may be related to the stage or severity of the disease or to other conditions. These syndromes include impaired fasting glucose, impaired glucose tolerance, gestational diabetes, previous abnormality of glucose tolerance, potential abnormality of glucose tolerance, and diabetes associated with certain other diseases.
   a. **Type 1 diabetes** affects 5%–10% of diabetic patients.
      (1) In type 1 diabetes, not only is insulin needed for optimal control of blood glucose, which also may be true for patients with type 2 disease, but **without exogenous insulin, patients are prone to the development of ketoacidosis.** This is thought to reflect a complete or almost complete absence of insulin in patients with type 1 diabetes, in contrast to the partial lack of insulin and the resistance to insulin characteristic of patients with type 2 diabetes.
      (2) Other key features of type 1 diabetes are its occurrence in children and young adults and its occurrence in individuals who are lean rather than obese.
   b. **Type 2 diabetes** commonly affects overweight individuals older than 40 years of age, although with the rising prevalence of obesity it is increasingly being diagnosed in children.
      (1) Because some insulin is produced by these patients, **ketoacidosis does not occur.**
      (2) However, insulin therapy may be necessary to prevent severe hyperglycemia.
   c. **Related syndromes**
      (1) **Impaired fasting glucose** or **impaired glucose tolerance.** This is a disorder of glucose metabolism in which blood glucose levels are higher than those of normal individuals but

TABLE 9–9 Major Types of Primary Diabetes Mellitus

	Type 1 Diabetes Mellitus	Type 2 Diabetes Mellitus
Prevalence	0.2%–0.5%; men = women	2%–4%; women > men
Age at onset	Usually < 25 years	Usually > 40 years
Genetics	< 10% of first-degree relatives affected; 50% concordance in identical twins	> 20% of first-degree relatives affected; 90%–100% concordance in identical twins
HLA	Associated with HLA-DR3, HLA-DR4, HLA-DQ	None
Autoimmunity	Increased prevalence of autoantibodies to islet cells and other tissues	None
Body build	Usually lean	Usually obese
Metabolism	Ketosis prone; insulin production absent	Ketosis-resistant; insulin levels may be high, normal, or low
Treatment	Insulin	Weight loss; oral agents (e.g., sulfonylureas, metformin, thiazolidinediones) or insulin

HLA = human leukocyte antigen.

lower than those of patients with diabetes. The risk of development of diabetes is increased in affected individuals.

(2) **Gestational diabetes.** Diabetes or impaired glucose tolerance develops in 2%–3% of pregnant, previously nondiabetic women, most often in the last trimester of pregnancy.
   (a) β-Cell reserve is apparently inadequate for the increased insulin requirements of pregnancy.
   (b) Careful screening for gestational diabetes and intensive treatment are essential because of an increased risk of neonatal morbidity.
   (c) The glucose tolerance of most patients returns to normal within a few weeks after delivery, although diabetes develops in many patients as long as 5–15 years later.

(3) **Previous abnormality of glucose tolerance.** This term refers to individuals with normal glucose levels who formerly were glucose intolerant or diabetic because of pregnancy, illness, obesity, or medications.

(4) **Potential abnormality of glucose tolerance.** This refers to individuals with an increased risk of future diabetes because of a history of having had large babies (>9 pounds), the presence of diabetes in an identical twin, or similar factors.

(5) Diabetes or impaired glucose tolerance **may occur secondary** to certain diseases that affect the production or action of insulin, such as **chronic pancreatitis, Cushing's syndrome, acromegaly, insulin receptor abnormalities,** and others.

(6) **The metabolic syndrome** (insulin resistance syndrome, syndrome X). Some metabolic and pathophysiologic abnormalities tend to cluster in certain patients. Insulin resistance may be a common abnormality, perhaps the primary one. Components of this syndrome include diabetes mellitus, obesity, hypertension, dyslipidemia, and atherosclerosis.

2. Etiology. The cause of diabetes mellitus is unknown. Many etiologic factors are suspected, with major differences between those factors that are etiologic for type 1 and type 2 diabetes.

a. Type 1 diabetes

(1) **Etiologic factors**

   (a) **Genetic factors**
      (i) Fifty percent of identical twins of patients with type 1 diabetes are diabetic.
      (ii) There is a strong association between type 1 diabetes and certain human leukocyte antigens (HLAs) [see Table 9–9].

   (b) **Autoimmune factors**
      (i) Antibodies to islet-cell antigens (insulin, glutamic acid decarboxylase, and insulin-associated protein 2) are commonly present in diabetic patients shortly after the disease is diagnosed, although they usually disappear within a few years.
      (ii) Antibodies against other tissues such as antithyroid antibodies also are increased.

   (c) **Environmental factors**
      (i) The concordance rate for diabetes in identical twins is 50% rather than 100%, which would be the rate predicted if the disease were totally genetic.
      (ii) Seasonal occurrence has been observed, with an increased diagnosis of new cases in the fall and winter.

(2) How these factors interact to cause diabetes is speculative. For example, a viral infection may trigger β-cell destruction in an individual with genetically determined susceptibility to such an infection and to autoimmune reactivity to islet-cell antigens.

b. Type 2 diabetes

(1) **Genetic factors** are even more important etiologically in type 2 than in type 1 diabetes. The concordance rate for diabetes in identical twins is 90%–100%.

(2) **Obesity** is a significant factor—80% of patients with type II diabetes are more than 15% above their ideal weight. Obesity is associated with resistance to the action of insulin both in diabetic and nondiabetic individuals; this resistance is caused mainly by abnormal insulin action beyond the receptor.

(3) Genetically susceptible individuals may be unable to sustain the increased insulin production needed to maintain carbohydrate homeostasis in the face of insulin resistance, with resulting diabetes.

3. **Pathophysiology**
   a. **Levels of insulin**
      (1) In **type 1 diabetes,** some insulin may be produced for a few years after the disease is diagnosed, but insulin production eventually ceases totally.
      (2) In **type 2 diabetes,** insulin levels vary and often are similar to the levels in nondiabetic individuals of similar weight. However, these insulin levels are low when considered in relation to the elevated blood glucose concentrations of diabetic patients, and these levels reflect a decrease in β-cell responsiveness to glucose.
   b. **Consequences of impaired insulin action.** Impaired insulin action may be caused by inadequate insulin secretion, by target-tissue resistance to the action of insulin, or both.
      (1) **Hyperglycemia.** Insulin increases the synthesis of glycogen in the liver and in muscle and increases the uptake of glucose in muscle and adipose tissue. In the absence of adequate insulin action, hepatic glucose production increases (with increased glycogenolysis and increased gluconeogenesis) and peripheral glucose use decreases. The result is hyperglycemia.
      (2) **"Glucose toxicity."** Hyperglycemia is thought to initiate a self-perpetuating cycle in which elevated glucose levels further impair both the ability of the β cells to produce insulin and the action of insulin on peripheral tissues, leading to a further rise in serum glucose levels.
      (3) **Other metabolic derangements**
         (a) Insulin normally acts as an anabolic, energy storage–promoting agent. In addition to the storage of glucose as glycogen, insulin stimulates the formation of fatty acids from glucose, the esterification of fatty acids to form triglycerides, and the storage of amino acids as protein.
         (b) Inadequate insulin action on target tissues causes inadequate disposal of ingested nutrients and excessive consumption of endogenous metabolic fuels. Blood fatty acids and lipids are increased because of decreased lipogenesis and increased lipolysis; blood amino acids are increased because of decreased protein synthesis and increased catabolism of muscle protein.
   c. **Levels of other hormones**
      (1) **Glucagon** levels are often elevated in diabetic patients. This may contribute to hyperglycemia through the action of glucagon in stimulating glycogenolysis.
      (2) **Epinephrine, cortisol, and GH** levels may be increased during periods of stress or poor diabetic control. This may contribute to hyperglycemia through the anti-insulin effect and diabetogenic action of these hormones.

4. **Clinical features**
   a. **Polyuria and polydipsia** usually occur. The most common symptom of hyperglycemia is increased urine volume, which is caused by glucose-induced osmotic diuresis. Increased fluid intake is a response to the resulting dehydration and thirst.
   b. **Weight loss** results from the loss of glucose in urine and the catabolic effects of the decrease in insulin action, despite increased food intake. Generalized weakness also reflects the metabolic derangements.
   c. **Infections of the skin, vulva,** and **urinary tract** are especially common in uncontrolled diabetes, because hyperglycemia decreases resistance to infection.
   d. **Blurring of vision** is caused by changes in the shape and refractive qualities of the optic lens that result from hyperglycemia-induced osmotic alterations.

5. **Diagnosis.** Diabetes mellitus is often suspected because of typical clinical manifestations such as polyuria and unexplained weight loss; however, a definitive diagnosis is based on **elevated glucose levels.**

a. **Glucose levels.** Diabetes mellitus is diagnosed if any one of the three abnormalities described in Table 9–10 is present. The diagnosis should be confirmed by obtaining the same results (or finding another abnormality) on a different day.

b. **Urine glucose levels.** Glucose appears in the urine only when the renal threshold of approximately 180 mg/dL is exceeded.

(1) This threshold varies widely and tends to increase with age. Therefore, urine glucose measurement is an insensitive and unreliable test for diabetes.

(2) However, urine glucose levels can be a rough guide to the presence or absence of marked hyperglycemia and occasionally may be of use in the day-to-day management of diabetes.

6. **Acute complications of diabetes.** Diabetic ketoacidosis, hyperosmolar nonketotic coma, and hypoglycemic coma are acute, life-threatening complications of diabetes mellitus; they cause rapid mental and physical deterioration and require prompt treatment. Because each of these complications may present with an alteration in mental status that often progresses to coma, and because each of these conditions requires different treatment, accurate diagnosis is essential.

a. **Diabetic ketoacidosis** occurs in patients with type 1 diabetes whose circulating insulin is insufficient to allow glucose use by peripheral tissue and to inhibit glucose production and tissue catabolism. Increased levels of glucagon and hormones that increase in response to stress (i.e., epinephrine, norepinephrine, cortisol, GH) contribute to the metabolic derangements.

(1) **Precipitating factors.** Ketoacidosis may occur after several days of worsening diabetic control or may appear suddenly within a few hours.

(a) Precipitating factors include any event that decreases insulin availability or causes stress that increases the need for insulin.

(b) Common factors are the omission of insulin doses, infections, injuries, emotional stress, excessive alcohol ingestion, and intercurrent illness.

(2) **Pathophysiology** (Figure 9–4)

(a) **Hyperglycemia.** Insufficient insulin reduces peripheral glucose utilization and, together with glucagon excess, increases hepatic production of glucose through the stimulation of gluconeogenesis and glycogenolysis and the inhibition of glycolysis. Protein breakdown in peripheral tissues provides a flow of amino acids to the liver as substrate for gluconeogenesis. Hyperglycemia is the result.

(b) **Osmotic diuresis.** This condition, which results from the elevated serum glucose (and ketone) levels, produces **hypovolemia, dehydration,** and **loss of sodium, potassium, phosphate, and other substances in the urine.** Volume depletion stimulates catecholamine release, which further opposes insulin action in the liver and contributes to lipolysis.

(c) **Ketogenesis.** The lipolysis that results from insulin lack and catecholamine excess mobilizes free fatty acids from their stores in adipose tissue. Instead of reesterifying

TABLE 9–10 Glucose Levels as Diagnostic Criteria for Diabetes Mellitus

Any one of the following three criteria must be met to make a diagnosis of diabetes mellitus. The diagnosis should be confirmed by obtaining the same results (or finding another abnormality) on a different day.

Fasting plasma glucose level ≥ 126 mg/dL (preferred test)*

Plasma glucose level ≥ 200 mg/dL 2 hours after a 75-g glucose load (oral glucose tolerance test)†

Casual plasma glucose level (i.e., without regard to food intake) 200 mg/dL or greater (valid only if symptoms such as polyuria, polydipsia, or weight loss are present)

*A fasting plasma glucose level > 110 mg/dL but <126 mg/dL indicates **impaired fasting glucose.**

†A plasma glucose level ≥ 140 mg/dL but < 200 mg/dL 2 hours after a 75-g glucose load indicates **impaired glucose tolerance.**

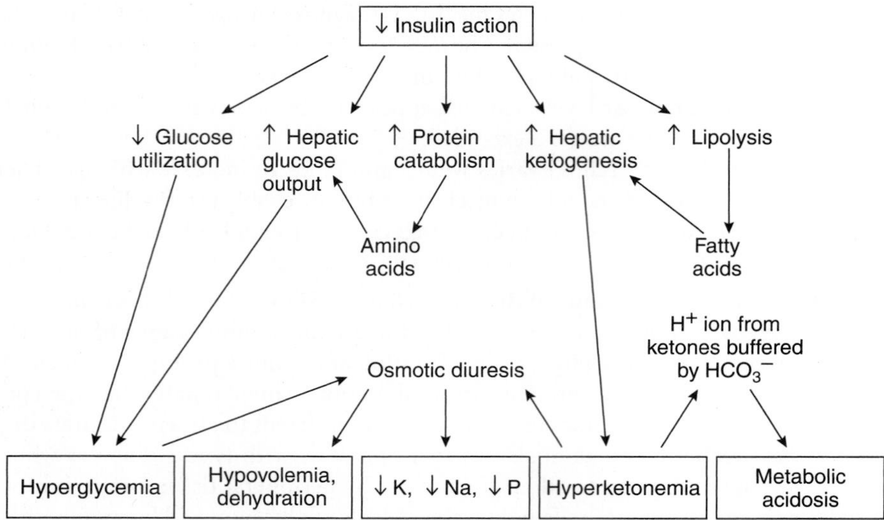

FIGURE 9–4 Pathogenesis of diabetic ketoacidosis. (From Adlin EV: *Endocrinology Science and Medicine.* Philadelphia, Lippincott Williams & Wilkins, 2001, p 80.)

the incoming fatty acids to form triglycerides, the liver shifts its metabolic pathways toward the production of ketone bodies.

- **(i)** Glucagon increases the hepatic level of carnitine, which enables fatty acids to enter the mitochondria, where they undergo β-oxidation to ketone bodies.
- **(ii)** Glucagon decreases the hepatic content of malonyl coenzyme A, an inhibitor of fatty acid oxidation.

(d) Acidosis. The increased hepatic production of ketone bodies (acetoacetate and β-hydroxybutyrate) exceeds the body's ability to metabolize or excrete them.

- **(i)** The hydrogen ions of the ketone bodies are buffered by bicarbonate, leading to a decrease in serum bicarbonate and pH.
- **(ii)** Arterial carbon dioxide tension ($Paco_2$) also decreases because of ventilatory compensation.
- **(iii)** The anion gap increases because of the elevated plasma levels of acetoacetate and β-hydroxybutyrate.
- **(iv)** The result is metabolic acidosis that is associated with an increased anion gap.

(3) Clinical features and diagnosis

(a) Physical findings

- **(i) Rapid, deep breathing (Kussmaul's respirations)** occurs as the body tries to compensate for metabolic acidosis by increasing carbon dioxide excretion.
- **(ii)** An **odor of acetone** is often detected on the breath.
- **(iii)** Marked dehydration is common, with **dry skin and mucous membranes** and **poor skin turgor. Orthostatic hypotension** may be present because of intravascular volume depletion.
- **(iv) Clouding of consciousness** is present in most cases, and approximately 10% of patients are **comatose.**

(b) Laboratory abnormalities

- **(i) Hyperglycemia.** Serum glucose levels in ketoacidosis may be only slightly increased, but more often they are markedly elevated, averaging approximately 500 mg/dL. Renal function affects the degree of hyperglycemia; glucose levels are greatly elevated only when urinary excretion of glucose is limited by volume depletion or renal abnormalities.

(ii) **Hyperketonemia.** Serum levels of acetoacetate, acetone, and β-hydroxybutyrate are greatly increased. The agent nitroprusside, in the form of tablets or reagent strips, is commonly used to measure serum and urine ketone bodies. It reacts only with acetoacetate. If the other ketone bodies are increased to a much greater or much lesser extent than acetoacetate, the results of the test may be misleading.

(iii) **Metabolic acidosis. The serum bicarbonate level is low** (usually <10 mEq/L). The **blood pH is low,** and the **anion gap is increased.**

(iv) **Glycosuria and ketonuria.** Urinary levels of glucose and ketone bodies are increased. The diagnosis of diabetic ketoacidosis can be made rapidly if marked glycosuria and ketonuria are present.

(v) **Other laboratory findings. Serum potassium concentration** may be increased initially in metabolic acidosis because of potassium ion movement from the intracellular to the extracellular space. Later, the serum potassium level is low because of both renal losses and the movement of potassium ions back into cells as the acidosis is corrected. **Serum sodium concentration** tends to be low, mainly because of dilution as the osmotic effect of the hyperglycemia increases extracellular water. **Serum osmolality** is high, usually greater than 300 mOsm/kg.

(4) **Therapy.** The treatment of diabetic ketoacidosis has four main components.

(a) **Insulin** is administered to increase glucose use in the tissues, to inhibit the flow of fatty acids and amino acids from the periphery, and to counter the effects of glucagon on the liver.

(i) **Route of administration.** If volume depletion and vascular collapse are present, poor tissue perfusion may impair the absorption of intramuscular or subcutaneous insulin, and insulin is usually administered intravenously.

(ii) **Dosage.** A priming dose of 0.1 U/kg regular insulin is given intravenously and is followed by the infusion of 0.1 U/kg/hr or approximately 5–10 U/hr. If the serum glucose level does not decrease (75–100 mg/dL/hr), the serum level of ketone bodies does not fall, and serum pH does not increase in a few hours, then larger doses of insulin must be given.

(iii) After the acidosis and hyperglycemia have resolved and the urine has become free of ketone bodies, treatment with intermediate-acting insulin is resumed.

(b) **Fluid replacement** corrects the dehydration caused by glucose-induced osmotic diuresis. The fluid deficit in patients with diabetic ketoacidosis averages 3–5 L, which must be promptly replaced.

(i) Approximately 1 L normal saline (0.9% NaCl) is given each hour for the first 2 hours, and then half-normal saline (0.45% NaCl) is given at a slower rate. When the serum glucose level falls to 200–300 mg/dL, 5% or 10% glucose is infused to prevent hypoglycemia.

(ii) Fluid replacement lowers serum glucose levels, even without insulin, by increasing urine flow (and hence, glycosuria) and by decreasing the levels of catecholamines and cortisol, which were increased by the stimulus of volume depletion.

(c) **Minerals and electrolytes must be replaced** because they are lost via osmotic diuresis.

(i) **Potassium** may be needed to replace low body stores. If initial serum potassium levels are elevated (due to severe acidosis), replacement is delayed; when the levels become normal or low, after therapy has been initiated, potassium chloride is infused at a rate of 20–40 mmol/hr. This can be given as potassium phosphate or potassium chloride, depending on the blood levels of calcium and phosphorus; too much phosphate replacement may cause hypocalcemia.

(ii) **Phosphate** must also be replaced. Approximately 10–20 mmol/hr may be given as potassium phosphate, for a total of 40–60 mmol.

(iii) **Bicarbonate** is given only when the arterial pH declines below 7.1 to maintain the pH above that level. Because diabetic ketoacidosis is corrected by fluids and insulin, excessive administration of bicarbonate may result in rebound alkalosis. Some physicians recommend bicarbonate administration only when the pH decreases below 6.9.

(d) **Treatment of precipitating factors and complications**

(i) Urinary tract infections as well as other infections must be investigated and treated.

(ii) Meningitis, stroke, and myocardial infarction should be considered, because they may escape detection in patients whose sensoriums are clouded by ketoacidosis.

(iii) If patients are unconscious and have been vomiting or have gastric dilatation, nasogastric aspiration should be performed.

(iv) If hypotension persists despite fluid replacement, blood or plasma expanders should be given.

b. Hyperosmolar nonketotic coma is less common than ketoacidosis but has a much higher mortality rate. It occurs primarily in elderly patients with type 2 diabetes, often in previously undiagnosed individuals.

(1) **Pathophysiology.** Often a precipitating factor (e.g., infection, increased glucose ingestion, omission of insulin, intercurrent illness) causes increasing hyperglycemia within a few days or weeks. Osmotic diuresis, without adequate fluid intake, causes dehydration and progressive decline in mental status. Ketoacidosis is mild or absent, presumably because sufficient insulin is present to inhibit hepatic ketogenesis.

(2) **Clinical features**

(a) The **hyperglycemia** tends to be more marked than it is in ketoacidosis, with average plasma glucose concentrations of approximately 1000 mg/dL.

(b) In the absence of ketoacidosis, the osmotic diuresis continues for a longer time before the diagnosis is made and therefore produces more severe **dehydration.**

(c) **Serum osmolality** is very high, averaging approximately 360 mOsm/kg. The dehydration and hyperosmolality may cause **mental obtundation, seizures,** and **focal neurologic signs.**

(d) Lactic acidosis may be present because of the hypovolemia and indicates a worse prognosis.

(3) **Therapy.** Treatment is similar to that for diabetic ketoacidosis. Fluid replacement and reversal of the hyperglycemia with insulin are the main goals.

(a) **Fluid replacement** in elderly patients with cardiovascular disease requires care to avoid volume expansion, which might precipitate heart failure.

(b) **Insulin** should not be started until fluid replacement is underway; a fall in plasma glucose levels may worsen the hypovolemia and precipitate shock due to the loss of the intravascular volume-expanding effect of the hyperglycemia.

c. Hypoglycemic coma must be rapidly differentiated from diabetic ketoacidosis and hyperosmolar nonketotic coma, because therapy is obviously quite different.

(1) **Etiology**

(a) Hypoglycemia in insulin-treated diabetic patients ("insulin shock") may be caused by **excessive insulin dosage, delay in the ingestion of a meal, and excessive physical activity.** Sulfonylureas may cause hypoglycemic reactions, but much less often than does insulin.

(b) Patients with type 1 diabetes may be susceptible to hypoglycemia because of **insufficient levels of the counterregulatory hormones** that normally limit the fall in serum glucose. The response of glucagon to hypoglycemia is frequently impaired in these patients, and epinephrine production may become impaired if autonomic neuropathy develops. (Epinephrine prevents severe hypoglycemia both by stimulating glucose production and by producing symptoms that alert the patient to hypoglycemia, prompting rapid glucose ingestion.)

(2) **Pathophysiology and clinical features.** Hypoglycemia produces symptoms through the following two mechanisms:

(a) A fall in the serum glucose concentration stimulates catecholamine production and sympathetic nervous system outflow. **Adrenergic stimulation** then causes sweating, tachycardia, palpitations, tremulousness, and muscular weakness.

(b) Prolonged hypoglycemia deprives the CNS of its main source of fuel, glucose. **CNS symptoms** of hypoglycemia usually occur later than the adrenergic symptoms, and they are potentially more serious. Mental changes may progress from **somnolence** and **confusion** to **coma.** Headache, slurred speech, focal neurologic signs, and seizures may occur.

(3) **Diagnosis.** The diagnosis of hypoglycemia is obvious if symptoms of sweating, palpitation, and tremulousness occur at the time of peak action of a recent insulin dose. Patients learn to recognize this reaction and treat it by drinking orange juice or eating candy. Less obvious is the cause of coma in diabetic patients who are brought to the emergency department. Clues that suggest hypoglycemia rather than ketoacidosis are the history of a missed meal or unusually vigorous exercise, the finding of profuse sweating rather than dehydration, and the absence of Kussmaul's respirations. A fingerstick blood glucose determination is useful for rapid confirmation of hypoglycemia.

(4) **Therapy**

(a) Patients who are unable to take glucose orally are given **50 mL 50% glucose intravenously** over 3–5 minutes, followed by a constant infusion of 5% or 10% glucose.

(i) Some patients regain consciousness immediately, others more slowly.

(ii) Glucose infusion may have to be maintained during the expected duration of action of the insulin or oral agent responsible for the hypoglycemia. If the hypoglycemia is caused by **chlorpropamide,** this may be several days.

(b) An intramuscular injection of 1 mg **glucagon** may increase the serum glucose level rapidly, allowing patients to regain consciousness and take oral glucose. Teaching patients' family members to inject glucagon may decrease the frequency of emergency department visits.

(c) After an episode of insulin-induced hypoglycemia, the insulin dosage, diet, or both should be readjusted to prevent subsequent attacks.

7. **Chronic complications of diabetes.** Patients with diabetes frequently develop microvascular disorders involving the small blood vessels of the eye, kidney, and muscle; macrovascular disease (i.e., atherosclerotic disease of the medium and large vessels), and diabetic neuropathy (i.e., abnormalities of the peripheral and autonomic nervous system).

a. **Pathogenesis**

(1) **Microvascular complications and neuropathy.** The Diabetes Control and Complications Trial, a 10-year randomized controlled trial involving 1441 patients with type 1 diabetes, has shown conclusively that better control of serum glucose levels reduces the incidence of retinopathy, nephropathy, and neuropathy. Several mechanisms have been proposed to explain how elevated glucose levels may cause these complications:

(a) Nonenzymatic glycosylation of proteins in capillary basement membranes and other tissues, similar to the process that produces glycosylated hemoglobin, may produce damage to these tissues that is related to the blood glucose levels.

(b) When glucose levels are elevated, the enzyme aldose reductase converts glucose to sorbitol, which may cause damage in nerve cells, the retina, and renal tissue.

(2) **Macrovascular complications.** Atherosclerosis, leading to coronary, cerebrovascular, or peripheral vascular disease, is associated with diabetes mellitus. Unlike the microvascular

complications, however, it is also associated with the lesser degree of glucose elevation known as impaired glucose tolerance.

b. Diabetic retinopathy. This condition is directly related to the duration and severity of diabetes. Prevalence increases from 3% at the time that diabetes is diagnosed to 20%–45% after 10 years. Of new cases of blindness in adults, 20% are caused by diabetes.

(1) Types

(a) Background (simple, nonproliferative) retinopathy makes up 90%–95% of all cases. Increased capillary permeability, vascular occlusion, and weakness of supporting structures lead to the findings on funduscopic examination of venous dilatation, exudates, hemorrhages, and microaneurysms.

(b) Proliferative retinopathy makes up 5%–10% of all cases. In response to vascular occlusion and ischemia, new vessels form on the surface of the retina (neovascularization) and may grow into the vitreous body of the eye.

(i) Preretinal or vitreous hemorrhage may lead to clot retraction and scar formation, with retinal detachment.

(ii) Vitreous hemorrhage may cause sudden blindness.

(2) Therapy

(a) Background retinopathy is less likely to progress if diabetic control is good. Annual screening for retinopathy is recommended, because blindness may be prevented by early treatment.

(b) Proliferative retinopathy may be treated with **laser-beam photocoagulation,** which is effective in obliterating new vessels. **Vitrectomy** is beneficial in selected cases.

c. Diabetic nephropathy. The renal lesion that is specific for diabetes is **intercapillary glomerulosclerosis (Kimmelstiel-Wilson disease).** Other renal diseases associated with diabetes are papillary necrosis, chronic interstitial nephritis, and arteriosclerotic disease.

(1) Incidence. Significant renal disease develops in approximately 40% of patients with type 1 diabetes and 20% of patients with type 2 diabetes. Nearly all patients with severe glomerulosclerosis also have retinopathy. Almost 33% of new cases of end-stage renal disease are caused by diabetes.

(2) Pathogenesis. Hyperglycemia may cause increased intraglomerular pressure, leading to damage to the basement membrane, deposition of protein in the mesangium, glomerulosclerosis, and renal failure. **Pathologic features** of diabetic glomerulosclerosis include an increase in the mesangial matrix and increased width of the glomerular basement membrane, hyaline arteriosclerosis of the afferent and efferent arterioles, and IgG and albumin deposits lining the tubular and glomerular basement membranes. Diabetic kidneys tend to be large, even when end-stage renal disease is present.

(3) Clinical features

(a) The first manifestation is usually **proteinuria,** which often progresses to the **nephrotic syndrome.**

(i) Microalbuminuria, which can be detected by special tests, predicts the later occurrence of renal failure.

(ii) The presence of **hypertension** is also associated with an increased risk of renal failure in diabetic patients.

(b) When renal failure occurs, the progression to **end-stage renal disease** is rapid; transplantation or dialysis usually becomes necessary within 3 years.

(4) Prevention. Progression of diabetic nephropathy can be prevented or delayed by intensive glycemic control and by control of coexisting hypertension. Angiotensin-converting enzyme (ACE) inhibitors slow the progression of renal disease by their antihypertensive effect and probably by an action independent of blood pressure control. A low-protein diet (0.6–0.89 g protein/kg body weight) may also slow the progression of renal disease.

d. Diabetic neuropathy. Older patients with a relatively long history of diabetes and severe hyperglycemia have an increased incidence of this common complication. Accumulation of sorbitol in Schwann cells, with subsequent cell damage, may play a causative role. Slowing of nerve conduction velocity occurs, with changes in Schwann cell function and eventual segmental demyelination and axonal degeneration.

(1) **Types**

(a) **Peripheral polyneuropathy** is the most common syndrome.

(i) Distal, bilateral sensory changes in the lower extremities predominate. Weakness and upper extremity involvement are less frequent. Neuropathic ulcers of the feet are a common manifestation of diabetic neuropathy and are more common than ischemic ulcers.

(ii) **Symptoms** include paresthesias and pain of the feet. Examination may show decreased reflexes, loss of vibratory sense, and loss of pain sensation.

(b) **Autonomic neuropathy** is less common than peripheral polyneuropathy, but usually it is seen in patients who have peripheral polyneuropathy. **Postural hypotension** is a major manifestation. Other clinically important problems are sexual impotence in diabetic men and urinary retention with abnormal bladder function. Abnormal gastrointestinal motility may result in delayed gastric emptying (diabetic gastroparesis), constipation, and diarrhea. The adrenergic symptoms of hypoglycemia may be decreased or absent, leading to delayed recognition and treatment of insulin reactions.

(c) Less common forms of diabetic neuropathy are **radiculopathy,** causing lancinating pain in a single dermatome, and **mononeuropathy,** involving cranial nerves or proximal motor nerves.

(2) **Therapy**

(a) Improved diabetic control may lessen the symptoms of peripheral polyneuropathy.

(b) Symptomatic treatment of painful neuropathy may be attempted with amitriptyline, phenytoin, carbamazepine, topical capsaicin, or gabapentin.

e. Atherosclerosis. The incidence of atherosclerosis is considerably increased in diabetic patients; that is, diabetes, like hypertension, smoking, hyperlipidemia, obesity, and a positive family history, is a major risk factor for the development of atherosclerosis.

(1) **Coronary artery disease** is twice as common in diabetic patients compared with non-diabetic patients. Small-vessel disease may contribute to myocardial ischemia.

(2) **Peripheral vascular disease,** which is common in diabetic patients, is most likely to affect the legs and feet. Small-vessel disease may play a major role—ischemic changes in a foot with a normal pedal pulse on examination is typical of diabetes. Foot infections, poorly healing ulcers, and eventual gangrene, resulting in amputation, are frequent complications.

8. Treatment of diabetes

a. Goals of treatment

(1) **Control of symptoms.** The polyuria, weight loss, increased incidence of infections, blurring of vision, and other symptoms of diabetes are related to the hyperglycemia. Return of serum glucose levels to normal brings relief of these symptoms.

(2) **Prevention of acute complications.** Diabetic ketoacidosis and nonketotic hyperglycemic coma are prevented by careful management of diabetes.

(3) **Prevention of long-term complications.** The Diabetes Control and Complications Trial and the United Kingdom Prospective Diabetes Study clearly showed that intensive therapy, with lowering of blood glucose below the levels needed to control symptoms and prevent ketoacidosis, delays or prevents the onset of retinopathy, nephropathy, neuropathy, and macrovascular complications.

b. Diet. Before insulin was available, severe restriction of carbohydrate intake was necessary to prolong life in patients with type 1 diabetes. In patients receiving insulin, the **regularity and**

timing of carbohydrate intake may be more important than the quantity. It is equally important to **avoid excessive fat intake,** which increases the risk of atherosclerosis. In seeking to balance these considerations, physicians recommend that caloric intake comprise 12%–20% protein, 50%–60% carbohydrate, and 20%–30% fat.

(1) **Specific objectives**

(a) **Type 1 diabetes.** The chief goals of dietary treatment are to provide adequate calories for growth and activity and to ensure day-to-day regularity of food intake so that the availability of insulin is coordinated with carbohydrate intake.

(b) **Type 2 diabetes.** The chief goal in most cases is to attain the patient's ideal weight by means of caloric restriction and regular exercise. Because many patients become normoglycemic with diet alone if significant weight loss is achieved, initial treatment should emphasize the importance of diet. However, most patients are not able to lose enough weight to control glucose levels through diet alone.

(2) **Diet calculation**

(a) **The ideal body weight should be estimated.**

(i) For men, the estimate is 106 pounds for the first 5 feet in height, and 6 pounds for each additional inch.

(ii) For women, the estimate is 100 pounds for the first 5 feet in height, and 5 pounds for each additional inch.

(iii) For heavy-framed individuals, 5–15 pounds may be added.

(b) The data in Table 9–11 can be used to determine the **daily caloric need,** which varies with the patient's activity level and need to gain or lose weight.

(c) **The protein, carbohydrate, and fat intake should be determined** by calculating 20% of the total calories as protein (4 kcal/g), 50% as carbohydrate (4 kcal/g), and the remaining 30% as fat (9 kcal/g).

(3) **Additional suggestions**

(a) Increased intake of monounsaturated and polyunsaturated fats and reduced intake of saturated fats and trans-fats are desirable. Cholesterol intake should not exceed 300–500 mg/day.

(b) For a balanced amino acid content, 50% of protein should be derived from the meat exchange list.

(c) Increased fiber intake, in the form of unprocessed bran, cereals, fruits, and vegetables, may lower blood glucose levels and decrease the need for insulin.

c. **Oral antihyperglycemic agents** (Table 9–12)

(1) **Sulfonylurea derivatives and meglitinides**

(a) **Mode of action.** These agents, which bind to receptors on the β-cell plasma membrane, result in closure of potassium channels, opening of calcium channels, and influx of calcium into the cell. The end result is an increase in insulin secretion by β cells.

TABLE 9–11 Daily Caloric Requirement*

	Activity Level		
Body Build	SEDENTARY	MODERATELY ACTIVE	VERY ACTIVE
Obese	20–25	30	35
Normal	30	35	40
Underweight	35	40	45–50

*Calories (kcal) required per kilogram of ideal body weight per day. These estimates are intended to produce weight loss in obese individuals, weight gain in underweight individuals, and maintenance of weight in normal individuals.

TABLE 9–12 Oral Antihyperglycemic Agents

Drug	Usual Starting Dose (mg/day)	Maximal Daily Dose (mg)	Timing of Dose
Sulfonylureas (second generation)			
Glimepiride	1	8	Once or twice daily
Glipizide	5	20	Once or twice daily
Glyburide	2.5	20	Once or twice daily
Meglitinides			
Repaglinide	1.5	16	15 minutes before each meal
Nateglinide	180	360	15 minutes before each meal
Biguanides			
Metformin	500	2500	Divided doses, with meals
Thiazolidinediones			
Rosiglitazone	4	8	Once or twice daily
Pioglitazone	15	45	Once daily
Alpha-glucosidase inhibitors			
Acarbose	25	300	Divided doses at the start of meals
Miglitol	25	300	Divided doses at the start of meals

(b) Use. The second-generation sulfonylureas listed in Table 9–12 have largely replaced the first-generation agents (tolbutamide, tolazamide, acetohexamide, chlorpropamide). Repaglinide and nateglinide have a mode of action like that of the sulfonylureas but differ in having a faster onset and shorter duration of action. They must be taken before each meal.

(c) Side effects. The primary side effect of sulfonylureas is hypoglycemia, which may result from excessive dosing, drug interactions, renal or hepatic disease, or inadequate food intake. With repaglinide and neteglinide, hypoglycemia may be less likely because of the close correspondence between the peak drug effect and peak glucose absorption after meals.

(2) Metformin

(a) Mode of action. The mechanism of action of this biguanide is not well understood, but metformin appears to decrease hepatic glucose output and increase peripheral glucose utilization. The drug does not affect β-cell function directly.

(b) Use. The starting dose is 500 mg once daily with breakfast or supper; this can be raised gradually to a maximum of 2500 mg daily in divided doses, with meals.

(c) Side effects. When metformin is used alone, hypoglycemia does not occur, because the drug does not stimulate insulin secretion.

(i) Gastrointestinal symptoms of anorexia, nausea, abdominal discomfort, and diarrhea are common, but they usually disappear or can be tolerated if the initial dose is low and increased slowly.

(ii) Lactic acidosis is a serious potential complication, but it is rare unless patients have a predisposing condition such as renal failure, liver disease, alcoholism, or any condition that may cause tissue hypoxia (e.g., heart failure or pulmonary disease). These conditions are strong contraindications to the use of metformin. Lactic acidosis has occurred when patients taking metformin have developed renal failure after the injection of radiocontrast dyes. Therefore, metformin should be stopped when such a procedure is performed and not resumed until normal renal function is documented—24–48 hours later.

(3) **Thiazolidinediones**

(a) **Therapeutic effect.** Rosiglitazone and pioglitazone increase the sensitivity to insulin in muscle and fat, and to a lesser extent, in the liver. They act by stimulating the peroxisome proliferator-activated receptor γ, a nuclear receptor that affects insulin-responsive genes.

(b) **Side effects**

(i) Hypoglycemia may occur, especially if thiazolidinediones are used with insulin or sulfonylureas.

(ii) Liver toxicity, which is sometimes fatal, has occurred in a small number of patients treated with these agents. Liver function tests should be performed every 2 months for the first year of treatment, and less often after that.

(iii) Other side effects associated with thiazolidinediones include weight gain that is partly attributable to fluid retention, increased plasma volume, edema, and possible exacerbation of congestive heart failure.

(4) **α-Glucosidase inhibitors**

(a) **Mode of action.** These drugs inhibit the action of enzymes in the brush border of the small intestine, decreasing the conversion of disaccharides and oligosaccharides to monosaccharides. This delays the absorption of carbohydrates, allowing more time for insulin to act and blunting the postprandial rise in plasma glucose.

(b) **Side effects.** The shifting of carbohydrate digestion to the distal small bowel and colon tends to cause symptoms of flatulence, abdominal discomfort, and diarrhea. To minimize these symptoms, these drugs are started at very low doses and increased very gradually.

d. Insulin

(1) **Preparations.**

(a) Insulin preparations are available with **short** (regular insulin, rapid-acting insulin analogs), **intermediate,** and **long durations of action** (Table 9–13).

(b) **Insulin lispro and insulin aspart** have earlier onset of action and shorter duration of action than regular insulin. They therefore can be injected immediately before meals rather than 15–30 minutes before meals and are less likely to have prolonged action that could cause hypoglycemia before the next meal.

(c) **Insulin glargine** is considered a "peakless" insulin because there is little variability in insulin blood levels over 24 hours if the insulin is injected once daily. This makes it an excellent agent to provide basal insulin levels during an entire 24-hour period.

TABLE 9–13 Insulin Preparations and Their Onset, Peak, and Approximate Duration of Action

Types	Onset of Action (hr)	Peak Effect (hr)	Duration of Action (hr)
Fast-acting			
Regular human insulin	½–1	2–4	5–8
Insulin lispro, insulin aspart	¼	½–1½	3–5
Intermediate-acting			
NPH human insulin	1–3	4–12	12–16
Lente insulin	1–4	8–12	14–18
70% NPH human, 30% regular human insulin	½–1	8	12–16
Long-acting			
Insulin glargine	–	Flat	24

NPH = isophane insulin suspension.

(d) NPH and similar intermediate-acting insulins are available in **premixed combinations** with regular insulin and insulins lispro and aspart. These combinations are 70% or 75% intermediate insulin and 30% or 25% short-acting insulin.

(2) **Insulin regimens**

(a) **Physiologic insulin secretion** consists of a relatively constant, low rate of production at night and between meals, with short bursts of glucose-stimulated insulin secretion at mealtime.

(b) This pattern of secretion can be mimicked by the use of long-acting insulin to provide **basal levels** (e.g., insulin glargine once daily or NPH insulin twice daily), and short-acting insulin before each meal to provide **prandial insulin coverage.** These regimens enable insulin coverage to be matched to individual patterns of diet and activity, but they require 4 or more daily injections.

(c) **Premixed combinations** of intermediate- and short-acting insulin, e.g., insulin 70/30, may be given before breakfast and before supper. This regimen provides basal and prandial coverage with only two daily injections, but there is less uniformity in coverage and less flexibility in dosage adjustment.

(d) If insulin 70/30 or insulin 75/25 is given before breakfast and before supper, the evening dose of NPH may have its peak effect during the night, causing nocturnal hypoglycemia. If the evening dose is split, giving the short-acting insulin before supper and the NPH at bedtime, the peak NPH effect may be more likely to occur during an early morning rise in glucose levels, with better glucose control (but a need for 3 instead of 2 daily injections).

(e) **Portable infusion pump.** The closest control of serum glucose levels is achieved by the constant infusion of regular insulin through a needle placed subcutaneously in the abdominal wall or thigh. A basal rate of approximately 12.5–15 mU/kg/hr is supplemented with pulse doses 15–30 minutes before each meal. The benefit of tighter glucose control with intensive therapy must be balanced against the increased risk of hypoglycemia and the inconvenience of the portable pump.

(3) **Factors affecting insulin requirements**

(a) **Intercurrent illness or other stress.** Insulin needs may increase as a result, perhaps because of increased levels of catecholamines. A temporary increase in the dose of insulin may be needed.

(b) **Exercise.** The increased glucose utilization may cause hypoglycemia unless the insulin dose is reduced or extra carbohydrate is ingested.

(c) **Somogyi effect.** Insulin-induced hypoglycemia causes release of counterregulatory hormones such as epinephrine and glucagon; this may then cause rebound hyperglycemia. If the cause of this hyperglycemia is not recognized, the insulin dose may be increased, leading to even more severe hypoglycemia. Hypoglycemia during the hours of sleep may be an unrecognized cause of increased morning fasting glucose levels; if this is the case, a decrease in the insulin dose may correct the morning hyperglycemia.

(4) **Complications of insulin therapy**

(a) **Local allergy.** Red, itchy lumps may form at the injection site minutes or hours after an insulin dose. This reaction tends to occur within a few weeks of initial insulin treatment and usually resolves in a few weeks or months.

(b) **Systemic allergy.** Generalized urticaria, angioedema, and anaphylaxis are rare but life-threatening reactions to insulin. Because a ketosis-prone patient cannot survive without insulin, that patient must be hospitalized and insulin desensitization must be performed. An initial intradermal dose of 1/10,000 U insulin is given and is increased every 30 minutes.

(c) **Antibody-mediated insulin resistance.** Insulin resistance is often defined as a need for more than 200 U daily, and it is more common in patients who have been exposed to insulin intermittently. IgG insulin-binding antibodies in the serum may cause the condition.

(i) Antibody-mediated resistance is often self-limited, resolving within 6 months.

(ii) Treatment consists of switching to human insulin (if not already in use) and cautious use of glucocorticoids if necessary (the sudden release of antibody-bound insulin in response to steroid therapy may cause hypoglycemia).

(d) Lipodystrophy

(i) **Lipohypertrophy.** Local swellings, composed of fibrous and fatty tissue, may occur at insulin injection sites, perhaps because of a local lipogenic effect of insulin on the fat cells. The swellings may regress if human insulin is used and the site of lipohypertrophy is avoided.

(ii) **Lipoatrophy.** Pits may form at injection sites because of the disappearance of subcutaneous fat. These may slowly disappear if human insulin is injected into the perimeter of the atrophic area.

e. Evaluation of glucose control

(1) **Home monitoring of capillary glucose levels,** using a glucose meter and test strips, is performed as often as necessary to evaluate glucose control. If satisfactory preprandial glucose levels are attained, the 2-hour postprandial glucose levels should be measured.

(2) **Goals of treatment** should be to achieve a fasting plasma glucose level below 120 mg/dL, a postprandial glucose level below 140–180 mg/dL, and an Hb_{A1C} level below 6%–7%.

(3) **Glycosylated hemoglobin measurements**

(a) The free amino acid groups of hemoglobin and other body proteins combine with glucose to form a reversible compound (Schiff base), which can then become a stable glycosylated protein (Amadori rearrangement). The extent of this nonenzymatic glycosylation is dependent on the concentration of glucose in blood; that is, the percentage of hemoglobin that is glycosylated depends on the blood glucose levels that were present during the life span of the currently circulating red blood cells (RBCs).

(b) The glycosylated hemoglobin level, therefore, reflects the degree of hyperglycemia during the preceding 6–12 weeks, and it may be useful in estimating the average control of serum glucose levels during this time.

f. Pharmacologic therapy of diabetes

(1) **Type 1 diabetes.** Patients with type 1 diabetes are dependent on insulin treatment. Oral antihyperglycemic agents are not indicated. Intensive insulin therapy, with multiple daily injections or the portable infusion pump, is increasingly being used.

(2) **Gestational diabetes.** If this condition cannot be controlled by diet, insulin must be used.

(3) **Type 2 diabetes**

(a) Oral antihyperglycemic agents should be tried first, although patients who present with severe hyperglycemia may require an initial period of insulin treatment to achieve prompt glycemic control. If control cannot be obtained with oral agents, insulin must be added.

(b) A scheme for the selection of oral agents and insulin in the treatment of type 2 diabetes is shown in Figure 9–5.

(i) Sulfonylureas (or meglitinides) or metformin are most commonly chosen as initial therapy. Metformin may be especially useful in obese patients because it does not cause further weight gain.

(ii) If two oral agents are used, it is reasonable that one is a promoter of insulin secretion (sulfonylurea or a meglitinide) and the other a promoter of sensitivity to insulin (metformin or a thiazolidinedione).

(iii) Sulfonylureas (or meglitinides) and metformin are usually recommended for initial treatment because they tend to have greater hypoglycemic efficacy as single drugs than the thiazolidinediones. The alpha-glucosidase inhibitors are

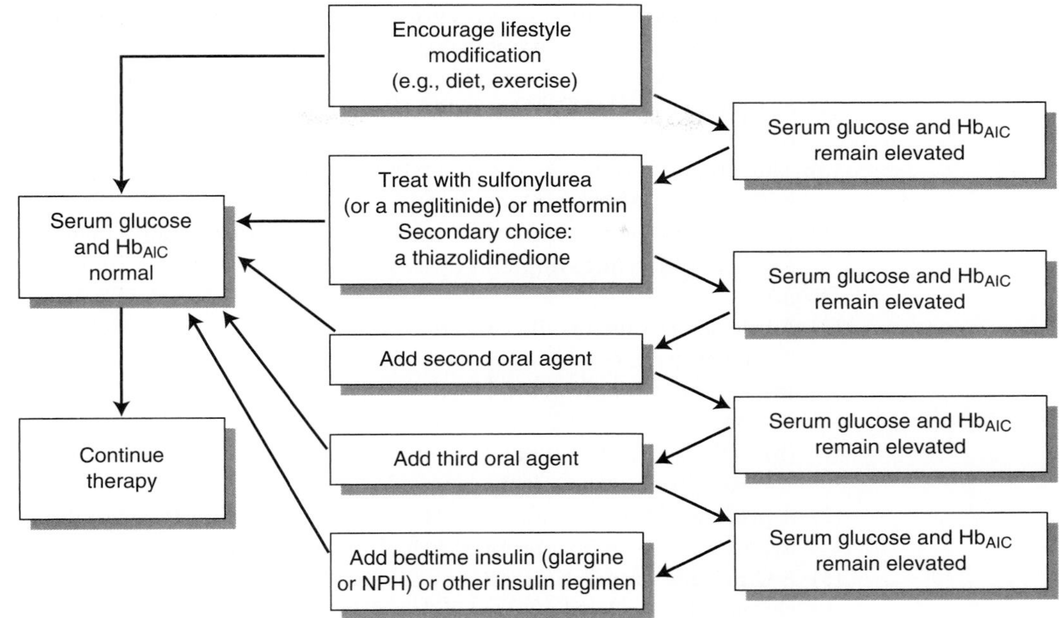

FIGURE 9–5 Treatment of type 2 diabetes mellitus. Factors that influence the selection of specific agents are described in the text (see IV A 8).

the least potent of these oral antihyperglycemic agents and have a secondary role in treatment.

(c) If insulin must be added because of failure to achieve adequate glucose levels, it is common practice to continue the oral agents.

(i) Sulfonylureas or meglitinides, because they stimulate glucose-dependent insulin secretion, may help provide the prandial insulin needs. (If a short-acting insulin is given before meals, sulfonylureas or meglitinides should be discontinued).

(ii) Metformin and thiazolidinediones, because they increase insulin sensitivity, may increase the effectiveness of exogenous insulin.

(d) When it becomes necessary to add insulin therapy, NPH insulin or insulin glargine may be added at bedtime to the oral agents. A starting dose of 10 units may be increased by 2 to 6 units every few days until fasting glucose levels fall below 120 mg/dL (or until nocturnal or daytime hypoglycemia occurs).

(e) If postprandial glucose levels cannot be controlled, a short-acting insulin may need to be added before one or more meals.

B Hypoglycemia There is no simple definition of hypoglycemia. Glucose levels less than 45 or 55 mg/dL may be associated with hypoglycemic symptoms, but some normal individuals have glucose levels lower than this without symptoms after several days of fasting or several hours after a glucose load, with resultant stimulation of insulin secretion. If the diagnosis is in doubt, **Whipple's triad** (i.e., symptoms of hypoglycemia, low serum glucose levels, and relief of the symptoms when normoglycemia is restored) may be used as a criterion.

1. **Insulinomas** are rare tumors that arise from the β cells of the islets of Langerhans. Most are single, benign adenomas, but approximately 10% of these tumors are multiple, and 10% are malignant. They occur with equal frequency in the head, the body, and the tail of the pancreas. β-cell hyperplasia occasionally may produce a similar syndrome.

a. **Clinical features.** Insulinomas produce excessive quantities of insulin, leading to **fasting hypoglycemia** (i.e., a category of hypoglycemia in which the lowest levels of serum glucose and the severest symptoms occur after prolonged periods without food intake).
   (1) Symptoms are most likely to occur in the early morning or late afternoon or after fasting or exercise.
   (2) The symptoms of hypoglycemia are the same as those that result from insulin overdose in diabetic patients [see IV A 6 c (2)].
   (3) Patients may gain weight before the diagnosis is made because they learn to relieve or avoid hypoglycemic symptoms by frequent snacking on carbohydrates.

b. **Diagnosis**
   (1) An **elevated serum insulin concentration** when the glucose level is low is strong evidence for the presence of an insulinoma, if an exogenous insulin source is excluded.
      (a) In normal individuals, insulin levels fall as glucose levels fall, and insulin levels become undetectable at glucose levels less than 30 mg/dL.
      (b) If the serum glucose concentration is less than 45 mg/dL, an insulin level higher than 10 mU/mL is abnormal.
   (2) A **prolonged fast,** extending for 24–72 hours, may be necessary to demonstrate fasting hypoglycemia with inappropriately high insulin levels.
   (3) A **C-peptide suppression test** may be used if prolonged fasting does not produce hypoglycemia but an insulinoma is still suspected. Hypoglycemia can be induced with the administration of exogenous regular insulin (0.1 U/kg intravenously over 1 hour).
      (a) The induced hypoglycemia suppresses endogenous insulin production in a normal individual but fails to suppress the autonomous insulin production by an insulinoma.
      (b) Serum insulin measurement cannot be used to evaluate endogenous insulin production because the injected insulin would be measured as well. However, C peptide, which is separated from the proinsulin molecule when the latter is cleaved to form insulin, can be measured. Because C peptide is not present in injected insulin, its concentration in serum reflects endogenous insulin production. A level of C peptide that is greater than 1.2 mg/mL after an insulin infusion suggests the autonomous insulin production of an insulinoma.
   (4) **Proinsulin,** the large precursor molecule of insulin, is produced in increased amounts by insulinomas. Proinsulin normally makes up 5%–20% of the total insulin in blood that is measured by radioimmunoassay; in patients with an insulinoma, proinsulin usually exceeds 25%.
   (5) **Diagnostic imaging** with MRI, CT, ultrasonography (including intraoperative ultrasound), and selective arteriography may be used to identify and localize an insulinoma. These tumors may be small, however, averaging 1–2 cm, and they often cannot be visualized.

c. **Therapy**
   (1) **Surgical removal** of an adenoma or partial pancreatectomy for multiple adenomas or β-cell hyperplasia is the treatment of choice.
   (2) **Medical therapy** is reserved for patients whose tumors cannot be completely removed because metastatic disease exists, previous surgical attempts have failed, or illness or patient refusal makes surgery infeasible.
      (a) **Diazoxide** inhibits the release of insulin from β cells. A dose of 200 mg daily, which can be raised as high as 800 mg if necessary, can prevent hypoglycemia in patients with an inoperable insulinoma.
      (b) **Streptozocin** is an antibiotic that specifically destroys β cells. It is used to treat malignant β-cell tumors.

2. **Factitious hypoglycemia** is caused by the surreptitious self-administration of insulin or an oral hypoglycemic drug, most often by an individual who is familiar with health care, such as a nurse

or medical technologist, or by a diabetic or relative of a diabetic. Differentiation from hypoglycemia caused by an insulinoma may depend on special studies.

a. **Serum C-peptide measurement** indicates the source of insulin secretion [see IV B 1 b (3)]. The low glucose and high insulin levels that are pathognomonic of an insulinoma should be accompanied by increased C-peptide levels; if the latter are low, indicating an exogenous source of the high insulin concentration, the disease is factitious.

b. Ingestion of a sulfonylurea, however, stimulates endogenous insulin production and the C-peptide level is high; therefore, **screening of blood or urine for sulfonylureas** is also necessary to rule out factitious disease.

3. **Extrapancreatic tumors** may cause hypoglycemia. These usually are large, intra-abdominal tumors, most often of mesenchymal origin (e.g., fibrosarcoma), although they may be hepatic carcinomas or other tumors. The mechanism of hypoglycemia is poorly understood; increased use of glucose by some tumors and production by others of an insulin-like substance have been observed.

4. **Ethanol-induced hypoglycemia** occurs in patients whose glycogen stores are depleted because of inadequate recent food intake, usually 12–24 hours after a bout of heavy drinking.

a. The oxidation of ethanol to acetaldehyde and acetate generates reduced nicotinamide-adenine dinucleotide (NADH) and decreases the availability of nicotinamide-adenine dinucleotide (NAD), which is needed for gluconeogenesis. When neither glycogenolysis nor gluconeogenesis is available to maintain hepatic glucose production in the fasting state, hypoglycemia results.

b. Prompt recognition and glucose administration are essential because the mortality rate is higher than 10%.

5. **Liver disease** may result in impairment of glycogenolysis and gluconeogenesis sufficient to cause fasting hypoglycemia. This is seen in fulminant viral hepatitis or acute toxic liver disease but not in the usual, less severe cases of cirrhosis or hepatitis.

6. **Other causes of fasting hypoglycemia** include cortisol deficiency, GH deficiency, or both, which may occur in **adrenal insufficiency** or **hypopituitarism.** Hypoglycemia may occur in patients with **renal failure** and **heart failure;** however, the causes are poorly understood.

7. **"Reactive hypoglycemia"** may occur as a result of another, smaller group of disorders, which cause hypoglycemia a few hours after the ingestion of carbohydrates. Insulinoma and the other conditions discussed previously most commonly produce hypoglycemia in the fasting state.

a. **Alimentary hypoglycemia** occurs in patients who have had a gastrectomy or other surgical procedure that leads to abnormally rapid movement of food into the small bowel. Rapid absorption of carbohydrate stimulates excessive insulin secretion, causing hypoglycemia several hours after a meal.

b. **Reactive hypoglycemia of diabetes** occurs in an occasional patient with early diabetes who may have a late but excessive release of insulin after a carbohydrate-containing meal. The glucose level is elevated after 2 hours but then decreases to hypoglycemic levels 3–5 hours after the meal.

c. **"Functional" hypoglycemia,** although commonly diagnosed in patients with chronic fatigue and anxiety, is probably a rare condition. Hypoglycemia is not a cause of chronic fatigue, depression, and lack of energy.

(1) **Clinical features.** Hypoglycemia, with adrenergic symptoms such as sweating and palpitations, occurs 2–5 hours after a carbohydrate-rich meal, presumably because of increased insulin production or insulin sensitivity.

(2) **Diagnosis**

(a) The overdiagnosis of functional hypoglycemia stems in part from misinterpretation of the 5-hour glucose tolerance test. One in four normal individuals has a serum glucose level less than 50 mg/dL 3–5 hours after the nonphysiologic stimulus of 75–100 g glucose, and some normal individuals have levels less than 35 mg/dL, without symptoms. These responses do not prove functional hypoglycemia.

(b) The diagnosis depends on finding hypoglycemia that coincides with the patient's typical symptoms and on finding relief of symptoms by carbohydrate ingestion.

(3) **Therapy** consists of eating four to six small meals daily that are low in carbohydrate and high in protein.

V DISORDERS OF THE ADRENAL GLAND

A General considerations

1. Diseases of the **adrenal cortex** are caused by the excessive production of cortisol (**Cushing's syndrome**), aldosterone (**primary aldosteronism**), and adrenal androgens (**congenital adrenal hyperplasia**), as well as by inadequate production of cortisol and aldosterone (**Addison's disease**).
2. Loss of the **adrenal medulla** does not cause illness, but **catecholamine overproduction by a pheochromocytoma** (a tumor of the adrenal medulla) causes a characteristic hypertensive syndrome.

B Cushing's syndrome is caused by excessive concentrations of cortisol or other glucocorticoid hormones in the circulation.

1. **Etiology**
   a. The most common cause of spontaneous Cushing's syndrome is **bilateral adrenal hyperplasia** (also known as **Cushing's disease**).* Bilateral adrenal hyperplasia is caused by increased secretion of ACTH by a corticotroph adenoma of the pituitary gland.
   b. **Adrenal adenomas and adrenal carcinomas** may cause Cushing's syndrome.
   c. **Ectopic ACTH** production by tumors such as oat cell carcinoma of the lung, carcinoma of the pancreas, bronchial carcinoid tumors, and others causes adrenal hyperplasia and Cushing's syndrome.
   d. **Iatrogenic Cushing's syndrome** is seen more often than the spontaneously occurring syndrome. It is an expected complication in patients receiving long-term glucocorticoid treatment for asthma, arthritis, and other conditions.
2. **Clinical features**
   a. **Central obesity** is caused by the effect of excess glucocorticoid levels on fat distribution. Fat accumulates in the face, neck, and trunk, while the limbs remain thin. The **"moon face," "buffalo hump"** (cervical fat pad), and **supraclavicular fat pads** contribute to the "cushingoid" appearance of affected individuals.
   b. **Hypertension** results from the vascular effects of cortisol as well as other actions of the hormone, including sodium retention.
   c. **Decreased glucose tolerance** is common; 20% of patients have overt diabetes. This is a result of the increased hepatic gluconeogenesis and decreased peripheral glucose utilization caused by elevated levels of glucocorticoid.
   d. **Symptoms of androgen excess** (e.g., oligomenorrhea, hirsutism, and acne) may occur in women with Cushing's disease because of stimulation by ACTH of adrenal androgen production.
   e. **Purple striae** are linear marks on the abdomen, where the thin, wasted skin is stretched by underlying fat.
   f. **Muscle wasting and weakness** reflect the catabolic effects of cortisol on muscle protein.
   g. **Osteoporosis** is a frequent result of cortisol excess. It is caused by increased bone catabolism and perhaps by the inhibitory effects of cortisol on collagen synthesis and calcium absorption.
   h. **Susceptibility to bruising** is probably caused by enhanced capillary fragility.
   i. **Psychiatric disturbances,** especially depression, are frequent results of cortisol excess.
   j. **Growth retardation** in children may be severe.

*Excess production of ACTH by the pituitary gland is Cushing's disease. Cushing's syndrome is a nonspecific designation that refers to increased glucocorticoid levels from any origin.

3. **Diagnosis.** Serum and urine cortisol levels are elevated in Cushing's disease and Cushing's syndrome, but overlap with normal values is common, and elevated levels are seen in normal persons at times of stress. Therefore, tests of the suppressibility of cortisol and other special tests are necessary. Figure 9–6 shows a scheme for the diagnosis of Cushing's syndrome that poses two questions. Is Cushing's syndrome present (Figure 9–6A)? If it is present, what causes its occurrence (Figure 9–6B)?
   a. **Nonspecific laboratory abnormalities** include leukocytosis, with a relatively low percentage of lymphocytes and eosinophils, and an elevation in the serum glucose level.
   b. The **serum cortisol** level in normal individuals is highest in early morning and decreases throughout the day, reaching a low point at about midnight. Although the morning level may be increased in patients with Cushing's syndrome, a loss of the normal diurnal variation and an increase in the evening level are more consistent findings.
   c. The **24-hour urinary free cortisol excretion rate** is increased in most patients with Cushing's syndrome. This test is the most useful indicator of daily cortisol secretion.
   d. **ACTH measurement** may help differentiate the causes of Cushing's syndrome.
      (1) ACTH levels are usually high-normal or slightly elevated in patients with Cushing's disease and may be markedly elevated in patients with ectopic ACTH production.
      (2) When an autonomously functioning adrenal tumor is the source of excess cortisol secretion, pituitary secretion of ACTH is suppressed because of the high levels of circulating cortisol, and the ACTH level is extremely low or undetectable.
   e. **Low-dose dexamethasone suppression tests**
      (1) The **overnight low-dose dexamethasone suppression test** is recommended as an initial screening procedure for any patient suspected of having Cushing's syndrome. The patient takes 1 mg dexamethasone orally at 11:00 PM, and the plasma cortisol level is measured at 8:00 AM the following morning.
         (a) The plasma cortisol level is less than 3 μg/dL in most individuals, indicating normal suppression of ACTH and cortisol by the dexamethasone. Because this test is very sensitive, the diagnosis of Cushing's syndrome is very unlikely in patients with a normal response.
         (b) Patients with Cushing's syndrome have cortisol levels greater than 3 μg/dL; they usually exceed 10 μg/dL. This result indicates that further study is needed. (The test is not very specific; mental or physical stress may produce a false-positive result.)
      (2) In the **standard low-dose dexamethasone suppression test,** the patient takes dexamethasone 0.5 mg every 6 hours for 48 hours, starting at 8:00 AM (eight doses). The morning plasma cortisol drawn after 48 hours is normally suppressed to less than 2 μg/dL.
   f. **High-dose dexamethasone suppression tests**
      (1) In the **overnight high-dose dexamethasone suppression test,** plasma cortisol is measured at 8:00 AM on two consecutive days, and dexamethasone 8 mg is taken at 11:00 PM on the first day. A decrease in the plasma cortisol level of less than 50% on the second day indicates failure of suppression. The high-dose test is designed to distinguish between the two primary causes of ACTH-dependent Cushing's syndrome.
         (a) Patients with Cushing's disease behave as though their feedback response to glucocorticoids is intact but set at a higher-than-normal level; they respond to high but not to low doses of dexamethasone.
         (b) Patients with ectopic ACTH secretion produce ACTH autonomously; their cortisol levels are not suppressed even by high doses of dexamethasone.
      (2) In the **standard high-dose dexamethasone suppression test,** 2 mg dexamethasone are taken every 6 hours for 48 hours (eight doses). A fall of 50% or more in the morning plasma cortisol at 48 hours indicates suppression.
   g. In **inferior petrosal sinus sampling,** ACTH concentrations are measured in venous blood obtained by catheterization of the inferior petrosal sinuses. Corticotropin-releasing hormone

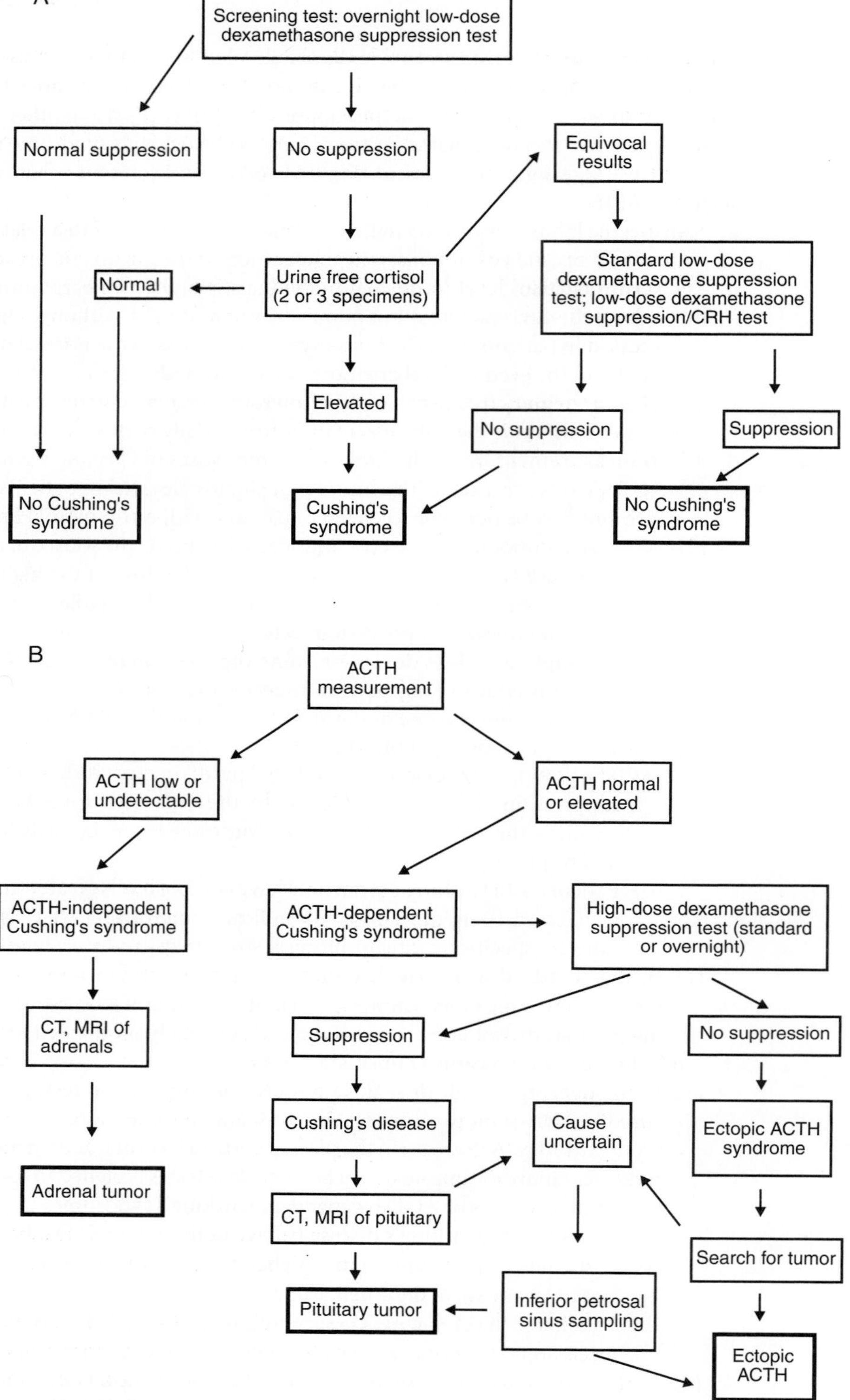

FIGURE 9–6 Algorithms to determine the diagnosis and etiology of Cushing's syndrome. (*A*) Steps to take to determine whether a patient has Cushing's syndrome (of any cause). (*B*) Steps to take to identify the cause of Cushing's syndrome (once the diagnosis has been made). *ACTH* = adrenocorticotropic hormone; *CRH* = corticotropin-releasing hormone; *CT* = computed tomography; *MRI* = magnetic resonance imaging.

(CRH) may be injected to stimulate ACTH secretion. A high concentration of ACTH compared with that in peripheral blood indicates that a pituitary adenoma is the cause of ACTH excess; if one superior petrosal sinus has a high ACTH concentration while the other has a concentration similar to peripheral blood, the adenoma is more likely to be on the side of the pituitary corresponding to the higher concentration.

h. A **combined standard low-dose dexamethasone suppression test and CRH test** may be used when other tests have failed to distinguish between true Cushing's syndrome and the "pseudo-Cushing's syndrome" sometimes seen with alcoholism or depression.
   (1) After the administration of 0.5 mg dexamethasone every 6 hours for 48 hours, CRH is injected intravenously, and plasma cortisol is measured 15 minutes later. Patients with Cushing's syndrome have cortisol levels greater than 1.4 μg/dL, whereas patients with "pseudo-Cushing's syndrome" have levels less than 1.4 μg/dL.
   (2) This combined test makes use of the following observations: patients with adrenal tumors or ectopic ACTH production are resistant to suppression of cortisol by dexamethasone, whereas patients with Cushing's disease have exaggerated responses to CRH. By combining these tests, it is possible to obtain a greater separation between the results seen in Cushing's syndrome and those seen in pseudo-Cushing's syndrome.

i. **Radiographic findings**
   (1) **Skull radiographs** show enlargement of the sella turcica in the 10% of patients with Cushing's syndrome who have **macroadenomas** but they do not reveal most of these tumors, which are **microadenomas** averaging 5–6 mm in diameter.
   (2) **CT scans with injection of contrast medium** detect approximately 50% of the pituitary adenomas that cause Cushing's disease. **MRI with gadolinium contrast,** however, reveals approximately 75% of these tumors and is the method of choice.
   (3) **CT scans of the adrenal gland** show most adrenal tumors. Uniform enlargement of both adrenal glands suggests an ACTH-dependent form of Cushing's syndrome, either Cushing's disease or the ectopic ACTH syndrome.

4. **Therapy**

a. **Adrenal adenomas** can usually be resected completely, often laparoscopically, with cure of the disease. Cortisol replacement may be needed for several months to a year postoperatively, until the remaining normal adrenal tissue, suppressed by the previous high cortisol levels, regains its ability to produce cortisol.

b. **Adrenal carcinoma** is often inoperable when first diagnosed because of metastases, usually to the liver and the lungs. Mitotane, metyrapone, and aminoglutethimide are drugs that block adrenal steroid production, and they may relieve the manifestations of excess cortisol production in patients with inoperable adrenal carcinoma. Prolonged survival of these patients is uncommon.

c. The **ectopic ACTH syndrome** can be cured by removal of the tumor, but this is not possible in many cases. The tumor causing the syndrome, rather than the Cushing's syndrome itself, is usually the primary problem.

d. **Cushing's disease** may be treated in several ways.
   (1) **Pituitary irradiation** is effective in many children, but it cures fewer than one third of affected adults; the reason for the difference in response between children and adults is unclear.
   (2) **Bilateral adrenalectomy** cures Cushing's disease but leaves the patient with **Addison's disease** and the need for lifelong steroid replacement. In addition, adrenalectomy is sometimes followed by the development of **Nelson's syndrome,** in which a pituitary adenoma undergoes rapid growth, perhaps because it is no longer inhibited by above-normal levels of cortisol.
   (3) **Transsphenoidal pituitary surgery is the treatment of choice.** Even when tumors cannot be seen on CT scan or MRI, transsphenoidal exploration may disclose a microadenoma.

Surgery is successful in 50%–95% of cases and is followed by normal pituitary and adrenal function as well as cure of Cushing's disease.

C Adrenal insufficiency (Addison's disease)

1. **Etiology**
   a. **Primary adrenal insufficiency**
      (1) **Idiopathic atrophy of the adrenal cortex** due to an autoimmune process is the most common cause of adrenal insufficiency.
      (2) **Tuberculosis** may involve the adrenal glands, with destruction of both the adrenal cortex and medulla.
      (3) **Iatrogenic causes**
         (a) **Bilateral adrenalectomy** for Cushing's disease results in adrenal insufficiency.
         (b) **Adrenal suppression following prolonged steroid therapy** may persist for up to 1 year or longer.
      (4) **Acquired immunodeficiency syndrome (AIDS)** sometimes leads to adrenal insufficiency through cytomegalovirus (CMV) and other infections of the adrenal glands.
      (5) **Adrenoleukodystrophy** is an X-linked disorder caused by a deficiency of very-long-chain acyl CoA synthetase. This leads to an accumulation of very-long-chain fatty acids in the adrenal glands, causing adrenal insufficiency, and in the CNS, causing a demyelinating syndrome.
      (6) **Less common causes** of adrenal destruction include **amyloidosis, fungal infections, syphilis, bilateral adrenal hemorrhage** (especially in patients receiving anticoagulants), and **metastatic malignancy.**
   b. **Secondary adrenal insufficiency** is due to pituitary disease and results from any of the causes of hypopituitarism (see I A 2 a).
2. **Clinical features.** The symptoms of adrenal insufficiency are caused by both cortisol and aldosterone deficiencies.
   a. **Cortisol deficiency**
      (1) **Hyperpigmentation of the skin** is caused by increased MSH activity that accompanies the increased pituitary secretion of ACTH. The latter is a feedback response to the cortisol deficiency.
         (a) Hyperpigmentation is most noticeable over exposed areas, on mucous membranes, and in skin creases and scars.
         (b) In secondary adrenal insufficiency (which is caused by pituitary disease), ACTH levels are low rather than elevated, and hyperpigmentation is absent.
      (2) **Hypotension,** often orthostatic, is caused by the absence of the pressor effect of cortisol on vascular tone and by a decrease in cardiac output.
      (3) **Gastrointestinal symptoms** include anorexia, nausea and vomiting, and weight loss.
      (4) **Hypoglycemia** is related to decreased cortisol-induced gluconeogenesis.
      (5) **Mental symptoms** may include lethargy and confusion. Psychotic manifestations occur on occasion.
      (6) **Intolerance to stress** may occur. Patients who cannot increase their cortisol output in response to severe stress risk an acute exacerbation of the symptoms discussed above, with life-threatening vascular collapse.
   b. **Aldosterone deficiency**
      (1) **Sodium loss** results from reduced aldosterone-mediated reabsorption of sodium in the distal renal tubules. **Hypovolemia, decreased cardiac output,** and **decreased renal blood flow with azotemia** as well as weakness, hypotension, and weight loss may be related to sodium depletion.
      (2) **Potassium retention** caused by aldosterone deficiency may lead to **hyperkalemia** and **cardiac arrhythmias.**

(3) Because **angiotensin II,** rather than **ACTH,** has primary control of aldosterone production, and the renin-angiotensin system is not affected by ACTH deficiency, there is usually no deficiency of aldosterone in secondary adrenal insufficiency.

3. **Diagnosis**
   a. **ACTH response**
      (1) The normal adrenal gland sharply increases its output of cortisol when stimulated by ACTH; absence of this response indicates adrenal insufficiency.
      (2) **ACTH test.** The serum level of cortisol is measured before and 1 hour after an intravenous or intramuscular injection of 0.25 mg (25 U) cosyntropin, a synthetic form of ACTH. The plasma cortisol should reach a level of 20 μg/dL or higher.
   b. **Laboratory findings**
      (1) Nonspecific laboratory abnormalities may include **hyponatremia, hyperkalemia, hypoglycemia,** and an **increased eosinophil count** (glucocorticoids lower the eosinophil count). Chest radiography may show a **small heart.**
      (2) **Plasma cortisol, urinary free cortisol, and urinary 17-hydroxycorticosteroid levels are low.** Baseline levels, however, may overlap with the values in normal individuals, which is why ACTH testing is necessary for a definitive diagnosis.

4. **Therapy**
   a. **Glucocorticoid replacement is needed in all patients.**
      (1) The usual dose of cortisol is 10–30 mg daily. A higher dose is usually given in the morning and a smaller dose in the evening, to mimic the normal diurnal variation. To avoid the potential harmful effects of excess cortisol, such as osteoporosis, the dose should be no more than is necessary to relieve the manifestations of cortisol deficiency.
      (2) The dose must be increased during times of stress. Typical doses would be twice the usual dose during minor stress (e.g., common cold or dental extraction), 3–5 times the usual dose during moderate stress (e.g., influenza or minor surgery), and "stress doses" of 200–300 mg during severe stress (e.g., major surgery or a serious infection or injury).
   b. **Mineralocorticoid replacement** is needed by most patients. **Fludrocortisone** (Florinef) is given in a daily dose of 0.05–0.2 mg. Persistence of low blood pressure, weakness, and low serum sodium and high serum potassium levels suggest that a higher dose of mineralocorticoid is needed; hypertension, edema, or hypokalemia suggest that the dose should be decreased.

5. **Adrenal crisis** (**Addisonian crisis**) is an acute, life-threatening complication of Addison's disease in which the manifestations of adrenal insufficiency are greatly exaggerated.
   a. **Clinical features. Fever, vomiting, abdominal pain, altered mental status,** and **vascular collapse** may occur if Addison's disease remains untreated, or it may occur in a treated patient during acute stress if additional glucocorticoid replacement is not provided.
   b. **Therapy.** Immediate intravenous administration of 100 mg cortisol over 5–10 minutes should be followed by an additional 300 mg in the next 24 hours. Intravenous saline is also needed, and mineralocorticoid replacement should be provided if hypotension and volume depletion persist.

D Primary aldosteronism

1. **Etiology.** Excessive adrenal production of aldosterone is usually caused by a single **small** (0.5–3.0 cm) **adrenal adenoma.** Less often (i.e., in 20%–40% of cases), there is bilateral hyperplasia of the adrenal cortex.
2. **Clinical features.** Aldosterone increases the reabsorption of sodium and the excretion of potassium and hydrogen ions in the distal renal tubules.
   a. **Sodium retention causes blood pressure elevation,** which is the chief clinical manifestation of this syndrome.

(1) The amount of sodium and water that are retained is limited by compensatory mechanisms that increase renal sodium excretion in response to extracellular fluid volume expansion; sodium balance is restored after 1–2 kg of fluid have accumulated.

(2) Although this amount of volume expansion does not cause edema, the long-term increase in cardiac output and, perhaps, other effects of mineralocorticoid excess lead to hypertension.

b. **Potassium loss causes hypokalemia,** which may produce **muscle weakness, paresthesias,** and **tetany** in severe cases.

(1) **Hypokalemic nephropathy** may cause polyuria.

(2) **Metabolic alkalosis** is a result of the renal loss of potassium and hydrogen ions.

3. **Diagnosis**

a. **Laboratory diagnosis**

(1) **Hypokalemia** in a hypertensive patient is often the clue that triggers the search for primary aldosteronism, although not all patients with aldosteronism have a low serum level of potassium.

(2) **Aldosterone** must be measured under standardized conditions because it is affected by sodium balance, diuretics, and other factors.

(a) Diuretics, angiotensin-converting enzyme inhibitors, and vasodilators should be discontinued at least 2 weeks before studies of aldosterone (and renin) are undertaken.

(b) Random aldosterone measurements in patients with primary aldosteronism may overlap those of normal individuals; sodium loading may be necessary to differentiate the aldosterone levels in affected patients (which are not suppressed by a sodium load) from the levels in normal individuals (which are suppressed by a sodium load). Two of the many ways that this procedure can be performed are as follows.

(i) The **24-hour urinary aldosterone excretion rate** can be measured after the patient has ingested more than 250 mEq sodium daily for at least 3 days. (This can be ensured by giving sodium chloride tablets.) Sodium loading may further lower serum levels of potassium; therefore, caution is necessary if the patient is hypokalemic. An elevated aldosterone level in a 24-hour urine sample that contains more than 250 mEq sodium indicates hyperaldosteronism.

(ii) **Plasma levels of aldosterone** can be measured after 2000 mL normal saline have been infused over 4 hours. Normally, the values are less than 8–10 ng/dL. Severe hypertension or congestive heart failure (CHF) are contraindications to saline infusion.

(3) **Plasma renin activity** is the most useful indicator of whether elevated aldosterone production is primary or secondary.

(a) **Secondary aldosteronism** is caused by conditions that originate outside the adrenal gland and that reduce the effective arterial blood volume, thus diminishing the pressure or tension sensed by the juxtaglomerular cells.

(i) Such conditions include heart failure, nephrosis, cirrhosis, volume depletion caused by diuretics, and renovascular disease.

(ii) Decreased pressure on the juxtaglomerular cells stimulates renin release, which increases angiotensin II and, in turn, aldosterone. Thus, **the high aldosterone level is accompanied by increased renin activity.**

(b) In **primary aldosteronism,** the enhanced aldosterone production is caused by an adrenal abnormality, not by increased renin activity; the resulting volume expansion suppresses renin production. This combination of **increased aldosterone production and reduced renin activity can be caused only by primary aldosteronism,** and it is a reliable indicator of this diagnosis.

(c) Suppression of renin activity is diagnosed with certainty only if levels remain low after manipulations that are known to stimulate renin in normal individuals such as dietary sodium restriction, several hours of upright posture, or furosemide administration.

(4) The **best screening test for primary aldosteronism** is measurement of the ratio of plasma aldosterone (ng/dL) to plasma renin activity (ng of angiotensin I/mL/hr) in a blood sample drawn with the patient upright. This ratio is increased both by the elevated aldosterone level and the suppressed renin level characteristic of the disease. An aldosterone-to-renin ratio greater than 25 indicates need for further study.

b. **Adenoma versus hyperplasia.** Primary aldosteronism due to an adenoma must be distinguished from primary aldosteronism due to hyperplasia, because the distinction affects treatment, which is usually surgical in cases of adrenal adenoma and medical in bilateral hyperplasia.

(1) The biochemical changes of primary aldosteronism—the hypokalemia, the increased aldosterone level, and the low renin activity—are more pronounced in cases caused by a unilateral adenoma than in cases caused by hyperplasia.

(2) The plasma aldosterone concentration may be measured at 8:00 AM, after 8 hours of recumbency, and again at noon, after 4 hours of ambulation.

(a) Levels are higher after ambulation in normal subjects and in patients with bilateral hyperplasia, because renin and angiotensin are stimulated by the upright posture and sympathetic outflow.

(b) However, patients with unilateral adrenal adenomas have a paradoxical fall in plasma aldosterone levels, presumably because when renin is profoundly suppressed, aldosterone is influenced mainly by the diurnal fall in ACTH.

(3) **Adrenal vein aldosterone concentrations** may be measured in blood samples obtained by selective catheterization. A very high level on one side indicates an adenoma; high levels on both sides indicate bilateral hyperplasia.

(4) **CT scans** and **MRI** sometimes show aldosterone-producing adenomas, but these tumors may be small and often cannot be visualized.

(5) An algorithm for the diagnosis of primary aldosteronism is shown in Figure 9–7.

4. **Therapy**

a. **Surgery**

(1) Removal of a unilateral adenoma results in cure of the hypertension in approximately 60% of cases and improvement in another 25%.

(2) In contrast, only 20%–50% of patients with bilateral hyperplasia are improved by surgery, even if bilateral adrenalectomy is performed. Medical therapy is preferable.

b. **Medical therapy. Spironolactone** inhibits the effects of aldosterone on the renal tubule. A dosage of 200–400 mg daily corrects the hypokalemia and often corrects the hypertension.

E Congenital adrenal hyperplasia

1. **Etiology and pathophysiology.** Congenital adrenal hyperplasia is caused by a defect in one of the enzymes that are necessary for the synthesis of cortisol. Cortisol deficiency stimulates ACTH, which causes hyperplasia of the adrenal cortex and overproduction of whatever ACTH-dependent steroids are not affected by the enzyme deficiency (mainly adrenal androgens).

2. **Clinical features**

a. **Androgen excess** is caused by increased adrenal production of dehydroepiandrosterone, androstenedione, and testosterone.

(1) If present during fetal development, this disorder may cause **ambiguous genitalia** in female infants. If androgen excess is manifested in the postnatal period, it may cause **virilization** in prepubertal girls or in young women.

(2) In male infants, the consequence of androgen excess during fetal development is macrogenitosomia. In the postnatal period, the consequence is **precocious puberty.**

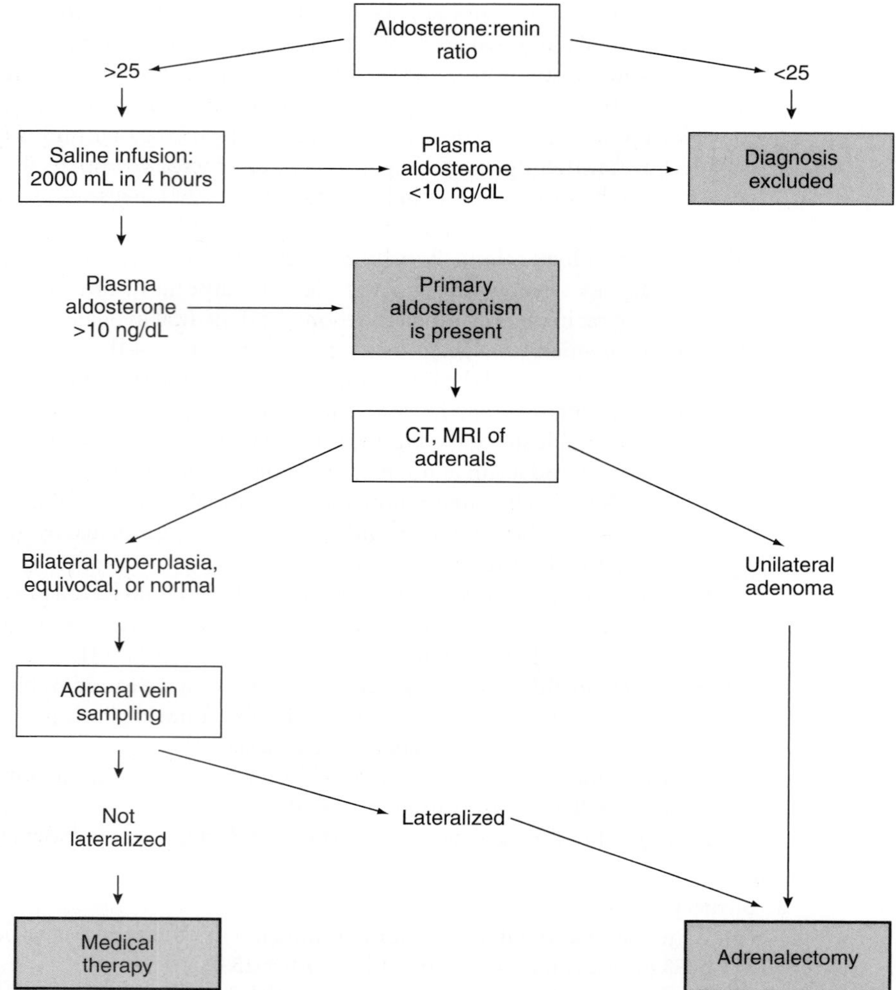

FIGURE 9–7 Algorithm for the diagnosis of primary aldosteronism. (From Adlin EV: *Endocrinology Science and Medicine.* Philadelphia, Lippincott Williams & Wilkins, 2001, p 123.)

b. The cortisol deficit usually does not cause major clinical manifestations because the ACTH stimulation and adrenal hyperplasia maintain cortisol levels in the low-normal range, despite the enzyme deficiency.

c. Other manifestations occasionally occur, depending on the specific enzyme affected.

(1) **21-Hydroxylase deficiency** accounts for 95% of cases of adrenal hyperplasia.

(a) In the mild (simple virilizing) form, only the androgen-excess symptoms are of importance.

(b) In the severe (salt-losing) form, the production of aldosterone is impaired as well as that of cortisol; mineralocorticoid deficiency leads to hyponatremia, hyperkalemia, dehydration, and hypotension.

(2) In **11-hydroxylase deficiency,** deoxycorticosterone, a mineralocorticoid, as well as adrenal androgens are overproduced. This causes hypertension through mechanisms that are similar to those causing hypertension in primary aldosteronism.

(3) In **17-hydroxylase deficiency,** deoxycorticosterone is overproduced, resulting in hypertension. However, because 17-hydroxylase is necessary for sex steroid synthesis, there is

androgen deficiency as well as estrogen deficiency. This causes the development of ambiguous genitalia in male infants and primary amenorrhea in women.

3. **Diagnosis.** Concentrations of adrenal androgens and precursors of cortisol are increased in blood and urine. The most useful measurements are of **blood testosterone, androstenedione, dehydroepiandrosterone,** and **17-hydroxyprogesterone** (a cortisol precursor) as well as **urinary 17-ketosteroids** and **pregnanetriol** (a metabolite of 17-hydroxyprogesterone).
4. **Therapy**
   a. **Medical therapy. Cortisol** administration suppresses the overproduction of ACTH and adrenal androgens. In the salt-losing syndrome, mineralocorticoid replacement with fludrocortisone may be necessary.
   b. **Surgery.** Reconstructive surgery of the external genitalia in female infants is done in the first few years of life.

F Pheochromocytoma This tumor is derived from **chromaffin cells,** the cells that synthesize and store catecholamines. Located primarily in the adrenal medulla, they also are located in sympathetic ganglia and elsewhere. The cells in the adrenal medulla produce epinephrine and norepinephrine; the extra-adrenal chromaffin cells make only norepinephrine.

1. **Epidemiology**
   a. **Incidence.** Pheochromocytoma is found in approximately 0.5% of patients with severe hypertension and in less than 0.05% of all hypertensive patients. However, because this tumor may cause a dramatic and debilitating syndrome, often with fatal complications if undetected, diagnostic efforts and awareness are required out of proportion to the frequency of occurrence.
   b. **Familial occurrence.** Pheochromocytomas may occur sporadically or may occur as part of one of several familial syndromes.
      (1) **Multiple endocrine neoplasia type II (Sipple's syndrome)** is characterized by multiple pheochromocytomas and medullary carcinoma of the thyroid; hyperparathyroidism is often present.
      (2) **Neurofibromatosis and von Hippel-Lindau disease** may be associated with pheochromocytoma.
2. **Pathology.** Most pheochromocytomas are single tumors of the adrenal medulla. However, 10%–20% are located outside of the adrenal gland, and 1%–3% are in the chest or neck. Approximately 20% are multiple and 10% are malignant.
3. **Clinical features.** The manifestations of pheochromocytoma (**Table 9–14**) are caused by increased levels of circulating catecholamines.
   a. **Hypertension** is paroxysmal in approximately 50% of cases and is sustained in the rest. The diagnosis is often suggested by the **paroxysmal nature of the symptoms,** caused by variations in the function of the tumor. Attacks typically last less than 1 hour and may be precipitated by exercise, induction of anesthesia, urination (suggesting a pheochromocytoma of the bladder), or palpation of the abdomen.
   b. **Other features** that suggest the presence of a pheochromocytoma are **hyperglycemia, hypermetabolism,** and **postural hypotension** in a hypertensive patient.
4. **Diagnosis.** Pheochromocytoma is suspected far more often than it is diagnosed. Many patients with symptoms of catecholamine excess prove to have normal hormone levels.

TABLE 9–14 Manifestations of Pheochromocytoma

Hypertension	Palpitations
Headache	Nervousness and tremor
Sweating	Weight loss

a. The levels of **urine catecholamines** and their metabolites are elevated in most confirmed cases.
   (1) The **24-hour urinary metanephrine excretion rate** may be the most useful screening test, but tests of **urinary free catecholamines** (i.e., epinephrine and norepinephrine) and **vanillylmandelic acid** concentrations are also of value.
   (2) Stressful illness can raise catecholamine levels twofold; greater than twofold elevations are more suggestive of pheochromocytoma.

b. **Serum catecholamine levels** are variable and are more difficult to interpret than the 24-hour urine measurements. Levels of **plasma free metanephrines** may prove to be a sensitive indicator of a pheochromocytoma.

c. The **clonidine suppression test** is useful in patients with mild catecholamine elevation. Three hours after an oral dose of 0.3 mg clonidine, the plasma level of norepinephrine is lowered into the normal range in most normal individuals, but it remains elevated in patients with pheochromocytoma.

d. **CT scans** or **MRI** of the abdomen detect as many as 90% of these tumors because they usually are greater than 1 cm in diameter.

e. **Adrenal scanning** with ^{131}I iodobenzylguanidine **(MIBG)** is especially useful for localizing extra-adrenal tumors.

5. **Therapy**

a. **Medical therapy**
   (1) The α- and β-adrenergic blocking agents are useful for inoperable tumors and for preparation for surgery.
      (a) **α-Adrenergic blocking agents** relieve the hypertension and adrenergic symptoms.
         (i) **Phenoxybenzamine** is given orally, starting with 10 mg twice daily and increasing to 40 mg twice daily, if necessary.
         (ii) **Phentolamine** can be given intravenously to treat acute severe elevations in blood pressure.
         (iii) **Prazosin, terazosin,** or **doxazosin** also can be given to produce sustained α-adrenergic blockade.
      (b) **β-Adrenergic blocking agents** should not be used alone, because unopposed α-adrenergic stimulation may lead to exacerbation of the hypertension. β-Blockers are sometimes useful in conjunction with α-blockers.
   (2) **Metyrosine,** which is an inhibitor of tyrosine hydroxylase, blocks the formation of norepinephrine and epinephrine and is an alternative agent for the relief of the symptoms of pheochromocytoma. It may be used when patients are intolerant of the adrenergic-blocking agents.

b. **Surgery. Surgical removal of the pheochromocytoma is the treatment of choice.** Careful exploration of the adrenal glands and the periaortic sympathetic chain should be performed.
   (1) **Complications** that frequently occur during and after surgery are extreme swings in blood pressure, cardiac arrhythmias, and shock. These are caused by the sudden removal of the source of excess catecholamine production and by the low blood volume that results from long-term constriction of the vascular compartment.
   (2) To prevent vascular instability during removal of a pheochromocytoma, patients are treated with α-blockers to maintain normal blood pressure for at least 1 week before surgery. β-Blockers may be added for a few days before surgery, especially if tachycardia or another arrhythmia is present.

VI FEMALE REPRODUCTIVE DISORDERS

Endocrine disorders that affect the female reproductive system usually cause menstrual abnormalities and include those disorders in which menarche does not occur **(primary amenorrhea)** and those disorders that cause cessation of menstrual periods after menarche (**secondary amenorrhea**). Androgen-excess syndromes are a common cause of reproductive abnormalities that also are considered in this section.

A **Primary amenorrhea** (Table 9–15)

1. **Gonadal dysgenesis (Turner's syndrome).** This condition occurs in 1 in 2500 live female births.
   a. **Etiology and pathophysiology.** Gonadal dysgenesis is caused by a **chromosomal abnormality** that is not familial and is not related to the mother's age. Patients have a chromatin-negative buccal smear and a 45,X karyotype.
   b. **Clinical features**
      (1) **Ovaries fail to develop;** only bilateral streaks of connective tissue are present, without germ cells. Estrogen deficiency, caused by the absence of ovarian tissue, results in **sexual infantilism,** with absence of breast development and other secondary sexual characteristics, and increased levels of LH and FSH.
      (2) **Somatic abnormalities** are associated with gonadal dysgenesis.
         (a) Most patients are short, between 48 and 58 inches in height.
         (b) Other features, present in varying numbers of patients, include a short, webbed neck, epicanthal folds, low-set ears, a shield-like chest with widely spaced nipples, cubitus valgus (wide carrying angle), and renal and cardiac abnormalities.
   c. **Therapy**
      (1) **Estrogen therapy** induces the development of secondary sexual characteristics. If estrogen is given cyclically with progesterone, regular menstrual bleeding occurs, but fertility is not possible because of the absence of ovaries.
      (2) **GH therapy,** if started early enough, may add 2–4 inches to the adult height.
      (3) **Removal of streak gonads** may be necessary. Gonadal dysgenesis may occur in patients with sex chromosome mosaicism in which one or more cell lines bear a Y chromosome. The frequency of gonadoblastoma and other gonadal tumors is increased in patients with these gonads, and their prophylactic removal is recommended.
2. **Testicular feminization syndrome.** Individuals with this syndrome are genetic males with a 46,XY karyotype, but they have normal female external genitalia and are raised as girls.
   a. **Pathogenesis.** The basic defect is resistance of target tissues to the action of androgens. The fetal testes produce testosterone, but because the wolffian ducts and genital tissues cannot respond to testosterone, female differentiation of the external genitalia takes place. The fetal testes also produce müllerian duct–inhibiting factor, which has its normal effect in inhibiting the müllerian anlage, and so the fallopian tubes, uterus, and upper vagina do not develop.
   b. **Clinical features.** The result is a phenotypic woman with a vagina that ends in a blind pouch, hypoplastic male ducts instead of the fallopian tubes and uterus, and testes located in the abdomen, inguinal canal, or labia majora. Endogenous estrogen stimulates normal breast

TABLE 9–15 Causes of Primary Amenorrhea

Gonadal causes	Extragonadal causes
Gonadal dysgenesis (Turner's syndrome)	Hypopituitarism
Testicular feminization syndrome	Hypogonadotropic hypogonadism
Resistant ovary syndrome	Delayed menarche
	Congenital adrenal hyperplasia
	Abnormalities of the uterus or vagina

development at puberty. The condition is suspected when menarche fails to occur or when a testis is felt as an abdominal mass, which is explored.

c. **Therapy.** The testes are prone to malignant degeneration and should be removed. Estrogen treatment is then given to maintain secondary sexual characteristics.

3. **Resistant ovary syndrome.** Inability of the ovaries to respond to normal or increased stimulation by gonadotropins may be a result of autoimmune destruction of the ovaries or other conditions.

4. **Hypogonadotropic hypogonadism**
   a. **Panhypopituitarism** due to destructive lesions of the hypothalamic–pituitary area (see I A 2 a) causes primary or secondary amenorrhea, depending on whether the problem is prepubertal or postpubertal in onset.
   b. **Isolated gonadotropin deficiency** is most often caused by defective hypothalamic production of GnRH, usually of unknown etiology. In **Kallmann's syndrome,** this defect is associated with anosmia.

5. **Delayed menarche.** This diagnosis should be considered when menstrual periods have not begun by 16 years of age.
   a. A diagnosis of delayed menarche, as opposed to that of primary amenorrhea, can only be made in retrospect, after spontaneous menstrual periods have begun. A family history of late pubertal development suggests that spontaneous menarche may yet be expected.
   b. If severe psychological stress is caused by the absence of sexual development, it may be necessary to give one or more 6-month courses of estrogen therapy, with long treatment-free periods to observe whether spontaneous puberty will occur.

B Secondary amenorrhea (Table 9–16)

1. **Hypothalamic** (also called **"psychogenic," "functional,"** and **"idiopathic") amenorrhea is** the **most common form of nonphysiologic secondary amenorrhea.** Obvious psychological stress may or may not be present. LH and FSH levels are low in some cases and normal in others. If the hypothalamic-releasing hormone GnRH is infused in physiologic fashion (pulse doses every 90–120 minutes), all abnormalities may be corrected—ovarian follicles mature, ovulation takes place, a corpus luteum develops and functions, and pregnancy may occur. This supports the clinical impression that most cases of functional or idiopathic amenorrhea are caused by abnormal hypothalamic GnRH production.

2. **Malnutrition** may play a role. Menarche seems to occur when a critical body weight is reached, and menstruation often ceases when the weight of a woman whose menstrual cycle was previ-

TABLE 9–16 Causes of Secondary Amenorrhea

Pregnancy	Ovarian causes
Menopause	Primary ovarian failure ("premature menopause")
Uterine causes	Oophorectomy
Intrauterine synechiae (Asherman's syndrome)	Radiation therapy, chemotherapy
Hysterectomy	Estrogen excess
Hypothalamic–pituitary causes	Ovarian tumors
Hypopituitarism	Prolactin excess
Hypothalamic ("psychogenic") amenorrhea	Pituitary tumors
Malnutrition, chronic illness	Androgen excess
Exercise	Polycystic ovary syndrome
Discontinuation of oral contraceptives	Overproduction of adrenal androgen
	Ovarian tumors

ously normal falls below this critical weight, whether because of food deprivation, chronic illness, excessive dieting, or anorexia nervosa.

3. **Exercise** may be a factor. Amenorrhea is present in up to 50% of female ballet dancers, runners, and athletes. Exercise-related weight loss is at least partially responsible; the risk of amenorrhea is much higher in women who have lost more than 10%–15% of their body weight. Levels of LH, FSH, and estrogen tend to be low, suggesting a hypothalamic abnormality.
4. **"Post-pill amenorrhea"** refers to a delay of more than 6 months in the return of menses after the discontinuation of oral contraceptive use. It occurs in fewer than 1% of oral contraceptive users. Other causes of amenorrhea must be excluded before contraceptive use is blamed.
5. **Primary ovarian failure ("premature menopause")** is similar to normal menopause; that is, ovarian function declines, estrogen levels decrease, and gonadotropin levels increase. However, primary ovarian failure occurs before 40 years of age. Autoantibodies against ovarian antigens have been found in some cases.
6. **Ovarian tumors** (e.g., granulosa–theca cell tumors) may inhibit normal menstrual cycling by producing excessive quantities of estrogen.
7. **Prolactin excess** is a common cause of secondary amenorrhea (see I A 4 b).
8. **Menopause**

   a. **Manifestations**

   (1) Menopause, or total cessation of menstrual periods, occurs in all women when the ovaries are depleted of follicles and ovulatory function and estrogen production cease. The average age of menopause in the United States is 51 years.

   (2) As follicular secretion of estradiol and inhibin (a suppressor of gonadotropins) falls at menopause, FSH and LH levels rise. Estradiol levels remain low, although some estradiol is formed by peripheral conversion of androstenedione produced by the adrenals and ovaries.

   (3) The most prominent symptoms of the menopause is the **hot flash,** a sensation of warmth that may last up to 5 minutes, sometimes followed by sweating and a cold sensation. Headache, palpitations, dizziness, and weakness may accompany the hot flash. These episodes occur irregularly and may interfere with sleep. Hot flashes usually disappear within a few years of menopause.

   (a) The hot flash seems to be related to a fall in estrogen levels. Feedback stimulation of GnRH-producing cells in the hypothalamus may affect nearby thermoregulatory centers.

   (b) Estrogen therapy is very effective in decreasing the frequency and severity of hot flashes.

   (4) Other symptoms associated with the menopause include genitourinary atrophy, vaginal dryness, urinary symptoms, insomnia, and depression.

   b. **Postmenopausal hormone replacement therapy**

   For many years it was widely accepted that replacement of estrogen after menopause had benefits that greatly outweighed its drawbacks. Recent studies have changed this perception, and the indications for postmenopausal hormone replacement therapy are being reconsidered.

   (1) **Effects of estrogen on cardiovascular disease**

   (a) Many observational studies showed that women who take estrogen after menopause have lower rates of cardiovascular disease. But large randomized controlled trials have recently shown that estrogen does not prevent cardiovascular disease, and may even, at the beginning of treatment, have slightly harmful effects in women who already have cardiovascular disease.

   (b) It appears that the earlier studies did not adequately account for socioeconomic and educational factors: the women who took estrogen also engaged in other health-promoting behaviors such as smoking cessation, exercise, blood pressure control, and healthier eating. Thus estrogen therapy was associated with, but not the cause of, cardiovascular benefit.

(2) **Benefits of estrogen therapy**

In addition to relieving the symptoms of hot flashes and genitourinary atrophy, estrogen replacement increases bone mineral density and reduces the risk of osteoporotic fractures. It also reduces colorectal cancer. A very large study, the Women's Health Initiative, found 5 fewer hip fractures and 6 fewer cases of colorectal cancer per 10,000 women per year among those taking estrogen.

(3) **Risks of estrogen therapy**

Estrogen is known to increase the risk of breast cancer, and to affect the clotting mechanism, increasing the risk of thromboembolic events. The Women's Health Initiative found 8 additional cases of breast cancer, 10 additional cases of deep vein thrombosis, and 8 additional cases of pulmonary embolism per 10,000 women per year in those taking estrogen.

(4) **Indications for hormone replacement therapy**

(a) Because the possible long-term harmful effects of estrogen replacement now appear to outweigh its benefits, long-term hormone replacement therapy is no longer recommended in most cases.

(b) Estrogen replacement therapy is indicated for short-term treatment of hot flashes in the perimenopausal period, but the smallest dose that relieves these symptoms should be used.

(5) **Estrogen administration**

(a) Estrogen therapy after menopause increases the risk of uterine cancer; this risk is minimized if progesterone is given along with the estrogen.

(b) Estrogen–progesterone combinations can be given cyclically or continuously. A typical cyclic regimen would be conjugated estrogens 0.625 mg daily from day 1 to day 25 each month, with 5 or 10 mg medroxyprogesterone acetate from day 16 to day 25. Bleeding is expected a few days after the hormones are stopped.

(c) Combined therapy also can be given daily. A typical regimen would be conjugated estrogens 0.625 mg and medroxyprogesterone acetate 2.5 mg once daily. This regimen has the advantage of causing amenorrhea after 6 months or more in a majority of women, but some women may continue to have unpredictable spotting.

(d) Other estrogen preparations include oral estradiol and ethinyl estradiol, and transdermal preparations of estradiol. Many other progestational agents are also available.

(e) In women who have had a hysterectomy, estrogen can be given daily without progesterone, because there is no risk of endometrial cancer.

C Androgen excess syndromes

1. **Polycystic ovary syndrome,** a disorder of unknown etiology, is characterized by a chronic lack of ovulation, associated with symptoms of androgen excess and often with obesity. It is present in 5%–10% of reproductive-age women.

a. **Pathophysiology.** In the cycle shown in Figure 9–8, the initiating event is uncertain, and it probably is not the same in all cases. Proposed primary defects include insulin resistance, primary ovarian disease, abnormal secretion of LH by the hypothalamic–pituitary axis, and adrenal disease.

(1) The ovary produces excess androgenic steroids, especially **androstenedione.** The androstenedione is converted to estrone, an estrogen, in fat and other peripheral tissues. The increased circulating and intraovarian levels of androstenedione and other androgens prevent the maturation of graafian follicles, causing **anovulation.**

(2) The increased circulating level of estrone has a positive feedback effect on pituitary production of LH and a negative effect on production of FSH. The **increased LH level** causes

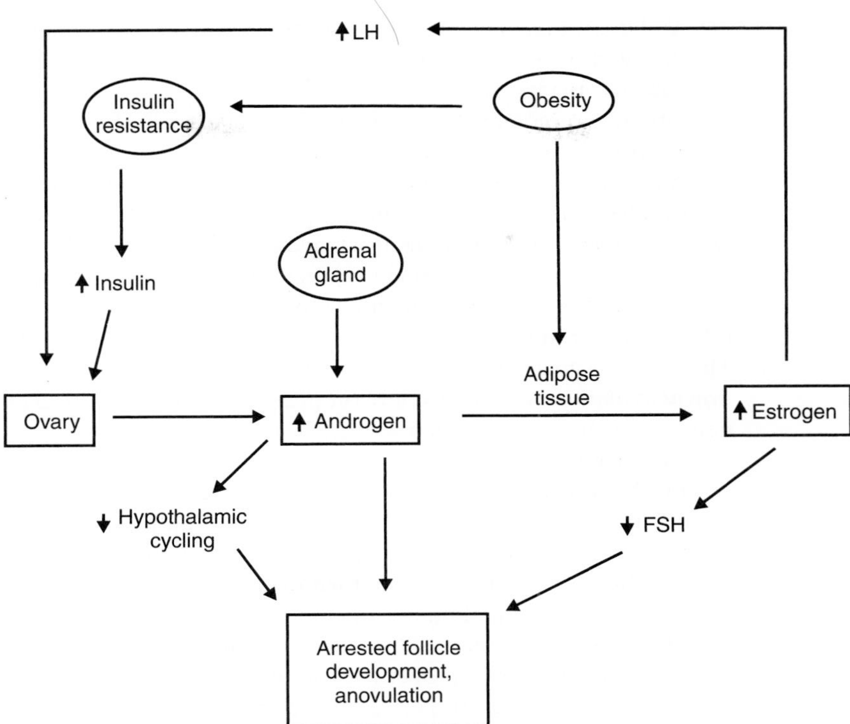

FIGURE 9–8 Proposed pathogenesis of the polycystic ovary syndrome. The oval-shaped blocks represent contributing factors; the rectangular blocks, key elements; and the unoutlined words, intermediate steps. *FSH* = follicle-stimulating hormone; *LH* = luteinizing hormone.

hyperplasia of ovarian thecal cells and stroma and increased androgen production. The **decreased FSH level** contributes to the lack of follicle maturation.

(3) **Obesity** may enhance the elevated levels of sex steroids by decreasing sex hormone–binding globulin, thus increasing the level of free testosterone, and by increasing the peripheral conversion of androstenedione to estrone.

(4) As a result of the **arrested follicle development,** the ovaries are enlarged, with thickened capsules and many small follicular cysts. Stromal and thecal hyperplasia are seen on microscopic examination.

(5) **Insulin resistance** is present in many women with the polycystic ovary syndrome; obesity accounts for some but not all of the insulin resistance. Insulin levels are elevated because of the tissue resistance to its action. That the hyperinsulinemia may be a primary cause (or at least a contributing cause) of the increased ovarian production of androgens is suggested by the clinical improvement that follows treatment with drugs that increase insulin sensitivity and thus return serum insulin levels to normal.

(6) Abnormalities of **adrenal androgen production** may be present; disappearance of the polycystic ovary syndrome has followed removal of an androgen-secreting adrenal adenoma in some cases.

b. Clinical features

(1) **Infertility and menstrual abnormalities** are the result of chronic anovulation. Most patients have amenorrhea or oligomenorrhea. The prolonged, noncyclic, unopposed estrogenic stimulation of the endometrium may cause functional bleeding and an increased risk of endometrial carcinoma.

(2) **Androgen excess** causes oiliness of the skin, acne, and hirsutism in most women with this syndrome. Signs of true virilization (e.g., deepening of the voice, enlargement of the clitoris) are rare.

(3) **Obesity** is present in approximately 40% of patients.

c. **Laboratory findings**

(1) An **increased LH-to-FSH ratio** (≥ 2) is a useful diagnostic finding. The LH level is usually elevated, and the FSH level is in the low end of the normal range (or the low-normal range).

(2) **Serum testosterone and androstenedione levels** are usually elevated. Increased levels of the androgens of predominantly adrenal origin (i.e., dehydroepiandrosterone, dehydroepiandrosterone sulfate) are found less often.

(3) **Serum estrone levels** are usually high, and estradiol levels are normal.

d. **Therapy.** The **goals of treatment are the relief of symptoms of androgen excess, the induction of ovulation and fertility, and the prevention of endometrial hyperplasia** due to excess noncyclic estrogen stimulation.

(1) **Androgen excess**

(a) **Metformin** and **thiazolidinediones,** drugs that increase the sensitivity of tissues to insulin, have lowered testosterone levels and improved the symptoms of hyperandrogenism and menstrual dysfunction in individuals with polycystic ovary syndrome. The efficacy of **metformin** in this syndrome makes it a reasonable choice for initial therapy, although it does not cause improvement in all cases.

(b) **Spironolactone,** an aldosterone antagonist that is used primarily for its diuretic and antihypertensive properties, has additional actions that make it useful in the treatment of hirsutism. This agent decreases ovarian and adrenal synthesis of androgens and inhibits androgen binding to receptors in hair follicles and other target tissues. A dose of 100 mg once or twice daily is often effective.

(c) **Estrogen–progestin combinations** may decrease androgen levels by feedback inhibition of pituitary LH production and by stimulation of hepatic synthesis of sex hormone–binding globulin, which decreases the unbound fraction of testosterone.

(d) **Glucocorticoids** (e.g., prednisone 5.0–7.5 mg daily) may decrease adrenal androgen production by suppressing ACTH. These agents may also lower ovarian androgen secretion, although the mechanism is unknown.

(e) The effects of medical therapy in diminishing the growth of unwanted facial and body hair are seldom dramatic and usually take place over a period of 3–6 months. **Mechanical methods of hair removal** are usually needed as well (e.g., shaving, electrolysis, laser treatment, bleaching, chemical depilatories, and wax treatments). **Vaniqa cream** (eflornithine hydrochloride) inhibits an enzyme in skin, ornithine decarboxylase, and may slow the rate of hair growth.

(2) **Infertility**

If metformin does not restore normal ovulatory menstrual cycles, other drugs may be used to treat infertility.

(a) **Clomiphene citrate** blocks the binding of estrogen to receptors in target tissues. By blocking the negative feedback effects of estrogen on the hypothalamus and pituitary gland, this drug stimulates LH and FSH production.

(i) If given on the fifth day through the ninth day after a menstrual period induced by progesterone, clomiphene citrate often stimulates follicle maturation and ovulation.

(ii) Ovulation can be induced with clomiphene citrate in approximately 80% of patients.

(b) **Human menopausal gonadotropin** has both FSH and LH bioactivity.

(i) It is injected daily until increasing serum estrogen levels and ultrasonography of the ovary indicate that follicle maturation has occurred.

(ii) Then human chorionic gonadotropin (hCG), which has primarily LH activity, is injected to induce ovulation. Because the risk of ovarian hyperstimulation and of multiple gestation is high, this therapy should be reserved for resistant cases of infertility.

(c) **GnRH,** when given intravenously or subcutaneously in pulse doses every 90–120 minutes, may induce ovulation without causing ovarian hyperstimulation.

(3) **Chronic anovulation and abnormal menstrual bleeding.** Unopposed noncyclic stimulation of the endometrium by estrogen may cause functional bleeding and may increase the risk of endometrial cancer. Persistent endometrial proliferation can be interrupted either with progestin treatment (e.g., 10 mg daily of medroxyprogesterone acetate for 10 days every 1–3 months) or with cyclic estrogen–progestin therapy.

2. **Androgen-producing ovarian tumors** are rare. Arrhenoblastoma, the most common of these tumors, makes up less than 1% of solid ovarian tumors; others are hilar cell tumors, adrenal rest tumors, and granulosa cell tumors.
   a. Testosterone levels tend to be higher than those in the polycystic ovary syndrome, and virilization occurs more frequently.
   b. Androgen levels are not suppressed by treatment with glucocorticoids or estrogen–progestin combinations, as they often are in the polycystic ovary syndrome.
   c. Diagnosis depends on detection of the tumor by pelvic examination (the majority are palpable) and on diagnostic imaging techniques.
3. **Hyperthecosis** of the ovary is probably a severe form of the polycystic ovary syndrome, but the androgen excess is more evident.
   a. **Diagnosis** depends on the histologic finding of luteinized thecal and stromal cells.
   b. **Medical therapy** is not effective, and oophorectomy may be necessary.
4. **Adrenal tumors,** either adenomas or carcinomas, may produce excess androgens with or without excess cortisol. High levels of adrenal androgens (urinary 17-ketosteroids, serum dehydroepiandrosterone) that cannot be suppressed by dexamethasone suggest this diagnosis; 24-hour urinary 17-ketosteroid levels greater than 50–100 mg strongly suggest adrenal carcinoma.
5. **Congenital adrenal hyperplasia** is discussed in the section on disorders of the adrenal gland (see V E).
6. **Idiopathic hirsutism** is a poorly understood but common condition in which hirsutism occurs in the absence of marked hormone abnormalities or menstrual dysfunction.
   a. The cause of idiopathic hirsutism is not known. It may have a familial occurrence, and it is more common in women of Mediterranean ancestry.
   b. Increased response of hair follicles to normal levels of testosterone is suspected.

VII MALE REPRODUCTIVE DISORDERS AND GYNECOMASTIA

A **Hypogonadism** in men affects two separate functions—the production of spermatozoa by the seminiferous tubules and the secretion of testosterone by the Leydig cells. The seminiferous tubule defect causes infertility; the testosterone deficiency leads to inadequate development and maintenance of secondary sexual characteristics.

1. **Physical and developmental effects**
   a. **Before puberty,** testicular failure prevents normal sexual development.
      (1) The penis and testes remain small, and spermatozoa are absent.
      (2) Facial and body hair are sparse.
      (3) The voice remains high-pitched, and muscle mass and strength are diminished.
      (4) Increased growth of long bones (because of delayed epiphyseal closure) produces the "eunuchoidal habitus," in which the arm span is more than 2 inches greater than the

height, and the floor-to-pubic symphysis distance is more than 2 inches greater than the symphysis-to-crown distance.

b. **After puberty,** loss of libido and sexual potency may be the first symptoms of testicular failure. Partial regression of secondary sex characteristics may occur gradually, with slowing of facial and body hair growth and decreased muscle mass.

2. **Clinical syndromes**

a. **Hypogonadotropic syndromes** (Table 9–17). The causes of hypogonadism are divided into **disorders of the hypothalamic–pituitary axis (hypogonadotropic hypogonadism) and disorders that originate with testicular damage,** with consequent feedback stimulation of LH and FSH (**hypergonadotropic hypogonadism).**

(1) **Hypogonadotropic (secondary) hypogonadism** is characterized by deficiency of LH and FSH, with resulting testosterone deficiency and eunuchoidism. **Kallmann's syndrome** is a form of hypogonadotropic hypogonadism that is associated with midline defects such as agenesis of the olfactory lobes, anosmia, and cleft palate. It is more common in men than in women. The basic hormonal defect is in the hypothalamus, rather than in the pituitary gland; this has been demonstrated by LH and FSH response to GnRH administration.

(2) **Delayed puberty** is a retrospective diagnosis. Puberty may occur spontaneously up to about 20 years of age; until this age, true hypogonadotropic hypogonadism cannot be diagnosed with certainty unless associated abnormalities such as anosmia are present. The diagnosis of delayed puberty is suggested by a family history of late maturation.

(a) If delayed puberty is suspected, a course of therapy with low doses of testosterone can be initiated to induce pubertal changes; true puberty may be induced by this treatment.

(b) Testosterone should be given for no more than 6 months at a time, with 6 months between courses, to avoid causing epiphyseal closure and limitation of ultimate height and to allow recognition of the onset of spontaneous puberty, if it should occur.

b. **Hypergonadotropic syndromes (primary hypogonadism)**

(1) **Klinefelter's syndrome,** in which the presence of two or more X chromosomes causes congenital testicular damage, occurs in approximately 1 in 400 male births.

(a) Approximately 80% of patients have a **47,XXY karyotype.**

(b) The testes are small (< 2 cm in length), with hyalinization of the seminiferous tubules and **azoospermia.**

(c) Leydig cell function is variable. Testosterone levels are deficient, and **eunuchoidism** is present in many, but not all, cases.

(d) **Gynecomastia** is present, and LH and FSH levels are elevated, even (for unknown reasons) in patients without testosterone deficiency.

TABLE 9–17 Causes of Hypogonadism in Men

Hypogonadotropic syndromes	**Hypergonadotropic syndromes**
Hypopituitarism	Klinefelter's syndrome
Hypogonadotropic eunuchoidism	Testicular agenesis
Kallmann's syndrome	Testicular injury
Delayed puberty	Mumps orchitis
	Other infections (e.g., gonorrhea)
	Trauma
	Surgery
	Radiation therapy
	Cancer chemotherapy
	Cryptorchidism
	Myotonic dystrophy

(e) **Mental deficiency** is an associated finding in 25% of patients.

(f) The only available treatment is **testosterone replacement** in those patients who require it.

(2) **Testicular agenesis** is recognized by failure of pubertal development and absence of testes in the scrotum or in the inguinal canals. Loss of the testes occurs after 7–14 weeks' gestation, because absence of testicular hormones before this stage would result in a female phenotype.

(3) **Mumps orchitis** affects mainly germinal cells; if the disease is bilateral, infertility may result, although this is uncommon. Testosterone production is usually unimpaired.

(4) **Cryptorchidism,** especially if it is bilateral, may be associated with hypogonadism because the undescended testes are damaged by trauma or torsion.

(a) An association between hypogonadism and cryptorchidism may exist because the cryptorchidism is sometimes a consequence of an intrinsic abnormality in the testes.

(b) Treatment with hCG or GnRH may induce testicular descent in some cases.

(5) **Myotonic dystrophy** is a syndrome consisting of myotonia, cataracts, and testicular atrophy.

3. **Therapy**

a. **Testosterone deficiency.** Although oral androgenic steroids are available, they do not provide fully virilizing blood levels of male hormones. Treatment of male hypogonadism is the injection of 200–400 mg of a long-acting testosterone preparation (e.g., Delatestryl or DEPO-Testosterone) every 2–4 weeks, or the use of skin patches (Testoderm, Androderm) or a gel (AndroGel, Testim) to provide transdermal testosterone absorption.

b. **Infertility.** Sperm production and fertility cannot be induced in individuals with primary testicular injury. In hypogonadotropic hypogonadism, spermatogenesis can sometimes be brought about by providing the testes with adequate gonadotropic stimulation.

(1) This can be done either by injections three times per week of hCG (which has LH activity) and human menopausal gonadotropin (which has FSH activity) or by administration via portable infusion pump of pulse doses of GnRH every 90–120 minutes.

(2) Both of these methods are expensive and impractical for long-term use, but they have been used successfully in some highly motivated men for the several months that are necessary to induce spermatogenesis.

B **Gynecomastia** is enlargement of the male breast. In true gynecomastia, firm, sometimes tender, glandular tissue is present. The disorders that cause gynecomastia are usually associated with increased levels of estrogens, decreased levels of androgens, or both.

1. **Pubertal gynecomastia** is not uncommon. At 12–15 years of age, approximately two thirds of normal boys have some degree of gynecomastia, usually a small, firm subareolar nodule that disappears in most cases within 1–2 years.

a. In the occasional boy with persistent breast enlargement, medical treatment with the antiestrogen **tamoxifen** may be tried.

b. If this is ineffective, however, **reduction mammoplasty** must be considered if psychological stress is severe.

2. **Hypogonadism,** either primary (hypergonadotropic) or secondary (hypogonadotropic), may be associated with gynecomastia.

3. **Refeeding after a period of starvation** often leads to transient gynecomastia, which may last for several months. Renewed secretion of previously inhibited gonadotropins and sex steroids and decreased hormone inactivation by the starved liver may be contributing factors.

4. **Liver disease,** especially alcoholic cirrhosis, is a common cause of gynecomastia.

a. Estrogen levels are increased because of accelerated conversion of androgenic precursors by peripheral tissues.

b. Also, alcohol inhibits the testicular production of testosterone and the pituitary production of gonadotropins and increases hepatic metabolism of testosterone.

5. **Chronic renal failure** is associated with gynecomastia, especially after the start of hemodialysis. The refeeding phenomenon may play a role, as may an increase in the ratio of estrogens to androgens in chronic renal failure.

6. **Drugs**
   a. **Estrogens,** commonly used to treat prostatic carcinoma, stimulate the breast directly.
   b. **Spironolactone, cimetidine,** and **digitalis** also produce gynecomastia. They are believed to inhibit androgen action by displacing dihydrotestosterone from its intracellular receptor.
   c. **Marijuana** binds to estrogen receptors and may cause gynecomastia through a direct estrogenic action.
   d. Other drugs that may cause this problem include **phenothiazines, tricyclic antidepressants, methyldopa, reserpine,** and **isoniazid.**

7. **Tumors** may cause gynecomastia.
   a. **Adrenal** and **testicular tumors** may cause gynecomastia through the production of estrogen.
   b. **Testicular choriocarcinomas** may cause gynecomastia through the secretion of hCG, which stimulates testicular estrogen production.
   c. Other malignant tumors may cause the condition through the ectopic production of gonadotropins.

8. **Hyperthyroidism** increases the conversion of androgens to estrogens in the peripheral tissues and increases the circulating level of sex hormone–binding globulin, which raises the estrogen-to-androgen ratio. These hormonal changes may cause gynecomastia in men with hyperthyroidism.

VIII METABOLIC BONE DISEASE

The metabolic bone diseases include osteomalacia, osteoporosis, osteitis fibrosa cystica, and other diseases. Osteitis fibrosa cystica is discussed briefly in the section on hyperparathyroidism (see III A 4 b).

A Osteomalacia

1. **Definition.** Osteomalacia is a **skeletal abnormality** in which there is **inadequate mineralization of bone matrix.** In children, this usually takes the form of rickets, caused by vitamin D deficiency. In adults, osteomalacia may be caused by many specific abnormalities of calcium, phosphorus, and vitamin D metabolism.

2. **Etiology**
   a. **Vitamin D deficiency**
      (1) Deficiency of vitamin D causes osteomalacia because its most active metabolite, 1,25-dihydroxyvitamin D_3, is essential for the absorption of calcium and phosphate from the gastrointestinal tract.
      (2) Deficiency of vitamin D is not rare in the United States. Although most Americans obtain the recommended dietary allowance of 400 U vitamin D from fortified foods, especially dairy products, dietary deficiency may still occur because of poverty, food faddism, eating disorders such as anorexia nervosa, or lack of sun exposure in elderly, debilitated patients.
      (3) Exposure to sunlight converts 7-dehydrocholesterol in the skin to vitamin D_3; this is an important source of the vitamin. Absence of sunlight may contribute to vitamin D deficiency.
   b. **Abnormal metabolism of, or response to, vitamin D**
      (1) **Liver disease,** when far advanced, may cause osteomalacia by interfering with the normal hepatic conversion of vitamin D to 25-hydroxyvitamin D_3.
      (2) **Anticonvulsant drugs** such as phenobarbital and phenytoin, if taken over a long period, may alter the metabolism of vitamin D by inducing hepatic microsomal enzymes.

Osteomalacia and decreased serum levels of 25-hydroxyvitamin D_3 have been described in patients receiving long-term treatment with anticonvulsants.

(3) **Vitamin D–dependent rickets type I** is an autosomal recessive disorder caused by impaired activity of renal 1α-hydroxylase, leading to inadequate conversion of 25-hydroxyvitamin D_3 to 1,25-dihydroxyvitamin D_3 (calcitriol). It is treated with small, physiologic doses (0.5–1.0 μg) of calcitriol.

(4) **Vitamin D-dependent rickets type II,** also autosomal recessive, is caused by resistance to the action of vitamin D because of altered structure or function of the calcitriol receptors. To overcome this resistance, large, supraphysiologic doses of calcitriol, along with calcium supplementation, must be used.

c. **Renal abnormalities**

(1) **Renal osteodystrophy** may occur in patients with chronic renal failure of any cause. Both osteomalacia, caused by impaired renal production of 1,25-dihydroxyvitamin D_3, and osteitis fibrosa cystica, caused by the secondary hyperparathyroidism of renal failure, are present in varying degrees.

(2) **X-linked hypophosphatemic rickets** and **autosomal dominant hypophosphatemic rickets** are X-linked dominant disorders in which the primary abnormality is renal loss of phosphate. They are caused by gene mutations that affect the proximal tubular reabsorption of phosphate. Relative deficiency of calcitriol production is also present. Supraphysiologic doses of calcitriol, together with phosphate, may raise the serum phosphate level, decrease the bony abnormalities of rickets, and increase growth.

(3) In **Fanconi's syndrome,** renal tubular defects may lead to the loss of phosphate as well as calcium, glucose, and amino acids, with resulting osteomalacia.

d. **Gastrointestinal disorders.** Any disease or surgical procedure that leads to malabsorption and steatorrhea may reduce the absorption of calcium, phosphate, and vitamin D; osteomalacia may result.

e. **Tumors** such as hemangiopericytomas and giant cell tumors of bone may produce a humoral substance that causes phosphaturia and osteomalacia; the syndrome (**"oncogenic osteomalacia"**) is cured by removal of the tumor.

3. **Pathophysiology**

a. The **common defect** in the various diseases associated with osteomalacia is the **lack of calcium and phosphorus for mineralization of bone matrix.**

(1) Circulating phosphate levels are usually low, because of either decreased gastrointestinal absorption or excessive renal excretion.

(2) Calcium levels may be low, but they are often normal because of compensatory parathyroid hyperactivity.

b. **Rickets is caused by defective mineralization of bone before closure of the cartilaginous growth plates.** Deformity occurs because of pressure on weakened growth plates and on the abnormally soft shafts of the long bones. After closure of the growth plates, only osteomalacia can occur, with defective mineralization of mature lamellar bone.

c. Histologically, bone biopsy shows an excess of unmineralized bone matrix, which is seen as an increase in the volume and thickness of osteoid seams covering the bone surfaces.

4. **Clinical features**

a. **Pain and tenderness** are common in affected areas of the skeleton, especially the spine, ribs, pelvis, and lower extremities.

b. **Muscle weakness** is common, affecting particularly the proximal muscles of the legs.

c. **Skeletal deformities and fractures** occur in severe cases.

(1) The long bones may bow because of the softening of the skeleton.

(2) Rickets in children is associated with widening of the epiphyses; swelling of the wrists, knees, ankles, and costochondral joints; bowlegs; and disturbances in growth.

5. **Laboratory findings**
   a. **Radiographs** may show **decreased bone density** and coarsening of the trabecular pattern. **Looser's zones** are radiolucent bands that are perpendicular to the periosteal surface, caused by pseudofractures.
   b. Although laboratory abnormalities depend on the cause and the severity of the osteomalacia, they often include **low serum phosphate, low or normal serum calcium, and increased serum alkaline phosphatase levels.**
6. **Therapy**
   a. **Treatment of the primary disorder** is sometimes possible (e.g., correction of a bowel disorder causing malabsorption or removal of a tumor causing osteomalacia).
   b. **Vitamin D** is usually the mainstay of treatment.
      (1) In simple vitamin D deficiency, a physiologic dose of 400 U vitamin D daily may be all that is needed.
      (2) Large doses of calcitriol, which does not require biochemical transformation to achieve full activity, may be needed in the uncommon syndromes caused by altered metabolism or action of vitamin D or renal wasting of phosphate.

B Osteoporosis

1. **Definition.** Osteoporosis is a decrease in total bone volume, with changes in bone microarchitecture, leading to an increased susceptibility to fractures. Both increased bone resorption and decreased bone formation have been observed.
2. **Etiology**
   a. **Decreased bone mass at maturity**
      (1) After reaching its peak at approximately 30 years of age, bone mass declines throughout the remaining years of life. A low total bone mass at maturity, a relatively rapid rate of bone loss, or both contribute to the development of "involutional" osteoporosis.
      (2) **Genetic factors** affect the bone mass at maturity.
         (a) Men and blacks have greater peak bone mass and less osteoporosis; women and individuals of northern European ancestry have less bone mass at maturity and more osteoporosis.
         (b) A familial tendency toward osteoporosis has been observed.
   b. **Calcium deficiency.** Evidence suggests that calcium intake in American women is less than is needed to maintain calcium balance.
      (1) More than 75% of women older than 35 years of age fail to ingest the recommended daily allowance of 1000 mg calcium. Also, calcium absorption decreases in later life.
      (2) The need to maintain normal serum levels of calcium may lead to increased bone resorption through the action of PTH. (The effect of PTH on bone is to increase the rate of calcium and phosphate resorption, and when serum calcium levels are low, the secretion of PTH increases.)
   c. **Hormone changes.** When estrogen levels decrease, whether because of ovarian disease, oophorectomy, or normal menopause, the rate of bone loss is accelerated.
      (1) Estrogen deficiency may result in less stimulation of osteoblastic activity and may increase the sensitivity of bone to the action of PTH.
      (2) The increased rate of bone loss persists for 5–10 years after menopause.
      (3) Hypogonadism in men is also a cause of bone loss and increased risk of fractures.
3. **Classification**
   a. **Two types** of osteoporosis have been described.
      (1) **Postmenopausal osteoporosis** primarily affects women within 15 years of menopause. The loss of trabecular bone is accelerated, and fractures of the vertebrae, which consist mainly of trabecular bone, are common.

(2) **Senile osteoporosis** affects men and women older than 75 years of age, causing loss of both cortical and trabecular bone. Fractures of the hip, which is largely cortical bone, occur, as do vertebral fractures.

b. Secondary osteoporosis may be associated with glucocorticoid therapy or spontaneous Cushing's syndrome, malabsorption syndromes or malnutrition, multiple myeloma, and prolonged immobilization, among other conditions.

4. Clinical features

a. Fractures

(1) **Vertebral compression fractures** typically affect T8 to L3 and occur more commonly in women. They may cause acute back pain that persists for several months or may occur gradually and painlessly.

(2) **Hip fractures,** characteristically in the neck and intertrochanteric regions of the femur, are common in both men and women older than 65 years of age. Loss of function frequently results, and, because of complications, mortality rates may be as high as 20% within 1 year.

(3) The **distal radius** and other areas also may be the site of fractures.

b. Pain and deformity. Back pain may persist long after an episode of vertebral fracture because of spinal deformity and alteration of spinal mechanics. Several inches may be lost from height, and severe kyphosis may be the result of multiple vertebral fractures.

5. Diagnosis

a. Radiography of the spine may indicate a decrease in bone density, with accentuation of the cortical outlines and prominence of the trabeculae.

(1) However, approximately 30% of bone tissue must be lost before these abnormalities appear on plain radiographs.

(2) Wedge-shaped deformities and compression fractures on spinal radiographs also suggest the diagnosis of osteoporosis.

b. Dual-energy absorptiometry (DEXA), the best method for evaluating bone mineral density, is the reference standard for the diagnosis of osteoporosis. The World Health Organization has suggested that a diagnosis of **osteopenia** be made when bone mineral density is reduced by more than 1 standard deviation (SD) but less than 2.5 SD below the mean bone density of young adults, and **osteoporosis** when it is reduced by 2.5 SD or more.

c. Screening for osteoporosis

(1) Precise guidelines are not available, but many agree that DEXA of the spine and hip should be performed in women older than 65 years, and in postmenopausal women younger than 65 if they have additional risk factors for osteoporosis.

(2) **Risk factors for osteoporosis** include:

(a) Small stature and slender build

(b) Family history of osteoporosis

(c) White ancestry, especially northern European

(d) Early age of menopause

(e) Smoking

(f) History of prior fractures

6. Therapy. Weight-bearing exercise and adequate intakes of calcium and vitamin D should be encouraged in everyone to help prevent osteoporosis, and these measures remain important in the treatment of osteoporosis. The most potent pharmacologic agents are the bisphosphonates and parathyroid hormone. Other treatments that may be of somewhat lesser value are estrogen replacement therapy, raloxifene, and calcitonin.

a. Calcium

(1) Patients with osteoporosis should ingest at least 1500 mg elemental calcium daily.

(a) Because the average American takes in only approximately 500 mg calcium in food, calcium supplements should be given. Calcium carbonate tablets (e.g., 500 mg Os-Cal two or three times daily) are usually well tolerated.

(b) Exogenous calcium may reduce the rate of bone loss and the fracture rate in patients with osteoporosis whose usual calcium intake is inadequate.

(2) Prevention of osteoporosis requires attention to calcium intake in healthy persons. Recommended daily calcium intake is 1000 mg in women who are premenopausal or taking estrogen replacement and in men younger than 65. A higher intake (1500 mg daily) is recommended in younger individuals who have not yet achieved their peak bone mass, in older men, and in estrogen-deficient women. Achieving these goals often requires calcium supplementation.

b. Vitamin D. Pharmacologic doses (>1000 U daily) have not proved effective in the treatment of osteoporosis. But physiologic doses (400–800 U daily) have decreased the fracture rate in elderly persons who may be deficient in vitamin D because of poor nutrition and lack of exposure to sunlight. Vitamin D supplementation of 400–800 U daily should be recommended in such individuals and in patients with osteoporosis.

c. Bisphosphonates.

(1) These agents bind to hydroxyapatite in bone and decrease osteoclastic bone resorption. Because osteoblastic bone formation continues for a time while resorption cavities in bone are filled in, bone density may increase by 5%–10% over the next 1–2 years. After this, the main effect of antiresorptive agents such as the bisphosphonates is to prevent the gradual decrease in bone density that might otherwise occur.

(2) **Alendronate (Fosamax)** is very effective in increasing bone mineral density and in decreasing the fracture rate.

(a) The dose is 10 mg once daily or 70 mg once weekly, which is equally effective.

(b) The primary side effects are gastrointestinal symptoms, especially esophageal irritation and in a few cases esophageal erosion. To prevent these complications and to maximize drug absorption, patients must take alendronate with a full glass of water on arising in the morning; 30 minutes before the first meal, beverage, or other medication; and they must not lie down for 30 minutes after they swallow the pill.

(3) **Risedronate (Actonel)** is similar in effectiveness to alendronate but may be less likely to cause gastrointestinal side effects. The dosage is 5 mg once daily or 35 mg once weekly.

d. Parathyroid hormone. When the skeleton is exposed to constantly elevated blood levels of PTH, as in patients with primary hyperparathyroidism, bone density is lost and fracture risk is increased (**see III A 4 b**). But, paradoxically, when low doses of PTH are injected once every 24 hours, the opposite effect occurs: bone density increases and fracture risk falls. Apparently the intermittent exposure of bone to PTH favors bone formation over bone resorption.

(1) It is possible that PTH initially causes resorption of bone, which releases growth factors such as IGF-1 and transforming growth factor beta, which then stimulate osteoblastic bone formation. This hypothesis is favored by the observation that PTH loses much of its bone-forming activity if given together with alendronate, an inhibitor of bone resorption.

(2) **PTH (teriparatide, Forteo)** is given once daily in a dose of 20 mg by subcutaneous injection. Side effects may include hypercalcemia (requiring dose reduction or discontinuation of PTH), dizziness, and leg cramps

(3) The role of PTH in the treatment of osteoporosis is not yet known. Its effects on bone density are quite favorable compared with other available agents, but it is expensive, it requires daily injections, and long-term experience is lacking. It should be considered for use in patients with severe osteoporosis who are at high risk for fractures and who have not responded well to other treatments.

e. Estrogen. Estrogen replacement therapy after menopause has been an important measure for the prevention and treatment of osteoporosis. Recent findings, however, suggest that the risks associated with estrogen therapy, especially breast cancer, thromboembolism, and cardiovascular disease, are greater than previously thought (**see discussion in VI B 8 b**). Because other very effective treatment for osteoporosis is available, such as bisphosphonates and PTH, estrogen replacement therapy is assuming a secondary role in treatment of osteroporosis.

f. **Raloxifene.** A group of compounds called selective estrogen receptor modulators (SERMs) has been developed. Raloxifene, one member of this group, has beneficial effects on the skeleton similar to estrogen (although less potent) but without the undesired estrogenic effects on the breasts and uterus.

g. **Calcitonin.** This hormone, which is secreted by the parafollicular cells of the thyroid, inhibits osteoclast activity and decreases the rate of bone loss and fractures in osteoporosis. It may be given by injection or nasal spray (Miacalcin). The nasal spray delivers 200 units of calcitonin, the daily dose, in one puff; the patient alternates nostrils each day because of possible nasal irritation.

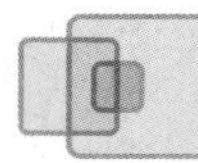

Study Questions

1. A 23-year-old man with gynecomastia is found to have a 47,XXY karyotype. This patient probably also has which of the following conditions?
   - A Abnormal liver function tests
   - B Low blood levels of luteinizing hormone (LH) and follicle-stimulating hormone (FSH)
   - C High blood levels of estrogen
   - D Azoospermia
   - E Enlargement of the testes

2. An 18-year-old woman is evaluated because she has never had a menstrual period. Pelvic examination is normal except that the vagina ends in a blind pouch. A karyotype is reported to be 46,XY. Which of the following diagnoses is most likely?
   - A Congenital adrenal hyperplasia
   - B Turner's syndrome
   - C Kallmann's syndrome
   - D Testicular feminization syndrome
   - E Polycystic ovary syndrome

3. A 55-year-old woman has been treated for type 2 diabetes with isophane insulin suspension (NPH), 35 U once daily before breakfast. Home glucose measurements on a typical day are 7:00 AM (fasting), 238 mg/dL; 11:00 AM, 155 mg/dL; 4:00 PM, 128 mg/dL; 8:00 PM, 125 mg/dL. Which of the following changes in insulin therapy would be reasonable?
   - A Increasing the dose of insulin
   - B Adding regular insulin to the dose of NPH
   - C Giving the dose in the evening instead of the morning
   - D Adding a dose of regular insulin before supper
   - E Adding a second dose of NPH insulin at bedtime

4. A 23-year old woman has noted a small amount of milk secretion from her nipples, and she has had no menstrual periods for the past 8 months. Serum prolactin is 78 ng/mL (normal, 5–25). Which test would be most sensitive for the diagnosis of a pituitary adenoma?
   - A Measurement of serum LH and FSH
   - B Visual field examination
   - C Computed tomography (CT) scan with contrast injection
   - D Magnetic resonance imaging (MRI) with gadolinium injection
   - E Insulin tolerance test

5. Successful treatment of primary hyperparathyroidism in a 60-year-old woman involves surgery to remove a single parathyroid adenoma. After surgery, she has a prolonged period of hypocalcemia, which requires continuous treatment with large doses of vitamin D and calcium. After 2–3 months, the need for vitamin D and calcium subsides, and she remains normocalcemic without treatment. This woman probably had which of the following conditions?
   - A Accidental destruction of the other three parathyroid glands
   - B Removal of the wrong parathyroid gland
   - C Severe pancreatitis caused by her hyperparathyroidism
   - D Unrecognized pseudohypoparathyroidism
   - E Severe bone disease

6. A 32-year-old woman is found on gynecologic evaluation to have multiple ovarian cysts. Which of the following findings would lead you to make the diagnosis of polycystic ovary syndrome?

A Deepening of the voice, enlargement of the clitoris, and a high testosterone level
B Oligomenorrhea, obesity, a high luteinizing hormone (LH) level, and a low follicle-stimulating hormone (FSH) level
C Amenorrhea, acne, a low LH level, and a low FSH level
D Facial hirsutism, acne, and increased urinary pregnanetriol, and 17-ketosteroids
E Facial hirsutism, normal menstrual periods, and normal levels of FSH, LH, and testosterone

7. A 58-year-old woman complains of fatigue, weight gain, and constipation. Examination shows puffy facial features and a slow return phase of the ankle reflex. Serum TSH is 52 mU/L (high), and free T_4 is 0.3 ng/dL (low). Treatment should be started with which of the following preparations?

A Thyroid extract
B Thyroglobulin
C Thyroxine (T_4)
D Triiodothyronine (T_3)
E T_4 and T_3

8. A 45-year-old woman complains of nervousness, palpitations, and a 10-pound weight loss. Her thyroid gland is enlarged twofold, and her heart rate is 108 beats/minute. Free T_4 is 3.6 ng/dL (high), and TSH is undetectable. You recommend radioiodine therapy, and the patient asks you about possible complications. What is the most common complication of radioiodine therapy?

A Thyroid storm
B Subacute thyroiditis
C Thyroid cancer
D Hypothyroidism
E Leukemia

9. A 60-year-old woman complains of headaches, and an MRI of the head is performed. This study shows a 9-mm microadenoma of the pituitary gland. Which of the following hormones is most likely to be elevated?

A Growth hormone (GH)
B Adrenocorticotropic hormone (ACTH)
C Prolactin
D Thyroid-stimulating hormone (TSH)
E Insulin-like growth factor I (IGF-I)

10. A 19-year-old woman complains of nervousness, a 5-pound weight loss, tremors, palpitations, and sweating for the past 4 weeks. The thyroid gland is slightly enlarged but not tender. The total T_4 level is 15.3 μg/dL (normal, 4.5–12.5), and T_3 uptake is 38% (normal, 25–35), and the TSH is undetectable. The best way to differentiate between the syndrome of painless thyroiditis and Graves' disease involves which of the following findings?

A Thyroid enlargement
B Low blood thyroid-stimulating hormone (TSH) levels
C Elevated blood thyroxine (T_4) levels
D Low radioactive iodine uptake
E Tenderness and pain involving the thyroid gland

11. A 23-year-old man is evaluated because of a diagnosis of hypogonadism. Which of the following findings would suggest primary testicular disease rather than hypothalamic or pituitary disease?

A Anosmia
B Increased levels of follicle-stimulating hormone (FSH) and luteinizing hormone (LH)
C Eunuchoidal habitus
D Loss of libido and sexual potency
E Decreased sperm number and motility

12. A 48-year-old man requires surgery to remove a tumor involving the hypothalamic area. The pituitary stalk is damaged by the surgery. Which pituitary hormone might be expected to increase rather than decrease in serum concentration?

A Adrenocorticotropic hormone (ACTH)
B Thyroid-stimulating hormone (TSH)
C Growth hormone (GH)
D Prolactin
E Luteinizing hormone (LH)

13. A 35-year-old woman has an MRI of the abdomen because of abdominal pain. Unexpectedly a 1-cm adenoma is seen in the left adrenal gland. In your evaluation of the patient, which of the following findings would be most compatible with a diagnosis of primary aldosteronism?

A Hyponatremia
B Acidosis
C Hypotension
D Hyperkalemia
E Suppressed plasma renin activity

Directions: *The response options for Items 14–16 are the same. You will be required to select one answer for each item in the set.*

A Graves' disease
B Hypothyroidism
C Pregnancy
D Subacute thyroiditis
E Nontoxic goiter

For each result of thyroid function tests, select the clinical condition with which it is most likely to be associated.

14. A 31-year-old woman complains of inability to sleep, weakness, heat intolerance, and sweating. The free T_4 is elevated, and the radioiodine uptake is low.

15. A 26-year-old woman with some fatigue is found to have an elevated total T_4 level and a low T_3 resin uptake.

16. A 21-year-old woman has noted weight loss and palpitations. Her free T_4 is increased, and the radioiodine uptake at 24 hours is 62% (normal, 10%–30%).

Directions: *The response options for Items 17–21 are the same. You will be required to select one answer for each item in the set.*

A Stimulation of an endocrine gland by autoimmune mechanisms
B Destruction of an endocrine gland by tumor, trauma, or infarction

C Destruction of an endocrine gland by autoimmune mechanisms
D Excessive production of hormone by an endocrine tumor
E Impaired sensitivity of peripheral tissues to normal circulating levels of a hormone

For each case, select the primary pathologic process most likely to cause the patient's disorder.

17. A 19-year-old woman has never had a menstrual period. On examination, it is found that her vagina ends in a blind pouch. She is a normal-appearing young woman, but her karyotype proves to be 46,XY.

18. A 55-year-old man complains of headaches, coarsening facial features and increasing shoe size. His growth hormone and IGF-1 levels are increased.

19. A 25-year-old woman has lost 15 pounds recently and is irritable and tremulous. Her free T_4 level and radioiodine uptake are elevated.

20. A 40-year-old man has noticed darkening of his skin in the past year, as well as weakness and generalized aching of his joints. An ACTH test is performed: baseline plasma cortisol is 5 μg/dL, rising to 6 μg/dL 1 hour after ACTH injection.

21. A 38-year-old woman has surgery to remove a pituitary macroadenoma that was causing visual impairment. Postoperatively she developed amenorrhea and fatigue, with low levels of LH, FSH, free T_4, and cortisol.

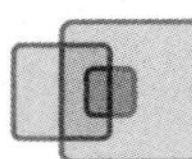

Answers and Explanations

1. **The answer is D** [VII A 2 b (1) (a)]. The 47,XXY karyotype indicates Klinefelter's syndrome. Elevation of gonadotropin levels, small testes, and gynecomastia also are common findings in Klinefelter's syndrome.

2. **The answer is D** [VI A 1 a, 2 b, C 1 b; VII A 2 a (1)]. Patients with the testicular feminization syndrome have a normal male karyotype, and testes (located in the abdomen or groin) that produce testosterone. But because there is resistance of the tissues to the effects of testosterone, the external genitalia develop as female during fetal life. Congenital adrenal hyperplasia is not associated with a short vagina and blind pouch, both of which are typical of testicular feminization. Turner's syndrome (gonadal dysgenesis) is characterized by a 45,X karyotype. Kallmann's syndrome is more common in men than in women and is often accompanied by anosmia and cleft palate. Polycystic ovary syndrome usually causes secondary, not primary, amenorrhea, and this patient has none of the other typical clinical features (e.g., oily skin, obesity, or hirsutism).

3. **The answer is E** [IV A 8 d (4) (b)]. The pattern of glucose levels suggests that the dose of isophane insulin suspension (NPH) is effective during the day but does not retain its effect until the next morning. Giving more insulin in the morning or adding regular insulin would risk causing hypoglycemia in the afternoon and evening when glucose levels are already at a satisfactory level. However, a second dose of NPH at bedtime would be expected to have its maximal action in the early morning, which is the time that an increased glucose-lowering effect is desired.

4. **The answer is D** [I A 1 b (3) (a), (4), c (1) (b)]. Magnetic resonance imaging (MRI) with gadolinium is the most sensitive test for the detection of pituitary adenomas. In fact, microadenomas may be seen in as many as 10%–20% of normal women. Oversecretion of LH and FSH is common, but many pituitary adenomas do not produce excessive amounts of these hormones. Impaired growth hormone (GH) response to insulin-induced hypoglycemia or visual field changes would occur only in those tumors that are large enough to interfere with normal pituitary function or to compress the optic chiasm. Computed tomography (CT) scans show very small adenomas, but MRI with gadolinium is even more sensitive.

5. **The answer is E** [III A 7 a (4)]. When primary hyperparathyroidism causes osteitis fibrosa cystica, the sudden correction of the primary hyperparathyroidism and consequent removal of the source of excessive parathyroid hormone (PTH) allows the skeleton to undergo rapid repair and remineralization, which creates a marked but self-limiting demand for calcium and phosphate. If the patient had hypoparathyroidism of this severity after surgery, the hypocalcemia would probably have been permanent, and the need for treatment would not have resolved.

6. **The answer is B** [VI C 1]. Polycystic ovary syndrome is characterized by a chronic lack of ovulation associated with symptoms of androgen excess and often with obesity. Severe virilization and marked testosterone elevation are more likely to be caused by an ovarian tumor or hyperthecosis. Neither a low luteinizing hormone (LH) level nor an increased urinary pregnanetriol concentration is characteristic of the polycystic ovary syndrome. Hirsutism without other clinical or laboratory abnormalities usually is diagnosed as "idiopathic hirsutism."

7. **The answer is C** [II B 4 a]. Thyroxine (T_4) is the agent of choice. Thyroid extract and thyroglobulin contain varying proportions of the two thyroid hormones, thyroxine (T_4), and triiodothyronine (T_3), making it difficult to adjust the dosage precisely. Preparations containing T_3 must be given several times

daily to maintain a normal blood level of T_3 because T_3 has a short half-life. However, T_4 has a long half-life and is converted to T_3 in the liver and elsewhere; hypothyroid patients taking the optimal dose of T_4 once daily have normal, stable blood levels of both T_4 and T_3.

8. The answer is D [II C 4 a (3) (c) (ii)–(iii)]. Hypothyroidism is present in 50% or more of patients treated with radioiodine 10–15 years after treatment. Thyroid storm and subacute thyroiditis are rare complications. No increased incidence of thyroid cancer, leukemia, or other malignancies has been attributed to radioiodine therapy.

9. The answer is C [I A 1 a (1), b (1), 4]. As many as 50% of all pituitary adenomas have been found to secrete prolactin, and blood prolactin levels should be measured in a patient suspected of having a pituitary tumor. Acromegaly due to growth hormone (GH) excess and Cushing's disease due to adrenocorticotropic hormone (ACTH) excess are considerably less common, and overproduction of thyroid-stimulating hormone (TSH) is rare. Insulin-like growth factor I is increased in acromegaly but is not elevated in most patients with pituitary tumors.

10. The answer is D [II D 3 a (2)]. Low radioactive iodine uptake is the most useful finding for distinguishing painless thyroiditis from Graves' disease. Inflammation and injury to thyroid cells, as well as a lack of thyroid-stimulating hormone (TSH), inhibit radioactive iodine uptake in painless thyroiditis, whereas the uninjured and immunoglobulin-stimulated thyroid cells in Graves' disease concentrate radioactive iodine at an increased rate. Enlargement of the thyroid gland and increased blood levels of thyroid hormone, with suppression of TSH, may occur in both Graves' disease and painless thyroiditis. The gland is not tender or painful in either condition.

11. The answer is B [VII A 1, 2]. Increased gonadotropin production indicates primary testicular failure with negative-feedback stimulation of the hypothalamic–pituitary axis. Anosmia is sometimes associated with hypothalamic failure to secrete gonadotropin-releasing hormone (GnRH). Hypogonadism, whether caused by hypothalamic–pituitary disease or testicular disease, is associated with loss of libido and potency and abnormalities of sperm production. A eunuchoidal habitus results from continued growth of long bones due to delay in testosterone-induced epiphyseal closure; therefore, eunuchoidal habitus can result from either primary testicular failure or hypothalamic–pituitary disease.

12. The answer is D [I A 4 a (2)]. Hypothalamic hormones reach the anterior pituitary gland through the portal vessels in the pituitary stalk, and injury to the stalk may remove the pituitary from the influence of the hypothalamus. Most of the hypothalamic factors are stimulatory: ACTH production is stimulated by corticotropin-releasing hormone (CRH), TSH by thyrotropin-releasing hormone (TRH), growth hormone by growth hormone-releasing hormone (GHRH), and LH by gonadotropin-releasing hormone (GnRH). But the main effect of the hypothalamus on prolactin production is inhibitory, through the action of dopamine. When injury to the pituitary stalk prevents dopamine and other hypothalamic factors from reaching the pituitary gland in high concentration, prolactin production increases, in contrast to the fall in levels of other pituitary hormones.

13. The answer is E [V D 2, 3 a (3) (b)]. Plasma renin activity suppression is a clinical feature of primary aldosteronism. Excess circulating levels of aldosterone increase the reabsorption of sodium, in exchange for potassium and hydrogen ions, in the distal tubules. The resulting expansion of extracellular fluid volume causes suppression of plasma renin activity and eventually causes hypertension. The loss of potassium and hydrogen ions causes a tendency toward metabolic alkalosis.

14–16. The answers are: 14-D [II D 1 c], **15-C** [II A 1 a], **16-A** [II C 3 d]. In subacute thyroiditis, injured thyroid follicular cells release thyroid hormone, raising the blood level of thyroxine (T_4). Radioactive iodine uptake is low, however, because the injured follicular cells are unable to trap iodine normally.

Also, thyroid-stimulating hormone (TSH) is suppressed by the increased level of circulating thyroid hormone, and this further reduces the radioactive iodine uptake.

In pregnancy, the high estrogen levels cause increased production of T_4-binding globulin. This raises the serum level of total T_4 and lowers the triiodothyronine (T_3) resin uptake. However, patients remain euthyroid, because the serum free T_4 level remains normal.

In Graves' disease, the follicular cells trap increased amounts of iodine and produce increased amounts of thyroid hormone. Therefore, both the radioactive iodine uptake and the serum T_4 level are elevated. This combination of findings indicates hyperthyroidism, caused either by Graves' disease or by toxic nodular goiter.

17–21. The answers are: 17-E [VI A 2 a], **18-D** [I A 3 a], **19-A** [II C 1 a], **20-C** [V C 1 a (1)], **21-B** [I A 2 a]. The testicular feminization syndrome results from the inability of tissue to respond to testosterone and other androgens. If not stimulated by androgens, the fetal external genitalia develop as female organs. Therefore, a genetic male infant with testes and normal male testosterone levels is born with female external genitalia and is considered to be a normal female.

The usual cause of acromegaly is a growth hormone (GH)–secreting pituitary adenoma. Rarely, GH-releasing hormone production by an islet-cell adenoma may cause acromegaly.

Graves' disease is caused by abnormal stimulation of the thyroid gland by thyroid-stimulating immunoglobulin. This immunoglobulin G (IgG) antibody binds to receptors for thyroid-stimulating hormone (TSH). This hormone then stimulates growth and hormone production by the thyroid follicular cells.

Addison's disease is most commonly caused by atrophy of the adrenal cortex. Antiadrenal antibodies are often present. Other evidence of autoimmunity such as antibodies against other tissues and the presence of other autoimmune diseases also are common findings. Hemorrhage into the adrenals and infectious agents (e.g., tuberculosis) are less common causes of Addison's disease.

Pituitary tumors may compress normal tissue, impairing its function. Surgical removal of the tumor may further damage the hypothalamus and pituitary gland. Ischemic infarction at childbirth (Sheehan's syndrome) and various destructive, infectious, and granulomatous lesions also cause hypopituitarism.

chapter **10**

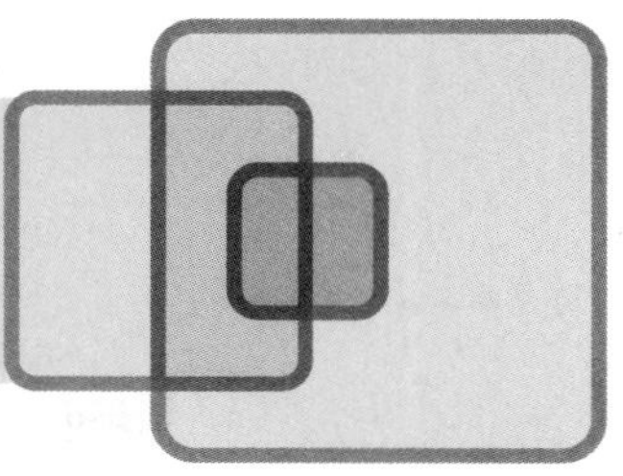

Rheumatic Diseases

S. CHRISTINE KOVACS, ALLEN R. MYERS, DONALD P. GOLDSMITH

I APPROACH TO THE PATIENT WITH JOINT PAIN

A A **thorough history and physical examination** are the cornerstone in the evaluation of patients with joint complaints (Figure 10–1).

1. **Step 1.** Is the pain joint-centered or localized in the periarticular tissues involving muscle, nerve, bursa, tendons, or ligaments?
2. **Step 2.** Is the arthritis inflammatory or noninflammatory? An important clue in making this distinction is the duration of morning stiffness. Morning stiffness lasting more than 1 hour is suggestive of an inflammatory arthritis (e.g., rheumatoid arthritis), whereas stiffness lasting less than 1 hour is suggestive of a noninflammatory arthritis (e.g., osteoarthritis).
3. **Step 3.** How many joints are affected? What is the pattern of joint involvement? The answers to these questions also provide important diagnostic clues. For example, if the pattern of joint involvement is asymmetric, it is more likely that the patient has a seronegative spondyloarthropathy, especially if there is associated inflammatory back pain. If the polyarthritis is symmetric, the differential diagnosis should include rheumatoid arthritis, systemic lupus erythematosus (SLE), polymyositis, and scleroderma.

B A variety of **laboratory tests** are helpful in making rheumatologic diagnoses. Some are also useful in assessing disease activity in individual patients.

1. **Acute phase reactants.** A heterogeneous group of proteins (e.g., fibrinogen) is synthesized in response to inflammation.
   a. **Erythrocyte sedimentation rate (ESR).** This indirect nonspecific measure of systemic inflammation is calculated by observing the distance in millimeters that red blood cells (RBCs) fall in a specific tube in 1 hour. A rise in acute phase reactants increases the dielectric constant of plasma, resulting in the dissipation of inter-RBC repulsive forces. This leads to increased aggregation of RBCs, which causes them to fall faster, thus elevating the erythrocyte sedimentation rate. Useful in the diagnosis of temporal arteritis and polymyalgia rheumatica (PMR), it can be helpful in assessing disease activity in these conditions as well as in rheumatoid arthritis. If the erythrocyte sedimentation rate is greater than 100 mm/hr, infection and malignancy should be considered in the differential diagnosis.
   b. **C-reactive protein (CRP).** The liver produces this pentameric protein as an acute phase reactant in response to interleukin-6 (IL-6) and other cytokines. C-reactive protein is more specific than the erythrocyte sedimentation rate; it rises and falls more quickly. A highly sensitive CRP assay also may reflect abnormalities that lead to atherothrombotic events and is used as a predictor of cardiovascular risk.
2. **Rheumatoid factor.** This antibody to the Fc portion of immunoglobulin G (IgG) can be in the IgG or IgA class, but it is usually in the IgM class. Only IgM rheumatoid factor is routinely measured by clinical laboratories. Although it is found in 75%–85% of patients with rheumatoid arthritis, it also occurs in other conditions characterized by chronic immune stimulation such as infection, malignancy, and hyperglobulinemic states. Rheumatoid factor is also present in some

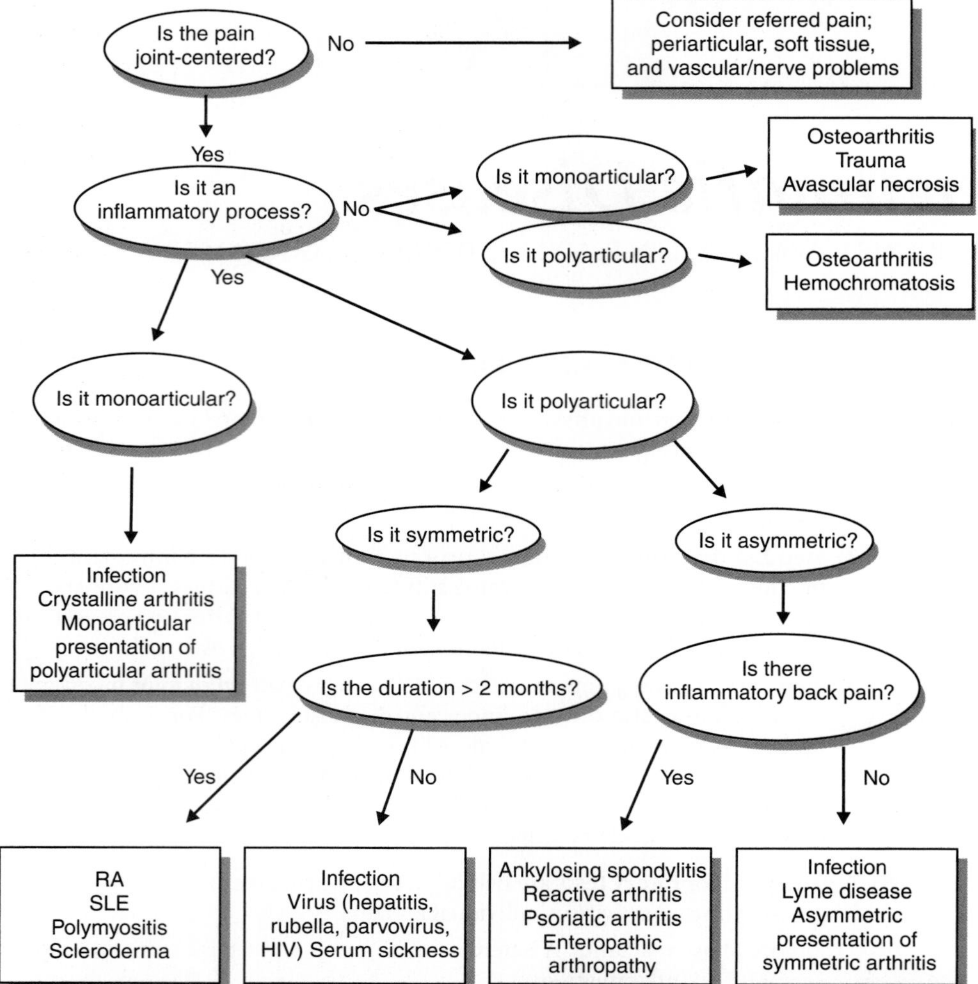

FIGURE 10–1 Approach to the patient with joint pain. The evaluation of chronic polyarthritis requires a careful history and physical examination for identification of systemic features typical of other illnesses that can cause arthritis. Selected laboratory and radiographic testing also can be helpful. *RA* = rheumatoid arthritis; *HIV* = human immunodeficiency virus; *SLE* = systemic lupus erythematosus.

normal individuals, typically those people over 70 years of age. Anti-cyclic citrullinated peptide (anti-CCP) [citrulline is an amino acid derived from arginine residues and is present in inflamed rheumatoid arthritis synovium] has an equivalent sensitivity as IgM rheumatoid factor (RF) in diagnosing rheumatoid arthritis but is more specific and may be more useful in the diagnosis of early rheumatoid arthritis.

3. **Antinuclear antibody (ANA).** These antibodies, which are directed against a variety of nuclear antigens, are characteristic of a number of connective tissue disorders.
   a. A positive ANA is found in 95% of patients with SLE and, to a lesser extent, in those with other conditions such as discoid lupus erythematosus, scleroderma, Sjögren's syndrome, rheumatoid arthritis, Raynaud's phenomenon, and vasculitis. Other inflammatory disorders associated with a positive ANA include chronic active hepatitis, interstitial pulmonary fibrosis, tuberculosis, human immunodeficiency (HIV) disease, and malignancy. Certain med-

ications such as procainamide, isoniazid, and hydralazine have been associated with ANA positivity and antihistone antibodies. ANA should not be performed as a screening test, because it is positive in approximately 5% of the normal population (usually in low titers).

b. A positive ANA must be interpreted in light of the patient's age, sex, and clinical and drug history. The level of the ANA titer is also important; titers of 1:160 or greater are associated with greater clinical significance than lower titers. Specific patterns of fluorescence are associated with certain antibodies (Table 10–1).

4. **Complement.** A measurement of activity (CH50) or antigens (C3 or C4) can be used as an indirect measure of immune complex formation. Serum complement may be decreased as a result of decreased production (hereditary deficiency or liver disease) or increased consumption [e.g., in SLE, vasculitis, mixed cryoglobulinemia, sepsis, subacute bacterial endocarditis (SBE)]. Typically, levels of C3 and CH50 are low in active SLE. In patients with angioedema, a low C4 may be a clue to the diagnosis of hereditary angioedema (C1 esterase inhibitor deficiency).
5. **Antineutrophil cytoplasmic antibody (ANCA).** This antibody, which is directed against specific proteins in the cytoplasm of neutrophils, is detected by indirect immunofluorescence. Two ANCA patterns exist: cytoplasmic (c-ANCA) characterized by diffuse staining and perinuclear (p-ANCA) with a perinuclear pattern. The protein recognized by the c-ANCA is proteinase-3, and the protein recognized by p-ANCA is most commonly myeloperoxidase.
   - **a. c-ANCA** is strongly associated with Wegener's granulomatosis, with a sensitivity of 30%–90% and a specificity of 98%. It has been shown to be helpful in following disease activity.
   - **b. p-ANCA** is associated with idiopathic crescentic glomerulonephritis, Churg-Strauss syndrome, microscopic polyangitis, polyarteritis nodosa, and other immunologic disorders.
6. **Antiphospholipid antibody.** Detection in serum involves an enzyme-linked immunosorbent assay (ELISA) for IgG or IgM anticardiolipin antibodies, positive lupus anticoagulant, or a false-positive Venereal Disease Research Laboratory (VDRL) test. A prolonged partial thromboplastin time (PTT) or prothrombin time (PT) may be a clue to the presence of antiphospholipid antibodies. Detection should be further evaluated by a mixing study, which should not correct

TABLE 10–1 Immunologic Specificity of Individual Antinuclear Antibodies (ANAs)

Antibody Reactivity to Antigen	Pattern	Disease Association
Antibody to dsDNA (measured by Farr assay)	Rim; homogeneous	Specific for SLE, useful for monitoring disease activity, especially lupus nephritis
Antibody to histones	Homogeneous	Drug-induced lupus, but also may be present in SLE
Antibody to extractable nuclear antigens	Speckled	
Smith		Specific for SLE but present in only 25% of patients
RNP		UCTD
SSA/SSB		Common in Sjögren's syndrome and SLE SSA associated with photosensitivity SSB associated with neonatal lupus and congenital heart block
Antibody to centromere	Centromere	CREST

RNP = Ribonucleoprotein; UCTD = Undifferentiated connective tissue disease; CREST = limited scleroderma with calcinosis, Raynauds, esophageal dysmotility; sclerodactyly, and telangiectasia.

with a 1:1 mix with normal plasma. Other tests for the lupus anticoagulant include a dilute activated PTT, the kaolin clotting time, and the Russell viper venom test. The anti-β_2 glycoprotein 1, which can be positive in patients with clotting abnormalities when other clotting tests are normal, is positive in patients with antiphospholipid antibody syndrome. Anticardiolipin antibodies have also been identified in patients with infections such as HIV and may be drug-induced, with no increase in the incidence of clotting.

7. **Cryoglobulin.** There are three major types of cryoglobulins, which are immunoglobulins or immunoglobulin complexes that spontaneously precipitate at low temperatures. **Type I** is associated with a single monoclonal immunoglobulin; **type II** is associated with a mixed cryoglobulin with a monoclonal component that acts as an antibody against polyclonal IgG; and **type III,** also associated with mixed cryoglobulins, is more difficult to detect because it is usually present in small quantities and precipitates more slowly. Mixed cryoglobulins are frequently present in patients with underlying connective tissue diseases. In addition, they have also been found in infections, lymphoproliferative diseases, liver diseases [hepatitis B (HBV) and hepatitis C (HCV)], and renal diseases such as proliferative glomerulonephritis.
8. **Lyme borreliosis antibody testing.** Measurement usually involves indirect immunofluorescence or ELISA. Because of the high frequency of false-positive results, the Western blot assay is ordered as a confirmatory test.
9. **Human leukocyte antigen (HLA).** A strong association of HLA-B27 has been noted in Caucasian individuals with seronegative spondyloarthropathies such as ankylosing spondylitis. Unfortunately, HLA-B27 is found in 3% of healthy African Americans and 8% of healthy Caucasians; thus, its diagnostic utility is limited. HLA determinations of the DR locus, specifically the DR4 alleles that mark more severe disease in rheumatoid arthritis, are currently only research tools, but may have broader applications in the future.
10. **Synovial fluid analysis.** Analysis of the synovial fluid is critical in the evaluation of arthritis. It is helpful in distinguishing an inflammatory arthritis from a noninflammatory arthritis, and it is essential in confirming the presence or absence of gout or pseudogout and in the evaluation of a possible septic joint.
    a. If only a small amount of fluid is obtained, it should be sent for Gram stain and culture. The leukocyte count can help classify the fluid into groups (Table 10–2). The finding of a hemarthrosis should raise suspicion for trauma, bleeding diathesis (e.g., anticoagulant use, hemophilia, tumors, scurvy), and pigmented villonodular synovitis.
    b. Compensated polarizing microscopy is an invaluable technique for examining synovial fluid. Needle-shaped monosodium urate crystals are strongly negatively birefringent, appearing yellow when their long axis is parallel to that of the compensator. Calcium pyrophosphate dihydrate (CPPD) crystals are usually rhomboid-shaped with blunt ends, and they appear blue when their long axis is parallel to that of the compensator.

TABLE 10–2 Synovial Fluid Categorization

Category	WBC Count (per mm^3)	Percent of PMNs	Associated Conditions
Normal	0–200	< 10 (> 50 monocytes)	
Noninflammatory	200–2000	< 20	Osteoarthritis, trauma
Inflammatory	2000–50,000	20–70	RA, gout, pseudogout, SLE
Pyarthrosis	> 50,000	> 70	Septic arthritis; but can be seen in gout, RA, and reactive arthritis

II APPROACH TO THE PATIENT WITH LOW BACK PAIN

A The low back comprises 5 lumbar vertebrae, the sacrum, the coccyx and the iliac bones. The lower nerve roots and lumbar sacral and pudendal plexuses arise from these areas. The spinal cord ends at L1, and below this level the cauda equina fills the canal down to the coccyx. In most patients with low back pain (LBP), the cause is benign, and neurologic impairment does not occur. Despite a thorough history and physical examination, an exact anatomic structure responsible for the pain often is not identified; however, the examination is crucial in ensuring that the cause is not something that requires emergent evaluation or specific treatment (Figure 10–2). Fortunately, most cases of acute LBP improve within a few days to a few weeks.

1. **Step 1.** Is the back pain originating from the spine and its supporting tissues or referred from a distant site? A list of the most common cause of referred LBP is shown in Table 10–3.
2. **Step 2.** Is the pain related to the **cauda equina syndrome?** This syndrome is characterized by LBP, bladder dysfunction (urinary retention or flow incontinence), saddle anesthesia, loss of sphincter tone, and lower extremity weakness. It may be associated with a tumor or a large central disc herniation and requires an emergent neurologic consultation and magnetic resonance imaging (MRI).
3. **Step 3.** Are other **warning signs** present to suggest an underlying systemic disease? In addition to the warning signs for the cauda equina syndrome, questions and examination should be directed with the consideration of a potential underlying malignancy, infectious process, or inflammatory spondyloarthropathy.
4. **Step 4.** The **pattern of pain radiation** is helpful in determining the etiology. Most patients with back pain will have pain without radiation. The pain in this case is often referred to as muscular or ligamentous "strain," although a precise anatomic diagnosis often cannot be made. Pain that radiated to the posterior thigh has a different differential than pain that radiates to the anterior thigh, and careful consideration of these entities (listed in the flow diagram) should be pursued when taking the history and doing the physical examination. Pain that radiates all the way down to the foot is most likely attributable to a radicular problem such as herniated disc. Often in these patients, the foot discomfort is more bothersome than the back pain.
5. **Step 5.** If there is no evidence of an underlying systemic disease, referred pain, or neurologic compromise, treatment should be aimed at pain relief with anti-inflammatory medications. Narcotics should be avoided. Data have shown that the addition of muscle relaxants can be used in breaking the pain-spasm-pain cycle. Bed rest is not indicated beyond the first 1 or 2 days. Physical therapy also may be helpful in the acute and chronic setting.
6. **Step 6.** If the pain persists beyond 6 weeks, further evaluation is indicated. Depending on the history and examination findings, further blood work such as a complete blood count (CBC), ESR, and alkaline phosphatase may help rule out systemic disease or an underlying inflammatory arthritis. Imaging studies with plain x-rays may be helpful but unfortunately are not very sensitive for identifying early metastatic disease or infection. At any point, if the index of suspicion is high for underlying pathology or if neurologic abnormalities are present, further imaging studies with CT, MRI, or bone scan are indicated. Electromyogram (EMG) also may help in delineating nerve injury.
7. **Nonorganic back pain** is often a difficult situation to deal with. Red flags that may alert the clinician to the presence of nonorganic back pain include physical examination findings that are inconsistent or change when the patient is distracted.

B **Imaging plays an important role in the evaluation process.**

1. **Plain x-rays** offer the advantage of being readily available and relatively inexpensive. Anteroposterior and lateral views are good for evaluating alignment, disc and vertebral body height. They also can provide a crude assessment of bone density. Oblique views can help evaluate for spondylolysis. The major disadvantage is the inability to evaluate the soft tissues, in addition to

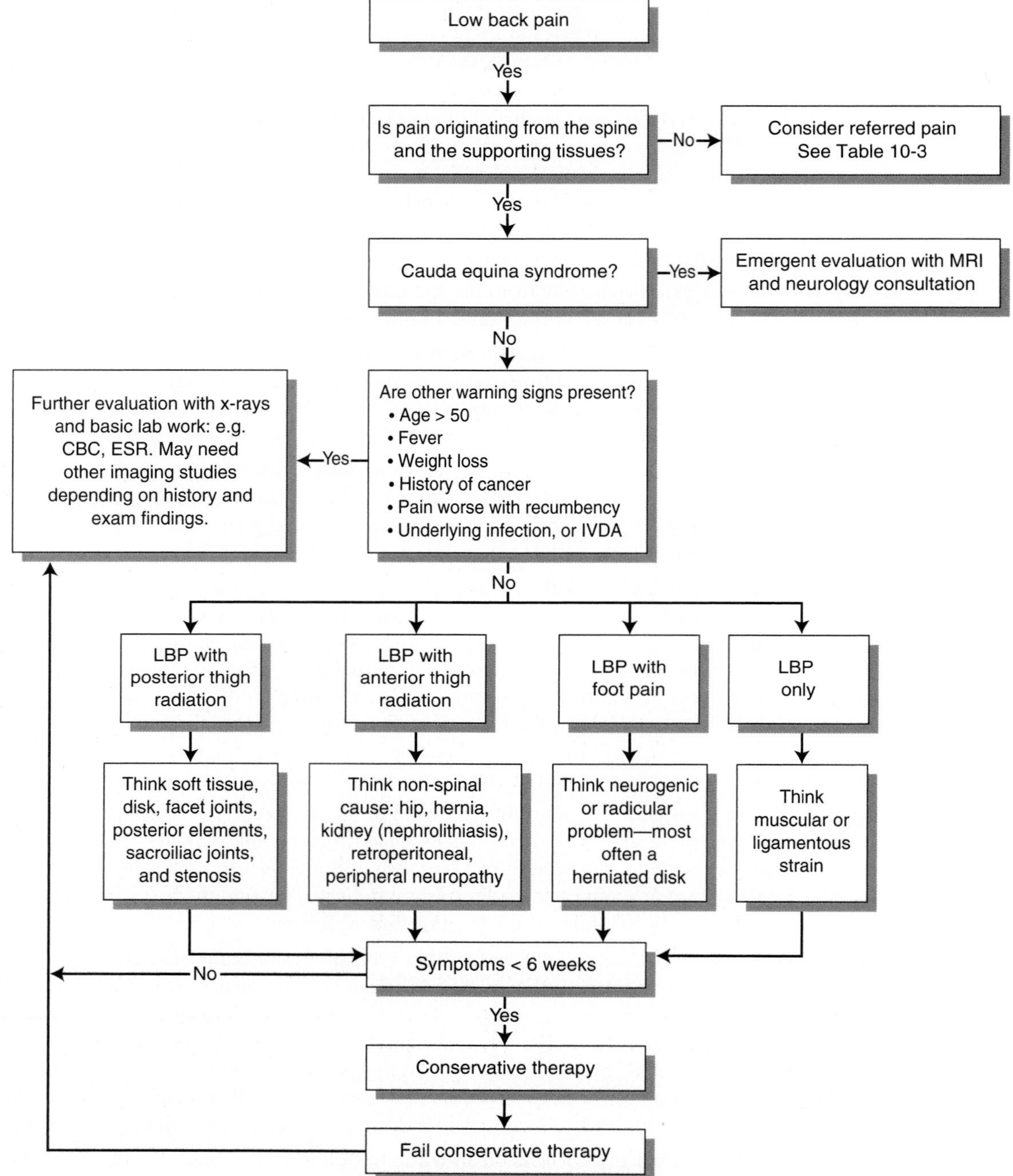

FIGURE 10–2 Approach to the patient with low back pain. LBP = low back pain; CBC = complete blood count; ESR = erythrocyte sedimentation rate.

TABLE 10–3 Causes of Referred Low Back Pain

Retroperitoneal
Tumors—lymphomas
Hematomas—especially in anticoagulated patients
Fibrosis
Renal—pyelonephritis, perinephric abscess, nephrolithiasis
Intra-abdominal
Pancreatitis
Cholecystitis
Perforated ulcer
Abdominal aortic aneurysm
Pelvic disease
Prostate—prostatitis, prostate cancer
Uterine—carcinoma, endometriosis

the fact that it may not reveal any abnormality in the early stages of an infectious process or malignancy. As with virtually any of the imaging modalities, plain x-rays may identify abnormalities that are not responsible for symptoms.

2. **Computed tomography (CT) scans** are good for evaluating the bony architecture. They may be helpful in evaluating nerve root impingement and spinal stenosis, especially if related to facet degenerative changes.
3. **Magnetic resonance imaging (MRI)** may be better than CT for spinal imaging given the better soft tissue contrast and better visualization of the ligaments, vertebral bone marrow, and the contents of the spinal canal. One of the strong advantages is the ability to detect early metastatic disease, and it is good at delineating the extent of an infection. Additionally, MRI can visualize the intrathecal and extrathecal nerve roots. The fact that MRI cannot directly visualize bone makes it not as useful in evaluating an acute fracture, especially of the posterior elements.
4. **Bone scan** imaging may be useful in detecting occult fractures, infections, and bony metastasis and in differentiating these changes from degenerative changes. It also may be helpful in determining the acuity of a suspected compression fracture. Triple phase bone scanning is routinely used to aid in the diagnosis of osteomyelitis.

C Common causes of back pain.

1. **Acute**
   a. **Strain** is a common diagnosis given to acute back pain in the absence of a precise anatomic diagnosis. It is usually related to overuse. The pain is typically localized, involving muscles or ligaments.
   b. **Disc herniation** usually results from abnormal forces on the spine. An inflammatory response with chemical irritation may occur in addition to compression of the nerve root with resultant radiculopathy. The pain is usually exquisite, extending from the back unilaterally down one leg. Depending on the exact location of the herniation, slight variations in lower extremity pain, numbness, and tingling occur.
   c. **Vertebral compression fracture** usually presents with acute intense localized pain with reduced spinal motion lasting up to 6 weeks. If the pain persists or is associated with constitutional symptoms, further evaluation for malignancy or myeloma should be considered.
2. **Chronic**
   a. **Spinal stenosis** is a narrowing of the neural canal, usually the result of degenerative changes such as bulging disc and hypertrophic osteoarthritis of the facet joints. As the patient attempts

to walk, the congestion in the affected region of the spinal cord results in compressed roots and impaired nerve function. Symptoms usually include progressive ambulation difficulties with associated leg heaviness, numbness, and associated leg or back pain. **Lower extremity claudication** and the presence of a **stooped forward posture** when walking are key findings. The physical examination is usually not that remarkable except for the absences of an S_1 reflex. Other conditions to exclude: diabetic neuropathy or vascular claudication.

i. **Central canal stenosis** is usually the result of osteophytes on the inferior articular process encroaching medially or the result of ligamentum flavum hypertrophy and annular bulging.

ii. **Neuroforaminal stenosis** occurs when osteophytes on the superior articular process enlarge anteriorly and medially, or osteophytes form at the vertebral margin, thus encroaching on the lateral nerve root canal.

b. **Degenerative arthritis and discogenic low back pain** present with chronic back pain that is worse with prolonged weight bearing or excessive use. There are typically no radicular findings.

c. **Spondylolisthesis** refers to the subluxation of one vertebra relative to the inferior vertebra. In many instances this is an anatomic x-ray finding not necessarily associated with pain.

d. **Ankylosing spondylitis** is an inflammatory arthritis affecting the axial skeleton and sacroiliac joints. The main feature is inflammatory back pain. (See section IV).

e. **Discitis.** A disc space infection should be considered in the chronically ill patient or the patient with a known systemic infection with associated back pain. Prompt treatment is indicated to prevent vertebral collapse and the formation of an epidural abscess.

III RHEUMATOID ARTHRITIS

A Definition

Rheumatoid arthritis is a chronic immunologically mediated inflammatory disorder of unknown cause that is typified by synovial cell proliferation and inflammation with subsequent destruction of adjacent articular tissue. The presentation is characterized by polyarticular, symmetrical joint involvement as well as characteristic extra-articular involvement. **Rheumatoid factor** frequently is present in the serum of affected individuals (see I B 2).

B Epidemiology

1. **Prevalence and sex distribution.** As many as 1% of adults may have rheumatoid arthritis, depending on the criteria used for diagnosis. Clinically meaningful forms of disease are less common—0.5% of women and 0.1% of men have forms of the illness that require ongoing treatment.

2. **HLA associations.** There is an increased prevalence of the B-cell alloantigen HLA-DR4 in patients with rheumatoid arthritis. Evidence also suggests that similar amino acid sequences coded by the third hypervariable region of the DR β chain may explain disease association with HLA-DR4, -DR1, -Dw4, -Dw14, and -Dw15. HLA-DR4 positivity also is a marker for more severe rheumatoid arthritis.

3. **Seropositivity for rheumatoid factor.** Patients who have rheumatoid factor in their serum appear to have a different illness from patients who are seronegative. Seropositive patients tend to have more severe disease, more erosions, and more extra-articular features.

C Etiology

No single factor or agent is known to cause rheumatoid arthritis. Presumably, an initial insult (possibly infectious) interacting with the host's genetically established immune responses determines whether an initial synovitis is suppressed or perpetuated.

1. **Extra-articular agent.** The earliest inflammatory changes in the rheumatoid joint involve inflammation and occlusion of small subsynovial vessels, suggesting that the agent is carried in the circulation to the joint.

2. **Infectious agent.** An infectious etiology is suggested because virus-like particles often are present in synovial biopsies early in the disease course and because polyarthritis occurs in association with

several human and animal bacterial or viral illnesses. However, no direct evidence of infection has been discovered. Symmetrical inflammatory arthritis can occur in patients who have parvovirus or rubella virus infections, although the joint findings are not typically persistent.

3. **Genetic factors.** A genetic susceptibility to altered immune responses probably is important in rheumatoid arthritis. There is no known association of HLA-A or HLA-B haplotypes with the disease, but a significant association exists between rheumatoid arthritis and the presence of HLA-DR4 and related alloantigens of the major histocompatibility complex (MHC). The presence of these and other genetically coded immune response alloantigens may be important in modulating the host's cellular and humoral immune responses to potential etiologic agents.
4. **Effects of Epstein-Barr virus on the immune response.** Rheumatoid arthritis patients have a defect in their ability to regulate B cells infected with Epstein-Barr virus. The virus may act as a polyclonal activator of B-cell autoantibody production in rheumatoid arthritis and, as such, may play a role in perpetuating (not initiating) the disease.

D **Pathogenesis** An unknown etiologic agent (an exogenous one or an "altered" endogenous one) initiates a nonspecific immune response. Most evidence supports the hypothesis that RA is a T-cell–driven disease (Figure 10–3). Not listed on the figure is the production of immunoglobulin (RF) from B cells and activation of vascular adhesion molecules. Once the T cells are activated, they infiltrate the synovium, which leads to vascular and synovial cell proliferation (pannus formation) and eventual resorption of cartilage and bone destruction. Immune-response genes also may be important in determining the type, intensity, and chronicity of the immune response.

1. **Synovial cell interactions** are important for maintenance of articular inflammation. Intercellular messages are transmitted by **cytokines** (small proteins that can amplify and perpetuate inflammation in the rheumatoid joint). In general, cytokines produced by macrophages and fibroblasts [IL-1, IL-6, granulocyte–macrophage colony-stimulating factor (GM-CSF), tumor necrosis factor-α (TNF-α)] are present at high concentrations in the rheumatoid synovium. **Lymphokines**

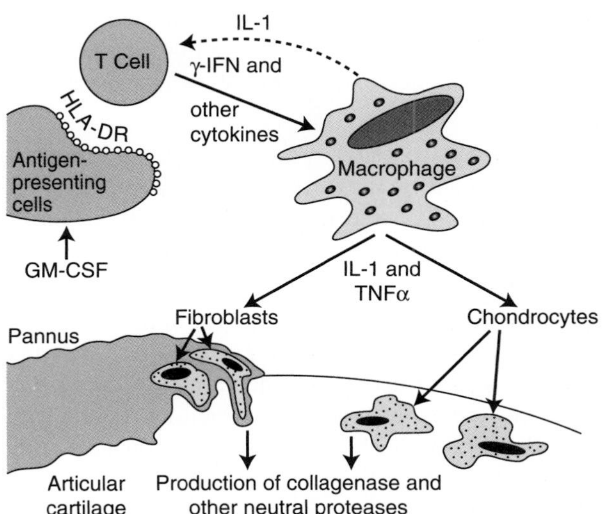

FIGURE 10–3 Stimulatory or agonist effects of cytokines on cell-cell interactions in rheumatoid synovitis. T cells, macrophages, and fibroblasts are all present in the rheumatoid pannus. Enzymes, such as collagenase and other neutral proteases, are secreted by synovial fibroblasts and chrondrocytes, and result in destruction of cartilage, bone, and periarticular structures. IL = 1-interleukin-1; γ-IFN = γ-interferon; GM-CSF = granulocyte-macrophage colony-stimulating factor; TNFα = tumor necrosis factor α. (From Arend W, Dayer J-M: Cytokines and cytokine inhibitors or antagonists in rheumatoid arthritis. *Arthritis Rheum* 1990;33(3):306.)

produced by T cells [IL-2, IL-3, IL-4, interferon-γ (IFN-γ)] are present at relatively low concentrations, apparently suppressed by substances secreted by macrophages.

a. **Macrophage–T cell.** Macrophage and helper T cell (Th) [CD4⁺ T-cell] interrelationships are central to the amplification of the immune response. Macrophages process antigen and present it (in association with class II MHC molecules) to the CD4⁺ T cells, which then become activated by the interaction. Certain bacterial toxins or retroviral proteins can function as **superantigens,** binding to HLA molecules or T-cell receptors directly, potentially amplifying the inflammatory response.

b. **Th cell–B cell.** Activated CD4⁺ T cells stimulate B cell proliferation and differentiation into antibody-producing cells. These B cells are factories for the production of **rheumatoid factor.**

c. **CD4⁺ T cell–synovial cell.** CD4⁺ T cells produce soluble mediators (lymphokines) that can modulate the function of synovial lining cells, both macrophage-like and fibroblast-like. The fibroblast-like lining cell produces collagenase and prostaglandins, and stimulates the growth of connective tissue; all of these effects may be important in the destructive effects of the synovial pannus.

d. **Macrophage–endothelial cell.** The ingrowth of capillaries is important to the propagation of synovitis and the later growth of the pannus. Macrophages signal capillary endothelial cells to migrate and replicate by heparin-binding growth factors.

2. **Synovial fluid phase**

a. In contrast to the mononuclear response in the synovium, the **neutrophil** is the predominant cell in rheumatoid synovial fluid inflammation. Numerous factors chemotactic for neutrophils are present in the inflamed joint [e.g., complement fragments, leukotriene B4 (LTB4), immune complexes with rheumatoid factor]. These neutrophils release oxygen-free radicals and hydrolytic enzymes that can destroy cartilage.

b. Bacterial, mycobacterial, and human **heat shock proteins** share many antigenic sequences and may cross-react with collagen or proteoglycan molecules; therefore, an infection could generate autoimmunity or localize an inflammatory response to a joint.

3. **Rheumatoid factor** (see I B 2). The synovium produces immunoglobulin, most of which consists of IgM and IgG rheumatoid factors. These immunoglobulins form complexes in synovial fluid, which activate complement. Rheumatoid factor aggregates also are ingested by macrophages (which secrete cytokines) and neutrophils (which release digestive enzymes); both actions amplify inflammation.

4. **Chronic proliferative lesion.** A mass of fibroblastic, vascular, and inflammatory cells (i.e., the **pannus**) accumulates at the margin of the synovial membrane–cartilage border. The destructive capacity of rheumatoid arthritis is associated with the formation of pannus and the production of monokines such as TNF, IL-1, and metalloproteinases. Together these abnormalities lead to the destruction of bone and cartilage.

5. **Joint destruction.** Destructive change is unpredictable, and counteracting anti-inflammatory cytokines [e.g., transforming growth factor-β (TGF-β)] can downregulate the effects of IL-1 and TNF-α, leading to cartilage repair and immunosuppression. Native IL-1 inhibitors perform similar functions. These compensatory mechanisms often are overwhelmed, and unimpeded synovial inflammation and proliferation lead to loss of cartilage and bone as well as anatomic distortion. Secondary degenerative joint disease results from the continued inflammation and alterations in biomechanical joint loading forces.

E Clinical features

1. **Synovitis**

a. **Articular involvement.** Fairly symmetrical, bilateral joint involvement is typical, often sparing the distal interphalangeal (DIP) joints of the hands. Metacarpophalangeal (MCP), proximal interphalangeal (PIP), and wrist joint involvement is so common as to be part of the American Rheumatism Association (ARA) revised criteria for disease diagnosis (Table 10–4).

b. **Tendon and ligament involvement.** Synovial linings outside joints can be involved as well.
   (1) **Palmar flexor tendinitis** can cause carpal tunnel syndrome.
   (2) **Rotator cuff tendinitis** can cause shoulder pain and limitation of motion.
   (3) **Atlantoaxial ligament involvement** in the cervical spine can lead to instability between the C1 and C2 vertebrae and potential neurologic complaints.

2. **Extra-articular features** (Table 10–5) more often exist in patients who are seropositive for rheumatoid factor and patients who have more severe and established disease.
   a. **Rheumatoid nodules** are the most common features of extra-articular disease and are found in 20%–25% of patients. These firm, subcutaneous masses typically are found in areas of repetitive trauma (e.g., the extensor surfaces of the forearm), although they also can appear in the viscera (e.g., lungs).
   b. **Eye involvement** also is common. **Keratoconjunctivitis sicca** is seen in 10%–15% of rheumatoid arthritis patients who have a secondary form of Sjögren's syndrome (see X). The often subtle inflammation of scleritis or episcleritis occurs less commonly.
   c. **Other organ involvement** is noted in Table 10–5.

F Diagnosis Rheumatoid arthritis is a sustained, inflammatory polyarthritis that typically is symmetrical in distribution. It is a diagnosis of exclusion of other forms of polyarthritis, which it may imitate. The patient must have arthritis for at least 6 weeks to eliminate viral syndromes or other causes of nonsustained polyarthritis. Finding rheumatoid factor in the serum is useful in patients who have

TABLE 10–4 The 1987 American Rheumatism Association Revised Criteria for the Classification of Rheumatoid Arthritis

Criterion	Definition
1. Morning stiffness	Morning stiffness in and around the joints, lasting at least 1 hour before maximal improvement
2. Arthritis of three or more joint areas	At least three joint areas simultaneously have had soft tissue swelling or fluid (not bony overgrowth alone) observed by a physician; the 14 possible areas are right or left PIP, MCP, wrist, elbow, knee, ankle, and MTP joints
3. Arthritis of hand joints	At least one area swollen (as defined above) in a wrist, MCP, or PIP joint
4. Symmetrical arthritis	Simultaneous involvement of the same joint areas (as defined in 2) on both sides of the body (bilateral involvement of PIPs, MCPs, or MTPs is acceptable without absolute symmetry)
5. Rheumatoid nodules	Subcutaneous nodules over bony prominences, or extensor surfaces, or in juxta-articular regions, observed by a physician
6. Serum rheumatoid factor	Demonstration of abnormal amounts of serum rheumatoid factor by any method for which the result has been positive in <5% of normal control subjects
7. Radiographic changes	Radiographic changes typical of rheumatoid arthritis on posteroanterior hand and wrist radiographs, which must include erosions or unequivocal bony decalcification localized in or most marked adjacent to the involved joints (osteoarthritis changes alone do not qualify)

For classification purposes, a patient is said to have rheumatoid arthritis if he or she has satisfied at least four of these seven criteria. Criteria 1 through 4 must have been present for at least 6 weeks. Patients with two clinical diagnoses are not excluded. Designation as classic, definite, or probable rheumatoid arthritis is **not** to be made. PIP = proximal interphalangeal; MCP = metacarpophalangeal; MTP = metatarsophalangeal. (Reprinted from Arnett FC, Edworth SM, Bloch DA, et al: American Rheumatism Association 1987 revised criteria for the classification of rheumatoid arthritis. *Arthritis Rheum* 1988;31:315.)

TABLE 10–5 Extra-articular Features of Rheumatoid Arthritis

Skin
Nodules (20%–25% of patients)
Vasculitis (purpura)
	Nerve
	Entrapment (carpal tunnel syndrome)
	Vasculitis
	  Distal sensory neuropathy
	  Mononeuritis

Eye Sicca complex (10%–15% of patients) Episcleritis Scleritis	**Blood** Anemia of chronic disease Thrombocytosis Felty's syndrome
Heart Pericarditis Myocarditis (rare) Valve dysfunction (rare)	**Metabolism** Amyloidosis

Lung
Pleural effusion
Interstitial fibrosis
Nodules
	Vessels
	Vasculitis
	  Skin
	  Nerve
	  Viscera (rare)

other features of inflammatory polyarthritis, but as many as 40% of patients with rheumatoid arthritis do not have this marker initially.

1. **History.** Patients with rheumatoid arthritis often have **prolonged** (> 1 hour) **morning stiffness. Pain in involved joints** typically is worse in the morning. **Constitutional complaints** (weight loss, anorexia, fatigue) are common.
2. **Physical examination.** Classically involved joints are the **wrists** and the **MCP** and **PIP joints of the hand;** DIP joints are typically spared, as is the axial skeleton except for the cervical spine. **Soft tissue swelling,** rather than bony enlargement, is typical around involved joints, unless secondary degenerative changes have occurred; limitation of joint motion and warmth may be noted. **Rheumatoid nodules** often are present in highly expressed disease; they can be found over extensor prominences, especially near the olecranon.
3. **Laboratory findings.** The complete blood count (CBC) may reveal a **normocytic, normochromic anemia** of chronic disease, leukocytosis, and thrombocytosis. These findings along with an increased erythrocyte **sedimentation rate** reflect chronic inflammation. **Rheumatoid factor** (see I B 2). Synovial fluid findings reflect mild-to-moderate inflammation; leukocyte counts are 5000–25,000/mm^3 and consist mainly of neutrophils.
4. **Radiographic findings.** Early characteristics include **soft tissue swelling** and loss of bone in periarticular areas **(periarticular osteopenia).** Signs of sustained inflammation include loss of bone at joint margins **(erosions)** and **joint space narrowing** as a result of cartilage loss.
5. **Differential diagnosis** (see Figure 10–1). Because rheumatoid arthritis is one of many illnesses characterized by chronic polyarticular inflammation, diagnosis relies on excluding other such illnesses and searching for symmetrical periarticular soft tissue swelling and inflammatory characteristics of rheumatoid arthritis.
   a. **Nonarticular disorders.** Fibromyalgia is a syndrome of generalized aching and tenderness in specific soft tissue areas, without joint involvement or inflammation. Tendon, neurologic, and vascular complaints also may mimic joint pain.
   b. **Noninflammatory disorders**
      (1) **Osteoarthritis** usually causes bony rather than soft tissue swelling, and the involved joints typically are the DIP and PIP joints of the hand, the hips, and the knees. The lumbar and

cervical spine can be involved as well. Constitutional and inflammatory complaints are absent, and synovial fluid leukocyte counts are less than 2000/mm^3.

(2) **Metabolic disorders** (e.g., CPPD, hemochromatosis, Wilson's disease) cause bony degenerative change in atypical joints (e.g., MCP joints).

c. **Axial joint inflammation.** Inflammation of the axial spine (especially the sacroiliac joints) is characteristic of the spondyloarthropathies, and inflammatory back pain due to **sacroiliitis** should be sought. Inflammatory back pain is insidious, day-after-day pain starting in the sacroiliac area and typically associated with prolonged morning stiffness. It is worsened with rest and improved by exercise, the opposite of mechanical low back pain. The absence of sacroiliac joint involvement does not rule out these disorders, but its presence makes spondyloarthropathy likely.

d. **Oligoarticular presentations.** Certain illnesses must be considered more strongly when the initial inflammatory presentation involves four or fewer joints and is asymmetrical. These disorders include crystal diseases, infectious arthritis (e.g., Lyme disease, gonococcemia, endocarditis, rheumatic fever), and spondyloarthropathies (e.g., reactive arthritis, psoriatic arthritis).

e. **Polyarticular presentations.** It also is important to consider inflammatory disorders that initially involve four or more joints and are fairly symmetrical. Although rheumatoid arthritis is the prototype, many other illnesses must be distinguished, based on clinical features or organ involvement not typical of rheumatoid arthritis. Detailed history and physical examination with basic laboratory data are critical in distinguishing among disorders that feature polyarthritis.

(1) **Other rheumatic diseases** (e.g., lupus, scleroderma, polymyositis/dermatomyositis, PMR, vasculitis) are distinguished by the features of the primary illness.

(2) **Viral disorders** (e.g., rubella, HBV, parvovirus infection) are distinguished by a typical rash, serologic markers, or organ involvement.

(3) **Malignancies** may manifest as long bone pain, digital clubbing, and periostitis mimicking polyarthritis (hypertrophic osteoarthropathy) or as paraneoplastic polyarthritis.

(4) **Sarcoidosis** exhibits mediastinal adenopathy on chest radiograph and usually erythema nodosum when it includes a polyarthritis.

(5) **Amyloidosis** is associated with Congo red–positive deposits in typical organs, subcutaneous tissue, and joints.

G Therapy In all patients with rheumatoid arthritis, an attempt is made to control pain and reduce inflammation without causing undesirable side effects. Preservation of joint function and the ability to maintain lifestyle are important long-term goals.

1. **Nonpharmacologic therapy**

a. **Patient education.** Educating patients about the disease process is particularly important in chronic diseases such as rheumatoid arthritis, in which compliance with instructions and drug treatment is critical to the outcome.

(1) **Description of the illness.** The various disease courses of rheumatoid arthritis must be described, emphasizing that most patients do well if they are appropriately treated. The chronicity and intermittency of symptoms must be discussed so that patients understand that spontaneous fluctuations in an extended disease course are normal. Patients must be educated about the systemic nature of the disease process, so that both they and their families understand that fatigue, malaise, and weight loss often accompany this illness.

(2) **Rest and exercise.** Patients should be advised to rest or splint acutely involved joints to reduce inflammation. Brief periods of bed rest may be useful in patients with severe polyarticular exacerbations, and regular naps may help patients deal with the fatigue of rheumatoid arthritis. Conversely, exercises to strengthen muscles surrounding involved joints should be encouraged when the arthritis is under good control. All joints should be put through a full range of motion once daily to prevent contractures.

b. Physical medicine

(1) Patients may benefit from coordination of their nonpharmacologic treatment by **physiatrists.**

(2) **Physical therapists** can help patients strengthen weakened muscle groups to protect damaged joints. They can show patients range-of-motion exercises that prevent joint contractures.

(3) **Occupational therapists** can help patients obtain devices to assist them, can construct splints for involved joints, and can aid in rehabilitating patients for activities of daily living and employment.

2. Pharmacologic therapy. Nonsteroidal anti-inflammatory drugs (NSAIDs) and corticosteroids are often used to provide relatively prompt control of pain and inflammation, but these drugs do not alter disease progression. Although the course of rheumatoid arthritis can be quite variable, most patients undergo a relentless progressive course requiring the use of disease-modifying antirheumatic drugs (DMARDs). Corticosteroids, which are not viewed as first- or second-line therapies, often are used intra-articularly for disease flareups or orally to help patients who are waiting for a DMARD to take effect.

a. NSAIDs. Aspirin is the prototypic drug of this class. Nonacetylated salicylates also have been developed, which cause less suppression of prostaglandin synthesis.

(1) **Mechanism of action.** The primary mechanism of action is the inhibition of cyclo-oxygenase, with a resultant decrease in prostaglandin production. More recent data have shown that cyclo-oxygenase exists in two isoforms: COX-1 and COX-2. COX-1 is expressed constituitively in monocytes/macrophages, the central nervous system (CNS), gastric mucosa, kidneys, and platelets, where it is responsible for many of the "housekeeping" activities. However, COX-2 is tightly regulated and produced during inflammation. Most of the available traditional NSAIDs inhibit both COX-1 and COX-2.

(2) **Use.** NSAIDs are used to control pain and inflammation by the mechanisms explained above. Most patients use them in combination with DMARDs.

(3) **Toxicity.** Because the majority of NSAIDs inhibit both COX-1 and COX-2, they are more likely to produce gastrointestinal ulceration. Typical toxicities include dyspepsia, peptic ulcers (primarily of the stomach), hypertension, renal dysfunction, and bleeding. Some patients are placed on misoprostol or omeprazole to reduce the risk of ulcers. Clinical hepatitis and bone marrow toxicity are very rare. The COX-2 agents have been shown to have a lower incidence of peptic ulceration and do not inhibit platelet function.

(4) **COX-2 inhibitors.** Celecoxib, rofecoxib, and valdecoxib are COX-2–specific inhibitors. These agents are purported to have a lower incidence of gastrointestinal ulceration compared with traditional NSAIDs, and, because of the lack of effect on platelets, can be used in patients on anticoagulation. They still must be used with caution in patients with renal insufficiency. They also may cause increased fluid retention (particularly rofecoxib); recent data have suggested an increased cardiovascular mortality in patients receiving rofecoxib. Sulfa-allergic patients should not take celecoxib.

b. Corticosteroids. These drugs have potent anti-inflammatory effects but equally potent and predictable toxicities. They are used most commonly in rheumatoid arthritis to control serious extra-articular manifestations (e.g., vasculitis).

(1) **Systemic administration.** In rare situations such as severe progressive disease, prednisone doses no higher than 5–10 mg once daily in the morning may be used to allow continued functioning. Continual attempts to taper the dosage should be made.

(2) **Local instillation.** Injectable corticosteroid preparations can be instilled into one or two joints inflamed "out of phase" with other involved joints. These injections should be performed only occasionally, because cartilage loss may result from frequent injections into the same joint.

c. **Traditional DMARDs.** **D**isease-**m**odifying **a**ntirheumatic **d**rugs are critical in the armamentarium in the treatment of rheumatoid arthritis. These agents need to be started early in the course of disease (ideally within 3 months). The hallmark of these agents is their ability to halt progression of disease, such as the development of erosions. Commonly used DMARDs in the treatment of rheumatoid arthritis are listed in Table 10–6. Although side effects of many of these medications may be serious, in most instances they are mild, predictable, and can be managed. In most cases, the risk of ongoing progressive disease outweighs the potential risk of medication toxicity. Each of the agents may be used alone or in combination.

(1) **Monotherapy.**

(a) **Methotrexate** is considered the gold standard for the treatment of rheumatoid arthritis, usually given as a weekly oral dose. At higher doses, subcutaneous injections of methotrexate may be given to improve absorption and diminish side effects. Concurrent daily folic acid administration helps prevent common side effects, including mucosal ulcers, dyspepsia and cytopenias. The use of leucovorin may be necessary if the side effects do not respond to the folic acid. The starting dose of methotrexate is 7.5–10 mg weekly, escalating to a maximum of 25 mg weekly. If a patient has

TABLE 10–6 DMARDS Used in the Treatment of Rheumatoid Arthritis

Agent	Mechanism of Action	Side Effects/ Potential Toxicity	Monitoring
Hydroxychloroquine sulfate	Unknown, but likely inhibits lysosomal enzymes and macrophage function	Macular damage	Eye examination every 6 months to 1 year
Methotrexate	Inhibits dihydrofolate reductase, thereby inhibiting purine (DNA) synthesis	Myelosuppression, hepatic fibrosis/cirrhosis, pulmonary inflammation/ fibrosis, stomatitis	CBC, AST, ALT, creatinine, albumin every month for 6 months then every 6–8 weeks. Baseline CXR and hepatitis profile
Leflunomide	Inhibits dihydro-orotate dehydrogenase, thereby inhibiting pyrimidine (DNA) synthesis	Diarrhea, elevated liver enzymes, alopecia, teratogenicity requiring elimination protocol with cholestyramine	Same as MTX but no baseline CXR
Sulfasalazine	Inhibits prostaglandins and chemotaxis	Gastrointestinal intolerance, hematologic cytopenias, hepatotoxicity, contraindicated if sulfa allergic	CBC every 2–4 weeks for first 3 months then every 3 months Baseline G6PD testing
Azathioprine	A prodrug converted to 6-mercaptopurine (6MP) subsequently converted into thiopurine nucleotides decreasing de novo synthesis of purines	Myelosuppression, hepatotoxicity, lymphoproliferative disorders; caution with concurrent use of allopurinol	CBC every 1–2 weeks with changes in dose and every 1–3 months thereafter
Cyclosporine	Inhibits T-cell activation	Renal insufficiency, anemia, hypertension hypertrichosis, paresthesias, gingival hypertrophy; caution—multiple medication interactions	Creatinine every 2 weeks until stable then monthly, periodic CBC, LFTs

underlying liver disease or pulmonary disease or uses alcohol, methotrexate may not be appropriate to use.

(b) **Leflunomide** acts similarly to methotrexate and requires essentially the same monitoring strategy except there is no risk of pulmonary toxicity; thus, it is often used when methotrexate cannot be used, such as in a patient with underlying pulmonary disease.

(c) **Sulfasalazine,** although not approved by the Food and Drug Administration (FDA) for use in rheumatoid arthritis, has been used because of its modest effectiveness and rather low incidence of toxicity. In Europe it is typically used as a first-line agent.

(d) Less commonly used agents as monotherapy in the treatment of RA include **gold, azathioprine, and hydroxychloroquine sulfate.**

(2) **Combination therapy** is used if patients have had a suboptimal response to monotherapy. Commonly used combinations are listed below.

(a) **Methotrexate and hydroxychloroquine sulfate**

(b) **Methotrexate and hydroxychloroquine sulfate and sulfasalazine**

(c) **Methotrexate and leflunomide**

(d) **Methotrexate and cyclosporine**

d. Biologic DMARDs. As the pathogenesis of rheumatoid arthritis and the various immune and inflammatory mediators have been identified, novel agents in the treatment of RA have been developed. These include the development of three tumor necrosis factor (TNF) antagonists in addition to anakinra, which binds to the interleukin-1 receptor. The common biologic DMARDs available for use are listed in Table 10–7.

(1) **TNF inhibitors.** TNF is a pro-inflammatory cytokine that is synthesized by a variety of cell types. Normally, small amounts of TNF are present, but overproduction triggers a cascade of inflammatory reactions. **Etanercept, infliximab,** and **adalimumab** are FDA-approved for the treatment of RA. Each of these agents has been shown to be effective in reducing signs and symptoms and inhibiting the progression of structural damage in rheumatoid arthritis. They may be used alone or in combination (usually with methotrexate).

TABLE 10–7 Biologic DMARDs Used in the Treatment of Rheumatoid Arthritis

Agent	Mechanism	Dose and Routine	Side Effects
Etanercept	Recombinant fusion protein binds to soluble TNF receptor and leukotriene (LT)	25 mg SQ twice weekly or 50 mg once weekly	Flu-like symptoms, injection site reactions, infections, exacerbation of heart failure, possible demyelination, unknown long-term malignancy risk, autoimmune phenomena
Infliximab	Chimeric monoclonal antibody that binds TNF	3 mg/kg IV over 2 hours every 8 weeks	Infusion may be associated with fever, nausea, flushing, hypertension or hypotension; infection, autoimmune phenomena, exacerbation of CHF, possible demyelination, unknown long-term malignancy risk
Adalimumab	Recombinant human IgG1 monoclonal antibody which binds TNF	40 mg SQ every other week	Injection site reactions, infections, lupus-like symptoms, unknown long-term malignancy risk
Anakinra	Binds to interleukin-1 receptors (IL-1RA)	100 mg SQ daily	Injection site reactions, infections, unknown long-term malignancy risk

(a) **Safety considerations.** Serious infectious and opportunistic infections (TB) have been seen with all of the TNF antagonists. TNF has been shown to be necessary in granuloma formation that is critical in the control of TB. Thus, inhibition of TNF has been associated with reactivation of TB. Screening for TB is recommended before initiating treatment with these agents.

(2) **Anti-cytokine therapy. IL-1RA (anakinra)** controls RA through a different mechanism than that of the TNF blocking agents but has similar safety concerns, including increased risk of infections (not TB), neutropenia, and the potential development of malignancies. No data as yet suggest higher risk of demyelination or development of congestive heart failure.

e. **Assessment of response.** The effectiveness of drug therapy is judged by assessing the reduction in a number of factors: morning stiffness, constitutional complaints, number of swollen and tender joints, and erythrocyte sedimentation rate. Sometimes improvement in anemia of chronic disease and resolution of thrombocytosis occurs. Indices that measure a patient's ability to perform activities of daily living (health assessment questionnaires) also are used.

f. As new therapies are being introduced, the treatment strategy has been evolving. In 2002, the American College of Rheumatology revised the management guidelines.

3. **Surgery.** Arthroplasties or total joint replacements may be appropriate to relieve pain or help restore function in structurally damaged joints.

H Prognosis

1. **Prognostic factors** (Table 10–8). Inability to control disease activity and the presence of several of these indicators suggests a poor prognosis and the need for more aggressive therapy, perhaps including combinations of second-line agents and low-dose oral glucocorticoids.
2. **Mortality.** Many patients with rheumatoid arthritis have a reasonably good prognosis if they respond well to treatment. Adequate early response to the use of NSAIDs or antimalarials, with or without corticosteroids, is a favorable prognostic sign. However, recent epidemiologic studies suggest that patients with severe and persistent disease have increased mortality rates. In those with the most highly expressed forms of rheumatoid arthritis, mortality rates approach those found in stage IV congestive heart failure (CHF) or stage IV Hodgkin's disease. The increase in mortality appears to be the result of organ compromise caused by extra-articular features (e.g., interstitial lung disease, cardiac complications, vasculitis), complications of drug therapy, and infection.

IV SPONDYLOARTHROPATHIES

A Unifying characteristics (Table 10–9) The spondyloarthropathies are a group of inflammatory arthritides distinct from rheumatoid arthritis, including ankylosing spondylitis, reactive arthritis,

TABLE 10–8 Indicators of Poor Prognosis in Patients with Rheumatoid Arthritis
Many persistently inflamed joints
Poor functional status (ascertained from health-assessment questionnaires)
Low formal education level
Rheumatoid factor positivity
HLA-DR4 positivity
Extra-articular disease
Persistently elevated acute phase reactants (e.g., erythrocyte sedimentation rate)
Radiographic evidence of erosions

TABLE 10–9 Distinguishing Characteristics of Spondyloarthropathies
Axial skeleton inflammation
Enthesis inflammation, often asymmetric
Characteristic extraskeletal features
Uveitis or conjunctivitis
Urethritis
Inflammatory bowel lesions
Psoriasis-like rashes
Association with HLA-B27
Absence of rheumatoid factor

psoriatic arthritis, and arthritis associated with inflammatory bowel disease. Typical distinguishing features include:

1. **Clinical features**
   a. **Skeletal**
      (1) **Axial.** As a group, the spondyloarthropathies prominently involve the axial skeleton, particularly the **sacroiliac joints.** With the exception of the cervical spine, the axial skeleton is not commonly involved in rheumatoid arthritis.
      (2) **Appendicular.** Inflammatory arthritis of the appendicular skeleton also occurs in these disorders, but the involvement tends to be oligoarticular and asymmetrical. In contrast, rheumatoid arthritis usually is polyarticular and symmetrical.
      (3) **Enthesis.** In both the axial and appendicular skeletons, inflammation of tendon and ligament sites of attachment to bone is common (e.g., costochondritis, Achilles tendinitis, plantar fasciitis). Tendon inflammation is less prominent in rheumatoid arthritis.
   b. **Extraskeletal**
      (1) **Nodules.** Rheumatoid nodules are not found in the spondyloarthropathies.
      (2) **Internal organ involvement.** The typical eye involvement in the spondyloarthropathies (conjunctivitis and anterior uveitis), cardiac involvement (aortitis), and genitourinary involvement (urethritis and prostatitis) are much different from the usual extra-articular features of rheumatoid arthritis.
   c. **Laboratory findings.** Several cardinal laboratory features of chronic inflammation (i.e., anemia, thrombocytosis, elevated gamma globulin levels) are not commonly present in the spondyloarthropathies as they are in rheumatoid arthritis. Although the erythrocyte sedimentation rate may be increased, it is not a good measure of disease activity. Rheumatoid factor typically is absent.
   d. **Radiographic findings.** The characteristic changes seen radiographically are those of periosteal new bone formation at the site of the enthesopathic lesions (see IV A 3), both at axial locations (in the form of **syndesmophytes**) and appendicular locations. Although erosive changes can occur, they occur most typically in the axial skeleton (in the hips, sacroiliac joints, and shoulders).
   e. **Therapeutic response.** Several second-line agents commonly used in treating rheumatoid arthritis (e.g., gold, hydroxychloroquine) have no proven role in the treatment of spondyloarthropathy, with the exception of psoriatic peripheral arthropathy. Sulfasalazine and methotrexate are used for both rheumatoid arthritis and the appendicular arthritis of the spondyloarthropathies.

2. **Genetic factors.** The strong association of the histocompatibility antigen **HLA-B27** with clinical expression of the spondyloarthropathies provides evidence for genetic transmission of these disorders. However, HLA-B27 is found in 8% of Caucasians, 3% of African Americans, and less than

1% of Asians, and all of these individuals do not develop spondyloarthropathies. Conversely, spondyloarthropathies are found in patients who are HLA-B27 negative (10%–20%).

a. This relationship also is a major reason for grouping these disorders. The independent correlation of HLA-B27 with specific features of spondyloarthropathies (e.g., sacroiliitis, aortitis, anterior uveitis) explains both the clinical overlap among these diseases and their familial clustering.

b. The role of the antigen in disease causation is not understood. However, transgenic rats can express HLA-B27 on cell surfaces and develop clinical features of spondyloarthropathies, so this gene product is clearly involved in disease causation or perpetuation.

c. Disease susceptibility is also associated with other unknown genes, perhaps T-cell receptor genes, accounting for the 10-fold increase in risk associated with HLA-B27 positivity in spondylitis families.

3. **Pathology**

a. The basic pathologic lesion in the spondyloarthropathies is an **enthesopathy**—an inflammation occurring at the site where ligaments and tendons attach to bone. This type of inflammation explains the frequency of sacroiliitis, ascending spinal lesions, and peripheral tendon lesions (e.g., Achilles tendinitis).

b. Although inflammatory synovitis that is indistinguishable from rheumatoid synovitis can be seen in these illnesses, it is not typically as widespread, chronically active, and potentially destructive as it is in rheumatoid arthritis (psoriatic arthritis mutilans is a notable exception).

4. **HIV-related spondyloarthropathic disease.** Some HIV-positive patients have spondyloarthropathic illness often with features of **reactive arthritis (Reiter's syndrome)** or **psoriatic arthritis.** However, most commonly, they have skin, joint, and tendon features that prevent easy classification into one illness or the other, suggesting that these spondyloarthropathic illnesses have a common pathogenesis (see XIV A 1).

B Specific disorders

1. **Ankylosing spondylitis**

a. **Definition.** Ankylosing spondylitis is the spondyloarthropathy that is most closely associated with inflammation of the axial skeleton. **Back pain** and **limited spinal mobility** caused by **sacroiliitis** and variable ascent of the inflammation up the spine dominate the clinical expression of this disease.

b. **Epidemiology**

(1) **Prevalence.** Ankylosing spondylitis may be as common as 1 in 1000 Caucasian individuals, because the frequency of disease parallels the prevalence of the HLA-B27 antigen in the population (see IV A 2). The frequency of ankylosing spondylitis is lower in African-American and Asian populations, paralleling the prevalence of the antigen in these groups.

(2) **Gender distribution.** Ankylosing spondylitis may be as prevalent in women as in men if radiographic findings of sacroiliitis are considered to be diagnostic of the disease. However, women tend to have somewhat milder disease with more peripheral joint manifestations.

(3) **Familial aggregation.** The risk of ankylosing spondylitis in an HLA-B27–positive family member of an affected proband is 20%, as compared to 1%–2% for the general population of those with HLA-B27.

c. **Etiology**

(1) The major histocompatibility antigen HLA-B27 occurs in 90%–95% of white patients with ankylosing spondylitis, but the association is less marked in nonwhite populations (40%–50% of African Americans with ankylosing spondylitis have HLA-B27).

(2) Because the gene coding for the expression of HLA-B27 resides on chromosome 6, autosomal transmission occurs. Thus, children of a proband who is heterozygous for the gene controlling HLA-B27 production have a 50% probability of eventual expression of the antigen on cell surfaces.

(3) The **presence of HLA-B27 on cell membranes** is thought to be important in the causation of ankylosing spondylitis. The disease is somehow caused or perpetuated by the presence of a short amino acid sequence in the peptide-binding cleft of the HLA-B27 molecule that is able to bind a unique arthritis-causing peptide.

(a) **Receptor theory** (Figure 10–4A). One current theory is that this marker is a receptor for an environmental factor (e.g., bacterial peptide antigen, virus), which then can cause disease. The **athritogenic peptide theory** is a variation in which an immune response to a bacterial peptide is increased because the peptide (after intracellular processing) is particularly well presented by HLA-B27.

(b) **Molecular mimicry theory** (Figure 10–4B). A bacterial or other environmental antigen presented on the cell surface with a different HLA molecule might share similar sequences with the HLA-B27 molecule. If this class I complex (non–HLA-B27 plus peptide) is recognized by the cytotoxic CD8+ T cell as HLA-B27, an immune response can be mounted against HLA-B27 (**autoimmunity**) or suppressed against the disease-causing peptide (**tolerance**). Either condition could lead to clinical disease expression.

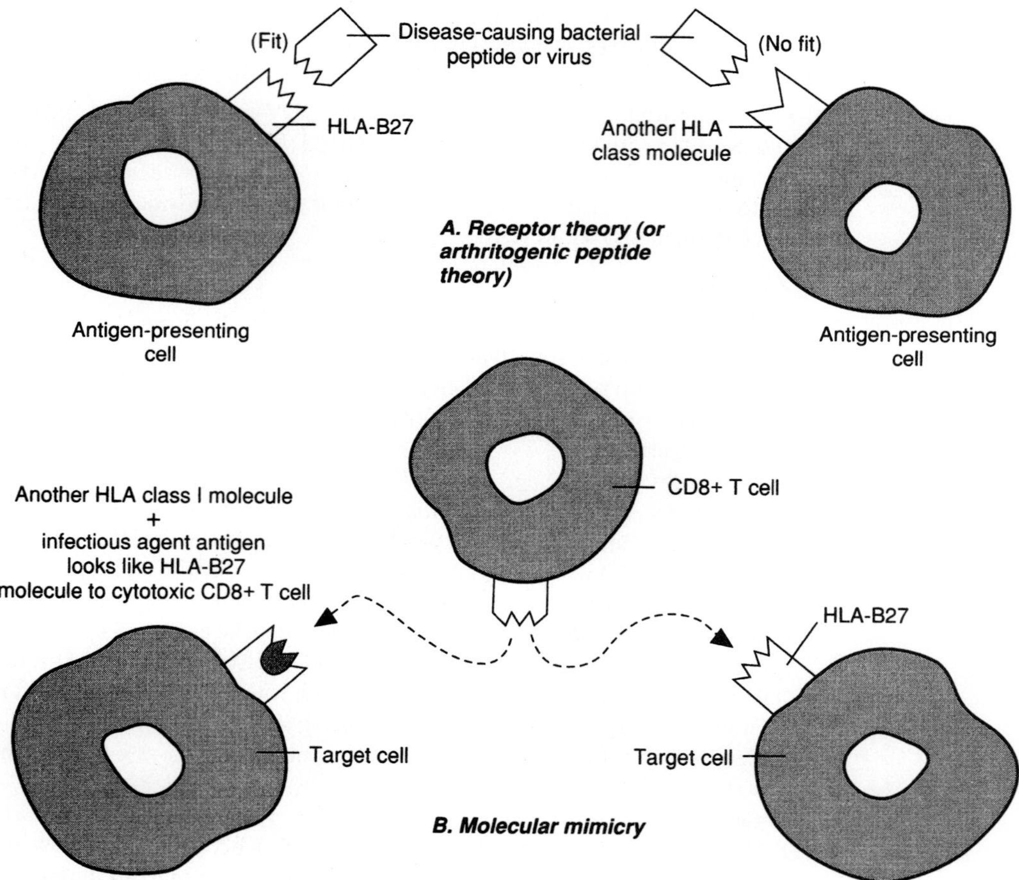

FIGURE 10–4 Human leukocyte antigen B27 (HLA-B27) as the cause of ankylosing spondylitis. (*A*) Receptor theory. A bacterial peptide or virus forms a complex externally with HLA-B27. The arthritogenic peptide theory, a variation of the receptor theory, maintains that the bacterial or viral peptide is processed intracellularly and only presented on the cell surface in association with the HLA-B27 molecule. (*B*) Molecular mimicry theory. An immune response is mounted against HLA-B27 (autoimmunity) or suppressed against the disease-causing peptide (tolerance) because the immune system cannot distinguish between their similar amino acid sequences.

(c) **Thymic selection theory.** HLA-B27 may function at the level of the thymus by allowing selection of **arthritogenic T cells.**

d. **Clinical features**

(1) **Disease onset.** The disease usually develops in the second or third decade of life (see XII E for a discussion of childhood disease).

(2) **Disease course.** The disease begins with the gradual onset of chronic sacral backache, which is associated with prolonged morning stiffness and which improves with exercise. Most patients have prolonged, unremitting low back pain for years. The disease may be mild and cause minimal interference with function, or it may be severe and deforming.

(3) **Manifestations of disease**

(a) **Axial skeletal involvement.** Symmetrical inflammation of the sacroiliac joints (sacroiliitis) is the most common presentation. Inflammation and consequent calcification of the spinal ligaments and the intervertebral zygoapophyseal joints can cause limited spinal mobility, and intercostal ligament enthesopathy can cause limitation of chest wall expansion.

(b) **Peripheral joint involvement.** This feature is typical of more severe ankylosing spondylitis. Erosive hip and shoulder involvement is not uncommon and may be severe. More distal synovitis is less common, although 35% of patients with ankylosing spondylitis have some evidence of peripheral joint disease.

(c) **Extraskeletal features.** Constitutional complaints, fatigue, and weight loss are not as common in ankylosing spondylitis as in rheumatoid arthritis, but they may occur. Anterior uveitis occurs in 25% of patients with ankylosing spondylitis, and sometimes occurs as an isolated clinical association of HLA-B27. Aortic root inflammation can occur, usually in patients with long-standing disease; this process can lead to aortic valve insufficiency or, if it extends into the conduction system, complete heart block. Upper lobe pulmonary fibrosis and chronic prostatitis are other uncommon extraskeletal features.

e. **Diagnosis.** Combining historical, physical, and radiographic evidence as well as excluding mechanical low back pain, other spondyloarthropathies, and other inflammatory arthritides, allows for diagnosis.

(1) **Historical information**

(a) **Inflammatory versus mechanical low back pain.** Inflammatory sacroiliitis has a gradual onset, in early adulthood, and is persistent for more than 3 months; the pain is associated with prolonged early morning back stiffness and is relieved by exercise and worsened by rest. In contrast, the onset of mechanical low back pain usually occurs later in life, with sudden, self-limited episodes that are worsened by exercise and improved by bed rest.

(b) **Familial association.** Patients with ankylosing spondylitis often have other affected family members.

(c) **Associated complaints.** Evidence of prior inflammatory eye symptoms, recurrent oligoarthritis, and inflammatory tendinitis should be sought.

(2) **Physical findings**

(a) **Musculoskeletal examination.** Each sacroiliac joint should be evaluated for tenderness, lumbar spinal mobility should be assessed in all directions, and chest expansion should be evaluated to assess severity of chest wall enthesopathic lesions.

(b) **General physical examination.** Evidence of associated abnormalities should be sought, including ocular erythema, aortic insufficiency murmurs, and peripheral arthritis and tendinitis.

(3) **Laboratory findings.** The only characteristic laboratory abnormality in ankylosing spondylitis is the variable presence of HLA-B27 in different population groups. In general, testing for this antigen is not necessary for the diagnosis.

(4) **Radiographic findings.** Sacroiliac involvement is best seen on an anteroposterior radiograph of the pelvis. Blurred joint margins, periarticular sclerosis, erosions, and joint space widening are characteristic, but total joint obliteration is typical of long-standing disease. If the illness is more severe or long-standing, ascending spinal involvement can occur, with flowing calcifications that bridge the intervertebral disk, culminating in a **bamboo-spine** appearance on a radiograph.

(5) **Differential diagnosis**

(a) **Nature of low back pain.** As previously mentioned, mechanical low back pain must be differentiated from inflammatory low back pain [see IV B 1 e (1) (a)].

(b) **Other disorders.** Sacroiliitis is highly unusual in nonspondylitic diseases. Characteristic skin lesions may suggest that a patient with sacroiliitis has psoriasis or reactive arthritis. Prominent urethritis in association with sacroiliitis may also suggest reactive arthritis, and prominent bowel complaints with sacroiliitis may suggest inflammatory bowel disease.

f. **Therapy.** Patient education and multidisciplinary treatment are important therapeutic components in ankylosing spondylitis, just as they are in rheumatoid arthritis. Short-term goals involve control of pain and reduction of inflammation without causing drug toxicity, and long-term goals are prevention of postural deformity and retention of employment.

(1) **Education**

(a) **Cigarette smoking.** Individuals with enthesopathic chest wall restriction or fibrotic lung disease should be discouraged from smoking.

(b) **Genetic counseling.** Patients should be made aware of the familial incidence of the illness so that it can be diagnosed early in children and treatment of spondylitic symptoms begun.

(c) **Protection of brittle spine.** Patients with extensive spinal involvement must understand that minimal trauma can cause a spinal fracture. Wearing a hard or soft collar should be recommended for automobile driving.

(2) **Exercise.** Spinal extension exercises and correct posture are important for prevention of deformity. Hard mattresses and small cervical pillows help prevent excessive spinal flexion during sleep.

(3) **Drug therapy.** Although many patients require DMARDS, NSAIDs are the mainstay of treatment. For persistent disease activity, TNF antagonists (e.g., infliximab or etanercept) may be used. Local joint or peritendinous instillation of a corticosteroid sometimes is beneficial in patients with prominent peripheral disease manifestations not controlled by NSAIDs.

g. **Prognosis.** Most patients with ankylosing spondylitis remain employable and continue to function well in society. The progression to severe, deforming disease cannot be predicted on the basis of HLA-B27 status or other criteria. Patients with severe spondylitis tend to have brittle spines, more cardiopulmonary disease, and other extraspinal complications; these patients may have shortened life spans.

2. **Reactive arthritis (Reiter's syndrome)**

a. **Definition.** Reactive arthritis, which is synonymous with Reiter's syndrome, is another spondyloarthropathy that is strongly associated with HLA-B27.

(1) Reiter's syndrome initially referred to the classic triad of nongonococcal urethritis, conjunctivitis, and arthritis that occurred after a diarrheal illness or genitourinary infection, usually with *Chlamydia trachomatis.* Many patients still have the classic disease triad, but the use of HLA-B27 typing has allowed "incomplete" forms (without the urethritis or conjunctivitis) to be identified.

(2) Reactive arthritis is a predominantly lower extremity oligoarthritis triggered by **urethritis, cervicitis,** or **dysenteric infection.** The variable features of the typical syndrome include **mucocutaneous lesions, inflammatory eye lesions,** and **sacroiliitis** or **peripheral arthritis.**

b. Epidemiology

(1) **Incidence.** Reactive arthritis occurs in 1%–3% of patients after nonspecific urethritis and 0.2% of patients after dysentery outbreaks caused by *Shigella flexneri.* HLA-B27 is present in 75%–80% of cases. Patients with the marker who develop nonspecific urethritis or *S. flexneri* dysentery have a 20%–25% chance of developing reactive arthritis.

(2) **Gender distribution.** Reactive arthritis is diagnosed in men much more often than in women, in part because cervicitis is less symptomatic than urethritis. However, the arthritis tends to be less severe in women as well.

c. Etiology and pathogenesis. Specific infections trigger the clinical expression of arthritis in susceptible patients, including chlamydial and mycoplasmal urethritis as well as dysenteric infections caused by certain serotypes of *Shigella, Salmonella,* and *Yersinia.* The presence of the organism may not be necessary for later exacerbations or chronic activity of the disease, although some polymerase chain reaction (PCR) and electron microscopic studies of inflamed synovium suggest the persistence of chlamydial organisms or fragments in reactive arthritis. The unusual severity of reactive arthritis in patients with acquired immunodeficiency syndrome (AIDS) suggests that the inflammatory response does not require functioning $CD4^+$ cells.

(1) **Exaggerated immune response.** Conceivably, infectious antigens cross-react with self antigens such as HLA-B27 and stimulate an exaggerated immune response that can include a noninfectious arthritis.

(2) **Suppressed immune response.** It is also conceivable that molecular mimicry between HLA-B27 and bacterial peptides prevents the host immune system from recognizing the pathogen, thus allowing dissemination and production of disease at widely varied sites. Evidence that suggests persistence of organisms or fragments at sites of chronic inflammation supports this theory.

(3) **Protected site of infection.** Persistent subclinical genitourinary or gastrointestinal infections (e.g., *Chlamydia, Shigella*) could cause recurrent shedding of organisms or bacterial antigens to joints. Persistent specific IgA responses to causative organisms and improvement with surgical stripping of the urethra in venereal onset of reactive arthritis supports this theory.

d. Clinical features

(1) **Disease onset.** Reactive arthritis begins most often in young adulthood. One to three weeks after an episode of urethritis or dysentery, any of the typical clinical features of the syndrome can occur. The disease often is misdiagnosed because these features tend to occur serially rather than simultaneously.

(2) **Manifestations of disease**

(a) **Musculoskeletal**

(i) **Arthritis.** A lower extremity oligoarthritis is the most common joint presentation. The arthritis may be acute and self-limited, but it is more commonly relapsing or chronic.

(ii) **Enthesopathy.** Inflammation of the tendons and ligaments are as much a part of reactive arthritis as they are of ankylosing spondylitis. Plantar fasciitis and Achilles tendinitis are most typical. **Dactylitis** (sausage toe), a lesion involving both joint and tendon inflammation in the same digit, is also a common feature.

(iii) **Sacroiliitis.** Asymmetrical involvement of sacroiliac joints occurs in approximately 20% of patients. Less frequently, asymmetrical ascending spinal disease occurs. The consequent back pain has typical inflammatory characteristics, but only rarely does the ascending spinal disease limit thoracic or cervical spinal mobility.

(b) **Genitourinary.** Symptomatic or asymptomatic **urethritis** is extremely common. Chronic **prostatitis** also is common, affecting as many as 80% of patients in some series.

(c) **Ocular.** Both **conjunctivitis** and **anterior uveitis** often occur. The conjunctival inflammation is an acute, usually self-limited manifestation, which may be recurrent. Anterior uveitis occurs in more established forms of disease; it may be chronic and require topical or systemic corticosteroids to prevent visual deterioration.

(d) **Mucocutaneous.** Fleeting and painless oral ulcers are the typical mucous membrane features. **Keratoderma blennorrhagica** is the characteristic scaling, plaque-like lesion found anywhere on the body, including the palms and soles. This lesion resembles pustular psoriasis clinically and pathologically. **Circinate balanitis** is a painless, erythematous erosion of the glans penis that may expand to surround the urethral orifice. Each of these skin lesions occurs in approximately 20%–30% of patients with reactive arthritis, although circinate balanitis is the most common.

(e) **Cardiovascular.** Early cardiovascular changes include transient **pericardial rubs** or **first-degree heart block.** In more severe, long-standing disease, an **aortitis** identical to that seen in ankylosing spondylitis can cause valvular insufficiency or conduction system lesions.

e. Diagnosis

(1) **General considerations.** Reactive arthritis can be difficult to diagnose when the onset of various clinical features is widely separated over time, but it is quite easy if **arthritis, dysentery** or **urethritis, conjunctivitis,** and **mucocutaneous lesions** appear simultaneously. A tentative diagnosis can be made when a seronegative asymmetrical oligoarthritis is associated with any of these extra-articular features. Because this form of arthritis is, strictly speaking, a "reactive" arthritis, the temporal appearance of arthritis after urethritis or a dysenteric illness is especially convincing. The mucocutaneous lesions, urethritis, and cervicitis, which often are asymptomatic, must be sought specifically while taking the patient history and during the physical examination.

(2) **Laboratory findings.** Eighty percent of whites with reactive arthritis have HLA-B27. The synovial fluid typically is mildly to moderately inflammatory, with neutrophil predominance and no important distinguishing characteristics.

(3) **Radiographic findings.** Asymmetrical, oligoarticular erosions, joint space narrowing, and periarticular osteopenia can be seen radiographically in established disease. Periosteal new bone formation is a characteristic feature of reactive arthritis, especially adjacent to the insertions of the Achilles tendon and plantar fascia. Sacroiliitis, if it occurs, typically is asymmetrical, and the occasional patient with spondyloarthropathy has asymmetrical, large syndesmophytes at scattered vertebral levels.

(4) **Differential diagnosis**

(a) **Diseases most likely to mimic acute reactive arthritis** are gonococcal arthritis and other infectious arthropathies, even Lyme disease. Thus, appropriate tissues should be cultured and serologies obtained. Crystal-mediated arthritis (i.e., gout and pseudogout) and the arthritis of rheumatic fever should be excluded.

(b) **Diseases most likely to mimic chronic recurring reactive arthritis** include other spondyloarthropathies, especially psoriatic arthritis and ankylosing spondylitis. Close attention to the symmetry and severity of sacroiliac and spinal involvement, to extraskeletal features, and to the presence or absence of infectious triggers may help differentiate these illnesses. Many cases of so-called **seronegative rheumatoid arthritis** may actually be cases of reactive arthritis. Typical clinical features as well as radiographic evidence of sacroiliac joint and periostitis should be sought. The presence or absence of HLA-B27 may be helpful in diagnosing particularly difficult cases.

f. Therapy

(1) **Goals of treatment** are essentially the same as in ankylosing spondylitis [see III B 1 f (1)].

(2) **Exercise.** Patients should be advised to rest to lessen inflammation and to perform appropriate exercises that allow preservation of joint function and prevention of contractures.

(3) **Drug therapy**

(a) **NSAIDs.** These agents are the mainstay of treatment. However, aspirin is relatively ineffective.

(b) **Corticosteroids.** Occasional intra-articular instillation may be useful in the management of particular joints that do not respond to treatment with NSAIDs.

(c) **Second-line agents.** Both azathioprine and methotrexate have been used to control particularly severe and chronic disease, and sulfasalazine is used for arthritis unresponsive to NSAIDs. The effects of these medications on disease course are not yet known. HIV testing should be considered for patients with reactive arthritis severe enough to require immunosuppressive medications.

(d) **Antibiotics.** Trials of tetracycline-like drugs, used for 3-month periods early in disease associated with urethritis, suggest that antibiotic treatment may lessen the severity and chronicity of arthritis.

g. **Prognosis.** Chronic or recurrent disease appears to be common. In 60%–80% of patients with reactive arthritis, skeletal complaints, extraskeletal complaints, or both, recur or become chronic. Perhaps as many as 25% of patients are functionally disabled by their illness. Long-term problems with aortic regurgitation and conduction disturbances are unusual but increase with the duration of the disease. Patients who have HLA-B27 antigen have more sacroiliitis and are more likely to have recurrent or chronic disease.

3. **Psoriatic arthritis**

a. **Definition.** Any form of inflammatory arthritis associated with psoriasis is called psoriatic arthritis. Rheumatoid factor generally is absent.

b. **Epidemiology**

(1) Psoriatic arthritis occurs much more commonly in patients who have a first-degree relative with the disorder.

(2) Psoriasis occurs two to three times more commonly in patients with arthritis than in the normal population. Conversely, as many as 10%–20% of patients with psoriasis may have an inflammatory arthritis.

c. **Etiology.** Although a hereditary etiology is apparent in psoriatic arthritis, its characteristics are not fully understood. HLA-B27 is highly associated with sacroiliitis in psoriasis, and HLA-B27, -B13, and -DR7 are independently associated with arthritis and psoriasis at an increased frequency. Unknown environmental factors also may be important in disease expression.

d. **Clinical features**

(1) **Disease onset.** Most patients with psoriatic arthritis develop the disease in their late thirties to early forties. Most patients develop skin lesions before the arthritis, but as many as 16% develop inflammatory arthritis before the psoriasis.

(2) **Patterns of arthritis.** Five patterns of psoriatic arthropathy have been distinguished, although the typical patient often has the skeletal manifestations of several of these patterns. Peripheral joint and tendon involvement may be more severe in the upper than in the lower extremities.

(a) **DIP arthritis** is the classic form of psoriatic arthritis. It is strongly associated with typical fingernail abnormalities as well as DIP joint redness, soft tissue swelling, and erosive changes seen radiographically in a clinical picture resembling primary erosive osteoarthritis.

(b) **Asymmetrical oligoarthritis.** Large and small joint oligoarthritis is another clinical form of psoriatic arthritis. **Sausage digits** are common in this form as a manifestation of joint and enthesis involvement of a single phalanx.

(c) **Symmetrical polyarthropathy.** A fairly symmetrical polyarthropathy can occur in conjunction with psoriasis, and it can be difficult to distinguish from rheumatoid arthritis. As many as 25% of these patients may be seropositive for rheumatoid factor.

(d) **Arthritis mutilans** is an unusually destructive form of psoriatic arthritis because of the severe periarticular bone resorption that occurs in the small finger joints. "Telescoping digits" characterize the end stage of this uncommon form of arthritis. Widespread joint ankylosis also can occur.

(e) **Sacroiliitis.** As many as 20% of patients with psoriatic arthritis can have clinical or radiographic evidence of sacroiliitis, usually asymmetrical. Ascending spinal syndesmophytes occur in an asymmetrical and patchy fashion.

(3) **Extra-articular features**

(a) **Skin.** Arthritis is more likely to occur in patients with severe skin involvement than in those with mild psoriasis, although it can occur in the presence of localized cutaneous lesions. Skin and joint flares of disease can occur in association with each other or independently in individual patients.

(b) **Nails.** Nail abnormalities most commonly occur in conjunction with DIP joint lesions; however, nail changes are noted more frequently in all of the peripheral forms of psoriatic arthritis in comparison to psoriasis uncomplicated by arthritis. Multiple **pitting,** transverse depressions, and **onycholysis** are the characteristic abnormalities found.

(c) **Ocular.** The only other extra-articular features that occur commonly in patients with psoriatic arthritis are conjunctivitis (in 20% of cases) and anterior uveitis (in 10% of cases).

e. **Diagnosis**

(1) **Clinical considerations.** An association should be made between the typical skin and nail lesions and the joint and spinal involvement to diagnose psoriatic arthritis. The skin manifestations may be subtle, so particular care must be taken to check the elbows, scalp, groin, navel, and buttock cleft.

(2) **Laboratory findings.** Laboratory indicators of chronic disease (e.g., anemia, thrombocytosis) typically are absent. Patients usually are seronegative for rheumatoid factor, although 25% of patients with symmetrical polyarthritis are seropositive.

(3) **Radiographic findings**

(a) **DIP joint erosions** can lead to joint space narrowing, and proximal phalangeal bone resorption can lead to a "pencil-in-cup" abnormality seen in arthritis mutilans. This severe destruction also can occur in more proximal joints.

(b) **Spinal involvement.** Asymmetrical sacroiliitis and asymmetrical patchy syndesmophytes are seen and are similar to those seen in reactive arthritis.

(c) **Enthesopathy.** Calcifications at tendon and ligament insertions occur.

(4) **Differential diagnosis**

(a) **Reactive arthritis** is distinguished from psoriatic arthritis by its characteristic extra-articular features and its tendency to involve the lower extremities more than the upper extremities. In psoriatic arthritis, upper extremity peripheral joint involvement is more common.

(b) **Rheumatoid arthritis.** Patients with psoriasis who present with symmetrical polyarthritis, seropositivity for rheumatoid factor, and rheumatoid nodules may be diagnosed with rheumatoid arthritis. Other overlapping presentations of the two diseases may be difficult to diagnose.

f. **Therapy.** Drug treatment for psoriatic arthritis is similar to that for the other spondyloarthropathies in that NSAIDs are the cornerstone of therapy. An important difference: gold can be administered intramuscularly to treat sustained manifestations of peripheral arthritis. Sulfasalazine also is effective. Methotrexate is often the first agent used if NSAIDs are not sufficient; it has been particularly successful in controlling both the skin disease and refractory arthritis. Other cytotoxic drugs (e.g., azathioprine) also have been used in treatment of severe skin and joint disease. Biological agents are also being used in refractory cases (see III G 2 d).

g. **Prognosis.** Most patients with psoriatic arthritis, except for the 5% or so who develop arthritis mutilans, can avoid significant deformity and remain employed.

4. **Enteropathic arthropathies**

a. **Definition.** Inflammatory arthritis associated with either Crohn's disease or ulcerative colitis is typified by a seronegative, migratory polyarticular involvement that waxes and wanes with the activity of the bowel disease. Sacroiliitis and spondylitis also can occur in affected individuals.

b. **Clinical syndromes**
   (1) **Peripheral arthritis.** In 10%–20% of patients with severe ulcerative colitis or Crohn's disease—usually those with other extra-intestinal manifestations—a predominantly lower extremity arthritis or tendinitis occurs in association with flareups of bowel disease. The arthritis often occurs abruptly and usually remits completely within weeks. There is no association with HLA-B27 in this peripheral arthritis. Treatment is directed at control of the bowel disease, although NSAIDs or local or systemic corticosteroids may help control the articular complaints.
   (2) **Spondylitis.** The spondylitis of inflammatory bowel disease is associated with HLA-B27 in about 50% of patients. The radiographic findings are typical of those found in primary ankylosing spondylitis (i.e., symmetrical sacroiliac joint changes and, less commonly, ascending symmetrical spondylitis without skin lesions). Approximately 5% of patients with inflammatory bowel disease develop sacroiliitis or spondylitis, but the activity of these lesions and that of the bowel disease are independent of one another. NSAIDs usually are effective in controlling symptoms but can cause increased bowel complaints; sometimes only nonacetylated salicylates can be tolerated by these patients.

c. **Differential diagnosis.** Whipple's disease can be confused with enteropathic arthropathies, because most patients manifest prominent bowel and joint complaints. In fact, sacroiliitis occurs in about 20% of cases. However, Whipple's disease is quite rare and most commonly manifests in middle-aged men as weight loss, skin hyperpigmentation, lymphadenopathy, fever, and symptoms of malabsorption.

V CRYSTAL-RELATED JOINT DISEASES

A Gout

1. **Definition.** Gout is a disorder of purine metabolism that is characterized by **serum uric acid elevation** (hyperuricemia) and **urate deposition** in articular or extra-articular tissues. Elevation of serum uric acid alone is not sufficient for the diagnosis of gout; in fact, only 10% of patients with hyperuricemia develop gout. Some unknown factor predisposes patients to urate deposition and articular inflammation in the setting of sustained hyperuricemia.

2. **Etiologic classification of hyperuricemia.** Gout is characterized by either episodic or constant **elevation of serum uric acid** concentration **above 7 mg/dL.** Patients with elevated serum uric acid can be classified as **overproducers** or **underexcreters** of uric acid, depending on the amount of uric acid excreted during a 24-hour period. Excessive dietary intake of purines can contribute to hyperuricemia in both types of patients.
   a. **Overproducers,** who make up approximately 10% of the gout population, excrete **more than 750–1000 mg** uric acid per day on an unrestricted diet. These patients synthesize greater than normal amounts of uric acid de novo from intermediates or via breakdown of purine bases from nucleic acids. The defect causing uric acid overproduction can be **primary** (associated with purine pathway enzymatic defects) or **secondary** (increased cell turnover associated with alcohol use, hematologic malignancies, chronic hemolysis, or cancer chemotherapy).
   b. **Underexcreters,** who constitute approximately 90% of the gout population, excrete **less than 700 mg** uric acid per day.
      (1) The most common causes of decreased uric acid excretion are **drug effects** (e.g., diuretics, alcohol, and low-dose aspirin interference with tubular handling of urate) and **renal disease** (e.g., chronic renal failure, lead nephropathy) [see Chapter 6, Part I: XII B 2 b]. Subtle renal tubular defects in urate handling also may be **inherited** and predispose to underexcretion.
      (2) This **group includes patients with combined defects,** because overproducers of uric acid also may be underexcreters. The decreased renal excretion of uric acid is the basis for hyperuricemia in these individuals.

(3) Multiple factors contribute to the occurrence of gout in **cardiac, renal, and liver transplant recipients.** Hyperuricemia develops in 75%–80% of patients who receive cardiac transplants. Underlying renal insufficiency, use of diuretics, and cyclosporine immunosuppressive therapy are the most common predisposing factors. Affected patients tend to have a rapidly progressive form of gout with the formation of extensive tophi.

3. **Associated conditions.** The following conditions occur more commonly in patients with gout but are not known to be causal.
   a. **Obesity.** Serum uric acid level rises with body weight. Gout is significantly more common in individuals who are more than 15% overweight, partly because of decreases in urate excretion.
   b. **Diabetes mellitus.** Impaired glucose tolerance is common in gout and may be a function of obesity.
   c. **Hypertension.** Although hypertension is common in patients with gout, no independent correlation exists between blood pressure and serum uric acid level. Obesity probably is responsible for a high rate of hypertension in patients with gout.
   d. **Hyperlipidemias** (types II and IV). Increased plasma concentrations of some lipids are common in patients with gout; however, diet, alcohol intake, and body weight seem to be more important associations.
   e. **Atherosclerosis.** Death in patients with gout is commonly attributable to cardiovascular or cerebrovascular diseases. However, the previously mentioned risk factors that commonly occur in gout patients seem to explain the tendency for accelerated atherogenesis.

4. **Clinical stages of gout**
   a. **Asymptomatic hyperuricemia** is characterized by an increased serum uric acid level in the absence of clinical evidence of deposition disease (i.e., arthritis, tophi, nephropathy, or uric acid stones).
      (1) **Hyperuricemia.** The risk of acute gouty arthritis or nephrolithiasis increases as the serum uric acid concentration increases. However, most patients do not develop either of these conditions.
      (2) **Hyperuricosuria.** The risk of uric acid stone formation in patients with hyperuricemia is most closely related to a urinary uric acid excretion exceeding 1000 mg/day. These patients also are at risk for **acute obstructive uropathy,** a form of acute renal failure occurring most often following combination chemotherapy for cancer. Large purine loads lead to sudden increases in serum uric acid levels, with subsequent precipitation of uric acid crystals in the collecting tubules and ureters.
   b. **Acute gouty arthritis,** the second stage and primary manifestation of gout, is an extremely painful, acute-onset arthritis.
      (1) **Typical patient.** Most patients (80%–90%) are middle-aged or elderly men who have had sustained asymptomatic hyperuricemia for 20–30 years before the first attack. Women seem to be spared until menopause, perhaps via an estrogen effect on uric acid clearance. Onset of acute gouty arthritis in the teens or twenties is unusual and most often associated with a primary or secondary cause of uric acid overproduction.
      (2) **Typical attack**
         (a) **Presentation.** A monoarticular, lower extremity presentation is most common with 50% of patients experiencing their first attack in the first metatarsophalangeal (MTP) joint (called **podagra**). Many attacks occur suddenly at night, with rapid evolution of joint erythema, swelling, tenderness, and warmth. Intense joint inflammation can extend into the soft tissues and mimic cellulitis or phlebitis. Fever can occur in severe attacks.
         (b) **Course.** Attacks usually resolve in a few days, although some can extend over several weeks. The joint usually returns to normal between attacks. Polyarticular involvement can occur in some cases, and a typical progression from monoarticular to polyarticular involvement occurs by extension to adjacent joints.

(3) **Pathogenesis of acute attacks** (see Figure 10–5)

(a) Sustained hyperuricemia or a rapid fluctuation in the level of serum uric acid (as occurs in the setting of dehydration, rapid rehydration, or with the initiation of uricosuric therapy), may lead to the development of **microtophi** (i.e., small crystal aggregates) in the synovial membrane and cartilage.

(b) Through several mechanisms, microtophi are disrupted and crystals are released into the joint space. Spontaneous urate crystallization can also occur in conditions of urate supersaturation of joint fluid. (Trauma, joint temperature changes, and fluctuations in serum or synovial fluid uric acid concentration are potential initiators of these processes.)

(c) Urate crystals are coated by **immunoglobulins** and **complement components.** These adherent proteins enhance phagocytosis by neutrophils.

(d) Phagosomes in the crystal-containing neutrophils fuse with lysosomes, and the lysosomal enzymes digest the protein coating of the crystals. The naked crystals then apparently disrupt the phagosomal membranes.

(e) Neutrophils are damaged by the crystals, and lysosomal enzymes are released into synovial fluid, potentiating inflammation.

(f) **Inflammatory mediators** (e.g., IL-6) can be released from synovial macrophages exposed to uric acid crystals and may be responsible for extension of inflammation to other joints and into soft tissues.

(g) **Lipoproteins** can enter inflamed synovial membranes and attach to the crystals, downregulating the inflammatory process.

c. **Intercritical gout,** the third stage of gout, is an asymptomatic period after the initial attack. This stage may be interrupted by new acute attacks.

(1) **Recurrence of monoarticular attacks.** About 7% of patients never experience a new attack of acute gouty arthritis after the first episode. However, 62% experience a recurrence within 1 year. Typically, patients are asymptomatic between attacks, but attacks eventually become more frequent and abate more gradually if urate deposition remains untreated over time.

(2) **Disease progression.** Attacks tend to become polyarticular and more severe over time. Some patients develop a chronic inflammatory arthritis without asymptomatic intervals—a condition that may be difficult to distinguish from rheumatoid arthritis. Tophaceous gout typically occurs over a 10- to 20-year period of untreated urate deposition.

d. **Chronic tophaceous gout,** which develops in untreated patients, is the final stage of gout. The tophus is a collection of urate crystal masses surrounded by inflammatory cells and variable fibrosis. Tophi tend to develop in areas that are lower in temperature, which diminishes the solubility of the crystals.

(1) **Typical locations of tophaceous deposits**

(a) The **pinna of the external ear** is a potential site of tophus development, although deposition here is uncommon.

(b) **Other common locations** are the surfaces of chronically involved joints and subchondral bone as well as extensor surfaces of the forearms, olecranon bursae, and the infrapatellar and Achilles tendons.

(2) **Pathogenesis of tophaceous gout**

(a) Although microtophi may form in joints early in the urate deposition phase, aggregates that are large enough to be palpable or to cause anatomic deformities take years to develop. The rate of tophus formation is directly related to the severity and duration of hyperuricemia in gout patients. Tophi do not occur in patients with asymptomatic hyperuricemia.

(b) Erosion of cartilage and adjacent subchondral bone occurs due to displacement of normal tissue by the tophus and by the inflammatory reaction to it.

e. **Renal complications** may arise at any stage of gout, but nephrolithiasis is the only common clinical presentation of renal involvement. Proteinuria and impaired ability to concentrate urine related to urate deposition in the renal interstitium have been described in gout patients (see Chapter 6, Part I: XII B 3).

5. **Diagnosis**
   a. **Acute gouty arthritis**
      (1) **Laboratory findings**
         (a) **Serum findings.** The serum uric acid value often is not helpful in the clinical diagnosis of acute gout. Serum uric acid concentration is normal in at least 10% of patients at the time of an acute attack, and an elevated serum uric acid level is not specific for acute gout.
         (b) **Synovial fluid findings.** The demonstration of **urate crystals,** especially intracellular crystals, in synovial fluid is diagnostic. These **crystals characteristically are needle-shaped and negatively birefringent** in red-compensated, polarized light, and they may be present in neutrophils during an acute attack. Synovial fluid white blood cell (WBC) counts of 10,000–60,000/mm^3 (predominantly neutrophils) also are common in acute attacks.
      (2) **Colchicine trial.** In a typical clinical setting (i.e., a middle-aged man with an acute attack of podagra), a good clinical response to colchicine treatment is reasonably specific for acute gout. Other forms of acute arthritis (e.g., sarcoid arthropathy, pseudogout) can respond to colchicine; therefore, this trial may not be as specific in less typical presentations.
   b. **Chronic tophaceous gout**
      (1) **Physical appearance.** Tophi are firm, movable, and cream-colored or yellowish if superficially located. If they ulcerate, a chalky material is extruded.
      (2) **Radiographic findings.** Tophaceous deposits appear as well-defined, large erosions (punched-out erosions) of the subchondral bone. These erosions are most common at the first MTP joint and at the bases and heads of phalanges; however, any articulation can be affected. Typical gouty erosions have an **overhanging edge** of subchondral new bone formation. Periarticular osteopenia is absent.
      (3) **Aspiration.** Tophi can be aspirated and crystals demonstrated by polarized microscopy.

6. **Therapy.** In all stages of gout, secondary causes of hyperuricemia (e.g., medications, obesity, excess dietary purine intake, alcohol intake, other disease) should be altered if possible.
   a. **Asymptomatic hyperuricemia.** In general, patients without evidence of urate deposition do not require treatment other than correction of underlying causes. Patients with uric acid elevations that chronically exceed 10 mg/dL have a greater than 90% chance of developing acute gout at some time, but most physicians wait for an acute attack to begin treatment.
   b. **Acute gouty arthritis.** Drug treatment of the acute attack is most effective when started very early after symptoms begin. As with any inflammatory arthritis, rest or immobilization of the involved joint is an important adjunct to treatment.
      (1) **Colchicine,** which inhibits neutrophil chemotaxis and inflammatory mediator release by suppressing phospholipase A_2, can be used intravenously to treat acute attacks. Caution is necessary in elderly patients and in those with renal or hepatic impairment due to increased bone marrow toxicity and neuromyotoxicity. Colchicine can be used orally for acute attacks, but nausea, vomiting, and diarrhea often appear before therapy is successful.
      (2) **NSAIDs** often are used in high but quickly tapered doses to treat acute attacks. Any of these agents can be used, although drugs that affect uric acid clearance (e.g., salicylates, diflunisal) should be avoided, because any fluctuation in serum urate can prolong acute attacks. Caution is warranted when using NSAIDs in the presence of gastrointestinal, hepatic, or renal disease. Indomethacin, if tolerated, appears to be the most acutely efficacious agent.
      (3) Intra-articular injections of **corticosteroids** can be used to treat acute gout of a single joint, particularly when the use of other agents is contraindicated.

(4) **Drugs that alter serum uric acid concentrations** (e.g., **allopurinol, probenecid**) should be avoided during acute attacks because raising or lowering serum uric acid can prolong attacks. In patients already taking such drugs, the dosage should not be altered.

c. **Intercritical gout.** Prophylactic treatment with small doses of colchicine (0.6 mg once or twice daily) or small doses of an NSAID can be used to forestall new attacks.

d. **Chronic or tophaceous gout.** Therapy for chronic gout centers on control of hyperuricemia. Drugs that increase renal uric acid excretion (uricosuric drugs) or that decrease uric acid production (xanthine oxidase inhibitors) are available. The aim of this treatment is to reduce serum urate below 6 mg/dL, to allow reduction in serum supersaturation by urate and mobilization of tissue uric acid deposits. Patients who have had a recent acute attack should receive low-dose colchicine or an NSAID to prevent new attacks caused by fluctuation in serum urate.

(1) **Uricosuric drugs** (e.g., **probenecid, sulfinpyrazone**) can be used in patients who excrete less than 700 mg uric acid daily, who have normal renal function, and who have no history of urinary stones.

(2) **Xanthine oxidase inhibitors** include **allopurinol,** which is an analogue of hypoxanthine. This drug inhibits de novo uric acid synthesis and competitively inhibits xanthine oxidase via enzymatic conversion to oxypurinol. Inhibition of uric acid synthesis with xanthine oxidase inhibitors is preferred in patients with urate excretion greater than 1000 mg/day, creatinine clearance less than 30 mL/min, tophaceous gout, or a history of nephrolithiasis. Dosages are reduced in the presence of renal failure to avoid toxicity. The most common side effects of allopurinol are dyspepsia, diarrhea, and rash, which occur in 3%–10% of patients. A full-blown hypersensitivity syndrome can occur rarely, with a mortality rate around 20%–30%.

(3) Important treatment issues:

(i) It is important to use colchicine, NSAID, or steroids while instituting allopurinol therapy to avoid an acute attack of gout induced by fluctuation in serum urate levels.

(ii) Can use colchicine chronically in patients unable to tolerate allopurinol.

(iii) Beware of use of colchicine in patients with renal insufficiency, because secretion is reduced and severe toxicity may occur.

(iv) May use chronic low-dose steroid treatment in patients with chronic gout and chronic renal insufficiency.

B Calcium pyrophosphate dihydrate (CPPD) deposition disease

1. **Definition.** Deposition of CPPD crystals in cartilage and periarticular connective tissues can cause a gamut of articular manifestations, ranging from asymptomatic deposition to acute and chronic inflammatory arthritis. The acute form of CPPD deposition disease is commonly called **pseudogout.**

2. **Etiologic classification**

a. **Hereditary CPPD disease.** A high prevalence of CPPD disease has been noted in many families, with autosomal dominant transmission the typical pattern. Secondary metabolic associations with CPPD disease typically are not present in these families.

b. **Osteoarthritis.** Chondrocalcinosis and CPPD crystals can occur as a result of severe osteoarthritis. CPPD disease also can cause osteoarthritis by damaging cartilage.

c. **CPPD disease associated with metabolic disorders.** Correction of underlying metabolic disorders, if possible, does not seem to alter the progression of CPPD disease.

(1) **Probable associations.** CPPD disease occurs at a higher-than-expected frequency in association with certain diseases and conditions. Potential abnormalities of calcium, phosphorus, or cartilage metabolism can explain the associations, which include:

(a) Hyperparathyroidism

(b) Hemochromatosis

(c) Hypothyroidism

(d) Hypophosphatasia
(e) Hypomagnesemia
(f) Wilson's disease

(2) **Possible associations.** CPPD disease may or may not occur at a higher than expected frequency in association with:
(a) Gout
(b) Diabetes mellitus
(c) Ochronosis

3. **Pathogenesis** (see Figure 10–5)

a. **Crystal deposition**

(1) **Site.** The initial site of CPPD deposition appears to be articular cartilage surrounding lacunae in the midzone. Later, deposition occurs in clefts of degenerated cartilage and in

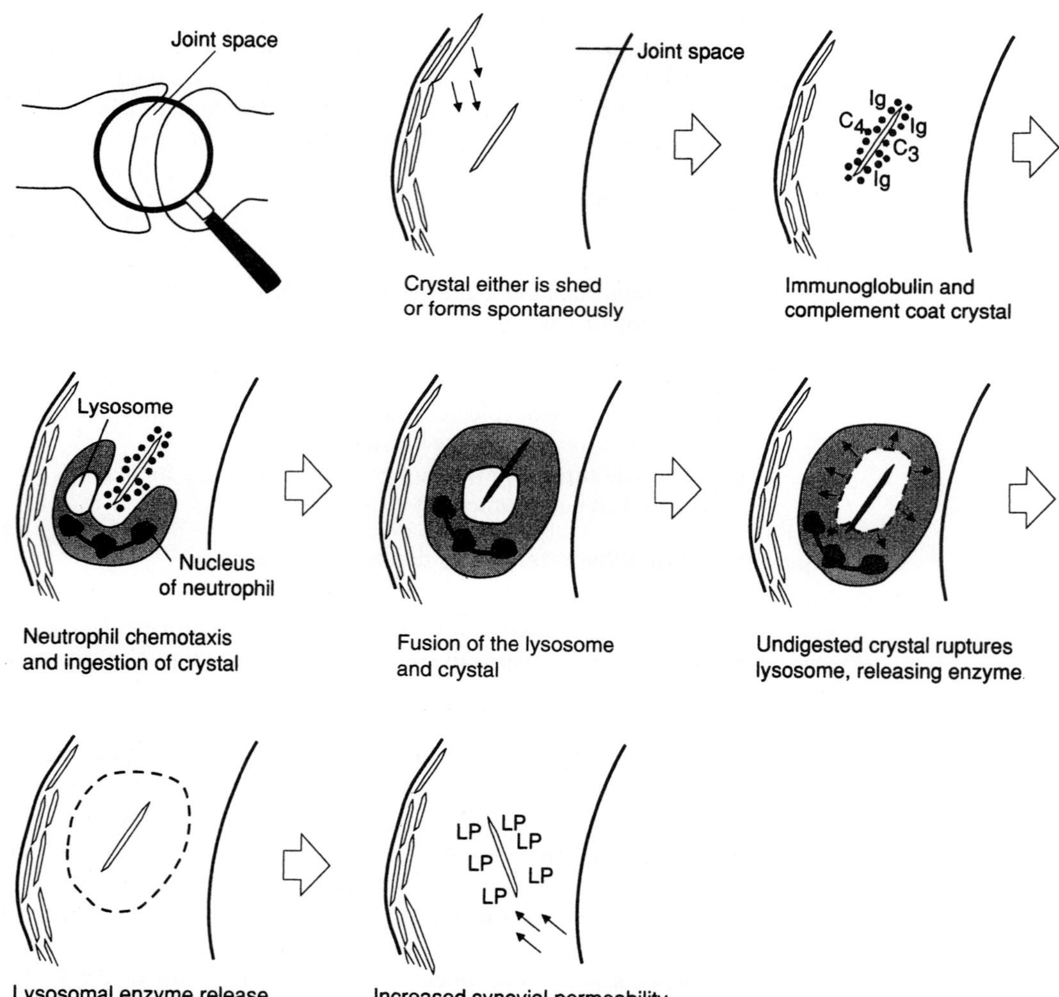

FIGURE 10–5 Postulated pathogenesis of crystal-induced joint inflammation. *Ig* = immunoglobulin; *C3* and *C4* = complement components C3 and C4; *LP* = lipoprotein.

scattered foci in the cartilage matrix and synovial membrane, eventually forming large crystalline masses.

(2) **Process.** An alteration of cartilage ground substance, the ionic composition of the matrix (i.e., calcium and pyrophosphate), or a combination of both is required for crystallization. Possibly, an altered condition of the matrix (e.g., removal of an inhibiting agent or addition of a nucleating agent) allows crystals to form in the microenvironment around the chondrocyte as pyrophosphate is released from the cell. A cell surface ectoenzyme, nucleoside triphosphate pyrophosphohydrolase (NTP-PPH), generates pyrophosphate in the process of scavenging extracellular adenosine triphosphate (ATP); the increased energy requirement of greater proteoglycan synthesis in osteoarthritis thus may lead to CPPD production.

b. Crystal-mediated joint damage. CPPD deposits stiffen the cartilage, impairing its weight-bearing properties and accelerating osteoarthritic change. The acute arthritic attacks are believed to be induced by the release of crystals from the cartilage into the joint space.

(1) **Factors mediating crystal release**

(a) **Matrix loosening.** CPPD crystals in cartilage exist in equilibrium with synovial fluid calcium and pyrophosphate concentrations. Decreases in serum calcium concentration can lead to decreases in synovial fluid pyrophosphate levels and solubilization of joint CPPD crystals as equilibrium is restored. Loss of marginal CPPD deposits may cause the entire deposit to loosen in the matrix, with subsequent release of abundant CPPD crystals into the joint space. Thus, fluctuations of serum calcium concentration in the setting of acute medical illness or during the perioperative period may initiate acute crystal release.

(b) **Loss of matrix.** Enzymatic erosion of cartilage due to an associated inflammatory arthritis (e.g., infectious arthritis) also may cause crystal release.

(c) **Biomechanical forces.** Impaired dissipation of weight-bearing forces on cartilage also may lead to crystal loosening and release into the joint space.

(2) **Factors affecting acute attacks**

(a) **Inflammatory response.** Neutrophils are attracted to crystals coated with IgG, complement, fibronectin, fibrinogen, or kininogen. Crystals are ingested, causing the release of inflammatory mediators such as prostaglandins and collagenase.

(b) **Degree of response.** CPPD crystals are somewhat less inflammatory than urate crystals. Generally, fewer are released in the acute attack, the crystals adsorb inflammatory proteins less well, and CPPD crystals are not membranolytic.

4. Clinical syndromes

a. Pseudogout accounts for 25% of cases of CPPD disease. Acute swelling, pain, stiffness, and erythema develop in previously asymptomatic joints. The knee is most commonly involved (50% of cases), but almost any synovial joint, including the first MTP joint, can be involved. Spread to adjacent joints can occur, and precipitation of attacks by acute medical or surgical illness is common, occurring in 10%–20% of cases. Systemic findings such as fever and leukocytosis may be present, especially in elderly patients. Joints typically return to normal between attacks, which may last days to weeks.

b. Pseudo–rheumatoid arthritis accounts for 5% of cases of CPPD disease. In some patients, a smoldering chronic arthropathy can occur. Subacute episodes of pain and swelling in one or more joints can be superimposed on a more chronic picture of prolonged morning stiffness, fatigue, synovial thickening, and progressive deformities.

c. Pseudo-osteoarthritis accounts for 50% of cases of CPPD disease. Affected patients present with a clinical and radiographic picture similar to that of degenerative joint disease, although about half have superimposed acute attacks of pseudogout. Flexion contractures are more common than in typical osteoarthritis, and bilateral knee varus deformities or isolated patellofemoral arthritis may occur more commonly than in osteoarthritis. A small percentage of these patients may have such severe joint destruction (e.g., of the shoulders or knees) that the clinical and radiographic appearance is that of a **neuropathic joint disorder,** even in the absence of underlying neurologic disease or apparent proprioceptive deficit.

d. Asymptomatic CPPD disease occurs in 20% of cases. These patients do not have joint pain; the disease typically is uncovered by the finding of asymptomatic chondrocalcinosis on radiography. The prevalence of this asymptomatic disease, as well as other clinically evident forms of CPPD disease, increases with age and is seen in as many as 7% of elderly people screened.

5. Diagnosis. The finding of typical crystals on synovial fluid analysis is diagnostic of pseudogout. Chondrocalcinosis seen on radiography is evidence for a diagnosis of CPPD deposition. However, chondrocalcinosis may be present in patients who never develop acute pseudogout.

a. Synovial fluid findings. Chunky, rhomboid **crystals that exhibit weakly positive birefringence** in red-compensated, polarized light are the hallmark of the acute arthritis syndromes associated with CPPD disease. These may be intracellular (in neutrophils) or extracellular, but they usually are much less prevalent than in a typical gout-involved joint. Synovial fluid leukocytosis of 10,000–20,000 cells/mm^3 (mostly neutrophils) is typical.

b. Radiographic findings

(1) Chondrocalcinosis. Calcification of articular hyaline cartilage, fibrocartilage (most commonly in the knee menisci, intervertebral disk annuli, symphysis pubis, and wrist triangular fibrocartilage), synovial membrane, tendons, and bursae can occur, usually in a stippled, linear fashion.

(2) Osteoarthritis. Osteoarthritic changes in atypical joints (e.g., wrist, elbow, and shoulder and MCP joints) suggest CPPD disease. Subchondral bone cysts may be more extensive in radiographs of joints affected by CPPD disease, and hook-shaped osteophytes characteristically are present with MCP involvement.

(3) Pseudoneuropathic joint. Radiographic findings typical of neuropathic joint disorders, including extreme joint disorganization and bone fragments, can be found in severe cases of CPPD disease.

c. Clinical diagnostic distinctions

(1) Clinical or radiographic evidence of osteoarthritis in joints not usually involved by osteoarthritis should suggest CPPD disease as an alternative diagnosis.

(2) Attacks of acute inflammatory arthritis in a setting of apparent osteoarthritis should suggest CPPD disease.

(3) Acute arthritis occurring shortly after a medical illness or surgical procedure should suggest a crystal-mediated arthritis such as gout or pseudogout.

(4) Radiographic changes more typical of osteoarthritis in patients thought to have rheumatoid arthritis should suggest CPPD disease as an alternative diagnosis.

(5) The **presence of diseases commonly associated with CPPD disease** (e.g., hyperparathyroidism, hemochromatosis) should suggest CPPD disease as a possible cause of any joint manifestations. In people younger than 55 years of age, or in those with recurrent, polyarticular disease, an associated metabolic disease is more likely. In these patients, determinations of calcium, magnesium, alkaline phosphatase, ceruloplasmin, and ferritin levels as well as liver and thyroid function tests should be considered.

(6) Neuropathic joint presentations should prompt investigation for CPPD disease as well as potentially associated neurologic disorders.

6. Therapy

a. Acute attacks. Typical treatment involves aspiration of inflammatory joint fluid, intra-articular injection of corticosteroid, and use of NSAIDs.

b. Prophylaxis. No clearly effective regimen is available, although NSAIDs and, rarely, low-dose colchicine are used.

C **Hydroxyapatite arthritis** Hydroxyapatite crystals, the typical complexed form of calcium in bone, also can cause several rheumatic syndromes.

1. **Clinical syndromes**
   a. **Crystal deposition in osteoarthritis.** Mineral formation in cartilage may be a result of abnormal cartilage metabolism in more severe forms of osteoarthritis. Joint effusions in these patients contain crystals of hydroxyapatite as often as they contain CPPD crystals.
   b. **Calcific periarthritis.** Hydroxyapatite deposition in bursae and tendon sheaths can cause episodes of acute inflammation (i.e., periarthritis and peritendinitis), with acute attacks of pain, swelling, and erythema. Discrete clumped deposits can be found radiographically around the shoulders, greater trochanters, wrists, elbows, and digits and in other periarticular areas. These deposits can be shown to disintegrate gradually on radiographs taken several weeks after the acute periarthritis.
   c. **Destructive arthritis.** Hydroxyapatite crystals can be associated with a chronic destructive arthropathy, which is characterized by erosive radiographic changes, large (usually noninflammatory) effusions, proliferative synovitis, synovial mineral deposition, and periarticular ligamentous instability. This syndrome occurs most often in the knee and shoulder (**"Milwaukee shoulder"**) of elderly patients. Synovial fluid analysis shows few WBCs (500–1000/mm^3), with monocytes predominating. High concentrations of neutral proteases and collagenases sometimes are present.
2. **Diagnosis.** Light microscopic examination of synovial fluid occasionally reveals brownish globules that are large clumps of hydroxyapatite crystals. Isolated crystals are too small to be seen with ordinary light or polarized light microscopy. A calcium stain, **alizarin red S,** can be used as a screening test for the presence of hydroxyapatite or CPPD crystals in effusions. Aspirates from bursae or tendon sheaths may yield milky or pasty material that contains high concentrations of these hydroxyapatite crystals.
3. **Associated conditions.** Disorders of calcium and phosphorus metabolism should be sought if multiple deposits are found.
4. **Therapy.** Mechanical splinting and NSAIDs are used to treat acute episodes of periarthritis. NSAIDs often are used in the chronic hydroxyapatite arthropathy as well. Periodic aspiration of the large synovial effusions that occur in the Milwaukee shoulder may help preserve ligamentous integrity and remove destructive enzymes. Corticosteroid injections may help treat acutely symptomatic joints.

VI OSTEOARTHRITIS

A **Definition** Osteoarthritis is traditionally defined as a noninflammatory joint disorder characterized by deterioration of articular cartilage and formation of new bone at the joint surfaces and margins. Emerging evidence recognizes the importance of biomechanical, biochemical, and cytokine-mediated changes in the pathogenesis of osteoarthritis.

B **Etiology** Both systemic and local factors contribute to the development of osteoarthritis. Systemic factors include age, sex, genetics, bone density, and nutritional elements, which may make the cartilage more vulnerable to injury and less efficient at repair. Local biomechanical components, in combination with systemic factors, have a synergistic effect on the process of cartilage breakdown.

1. **Age.** The prevalence and incidence of osteoarthritis in all joints correlates with increasing age. Aging is associated with the following changes:
   a. Decreased responsiveness of chondrocytes to growth factors that stimulate repair
   b. Increased laxity of ligaments, which makes the joints more unstable and susceptible to injury
   c. Failure of shock absorbers or protectors of the joint, which includes decreases in muscle strength and neurologic responses

d. Development of a thinner rim of noncalcified cartilage, which leads to an increased shear stress at the basal cartilage level

2. **Race.** No clear racial predilection has been documented. The prevalence of osteoarthritis of the hip is very low in Asians.

3. **Sex.** Gender appears to be particularly important in the development of **erosive osteoarthritis** of the DIP and PIP joints. This variant is 10 times more common in women than men; it is autosomal dominant in women and recessive in men.

4. **Genetics.** Researchers have discovered a defect in the gene coding for **type II collagen synthesis,** which allows for early degeneration of the type II collagen. The presence of this abnormal gene is associated with a type of premature polyarticular osteoarthritis and mild epiphyseal dysplasia seen in several families.

5. **Inflammation.** Despite the noninflammatory nature of the synovial membrane and synovial fluid in osteoarthritis, evidence indicates that inflammatory mediators produced by synovial tissues and cartilage play a significant role. Cytokines such as IL-1 as well as other inflammatory mediators such as nitric oxide and prostaglandins are important in the autodestructive processes that promote cartilage degeneration. These mediators, sequestered within avascular and aneural hyaline cartilage, do not provoke the classical signs of inflammation.

6. **Obesity and abnormal stresses.** An association exists between obesity and osteoarthritis of the knee, but interestingly, the same association does not exist with osteoarthritis of the hip. Abnormal mechanical loading contributes to disease progression by altering the metabolism of osteocytes within subchondral bone and chondrocytes within articular cartilage. In addition, abnormal biomechanical forces can increase the expression of mechanoresponsive genes, with the resultant release of proteolytic enzymes, growth factors, and mediators.

7. **Neuropathy.** Muscle tone around a joint modulates the forces of joint impact loading. If proprioceptive input to the joint is impaired, abnormal muscle tone may result in osteoarthritis by transferring abnormal forces to the joint.

8. **Deposition diseases** (e.g., hemochromatosis, ochronosis, Wilson's disease, crystal deposition diseases). These conditions, which cause deposition of substances in the cartilage matrix, can result in direct chondrocyte injury or can impair the ability of the matrix to dissipate loading forces.

C Pathogenesis Osteoarthritis is a metabolically active condition, not a degenerative one. Repair and synthesis counteract the destructive processes until the repair processes are overwhelmed late in the disease course.

1. **Initial insult.** Chondrocytes in hyaline cartilage are responsible for maintaining the extracellular matrix by balancing catabolic and anabolic functions. Synthesis of the matrix is synchronized with their degradation by proteolytic enzymes. Two factors may contribute to the initiation of osteoarthritis.
   a. A region of highly focal mechanical stress
   b. An intrinsic defect in the cartilage matrix, as single-base mutation in the type II procollagen gene (COL2A1) renders collagen fibrils prone to fragmentation and thus early osteoarthritis (see VI B 3 b)

2. **Progression**
   a. **Early.** Synthesis of proteoglycan and collagen is increased, with some degree of degradation.
   b. **Late.** As osteoarthritis develops further, proteoglycan synthesis decreases, resulting in a net loss of matrix protein. Structural changes in the proteoglycan molecules include degradation of the core protein, reduction in the size of the proteoglycan aggregates, and reduction in the hyaluronic acid content. In addition, synthesis of different collagen gene products, which alter the collagen fiber network, characterizes this late phase.

3. **Factors involved**
   a. **Proteolytic enzymes.** Chondrocytes secrete degradative enzymes (e.g., metalloproteinases). Metalloproteinase activity is controlled by inhibitors and activators. In osteoarthritis, the production of metalloproteinases exceeds the amount of so-called tissue inhibitors of metalloproteinase (TIMPs).
   b. **Cytokines and inflammatory mediators**
      (1) **Catabolic:** IL-1, IL-6, and IL-8; TNF; nitric oxide; and prostaglandin E_2 (PGE_2). IL-1 stimulates the production of proteases while suppressing the synthesis of proteoglycan and type II collagen. In addition, IL-1 induces chondrocyte production of other detrimental cytokines as well as nitric oxide and PGE_2.
      (2) **Anabolic:** growth factors such as TGF-β and insulin-like growth factor (IGF-1). TGF-β antagonizes the action of IL-1, and IGF-1 is the major regulator of proteoglycan synthesis.

D Pathology

1. **Cartilage changes**
   a. Early in osteoarthritis, cartilage changes in **color** from blue to yellow due to loss of proteoglycan.
   b. Localized areas of **softening** are the earliest pathologic changes in osteoarthritis.
   c. Superficial **chipping and flaking** of cartilage signifies more advanced disease.
   d. Vertical **fibrillations** in the cartilage indicate further progression.
   e. If the healing forces are overwhelmed by destructive forces, confluent **erosions** eventually progress to full-thickness cartilage loss.
2. **Bone changes**
   a. **New bone formation** can occur under the cartilage (seen as eburnation on a radiograph) or at the joint margin (seen as osteophytic spurs on a radiograph).
   b. **Subchondral cysts.** Large pseudocystic areas can form in the juxta-articular bone due to transmission of increased mechanical forces to bone; presumably, these cysts fail to heal because of impaired perfusion from subchondral microfractures.

E Classification (Table 10–10)

1. **Primary osteoarthritis** has no underlying cause for joint damage. It typically involves the DIP and PIP joints and the first carpometacarpal joints. Knees, hips, and first MTP joints often are involved

TABLE 10–10 Classification of Osteoarthritis

Primary osteoarthritis	Secondary osteoarthritis
Primary osteoarthritis (multiple sites)	**Secondary osteoarthritis**
Heberden's nodes	Congenital (e.g., hip dysplasia)
Generalized osteoarthritis	Deposition disease
"Erosive" osteoarthritis	Ochronosis
Diffuse idiopathic skeletal hyperostosis	Wilson's disease
	Hemochromatosis
Primary osteoarthritis (local)	Gout
Cervical spine	Calcium pyrophosphate deposition disease
Hip	Neuropathic joint (e.g., diabetes mellitus, syphilis)
First carpometacarpal joint	Endocrine/metabolic (e.g., acromegaly)
Distal interphalangeal joints	Osteonecrosis (especially hips, knees)
Lumbar spine	Infection (tuberculosis)
Knee	Inflammation (rheumatoid arthritis)
First metatarsophalangeal joint	
Proximal interphalangeal joints	

as well as cervical and lumbar spine facet joints. The joint involvement may be **generalized** or it may occur in an isolated, **sporadic** fashion. **Erosive** osteoarthritis is a unique subset that occurs predominantly in middle-aged women and has autosomal dominant, sex-influenced characteristics. Episodic erythema, swelling, and tenderness occur in involved joints, especially the DIP and PIP joints of the hands. Characteristic radiographic abnormalities include bone erosions and ankylosis, which are unusual in typical osteoarthritis. **Diffuse idiopathic skeletal hyperostosis** is noninflammatory axial and peripheral enthesis hyperostosis manifested by radiographic "whiskering" at tendon or ligament insertion and flowing osteophytes adjacent to vertebral disks.

2. **Secondary osteoarthritis** exhibits an underlying cause for degenerative joint disease and may involve joints not typically affected by primary osteoarthritis (e.g., elbow, wrist). A primary metabolic, inflammatory, or mechanical process leads secondarily to osteoarthritis (see Table 10–10).

F Clinical features

1. **Symptoms** vary with the joint involved and the severity of the disease.
   a. **Pain.** Most patients experience the gradual onset of a deep, aching pain, which worsens with activity and is relieved by rest. With more severe disease, pain can occur even at rest and interfere with sleep.
   b. **Morning stiffness** is brief (< 30 minutes) in contrast to that occurring in inflammatory rheumatic conditions, which generally lasts much longer.
   c. **Gelling phenomenon** refers to the sensation of renewed stiffness in osteoarthritic joints after prolonged inactivity.
2. **Signs**
   a. **Tenderness.** Mild or moderate tenderness can be present in involved joints.
   b. **Painful range of motion** in large joints (e.g., knees, hips) is the equivalent of tenderness in small joints.
   c. **Crepitus** (i.e., a grinding sound or sensation) can be felt and sometimes heard when a joint is put through a full range of motion. Crepitus is caused by surface incongruities in the joint.
   d. **Warmth.** Involved joints usually are cool but can feel warm with flare-ups of disease activity.
   e. **Joint enlargement.** Soft tissue swelling may occur if an effusion is present. More commonly, bone enlargement occurs in the form of osteophytes.
   f. **Deformity. Varus** (medial) or **valgus** (lateral) **angulation** of joints can occur late in the disease. Gross bone enlargement and joint subluxation also can occur in severe disease.
      (1) **Heberden's nodes** specifically refer to enlargement of the DIP joints of the hand.
      (2) **Bouchard's nodes** specifically refer to enlargement of the PIP joints of the hand.

G Diagnosis

Patient history combined with physical, laboratory, and radiographic findings form the basis for diagnosis.

1. **Joint involvement**
   a. The **distribution of the involved joints** should suggest whether the osteoarthritis is primary or related to an underlying disorder (see VI E 1–2).
   b. **Joint swelling** is typically **bony,** sometimes with superimposed **fluid.**
2. **Laboratory findings**
   a. **Hematologic findings.** Results, including the erythrocyte sedimentation rate, are generally normal.
   b. **Synovial fluid findings.** Typical osteoarthritic synovial fluid is slightly turbid, contains no crystals, and has a WBC count that is only mildly inflammatory (i.e., < 2000 cells/mm^3 and < 25% neutrophils).
3. **Radiographic findings.** Radiographic evidence is common after age 40 in joints typically affected by osteoarthritis, and it often is asymptomatic.

a. **Findings typically present**
   (1) Joint space narrowing (due to loss of cartilage)
   (2) Subchondral sclerosis (increased subchondral bone density)
   (3) Marginal osteophytes
   (4) Subchondral cysts

b. **Findings typically absent**
   (1) Periarticular osteopenia
   (2) Marginal erosions (except in the distal DIP and PIP joints in the erosive osteoarthritis variant)

c. **Clinical correlates**
   (1) **Comparison views** of the contralateral joint can be helpful.
   (2) **Standing views** best demonstrate the amount of cartilage loss in knees.

4. **Differential diagnosis**

a. **Monoarticular problems**
   (1) **Periarticular abnormality.** Patients may complain of pain in a joint yet have involvement of a periarticular structure such as a tendon, ligament, or bursa as the real cause of symptoms.
   (2) **Other causes.** Bacterial infections and crystal-mediated problems must always be considered if only one joint is involved. Trauma, hemorrhage, and monoarticular presentations of inflammatory diseases also can be confused with osteoarthritis.

b. **Polyarticular problems**
   (1) **Inflammatory rheumatic disease.** Systemic complaints (e.g., anorexia, weight loss, fatigue, fever), prominent morning stiffness, and findings of inflammatory rheumatic diseases should be sought.
   (2) **Soft tissue syndromes.** Disorders associated with regional aching (regional myofascial pain) or generalized aching (e.g., fibromyalgia, PMR) also should be considered in polyarticular presentations.

H Therapy

1. **Nonpharmacologic therapy**

a. **General advice to patients.** Joint overuse or repetitive trauma must be avoided. **Weight loss** may be beneficial in arthritis of weight-bearing joints such as the knees. Osteoarthritic pain improves with rest, so **joint rest** is particularly important when pain is prominent.

b. **Supports**
   (1) A **knee cage or brace** sometimes is used when knee ligamentous instability coexists with osteoarthritis.
   (2) A **soft cervical collar** may be used for symptomatic flare-ups of cervical spine osteoarthritis.
   (3) A **lumbar corset** (back brace) sometimes is used to buttress sagging abdominal or back muscles in patients with low back pain.
   (4) A **cane** may be helpful in supporting a patient with unilateral hip or knee osteoarthritis.
   (5) **Arch supports (orthotics)** or cushioned shoes may decrease the transmission of weight-bearing forces to the hips and knees.

c. **Exercise. Isometric strengthening** of supporting muscles around joints may be helpful (e.g., quadriceps-setting exercises in knee arthritis). Swimming and water aerobics are the best form of **aerobic exercise** for a patient with osteoarthritis of the hips or knees; running should be avoided by these patients.

d. **Heat/cold modalities.** Application of moist heat or heating pads, or even ice, often can temporarily lessen the pain of osteoarthritis.

e. **Nutrition.** Research on deficiencies of vitamins C and D are ongoing. The value of nutritional supplements is still controversial.

2. **Pharmacologic therapy**
   a. **Analgesics**
      (1) **Topical.** Direct application of **capsaicin** (substance P inhibitor) to the skin overlying a painful joint can relieve pain.
      (2) **Systemic.** Pain-relieving medications such as **acetaminophen** often are effective in moderate-to-high doses for mild-to-moderate osteoarthritis. Narcotics should only be used under extenuating circumstances.
   b. **NSAIDs.** Pain relief with low-to-moderate doses of aspirin or other NSAIDs may be useful. Elderly patients have more gastrointestinal and renal side effects from these drugs and, thus, should be carefully monitored when receiving such treatment. The selective COX-2 blocking agents have been shown to have similar efficacy, but with less gastrointestinal toxicity (see II G 2).
   c. **Corticosteroids.** Oral steroids have no place in the management of osteoarthritis. Occasional **intra-articular** injections of corticosteroids may be of temporary benefit in flare-ups, but repeated use of steroids carries the risk of possible acceleration of the disease process.
   d. **Viscosupplementation therapy with intra-articular hyaluronic acid.** Two formulations of intra-articular hyaluronic acid are available for use in the treatment of early (mild) osteoarthritis of the knee. Studies have shown these agents to be effective in modulating pain originating from the osteoarthritic knee joint and have demonstrated that these agents may have a positive effect on articular cartilage biology.
   e. **Ongoing research**
      (1) **Metalloproteinase inhibitors** (see VI C 3)
      (2) **Biological agents.** Agents such as proinflammatory cytokine inhibitors, cytokine soluble receptors, and anti-inflammatory cytokines. These agents have potential beneficial therapeutic properties.
      (3) **Cartilage transplantation.** Once perfected, this technique likely will be restricted to younger patients with cartilage lesions in the absence of bony changes.
      (4) **Surgery.** In advanced disease of the knee or hip, **total joint replacement** can be dramatically effective in alleviating pain and restoring function. **Angulation osteotomy** is still performed in osteoarthritis of the knee to treat unicompartmental disease. The development of new biomaterials and expanding knowledge on the biology of prosthesis loosening should help lower the failure rate.

VII BACTERIAL (SEPTIC) ARTHRITIS

Bacterial arthritis is a serious inflammatory arthritis of one or more joints that can lead to rapid joint destruction if untreated. Numerous organisms can cause a septic arthritis syndrome.

A Epidemiology (Table 10–11) Otherwise healthy individuals can develop bacterial arthritis by direct inoculation or by blood-borne invasion of a joint, but certain people are at higher risk.

1. **Joint damage.** Patients with joints damaged by osteoarthritis, rheumatoid arthritis, or other destructive joint processes are more at risk for infection in the already damaged joints. Perhaps joint structural disorganization impairs efficient processing and removal of pathogenic organisms.
2. **Immunosuppression.** Patients with immune deficiencies are at greater risk for bacterial arthritis, particularly if those defects involve neutropenia or impaired phagocytosis.
3. **Inoculation.** Repeated septicemia (e.g., in the setting of intravenous drug abuse) presents the greatest risk. Most medical procedures involving potential direct inoculation (e.g., joint aspira-

TABLE 10–11 Epidemiology of Bacterial Arthritis

Risk Factor	Clinical Setting	Organism
Prior joint damage	Rheumatoid arthritis, osteoarthritis	*Staphylococcus aureus*
Immunosuppression	Diabetes mellitus, alcoholism, chronic renal failure, cytotoxic drugs, SLE, cancer, AIDS	*S. aureus,* gram-negative rods
Joint aspiration or injection	Damaged or inflamed joint (rare)	*Staphylococcus epidermidis, S. aureus*
IV drug abuse	Axial joint (acromioclavicular, sternoclavicular, sacroiliac) involvement	*S. aureus,* gram-negative rods, *Pseudomonas aeuruginosa*
Sickle cell arthropathy	Joint infection or osteomyelitis	*Salmonella* and *Staphylococcus* species, *Streptococcus pneumoniae,* gram-negative rods
Prosthetic joint	Perioperative period	*S. epidermidis*
	Postoperative period	*S. aureus,* gram-negative rods or anaerobes

tion and injection) are performed aseptically and only minimally increase the risk of organism introduction into the joint.

4. **Prosthetic joint.** Replacement of a joint with a prosthesis removes the normal defenses against joint infection, and prosthetic materials are difficult to sterilize once infected.

B **Etiology** Infectious arthritis is best classified as **gonococcal** or **nongonococcal.** Gonococcal infections account for at least half of cases of bacterial arthritis in adults, are much less destructive, and are very responsive to treatment.

1. ***Neisseria gonorrhoeae.*** This gram-negative intracellular diplococcus causes **disseminated gonococcal infection (DGI).** Typically sexually transmitted, *N. gonorrhoeae* can cause **septic arthritis** or a **periarthritis–dermatitis syndrome.**
2. ***Staphylococcus* species.** Clusters of gram-positive cocci on Gram stain suggest a staphylococcal infection.
   a. ***Staphylococcus aureus*** is the most common nongonococcal cause of septic arthritis, which typically arises from a skin source and can be especially rapid in causing joint destruction.
   b. ***Staphylococcus epidermidis*** also typically arises from a skin source. Although usually less virulent than *S. aureus, S. epidermidis* is becoming a more common cause of joint infection in prosthetic joints and in the setting of intravenous drug abuse.
3. ***Streptococcus species***
   a. **Group A β-hemolytic streptococci** remain the most common cause of infection associated with gram-positive chains on Gram stain and arise from skin or respiratory tract sources.
   b. **Non-group A streptococci** arising from skin or urinary tract sources are being seen more often in immunocompromised patients, those with prosthetic joints, and those who use intravenous drugs.
4. **Nongonococcal gram-negative organisms**
   a. **Gram-negative enteric pathogens.** Skin colonization with gram-negative organisms is a potential source of joint infection in elderly or immunocompromised individuals, particularly those in hospitals or chronic care institutions. Urinary tract sources also are common in these patients.

b. ***Haemophilus influenzae.*** This gram-negative coccobacillus remains a major respiratory pathogen in infants. The potential for dissemination to joints is greatest between 6 months and 2 years of age, when infants are without protective maternal antibodies and have not developed their own.

c. ***Neisseria meningitidis.*** This gram-negative intracellular diplococcus, similar to *N. gonorrhoeae,* arises from an upper respiratory tract source. It is a much less common cause of a disseminated periarthritis–dermatitis infection, which is typically characterized by more skin lesions than are seen in DGI.

5. **Anaerobic and polymicrobial infections** are uncommon; they typically arise in the setting of prosthetic joint infection or severe immunocompromise.

C Pathophysiology

1. **Entry.** Bacteria enter the joint via the bloodstream (septicemia) or direct inoculation (synovial aspiration, trauma, surgery).
2. **Early events.** Once inside the joint, the presence of bacteria elicits synovial lining cell hyperplasia and neutrophil chemotaxis.
3. **Acute destructive process.** Synovial cells and neutrophils release **proteolytic enzymes,** which damage cartilage and subchondral bone as well as killing the bacteria. Dying bacteria release **lipopolysaccharides** that can either directly degrade cartilage or indirectly degrade it by stimulating the release of **IL-1 or IL-1–like factors** that cause chondrocytes to release **collagenases** and **prostaglandins.**
4. **Chronic destruction.** Granulation tissue acts similarly to **rheumatoid pannus** in degrading cartilage and bone.

D Clinical features

1. **Gonococcal arthritis.** Patients with DGI typically have genital infection without symptoms of arthritis or pelvic inflammatory disease; changes in the endometrium or cervical mucus may allow causative strains to disseminate during menses. The lack of genitourinary complaints delays treatment before dissemination.

   a. **Periarthritis–dermatitis syndrome.** Most patients exhibit **migratory or additive polyarthralgias** for several days, followed by **fever, tenosynovitis,** and often **dermatitis.** The skin lesions can be **maculopapular** or **vesicular,** with the vesicles becoming **vesiculopustular** over time.

   b. **Monoarthritis.** Twenty-five to fifty percent of patients with DGI develop an infectious mono- or oligoarthritis with purulent joint effusions. These "septic joints" can occur with or without preceding **periarthritis–dermatitis syndrome.**

2. **Nongonococcal arthritis.** Patients typically present with acute pain, tenderness, swelling, and severe limitation of motion in the affected joint(s). Warmth and erythema are sometimes present, and some patients have evidence of a source (e.g., skin, urinary tract, pharynx, lung, cardiac valve) responsible for septicemic joint inoculation.

E Diagnosis

1. **Making a presumptive diagnosis**

   a. **Gonococcal arthritis.** History of recent sexual contact should be sought and cultures from appropriate sites (pharynx, skin lesions, joint fluid, blood, rectum, urethra, cervix) taken in patients who have suspicious skin lesions or tenosynovitis. A sexually active adult who has an acute monoarthritis without crystals or other known cause should be cultured and treated for DGI, until other information suggests a more appropriate course.

   b. **Nongonococcal arthritis.** Synovial fluid should be aspirated and sent for Gram stain, glucose, WBC count and differential, and culture and sensitivity. A synovial fluid WBC count greater than 50,000/mm^3 with more than 90% neutrophils is highly suggestive of bacterial infection. Infected fluids can sometimes have less striking WBC elevations (10,000–20,000/mm^3).

2. **Differential diagnosis.** Other causes of infectious and noninfectious arthritis should be considered when making a presumptive diagnosis of bacterial arthritis. **Periarticular bone and soft tissue infections** should also be sought.
   a. **Other infections.** Patients with monoarticular arthritis may have another infection.
      (1) **Lyme disease.** This condition should always be considered in patients living in endemic areas who have a mono- or oligoarticular inflammatory arthritis, especially when the arthritis is accompanied by one or more of the dermatologic, cardiac, or neurologic features of the disorder.
      (2) **Tuberculous or fungal arthritis.** These infections generally are more indolent; they typically are associated with lower synovial fluid WBC counts and lower percentages of neutrophils than are seen in bacterial infections. Synovial biopsy may be required for diagnosis because joint fluid cultures are frequently negative.
   b. **Inflammatory arthritis.** Disorders such as rheumatoid arthritis, acute rheumatic fever (ARF), reactive arthritis, and psoriatic arthritis can manifest as severe monoarticular involvement looking like an infection, sometimes with WBC counts exceeding 50,000/mm^3 and more than 90% neutrophils. In some instances, patients with these diseases must be treated with antibiotics for 48 hours until joint fluid cultures are known to be negative. Gout and pseudogout can cause acute monoarthritis, so synovial fluid must be examined under polarized light microscopy for the causative crystals.
   c. **Infection outside joints**
      (1) **Osteomyelitis** near a joint can cause fever and a sterile, inflammatory effusion mimicking septic arthritis.
      (2) **Subcutaneous bursae** next to joints (e.g., prepatellar, olecranon) can be inflamed or infected and mimic an infection of the adjacent joint. The physical appearance and location of the swollen bursa should be distinctive.

F Therapy

1. **Antibiotics**
   a. **Choice of therapy**
      (1) **Empiric treatment.** Because bacterial arthritis is so rapidly destructive, presumptive antibiotic therapy must be started before results of definitive cultures are known. The particular antibiotic regimen is tailored to the organisms most likely in a particular individual (see Table 10–11) and particular age group (Table 10–12). In adults, gonococcal coverage is appropriate unless sexual contact can be excluded. Otherwise, coverage for *S. aureus* and streptococci typically is included. Gram-negative coverage is added in patients who are immunocompromised or who are intravenous drug abusers.

TABLE 10–12 Bacterial Arthritis: Age Groups and Common Organisms

Age Group	Organism
< 2 years	*Haemophilus influenzae**, *Staphylococcus aureus,* group A streptococci, Enterobacteriaceae
2–6 years	*S. aureus,* group A streptococci, *H. influenzae*
6 years to adult	Sexually transmitted: *Neisseria gonorrhoeae*†
	Non-sexually transmitted: *S. aureus,* group A streptococci, Enterobacteriaceae

*Young children at risk after loss of maternal antibody.
†In adults, *N. gonorrhoeae* is implicated twice as often as all other agents combined.

(2) **Directed therapy.** Positive results on synovial fluid Gram stain or positive culture results from blood, synovial fluid, or other sources allow more specific treatment of the causative organism.

b. **Route and duration of therapy**

(1) **Gonococcal arthritis.** The gonococcus is so sensitive that 3 days of intravenous antibiotic followed by 7 more days of oral antibiotic usually is sufficient treatment.

(2) **Nongonococcal arthritis.** Antibiotics typically are given intravenously for at least 2 weeks in nongonococcal bacterial arthritis, longer if clinical improvement is slow. Oral medication is given for 2 additional weeks.

2. **Drainage**

a. **Closed-needle aspiration.** Daily drainage of any effusion is imperative to remove organisms and inflammatory debris, which can destroy cartilage and subchondral bone. Closed-needle aspiration usually is appropriate, because open surgical drainage prolongs immobilization and delays return of effective function.

b. **Open surgical drainage.** Hip infections are best handled by immediate open drainage, especially in children. Joints that do not respond to needle drainage are treated either by open drainage or by arthroscopy.

c. **Arthroscopic drainage.** Arthroscopy is an attractive alternative to open drainage, because lysis of adhesions and removal of inflamed synovium can often be accomplished without the prolonged immobilization of open drainage.

3. **Other ancillary measures. Continuous passive motion** early in treatment is somewhat more effective than complete immobilization at preventing loss of cartilage and subchondral bone. The avascular cartilage depends on joint motion for nutrition. **Weight-bearing and ambulation of involved joints should be avoided** until effusions are gone; otherwise, **postinfectious inflammatory arthritis** can delay recovery.

4. **Response to treatment**

a. Trends in the following clinical and laboratory parameters allow assessment of therapeutic progress:

(1) Resolution of fever
(2) Resolution of synovial effusion
(3) Improvement in joint pain, tenderness, and range of motion
(4) Resolution of leukocytosis (blood, synovial fluid)
(5) Sterility of synovial fluid cultures

b. **Failure of improvement** should lead to reconsideration of diagnosis, reconsideration of choice or dosage of antibiotic, and consideration of open or arthroscopic drainage.

VIII SYSTEMIC LUPUS ERYTHEMATOSUS (SLE)

A Definition

SLE is a chronic immune disorder characterized by multisystem involvement and clinical exacerbations and remissions. **Circulating immune complexes** and **autoantibodies** cause tissue damage and organ dysfunction. Manifestations involving the skin, serosal surfaces, CNS, kidneys, and blood cells are particularly characteristic. Evidence for the autoimmune nature of this disorder lies in the laboratory finding of ANAs, demonstration of immune complexes in tissues, and utilization of complement.

B Epidemiology

1. The overall **prevalence** of SLE is approximately 15–50 cases per 100,000 population. The prevalence in young women of childbearing age is approximately eight to ten times that in men. African-American women are affected approximately three times as often as Caucasian women.

2. The frequency of occurrence of lupus is higher in the relatives of affected individuals than in the general population, and the disease concordance rate in identical twins approaches 50%.

C Etiology No single cause of lupus has been discovered. Complex interrelationships among environmental factors, genetically determined host immune responses, and hormonal influences probably are critical in the initiation as well as the expression of the disease.

1. **Environmental factors.** Viruses and drugs or toxins have been pursued as causative agents, but neither has been shown to cause idiopathic SLE. Microbial toxins and viral (particularly retroviral) products can function as **superantigens,** binding to the helper T-cell receptors and MHC class II molecule complexes nonspecifically. Binding to B-cell MHC class II molecules might activate helper T cells to generate **autoimmune responses.**
2. **Genetic factors.** Twin and family studies suggest a genetic predisposition to SLE. The disease occurs commonly in families with hereditary deficiencies of early complement components. The histocompatibility antigens HLA-DR2 and HLA-DR3 are present much more commonly in SLE patients than in controls. Some of the HLA-DR3 association may be due to linkage with a deletion for a C4a gene. Specific combinations of histocompatibility antigens may be associated with the production of specific autoantibodies (e.g., HLA-DR or HLA-DQ associations with Ro and La antibodies).
3. **Autoimmunity.** Loss of tolerance to autoantigens is central to the pathogenesis of SLE, and genetic tendencies toward the development of autoantibodies, B-cell hyperactivity, and T-cell dysfunction are evident in patients with the disease. The tendency to develop autoimmunity in SLE is not MHC-linked but may be caused by genes outside the histocompatibility loci.
4. **Apoptosis.** Programmed cell death, or apoptosis, leads to the orderly replacement of old cells in all organs, including the B and T lymphocytes of the immune system. Defects in apoptosis genes have been discovered in lupus mouse kindreds, resulting in the development of autoimmunity, perhaps related to failure to delete autoreactive T cells or autoantibody-producing B cells.
5. **Hormonal influences.** Lupus is predominantly a disease of women of childbearing age, but hormonal factors probably are more important in modulation of the expression of disease than in causation. Estrogen may be a permissive factor in polyclonal B-cell activation.

D Pathogenesis All of the clinical features of SLE are manifestations of cellular and humoral immune dysfunction; however, **atherosclerosis** can be a secondary effect of vascular damage that leads to further organ ischemia.

1. **Immune complexes.** Circulating antigen–antibody (immune) complexes are deposited in blood vessels and the renal glomerulus, initiating a pathologic response that damages these tissues. These complexes are characteristic features of active disease, and their size, solubility, concentration, and complement-fixing properties as well as vessel hydrostatic forces are important in determining tissue deposition.
2. **Reticuloendothelial dysfunction.** The chronic circulation of immune complexes seems to be important in their pathogenicity, as occurs in a chronic serum sickness reaction. At times, the ability of the reticuloendothelial system to remove immune complexes from the circulation may be overwhelmed. Patients with C4a gene deletions more commonly have SLE, perhaps as a result of impaired immune complex clearance.
3. **Autoantibodies** are produced either in the setting of specific, antigen-driven, induction of autoreactive lymphocyte clones or polyclonal activation of different B-cell lineages. These autoantibodies can cause the following conditions:
   a. **Tissue damage.** Antibodies to RBCs, WBCs, or platelets can cause immune cytopenias.
   b. **Cellular dysfunction.** Antibodies to lymphocytes can impair lymphocyte function and intercellular signaling; antineuronal antibodies crossing a breached blood–brain barrier can impair neuron function.

c. **Immune complex formation.** Complexes of antibodies and double-stranded DNA are important in mediation of autoimmune renal disease.

4. **Lymphocyte dysfunction.** B-cell hyperactivity, impaired $CD8^+$ cell function, and augmented $CD4^+$ cell activity are present in various combinations in lupus patients, leading to autoantibody production and increased generation of immune complexes.

E Pathology

1. **Characteristic microscopic changes**
   a. **Hematoxylin bodies.** Amorphous masses of nuclear material bound with immunoglobulin can be found in connective tissue lesions that become purple–blue when stained with hematoxylin. Neutrophils that ingest these bodies in vitro are called **LE cells.**
   b. **Fibrinoid necrosis.** In SLE, immune complexes of DNA, antibody to DNA, and complement may stain with eosin (which can stain immune complexes as well as fibrin) in vessel walls and connective tissue, demonstrating so-called "fibrinoid necrosis."
   c. **Onion-skin lesions.** Lesions characteristic of SLE in splenic arteries are called onion-skin lesions because of the concentric deposition of collagen around them, presumably formed as vasculitic lesions heal.
2. **Tissue changes**
   a. **Skin.** Although some of the milder skin lesions in SLE have only nonspecific lymphocytic infiltration in perivascular locations in the dermis, more typical lupus lesions show **dermal–epidermal junction deposits of immunoglobulins** and complement as well as necrosis. Classic discoid lesions show follicular plugging, hyperkeratosis, and the loss of skin appendages. Frank vasculitic lesions also can occur in small dermal vessels.
   b. **Kidney.** Immune complex deposition in the kidney can lead to various histologic pictures of inflammation. A cardinal characteristic of renal pathology in SLE is the tendency of these pathologic pictures to change over time, based either on changes in disease activity or therapy. Biopsy specimens are graded with regard to activity (active inflammation) and chronicity (glomerular sclerosis and fibrotic interstitial change); the most treatable lesions have high activity and low chronicity.
      (1) **Mesangial disease** refers to **mesangial hypercellularity** caused by the presence of immunoglobulin deposits and is the most common renal pathologic lesion in SLE.
      (2) **Focal proliferative nephritis** involves cellular proliferative change only in **segments of glomeruli** and in **less than 50% of glomeruli.**
      (3) **Diffuse proliferative nephritis** involves cellular proliferation in **most of the segments** of the glomerulus and in **more than 50% of glomeruli.**
      (4) **Pure membranous nephritis** consists of **subepithelial** glomerular basement membrane immunoglobulin deposits without glomerular hypercellularity (called **wire looping** on light microscopy), although patients may have overlapping combinations of proliferative and membranous forms on biopsy.
      (5) **Interstitial inflammation** can also occur in all of the above pathologic pictures.
   c. **CNS.** Large vessel vasculitic lesions can occur (although they are uncommon) in focal presentations of the disease, but focal areas of perivascular small vessel inflammation, microinfarction, or microhemorrhages are more typical and do not correlate well with abnormalities found on imaging studies [computed tomography (CT) or magnetic resonance imaging (MRI) scans] or the neurologic examination. The **phospholipid antibody syndrome** may be associated with the small vessel occlusive lesions.
   d. **Vasculitis.** Inflammatory lesions of capillaries, venules, and arterioles, caused by immune complex deposition and variable cellular infiltration, are responsible for much of the tissue destruction and damage seen in SLE.
   e. **Other tissue lesions.** Nonspecific mild synovitis and lymphocytic infiltration of muscles occur frequently. Nonbacterial endocarditis often is present but typically is asymptomatic.

F Clinical features and laboratory findings (Table 10–13)

1. **Manifestations of SLE.** Fatigue, weight loss, and fever are prominent **systemic complaints.**
   a. **Skin.** The **butterfly rash** (i.e., facial erythema over the cheeks and nose) and the chronic, potentially scarring, **discoid lesions** (i.e., coin-shaped lesions with hyperemic margins, central atrophy, and depigmentation) are the most classic. Less commonly, bullous and maculopapular eruptions can occur. Nonscarring, psoriasiform lesions **(subacute cutaneous lupus)** occur and are associated with the Ro antibody. Recurrent mucous membrane ulceration, generalized or focal alopecia, digital vasculitis, and photosensitivity also are potential dermatologic features.
   b. **Nerve**
      (1) **CNS.** Focal or diffuse neurologic disorders occur in approximately 50% of patients. **Generalized manifestations** include severe headache, reactive depressions, psychoses, cognitive disturbances, and seizures. Psychosis in some lupus patients correlates with the presence of antibody to ribosomal P protein. **Focal seizures** also have been described, and hemiparesis, cranial nerve deficits, transverse myelitis, and movement disorders may pinpoint discrete areas of involvement. Lumbar puncture (LP), electroencephalography (EEG), and CT scanning often are unrevealing. However, MRI scanning reveals CNS lesions in many patients, especially those with focal presentations.
      (2) **Peripheral nervous system.** Some patients have sensory or sensorimotor neuropathies, and those with vasculitis of the vasonervorum may manifest as mononeuritis multiplex.
   c. **Heart.** Symptomatic **pericarditis** occurs in approximately 20% of SLE patients and pericardial effusions on echocardiography in as many as 50%, but tamponade is uncommon. **Myocarditis** (conduction abnormalities, arrhythmias, and CHF) is less common and may be reversible if treated promptly with corticosteroids. Although **coronary vessel vasculitis** can occur in fulminant cases, premature atherosclerosis in steroid-treated patients is a more common cause of myocardial infarction (MI) in lupus patients. **Nonbacterial endocardial lesions** (Libman-Sacks endocarditis) can be associated with embolic CNS events, valvular dysfunction, the antiphospholipid antibody syndrome, or infective endocarditis.
   d. **Lung.** At some time in the disease course, approximately 30% of SLE patients have symptomatic **pleuritis,** and fewer have friction rubs or actual effusions apparent on ultrasonography. Diaphragmatic fibrosis or diaphragm dysfunction may manifest as **"shrinking lung syndrome,"** with a restrictive picture on pulmonary function testing. Parenchymal involvement **(lupus pneumonitis)** can be difficult to distinguish from acute infections; lupus infiltrates may be unilateral or bilateral, tend to be fleeting, occur with active disease, and lack purulent sputum. **Hemoptysis** occurs as a feature of pulmonary vasculitis and the **acute pulmonary hemorrhage syndrome. Diffuse interstitial lung disease** is recognized, albeit uncommonly. **Pulmonary hypertension** as a result of isolated pulmonary vascular involvement also occurs.
   e. **Gastrointestinal tract.** Although symptoms of nausea, vomiting, and abdominal pain are common, diagnostic testing often is unrevealing. Overt **intestinal vasculitis** can lead to bowel infarction, perforation, and hemorrhage. Lupus- or corticosteroid-related **pancreatitis** and reversible gastric damage or hepatitis induced by NSAIDs can occur as well.
   f. **Kidney.** Most lupus patients have some clinical and pathologic evidence of renal involvement. Active disease often is announced by abnormalities in the urinary sediment (i.e., RBCs, WBCs, or cellular casts formed in the absence of acute bacterial infection). Other clinical laboratory features typically associated with active renal disease are elevations in serum creatinine and blood urea nitrogen (BUN) levels, decreased levels of serum complement components or increased titers of antibodies against double-stranded DNA. The renal biopsy often can aid in treatment decisions and the determination of prognosis, although the biopsy pathology may change with disease course or therapy.
      (1) **Mesangial disease** is the most common and mildest form of renal involvement and may be asymptomatic. Many patients have mild proteinuria or RBCs or WBCs on urinalysis. Treatment usually is not required.

TABLE 10–13 Criteria for the Classification of Systemic Lupus Erythematosus

Criterion	Definition
1. Malar rash	Fixed erythema, flat or raised, over the malar eminences, tending to spare the nasolabial folds
2. Discoid rash	Erythematous raised patches with adherent keratotic scaling and follicular plugging, atrophic scarring may occur in older lesions
3. Photosensitivity	Skin rash as a result of unusual reaction to sunlight, by patient history or physician observation
4. Oral ulcers	Oral or nasopharyngeal ulceration, usually painless, observed by a physician
5. Arthritis	Nonerosive arthritis involving two or more peripheral joints, characterized by tenderness, swelling, or effusion
6. Serositis	a) Pleuritis—convincing history of pleuritic pain or rub heard by a physician or evidence of pleural effusion OR b) Pericarditis—documented by ECG or rub or evidence of pericardial effusion
7. Renal disorder	a) Persistent proteinuria greater than 0.5 g/day or greater that 3+ if quantitation not performed OR b) Cellular casts—may be red cell, hemoglobin, granular, tubular, or mixed
8. Neurologic disorders	a) Seizures—in the absence of offending drugs or known metabolic derangements; e.g., uremia, ketoacidosis, or electrolyte imbalance OR b) Psychosis—in the absence of offending drugs or known metabolic derangements; e.g., uremia, ketoacidosis, or electrolyte imbalance
9. Hematologic disorder	a) Hemolytic anemia—with reticulocytosis OR b) Leukopenia—less than 4000/mm^3 total on two or more occasions OR c) Lymphopenia—less than 1500/mm^3 on two or more occasions OR d) Thrombocytopenia—less than 100,000/mm^3 in the absence of offending drugs
10. Immunologic disorder	a) Anti-DNA: antibody to native DNA in abnormal titer OR b) Anti-SM: presence of antibody to SM nuclear antigen OR c) Positive finding of antiphospholipid antibodies based on (1) an abnormal serum level of IgG or IgM anti-cardiolipin antibodies, (2) a positive test result for lupus anticoagulant using a standard method, or (3) a false-positive serologic test for syphilis known to be positive for at least 6 months and confirmed by *Treponema pallidum* immobilization or fluorescent treponemal antibody absorption test
11. Antinuclear antibody	An abnormal titer of antinuclear antibody by immunofluorescence or an equivalent assay at any point in time and in the absence of drugs known to be associated with "drug-induced lupus" syndrome

a. This classification is based on 11 criteria. For the purpose of identifying patients in clinical studies, a person must have SLE if any four or more of the 11 criteria are present, serially or simultaneously, during any interval of observation.

b. The modifications to criterion number 10 were made in 1997.

Adapted from Tan EM, Cohen AS, Fries JF, et al: The 1982 revised criteria for the classification of systemic lupus erythematosus (SLE). *Arthritis Rheum* 1982;25:1271–1277, with permission from the American College of Rheumatology.

Adapted from Hochberg MC: Updating the American College of Rheumatology revised criteria for the classification of system lupus erythematosus [letter]. *Arthritis Rheum* 1997;40:1725, with permission of the American College of Rheumatology.

(2) **Focal proliferative nephritis** often has a good prognosis as well and typically requires treatment with corticosteroids alone; however, its more severe presentations blend with diffuse proliferative nephritis clinically and prognostically.

(3) **Diffuse proliferative nephritis** is the most severe pathologic lesion and usually is associated with hypertension, severe proteinuria, and some degree of renal insufficiency. The most severe cases can be associated with **crescents** and the rapid development of severe renal insufficiency. Corticosteroids and cytotoxic agents typically are required for preservation of renal function.

(4) **Membranous glomerulopathy** classically manifests as large amounts of protein in the urine and nephrotic syndrome, usually with relatively few cells in the urine. Corticosteroid therapy may help control protein loss. Slowly progressive renal insufficiency may develop over time; it is not clear whether the addition of cytotoxic agents retards this progression.

g. **Muscle and bone. Arthralgia** and **symmetrical arthritis** often are features of acute SLE, but the rare joint deformities (**Jaccoud's arthropathy**) that occur are a function of tendon or ligament laxity rather than erosive joint disease. Inflammatory muscle involvement usually is subclinical, but clinical inflammatory myopathy can occur.

h. **Other.** Photosensitivity can trigger systemic symptoms as well as skin manifestations. Raynaud's phenomenon and secondary Sjögren's syndrome each occur in approximately 25% of patients.

2. **Laboratory findings**

a. **Hematologic findings.** Anemia is common during active disease and more often is the anemia of chronic disease than hemolytic anemia. Antibodies to leukocytes also occur, with autoimmune lymphopenia a common feature of active disease; neutropenia is less common. Antibodies to platelets can cause chronic immune thrombocytopenia or more acute falls in the platelet count with active disease. Elevation of the erythrocyte sedimentation rate is common and correlates with disease activity in some patients.

b. **Coagulation parameters.** Antibodies to the phospholipid components of individual clotting factors can interfere with coagulation testing, causing prolongation of the PTT not correctable by the addition of normal plasma. Paradoxically, patients with the PTT prolongation (the **"lupus anticoagulant"**) have a higher frequency of thrombosis than bleeding.

c. **Serologic findings.** Phospholipid antibodies also can cause false-positive test results for syphilis, more often by interference with reagin [e.g., rapid plasma reagin (RPR) or VDRL] testing than with antitreponemal [e.g., fluorescent treponemal antibody absorption (FTA-ABS)] testing.

d. **Immunologic findings.** Lupus patients commonly have **low complement component (C3 and C4) levels** as a result of immune complex activation; in many patients, falls in serum complement levels parallel disease flare-ups if complement synthesis is unchanged.

(1) **Hypergammaglobulinemia** reflects B-cell hyperactivity. By far the most significant immunologic findings in SLE patients are **autoantibodies.**

(2) **ANAs.** Approximately 99% of patients with SLE have ANAs. These antibodies are detectable by an immunofluorescence technique that involves human epithelial cell lines (e.g., HEp-2 cells). When the test serum is applied to the epithelial cells that have been frozen and cut to expose nuclear components, the patient's ANAs interact with the nuclear material, and this interaction can be detected by fluorescence microscopy. A **diffuse** or **homogeneous** immunofluorescent staining **pattern** is most common in SLE, although **speckled, nucleolar,** and **rim patterns** also can be seen (see I B 3).

G Diagnosis Careful consideration of the historical and physical findings that suggest this multisystem disease is necessary. Systemic illness with characteristic rash, polyarthritis, and serositis is a common presentation, but the possibility of lupus should be entertained even when patients present with seemingly isolated hematologic cytopenias, CNS disease, or glomerulonephritis. In suspicious settings, physicians should seek laboratory evidence of autoimmunity and attempt to exclude other illnesses.

1. **Diagnostic criteria** (Table 10–13). The 1997 ARA revised criteria for the diagnosis of SLE are useful when the disease is suspected, and the presence over time of any **four** of the eleven criteria strongly suggests the diagnosis. Although findings such as alopecia, periungual vasculitis, and low serum complement levels are not among the criteria, they may be supportive evidence in individual patients.
2. **Differential diagnosis.** Physicians must be careful to exclude other chronic rheumatic diseases, especially rheumatoid arthritis, overlap syndromes (inflammatory myopathies or scleroderma overlapping with SLE), and vasculitic syndromes in arriving at the diagnosis of SLE. The following syndromes also should be considered in the setting of possible SLE:
   a. **Undifferentiated connective tissue disease** (UCTD). This disorder is used to describe patients with clinical features of several connective tissue diseases and high titers of antibody to U_1RNP. Patients with UCTD may have cutaneous features of SLE, dermatomyositis, or scleroderma; inflammatory muscle disease; and a destructive form of arthritis more typical of rheumatoid arthritis. Furthermore, the severe renal and CNS manifestations of SLE usually are not present. When followed for prolonged periods, most patients with this disease more closely resemble patients with scleroderma or SLE.
   b. **Drug-induced lupus.** Chronic ingestion of several drugs can precipitate a syndrome of **polyserositis, arthritis,** and **antihistone ANAs.** The drugs most commonly associated include hydralazine, procainamide, penicillamine, isoniazid, and phenytoin. Renal disease is rare in this syndrome, and dermal and CNS features are less common than in idiopathic SLE. Drug-induced SLE typically resolves on discontinuation of the drug. Hepatic acetylation of drugs such as hydralazine, isoniazid, and procainamide is apparently slow in patients who develop this syndrome, although these drugs typically are tolerated well by patients with SLE.
   c. **Discoid lupus.** Patients can have typical skin manifestations of SLE without systemic disease. Fifteen percent of these patients have positive ANAs. These patients should be considered to have SLE when other disease features are present.
3. **Associated syndromes**
   a. **Neonatal lupus syndrome** can develop in infants of mothers who have high-titer **IgG antibodies** to **Ro.** The maternal antibodies apparently cross the placenta, bind to fetal tissue, and cause immunologic injury. The most typical features include evanescent lupus skin lesions, but transient thrombocytopenia or hemolytic anemia can occur. The most serious clinical presentation occurs in pregnant women when the antibody to Ro binds to fetal cardiac tissue and causes congenital heart block, which can require permanent pacing. Most mothers of affected infants develop a mild version of some autoimmune disease over time, often SLE.
   b. **Phospholipid antibody syndrome** can occur as a mimic of SLE or as part of the disease. One-third to one-half of lupus patients exhibit phospholipid antibody if tested, although the associated clinical syndrome occurs less commonly.
      (1) Manifestations most commonly include **venous or arterial thromboses,** sometimes of large vessels, and can also include **episodic thrombocytopenia. Pregnant patients may experience fetal death** after the first trimester or premature birth, and these problems may recur in successive pregnancies. Some of these patients exhibit placental thrombosis, infarction, or insufficiency, but the cause of fetal death is not always clear.
      (2) Testing for antibodies to phospholipids is involved (see I B 6).
      (3) **Management** primarily involves **chronic anticoagulation therapy,** typically with warfarin, after the first episode of clinical thrombosis.

H Therapy Treatment must be individualized to the features that a particular patient exhibits, and it need not always include corticosteroids. Patients must understand that the prognosis in this chronic disease generally is better than they fear and that their compliance with medication regimens and avoidance of disease precipitants (e.g., ultraviolet light, emotional stress) often can favorably affect the disease course. Physicians must be alert to disease flare-ups related to surgery, antecedent infections, or the postpartum period. Sulfonamides and oral contraceptives may precipitate flare-up of disease in some patients.

1. Topical **sunscreens** containing *para*-aminobenzoic acid (PABA) or benzophenones are effective in protecting the one-third of lupus patients who are photosensitive.
2. **NSAIDs** are used in full anti-inflammatory doses for fever, joint complaints, and serositis. Mild elevation in transaminase levels often develops in SLE patients on these drugs, and aseptic meningitis has been reported in lupus patients on ibuprofen, tolmetin, and sulindac.
3. **Antimalarial drugs** (e.g., hydroxychloroquine, chloroquine) often are used to treat fatigue, skin disease, and arthritis in SLE. Retinal pigmentary deposition leading to blindness is a rare complication of antimalarial treatment since hydroxychloroquine replaced chloroquine. Patients should be screened by an ophthalmologist every 6 months to 1 year.
4. **Corticosteroids**
   a. **Topical preparations.** Some of the skin manifestations are improved by treatment with topical glucocorticoids, although discoid lesions usually require additional treatment with antimalarial agents.
   b. **Systemic corticosteroids**
      (1) **Glucocorticoids** in varying doses are often required to control severe manifestations of SLE and less severe symptoms when they are persistent and disabling. These drugs should be used cautiously, because long-term treatment usually is needed and typical side effects ensue. **Chronic arthritis** and **serositis** may require glucocorticoids if NSAIDs are not sufficient. Severe **hemolysis,** life-threatening **thrombocytopenia, pneumonitis, CNS** or **peripheral nervous system disease,** clinically evident **cardiac** or **skeletal muscle disease, renal disease,** and **vasculitis** are typical indications for systemic glucocorticoids. Usually the drug dosage selected is proportionate to the severity of the illness; the dosage is tapered as manifestations subside. Alternate-day therapy is ideal for patients with only nephritis, but patients who are systemically ill typically require daily doses.
      (2) **"Pulse" corticosteroids** may be necessary. Large doses of corticosteroids sometimes are administered intravenously for particularly severe cases of SLE. Serious **renal** and **CNS manifestations** have been the typical indications for pulse treatment, but dangerous **cardiopulmonary** and **hematologic involvement** also might warrant this aggressive treatment.
5. **Cytotoxic agents** (e.g., azathioprine, cyclophosphamide) sometimes are used to treat severe, refractory features of lupus, particularly **renal disease.** Intravenous "pulse" use of cyclophosphamide has become popular for the treatment of diffuse proliferative glomerulonephritis and acute severe manifestations of lupus refractory to corticosteroids.
6. **Mycophenylate mofetil** is a reversible inhibitor of inosine monophosphate dehydrogenase and blocks proliferation of B and T cells. It has been used successfully in renal allograft rejection. It also has been used in the treatment of lupus nephritis, with encouraging results.
7. **Intravenous immunoglobulin** may be effective. Large doses of immunoglobulin have been given intravenously to treat refractory manifestations of lupus, particularly **immune-mediated thrombocytopenia** or **hemolytic anemia.** Typical doses are 400 mg/kg administered daily for 5 days. This therapy is expensive, often must be given monthly, and **cannot be given to IgA-deficient patients** because of the risk of anaphylaxis.
8. **Ancillary drugs** are important in managing particular features of the disease. Phenytoin and phenobarbital are useful in the control of seizure disorders, and antipsychotic agents with or without corticosteroids help treat acute or chronic psychoses.

I **Prognosis** Outcomes are clearly better today than in the presteroid era; milder forms of disease are recognized and, presumably, appropriate drug treatment improves morbidity and mortality rates.

Renal disease and **infectious complications** are still major causes of death, and prominent **CNS disease** can lead to severe disability. The mortality rate is higher in patients of lower socioeconomic status and educational attainment, a characteristic common to many chronic illnesses. Steroid-related complications can be crippling (e.g., avascular necrosis of the femoral head and osteoporotic vertebral fractures) or fatal (e.g., premature coronary atherosclerosis).

IX SCLERODERMA

A Definition Scleroderma (systemic sclerosis) is a connective tissue disease characterized by widespread **small vessel obliterative disease** and **fibrosis of the skin** (especially distal, digital skin) and **multiple internal organs,** including the heart, lungs, kidneys, and gastrointestinal tract. The description best fits the diffuse form, but localized forms also exist. These latter forms involve patches of skin and subcutaneous tissues but do not include digital skin involvement, Raynaud's phenomenon, or internal organ changes.

B Epidemiology Scleroderma is a relatively rare disease; familial clustering is uncommon. The disease is three to four times more common in women than in men. Coal miners are at a higher risk for the disease, possibly as a result of exposure to silica dust.

C Etiology The etiology of scleroderma is unknown. In some cases it seems likely that an environmental agent (e.g., toxin, virus) causes vascular endothelial injury, with later immunologic responses leading to continued endothelial damage and tissue fibrosis. Supportive evidence includes the initiation of a fibrosing syndrome in patients with polyvinyl chloride exposure, Spanish "toxic oil" syndrome, and L-tryptophan–related eosinophilia myalgia syndrome.

D Pathogenesis Whether the initiating event is environmental or immunologic, the early lesion seems to be one of **vascular endothelial damage,** especially in small vessels. There is evidence of T-cell activation in the blood, skin, and lungs. Unregulated immunologic processes appear to be responsible for continuing vascular damage and widespread **dermal** and **internal organ fibrosis.**

1. **Vascular endothelial damage. Intimal hyperplasia** of small vessels in skin and internal organs occurs at the earliest stage of disease. **Luminal narrowing** from this endothelial fibrotic process can lead to tissue ischemia; this process is enhanced by release of the potent vasoconstrictor, endothelin, from damaged vessels. **Physiologic vasoconstrictive stimuli** (e.g., cold, emotion, platelet-derived thromboxane A_2, serotonin) can result in further narrowing and symptomatic **Raynaud's phenomenon** in skin or internal organs. Local release of the physiologic vasodilators nitric acid and endothelium-derived relaxation factor (EDRF) is diminished in damaged vessels. In patients with renal vascular involvement, increased renin–angiotensin production can cause a vicious circle of vasoconstriction, which is the presumed mechanism for **renal crisis** in this illness.
2. **Tissue fibrosis** may be caused by the healing of ischemic lesions from small vessel injury and from immune processes causing increased fibroblastic activity. **Cytokines** and **growth factors** secreted by lymphocytes, monocytes, and platelets [e.g., platelet-derived growth factor (PDGF), TGF-β] lead to increased secretion of collagen and ground substance by fibroblasts with the consequent development of fibrotic lesions. Mast cells are present in increased amounts in scleroderma skin and may interact with lymphocytes in cytokine-driven fibroblast activation.
3. **Autoantibodies.** Scleroderma patients often demonstrate ANAs; their relationship in scleroderma patients to disease pathogenesis is unknown, but these antibodies may help distinguish subsets of the illness (see IX E 2).

E Clinicopathologic features

1. **Organ involvement.** The degree of skin change and the type and progression of internal organ involvement are different in the **limited form** as compared to the **diffuse form** of scleroderma. Also, spontaneous fluctuations in disease activity can occur.

a. Skin involvement. Skin changes occur in **95% of patients** with scleroderma. An early **edematous phase** of small vessel endothelial injury and increased permeability may progress through an **indurative phase** as increasing amounts of collagen are produced in the subcutaneous tissue. Epidermal and skin appendage atrophy may occur in late forms of the disease (**atrophic phase**) as the skin becomes progressively bound to underlying tissue.

(1) **Distribution.** Changes most often begin in the fingers and hands and may spread to involve more proximal tissues, including the trunk and face. The lower extremities often are less severely involved.

(2) **Associated features**

(a) **Raynaud's phenomenon** occurs in **95% of patients** with scleroderma. Episodic vasospasm of the damaged small vessels in the digits results in a **triphasic color change** of the involved area as blood flow ceases (white), returns sluggishly (blue), and exhibits reactive hyperemia (red).

(b) **Telangiectasias** can occur in involved areas as well as on mucous membranes.

(c) **Subcutaneous calcifications** can occur, especially in finger tips.

(d) **Salt-and-pepper changes may occur,** in which the skin can become taut, shiny, and immobile, and hyperpigmented areas can alternate with depigmented areas.

(e) **Microcapillary abnormalities** may be present. The distal nail bed proliferates and the capillary bed becomes visibly abnormal, with dilatation, tortuosity, and loss of vessels. These abnormalities can be seen by examining the proximal nail beds with wide-field microscopy.

(f) **Skin ulcers** are possible. Distal digital ulcers and finger tapering occur due to distal infarctions and consequent loss of digital pulp, sometimes resulting in infection.

b. Gastrointestinal tract

(1) **Esophageal dysfunction** is the most common manifestation of internal organ involvement. **Esophageal motility dysfunction** and **reflux** develop as collagen replaces smooth muscle in the lower two-thirds of the esophagus; striated muscle in the upper one-third of the esophagus is relatively unaffected. **Esophageal strictures** can result from the constant reflux, and **ulceration** can occur at the gastroesophageal junction. Barium swallow and esophageal manometry may be helpful in documenting disease extent. Upper gastrointestinal endoscopy is helpful in evaluating the extent of involvement and possible Barrett's esophagus [see Chapter 5 I B 1 c (5)].

(2) **Similar small bowel involvement** leads to intestinal hypomotility and intermittent cramping, diarrhea, and **bacterial overgrowth malabsorption syndrome. Wide-mouth diverticuli** can be seen in the transverse and descending colon in areas of patchy muscularis involvement. Lower gastrointestinal contrast radiographic studies or malabsorption testing may demonstrate small bowel or colonic involvement.

c. Lung. Widespread small pulmonary arterial narrowing and fibrotic change eventually can lead to **isolated pulmonary hypertension.** More commonly, a fibrotic proliferation in the peribronchial and perialveolar tissues leads to progressive **interstitial lung disease.** Patients with interstitial lung disease present with symptoms of progressive dyspnea on exertion and demonstrate a restrictive pattern on pulmonary function testing, a better disease indicator than chest radiographic changes. High-resolution CT (HRCT) scanning of the lung can reveal the character and distribution of fine structural abnormalities not visible on chest radiography. Studies with bronchoalveolar lavage (BAL) have shown that a significant proportion of patients with scleroderma have an alveolitis, and aggressive chemotherapy may be indicated in this subset of patients. Pleuritis is uncommon in scleroderma as compared with other rheumatic diseases (e.g., rheumatoid arthritis, SLE).

d. Heart. Clinical cardiac involvement can take several forms. Clinically, acute and chronic pericarditis are unusual, but effusions often can be seen on ultrasonography and are associated with myocardial involvement. If interstitial myocardial disease is extensive, frank **cardiomyopathy** can result, producing CHF, arrhythmias, and conduction disturbances. Angina can be a result of fibrotic involvement of small myocardial vessels. Ambulatory electrocardiogram (ECG) monitoring or exercise stress testing can help to uncover dangerous arrhythmias or subtle ischemia in need of treatment.

e. **Kidney.** Sudden renal failure **(scleroderma renal crisis)** can occur often as a combination of interlobular artery fibrotic damage and some vasoconstrictive stimulus (e.g., diuresis, blood loss, surgery). Massive renin–angiotensin release in response to decreased renal perfusion worsens the vasoconstriction, and acute renal failure can occur. **Malignant hypertension** and **microangiopathic hemolytic anemia** often accompany these renal events. **Chronic renal failure** and **death** occur unless emergent treatment restores renal perfusion. Some but not all patients demonstrate new hypertension, urinary protein, or elevated serum creatinine testing before acute renal decompensation, so these features should be monitored periodically.

f. **Muscle.** In many patients, a mild indolent myopathy manifested by minor enzyme elevations and perhaps mild weakness occurs but does not require treatment. In some patients, an overt **inflammatory myopathy** identical to polymyositis can occur **("overlap" presentation).**

g. **Joint and tendon.** More than 50% of patients with scleroderma develop swelling, stiffness, and pain in finger, wrist, and knee joints. Mild, self-limited inflammatory arthritis can occur early in the disease, but typical joint involvement is limited to synovial fibrosis and impaired range of motion due to the generalized restriction of the fibrotic process. Tendon sheath involvement is not unusual; carpal tunnel syndrome can result from extensive tendon sheath fibrosis in the wrist.

h. **Nerve.** Neurologic involvement typically is limited to fibrotic **entrapment neuropathies** of the median and trigeminal nerves.

2. **Clinical syndromes.** Classification of the disease into **limited** and **diffuse forms** is important because of differences in organ involvement and, thus, prognosis. In general, the more widespread visceral involvement of the diffuse form gives it a poorer prognosis than the limited variant. Scleroderma can also exist in **overlap forms,** the most distinct of which is **UCTD.**

a. **Diffuse scleroderma** is typified by **proximal skin involvement** (skin proximal to the MCP joints or forearms in various definitions) and the presence of **Scl-70 antibodies** or **antinucleolar ANAs.** Visceral organ involvement in this form typically occurs earlier than in the limited variant. Renal involvement is much more common than in the limited form, and pulmonary fibrosis occurs earlier and more quickly.

b. **Limited scleroderma** typically has skin involvement limited to the distal extremities and face, and also is known as the **CREST variant** (involving the coexistence of subcutaneous **calcinosis, Raynaud's phenomenon, esophageal motility dysfunction, sclerodactyly,** and **telangiectasia**). **Anticentromere antibody** is most closely associated with this form, and visceral involvement is usually more slowly progressive than in the diffuse form. One exception is the early development of **pulmonary vascular hypertension** in this form due to obliterative changes in pulmonary arterioles. The pulmonary fibrosis so typical of the diffuse variant occurs more slowly in this form but can become severe after several decades of disease.

c. **Undifferentiated connective tissue disease** (UCTD) is a rheumatic syndrome that can include clinical features of scleroderma, SLE, and polymyositis in association with the presence of high titers of **antibody** to **U_1RNP.** Most cases evolve into more typical scleroderma or SLE over time.

F Diagnosis

1. **Clinical approach.** A diagnosis of scleroderma should be entertained in the presence of symptoms of **Raynaud's phenomenon, distal skin thickening,** and **visceral organ involvement.** Physicians should evaluate distal nail beds for the suggestive capillary abnormality and attempt to document the location and extent of the skin thickening to differentiate local from generalized forms. In addition, they should look for evidence of internal organ change. Characteristic ANA test results also may be useful in classifying patients.

a. **Raynaud's phenomenon.** The abnormal vascular response to cold or emotional stimuli is present in most patients with the diffuse or limited form of scleroderma, but most patients with Raynaud's phenomenon do not have scleroderma or another form of connective tissue disease. As many as 5%–10% of nonsmoking women in population surveys may have Raynaud's phenomenon; typical screening procedures for scleroderma would include examination for finger edema, fingernail-fold capillary abnormalities, and ANAs. Patients with none of these features are unlikely to develop scleroderma. Because patients can have Raynaud's phenomenon in association with other connective tissue diseases (SLE, polymyositis), a clinical search for these illnesses should be made as well.

b. **Distal skin thickening.** Such epidermal thickening is a diagnostic feature of both the diffuse and limited forms of scleroderma. Patients with diffuse scleroderma also have more proximal involvement, typically of the upper arms, upper legs, or trunk. Fewer than 5% of patients may have visceral involvement typical of scleroderma without skin thickening (**scleroderma sine scleroderma**).

c. **Laboratory findings.** Differences in ANA testing may discriminate between diffuse and limited forms of scleroderma. Patients with the diffuse form often have **Scl-70 antibodies** or **antinucleolar ANAs.** Patients with the more limited forms often have **anticentromere antibodies.**

d. **Visceral involvement.** Typical internal organ involvement (see IX E 1) lends further support to scleroderma diagnosis and helps discriminate between diffuse and limited forms.

2. **Differential diagnosis.** Skin thickening can be seen in other illnesses besides scleroderma. Typically, Raynaud's phenomenon, characteristic distal hand involvement, and visceral organ changes of scleroderma are absent.

a. **Local scleroderma.** Two forms of purely local disease, **morphea** and **linear scleroderma,** have similar clinical and pathologic appearance to sclerodermatous skin. These forms manifest as localized fibrotic plaques (morphea) or as longitudinal bands (linear scleroderma).

(1) **Morphea** may occur at any age (it is more common in childhood) as a disease characterized by small circumscribed skin lesions **(guttate morphea)** or larger patches **(morphea en plaque).**

(2) **Linear scleroderma** occurs most commonly in children and young adults. Facial involvement **(coup de sabre)** can be extremely disfiguring. The principal impact of linear scleroderma can be interference with function or growth of underlying muscle or bone leading to extremity wasting or contractures.

b. **Eosinophilic fasciitis.** Pain, swelling, and tenderness develop in one or more extremities, sometimes after an episode of vigorous exercise. Induration of involved skin and subcutaneous tissue develops, but without Raynaud's phenomenon or sclerodactyly. Patients often have marked peripheral blood eosinophilia, and a full-thickness skin biopsy (including underlying fascia and muscle) is required to demonstrate the deep fascial eosinophils and chronic inflammatory cell infiltrate.

c. **Eosinophilia–myalgia syndrome.** A clinical syndrome related to the ingestion of **L-tryptophan dietary supplements** can be confused with scleroderma (due to the skin thickening in some cases) and may be responsible for some cases of eosinophilic fasciitis. Patients who take L-tryptophan likely have ingested a toxic contaminant generated by the synthetic process, although some may metabolize L-tryptophan abnormally. The cornerstones of diagnosis are **eosinophilia (> 1000/mm^3) and severe myalgia** found in the absence of other possible causes. Variable features include skin rashes and induration, interstitial pulmonary infiltrates, and polyneuropathy. Elevation of muscle enzymes [aldolase, not creatine kinase (CK)] and hepatic enzymes also can occur.

G Therapy

1. **General.** No therapy is of proven value in scleroderma. Trials of **D-penicillamine** suggest possible effectiveness in slowing skin and internal organ involvement.

2. **Specific disease features**
   a. **Skin involvement.** D-Penicillamine appears to be effective in slowing or reversing skin involvement in the diffuse form, particularly when used early in disease. **Nitroglycerin ointment** applied directly to fingertip ulcerations may help heal them. **Colchicine** helps prevent painful inflammatory episodes related to subcutaneous calcinosis.
   b. **Raynaud's phenomenon.** Patients should understand the need to cover their head, ears, hands, feet, and trunk in cold weather to minimize reflex vasoconstriction, and smoking should be discouraged. **Calcium channel blocking agents** are the most useful vasodilating agents in the treatment of scleroderma. Patients should avoid nonselective β-blockers that can also contribute to vasoconstriction. **Intravenous prostaglandin infusions** have been used with success for treating refractory vasospastic episodes and for healing skin ulcerations. Antiplatelet therapy with low-dose aspirin should be considered.
   c. **Esophageal involvement.** Reflux esophagitis, often severe, requires the use of proton-pump inhibitors (e.g., omeprazole, lansoprazole). Antireflux measures (e.g., head-of-bed elevation, frequent small feedings) are helpful as well.
   d. **Pulmonary involvement.** For interstitial pulmonary disease, **corticosteroids** or **D-penicillamine** may be used, but neither treatment is clearly efficacious. A 6-month regimen of daily **oral cyclophosphamide with prednisone** may be the most effective therapy for progressive pulmonary fibrosis. Tobacco smoking may be synergistic in pulmonary injury. No treatment is known to be effective for the primary pulmonary hypertension-like syndrome, although **vasodilators** and continuous **intravenous prostaglandins** often are used. Anticoagulation in combination with vasodilators improves survival, which probably relates to the high incidence of in situ microthrombi or pulmonary emboli. Bosentan, an orally active endothelin receptor blocker, has shown promise in reducing pulmonary hypertension.
   e. **Lower gastrointestinal involvement.** Bacterial overgrowth malabsorption may be improved by intermittent treatment with **broad-spectrum antibiotics** (e.g., tetracycline). **Prokinetic agents** (e.g., octreotide, cisapride) help constipation and bloating related to lower gastrointestinal motility dysfunction.
   f. **Muscle involvement.** When inflammatory myositis occurs in overlap syndromes, **corticosteroids** are used, as in polymyositis. **NSAIDs** may be used in treating articular symptoms, taking care to monitor renal function closely.
   g. **Renal involvement.** Aggressive control of hypertension is best. The **angiotensin-converting enzyme (ACE) inhibitors** (e.g., captopril, enalapril) are major advances in controlling blood pressure in patients with scleroderma and may help reverse the angiotensin-dependent vasoconstrictive state of scleroderma renal crisis. The avoidance of hypovolemia in diuresis and in the perioperative state is important.
   h. **Cardiac involvement.** Medications useful for control of angina, CHF, and arrhythmias are used when these complications occur.

X INFLAMMATORY MYOPATHIES (POLYMYOSITIS AND DERMATOMYOSITIS)

A Definition **Polymyositis** is an idiopathic inflammatory muscle disease associated with prominent proximal muscle weakness, muscle enzyme elevations, characteristic myopathic electromyogram (EMG) patterns, and inflammatory infiltrates on muscle biopsy. When this complex is accompanied by a characteristic rash it is called **dermatomyositis.** Dermatomyositis is much more common than polymyositis in children.

B Epidemiology Polymyositis is a rare disease, occurring in approximately 1 in 200,000 individuals, with a peak incidence in childhood and in late adulthood. It is twice as common in females as in males and may be associated with malignancy in the adult-onset form.

C **Etiology and pathogenesis** The basic cause of polymyositis is unknown. However, it is believed that an initiating viral infection and altered immune responses are potentially important in causation and pathogenesis. Lymphocyte-mediated muscle cell damage is thought to be the central pathogenetic factor in this disease, although small vessel damage is also an important factor in dermatomyositis.

1. **Infections** can cause acute myositis.
   a. **Elevated titers of antibodies to picornaviruses** (e.g., coxsackievirus B) have been found in some juvenile dermatomyositis patients, and high titers of antibodies to *Toxoplasma gondii* have been found in some adult polymyositis patients.
   b. Isolation of these organisms from muscle of patients with polymyositis or dermatomyositis has not been accomplished, and antibiotic treatment for toxoplasmosis has not improved myositis in patients with high titers of antibody to *T. gondii.*
2. **Autoimmunity**
   a. **Humoral.** Most patients with inflammatory myopathies demonstrate autoantibodies when human tumor cell lines [i.e., human epithelial cells (**HEp-2**)] are used as testing substrate, but it is not known whether these antibodies interfere with the normal physiologic function of their antigens. **Molecular mimicry** may be important in polymyositis/dermatomyositis, because autoantibodies directed against tRNA synthetases are found in some patients, perhaps resulting from mimicry between a virus and an epitope on the intracellular enzyme. Vascular deposits of immune complexes and complement are associated with endothelial cell injury and small vessel obstruction in dermatomyositis, especially in juvenile dermatomyositis.
   b. **Cellular**
      (1) **Polymyositis.** Peripheral blood lymphocytes from polymyositis patients produce a lymphotoxin that is cytotoxic to muscle cells. In addition, cytotoxic $CD8^+$ T cells are the predominant cell type found in the inflammatory infiltrate in muscle, apparently attacking muscle cells expressing increased numbers of class I MHC-restricted markers.
      (2) **Dermatomyositis.** Some studies suggest that $CD4^+$ T cells and B cells are predominant in dermatomyositis infiltrates, in contrast to the predominantly $CD8^+$ T-cell infiltrates in polymyositis. Perhaps humoral mechanisms are relatively more important in dermatomyositis than in polymyositis.

D **Pathology** The major sites of inflammation are skeletal muscle and, less commonly, cardiac muscle. Skin involvement is a minor pathologic feature.

1. **Inflammatory infiltrate.** Lymphocytes and plasma cells are the predominant inflammatory cells, although macrophages, eosinophils, and neutrophils also can be seen in muscle tissue. $CD8^+$ cells infiltrate muscle fibers in polymyositis. In dermatomyositis, $CD4^+$ cells and B cells often are clustered around small blood vessels within the muscle.
2. **Muscle fiber damage.** Spotty muscle fiber necrosis and degeneration occur, with loss of cross striations and variation in the size of surviving fibers. Increased numbers of muscle nuclei and enhanced basophilic staining of fibers indicate regeneration in the midst of cell death. Interstitial fibrotic infiltrates occur in chronic cases.

E **Clinical features and laboratory findings** Inflammatory myopathies are clinically grouped into specific syndromes, depending on specific organ manifestations and results of laboratory tests.

1. **Organ involvement**
   a. **Skin.** The rash of dermatomyositis consists of erythematous patches, which sometimes are scaling or atrophic and are distributed over the face, neck, upper chest, and extensor surfaces. Only scattered inflammatory infiltrates in the dermis are evident on biopsy.
      (1) Pathognomonic skin findings include **heliotrope rash** (a violet discoloration and swelling of the eyelids) and **Gottron's sign** (heaped-up erythematous papules over the MCP or PIP joints).

(2) Other significant findings include **mechanic's hands** (roughened erythematous skin and hypertrophic changes of the palms and fingers) as well as the erythematous **V sign** (anterior chest) and **shawl sign** (neck and upper back).

b. **Lung.** Chronic interstitial lung disease can occur, especially in association with antisynthetase antibodies. Aspiration pneumonitis and ventilatory insufficiency also can occur.

c. **Joint.** A mild, symmetrical inflammatory arthritis occurs uncommonly and rarely is destructive; it is seen most often in patients with the synthetase antibodies [see X E 2 b (2) (a)].

d. **Muscle.** Most patients have gradual but steady progression of muscle weakness; however, some patients have such fulminant courses that **acute respiratory failure** or **myoglobinuric renal failure** can ensue.

(1) **Skeletal muscle weakness** is the primary manifestation of polymyositis.

(a) **Symmetrical, proximal, upper and lower extremity weakness** occurs, causing difficulty with rising from a chair, sitting up in bed, or combing hair.

(b) **Pharyngeal muscle involvement** can lead to swallowing difficulties and aspiration, and respiratory muscle dysfunction can lead to respiratory failure.

(2) **Cardiac muscle involvement** is not as common, but when it occurs it manifests as cardiomyopathy with CHF, arrhythmias, and conduction disturbances.

2. **Laboratory findings**

a. **Muscle enzymes.** An increased concentration of enzymes typically present in skeletal muscle is prominent in polymyositis. **CK** and **aldolase** are routinely measured, and CK fractionation may suggest myocardial involvement if the **MB fraction** (i.e., the CK isoenzyme found mainly in myocardium but also in regenerating skeletal muscle) is increased. However, in most patients, CK elevation is caused by the **MM band** (i.e., the fraction most prevalent in skeletal muscle). Serum **myoglobin** levels are also elevated in most patients and may be more sensitive than CK levels in some myositis patients. Enzyme elevations usually correlate with activity of the muscle disease and are used as a parameter to evaluate treatment response.

b. **Autoantibodies.** Most patients with polymyositis/dermatomyositis (80%–90%) have antibodies to nuclear or cytoplasmic antigens. Routine ANA testing against HEp-2 cells is performed; other myositis-specific antibodies require specialized testing (e.g., immunoprecipitation).

(1) **Nonspecific autoantibodies.** ANAs, particularly **speckled-pattern ANAs,** are the most common autoantibodies in the inflammatory myopathies, occurring in more than 50% of patients. Other antibodies also can be seen, including **Ro antibodies, La antibodies, PM/Scl antibodies,** and **Ku antibodies.**

(2) **Specific autoantibodies.** Several autoantibodies are formed only in inflammatory myopathies; they target cytoplasmic or nuclear constituents of myocytes. The appearance of these antibodies, which seem to correlate with clinical patterns of involvement, may be more useful in classifying patients.

(a) **Synthetase antibodies (anti-aminoacyl–tRNA synthetases)** are directed against cytoplasmic enzymes involved in specific amino acid attachment to tRNA. **Jo-1 antibody,** found in 20% of myositis patients, is the most common, directed against histidyl–tRNA synthetase. Patients with these antibodies may be considered to have the antisynthetase syndrome, which is associated with DR3 and DRw52 haplotypes. This condition, which usually occurs in the spring, is characterized by acute onset of arthritis, interstitial lung disease, fever, mechanic hands, and Raynaud's phenomenon. Affected patients have a 5-year survival rate of 70%.

(b) **Signal recognition particle antibodies (SRP antibodies)** recognize one of the components of the SRP, a cytoplasmic protein complex involved in polypeptide transfer across the endoplasmic reticulum. Immunogenetic data indicate a DR5 and DRw52 association. Patients tend to have an acute onset of severe myalgia and significant cardiac problems such as palpitations. Prognosis is very poor, with a 5-year survival rate of only 25%.

(c) **Mi-2 antibodies** target a nuclear protein of unknown function, in contrast to the cytoplasmic proteins of the other myositis-specific antibodies. This antibody pattern is found in patients with classic dermatomyositis. The 5-year survival is nearly 100%.

3. **Clinical syndromes.** The traditional classification scheme is given below. However, in the future, it may be more useful to use the previously listed myositis-specific antibody groups for prognostic and therapeutic purposes [see X E 2 (b) (2)].

   a. **Polymyositis.** Characteristic features include upper and lower extremity proximal muscular weakness and elevated muscle enzymes. All organ manifestations listed in X E 1 can occur, except the skin findings. Patients with polymyositis tend to have disease that is less responsive than dermatomyositis to therapy. The treatment-resistant, acutely severe disease is often associated with cardiac muscle involvement, a finding more prominent in patients with **SRP antibodies.** Patients with polymyositis who have **PM/Scl antibodies** tend to do relatively well.

   b. **Dermatomyositis.** Characteristic features include the muscle weakness, elevated muscle enzymes, and organ manifestations seen in polymyositis, but the distinct feature of this syndrome is the presence of **skin involvement.** In general, dermatomyositis patients respond reasonably well to therapy.

   c. **Polymyositis or dermatomyositis associated with malignancy.** Visceral malignancies occur in approximately 10%–25% of cases, especially in elderly individuals with late-onset inflammatory myopathy. The incidence of malignancy is thought to be higher in patients with dermatomyositis than in those with polymyositis. The most common malignancies are those that are typical in middle-aged or elderly individuals (i.e., cancers of the lung, gastrointestinal tract, breast, uterus, and ovaries). Removal of the malignancy occasionally results in remission of the muscle disease, but the prognosis in general for these patients is poor; they die of their malignancy or uncontrollable muscle disease.

   d. **Juvenile dermatomyositis.** Most children have dermatomyositis rather than polymyositis. Late in the disease course, young patients may develop muscle contractures from calcific deposits in the chronically damaged muscle. A widespread small artery and capillary vasculitis may lead to skin, muscle, and bowel ischemic lesions. Otherwise, prognosis is similar to that in adult forms of inflammatory myopathy.

   e. **Overlap syndromes.** Muscle disease that is identical to polymyositis can occur in SLE, rheumatoid arthritis, systemic sclerosis, and Sjögren's syndrome. Patients often have milder muscle disease that is responsive to therapy, and prognosis is determined by the features of the underlying disease more than the muscle findings.

   f. **Inclusion body myositis.** This syndrome is considered a subset of inflammatory myopathies because of the associated $CD8^+$-cell cytotoxicity directed against muscle fibers. The syndrome tends to affect **older men** and has a gradual disease onset and progression. Although patients have muscle weakness, CK elevations, and myopathic EMGs, they are distinguished from typical polymyositis patients by having **distal as well as proximal weakness,** typical **absence of autoantibodies,** and a **characteristic muscle biopsy** showing vacuolar changes and distinctive electron microscopic findings. The clinical features often are poorly responsive to immunosuppressive therapy, but patients have an excellent 5-year survival rate because of the slow progression of the disease.

F Diagnosis

1. **Approach**

   a. **Distinctive muscle findings.** A clinical diagnosis of inflammatory myopathy typically is considered when patients present with **proximal muscle weakness or increased muscle enzymes** (e.g., CK, aldolase). True proximal muscle weakness must be distinguished from generalized fatigue, distal weakness more typical of neuropathy, and pain-related weakness (i.e., joint or tendon pain that prevents full muscle contraction). Patients with true proximal muscle weakness complain of being unable to comb their hair or to rise from a squatting or sitting position. If true proximal weakness appears likely from the history and physical examination, CK testing is performed and EMG and biopsy of symptomatic deltoid or quadriceps muscle should be considered. MRI may also be useful in localizing the best biopsy site. The diagnosis of polymyositis is likely if a patient has three of the following muscle criteria:

(1) Characteristic proximal muscle weakness
(2) Inflammatory cell infiltrate and myofibril degeneration on muscle biopsy
(3) Increased muscle enzyme levels
(4) Myopathic EMG changes

b. **Supportive findings**

(1) The **characteristic skin findings,** if found, are supportive evidence and sometimes precede clinical evidence of muscle involvement.
(2) Because 90% of polymyositis patients have autoantibodies when their serum is tested against HEp-2 cells, the presence of a positive test for autoantibodies also is supportive evidence for the disease, particularly if a **myositis-specific antibody** is found.

2. **Consideration of malignancy.** A search for a malignancy is warranted in middle-aged or elderly polymyositis/dermatomyositis patients. Thorough physical examination, including a careful pelvic evaluation in women, chest radiograph, routine hematologic and biochemical testing, urinalysis and stool testing for occult blood should be performed. Abnormalities found should be pursued through additional testing.

3. **Differential diagnosis.** Other entities should be considered in making a diagnosis of inflammatory myopathy, especially when the presentation is somewhat atypical. Some disorders can be eliminated on clinical grounds; others require laboratory testing, EMG, or muscle biopsy.

a. **Endocrine disorders**

(1) **Hypothyroidism** can manifest as proximal muscle aching, weakness, and mild-to-moderate CK elevation.
(2) **Hyperthyroidism** can manifest as diffuse weakness; CK levels typically are normal.
(3) **Cushing syndrome** patients may have lower more than upper extremity proximal muscle weakness; muscle enzymes are normal.

b. **Drugs.** Numerous drugs and toxins can cause muscle weakness and sometimes CK elevation; these effects usually resolve when the agent is removed. Some of the most common of these agents include alcohol, cholesterol-lowering drugs (e.g., clofibrate, gemfibrozil, lovastatin), colchicine, chloroquine, corticosteroids, D-penicillamine, and zidovudine.

c. **Muscle diseases.** Muscular dystrophies and metabolic muscle diseases can be distinguished by careful family history, distinguishing patterns of weakness, and lack of inflammation on muscle biopsy. Some require exercise testing with venous lactate determinations or electron microscopic examination of muscle.

d. **Neurologic diseases.** Early in the disease course, illnesses such as myasthenia gravis or amyotrophic lateral sclerosis (ALS) can mimic inflammatory myopathy. The presence of ocular muscle involvement or characteristic EMG or nerve conduction velocity (NCV) findings can help in diagnosing these diseases.

e. **Infections**

(1) **Bacterial.** Some cases of Lyme disease are associated with myopathy.
(2) **Viral.** Acute and convalescent serologies can distinguish viral illness. Common causes include coxsackievirus, echovirus, influenza virus, and HIV.
(3) **Parasitic.** Serologic testing can help distinguish toxoplasmosis or trichinosis from polymyositis.

f. **Sarcoidosis.** Inflammatory muscle involvement, which can be distinguished by characteristic organ involvement and finding noncaseating granulomas on muscle biopsy, may occur.

G Therapy

1. **Corticosteroids.** Large doses of corticosteroids appear to be effective in controlling the muscle disease in most patients. Prednisone usually is begun at a dose of 60 mg/day and is reduced gradually over several months as muscle strength improves and CK level falls. Alternate-day regimens can be used to prevent steroid toxicity but only after the normalization of CK level and return of muscle strength.
2. **Immunosuppressive agents.** Patients who do not respond to the previously mentioned corticosteroid schedules within 3 months are considered to be nonresponders to treatment. Frequently, the addition of methotrexate or azathioprine allows control of the muscle disease and gradual tapering of the steroids. The $CD4^+$ cell-specific drug cyclosporine also has been effective in some patients who do not respond to general immunosuppression.
3. **Physical therapy.** When the disease process has been clinically controlled (i.e., CK levels normalized and muscle strength improved), muscle strengthening exercise and aerobic training can be initiated. Mild exercise and passive stretching to prevent contractures should be used in active disease.
4. **Hydroxychloroquine.** This agent may help control the rash of dermatomyositis.
5. **Intravenous immunoglobulin.** This agent has been helpful in some steroid-resistant patients.

XI SJÖGREN'S SYNDROME

A Definition Sjögren's syndrome (also called **sicca syndrome**) is an idiopathic, autoimmune disorder characterized by dry mouth (**xerostomia**) and dry eyes (**keratoconjunctivitis sicca**). Variable **lacrimal** or **salivary gland enlargement** can occur (related to lymphocytic infiltration of lacrimal and salivary glands).

B Classification Sjögren's syndrome is divided into primary and secondary forms. The two forms can be distinguished on the basis of clinical features and HLA associations.

1. **Primary Sjögren's syndrome** has characteristic organ and exocrine glandular features and a significantly increased association with **HLA-DR3.** Patients can present with a variety of clinical manifestations that are uncommon in the secondary form, mainly due to a wider attack on exocrine glands in the primary form. Specific organ involvement is as follows:
   a. **Skin:** dry skin and vagina, Raynaud's phenomenon, and purpura (vasculitis)
   b. **Lung:** recurrent infections and interstitial fibrosis
   c. **Gastrointestinal tract:** angular cheilitis, oral candidiasis, beefy red tongue, recurrent parotitis, dysphagia, atrophic gastritis, chronic active hepatitis, biliary cirrhosis, and pancreatitis
   d. **Kidney:** renal tubular acidosis and interstitial nephritis
   e. **Muscle:** indolent myositis
   f. **Nerve:** CNS involvement (possibly vasculitis, with clinical manifestations similar to CNS lupus) and peripheral neuropathy
   g. **Hematologic system:** splenomegaly with neutropenia, lymphomas, and pseudolymphomas
   h. **Joint:** arthralgias or mild inflammatory arthritis
   i. **Endocrine system:** chronic thyroiditis [increased thyroid-stimulating hormone (TSH) levels and antithyroid antibodies, perhaps in as many as 50% of patients]
   j. **Vasculitis** (polyarteritis-like)
2. **Secondary Sjögren's syndrome** occurs in the setting of another rheumatic disease (e.g., rheumatoid arthritis, SLE, scleroderma) and has an increased association with **HLA-DR4.** Patients usually

have symptoms that are limited to lacrimal and salivary gland abnormalities, although they also have typical features of a primary rheumatic disease.

C Diagnosis

1. **Clinical approach.** Patients are most commonly evaluated for Sjögren's syndrome when they have complaints of **dry eyes, dry mouth,** or **salivary gland enlargement.** Primary Sjögren's syndrome also should be considered in the setting of **cutaneous vasculitis** (purpura), **CNS dysfunction** similar to that which occurs in SLE (either focal neurologic abnormalities or diffuse features such as depression, psychosis, or cognitive dysfunction), or the conspicuous presence of other clinical features listed in XI B 1.
   a. Complaints of **gritty eyes and dry mouth** can be investigated in the following way:
      (1) **Ophthalmologic slit-lamp examination** with fluorescein or Rose Bengal staining can be used to examine for the punctate staining of keratoconjunctivitis. The **Schirmer test,** which measures the degree of tear wetting on filter paper, is a supportive test; limited wetting suggests that keratoconjunctivitis found on staining is sicca-related.
      (2) **Lip biopsy** of the lower lip mucosa can be used to search for characteristic lymphocytic infiltration of the minor salivary glands in that location.
   b. **Salivary gland enlargement** can be evaluated with an MRI of the parotid gland. A nonhomogeneous density, which can be distinguished from parotitis, tumor, and normal glandular tissue, may be evident.
   c. **Salivary flow rate tests** (**sialometry**) and **radiographic studies** (**sialography**) are sensitive but nonspecific tests and are not often used.
   d. Many **laboratory abnormalities** occur and may offer suggestive evidence; however, no specific laboratory test is diagnostic.
      (1) **Tests suggesting chronic inflammation.** Anemia of chronic disease, elevated erythrocyte sedimentation rate, hypergammaglobulinemia, and rheumatoid factor often are found in Sjögren's syndrome, whether primary or secondary.
      (2) **Autoantibody findings.** ANAs are seen frequently in Sjögren's syndrome; antibodies to the small RNA protein **Ro** are found in **70%** of patients and antibodies to the protein **La** are found in **40%** of patients. La antibodies rarely are found without Ro antibodies, and the presence of both is relatively specific for Sjögren's syndrome. Salivary duct antibodies are common only in the secondary form.
2. **Differential diagnosis**
   a. **Salivary gland enlargement** also may be caused by a lymphoid or parotid gland neoplasm, granulomatous infiltration (sarcoidosis), alcohol use, cirrhosis, starvation, diabetes, amyloidosis, graft-versus-host disease (GVHD), hyperlipidemias, or infection (e.g., bacterial infections, mumps, HIV).
   b. **Dry mouth** may be caused by the use of certain drugs, including tricyclic antidepressants, phenothiazines, and antihistamines.
   c. **Dry mouth and dry eyes** are common in the geriatric population, and they often are present without any other features of Sjögren's syndrome.

D Therapy

1. **General considerations**
   a. **Scrupulous oral hygiene** is important to prevent rampant dental caries.
   b. Patients with primary Sjögren's syndrome who demonstrate salivary gland or lymphoid tissue enlargement must be considered **at risk for lymphoma,** because non-Hodgkin's lymphomas occur at 40 times the normal rate in these patients.
2. **Symptomatic treatment**
   a. **Xerostomia.** Avoidance of drugs that dry out the mouth and frequent drinks of water or other liquids to keep the mouth wet are the usual symptomatic measures for this condition. Artifi-

cial salivas are commercially available, which may help with mouth wetting and dental caries prevention. Pilocarpine hydrochloride, a cholinergic agonist, is available for oral use and can increase secretion by the exocrine glands increasing salivary flow.

b. **Keratoconjunctivitis sicca.** Artificial tears (methyl cellulose) are used as often as needed to keep the eyes lubricated. Refractory symptoms may respond to punctal insertion of silicone plugs.

c. **Features of severe disease. Progressive pneumonitis, vasculitis, neuropathy,** and **CNS involvement** may require anti-inflammatory treatment with corticosteroids and immunosuppressive drugs.

E Prognosis Outcome for patients with primary Sjögren's syndrome depends on the severity of involvement of organs other than the salivary glands, particularly the CNS. Also, the risk of lymphoma is higher in more severe cases. Features of the primary rheumatic disease determine the prognosis for patients with secondary Sjögren's syndrome.

XII VASCULITIS

A Definition Vasculitic syndromes are a group of clinically disparate disorders characterized by **necrosis and inflammation of blood vessel walls.** Vasculitis can exist as the primary feature of an idiopathic condition or as a secondary manifestation of infectious, malignant, or rheumatic disease.

B Etiology Most of the vasculitic syndromes are idiopathic. Hepatitis B surface antigen (HBsAg) and HCV have been found in immune complexes of several different syndromes, including some cases of polyarteritis nodosa and essential mixed cryoglobulinemia. HIV, parvovirus, and cytomegalovirus (CMV) have been associated with vasculitic diseases, particularly polyarteritis. Methamphetamine abuse also has been implicated in the causation of vessel lesions in some cases of polyarteritis.

C Pathogenesis Individual syndromes often demonstrate features of disordered humoral and cellular immunity.

1. **Disordered humoral immune response.** In some vasculitic syndromes (e.g., leukocytoclastic vasculitis perhaps polyarteritis nodosa), soluble immune complexes form and deposit in vessel walls, fix complement, and attract inflammatory cells, which cause damage. Antibodies may also react directly with neutrophils or endothelial cells to cause vessel damage (e.g., Wegener's granulomatosis and ANCAs). The site and degree of damage are determined by many variables, including:
   a. Physical and biochemical characteristics of the immune complexes
   b. Variations in blood pressure (hydrostatic forces)
   c. Changes in blood vessel size and permeability
   d. Endothelial cell adhesive properties
   e. Effectiveness of reticuloendothelial system removal of immune complexes
   f. Degree of turbulence in vessels (e.g., immune complexes deposit at branch points)
   g. Degree of persistence or recurrence of antigen exposure (e.g., toxin versus HBV)
   h. Variations in host immune response (e.g., ANCA in patients with Wegener's granulomatosis). An inhaled antigen or other immune system challenge may activate neutrophils, which in the presence of ANCA, degranulate, recruit T cells and monocytes, and damage vessel walls.
2. **Disordered cellular immune response.** Disorders involving granuloma formation are the best examples of the contributions of the cellular immune response to vasculitic processes. Interactions between macrophages and $CD4^+$ T cells in response to unknown antigens lead to granuloma formation in and around vessel walls. In giant cell arteritis, age-related vessel degeneration in large arteries may expose antigens typically hidden to the immune system, which then elicit a cellular immune response; there also may be an HLA-DR4 association with this disease and proliferation of specific T-cell clones in vessel lesions.

D Classification The current systems for classifying vasculitic syndromes use clinical features, size of the involved vessel, and type of cellular infiltrate to separate the syndromes (Table 10–14).

TABLE 10–14 Major Vasculitic Syndromes: Clinicopathologic Distinctions

Syndrome	Clinical Features	Pathology		Diagnosis	Therapy
		VESSEL SIZE	CELLULAR INFILTRATE		
Hypersensitivity vasculitis (serum sickness; drug reactions; Henoch-Schönlein purpura; mixed essential cryoglobulinemia)	Skin involvement predominant Visceral involvement typically minimal and self-limited	Small (capillaries; venules; arterioles)	Leukocytoclastic vasculitis with all lesions at the same developmental stage	Skin biopsy	Supportive Corticosteroids for serious vessel involvement
Polyarteritis nodosa	Multisystem illness Major arterial ischemic lesions that spare lungs and spleen Nodose skin lesions uncommon	Small and medium-sized arteries	Necrotizing arteritis at vessel branch points Simultaneous lesions at various stages	Biopsy of involved organ Visceral angiography	Corticosteroids; cytotoxic agents added if no response
Allergic angiitis (Churg-Strauss disease)	Prominent allergic, asthmatic history Lung involvement Blood eosinophilia common	Varying (capillaries; venules; small arteries)	Granulomatous infiltrates with eosinophils	Biopsy of involved organ, typically lung	Corticosteroids; cytotoxic agents added if no response

Wegener's granulomatosis	Upper and lower respiratory tract involvement Prominent renal abnormalities	Small (arteries; veins)	Necrotizing granulomas in upper and lower airways Focal necrotizing arteritis in lungs Necrotizing glomerulonephritis in kidneys	Lung biopsy (sinus biopsy usually nondiagnostic) c-ANCA	Cyclophosphamide; corticosteroids added if disease is fulminant; switch to methotrexate may lessen cyclophosphamide toxicity after induction
Giant cell arteritis (temporal arteritis)	Polymyalgia rheumatica in 50% Occurs in patients older than 50 Signs and symptoms of cranial artery involvement High erythrocyte sedimentation rate	Large arteries (especially temporal artery)	Giant cell and chronic mononuclear infiltrates in vessel walls	Temporal artery biopsy	Corticosteroids
Takayasu's arteritis	Large vessel claudication Occurs in young (often Asian) women	Large arteries (aortic arch)	Giant cell and chronic mononuclear infiltrates in vessel walls	Angiography Chest MRI Neck ultrasonography	Corticosteroids Large vessel reconstructive surgery

ANCA = antineutrophil cytoplasmic antibody; c-ANCA = cytoplasmic ANCA; MRI = magnetic resonance imaging.

Nonspecific hematologic and immunologic abnormalities (e.g., anemia, leukocytosis, elevated erythrocyte sedimentation rate, hypocomplementemia) often exist in many of these syndromes, but these are not noted in Table 10–14 unless they are specifically important for the diagnosis of a particular syndrome. It is important to understand that these syndromes often blur and overlap in actual patients.

E Vasculitic syndromes

1. **Hypersensitivity vasculitis**
   a. **Typical hypersensitivity vasculitis syndrome.** Hypersensitivity vasculitis (also called **leukocytoclastic vasculitis** or **cutaneous vasculitis**) is immune complex–mediated inflammation of small vessels (arterioles, capillaries, venules). The cause often is unclear. In many cases, hypersensitivity vasculitis seems to occur as an exaggerated immune response to a **drug** (e.g., penicillin) or **infection** (viral or bacterial antigen), causing a self-limited immune complex vasculitis. The skin almost always is involved, with palpable purpura, urticaria, or ulcers. Polyarticular arthritis is common. Distinct organ involvement may allow further classification.
   b. **Distinctive subsets**
      (1) **Henoch-Schönlein purpura** is a systemic, small vessel vasculitis that occurs primarily in children, often following a streptococcal pharyngitis.
         (a) **Clinical features.** Palpable purpura, polyarticular arthralgias or inflammatory arthritis, abdominal pain or gastrointestinal bleeding due to mesenteric vessel involvement, and immune complex–mediated glomerulonephritis typically occur. A distinctive feature is **IgA deposition** in the vascular lesions.
         (b) **Course.** Most cases of Henoch-Schönlein purpura resolve spontaneously over a period of days to weeks. Patients with severe renal or gastrointestinal involvement may require steroids.
      (2) **Serum sickness** is an immune complex vasculitis that often follows a drug (e.g., penicillin, sulfonamide) or foreign protein exposure by 7–10 days. Antilymphocyte globulin now is one of the most common causes. HBV arthritis–dermatitis syndrome is a serum sickness–like response to HbsAg.
         (a) **Clinical features.** Urticaria, purpura, arthritis, and arthralgias are characteristic, and lymphadenopathy and immune complex glomerulonephritis are common.
         (b) **Course.** Resolution is typical following removal of the inciting agent.
      (3) **Hypocomplementemic urticarial vasculitis**
         (a) **Clinical features.** Patients with this form of vasculitis exhibit urticaria, typically lasting longer than 24 hours and, sometimes, arthritis, glomerulonephritis, or gastrointestinal involvement. **Hypocomplementemia** is a consistent feature, apparently related to antibodies directed against C1q; the degree of complement depression typically parallels disease activity.
         (b) **Course.** The disease follows a relapsing, remitting course and may require corticosteroids for the more disabling manifestations.
      (4) **Mixed essential cryoglobulinemia** is an idiopathic disorder caused by cold-precipitated immunoglobulin (cryoglobulin) complexes, which produce a vaso-occlusive or inflammatory injury. The syndrome typically occurs in patients who have type II (mixed) cryoglobulin. Many patients have been found to have HCV or less often, HBV, in the immune complexes.
         (a) **Clinical features.** Recurrent attacks of palpable purpura, Raynaud's phenomenon, arthralgia, and immune complex glomerulonephritis may occur. Gastrointestinal, hepatic, and pulmonary dysfunction are occasional features.
         (b) **Course.** Severe renal involvement is the most common reason for treatment, which may include corticosteroids, cytotoxic agents, or removal of the cryoglobulin by apheresis. IFN-α may help when the disease is associated with HBV or HCV.

2. **Polyarteritis nodosa** is a necrotizing vasculitis of small and medium-sized arteries, which manifests as a multisystem illness. Ischemic arterial lesions are caused by vessel wall inflammation, in some cases associated with immune complex deposition.
   a. **Clinical features. Constitutional complaints** (e.g., fever, weight loss, anorexia) are common, and **multiorgan ischemic dysfunction** is the rule. The lungs and spleen typically are spared.
      (1) **Renal involvement** is most common and manifests as severe hypertension, proteinuria and active sediment from glomerulonephritis, or renal insufficiency.
      (2) **Other common features** include arthralgias, myalgias, peripheral nervous system abnormalities (sensory polyneuropathies, mononeuritis multiplex), and skin lesions (infarctions, nodose lesions). Insidious CHF, diffuse or focal CNS dysfunction, and gastrointestinal involvement also can occur, depending on the size of the ischemic lesions.
      (3) **Microscopic polyarteritis** is a clinical variant typified by prominent lung involvement and segmental glomerulonephritis, sometimes rapidly progressive. The vessels involved tend to be smaller (capillaries, arterioles, and small arteries). **p-ANCA** is commonly found (50%–80% of patients) and abdominal angiography is typically negative (because the smaller vessels are involved).
   b. **Course.** Treatment with corticosteroids, cytotoxic agents, or both is necessary; the illness typically is fatal if untreated. IFN-α may help in HBV- or HCV-associated cases.
3. **Allergic angiitis (Churg-Strauss disease)** is a granulomatous vasculitis that typically occurs in patients with asthma.
   a. **Clinical features.** Allergic angiitis is typically a triphasic disease. **Asthma** occurs first, often associated with **blood eosinophilia. Tissue infiltrates,** especially **pulmonary** ones, occur next; eosinophils are often present in these lesions, sometimes in granulomas. **Vasculitis** of small or medium-sized vessels occurs last, commonly involving skin, nerve, or muscle lesions.
   b. **Course.** The farther apart in time the three phases of illness occur, the milder the disease; the closer together, the more explosive. Catastrophic lung, gastrointestinal tract, cardiac, or nerve lesions may mandate aggressive intravenous corticosteroid and cytotoxic therapy, but more indolent forms are often easily controlled with moderate corticosteroid doses.
4. **Wegener's granulomatosis** is a granulomatous, small vessel vasculitis that typically involves the upper and lower respiratory tract and kidney.
   a. **Clinical features**
      (1) **Respiratory tract.** Pulmonary features typically include upper airway complaints (e.g., sinusitis, rhinitis) as well as lower airway symptoms (e.g., cough, shortness of breath, hemoptysis). Cavitary or multiple infiltrates may be seen on chest radiography.
      (2) **Kidney.** Renal involvement is characterized by abnormal sediment or renal functional impairment.
      (3) **Organs.** Other, less classical features include skin lesions (palpable purpura), arthritis, ocular or orbital inflammation (typically with proptosis), cardiac lesions, and CNS or peripheral nervous system involvement.
      (4) **Presence of c-ANCA.** c-ANCA is often found in patients with active, multiorgan disease. In these patients, the presence of c-ANCA may be a relatively specific diagnostic test and may help monitor disease activity.
   b. **Course.** Although corticosteroids may be used initially, cytotoxic agents such as cyclophosphamide are uniformly required to prevent death. Methotrexate may play a role in maintaining disease remission.
5. **Takayasu's arteritis** is a granulomatous inflammation of the vessels of the aortic arch that is characterized pathologically by a panarteritis containing mononuclear and giant cells. Young, often Asian, women are at highest risk for this disorder.
   a. **Clinical features**
      (1) **Generalized aching** similar to PMR often occurs early in the illness. Features of **large artery ischemia** develop weeks to months later and may include upper extremity claudication,

angina, and CHF from cardiac or aortic involvement. Pulmonary and mesenteric vessels also can be involved.

(2) **Findings on physical examination** include arterial bruits, pulse deficits, and blood pressure differences between extremities.

b. **Course.** Patients may require steroids early in the course of the illness; later, vascular reconstruction may be required for occlusive lesions. Cytotoxic agents are typically added if steroids do not control inflammatory disease.

6. **Giant cell (temporal) arteritis** usually is a granulomatous inflammation of the carotid artery and its branches, but it sometimes can involve the vertebral artery or other aortic branches. The pathology is indistinguishable from that of Takayasu's arteritis.

a. **Clinical features.** The disease rarely occurs in patients younger than age 50.

(1) Approximately 50% of patients have **PMR** (i.e., aching and stiffness of shoulder and hip girdles associated with an erythrocyte sedimentation rate > 50 mm/hr, age > 50 years, and constitutional complaints such as fever, malaise, and weight loss), and most patients have features related to ischemia in the carotid artery region (i.e., headache, visual symptoms, jaw claudication, scalp tenderness, neurologic complaints).

(2) **Superficial temporal artery involvement** is common but often is clinically silent. Potential clinical features include tenderness, nodules, or erythema. Even when the artery is clinically normal, temporal artery biopsy typically reveals pathology.

b. **Course.** Patients require steroids early and in high doses to prevent **blindness,** the most serious complication of this illness. Patients should be started immediately on at least 1 mg/kg prednisone to prevent blindness. A temporal artery biopsy may still be diagnostic up to 1 week after the initiation of steroids. A contralateral temporal artery is necessary for diagnosis if the original biopsy specimen is negative.

7. **Other vasculitic syndromes** do not fit into the major categories of vasculitis due to distinct clinical or overlapping pathologic features.

a. **Vasculitis as a secondary feature of a primary disease.** Certain diseases can exhibit vasculitic inflammation as a secondary feature. The vasculitis typically is small vessel, cutaneous vasculitis but sometimes can overlap with polyarteritis-like vessel involvement, especially in **rheumatoid arthritis** and **lupus.** Dermal and CNS vasculitic lesions are recently recognized secondary features of **Sjögren's syndrome. Hematologic malignancies** and bacterial and viral **infections** also can include vasculitic features, usually with the skin the predominant organ involved.

b. **Behçet's syndrome.** The presence of recurrent oral and genital ulcers defines this syndrome. Patients also may have eye inflammation, **pathergic skin lesions** (lesions occurring at sites of skin injury), and vasculitis of the CNS or other organs.

c. **Kawasaki disease (mucocutaneous lymph node syndrome).** This febrile illness of infants and young children is characterized by conjunctival injection; diffuse maculopapular rash with associated edema, erythema, and eventual desquamation of the hands and feet; cracked lips; "strawberry tongue"; and cervical adenopathy. Coronary vasculitis can develop in 25% of patients and lead to aneurysm, MI, and sudden death. However, the incidence of this vasculitis has greatly decreased since the advent of intravenous immunoglobulin therapy, which, along with aspirin, is the treatment of choice in this disease.

d. **Isolated CNS vasculitis.** This condition is a granulomatous inflammation of small or medium-sized arteries of the brain. Typically, patients do not have clinical or laboratory evidence of inflammation elsewhere. Presenting features often are combinations of diffuse CNS complaints (headache, altered mental status, poor memory) and more focal ones (cranial nerve defects, hemiparesis). A chronic meningitis picture, with pleocytosis and increased protein, typically is found on LP. An enhanced MRI scan of the brain is a sensitive but nonspecific indication of possible involvement.

F Diagnosis

1. **Recognizing a possible vasculitis.** Combinations of clinical features suggest the possibility of a vasculitis.
   a. **Specific clinical data.** The history and physical examination should be performed with attention to signs of organ ischemia or vessel abnormalities. Laboratory data may suggest a general inflammatory process or point to a specific syndrome (Table 10–15).
   b. **Syndrome recognition.** The diagnostic investigation should aim to identify patterns of organ involvement or distinct clinical features that suggest a vasculitic process. Overlap between vasculitic categories may blur the diagnosis.
2. **Confirming the diagnosis.** If the clinical evaluation suggests a reasonable chance of vasculitis, the appropriate approach to making a diagnosis usually lies in biopsy of involved tissue or visceral angiography; ANCA testing may be helpful when microscopic polyarteritis or Wegener's granulomatosis are suspected.
   a. **Biopsy of a fresh lesion.** Biopsy from clinically involved tissues is the preferred method of diagnosing vasculitis; if involved, the skin often is the easiest tissue to obtain.
      (1) Diagnosis of **Wegener's granulomatosis** often relies on open lung biopsy demonstration of granulomatous vasculitis, because paranasal sinus tissue typically shows nonspecific inflammation and renal tissue shows only glomerulonephritis.
      (2) Diagnosis of **temporal arteritis** requires examination of a 3- to 6-cm segment of the superficial temporal artery in multiple sections; biopsy of the contralateral side may be needed if the first biopsy is negative and clinical suspicion remains high.
      (3) Biopsy of leptomeninges and clinically involved brain tissue may be needed when **isolated CNS vasculitis** is strongly suspected.

TABLE 10–15 Clinical Data Suggesting Vasculitis

History	Physical Examination	Laboratory Studies
Constitutional complaints	**Vessel findings**	**Nonspecific tests** (chronic inflammation)
Malaise	Blood pressure/pulse deficits	Anemia (chronic disease)
Anorexia	Hypertension (sudden onset)	Thrombocytosis
Fever	Vessel tenderness, nodules, bruits	Increased erythrocyte sedimentation rate
Weight loss	**Skin findings**	Increased gamma globulins
Drug exposure (prescribed or illicit)	Palpable purpura	**Test indicating potential ischemia**
Infection	Infarctions	Abnormal renal function (↑ creatinine, BUN)
Human immunodeficiency virus (HIV)	Ulcers	Abnormal muscle/liver enzymes (↑ CK, AST, ALT)
Hepatitis B or C virus	**Muscle findings**	Electrocardiogram
Organ ischemic complaints	Tenderness, cramping	**Tests pointing toward specific diagnoses**
Angina	**Nerve findings**	HIV (several syndromes)
Extremity or jaw claudication	Sensory/motor neuropathies	HBsAg (20%–30% of polyarteritis patients)
Visual complaints	Focal/diffuse CNS dysfunction	Hepatitis C RNA
Transient ischemic attacks	**Testis**	ANA (SLE more likely)
Stroke	Tenderness	c-ANCA (Wegener's granulomatosis)
		p-ANCA (microscopic polyarteritis)
		Cryoglobulins (mixed essential cryoglobulinemia)
		Anti-Ro (Sjögren's syndrome, SLE)

b. **Visceral angiography.** When polyarteritis is suspected and appropriate tissue cannot be obtained for biopsy or when the biopsy is unrevealing, abdominal three-vessel angiography may show aneurysms or arteriopathy (discrete narrowing) suggestive of small to medium-sized artery vasculitis. Aortic arch and large vessel angiograms, carotid ultrasonography, and MRI studies of the chest are useful in Takayasu's arteritis and giant cell arteritis, because the involved vessels often cannot be safely subjected to biopsy. CNS angiograms may be warranted when isolated CNS vasculitis is suspected.

c. **Presence of ANCA.** ANCA are typically IgG antibodies directed against cytoplasmic components of neutrophils and monocytes (see I B 5).

3. **Differential diagnosis.** Numerous conditions should be considered in the differential diagnosis of vasculitis. Important disorders and the tests used to eliminate them include:
   a. **Bacterial endocarditis** (blood culture)
   b. **Left atrial myxoma** (two-dimensional or transesophageal echocardiogram)
   c. **Cholesterol embolism** syndrome (biopsy showing refractile crystals)
   d. **Thrombotic diseases** such as **antiphospholipid syndrome** (antiphospholipid antibody) and **disseminated intravascular coagulation (DIC)** or **thrombotic thrombocytopenic purpura** (TTP) [PT, PTT, platelet count, fibrinogen, fibrin split products]

G **Therapy** The management of patients with vasculitis is complex. In all patients with known vasculitic disease, it is important to record the extent of disease initially and to monitor organ involvement (in terms of clinical, biopsy, and angiographic evidence). The tempo of disease progression also should be gauged to determine the best treatment.

1. **Antigen removal.** Drugs that may be causing vasculitic processes should be stopped; plasmapheresis has been used in attempt to remove known antigens (HBsAg, HCV) and unknown antigens (cryoglobulin).
2. **Treatment of primary disease.** Control of any primary rheumatologic, infectious, or malignant process generally is the most effective way to control vasculitis that is a secondary feature.
3. **Immunosuppressive treatment.** Vasculitic syndromes that are not related to a removable antigen or treatable primary disorder often should be controlled with immunosuppressive agents—either **corticosteroids, cytotoxic drugs,** or a combination of both. **Cyclosporine,** working specifically on activated $CD4^+$ T cells, has been used in some vasculitis diseases, particularly to counteract eye involvement in Behçet's syndrome and some cases of refractory small vessel vasculitis.
   a. **Corticosteroids** alone should be attempted as first-line pharmacologic treatment in all patients except those with Wegener's granulomatosis. Daily dosing usually is required, although alternate-day dosing may be sufficient once systemic features of the illness are controlled. **Low-dose aspirin therapy** is often added to treatment of vasculitic disorders to counteract the potential **vaso-occlusive** effects of glucocorticoids.
   b. **Cytotoxic drugs** (e.g., cyclophosphamide)
      (1) **Wegener's granulomatosis** almost always is fatal without cytotoxic therapy; thus, patients should be started on a combination of one of these agents and corticosteroids.
      (2) **Polyarteritis nodosa and allergic angiitis** also often require cytotoxic drugs in addition to steroids for control of disease manifestations, although recent prospective studies have shown benefit in decreasing disease recurrences but not in preventing mortality.
      (3) In other disorders, cytotoxic drugs typically are added to corticosteroid therapy if the steroid doses cannot be easily lowered without the disease flaring.
4. **Other drugs** such as dapsone, colchicine, NSAIDs, hydroxychloroquine, and H_1- or H_2-blocking antihistaminic agents have been used, particularly in refractory small vessel vasculitis.
5. **Plasmapheresis,** which removes antibodies and immune complexes from plasma, has not been shown to improve outcome in systemic necrotizing vasculitis (e.g., polyarteritis, allergic angiitis).

In **mixed cryoglobulinemia,** whether or not it is related to HBV or HCV infection, plasmapheresis may improve disease features, at least temporarily.

XIII JUVENILE RHEUMATOID ARTHRITIS (JUVENILE IDIOPATHIC ARTHRITIS)

A Definition Juvenile rheumatoid arthritis—or juvenile idiopathic arthritis, as it is now more commonly called—is a **chronic inflammatory arthritis** that begins before age 16 years. Before considering a diagnosis of juvenile rheumatoid arthritis, arthritis should be present in one or more joints for more than 6 weeks, and other rheumatic diseases should be excluded.

B Epidemiology Annual incidence may be as high as 0.01%. Although the apparent HLA associations suggest that the altered immune responses are genetically transferable, familial aggregation of cases is uncommon.

C Etiology and pathogenesis The same factors important in the development of adult rheumatoid arthritis also apply to juvenile rheumatoid arthritis (see III C–D). Etiologic factors are unknown but may include infectious agents. **Immune system dysfunction** is apparent in the prolongation and maintenance of synovitis. A subset of patients with juvenile rheumatoid arthritis have selective IgA deficiency which may be important in disease pathogenesis.

D Pathology The **synovial lesions** cannot be distinguished histologically from those in adult rheumatoid arthritis. Inflammatory changes contiguous to the growth plate may lead to premature epiphyseal closure and shortened limbs or digits. Chronically involved joints exhibit **fibrous ankylosis** more often than in adult rheumatoid arthritis. **Pannus formation** can occur, although typically later in the disease course than in adults with rheumatoid arthritis. As a consequence, destructive joint disease also is much less common in juvenile rheumatoid arthritis.

E Classification Three primary subtypes of juvenile rheumatoid arthritis (i.e., systemic-onset juvenile rheumatoid arthritis, pauciarticular arthritis, and polyarticular arthritis) can be distinguished in the first 6 months of illness. It is important prognostically and therapeutically to distinguish between subtypes of illness. Important classification features are the **presence or absence of prominent systemic features** and the **total number of involved joints.**

1. **Systemic-onset juvenile rheumatoid arthritis,** also called **Still's disease,** occurs in approximately 10%–20% of patients and is characterized by an early pattern of **prominent systemic complaints** and **extra-articular involvement.** Boys are affected as commonly as girls, and a peak age of incidence is not evident.
   a. **Clinical features**
      (1) **Typical features of the early disease course** are **high spiking fevers** and marked **constitutional complaints.** Overt arthritis may not be part of the early course but develops within weeks to months of the onset of illness. A characteristic **nonpruritic, fleeting, maculopapular rash** occurs in 90% of patients and is most apparent with fever spikes.
      (2) **Common features of active disease** include lymphadenopathy, hepatosplenomegaly, and pericarditis. Accompanying myocarditis is rare.
      (3) The most serious manifestation of systemic-onset juvenile arthritis is macrophage activation syndrome. Activated macrophages in multiple organs leads to leukopenia, thrombocytopenia, CNS and liver dysfunction, and possible multiorgan failure and death.
   b. **Laboratory findings**
      (1) **Hematologic findings** include a strikingly elevated erythrocyte sedimentation rate, prominent leukocytosis, and thrombocytosis, and moderate-to-severe anemia of chronic disease, although there often is striking microcytosis.
      (2) **Serologic findings** only rarely include rheumatoid factor and ANAs.

c. **Disease course.** Disease flare-ups are punctuated by relatively symptom-free intervals. Polyarticular arthritis becomes evident at some point in the first 6 months of illness. Systemic symptoms most often decrease within 9 months after onset.

(1) Approximately 50% of patients may begin to develop symptoms of disease that resemble the polyarticular arthritis subset, with progressive joint involvement determining disease outcome.

(2) The remaining 50% of patients eventually recover completely.

2. **Polyarticular arthritis** occurs in approximately 30%–40% of patients and **involves five or more joints** in the first 6 months of illness. **Systemic features are not present.** Girls are affected much more often than boys. Polyarticular arthritis can be further separated into **rheumatoid factor–positive or –negative subsets.** Patients who are positive for rheumatoid factor present most often in late childhood; a peak age of incidence is not evident for patients who are negative for rheumatoid factor.

a. **Clinical features**

(1) Typically, inflammatory polyarticular arthritis may have an acute or a gradual onset similar to the presentation of adult rheumatoid arthritis. Symmetrical large and small joint involvement also is typical. Prominent features may include cervical spine, and temporomandibular joint (TMJ) disease.

(2) Rarely, patients have symptoms and signs of anterior uveitis.

(3) Patients who are positive for rheumatoid factor can have subcutaneous nodules as in adult-onset rheumatoid arthritis.

b. **Laboratory findings**

(1) **Hematologic findings** frequently include moderate elevation of erythrocyte sedimentation rate, leukocyte count, and platelet count. Patients usually develop a mild normochromic, normocytic anemia of chronic disease.

(2) **Serologic findings** include rheumatoid factor in 10%–20% and ANAs in 20%–40% of patients.

c. **Disease course.** Polyarticular arthritis can be chronic and persistent or can pursue a more intermittent, relapsing course.

(1) Patients who are positive for rheumatoid factor are at greatest risk for chronic, erosive, and severe arthritis and significant disability. These patients have disease that is very similar to adult-onset rheumatoid arthritis.

(2) Patients who are negative for rheumatoid factor less often have severe disease or disease that lasts into adulthood.

3. **Pauciarticular arthritis** occurs in approximately 50% of patients and involves **four or fewer joints** in the first 6 months of illness. This patient group is composed of three subsets.

a. **Oligoarthritis and anterior uveitis** affect girls more often than boys, and peak incidence is in early childhood.

(1) **Clinical features**

(a) Typically, the arthritis is asymmetrical, mild, and involves the knee. Other peripheral joints also can be involved, but the axial skeleton usually is spared.

(b) Systemic symptoms and signs are mild or absent.

(c) Potentially serious **anterior uveitis** unrelated to arthritis activity can develop in up to 25% of patients. This usually chronic eye lesion can be asymptomatic and can lead to **blindness** if unrecognized or inadequately treated.

(2) **Laboratory findings**

(a) **Hematologic findings** usually do not include anemia, thrombocytosis, and leukocytosis. The erythrocyte sedimentation rate is normal or only minimally elevated.

(b) **Serologic findings** include ANA positivity in 60% of patients, which identifies those at higher risk for chronic uveitis. Rheumatoid factor typically is not present.

(3) **Disease course.** Most patients have pauciarticular involvement that is manageable and not disabling. In approximately one third of patients, the disease eventually involves more than four joints, and is further subdivided as extended pauci-articular arthritis.

b. Axial skeleton oligoarthritis predominantly affects boys, with disease onset usually beginning in late childhood.

(1) **Clinical features.** Asymmetrical knee, ankle, or mid-tarsal arthritis is most common, followed by the sacroiliac hip joints. Acute anterior uveitis can occur as in adult spondyloarthropathies, but this feature is not the chronic and sight-threatening form seen in the other pauciarticular subset.

(2) **Laboratory findings**

(a) **Hematologic findings** are not distinct.

(b) **Serologic findings** indicate that 50% of these patients have HLA-B27, but few have rheumatoid factor.

(3) **Disease course.** Many of these patients develop features of ankylosing spondylitis, psoriatic arthritis, or reactive arthritis in later life.

c. Oligoarthritis with prominent dactylitis is a third presentation seen most frequently in girls of any age. **Psoriasis** commonly affects these patients and their families.

F Diagnosis

1. Difficulties in diagnosis. Diagnosing arthritis in children may be difficult. Children may avoid using an involved joint instead of complaining of pain. They may respond to the pain of an inflamed joint by displaying irritability, regressive behavior, or emotional withdrawal. Once joint involvement has been discovered, disease should be present for at least 6 weeks before a diagnosis of juvenile rheumatoid arthritis is seriously considered. Within the first 6 months, an attempt should be made to classify patients into a clinical subset.

a. The **synovial fluid** usually is mildly inflammatory (i.e., a WBC count of 10,000–20,000/mm^3); however, the number of WBCs present may not parallel disease activity. Joint fluid culture and analysis are especially important in more acute pauciarticular forms to exclude infection (bacterial or mycobacterial).

b. Radiographic findings are nonspecific.

(1) **Early findings** may include only soft tissue swelling and periarticular demineralization.

(2) **Late findings** include epiphyseal changes (either premature closure or overgrowth, depending on epiphyseal activity at the time of involvement) and articular erosion or joint space narrowing.

(3) **Distinctive long bone periosteal elevation in leukemia** may allow differentiation from juvenile rheumatoid arthritis. Localized joint abnormalities (e.g., osteonecrosis, osteochondritis) may have distinct radiographic presentations.

(4) **Cervical spine involvement,** particularly with ankylosis at C2–C3, is common in juvenile rheumatoid arthritis.

2. Differential diagnosis

a. A variety of **genetic or inborn metabolic disorders** as well as nonrheumatic conditions can superficially resemble juvenile rheumatoid arthritis. It is specifically important to rule out **infectious etiologies** (e.g., Lyme disease, tuberculosis) and **malignancies** (e.g., leukemia) as causes of childhood arthritis.

b. Other rheumatic diseases (e.g., rheumatic fever, SLE, undifferentiated connective tissue disease) may require a period of observation for characteristic extra-articular features to evolve.

G Therapeutic approach

1. Education of patients and parents about inflammatory arthritis is important, and the generally favorable course of juvenile rheumatoid arthritis should be emphasized. Long-term goals of suppression of disease activity and prevention of deformity should be instituted, and children's psychological and emotional development should not be neglected.

2. The use of appropriate **therapy** is important in relieving pain and maintaining function. Parents should be urged to perform active roles in giving physical therapy and medications, encouraging school attendance, and maintaining children's ability to be self-sufficient.
   a. **Pharmacologic therapy**
      (1) **Salicylates.** These agents are no longer the primary drugs used in the treatment of juvenile rheumatoid arthritis because of concerns about the potential precipitation of Reye's syndrome by aspirin.
      (2) **Other NSAIDs.** Currently, naproxen and ibuprofen are most often prescribed as initial treatment. Although indomethacin and nabumetone are not FDA-approved for children, they are also effective.
      (3) **Second-line agents.** Methotrexate, the most commonly used second-line agent, is effective. Oral gold, hydroxychloroquine, and D-penicillamine also are now rarely used in the treatment of juvenile rheumatoid arthritis. Sulfasalazine is also used because it has rapid onset of effect (<2 months), infrequent serious toxicity, and relatively good efficacy. A recent trial of leflunomide was effective.
      (4) **Biologic agents.** Etanercept, a genetically engineered fusion protein of recombinant TNF and human IgG, is approved for use in children. This agent is most often indicated in juvenile rheumatoid arthritis of a polyarticular course that is unresponsive to methotrexate. Infliximab, although not yet FDA-approved for children, appears to be effective. Neither of these biologic agents is particularly effective for systemic juvenile rheumatoid arthritis.
      (5) **Corticosteroids**
         (a) In **patients with systemic complaints who have life-threatening manifestations** (e.g., pericarditis), moderate-to-high–dose systemic corticosteroids may be required.
         (b) In **nonambulatory children with polyarticular disease,** a small, every-other-day dose of corticosteroids may promote weightbearing. The consequences of being nonambulatory in childhood outweigh possible corticosteroid complications in this clinical situation.
         (c) Local corticosteroid injections often are effective in managing **pauciarticular disease** or more **severely involved joints in polyarticular disease.** In some children with limited pauciarticular disease, intra-articular steroid therapy at onset may lead to complete remission.
         (d) In the treatment of **chronic uveitis,** systemic corticosteroids may be needed if initial treatment with topical or local corticosteroids and dilating agents is not effective. Recent clinical trials with infliximab are very encouraging. Patients at high risk for chronic uveitis (oligoarticular subgroup) should be evaluated every 3 months to determine treatment effectiveness.
      (6) **Intravenous infusions of gamma globulin.** This agent has been used to control severe systemic-onset or polyarticular disease.
   b. **Surgery.** Correction of deformities and total joint replacements may be needed in chronic, severe disease. Jaw implants have been used for micrognathia.
   c. **Physical and occupational therapy.** Such treatment is especially important in juvenile rheumatoid arthritis. Children must learn and practice exercises that maintain muscle tone and prevent joint contractures. Night splints may help minimize the evolution of joint contractures; serial splinting may improve existing joint contractures.

H Prognosis

1. **Disability.** Between 50% and 75% of patients recover completely by adulthood. Approximately 10% develop severe functional deformities.

2. **Specific complications**
   a. **Joint deformities.** Patients with polyarticular arthritis are most likely to develop chronic, erosive arthritis and subsequent joint deformities, especially those children with rheumatoid factor, who resemble patients with adult rheumatoid arthritis.
   b. **Chronic uveitis.** As many as 15% of patients with oligoarticular disease who have chronic uveitis develop some visual impairment, even if the problem is carefully treated.
   c. **Growth retardation**
      (1) **General growth retardation** can occur in patients with persistent, widespread inflammatory activity and in those treated with systemic corticosteroids.
      (2) **Local growth abnormalities** from the inflammatory process can lead to **micrognathia** as well as to **leg and finger length discrepancies** in some patients.
3. **Death.** Macrophage activation syndrome may be life-threatening and in rare cases, patients with particularly severe and protracted disease develop progressive **amyloidosis** or die of secondary infection. Rarely, overwhelming **myocarditis** in systemic-onset juvenile rheumatoid arthritis can lead to CHF and death.

XIV MISCELLANEOUS SYNDROMES

A Rheumatic manifestations of human immunodeficiency virus (HIV) Musculoskeletal complaints are relatively common during the course of HIV infection. The clinical spectrum is varied, ranging from arthralgias to distinct rheumatic disorders. Arthralgia and myalgias, the most common rheumatic manifestations, occur in 10%–20% of patients, usually with the initial infection. Other manifestations can be classified into the following groups:

1. **Spondyloarthropathy** (reactive arthritis, psoriatic arthritis, and undifferentiated spondyloarthropathy). In young persons with seronegative arthritis, it is important to consider HIV.
2. **HIV-associated arthritis.** The usual presentation is an oligoarticular asymmetric peripheral arthritis affecting the knees and ankles. A symmetrical polyarticular erosive form, which can also occur, may be difficult to distinguish from rheumatoid arthritis. This form is usually responsive to treatment with NSAIDs.
3. **Painful articular syndrome.** This poorly understood syndrome, which affects 10% of HIV-infected patients, is characterized by severe joint pain of abrupt onset that lasts a few hours to 2 days. Laboratory studies and imaging results usually are normal.
4. **Septic arthritis.** This condition is usually seen more frequently in patients with a history of intravenous drug abuse and in hemophiliacs. Both the usual and opportunistic organisms are implicated. In intravenous drug abusers, the most common pathogens are *S. aureus* and *Streptococcus pneumoniae.* Of the opportunistic organisms, *Candida albicans* is the most common. Axial joints are affected more frequently than peripheral joints.
5. **Diffuse infiltrative lymphocytosis syndrome** (DILS). This syndrome consists of dry eyes and mouth with a positive Schirmer test and salivary gland enlargement. DILS differs from classic Sjögren's syndrome in that it usually affects males and is not characterized by arthritis or autoantibody production (SS-A, SS-B, and rheumatoid factor).
6. **Myopathies.** Significant muscle weakness may be the presenting complaint. Such conditions may be the result of HIV myopathy, zidovudine myopathy, HIV wasting syndrome, rhabdomyolysis, or pyomyositis.
7. **Avascular necrosis and osteopenia/osteoporosis.** Recently, avascular necrosis has been reported in HIV patients. The etiology is unclear. Osteopenia and osteoporosis likewise are newer findings in this patient group. HIV therapy may be implicated.

B Hepatitis and cryoglobulinemia Both HBV and HCV can be linked with arthritis. HBV is associated with sudden-onset symmetric arthritis occasionally found with urticaria. HCV is often associated with type II cryoglobulinemia and can manifest as a combination of arthritis, palpable purpura, and cryoglobulinemia.

C Acute rheumatic fever (ARF) Skin infections do not cause ARF. The disorder occurs following a group A streptococcus (*S. pyogenes*) pharyngeal infection. In one third of patients, the triggering infection is silent, but it can be identified serologically. The incubation period from pharyngitis to infection is 2–3 weeks. According to the revised Jones Criteria (1992) for the diagnosis of ARF, if a patient has supportive evidence of preceding infection, the presence of two major or one major and two minor manifestations suggests a high probability of ARF.

1. **Major manifestations** are carditis, polyarthritis, chorea, erythema marginatum, and subcutaneous nodules. The arthritis is usually migratory, preferentially affecting the large joints of the lower extremities. Pain in affected joints may be out of proportion to physical examination findings of inflammation.
2. **Minor manifestations** are arthralgias, fever, elevated erythrocyte sedimentation rate, and a prolonged P-R interval.
3. **Supporting evidence of preceding group A streptococcal infection** includes a positive throat culture, elevated or rising antistreptolysin-O titer, or rapid streptococcal antigen test.

D Avascular necrosis This condition, which is also referred to as **osteonecrosis,** is used to describe the death of cellular components of bone as the result of diminished arterial blood supply. It may be idiopathic or occur in a variety of settings associated with certain medications (steroids, cytotoxic agents), underlying connective tissue diseases, hematologic disorders, infiltrative disorders, embolism, alcohol, and trauma. Involvement of the epiphysis of long bones such as the femoral heads is usually characteristic, but other bones can be affected. In the earliest stages, diagnosis can be made by MRI, but at later stages, findings can be identified on plain films. Blood stasis, hypercoagulability, and damage to endothelial cells are important.

E Fibromyalgia This common noninflammatory condition is characterized by diffuse pain. The etiology remains unclear, but affected patients tend to have disruption of non–rapid-eye movement (REM) stage IV sleep. In addition to diffuse pain, patients often report problems with insomnia, irritable bowel, tension headaches, migraines, and depression. Examination reveals multiple tender points (pain on palpation) over the following muscle regions: suboccipital muscle insertion; trapezius; supraspinatus; gluteal; greater trochanter; low anterior cervical; second costochondral junction, 2 cm distal to the lateral epicondyles; and the medial fat pad of the knees, proximal to the joint line. Laboratory investigation should include studies to rule out metabolic disorders (e.g., hypothyroidism, hyperthyroidism); electrolyte disturbances (e.g., low magnesium, calcium, or phosphorus); liver disease (e.g., viral hepatitis); connective tissue disease (e.g., PMR, SLE); and primary myopathy as clinically indicated. Treatment is aimed at improving the quality of sleep. Amitriptyline or low-dose muscle relaxants, in addition to regular physical exercise, are commonly used. If depression is a major component, referral to psychiatry is indicated.

F Amyloidosis The three main forms of amyloid deposition disorders that present with an arthropathy are AL amyloid, B2 microglobulin amyloid, and AA amyloid.

1. **AL amyloid** usually manifests as proteinuria/renal failure, a cardiomyopathy, or a variety of neuropathic symptoms. Other findings include edema, hepatomegaly, macroglossia, and purpura. Periarticular amyloid deposition can present as a pseudoarthritis, but joint effusions with amyloid fibrils may also be found. The characteristic finding may be a soft tissue "shoulder pad sign."
2. **B2 microglobulin** amyloid is the second most common form of amyloid deposition. Most patients who develop this form of amyloidosis have been on renal dialysis for prolonged periods and present with joint pain, carpal tunnel syndrome, and osteonecrosis.

3. **AA amyloid** is found in patients with rheumatoid arthritis and familial Mediterranean fever. It is also referred to as a secondary (reactive) amyloid, because it can occur in any chronic inflammatory disorder, including infections, neoplasia, or other rheumatic conditions.

G **Parvovirus B19 infection.** Parvovirus or Fifth's disease is endemic in school-age children. It manifests as fever, constitutional symptoms, and a "slapped cheek" appearance with striking erythema on the child's face. Adults typically present with arthralgias or a symmetrical arthritis that may mimic rheumatoid arthritis. Testing for Parvovirus serology early in the course of the disease can be diagnostic (positive IgM antibody). The course is self-limited and responds to anti-inflammatory pain medications.

H **Relapsing polychondritis** is a condition characterized by inflammation of cartilage. It can affect any cartilage in the body, but most commonly affects the cartilaginous portion of the nose and external ear, presenting as sudden pain, redness, and swelling with eventual destruction if untreated. The etiology is unclear, but autoimmune mechanisms may be involved. It is sometimes associated with other connective tissue disorders as well as malignancies.

I **Autoinflammatory diseases** These disorders are delineated most often by cycles of clinical inflammation without the presence of antigen-specific T cells or characteristic autoantibodies. Several of these diseases previously have been categorized as periodic fever syndromes. Over the last 5 years, the genetic basis for most of these disorders has been determined, and DNA sequencing to detect specific mutations is available in commercial laboratories (see Table 10–16).

1. **Familial Mediterranean Fever (FMF).** This disorder usually presents before age 20 with periodic 1- to 3-day episodes of fever, pleuro-peritoneal pain, and arthritis. A majority of patients, particularly those not treated with colchicine, develop amyloidosis.
2. **Tumor Necrosis Factor–Associated Periodic Syndrome (TRAPS).** This syndrome also presents primarily before age 20, but patients experience longer and less regular episodes of fever and also develop tender deep erythematous patches, and painful conjunctival injection.
3. **Hyper IgD Syndrome (HIDS).** Clinical symptoms usually start within the first 6 months of life. Along with fever, there is significant abdominal pain, often with diarrhea, cervical lymphadenopathy, maculopapular rash, and oligoarthritis.
4. **Familial Cold Autoinflammatory Syndrome (FCAS).** Symptoms start during infancy with a short-lived (<24 hours) maculopapular rash, conjunctival injection, and irritability without fever, all of which is usually triggered by exposure to cold temperatures.
5. **Muckle Wells Syndrome (MWS).** Clinical manifestations include an urticarial-like but not pruritic eruption, severe distal limb pains, and the gradual development of sensorineural deafness.
6. **Neonatal-Onset Multisystem Inflammatory Disease (NOMID).** This disorder not uncommonly presents during the neonatal period with an urticaria-like rash, the gradual development of severe arthropathy with extensive cartilage overgrowth, chronic meningitis, and sensorineural hearing loss.

FCAS, MWS, and NOMID are now considered to be a family of disorders with a spectrum of progressive clinical severity and common mutations of the CIAS1 gene at the q44 locus of chromosome 1.

TABLE 10–16 Auto Inflammatory Diseases

Features	FMF	TRAPS	HIDS	FCAS	MWS	NOMID
Major Ancestry	Jewish, Turkish, Arab, Armenian	Scottish, Irish	Dutch, French	No pattern	No pattern	No pattern
Genetic Pattern	Autosomal Recessive	Autosomal Dominant	Autosomal Recessive	Autosomal dominant	Autosomal dominant	Rarely autosomal dominant
Chromosomal Location	16p13	12p13	12q24	1q44	1q44	1q44
Gene Involved	MEFV	TNFRSFIA (type I TNF receptor)	Mevalonate Kinase	CIAS1	CIAS1	CIAS1
Age at Onset	90% by age 20	100% by age 20	6 months median	95% < 6 m	85% < 20 Y	Most within 6 m
Duration of Attacks	1–3 days	Days to weeks	3–7 days	<24 hours	2–3 days	Continuous
Abdominal	Peritoneal Irritation (95%)	Pain–nonspecific	Pain–diarrhea and vomiting	None	None	None
Pleuritic	Frequent	Frequent	None	None	None	None
Cutaneous	Occasional: erysipeloid erythema	Frequent: tender erythematous patches	Common: macules, papules, purpura	Maculopapular	Urticarial (not pruritic)	Urticarial (not pruritic)
Rheumatologic	Monarthritis: large joints (75%)	Localized myalgia: arthralgias	Oligosymmetric arthritis	Polyarthralgias	-Poly arthralgias-lancinating distal limb pains	Progressive destructive changes, massive cartilage over growth
Conjunctivitis	Absent	Frequent, (painful)	Absent	Very frequent	None	Anterior and posterior uveitis
Lymphadenopathy	Uncommon	Common	Very common (Cervical)	None	None	Uncommon
Cold Exposure Exacerbations	None	None	None	Consistent	Rare	None
Sensorineural Deafness	None	None	None	None	Common	Common
CNS	None	None	None	None	None	Chronic meningitis
Amyloidosis	Common	25%	None	None	None	None
Labs	Low C5a inhibitor in serosal fluids	↓ Serum type I TNF receptor (< 1 ng/mL)	↑ IgD (> 100 IU/mL); may be normal below age 3	↑ WBC, ESR	↑ WBC, ESR	↑ WBC, ESR
Treatment	Colchicine	Etanercept, Corticosteroids	None effective ?Statins	?NSAIDs	?NSAIDs	?IL–1 antagonists

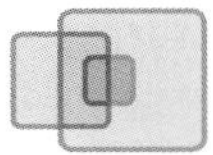

Study Questions

1. A 56-year-old women presents to your office with pain and stiffness in her hands. She states that the stiffness seems to last the entire morning. Which of the following joint findings is most suggestive of an inflammatory arthritis, rather than osteoarthritis, as the cause of her joint pain?

   [A] Painful range of motion
   [B] Crepitus
   [C] Bony articular enlargement
   [D] Swelling and warmth
   [E] Instability

2. A 45-year-old man with a history of hypertension complains of left great toe pain of 24 hours' duration. He has had a low-grade fever and chills. He has no history of joint problems. The examination is notable for a red, warm, swollen, left great toe. No other joints are involved. There are no tophi. How is a definitive diagnosis made?

   [A] Obtain an X-ray
   [B] Obtain fluid for synovial analysis
   [C] Obtain a serum uric acid level
   [D] Obtain blood cultures
   [E] Obtain HLA-B27

3. Which of the following forms of juvenile rheumatoid arthritis is most likely to be associated with serious eye complications?

   [A] Polyarticular arthritis that is seropositive for rheumatoid factor
   [B] Polyarticular arthritis that is seronegative for rheumatoid factor
   [C] Oligoarticular arthritis without axial spine involvement
   [D] Oligoarticular arthritis with axial spine involvement
   [E] Systemic-onset juvenile rheumatoid arthritis

An 18-year-old woman comes to the emergency department complaining of severe right knee, right wrist, and left ankle pain. She has several skin lesions on her arms and legs; some are petechial and others are vesiculopustular. Physical examination also reveals tenderness and swelling of tendons around the involved joints but no actual joint swelling.

4. Which of the following tests is most likely to yield the diagnosis?

   [A] Pelvic examination and cervical culture
   [B] Joint fluid aspiration
   [C] Antinuclear antibody (ANA) testing
   [D] Rheumatoid factor testing
   [E] Streptococcal enzyme testing

5. While awaiting results of laboratory testing, the patient in question 4 should receive which of the following treatments?

   [A] Corticosteroids
   [B] Nonsteroidal anti-inflammatory drugs (NSAIDs)
   [C] Antibiotics
   [D] Local care of skin lesions
   [E] Splinting of painful joints

6. A 50-year-old woman complains of a 2-month history of her hands becoming painful and turning white or blue in the cold; progressive skin tightness and thickening of fingers, hands, and forearms; shortness of breath on exertion; and a sensation of lower chest burning and food sticking on swallowing. Antibody testing shows the presence of antinuclear antibody (ANA) and elevated titers of antibody to Scl-70. Which of the following pathogenetic explanations best fits this patient's illness?

   A Infiltration of mucopolysaccarides into underlying subepithelial tissues
   B Unregulated fibroblastic collagen synthesis
   C Raynaud's phenomenon leading first to ischemia and later to tissue fibrosis
   D Vascular endothelial damage and immunologically mediated tissue fibrosis
   E Carcinomatous paraneoplastic process

7. Which of the following manifestations is more likely to be found in the diffuse form of systemic sclerosis than in the CREST variant?

   A Esophageal motility dysfunction
   B Pulmonary involvement
   C Distal skin thickening
   D Renal disease
   E Telangiectasias

8. Which of the following therapies is essential for treating polymyositis?

   A Antimalarial drugs
   B Nonsteroidal anti-inflammatory drugs (NSAIDs)
   C Corticosteroids
   D Bed rest
   E Aerobic exercise

9. A 32-year-old man presents with back pain with prominent stiffness lasting several hours, in addition to a painful swollen left ankle. The examination shows limited motion of the spine and a left Achilles tendinitis. You are considering a spondyloarthropathy as a unifying diagnosis. Which of the following clinical features is typical of all spondyloarthropathies?

   A Enthesopathic inflammation
   B Urethritis
   C Skin lesions
   D Bowel inflammation
   E Oral ulcers

10. A 57-year-old previously well man has been ill for 2 months with fatigue, malaise, dyspnea on exertion, abdominal pain, and progressive numbness in his feet. He has lost 20 pounds during this period. Recently, he developed mild inflammatory polyarthritis of the hands and has physical signs suggesting a mononeuritis in the right median nerve distribution. Chest radiograph shows cardiomegaly and findings of early pulmonary edema. Which of the following is the most likely diagnosis?

    A Hypersensitivity vasculitis
    B Rheumatoid arthritis
    C Systemic lupus erythematosus (SLE)
    D Polyarteritis nodosa
    E Churg-Strauss syndrome

11. A 64-year-old woman presents with gradually increasing right knee pain. The pain is worse with

weight bearing and relieved with rest. The knee is cool to touch. There is marked crepitus on range of motion, with a trace effusion. Which of the following would help confirm the diagnosis?

[A] Joint aspiration
[B] Trial of oral corticosteroids
[C] X-ray with weight-bearing views
[D] CBC, ESR
[E] Bone scan

12. A 70-year-old man complains of increasing back pain. He has no other history of arthritis or preceding trauma. He can walk about 2 blocks then has to stop because of the low back pain with an associated numbness and tingling extending into his buttocks and left thigh. His examination shows a well-appearing man. His peripheral pulses were normal. There was no spinal tenderness. His straight leg test was negative. His left lower extremity strength, range of motion, sensation, and reflexes were normal. What is the most likely diagnosis?

[A] Spondyloarthropathy
[B] Herniated disk
[C] Spinal stenosis
[D] Osteoarthritis of the left hip
[E] Muscular strain

Directions: *The response options for Items 13–15 are the same. You will be required to select one answer for each item in the set.*

[A] Rheumatoid arthritis
[B] Lyme disease
[C] Gonococcal arthritis
[D] Systemic lupus erythematosus (SLE)
[E] Polymyositis
[F] Sjögren's syndrome
[G] Polymyalgia rheumatica (PMR)
[H] Reactive arthritis (Reiter's syndrome)
[I] Pseudogout

For each of the following case descriptions, select the most appropriate diagnosis.

13. A 20-year-old woman complains of 2 weeks of fever, pleuritic chest pain, stiffness and swelling in wrists and metacarpophalangeal (MCP) and proximal interphalangeal (PIP) joints, an erythematous rash over both cheeks, and bilateral pretibial edema.

14. A 50-year-old man complains of a gritty sensation in his eyes and dry mouth, which he has experienced for several months. He has vague arthralgias in his hands and knees but only bulge signs (small amount of synovial fluid) in the knees on physical examination. He has scattered purpuric lesions over both calves and ankles.

15. An 80-year-old man complains of right knee pain and swelling. He has bony enlargement of the second and third metacarpophalangeal (MCP) joints bilaterally as well as wrist, proximal interphalangeal (PIP), and distal interphalangeal (DIP) joints. His knee is swollen, and range of motion is moderately limited by pain. A radiograph shows only flecks of calcium in the meniscal cartilage of the knee.

16. A 25-year-old woman presents to your office with a month history of fatigue, generalized arthralgias, and photosensitivity. Her examination shows an erythematous rash sparing her nasolabial folds. Her lab tests indicated a normal CBC and comprehensive metabolic profile. Her ESR was elevated at 40, ANA was positive at 1:320 speckled, SSA was borderline positive. Her urinalysis was normal. The best treatment now would be

- A Hydroxychloroquine
- B NSAIDs
- C Steroids
- D Sunscreen
- E Cyclophosphamide

17. A 35-year-old preschool teacher presents with a 2 -week history of malaise, low-grade fever, and a symmetric polyarthritis. Her examination shows synovitis affecting her wrists, MCPs, and PIPs bilaterally. Her CBC and comprehensive metabolic profile are normal. The ANA and RF are negative. The most likely diagnosis would be

- A Parvovirus B19 infection
- B Polymyalgic rheumatica (PMR)
- C SLE
- D Scleroderma
- E Osteoarthritis

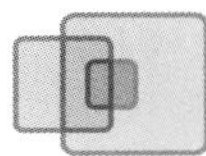

Answers and Explanations

1. The answer is D [V F; II F 1–2]. A swollen and warm joint is more likely to be affected by an inflammatory arthritis than by osteoarthritis. The presence of synovial fluid is more commonly associated with inflammatory arthritis than osteoarthritis, and warmth suggests some degree of inflammation. Osteoarthritis typically is associated with bony joint enlargement in response to cartilage and subchondral bone injury. Painful joint range of motion, joint crepitus, and joint instability could occur in either an inflammatory or osteoarthritic joint problem.

2. The answer is B [V A 5; V A 6 a]. The likely diagnoses are gout or pseudogout. The only way to make a definitive diagnosis is to perform a diagnostic arthrocentesis and evaluate the fluid under the polarized microscope for the presence of crystals. X-rays in patients with long-standing symptoms can have erosions characteristic of gout, but they are usually normal in this setting, with this being his first attack. Hyperuricemia can be a risk factor for gout, but not everyone with hyperuricemia develops gout. Additionally, during an acute attack the uric acid level may be falsely low. Thus, in this patient with acute symptoms, the uric acid level would not be that helpful. The toes can be involved in the presentation of a spondyloarthropathy, but usually as a sausage digit. He has no other features of spondyloarthropathy. HLA-B27 testing would not be helpful.

3. The answer is C [V E 3 a (1) (c)]. Patients with oligoarticular arthritis without axial spine involvement are most likely to develop chronic and potentially severe anterior uveitis, which can be clinically quite subtle even as it leads to progressive visual loss. Up to 25% of patients in this subset may develop anterior uveitis, and the group that is antinuclear antibody (ANA)–positive appears to be at highest risk. Patients with axial spine involvement can also develop anterior uveitis, but this tends to be acute, self-limited, and easily treatable.

4–5. The answers are: 4-A [VI D 1 a, E 1 a], **5-C** [VI F 1]. This patient has clinical features suggestive of gonococcal periarthritis–dermatitis syndrome. In this setting, the cervix would be the most likely site for a positive culture. Joint fluid aspiration could yield a positive culture, but the patient does not have joint effusions. Antinuclear antibody (ANA) testing would be helpful if the findings were more consistent with systemic lupus erythematosus (SLE) than gonorrhea. A patient with rheumatoid arthritis would be unlikely to have the skin findings, so rheumatoid factor is not a helpful test. Different skin and articular findings would be present in rheumatic fever, so streptococcal enzyme testing would be unlikely to yield a diagnosis.

Because gonorrhea is the most likely diagnosis, antibiotic treatment is required. Corticosteroids are contraindicated. Nonsteroidal anti-inflammatory agents (NSAIDs), local skin care, and splinting of joints may be useful ancillary measures but do not treat the primary problem of a bacterial infection.

6. The answer is D [VIII D]. This patient presents with characteristic features of scleroderma, a chronic illness in which unregulated immunologic processes (perhaps triggered by unknown environmental antigens) cause small vessel endothelial damage and widespread dermal and internal organ fibrosis. The small vessel endothelial damage leads to secondary vascular reactivity (Raynaud's phenomenon) and, possibly, ischemic tissue damage. The increased collagen synthesis by tissue fibroblasts, which leads to widespread fibrosis, is not unregulated; rather, it is caused by cytokine and growth factor secretion from lymphocytes, mast cells, and platelets. There is no evidence that scleroderma patients have tissue mucopolysaccharide infiltration or that there are tumors responsible for paraneoplastic dermal fibrosis.

7. The answer is D [VIII E 2 a]. Of the clinical manifestations listed, only renal disease is more likely to be found in diffuse systemic sclerosis than in the CREST syndrome, which involves the coexistence of subcutaneous **c**alcinosis, **R**aynaud's phenomenon, **e**sophageal motility dysfunction, **s**clerodactyly, and **t**elangiectasia. Also, pulmonary interstitial fibrosis typically worsens faster in the diffuse form. Both forms are characterized by esophageal motility dysfunction, distal skin thickening, and Raynaud's phenomenon. Telangiectasias also can occur in both forms of scleroderma, although they are more common and widespread in the CREST syndrome.

8. The answer is C [IX G 1]. Oral corticosteroids are the typical initial treatment for inflammatory myopathy. Nonsteroidal anti-inflammatory agents (NSAIDs), antimalarial drugs, bed rest, and aerobic exercise are not recognized treatments for polymyositis, although NSAIDs might help associated joint complaints and antimalarial drugs have been used for the skin features of dermatomyositis. Aerobic exercise is appropriate for patients with controlled disease but might be detrimental to those with active disease.

9. The answer is A [IV A 1 a (3)]. Enthesopathic inflammation (i.e., inflammatory lesions at ligamentous, cartilaginous, and tendinous attachments to bone) is a characteristic feature of all spondyloarthropathies. Urethritis and oral ulcers are typical of reactive arthritis (Reiter's syndrome), and skin lesions are seen in reactive and psoriatic arthritis. Some patients with inflammatory bowel disease also have skin lesions (e.g., pyoderma gangrenosum), but the most typical feature other than rheumatic complaints is bowel inflammation.

10. The answer is D [XI E 2 a]. This patient suffers from constitutional complaints (fatigue, malaise, 20-lb weight loss) and has clinical evidence of impaired functioning of multiple organs; these findings make vasculitis a distinct diagnostic possibility. Mononeuritis is an even more specific finding, suggesting a small to medium-sized vasculitis of vasa nervorum. The other clinical findings are compatible with vasculitic organ impairment as well and are typical of polyarteritis nodosa. Hypersensitivity vasculitis is unlikely, because patients with this disorder of the very small vessels almost always have distinct skin findings (e.g., palpable purpura) to support the diagnosis. Both rheumatoid arthritis and systemic lupus erythematosus (SLE) are systemic illnesses that can be complicated by a small to medium-sized vessel vasculitis, but the only findings supporting these diagnoses are the mild joint complaints. The absence of allergic history, eosinophilia, and chest radiograph infiltrate distinct from pulmonary edema makes Churg-Strauss syndrome unlikely.

11. The answer is C [VI G 3]. The patient has classic findings of osteoarthritis of her knee. The best test to confirm the diagnosis would be an x-ray, which usually shows joint space loss, bony sclerosis, and degenerative spurs. Although the patient does have an effusion, the knee has no associated warmth; thus, an aspiration in not necessary. If there is concern about a crystalline disease or infection, then joint fluid analysis would be helpful. Laboratory studies such as CBC and ESR would not be indicated in this patient, because there are no constitutional symptoms, or inflammatory signs or symptoms. A bone scan will likely show degenerative changes, but is more costly and time consuming. Only if an occult fracture, avascular necrosis, infection, malignancy, or an inflammatory arthritis is suspected would a bone scan be helpful. Oral steroids have no role in the treatment of this disorder.

12. The answer is C [II C 2 a]. The patient presents with classical symptoms of spinal stenosis. Pseudoclaudication is the most common symptom, with pain worsened by erect posture, improved by forward flexion, and associated numbness and weakness. Spondyloarthropathies usually present in younger individuals with associated inflammatory back pain (pain lasting more than 1 hour). The lack of a positive straight leg test helps eliminate sciatica/herniated disk. Although underlying osteoarthritis of his hip may be contributing to his left thigh discomfort, it does not explain his back symptoms. Additionally, on examination he has good range of motion of his hip, making hip pathology less likely. His symptoms are not consistent with simple strain, because most strain syndromes improve in 6–8 weeks.

13–15. The answers are: 13-D [VII G 1; Table 10–10], **14-F** [X B], **15-I** [IV B 4 d, 5]. This young woman has the sudden onset of a systemic febrile illness that includes findings suggestive of serositis (pleuritic chest pain), arthritis, and a facial skin rash (possibly a butterfly rash). New pretibial edema suggests the possibility of urinary protein loss from renal involvement (glomerulonephritis or nephrotic syndrome). Although laboratory data [including positive antinuclear antibodies (ANAs)] or radiographic support are necessary to confirm possible organ abnormalities, systemic lupus erythematosus (SLE) is the most likely cause of these findings.

This man likely has primary Sjögren's syndrome. The dry eyes and dry mouth suggest lacrimal and salivary gland involvement in this disorder, and further ophthalmologic evaluation or labial salivary gland biopsy could confirm these suspicions. Arthralgias are a common feature of primary Sjögren's syndrome; the arthritis of rheumatoid arthritis should have more actual joint findings (tenderness, swelling, or limitation of motion) to be considered as a primary disease accompanied by a secondary form of Sjögren's syndrome. The purpuric lesions on the calves suggest the possibility of a small vessel vasculitis, a common skin feature of primary Sjögren's syndrome.

The man's presentation is most consistent with a chronic degenerative arthritis and a superimposed acute inflammatory arthritis. The degenerative, bony changes involve unusual joints [wrist, metacarpophalangeals (MCPs)] and include an unusual feature (chondrocalcinosis on knee radiograph). These findings are most compatible with calcium pyrophosphate deposition (CPPD) disease causing atypical degenerative arthritis, and the superimposed acute knee inflammation (pseudogout) is likely caused by release of the CPPD crystals into the knee joint. Finding positively birefringent crystals under red-compensated, polarized light examination of synovial fluid would be diagnostic.

16. The answer is A [VIII H 3]. The patient has SLE, with the main manifestations being fatigue, arthralgias, and the malar rash and photosensitivity; all of which would respond to hydroxychloroquine. Although NSAIDs may improve her joint symptoms, they have no effect on the rash. Likewise, sunscreen would be helpful in controlling the skin disease and possibly preventing disease flares, but would not directly improve her fatigue or arthralgias. There is no evidence of major organ involvement; thus, steroids or cytotoxic therapy have no role in this patient at this point.

17. The answer is A [XIV G]. Given that the patient is exposed to young children and has an acute (less than 6 week) symmetric polyarthritis, Parvovirus B19 is the most likely diagnosis at this point. Polymyalgic rheumatica usually presents with proximal shoulder and pelvic girdle pain and stiffness and does not occur in this age group. SLE could be a consideration if her symptoms were to persist, but the fact that her ANA is negative makes SLE very unlikely. She has no features of scleroderma. Osteoarthritis would be unlikely based on her age and the fact that she has inflammatory joint findings on examination (synovitis).

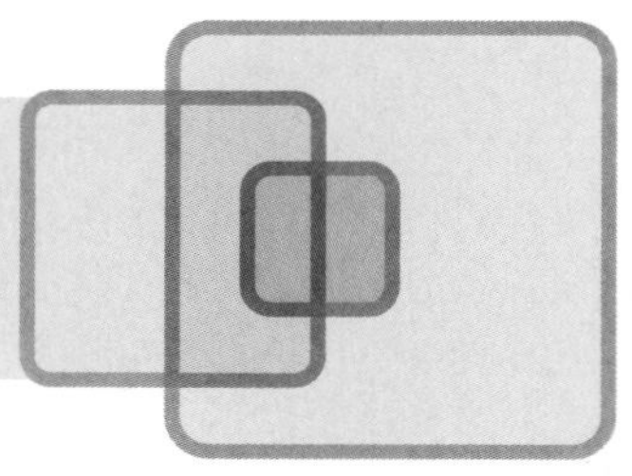

chapter 11

Neurologic Disorders

BARNEY J. STERN

I APPROACH TO THE PATIENT WITH A NEUROLOGIC COMPLAINT

A Patient history The patient history is the cornerstone of neurologic assessment.

1. **Key questions.** Questions that may help direct the patient interview include:
   - a. Was the onset of symptoms gradual or sudden?
   - b. Are the symptoms static, intermittent, or progressive?
   - c. Has the problem remained limited in scope, or have new features been introduced over time?
   - d. What concurrent problems does the patient have, and what medications or drugs are being used?
   - e. Is there a family history of the disorder or predisposing conditions?
   - f. What habits and toxin exposures might the patient have?
2. **Review of symptoms.** Depending on the clinical complaint, a patient should be asked whether there is any history of:
   - a. Headache or trauma to the head, neck, or spine
   - b. Loss of consciousness, convulsive activity, mood alterations, confusion, or memory disturbances
   - c. Impaired or double vision, facial numbness or weakness, impaired hearing or swallowing, or abnormal speech
   - d. Arm or leg weakness or heaviness, slowness of movement, altered limb sensation, discomfort or tingling in the extremities
   - e. Clumsiness, falling, or dizziness
   - f. Bowel or bladder disturbances or sexual dysfunction

B Neurologic examination From the patient history, the physician can generate a series of diagnostic hypotheses that can be tested with a focused neurologic examination. Anatomic localization of the pathology within the nervous system is essential to this process (Figure 11–1).

1. **Mental status.** If the patient's mental status is abnormal, the history and those components of the physical examination that depend on patient cooperation must be approached within the proper context. For example, if the patient is confused, the sensory examination may be unreliable.
   - a. The patient's level of arousal, orientation, short- and long-term memory, affect (i.e., mood), concentration and attention, fund of knowledge, insight, judgment, and constructional ability should be assessed.
   - b. Linguistic abilities are evaluated by examining comprehension, repetition, fluency, naming, reading, and writing.
   - c. The integrity of other cortical functions (e.g., graphesthesia, stereognosis, two-point discrimination, right–left orientation) should be examined if parietal lobe dysfunction is suspected. A search for extinction to double simultaneous visual and sensory stimulation, as evidence of neglect phenomena, should be made. (Patients with neglect may be unaware of their neurologic deficits.)
2. **Cranial nerves.** Examination of cranial nerves I–XII is necessary (Table 11–1).

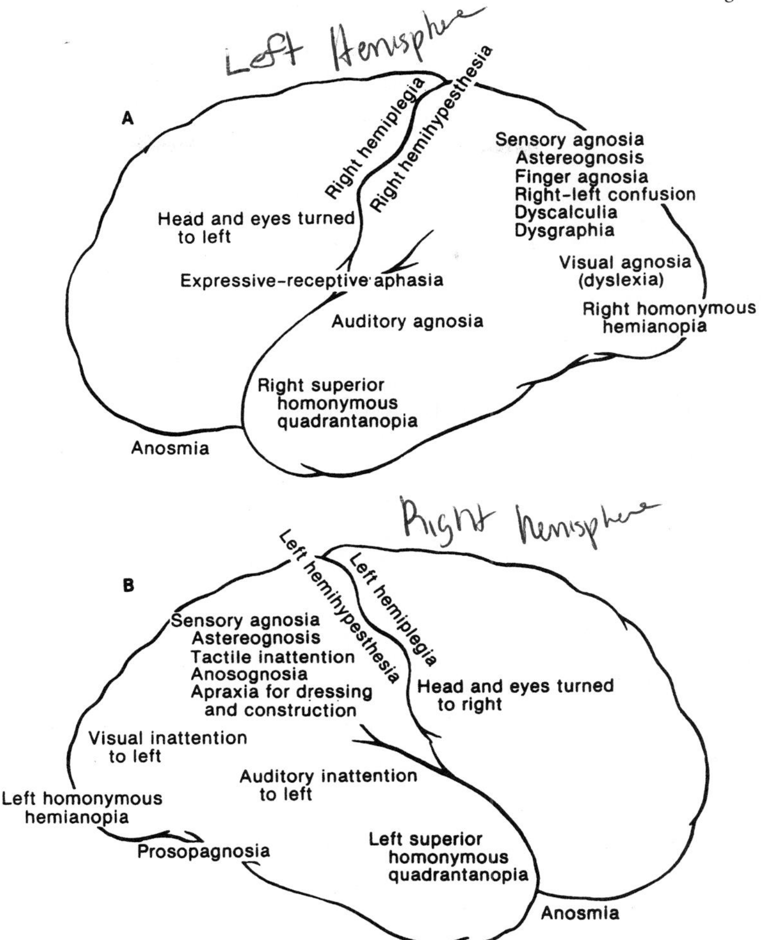

FIGURE 11–1 Summary of some of the outstanding neurologic signs and symptoms that occur with focal destructive lesions in the right or left cerebral hemisphere as detected on neurologic examination. (*A*) Lateral view of the left cerebral hemisphere. (*B*) Lateral view of the right cerebral hemisphere. (Reprinted from NMS *Neuroanatomy*. Malvern, PA, Harwal Publishing, 1988, p 314).

   a. In particular, visual acuity and fields should be checked; the optic nerve should be examined; and abnormalities of ocular motility, including nystagmus and dysmetria, should be documented (Table 11–2).
   b. Abnormalities of facial sensation (including the corneal reflex) and movement also should be investigated.

3. **Sensory system.** Regions of abnormal touch, pain (estimated by pinprick), temperature, vibration, and proprioception should be defined.
   a. Are the findings confined to one side of the body, the distribution of one or more dermatomes, or the territory of one or more peripheral nerves?
   b. Are the sensory changes found in a "stocking–glove" distribution?
4. **Motor system**
   a. The patient's **strength** should be defined as it pertains to individual muscles or groups of muscles. One conventional method of grading muscle strength for purposes of comparison and description is shown in Table 11–3.
   b. The presence of **atrophy, fasciculations, spasticity,** and **rigidity** should be noted.

TABLE 11–1 Twelve Cranial Nerves

Number	Name	Summary of Function
I	Olfactory	Smells
II	Optic	Sees
III	Oculomotor	Moves eyeball and constricts pupil
IV	Trochlear	Moves eyeball
V	Trigeminal	Feels front half of head and chews
VI	Abducens	Moves eyeball
VII	Facial	Moves face; tears, tastes, and salivates
VIII	Vestibulocochlear	Equilibrates and hears
IX	Glossopharyngeal	Tastes, salivates, and swallows and monitors carotid body and sinus
X	Vagus	Tastes, swallows, lifts palate, and phonates; sensorimotor to thoraci coabdominal viscera
XI	Spinal accessory	Turns head and shrugs shoulders
XII	Hypoglossal	Moves tongue

Adapted from NMS *Neuroanatomy*. Malvern, PA, Harwal Publishing, 1988, p 139.

TABLE 11–2 Innervation of the Eye by Its Six Nerves

Number and Name of Nerve	Innervation	Clinical Effects of Interruption of Nerve
Efferent		
CN III (oculomotor nerve)	Striated muscle: superior, medial, and inferior recti; inferior oblique	Diplopia, eye abducted and turned down
	Levator palpebrae	Ptosis (paralysis of volitional lid elevation)
	Smooth muscle: pupilloconstrictor	Pupil dilated and fixed to light
	Ciliary muscle	Loss of lens thickening
CN IV (trochlear nerve)	Striated muscle: superior oblique	Diplopia, most severe on looking down and in; eye extorted; head tilted to side opposite paralyzed eye
CN VI (abducens nerve)	Striated muscle: lateral rectuus	Diplopia, most severe on looking to side of paralysis; eye turned in (abducted)
Carotid sympathetic nerve	Smooth muscle; superior tarsal and pupillodilator	Horner's syndrome (ptosis, miosis, hemifacial anhidrosis, vasodilation)
Afferent		
CN II (optic nerve)	From retina	Blindness
CN V (trigeminal nerve)	Corneal/conjunctival afferents	Anesthesia of cornea with loss of corneal reflex

Adapted from NMS *Neuroanatomy*. Malvern, PA, Harwal Publishing, 1988, p 219.

TABLE 11–3 Medical Research Council of Great Britain Muscle Strength Grading Scale

Grade	Equivalent Patient Ability
5/5	Normal ability
4/5	Ability to overcome gravity and some resistance imposed by the examiner
3/5	Ability to overcome gravity only
2/5	Ability to move with gravity eliminated
1/5	Only a flicker of movement
0/5	Complete inability to move

   c. The patient's ability to perform **rapid alternating and other complex maneuvers** should be determined.
   d. The patient's **stance and gait** should be evaluated (Table 11–4).
5. **Coordination.** Finger-to-nose and heel-to-shin testing should be performed. The physician should look for **Romberg's sign** (i.e., swaying or falling when standing with eyes closed and feet close together).
6. **Muscle stretch reflexes.** The activity and symmetry of the brachioradialis (C5, C6), biceps (C5, C6), triceps (C7, C8), knee (L3, L4), and ankle (S1, S2) reflexes should be determined. The presence of the **Babinski response** should be assessed with plantar stimulation.

C Neurodiagnostic studies

1. **Cerebrospinal fluid (CSF) evaluation**
   a. **Indications.** Study of the CSF can provide information about intracranial pressure (ICP) and infection, bleeding, malignancy, and sterile inflammation within the central nervous system (CNS).
   b. **Specific measurements and assays**
      (1) **Pressure.** The opening pressure should be determined. Pressure exceeding 180 mm H_2O is abnormal when a patient is relaxed and in a lateral decubitus position.
      (2) **Protein.** An elevated CSF protein level is a nonspecific indicator of inflammation or breakdown of the blood-brain barrier.
      (3) **Glucose. Hypoglycorrhachia** (i.e., CSF glucose < 40 mg/dL or a simultaneous CSF–blood glucose ratio of < 0.6) suggests infection or sterile inflammation.
         (a) Relatively common causes of hypoglycorrhachia include bacterial, fungal, or tuberculous infection; carcinomatous meningitis; and hypoglycemia.
         (b) Less common causes include mumps, herpes simplex virus (HSV) or zoster infection, subarachnoid hemorrhage (SAH), sarcoidosis, syphilitic meningitis, and systemic lupus erythematosus (SLE).
      (4) **White blood cell (WBC) count.** A WBC count exceeding 5 cells/mm^3 is considered abnormal.
         (a) **Excess neutrophils** suggest infection or, on occasion, sterile inflammation.
         (b) **Excess mononuclear cells** suggest a viral infection, an indolent nonviral infectious process, or sterile inflammation.
      (5) **Blood.** Blood may appear in the CSF as a result of the local trauma of a lumbar puncture (LP) or by CNS hemorrhage from multiple causes.
         (a) A traumatic LP is suspected if gross blood exudes from the needle and then clears quickly, or if a large discrepancy exists between the number of red blood cells (RBCs) in the first drops of CSF obtained as compared with a later aliquot.
         (b) A traumatic LP should not reveal a xanthochromic (yellow-tinged) CSF, because sufficient time would not have elapsed to cause breakdown of RBCs.
      (6) **Culture and Gram staining.** These studies are indicated to evaluate the possibility of infection. A CSF Venereal Disease Research Laboratory (VDRL) test is indicated if CNS syphilis is a diagnostic consideration.
      (7) **Cytology.** Cytologic examination is useful if malignancy is suspected.
      (8) **Intrathecal immunoglobulin production.** This can be determined using the immunoglobulin G (IgG) index:

$$\frac{\text{CSF IgG/serum IgG}}{\text{CSF albumin/serum albumin}}$$

or through CSF electrophoresis, which reveals the presence of oligoclonal bands (discrete immunoglobulin aggregates). An elevated IgG index or oligoclonal bands are found in CNS inflammatory disorders such as multiple sclerosis (MS) and infections.

TABLE 11–4 Classification of Gait Disorders

Gait Disorder	Disequilibrium (Impaired Balance)	Gait Ignition Failure (Start/Turn Hesitation) (Freezing)	Wide Base	Shortened Stride	Associated Findings
Cautious gait	Mild	Absent	Mild	Mild to moderate	. . .
Subcortical disequilibrium	Severe	Variable	Variable	Variable	Occasional parkinsonism; pyramidal signs
Frontal disequilibrium	Severe	Variable	Variable	Variable	Dementia, frontal release signs, and urinary incontinence; occasionally apraxia, parkinsonism, and pyramidal signs
Isolated gait ignition failure	None	Severe	Absent	Absent*	. . .
Frontal gait disorder	Moderate	Moderate to severe	Variable	Mild to moderate	Dementia, frontal release signs, and urinary incontinence; occasionally apraxia, parkinsonism, and pyramidal signs

Apraxia may be gauged by asking the patient to mime gestures with the arms or legs. Frontal release signs include gegenhalten hand and foot grasp reflexes, and rooting responses.
In this table, "parkinsonism" refers to hypokinesia and difficulty executing rhythmic and repetitive alternating or sequential movements.
(Adapted from Nutt JG, Marsden CD, Thompson PD: Human walking and higher-level gait disorders, particularly in the elderly. *Neurology* 1993;43:272.)
*Steps would be of normal size and rhythm once walking was underway.

c. **Contraindications** to the performance of an LP
   (1) A **mass effect** sufficient to cause distortion of the lateral or third ventricles or a midline shift
   (2) A **posterior fossa mass**
   (3) A **coagulopathy** [e.g., a prothrombin time (PT) > 3 seconds over control or a platelet count of < 50,000/mm^3].

2. **Electroencephalography** (EEG) and **evoked potentials (EPs)**
   a. **EEG** is indicated in the evaluation of **seizure disorders, encephalopathies, sleep disorders,** and **brain death.** Prolonged video EEG monitoring is the **gold standard** for evaluating seizure problems that are difficult to diagnose or treat.
   b. **EPs** are repetitive afferent stimuli presented to the eye, ear, peripheral sensory nerves, or cerebral cortex that cause stereotypic wave forms that can be analyzed by computerized signal averaging methodology.
      (1) **Visual, brain stem–auditory,** and **somatosensory EPs** can detect lesions, which are often clinically silent, in the anatomic pathways subserving these sensory systems.
      (2) **Motor EPs,** which can be elicited by transcranial magnetic stimulation of the motor pathways, provide information about the integrity of the motor system.

3. **Imaging studies**
   a. **Computed tomography** (CT) **scanning** provides an image of the brain that allows definition of **hemorrhage, edema, atrophy, mass lesions,** and **ventricular size.**
      (1) Intravenous contrast can be administered to define **regions where the blood-brain barrier is not intact.**
      (2) CT scanning can also visualize **the spinal cord** and **surrounding bony structures;** transverse images are especially well represented.
   b. **Magnetic resonance imaging** (MRI) provides excellent **anatomic depiction of the brain,** especially the posterior fossa, **and the spinal cord.** Disease of the cerebral white matter is particularly well defined. Intravenous contrast can detect sites of a disturbed blood-brain barrier. Diffusion weighted imaging can detect regions of cerebral ischemia, as reflected by an area of decreased free water diffusion.
   c. **Single-photon emission computed tomography** (SPECT) provides an image-based estimate of **cerebral blood flow** after intravenous injection of a radioactive tracer.
   d. **Noninvasive vascular studies**
      (1) **Duplex scanning** provides an ultrasound image of the extracranial carotid and vertebral arteries together with a Doppler description of flow patterns.
      (2) **Transcranial Doppler** (TCD) defines intracranial large artery flow patterns.
      (3) **Magnetic resonance angiography** (MRA) uses magnetic resonance technology to image the vascular anatomy.
      (4) **Computed tomography angiography** (CTA) uses computed tomography technology with intravenous contrast administration to image the vascular anatomy.
   e. **Angiography.** The vascular anatomy is best defined with cerebral angiography. This study is useful for identifying an aneurysmal source of SAH, evaluating occlusive cerebrovascular disease (especially if surgery is contemplated), defining vasculitis, and assessing arteriovenous malformations.

4. **Nerve conduction velocity** (NCV) **studies and electromyography** (EMG)
   a. **NCV studies** can place peripheral nerve disease into sensory, motor, or sensorimotor categories; define primarily demyelinating or axonal dysfunction; and identify sites of conduction block. These distinctions help in making a diagnosis.
   b. **EMG** can differentiate problems affecting muscle so that they can be divided into broad categories such as denervation and myopathy.
      (1) The **distribution of the observed changes** helps determine whether the problem is myotomal (i.e., limited to a few nerve roots) or diffuse.

(2) The **pattern of wave forms** provides information pertaining to ongoing muscular denervation and reinnervation.

II LOSS OF CONSCIOUSNESS

A Syncope

1. **Definition.** Syncope refers to a transient loss of consciousness that typically follows insufficient blood supply to the brain for more than a few seconds.
2. **Clinical signs.** Patients are transiently unresponsive, with diminished muscle tone. A few generalized tonic spasms may occur, especially if patients are prevented from lying down.
3. **Etiology.** Cardiac and circulatory causes of syncope are discussed in Chapter 1 IX. Most patients with syncope have a cardiac or circulatory basis for the event, although neurologic conditions need to be considered if the diagnosis remains elusive.
   a. **Circulatory disturbances** are particularly common.
      (1) **Vasovagal syncope,** which is often seen in young people, is commonly associated with emotional stress, fear, or pain.
      (2) **Postprandial syncope,** which frequently affects the elderly, often occurs following meals in which alcohol was consumed.
      (3) Syncope can occur in diverse settings that have in common a **preceding Valsalva** or **straining maneuver** that decreases venous return and promotes parasympathetic tone.
   b. **Cardiac output disturbances,** other than arrhythmia or mechanical obstruction, should be considered.
      (1) **Vasodepressor (neurocardiogenic) syncope** is caused by undue stimulation of afferent cardiac mechanoreceptors because of cardiac distention or strenuous contractions. This causes a decrease in sympathetic activity and an increase in parasympathetic activity that leads to vasodilatation, bradycardia, and subsequent hypotension.
      (2) **Carotid sinus hypersensitivity** can lead to bradyarrhythmias and hypotension. Because carotid sinus hypersensitivity is present in many older men, it should be considered responsible for syncope only if other causes have been excluded.
         (a) **Atropine** may be used to treat **cardioinhibitory** carotid sinus hypersensitivity.
         (b) **Epinephrine** blocks the effects of **cardiodepressor** carotid sinus hypersensitivity.
         (c) Patients can exhibit both types of carotid sinus hypersensitivity.
   c. **Hypoglycemia** causes a lack of nutrient supply to the brain and can lead to syncope. Hypoglycemia as a cause of syncope is particularly likely in patients with type 1 (insulin-dependent) diabetes. Therapy involves the administration of glucose.
   d. **Neurologic disorders** are relatively uncommon causes of syncope. Several conditions are important because they can lead to unresponsiveness and are therefore often considered during the evaluation of a patient with transient unresponsiveness.
      (1) **Seizures** (see also IX A–B) are a cause of unresponsiveness that must be differentiated from syncope.
         (a) Patients are rarely limp during seizures. Many seizures cause intermittent, relatively rhythmic limb contractions (clonic activity) or sustained limb extension (tonic activity).
         (b) Atonic seizures are rare in adults but do cause sudden collapse. Absence seizures, conversely, do not result in a fall.
         (c) Because some patients with syncope can exhibit involuntary movements, the possibility of a primary seizure is a consideration. However, in most cases, the tonic or

myoclonic activity tends to occur several seconds after consciousness is lost and merely reflects cerebral hypoperfusion, not a primary seizure disorder.

(2) **Focal cerebral ischemia** is rarely a cause of syncope.

(a) Rarely, ischemia to the ascending **reticular activating system (RAS),** as found in the top-of-the-basilar syndrome, can cause transient unresponsiveness.

(i) Cardiogenic emboli or extracranial or intracranial large artery occlusive disease may compromise perfusion.

(ii) Sometimes, obstruction of small penetrating arteries arising from the rostral basilar artery can be responsible for transient unresponsiveness.

(iii) Patients with vertebrobasilar occlusive disease may experience transient unresponsiveness as a result of focal ischemia. These patients typically have other symptoms and signs referable to focal ischemia (see VIII B 1 b).

(b) Generally, unilateral carotid territory ischemia does not result in syncope.

(3) **SAH** can transiently increase ICP, compromising global cerebral perfusion. Clues to the diagnosis include persistent headache, meningismus, and papilledema.

(4) **Basilar artery migraine** (a unique type of migraine with aura) is a rare cause of unresponsiveness. A history of recurrent headache, recurrent episodes of unresponsiveness, and associated symptoms (e.g., visual distortion, dizziness) should lead to consideration of this condition. In most instances, other causes of vertebrobasilar ischemia should be sought before assigning a diagnosis of basilar artery migraine.

(5) An **Arnold-Chiari malformation** (characterized by extension of the cerebellum into the spinal canal and brain stem distortion) can occasionally cause transient symptomatic hydrocephalus or compromised medullary function, leading to a brief loss of consciousness.

(6) **Narcolepsy** can cause episodes of sleep or cataplexy that can be mistaken for syncope.

(7) **Glossopharyngeal neuralgia** can cause bradycardia and vasodilation. Patients have paroxysms of pain in the pharynx or external auditory canal.

(8) A **colloid cyst of the third ventricle** can cause sudden obstructive hydrocephalus, leading to increased ICP and hypoperfusion.

e. Psychogenic unresponsiveness can be associated with anxiety, panic attacks, or hyperventilation, as well as somatoform (conversion) disorder.

4. Diagnosis. A history and physical examination often can provide clues to the proper diagnosis. If no clues are evident, it is generally appropriate to proceed with a cardiovascular evaluation as outlined in Chapter 1 IX D.

a. Neurologic testing frequently includes an EEG. Rarely is a CT scan diagnostic. In some patients, an MRI or an imaging study of the vascular system can be informative.

b. Upright tilt testing, possibly with isoproterenol infusion, can provide evidence for a diagnosis of vasodepressor (neurocardiogenic) syncope, especially if the characteristic hemodynamic changes occur in less than 15 minutes without isoproterenol infusion.

5. Therapy. Treatment depends on the underlying diagnosis. First-line therapy of neurocardiogenic syncope is treatment with β-adrenergic blockers.

B Coma

1. Definition. Coma is a state in which a patient is unresponsive to environmental stimuli and unable to communicate in any manner. Coma is associated with extensive structural or physiologic damage to both cerebral hemispheres or to the ascending RAS in the diencephalon, mesencephalon, or pons.

2. Etiology. The many causes of coma can be broadly grouped as shown in Table 11–5.

TABLE 11–5 Causes of Coma

Category	Possible Etiologic Factors
Supratentorial (hemispheric) lesions	Epidural or subdural hematoma Intraparenchymal hemorrhage Large ischemic infarction Tumor Abscess Trauma
Infratentorial lesions	Pontine or cerebellar hematoma Basilar artery thrombosis Ischemic cerebellar infarction Tumor Abscess
Diffuse diseases, metabolic disorders, and toxins	Subarachnoid hemorrhage Meningitis Encephalitis Hydrocephalus Drugs (e.g., narcotics, alcohol, barbiturates, benzodiazepines) Hypo- or hyperglycemia Ischemic or hypoxic encephalopathy Hypercarbia Myxedema Hypothermia Hepatic or renal failure Thiamine deficiency
Psychogenic	

3. **Approach to the patient.** Complete and rapid assessment is critical for optimal care.
   a. **Patient history.** The physician should ascertain the following information:
      (1) **Past medical status,** especially if there is a preexisting neurologic, cardiac, pulmonary, hepatic, or renal condition
      (2) **Prescription** and **over-the-counter drugs** used by the patient
      (3) History of **drug abuse,** if applicable
      (4) **Recent patient complaints**
      (5) **Details regarding the site** where the patient was found (e.g., presence of empty drug vials, evidence of a fall)
   b. **Physical examination.** The **examination** should be thorough. Extremes of blood pressure, pulse, or temperature, abnormal breathing patterns, evidence of head or neck trauma, and the presence of meningismus should be noted carefully. The skin should be inspected for signs of trauma or needle tracks. Special attention should be directed to the patient's:
      (1) **Pupils.** Pupillary size and reactivity are dependent on sympathetic and parasympathetic innervation. Brain stem reflexes such as the pupillary reaction to light offer clues to the location of the lesion responsible for the coma.
         (a) **Large, nonreactive pupils** result from the disruption of the parasympathetic pupilloconstrictive impulses that arise from the mesencephalic Edinger-Westphal nucleus and travel as a component of the third cranial nerve to the eye.
         (b) **Small, reactive pupils** result from the disruption of the sympathetic pupillodilatory impulses that arise in the hypothalamus and course caudally through the periaqueductal gray matter and cervical spinal cord before travelling rostrally with the internal carotid artery toward the eyes.

(2) **Ocular motility.** Analysis of ocular motility allows assessment of damage to the brain stem and the cranial nerves that control eye movement.

(a) The eyes should first be examined in the resting position for spontaneous motion of the eyeballs. Although the eyes of comatose patients may move spontaneously, they do not fixate or track in a purposeful manner.

(b) If the eyes are immobile, movement can be elicited through the **vestibulo-ocular reflex** by moving the patient's head side to side (the **"doll's head"** or **oculocephalic maneuver**) or by elevating the patient's head 30° and irrigating the external auditory canal with ice water.

(i) **Conjugate deviation** of the eyes bilaterally implies intact brain stem circuitry.

(ii) **Failure of an eye to abduct** in response to these maneuvers implies dysfunction of pontine structures or sixth nerve compromise.

(iii) **Failure of an eye to adduct** implies dysfunction of the medial longitudinal fasciculus or oculomotor nucleus or nerve.

(iv) The presence of **conjugate nystagmus** contralateral to the side of ice water irrigation suggests psychogenic coma.

(3) **Motor functions.** Quadriparesis, hemiparesis, or monoparesis may occur in comatose patients.

(a) **Quadriparesis and flaccidity** suggests pontine or medullary compromise or a high cervical spinal cord insult.

(b) **Decorticate posturing** (i.e., leg extension with flexion of the arm, wrist, and fingers) can be unilateral or bilateral and suggests a hemispheral or diencephalic lesion.

(c) **Decerebrate posturing** (i.e., leg and arm extension) also can be unilateral or bilateral and suggests midbrain or pontine compromise.

4. **Clinical features.** Once global brain stem dysfunction has developed, differentiation between supratentorial and infratentorial causes of coma cannot be made without diagnostic testing unless a history and serial observations of the patient's clinical course can be documented.

a. **Supratentorial causes of coma** are often characterized by pathologic processes that result in **swelling of a cerebral hemisphere.**

(1) This mass effect causes a midline shift of the affected hemisphere toward the contralateral side, compression of the ipsilateral third nerve as it courses near the medial temporal lobe (uncus), herniation of the medial temporal lobe below the tentorial notch (uncal herniation), distortion of the mesencephalon, and herniation of the cingulate gyrus under the midline falx (subfalcial herniation).

(2) Typically, there is a progressive clinical deterioration characterized by increasing unresponsiveness, development of a third nerve palsy ipsilateral to the swollen hemisph… and, ultimately, midbrain compromise (reflected by bilaterally nonreactive, dilated …

b. **Infratentorial causes of coma** can be suspected if ataxia, multiple asymmetric cr… palsies, and unilateral or bilateral limb weakness or sensory loss develop befo… ment of more global, severe impairment of brain stem function (characteri… pupils, absent ocular motility, and absent corneal and gag reflexes).

c. **Diffuse, toxic, or metabolic causes of coma** can be suspected if pupi… ocular motility is preserved, corneal reflexes can be elicited, a gag … movement in response to noxious local stimuli is observed. If pupi… even when other brain stem and limb function is lost, a metab… considered.

d. **Psychogenic coma** should be suspected if the patient has a … the findings on physical examination are nonphysiolo… responses in a "comatose" patient include:

(1) The presence of **nystagmus** when the patient's ears a…

(2) Adversive head and eye movements

(3) Failure of the patient's arm, when held by the examiner over the patient's face, to fall on the face when released by the examiner
(4) Resistance to having the eyelids opened

5. **Therapy.** Ideally, care of the comatose patient is intertwined with the initial assessment and the development of etiologic hypotheses.
   a. **Initial therapy.** Maintaining an **adequate airway, optimal ventilation,** and **appropriate blood pressure** are priority concerns.
      (1) If **cervical fracture** is a possibility, **immobilization of the neck** is of great importance.
      (2) **Endotracheal intubation** is usually indicated to protect the airway.
      (3) **Blood samples** for a complete blood count (CBC), electrolytes, glucose, renal and liver function studies, coagulation profiles, blood gases, and toxicology should be obtained.
      (4) **Intravenous thiamine** (100 mg), one ampule of $\mathbf{D_{50}W}$, and **naloxone** (0.4 mg) are often administered. **Flumazenil** can be given if benzodiazepine or hepatic coma is suspected.
   b. **Management**
      (1) **Imaging.** If the patient's general medical condition permits, and if the cause of coma is not clearly cerebral anoxia after cardiopulmonary arrest or a drug overdose, most patients should have a brain **CT scan** to define the presence of an **intracranial mass, cerebral edema,** or **hydrocephalus.** Further management depends on the etiology of the coma.

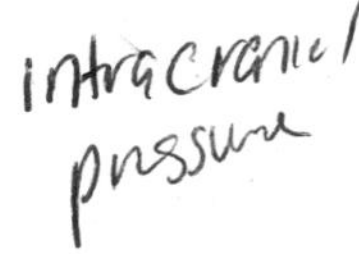

      (2) **ICP evaluation and management**
         (a) **ICP evaluation.** Consideration of the patient's ICP is intimately tied to the evaluation of coma. The intracranial cavity has a finite volume and compliance.
            (i) Normally, modest volume additions to the intracranial contents (e.g., from a small intraparenchymal hematoma) cause only a small rise in ICP.
            (ii) With progressive incremental increases to the intracranial volume (e.g., from massive cerebral edema, a hematoma, or a tumor), the intracranial compliance decreases, and the ICP markedly increases.
            (iii) Because cerebral perfusion pressure is the result of the mean arterial pressure minus the ICP, an **excessive rise of the ICP** is associated with **impaired cerebral perfusion** and **progressive neurologic deterioration.**
         (b) **ICP management.** If a pathologic process associated with elevated ICP is suspected, emergency management should include steps to decrease the pressure, or at the very least, avoid increasing it. If possible, the cerebral perfusion pressure should be kept at greater than 60 mm Hg and the ICP at less than 20 mm Hg. Optimal management of increased ICP often requires direct ICP monitoring as well as determination of hemodynamic parameters.
            (i) Patients can be hyperventilated with an Ambu bag before intubation. Intubation and endotracheal suctioning should be performed carefully to minimize elevation of ICP.
            (ii) Fever and agitation should be minimized.
            (iii) The patient's head should be elevated 30° and kept in midposition to optimize venous drainage.
            (iv) Osmotic therapy is used to dehydrate the brain and decrease the ICP. Patients are kept euvolemic, and intravenous mannitol or hypertonic saline is administered to achieve a hyperosmotic state.
            (v) **Durotomy and hemicraniectomy can be used to decompress swollen brain.**

C Vegetative state

1. **Definitions**
   a. The **vegetative state** is characterized by the unawareness of self or external stimuli. Patients cannot interact with others in a meaningful fashion. Autonomic functions are relatively well maintained, and a sleep–wake cycle exists. Patients can survive with medical and nursing support.

b. A **persistent vegetative state** is defined as a vegetative state that persists for at least 1 month after the initial brain insult. If, with continued observation (usually 3 months for nontraumatic injury), there is no meaningful recovery, the likelihood of functional recovery can be judged to be nil; the patient can be said to be in a **permanent vegetative state.**

2. **Therapy.** The family and physician should determine the level of treatment appropriate for the patient in a persistent vegetative state.

D Brain death

1. **Definition.** Death is recognized as occurring when there is irreversible cessation of all brain function. A brain insult sufficient to cause complete loss of cerebral function should be documented, if possible.
2. **Approach to the patient**
   a. **Physical examination.** Patients are completely unresponsive to external visual, auditory, and tactile stimuli and are incapable of communication in any manner.
      (1) Pupillary responses are absent, and eye movements cannot be elicited by the vestibulo-ocular reflex or by irrigating the ears with cold water.
      (2) The corneal and gag reflexes are absent, and there is no facial or tongue movement.
      (3) The limbs are flaccid, and there is no movement, although primitive withdrawal movements in response to local painful stimuli, mediated at a spinal cord level, can occur.
   b. **Apnea test.** Patients have no respiratory function. An apnea test should be performed to ascertain that no respirations occur at a $Pa{CO_2}$ level of at least 60 mm Hg. The oxygenation should be maintained as the $Pa{CO_2}$ is allowed to rise. The inability to develop respiration is consistent with medullary failure.
   c. **Exclusionary criteria.** A diagnosis of brain death cannot be made in the setting of drug intoxication, hypothermia (defined as a core temperature of $< 32°C$), severe hypotension (i.e., shock), or drug-induced paralysis.
   d. **Confirmatory tests.** These tests are usually not necessary to diagnose brain death but can be used if doubt exists or if local statutes require them.
      (1) An **EEG** does not demonstrate any physiologic brain activity.
      (2) **Tests to assess cerebral blood flow** fail to show cerebral perfusion.
   e. **Period of observation.** Periodic evaluation is necessary before a diagnosis of brain death can be made, unless there is gross evidence of a nonsurvivable insult to the brain.
      (1) Two evaluations (at 6 and 12 hours) are usually sufficient to support a diagnosis of brain death.
      (2) In the presence of anoxic brain damage, 24 hours of observation are appropriate befor declaring brain death.

III ALTERATION IN BEHAVIOR

A Delirium

1. **Definition.** Delirium is a disorder of brain function affecting behavio attention and cognition, motor hyper- or hypoactivity, altered sleep- states of arousal. It is often acute, reversible, and secondary to a med
2. **Etiology.** Generalized or focal causes of cerebral dysfunction are p
   a. **Generalized brain dysfunction.** Causes include the followin
      (1) **Drugs,** including anticholinergics, antiparkinsonians, benzodiazepines, antidepressants, and illicit substan drawal from alcohol, barbiturates, and benzodiazepir The **serotonin syndrome** consists of delirium and disc tion; it results from overstimulation of serotonin recep

syndrome causes delirium in association with fever, rigidity, tremulousness, and occasionally myoglobinuria.

(2) **Metabolic alterations,** including hypoxia, hypercarbia, hyponatremia, uremia, hepatic failure, hyperglycemia, hypoglycemia, sepsis (septic encephalopathy), fever, dehydration, hypercalcemia, myxedema, hyperthyroidism, porphyria, anti-thyroid antibodies (Hashimoto's encephalopathy), and thiamine and niacin deficiencies, can cause delirium.

(3) **Diffuse insults to the brain** such as meningitis, encephalitis, fat emboli, and disseminated intravascular coagulation (DIC) are associated with cognitive impairment.

(4) **Nonconvulsive status epilepticus,** including absence or complex partial seizures, may cause delirium. Postictal patients may also be delirious.

b. **Focal cerebral disease.** Differentiating a global cerebral disorder from a focal brain disease that also may cause altered behavior presents a clinical challenge. For example, focal brain disease can cause a subtle aphasia, which may be misinterpreted as delirium. Appropriate laboratory and neurodiagnostic tests should be performed based on the clinical presentation.

(1) **Focal cerebral disease,** typically caused by stroke, involves the nondominant temporoparietal area, frontal lobes, head of the caudate nucleus, thalamus (the top-of-the-basilar syndrome), or occipital lobes, which may cause blindness. Patients suffering from a focal cerebral disease may be agitated and experience hallucinations.

(2) **Mass lesions** also can cause a confusional state, especially if they are located in the frontal lobes.

3. **Therapy.** The aim of therapy is identification and treatment, when possible, of the causes of delirium. An offending agent may have to be withdrawn. Adequate nutrition should be maintained and the safety of the patient ensured. If necessary, sedation with a low dose of haloperidol or a newer neuroleptic such as risperidone, quetiapine, or olanzapine can be helpful.

B Dementia

1. **Definition.** Dementia is a progressive mental disorder characterized by compromised abstract thinking ability, memory, and judgment. Unlike delirium, dementia is usually chronic and often results from primary degenerative brain disease or from a host of other conditions such as multiple strokes.

2. **Etiology.** The causes of dementia are many. Identification of a treatable condition masquerading as a degenerative process is critical.

a. Some **causes of dementia** include Alzheimer's disease, Parkinson's disease, multiple cerebral infarcts, Huntington's disease, frontotemporal degeneration including Pick's disease, dementia with Lewy bodies, human immunodeficiency virus (HIV) infection, and Creutzfeldt-Jakob disease.

b. **Potentially treatable conditions that can manifest as dementia** include depression (pseudodementia), normal pressure hydrocephalus (NPH), subdural hematoma, tumor, adverse drug effects, thyroid disease, vitamin B_{12} deficiency, thiamine deficiency, syphilis, heavy metal intoxication, and conditions causing hypersomnia (e.g., sleep apnea syndrome).

3. **Alzheimer's disease.** This condition is the **most common cause** of chronic dementia.

a. **Definition.** Alzheimer's disease is a clinicopathologic entity characterized by progressive memory loss and other cognitive deficits. Onset commonly is late in life, although patients may be affected in middle age.

(1) The disease usually arises spontaneously, but genetic factors have been identified. Familial cases have been associated with mutations of the genes for amyloid precursor protein, presenilin 1, and presenilin 2.

(2) There is an association between the age of onset of Alzheimer's disease and the apolipoprotein E genotype. Patients with the APOE4/4 genotype have the greatest risk for Alzheimer's disease at a given age.

b. Prevalence. Alzheimer's disease is a burgeoning public health problem. It is estimated that 60%–80% of demented patients have Alzheimer's disease. The prevalence increases sharply with age, affecting 5%–15% of people over age 65 and about three times as many people age 85 and older (the fastest-growing segment of the population).

c. Pathology. Although the cause and pathogenesis are unknown, Alzheimer's disease has a characteristic pathology consisting of **intracellular neurofibrillary tangles** and **extracellular neuritic plaques.**

(1) The tangles are composed primarily of abnormally phosphorylated, microtubule-associated tau proteins.

(2) The amyloid protein, Aβ, is derived from amyloid precursor protein and is deposited in senile plaques and blood vessels. The gene for amyloid precursor protein resides on chromosome 21 and may be involved in familial cases.

(3) Associated pathologic processes disturb many neurotransmitters, particularly the cholinergic system.

d. Diagnosis

(1) The **clinical diagnosis** of **senile dementia of the Alzheimer's type (SDAT)** can be made if an otherwise alert patient exhibits progressive memory loss and other cognitive deficits such as disorientation, language difficulties, inability to perform complex motor activities, inattention, visual misperception, poor problem-solving abilities, inappropriate social behavior, and, occasionally, hallucinations.

(a) The **intellectual decline** should be present in two or more domains of cognition and be documented by clinical examinations such as the **mini mental state examination.** The original examination was published in "Mini-Mental State." A Practical Method for Grading the Cognitive State of Patients for the Clinician. *J Psychiatr Res* 12(3):189–198, 1975. Table 11–6 shows sample test items and where the test currently may be obtained.

(b) **Formal neuropsychologic testing** can confirm the clinical impression and document progression of the disease. Tests that address recall (with or without cues) and delayed recall are especially sensitive for documenting early memory impairment.

(c) Other systemic and neurologic diseases that could produce cognitive decline should be absent.

TABLE 11–6 MMSE Sample Items

Orientation to Time
"What is the date?"

Registration
"Listen carefully, I am going to say three words. You say them back after I stop.
Ready? Here they are . . .
HOUSE (pause), CAR (pause), LAKE (pause). Now repeat those words back to me." [Repe
but score only the first trial.]

Naming
"What is this?" [Point to a pencil or pen.]

Reading
"Please read this and do what it says." [Show examinee the words on the sti
CLOSE YOUR EYES

(2) **Differential diagnosis**

(a) Patients with **pseudodementia (depression)** can exhibit many of the features of Alzheimer's disease. To complicate matters further, patients with Alzheimer's disease may present with depression. Identification of patients with pseudodementia is important, because treatment of the depression can restore cognitive function.

(i) A careful history and neuropsychological evaluation often can determine the proper diagnosis.

(ii) If doubt remains as to the role of depression in the clinical presentation, appropriate treatment for depression is warranted.

(b) **Mild cognitive impairment**

(i) Individuals with mild cognitive impairment have a memory impairment beyond that expected for normal aging. However, these individuals do not yet meet criteria for Alzheimer's disease.

(ii) People with mild cognitive impairment evolve to Alzheimer's disease at a rate of 10%–15% annually, compared with 1%–2% annually for normal individuals.

(c) **Other types of dementia**

(i) **Pick's disease** is a frontotemporal dementia characterized by personality changes, disinhibition, hyperorality, and frontotemporal atrophy on imaging studies. Hyperphosphorylated tau protein that accumulates in the cerebral cortex is associated with the disease.

(ii) **Dementia with Lewy bodies** is characterized by cognitive impairment that can fluctuate, hallucinations, and early parkinsonian features.

(iii) **Frontotemporal dementia with parkinsonism linked to chromosome 17 (FTDP-17)** is characterized by the same behavioral characteristics as the frontotemporal dementia described for Pick's disease. It is associated with abnormal tau protein.

d. **Therapy**

(1) **Medical therapy** is useful in treating insomnia, agitation, and depression.

(a) In general, drugs should initially be given at a low dose; the dose can be adjusted upward slowly as clinically indicated.

(b) Medications with a short half-life and few anticholinergic side effects are best tolerated.

(c) Cholinesterase inhibitors such as donepezil, galantamine, and rivastigmine may improve cognitive and behavioral function.

(2) **Day care centers** (including day hospitals) and **respite care** are useful adjuncts to family supervision of the patient with Alzheimer's disease and other dementing disorders.

4. **Normal pressure hydrocephalus (NPH)**

a. **Definition.** NPH is a condition characterized by cognitive impairment, urinary incontinence, and gait apraxia (i.e., impaired ambulation without evidence of primary motor, sensory, or cerebellar dysfunction).

b. **Etiology.** In most patients, the cause of NPH is unknown. However, NPH can follow SAH or meningitis, sometimes even years later.

c. **Diagnosis.** NPH should be suspected in patients who present with the clinical features noted in III B 4 a. The following tests may help confirm the diagnosis.

(1) **Imaging studies**

(a) **CT or MRI** reveals ventricular enlargement with relatively little cortical atrophy (Figure 11–2).

(b) **Cisternography** involves injecting a radionuclide into the lumbar thecal sac and then taking serial determinations of the flow pattern of the radioactive bolus. In the presence of NPH, cisternography demonstrates persistent activity of the radionuclide in the lateral ventricles after 48 hours.

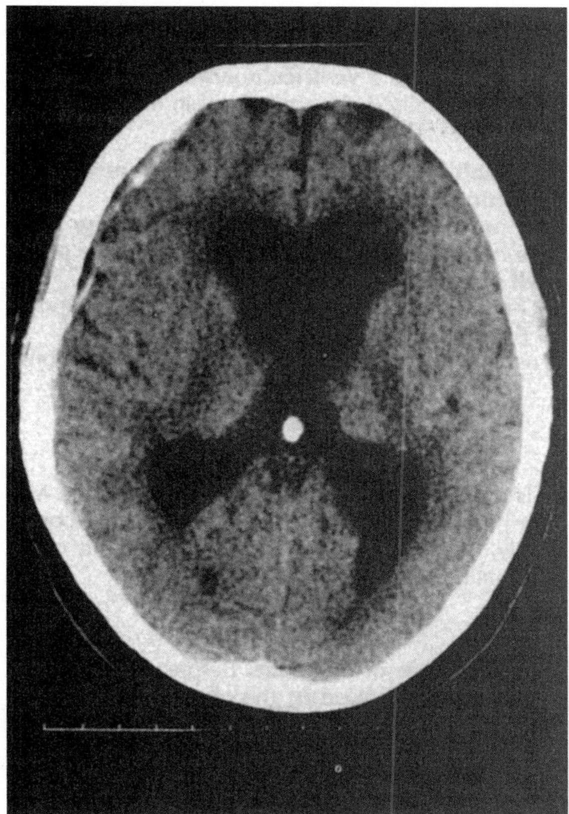

FIGURE 11–2 A nonenhanced computed tomography (CT) scan showing hydrocephalus consistent with normal pressure hydrocephalus (NPH). Note the lack of cortical atrophy (sulcal effacement).

(2) **ICP monitoring** for 24–48 hours can reveal transient pressure increases, if the diagnosis is in doubt.

d. **Therapy.** Insertion of a **ventriculoperitoneal shunt** can improve the patient's condition, especially if performed within 6 months of the onset of the problem.

5. **Creutzfeldt-Jakob disease.** This progressive, degenerative illness is caused by **prions** (i.e., infe tious proteinaceous particles) and is associated with a **spongiform encephalopathy.**
   a. The gene for the prion protein is on **chromosome 20;** approximately 10% of cases itary. Illness can develop because of **infection** or **somatic** and **germ cell mutati** 14-3-3 protein is a marker for Creutzfeldt-Jakob disease. **"Mad cow diseas** resents transmission of prion disease from infected cows to humans vi food products.
   b. Patients may exhibit **myoclonus.** The **EEG** often demonstrates **pe** abnormal background rhythm.
   c. **Death** usually occurs within several months of the onset of the

IV HEADACHE

Many patients are concerned that their headaches are caused by a brain tumor. Fortunately, this is rarely the case, but complaints of h mon, always deserve further evaluation.

A Etiology

1. **Non-neurologic causes.** Before assuming that cephalic discomfort is caused by an intracranial disorder, the physician should consider the possibility of a non-neurologic cause. Disorders of the head and neck such as sinus disease, glaucoma, dental infections, temporomandibular joint (TMJ) disease, ear pathology, muscular injury, or cervical spine problems can cause headache.
2. **Intracranial stimulation of pain-sensitive structures.** Problems that affect the meninges or distort the larger blood vessels cause pain.
3. **Life-threatening causes**
   a. An **intracranial mass** causes a headache that typically develops insidiously and progressively worsens.
      (1) **Clinical features.** The **pain** is unlike any the patient has experienced and **may awaken the person** from sleep. Occasionally, the headache is worse early in the day. With time, **associated symptoms** (e.g., **nausea, vomiting, exacerbation with lifting** and **straining**) can develop. On examination, evidence of **focal CNS disease** is typically apparent.
      (2) **Therapy.** Treatment is directed at the underlying lesion.
   b. A **"sentinel" SAH** causes the apoplectic onset of headache in previously healthy individuals or the sudden occurrence of headache that is of unique character in a chronic headache sufferer (see also VIII C 1).
      (1) **Clinical features.** The possibility that a headache is a result of SAH is strengthened if the cephalic discomfort cannot be easily attributed to any of the usual causes of head pain. No neurologic findings may be present on examination, and meningismus may be absent.
      (2) **Diagnosis.** Given the potential seriousness of the condition, patients should have a **cranial CT scan.** If this is unrevealing, an **LP** documents the presence of subarachnoid bleeding.

B Headache syndromes

1. **Migraine**
   a. **Etiology.** The cause of migraine is unknown, but several common precipitants have been observed.
      (1) A **family history** of migraine often exists.
      (2) Headaches can be related to **stress, altered sleep patterns, menses, oral contraceptives, alcohol use, caffeine withdrawal, monosodium glutamate (MSG) intake,** and various **foodstuffs** (e.g., chocolate, nuts, aged cheeses, and meats containing nitrates).
      (3) Migraine can develop **after seemingly minor head trauma;** recognition and treatment may prevent prolonged disability.
   b. **Pathophysiology.** Hypotheses center around the idea that a migraine attack is brought on by neurovascular disturbances.
      (1) The classic **vasospasm–vasodilation theory** arose from clinical observations. Recent data suggest that oligemia, secondary to a slowly spreading area of **neuronal depolarization** (the cortical depression of Leão), occurs during a headache prodrome and persists into the headache phase. Hyperemia occurs subsequently and can persist after the headache subsides.
      (2) Current theory maintains that **dysfunction** of the **trigeminovascular system,** resulting in the perivascular release of substance P and other neurotransmitters and inflammatory markers, leads to migraine.
   c. **Migraine syndromes**
      (1) **Migraine without aura (common migraine)** is an **intermittent** syndrome characterized by generalized or hemicranial **pulsatile** cephalic discomfort. Nausea, vomiting, photophobia, sonophobia, and anorexia may accompany the headache.
      (2) **Migraine with aura (classic migraine)** presents with an aura, often a **vivid visual array** of colors in a geometric pattern involving one visual hemifield.

(a) The **throbbing headache** is often **contralateral to the visual display,** and nausea, vomiting, photophobia, sonophobia, and anorexia may be present.

(b) Migraine with aura also can be associated with transient neurologic deficits such as visual field deficits and hemisensory loss.

(c) On very rare occasions, stroke is a complication of migraine.

d. Therapy. Treatment should first involve removal of inciting agents when possible.

(1) **Abortive therapy for migraine**

(a) **Ergotamine,** available in oral, sublingual, nasal, and suppository forms, is a serotonin (5-HT_1)-receptor agonist that decreases substance P release at the trigeminovascular junction. Intravenous ergotamine [dihydroergotamine (DHE 45)] also has proved to be efficacious; pretreatment with metoclopramide or prochlorperazine prevents nausea.

(b) **Aspirin, nonsteroidal anti-inflammatory drugs (NSAIDs), and isometheptene** can abort a migraine. Analgesics may be administered for symptomatic relief as well.

(c) **Triptans,** a family of serotonin 5-HT_1–receptor agonists, are effective.

(2) **Prophylactic measures** include drug regimens and changes in patient behavior referable to headache precipitants.

(a) **Medications** such as β-blockers, tricyclic antidepressants, calcium channel blockers, NSAIDs, gabapentin, topiramate, or valproic acid may be used to prevent migraines. Prophylactic medications, although of seemingly diverse types, all have a tendency to alter CNS serotonin activity.

(i) The choice of medication is guided, in part, by the need to avoid or exploit a particular drug action (aside from the antiheadache effect).

(ii) Initially, a low dose should be administered, and the therapeutic benefits and undesirable side effects should be monitored as the dose is increased. The dose can be increased until either a beneficial response is achieved or adverse side effects develop. A maximal dose is best maintained for several weeks before concluding that an agent is not effective.

(b) **Biofeedback therapy** may enable patients to lessen migraine events by helping them deal more effectively with stress.

2. A **muscle contraction,** or **tension, headache** is characterized by a band-like discomfort about the head.

a. Clinical features. This type of headache often develops during the course of the day and may be associated with emotional stress. Posterior cervical and occipital muscles are often tender and may be in spasm. The distinction between this type of headache and migraine without aura can be difficult.

b. Therapy. Treatment involves reassurance, NSAIDs, muscle relaxants, moist heat, ar occasion, antidepressant drugs and psychotherapy.

3. **Chronic daily headache**

a. Etiology. Patients with migraine or tension headache can develop chron spontaneously or as a result of excessive use of analgesics or ergotamin

b. Therapy. Treatment consists of **withdrawal from excessive medicati** 45 given for 2–3 days can help break the headache cycle. **Prophyla** help prevent a headache recurrence.

4. **Cluster headache**

a. Clinical features. Cluster headaches are severe periorbital hea tion, that occur once or several times daily over a period of s lateral pain may be accompanied by ipsilateral lacrima congestion, and Horner's syndrome. The typical patient i cluster headaches often pace, as opposed to migraineurs, wi

b. **Therapy**
   (1) **Abortive and symptomatic treatment** includes the administration of 100% oxygen, ergotamines, analgesics, or sumatriptan.
   (2) **Prophylactic therapy** incorporates lithium, calcium channel blockers, or corticosteroids.

5. **Temporal (giant cell) arteritis** (see also Chapter 10 XI E 6)
   a. **Clinical features.** Patients over the age of 50 years who complain of a headache centered about one temple or located in the occipital area should be evaluated for giant cell arteritis. Associated symptoms include visual disturbances, jaw claudication, fever, arthralgias and myalgias, and weight loss. Polymyalgia rheumatica (PMR) is also present in approximately 50% of patients who suffer from giant cell arteritis.
   b. **Diagnosis.** The erythrocyte sedimentation rate is typically greater than 40 mm/hr, and the c-reactive protein level is elevated. Biopsy of a temporal artery confirms the diagnosis.
   c. **Therapy. Corticosteroid treatment** can bring rapid relief.

6. **Benign (idiopathic) intracranial hypertension (pseudotumor cerebri)** has no known cause but is associated with obesity, pregnancy, oral contraceptives, SLE, cranial venous sinus thrombosis, and a host of other conditions.
   a. **Clinical features.** The development of a relatively constant, generalized headache in patients with a clear sensorium, papilledema, and an otherwise normal neurologic examination is suggestive of benign intracranial hypertension. Visual obscurations can occur, and visual loss is the most serious complication.
   b. **Diagnosis.** The diagnosis is suggested by a CT or MRI scan, which is normal. The diagnosis can be confirmed by finding an elevated CSF opening pressure and an otherwise normal CSF analysis.
   c. **Therapy**
      (1) Visual acuity and fields should be monitored.
      (2) **Serial LPs** can relieve the syndrome.
      (3) **Corticosteroids, acetazolamide, or furosemide** may be administered.
      (4) Refractory disease has been managed with **lumboperitoneal shunting of CSF** or **optic nerve sheath fenestration.**

7. **Trigeminal neuralgia (tic douloureux)** is a syndrome that most often is idiopathic but has been associated with MS, neoplasia, and vascular "loops" that impinge on the trigeminal nerve.
   a. **Clinical features.** Lightning-quick, severe facial pain, often associated with a trigger point, is suggestive of trigeminal neuralgia. The painful jabs are usually restricted to one or two divisions of the trigeminal nerve. There is no loss of facial sensation.
   b. **Therapy.** Therapeutic modalities include **carbamazepine, baclofen, gabapentin, surgical intervention,** and **stereotactic radiation therapy.**

8. **Indomethacin-responsive headaches** are characterized by severe, unilateral pain that may be relieved by treatment with indomethacin.
   a. **Chronic paroxysmal hemicrania** is characterized by painful, multiple attacks (up to 40 daily) that last from 2 minutes to 2 hours with nocturnal awakenings and associated autonomic features. Alcohol can precipitate the attacks.
   b. **Episodic paroxysmal hemicrania** is characterized by painful, multiple attacks (6–30 daily) that last up to 30 minutes and are associated with nocturnal awakenings and other autonomic features. Remissions lasting months to years can occur.

9. **Low pressure–volume headache** is characterized by a headache that substantially worsens when in the upright position and conversely improves with a supine posture.
   a. **Etiology.** Postural headaches typically occur after LP but can develop spontaneously or in association with a defect in the integrity of the dura.

b. **Diagnosis.** MRI shows generalized dural enhancement. The cerebellar tonsils may have descended below the level of the foramen magnum, and the brain stem may be "kinked."
c. **Therapy.** Treatment consists of a **blood patch** (injection of autologous blood into the lumbar epidural space).

V WEAKNESS

Many disorders can cause weakness. To pinpoint the causative disorder, the physician must first determine which part of the nervous system is diseased.

A Anatomic and functional approach

Weakness can result from dysfunction at various points in the CNS or peripheral nervous system. Localization of the site of the lesion depends on associated findings and the pattern of weakness.

1. **Upper motor neuron disorders.** Dysfunction of the descending corticospinal tracts (i.e., the cortical pyramidal cells and their axonal processes) results in a pattern of weakness such that the muscle flexor groups in the upper extremities tend to be stronger than the extensor muscles, whereas in the lower extremities, the extensor muscles remain stronger than the flexors.
   a. **Spasticity and hyperreflexia** are associated with upper motor neuron disorders, and often an extensor plantar response (Babinski's sign) may be elicited.
   b. Because of the relatively greater spatial dispersion of pyramidal cells and their axons rostral to the internal capsule, a large lesion in this area is necessary to cause widespread contralateral weakness; small lesions may produce somewhat restricted areas of weakness.
   c. Because of the relatively restricted spatial dispersion of the corticospinal tracts in the internal capsule and caudally, a small lesion targeting the corticospinal tracts can cause widespread contralateral weakness.
2. **Lower motor neuron disorders.** Dysfunction of the lower motor neurons, which, as part of a motor unit, innervate the skeletal muscles, causes a pattern of segmental (e.g., as seen in poliomyelitis) or, in some cases, widespread weakness [e.g., as seen in amyotrophic lateral sclerosis (ALS)]. Muscle fasciculations, diminished muscle tone and bulk, and hyporeflexia often accompany lesions of the lower motor neurons.
3. **Nerve root and peripheral nerve disorders.** Pathologic processes involving the nerve roots or peripheral nerves (e.g., herniation of an intervertebral disk, carpal tunnel syndrome) cause selective patterns of weakness referent to the unique pattern of innervation of the impaired motor root or nerve.
   a. **Fasciculations** and **diminished muscle bulk** and **stretch reflexes** may occur.
   b. More widespread weakness may be present, as in the **Guillain-Barré** syndrome.
4. **Dysfunction of the neuromuscular junction** (e.g., as in myasthenia gravis or botulism dysfunction results in either widespread or restricted weakness. Usually, reflexes are and there is no decrease in muscle bulk. Fasciculations do not occur.
5. **Muscle disease.** Patients with weakness attributable to muscle disease (e.g., po present with symmetric, proximal loss of strength. Muscle bulk may be stretch reflexes depressed in proportion to the degree of weakness.

B Selected disorders characterized by weakness

1. **Facial weakness**
   a. **Upper motor neuron (central) facial weakness** (e.g., as cau by preservation of forehead movement with accompanying
      (1) **Etiology.** Any process affecting the facial upper moto cause the pattern of central facial weakness. This pa

innervation of forehead muscles and predominantly contralateral innervation of lower facial muscles.

(2) **Therapy.** Treatment depends on the underlying cause.

b. **Lower motor neuron (peripheral) facial weakness** is characterized by weakness involving the forehead and lower face. A peripheral facial palsy may be accompanied by impaired tearing (decreased lacrimal gland function), hyperacusis (impaired stapedius muscle function), or impaired taste (chorda tympani dysfunction).

(1) **Etiology.** Some cases are idiopathic (e.g., Bell's palsy). Others may be associated with Lyme disease, herpes zoster, trauma, otitis media, HIV infection, syphilis, sarcoidosis, diabetes, or neoplasia. Bell's palsy is being increasingly associated with herpes zoster virus infection.

(2) **Therapy**

(a) Because the patient's ability to protect the cornea is impaired, the exposed eye should be frequently lubricated and gently taped closed during sleep.

(b) Corticosteroid therapy and antiherpesvirus agents are often used to treat an idiopathic peripheral facial palsy, barring any contraindications.

2. **Amyotrophic lateral sclerosis (ALS)** occurs in approximately 1 in 100,000 people. Half of affected patients die within 3 years of the onset of the disease.

a. **Etiology.** The cause is unknown.

(1) 5%–10% of ALS cases are familial. Mutations in the superoxide dismutase gene have been found in some of these families.

(2) An **excess of the excitatory amino acid glutamate** may play a role in the pathogenesis. Synaptic reuptake of glutamate may be impaired.

b. **Diagnosis**

(1) **Clinical features.** The **hallmark of ALS is progressive weakness.**

(a) Patients typically exhibit signs of **both upper and lower motor neuron dysfunction.** Rarely, patients have a preponderance of upper (primary lateral sclerosis) or lower (primary muscle atrophy) motor neuron features.

(b) Loss of strength early in the course of the disease is usually focal and may only compromise speech, swallowing, or the use of one extremity.

(2) **Differential diagnosis.** Other conditions may masquerade as ALS. Therefore, it is essential to evaluate patients for the following conditions:

(a) Cervical myelopathy or radiculopathy associated with cervical spondylosis

(b) A mass lesion at the craniocervical junction

(c) Thyrotoxicosis

(d) Disorders of calcium metabolism

(e) Multifocal motor neuropathy, a potentially treatable condition characterized by slowly progressive asymmetric weakness with multifocal demyelination and often associated with anti-GM_1 ganglioside antibodies

(f) Diabetic amyotrophy

(g) Postpolio syndrome

(h) Lead intoxication

(i) Hexosaminidase A deficiency

(j) Spinocerebellar degeneration or multiple-system atrophy presenting with motor neuron dysfunction

(k) Lower motor neuron dysfunction as a result of infection with polio, coxsackievirus, or West Nile virus.

c. **Therapy.** Treatment is supportive; there is no cure. Particular attention should be paid to supporting breathing and swallowing functions.

(1) **Riluzole,** a glutamate antagonist, minimally slows disease progression and prolongs life for a few months.

(2) Issues related to palliative care, including advance directives, should be discussed with the patient and family.

3. The **postpolio syndrome** occurs in patients two to three decades after an attack of poliomyelitis. Previously stable patients experience fatigue and further worsening of their lower motor neuron syndrome. Strengthening exercises may be beneficial.

VI DISEQUILIBRIUM AND DIZZINESS

A **Clumsiness** can be caused by cerebellar dysfunction or disorders of the motor or sensory system.

1. **Cerebellar dysfunction.** In addition to clumsiness and limb or truncal instability, as manifested by incoordination and impaired stance and gait, patients may exhibit hypotonia and ocular dysmetria.
   a. **Acute cerebellar dysfunction** (e.g., stroke, MS, neoplasia) typically manifests with unilateral findings.
   b. Causes of relatively symmetric **subacute** or **chronic cerebellar dysfunction** include alcoholic cerebellar degeneration; drug intoxication (e.g., phenytoin); hypothyroidism; cerebellar or spinocerebellar degenerations; and paraneoplastic, immune-mediated degeneration.
2. **Motor or sensory disorders.** Patients with strength in the 2/5–4/5 grade range (see Table 11–3) may appear clumsy, as may patients with a sensory neuropathy, dorsal root ganglion disease, posterior column dysfunction, or parietal lobe disease (parietal ataxia).

B Dizziness

1. **Approach to the patient**
   a. **History.** Obtaining a thorough history aids in patient evaluation. By paying special attention to associated symptoms, the physician may be able to identify pathology of the inner ear, eighth cranial nerve, or CNS as the cause of the dizziness.
   b. **Physical examination.** The physician uses several screening techniques to search for evidence of structural disease.
      (1) **Nystagmus** is present in many patients who suffer from vertigo. The nystagmus can be observed spontaneously (when the patient gazes straight ahead, laterally, or vertically), or it may be elicited by using Fresnel lenses to block visual fixation, by having the patient shake his or her head during ophthalmoscopy, or by covering the contralateral eye during ophthalmoscopy (to decrease visual fixation).
         (a) **Horizontal or vertical nystagmus** is characterized by a slow eye drift and a rapid shift in the opposite direction.
         (b) **Torsional nystagmus** is characterized by a slow clockwise or counterclockwise rotation and a rapid movement in the opposite direction.
         (c) The direction of nystagmus refers to the direction of the fast component of eye movement.
      (2) **Gaze mechanisms** should be tested, including **saccadic speed** and **accuracy,** and the integrity of **smooth pursuits.** The presence of **ocular dysmetria** and **visual acuity** while shaking the head should be noted. **Suppression of the vestibulo-ocular reflex** (which may be tested by asking the patient to fixate on a target moving synchronously with the head) should be noted as well. The **head thrust maneuver** may demonstrate abnormal corrective saccades.
      (3) The physician should check for the presence of **benign paroxysmal positional vertigo (BPPV)** by performing the Nylen-Bárány maneuver (i.e., by hyperextending the patient's neck and rotating the patient's head laterally as the patient is rapidly moved from a seated to a supine position.) Rotary nystagmus with a linear component that appears after a several-second latency period suggests BPPV.

(4) Vertigo that worsens when pressure is applied to the tragus may suggest a perilymphatic fistula.

2. **Selected causes of dizziness**
   a. **Labyrinthitis (vestibular neuronitis)** is characterized by the acute onset of a spinning sensation (vertigo), exacerbated by movement, and associated with nausea and vomiting.
      (1) **Etiology.** The **etiology is often viral,** but labyrinthitis may also be caused by **trauma or inflammatory and vascular diseases.**
      (2) **Physical examination.** Nystagmus is away from the affected ear (i.e., slow phase of eye movement is toward the side of the lesion). It is often of a mixed horizontal and torsional type.
   b. **Meniere's disease** is characterized by episodic vertigo accompanied by nystagmus, tinnitus, fluctuating hearing loss, and aural discomfort.

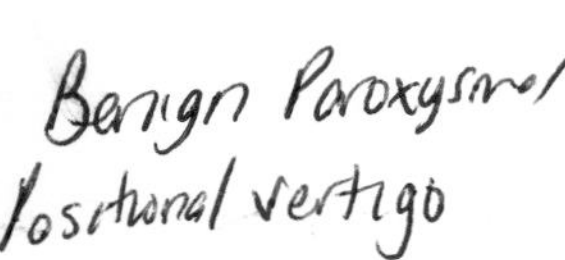

   c. **BPPV** occurs when the patient moves his or her head (e.g., by rolling over in bed, looking up, or standing up). This condition is usually idiopathic in nature but can be caused by trauma, viral or ischemic injury, or drug toxicity. A unique physical therapy technique that can be used to decrease symptoms of BPPV has been developed.
   d. **Drug-induced vestibulopathy** can be caused by gentamicin, streptomycin, furosemide, and cisplatin.
   e. **Eighth cranial nerve disease** can be associated with hearing loss. Causes include acoustic neuroma, metastatic disease, vasculitis, and basilar meningitis associated with infectious and inflammatory processes.
   f. **Lateral medullary syndrome (Wallenberg's syndrome)** is due to occlusion of the vertebral or posterior inferior cerebellar artery.
      (1) Patients often feel that the external world is "tilting" and complain of feeling propelled toward one side (usually the side of the lesion).
      (2) Physical examination can indicate nystagmus (often horizontal–torsional and away from the lesion), ipsilateral ataxia, ipsilateral Horner's syndrome (characterized by ptosis, miosis, and anhidrosis), and ipsilateral facial sensory impairment with contralateral body sensory loss.
   g. **Cerebellar disease** can be caused by stroke, tumor, infection, or degenerative and inflammatory disease (see XVIII H). Paraneoplastic cerebellar degeneration is associated with anti-Yo antibodies (leading to Purkinje cell loss) and anti-Ri (antineuronal) antibodies. Physical examination indicates ataxia and postural instability and many types of nystagmus. Opsoclonus is associated with anti-Ri antibodies.
   h. **Brain stem lesions** are typically associated with cranial nerve, motor, sensory, and cerebellar dysfunction.
   i. **Other causes of dizziness** include postural hypotension, hyperventilation, hypoglycemia, hypothyroidism, epilepsy, migraine, psychiatric disorders (e.g., depression, anxiety, somatization disorders), and multisensory impairment (i.e., poor vision and positional sense).

3. **Therapy**
   a. Dizziness may be relieved by **treating the underlying disease.**
   b. If the underlying disease is unknown or otherwise untreatable, **acute symptomatic therapy** includes the use of meclizine, prochlorperazine, promethazine, topical scopolamine, and diazepam.
   c. **Vestibular and gait exercises** may help habituate the vestibular pathways to the abnormal influences of the disease.
   d. **Chronic, poorly defined causes** of dizziness can be managed by withdrawing the patient from drugs that affect the vestibular system. This action may allow a better reevaluation of the patient. Treatment with a **low dose** of a **benzodiazepine** and **vestibular and gait exercises** may be effective.

VII PAIN SYNDROMES

When patients complain of pain, it is important to explore whether the pain is new-onset, long-standing, or intermittent, and whether it is static or progressive. Patients should be asked to identify exacerbating and alleviating factors as well as associated symptoms such as weakness or numbness.

A Pain originating from the lower back

1. **Etiology**
   a. Diagnostic considerations include local muscular strain, traumatic conditions of the spine, degenerative and inflammatory arthritides, neoplastic and infectious processes, and nerve root irritation.
   b. Neurologic dysfunction commonly develops from impingement on nerve roots by disk material, bony overgrowth, or thickened ligaments.
2. **Disorders associated with low back pain**
   a. **Sciatica** denotes a syndrome of sharp pain radiating from the low back to the buttock, down the back of the thigh to the calf, and, at times, over the bottom or top of the foot. Sciatica is commonly associated with disk herniation but can result from other conditions that irritate nerve roots L4, L5, or S1.
      (1) **Clinical features.** Myotomal weakness and dermatomal numbness, along with appropriate muscle stretch reflex changes and pain that increases when the examiner raises the patient's extended leg, can occur.
      (2) **Diagnosis.** Persistent symptoms and neurologic deficits warrant in-depth investigation, which commonly includes the use of lumbosacral radiographs, lumbar MRI, and EMG. CT myelography may be indicated for better definition of the bony anatomy.
      (3) **Therapy.** Acute low back pain should be evaluated carefully. Treatment should be directed at the underlying disorder if possible.
         (a) Unless tumor or infection is the likely cause for sciatica, initial therapy should include **bed rest** and treatment with **NSAIDs.** If patients show signs of a **cauda equina syndrome** (i.e., a flaccid bladder, rectal dysfunction, and bilateral lower motor neuron leg weakness), **emergency surgery** is usually required.
         (b) **Long-term therapy** may be appropriate. As the acute syndrome remits, a regimen of **back-strengthening exercises** and **weight loss** (if applicable) can be helpful. Surgery (e.g., **laminectomy**) may be necessary to relieve persistent symptoms.
   b. **Lumbar stenosis** is another common condition resulting in low back pain. Patients often have a congenitally small lumbar canal. Over time, bony and ligamentous overgrowth and disk protrusions may further encroach on the neural and vascular contents of the canal and foramina.
      (1) **Clinical features.** Patients develop pain and, occasionally, **sensory loss** and **weakness** with **ambulation** and **prolonged standing,** but they are relatively comfortable at rest. The neurologic examination of resting patients is often quite normal.
      (2) **Therapy.** It is necessary to differentiate pain caused by lumbar stenosis from that caused by vascular insufficiency. If symptoms are severe, **decompression surgery** is often pursued for treatment of lumbar stenosis.

B Pain originating from the neck

1. **Etiology.** Neck pain is often due to trauma (e.g., "whiplash"). Degenerative and inflammatory bone and disk disease can lead to nerve root irritation and is also a common source of neck pain. Local infection should be considered for acute symptoms; neoplasia may be the culprit when subacute symptoms exist.
2. **Disorders associated with neck pain**

a. **Cervical radiculopathy.** Pain can radiate in a dermatomal pattern with a parallel loss of sensation. Weakness may be in a myotomal distribution with a corresponding loss of muscle stretch reflexes.

b. **Arthritis.** The cervical radiculopathy associated with cervical arthritis (spondylosis) can often be treated with a **soft cervical collar, NSAIDs, muscle relaxants,** and, occasionally, **surgery.**

C Selected pain syndromes

1. **Herpes zoster**

a. **Acute syndrome. "Shingles"** is a painful condition caused by the activation of a latent herpes zoster infection, which affects the nerves that supply the skin. Although most common in the elderly, shingles can occur in immunosuppressed patients as well.

(1) **Clinical features.** The rash, characterized by painful vesicles on an erythematous base, may be preceded by discomfort. The pain often abates when the skin lesions heal but may persist and lead to postherpetic neuralgia.

(2) **Therapy**

(a) **Corticosteroids** may lessen the risk of postherpetic neuralgia in nonimmunosuppressed patients older than 60 years.

(b) **Famciclovir** decreases the duration of postherpetic neuralgia in **immunocompetent patients.**

(c) **Acyclovir** should be given to **immunosuppressed patients** to hasten recovery.

(d) **Analgesics, tricyclic antidepressants, gabapentin, and topiramate** treat pain during the acute phase of the illness.

b. **Chronic syndrome**

(1) Once the vesicles have healed, residual discomfort can be managed with capsaicin ointment, vapo-coolant spray, or tricyclic antidepressants.

(2) Tricyclic antidepressants, carbamazepine and other anticonvulsant medications, vapo-coolant spray, transcutaneous electrical nerve stimulation, and, occasionally, surgical intervention may be effective.

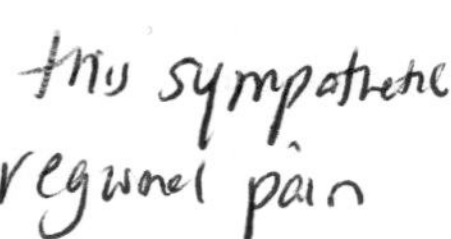

2. **Complex regional pain syndrome** (Reflex sympathetic dystrophy; sympathetic maintained pain). This chronic painful condition can occur idiopathically or develop after trauma to a limb. At times the severity of the initial injury can be quite trivial.

a. **Clinical features.** The affected limb is painful, with altered sensory perceptions, vasomotor tone, and temperature. The skin is often discolored.

b. **Diagnosis.** To make a diagnosis, other local conditions that can cause pain must be eliminated. A differential nerve block via infiltration of paravertebral nerves with varying doses of local anesthesia helps differentiate between local somatic nerve hyperexcitability and the autonomic sympathetic dysfunction attributable to sympathetic mediated pain. Intravenous phentolamine blockade can also provide evidence for sympathetic mediated pain.

c. **Therapy.** Treatment includes **paravertebral sympathetic ganglion blocks** and **aggressive physical therapy.** Administration of tricyclic antidepressants, anticonvulsants, or topical capsaicin or lidocaine are useful adjuvant therapies.

D Chronic pain syndromes

Nonmalignant pain syndromes, when chronic, can be especially difficult to evaluate and manage.

1. Care should be taken to assess patients fully for remedial problems (e.g., lumbar stenosis). An **interdisciplinary team approach** is best.

2. Use of **antidepressants** and **supportive psychotherapy,** coupled with **attempts to improve the patient's functional status,** can be beneficial. In selected instances, **chronic opiate** therapy can be beneficial.

VIII STROKE

This neurovascular disorder is the most common neurologic disease causing serious morbidity and mortality.

A Introduction

1. Disease of the vascular system can disrupt blood supply to the CNS, leading to **neuronal dysfunction.** Stroke syndromes can be broadly classified into predominantly **ischemic** or **hemorrhagic processes.** Asymptomatic lesions in either category of stroke syndrome can predispose patients to future disease.
2. **Optimal management** requires precise diagnosis for effective therapy.
   a. **General principles of management** of symptomatic patients include monitoring for signs of clinical deterioration, ensuring adequate oxygenation, maintaining euvolemia, avoiding extremes of blood pressure without excessively lowering high blood pressure, treating infection and fever, and using normal saline (rather than glucose solutions) for intravenous hydration. Efforts should be made to prevent deep venous thrombosis and decubiti, avoid aspiration, maintain nutrition, and attend to bowel and bladder function.
   b. **Rehabilitation** of patients with persistent neurologic defects is important.
      (1) Multidisciplinary therapy involving physical, occupational, and speech therapy can be pursued on an inpatient or outpatient basis.
      (2) Depression occurs frequently and may be treated medically.

B Ischemic stroke

1. **Introduction**
   a. **Etiology.** Causes include cardiogenic emboli, extracranial and intracranial large artery disease, small artery disease, and various systemic and hematologic disorders.
   b. **Clinical signs**
      (1) Impaired carotid territory circulation produces symptoms of contralateral weakness and sensory loss and aphasia or neglect syndromes and ipsilateral transient monocular blindness (amaurosis fugax). Typically, the weakness or numbness is greatest in the facial area, less pronounced in the arm, and still less pronounced in the leg.
      (2) A diagnosis of vertebrobasilar disease is fairly certain if there is transient binocular blindness or other bilateral visual disturbances, diplopia, ataxia, quadriparesis, or vertigo associated with other neurologic symptoms.
   c. **Therapy.** New treatments for acute ischemic stroke are under investigation, driven by the evidence that there is at least a 3- to 6-hour "therapeutic window" during which intervention may lessen brain damage.
      (1) **Thrombolytic agents** may be administered with an acceptable incidence of hemorrhagic infarction and intraparenchymal hematoma. A randomized, double-blind trial of intravenous recombinant **tissue plasminogen activator (t-PA)** administered no more than 3 hours after the onset of an acute ischemic stroke at a dose of 0.9 mg/kg (with 10% of the dose given as a bolus and the remainder infused over 1 hour) resulted in an improved clinical outcome at 3 months in patients treated with the active drug. Patients treated with t-PA were more likely to sustain a symptomatic intracerebral hemorrhage during the first 36 hours; however, there was no significant difference in mortality between treated and untreated patients.
         (a) Treatment with t-PA appears to be beneficial for patients with small or large artery occlusive disease or cardioembolic stroke. Because there is such a narrow window of opportunity for the administration of t-PA, rare patients destined to have a transient

ischemic attack (TIA; see VIII B 2) will be inadvertently treated. However, this treatment is most suitable for ischemic stroke patients.

(b) Patients to be treated with t-PA must meet strict criteria to minimize the risk of hemorrhagic complications. In addition, no anticoagulants or antiplatelet agents should be administered for 24 hours after t-PA treatment, and blood pressure elevations should be treated. **Contraindications** include:

(i) A rapidly improving neurologic deficit or minor symptoms

(ii) A baseline CT scan showing evidence of intracranial hemorrhage

(iii) A systolic blood pressure >185 mm Hg or a diastolic blood pressure >110 mm Hg

(iv) A medication-induced or disease-related coagulopathy

(v) A history of hemorrhagic stoke, recent surgery, or another invasive procedure

(2) Though not yet "standard of care," there is increasing experience with intra-arterial thrombolysis and several mechanical approaches to intra-arterial clot lysis for patients acutely presenting with large artery thromboembolic occlusions. A variety of imaging techniques, including CT and MR perfusion scans, MR diffusion, and CT or MR angiography may assist in patient selection.

2. Transient ischemic attacks (TIAs) are short-lived neurologic deficits, typically lasting minutes. A recent recommendation is that the maximal duration of a TIA be revised downward to 1 hour, in contradistinction to the classic definition of up to 24 hours. Symptoms are attributable to ischemia in the carotid or vertebrobasilar arterial distributions. The distinction between a TIA and a stroke is arbitrary, and even a brief symptomatic episode of cerebral ischemia, in conjunction with an abnormal diffusion weighted imaging (DWI) scan, might be construed as representing a stroke. Both warrant complete evaluation to determine the underlying pathophysiology and decrease the risk of subsequent ischemic events.

a. Etiology. Although TIAs often result from atherosclerotic large vessel disease, other diagnostic possibilities deserve consideration, including cardiogenic emboli, aortic arch atherothrombotic emboli, other large artery disorders such as dissection and fibromuscular dysplasia, small artery disease, hematologic disorders, and migraine. Other disease entities such as seizures, tumors, subdural hematomas, and MS sometimes masquerade as a TIA.

b. Diagnosis. Diagnostic studies should include a CBC, syphilis serology, a coagulation profile, and a CT scan or MRI. A transthoracic or transesophageal echocardiogram and 24-hour ambulatory electrocardiography (ECG) monitoring may be indicated.

(1) A duplex examination of the extracranial carotid artery territory is often informative.

(2) TCD studies, MRA, and CTA can provide insight into the extracranial and intracranial arterial circulation.

(3) Conventional interventional angiography is the definitive test to outline the vascular anatomy.

(4) Patients with an unrevealing cardiac evaluation who are thought to have an embolus may benefit from a transesophageal echocardiogram.

(5) If clinical suspicion exists, an LP can be used to evaluate the possibility of CNS inflammation.

c. Therapy. If atherosclerosis is suspected as the cause transient cerebral ischemia, control of risk factors for atherosclerosis is essential (see Chapter 1 III A 2). An evaluation for coronary artery disease is also appropriate.

(1) Extracranial carotid artery disease. Carotid endarterectomy is superior to medical therapy in the prevention of ischemic stroke in patients experiencing a TIA ipsilateral to an angiographically demonstrated 50%–99% stenosis at the internal carotid artery origin.

(a) Patients with less severe stenosis should be treated with aspirin. Clopidogrel and aspirin combined with slow-release dipyridamole are also effective in preventing stroke.

(b) Risk factor management pertinent to atherosclerosis is appropriate.

(2) **Intracranial large artery disease.** A TIA can result from large artery stenosis or occlusion. Recent evidence suggests that aspirin therapy is safer than, and equally effective as, anticoagulatin therapy for symptomatic intracranial large artery stenosis.

(3) **Other causes of TIA.** Therapy should be directed at the appropriate pathophysiologic process. For instance, anticoagulants are frequently used in patients with a source of cardiogenic emboli.

3. Cardiogenic embolic stroke

a. Etiology. The most common cause of embolic stroke is nonvalvular atrial fibrillation.

(1) Other conditions associated with cardiogenic emboli include recent myocardial infarction (MI), an akinetic ventricular segment, dilated cardiomyopathy, a prosthetic heart valve, infective and nonbacterial thrombotic endocarditis, left heart myxoma, left atrial spontaneous contrast echo, and atrial septal aneurysm.

(2) A patent foramen ovale (PFO) or atrial septal defect predisposes patients to paradoxical emboli, especially if there is a documented venous thrombosis. Patients less than 55 years of age with a PFO and an associated atrial septal aneurysm may be at particularly high risk for embolic stroke.

(3) Other cardiac conditions such as mitral valve prolapse or a hypokinetic ventricular segment are rarely associated with a cardiogenic embolus.

b. Diagnosis. The diagnosis is most certain if there is an abrupt onset of neurologic dysfunction, an underlying cardiac condition known to predispose to emboli, strokes in multiple vascular territories, hemorrhagic arterial infarction, systemic emboli, an absence of concurrent conditions known to cause stroke, and angiography demonstrating (potentially transient) vessel occlusions in the absence of an intrinsic vasculopathy. Patients suffering from a cardiac embolism rarely present with all of these conditions.

c. Therapy. An ischemic infarction caused by a cardiogenic embolus may develop into a hemorrhagic infarction, especially if reperfusion occurs or the infarction is large. Therefore, care must be taken to lessen the risk of parenchymal hemorrhage in acutely ill patients while simultaneously taking measures to protect them from another embolic stroke.

(1) If the patient has had a relatively small ischemic embolic infarction, a CT scan should be obtained. If no blood is present, a continuous infusion of heparin is administered. A partial thromboplastin time (PTT) greater than twice the control value should be avoided to minimize the risk of hemorrhagic conversion of the ischemic infarction and clinical worsening.

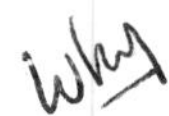

(2) If the patient has had a large ischemic embolic infarction, anticoagulation therapy should be withheld for 5–7 days. If the patient is recovering and a subsequent CT scan reveals no blood, heparin may be administered.

(3) Subsequent treatment with oral anticoagulants depends on the underlying disease process and the patient's general condition.

4. Large artery disease

a. Aortic arch atheromas or **thrombi.** These thrombi, which are visualized by transesophageal echocardiography, can embolize to the cerebral circulation and cause stroke. Optimal management is yet to be defined but usually involves antiplatelet or anticoagulation therapy, with the latter being used for mobile, pedunculated thrombi.

b. Asymptomatic cervical bruit and carotid stenosis. The combination of an internal carotid artery bruit and atherosclerosis at the internal carotid artery origin is a marker for coronary artery disease as well as cerebrovascular disease. Approximately 2% of these patients will suffer an ischemic stroke each year. Patients with a hemodynamically significant or progressive stenosis are at increased risk for cerebral infarction.

(1) **Etiology.** A midcervical bruit can be caused by a hyperdynamic circulation (e.g., as in anemia, pregnancy, and thyrotoxicosis), an external carotid artery stenosis, an internal carotid artery stenosis, or a venous hum.

(2) **Diagnosis.** Noninvasive vascular testing (see I C 3 d) is helpful in determining whether the bruit originates from atherosclerotic internal carotid artery disease and whether the lesion is hemodynamically significant. Angiography is usually used if the patient is a surgical candidate.

(3) **Therapy**

(a) **Control of risk factors for atherosclerosis** (see Chapter 1 III A 2). Antiplatelet therapy (aspirin, clopidogrel, or aspirin combined with slow-release dipyridamole) is often prescribed, and a careful coronary artery evaluation is warranted.

(b) **Medical treatment.** Patients with less than a 60% internal carotid artery stenosis should be managed medically.

(c) **Carotid endarterectomy**

(i) Patients with a 60%–99% stenosis who undergo **carotid endarterectomy** have less of a risk of ipsilateral stroke than patients managed medically if surgery can be achieved with less than a 3% risk of complications.

(ii) **Prophylactic carotid endarterectomy** for unilateral, slightly or moderately stenotic, asymptomatic internal carotid artery disease before major cardiac or vascular surgery is **usually inadvisable.**

c. **Ischemic infarction.** An understanding of neuroanatomy is essential to localize the compromised area of the brain and to correlate this information with a likely site of vascular disease.

(1) **Etiology**

(a) **Large artery occlusive disease** can cause ischemic infarction, either by being a source of artery-to-artery emboli or by causing hypoperfusion distal to a hemodynamically significant vascular stenosis. Large artery disease can involve the extracranial or intracranial portions of the cerebrovascular circulation.

(b) Vascular conditions other than atherosclerosis (e.g., **arterial dissection, arteritis, Takayasu's syndrome, fibromuscular dysplasia,** and **radiation-induced vasculopathy**) should be considered.

(2) **Diagnosis.** Diagnostic studies are pursued to define the vascular anatomy. CTA, MRA, carotid duplex, TCD, and conventional angiography can be used. The scope of testing is determined, in part, by the clinical condition of the patient and whether carotid endarterectomy or antithrombotic therapy are primary therapeutic considerations. The more accurate the definition of the underlying cause of the infarction, the more precise the determination of prognosis and treatment.

(3) **Therapy**

(a) **Extracranial carotid artery disease.** If the patient has sustained a minor infarction with a functional recovery and has a 50%–99% atherosclerotic stenosis of the ipsilateral origin of the internal carotid artery, carotid endarterectomy is superior to medical therapy for prevention of subsequent stroke. If the stenosis is less than 50%, therapy with antiplatelet drugs is appropriate.

(b) **Intracranial large artery disease**

(i) If the infarction is caused by a severe stenosis or occlusion of a large intracranial artery, recent evidence suggests that aspirin therapy is safer than, and equally effective as, anticoagulation therapy.

(ii) Some physicians use anticoagulation agents if the patient has new symptoms.

5. **Small artery disease.** The infarctions resulting from small artery disease typically are deep in the hemispheres or the pontomesencephalic region and are known as **lacunae.** The lesions are less than or equal to 15 mm in diameter.

a. **Etiology.** The underlying vascular lesion is usually hypertension-associated lipohyalinosis. Diabetes mellitus is also associated with lacunar infarcts. A small atheromatous plaque blocking the ostium of an arteriole may, on occasion, be the cause of some occlusions, as may infectious or sterile inflammation, cardiogenic emboli, and large artery occlusive disease.

b. Diagnosis

(1) Ischemic events from small artery disease cause stereotypic syndromes such as pure motor or sensory stroke, sensorimotor stroke, clumsy hand–dysarthria syndrome, and ataxic hemiparesis.

(2) Patients should be screened for the possibility of cardiogenic emboli, large artery occlusive disease, and hematologic and inflammatory disorders (see VIII B) if they are not hypertensive or if their history, examination, or routine diagnostic tests suggest a cause other than hypertension.

c. Therapy is directed at controlling hypertension. If another condition is defined as the cause of the infarction, appropriate intervention should be pursued. Antiplatelet therapy may be administered to decrease the likelihood of subsequent ischemic stroke.

6. Hematologic and systemic conditions. These disturbances are associated with ischemic infarction.

a. Associated conditions. Sickle cell disease, hyperviscosity associated with polycythemia and paraproteinemias, and hypercoagulability are conditions associated with ischemic stroke.

b. Etiology. Hypercoagulability is associated with antiphospholipid antibodies (including anticardiolipins and the lupus anticoagulant syndrome), hyperhomocysteinemia, deficiency of proteins C and S, activated protein C resistance, antithrombin III deficiency, malignancy, nephrotic syndrome, and pregnancy, as well as several other conditions.

7. The young ischemic stroke patient. Patients younger than 45 years of age who present with stroke are often diagnostic challenges. The potential etiologies are vast and include, but are not limited to, the following conditions:

a. Drug (especially cocaine) and alcohol abuse
b. Hypercoagulable states
c. Cardiogenic emboli
d. Migraine
e. Vasculitis and other rare arterial lesions
f. CNS infection, including HIV-associated conditions
g. Cancer
h. Disorders of homocysteine metabolism
i. Familial conditions [e.g., neurofibromatosis (NF), von Hippel-Lindau disease)]
j. Pregnancy and the postpartum state

8. The deteriorating ischemic stroke patient

a. Pathophysiology

(1) The patient's condition may deteriorate as a result of progressive occlusion of arteries from clot propagation or artery-to-artery emboli or because of subsequent cardiogenic emboli. Deterioration also may result from excessive lowering of blood pressure or inadequate anticoagulation therapy.

(2) Hemorrhagic infarction or a parenchymal hematoma can occur spontaneously or as a result of thrombolytic or anticoagulation therapy.

(3) If heparin is being used as treatment, the possibility of heparin-induced thrombosis (with associated thrombocytopenia) should be considered.

(4) Cerebral edema can develop, causing shifting of brain structures and an increase in the ICP.

b. Approach to the patient. Ideally, continuing efforts should be made to define the pathophysiology of the stroke.

(1) The blood pressure and degree of hydration should be checked.

(2) A CT scan should be obtained to define mass effect and hemorrhagic complications.

(3) A hematocrit, platelet count, and clotting profile should be obtained as appropriate.

c. Therapy. Patients should be confined to bed, and extremes of blood pressure should be avoided.

(1) Appropriate hydration should be maintained with normal saline, and increases in ICP should be treated as necessary.

(2) Consideration can be given to novel, interventional neuroradiologic techniques such as intra-arterial thrombolysis and angioplasty, depending on the degree of neurologic impairment, the time course of the illness, and the availability of resources.

C Hemorrhagic disorders

1. Subarachnoid hemorrhage (SAH)

a. **Etiology.** The most common causes of SAH are **trauma** and **ruptured berry aneurysms.**

(1) Other causes include coagulopathies, mycotic aneurysm, arteriovenous malformation, vasculitis, and sympathomimetic drugs.

(2) **Aneurysms** may be familial and are associated with polycystic kidney disease, coarctation of the aorta, fibromuscular dysplasia, moyamoya disease, polyarteritis nodosa, pseudoxanthoma elasticum, and Marfan and Ehlers-Danlos syndromes.

b. **Diagnosis**

(1) **Clinical signs.** Patients suffering from a ruptured berry aneurysm complain of an excruciating headache, but examination may not reveal many objective findings. Other patients can present with meningismus, altered states of arousal, and focal neurologic findings. A partial third nerve palsy with pupillary dilatation is suggestive of a posterior communicating artery aneurysm.

(2) **Diagnostic studies.** A **CT scan** reveals the presence of subarachnoid blood in most patients (Figure 11–3). If the index of suspicion for an SAH is high, but a CT scan is un-

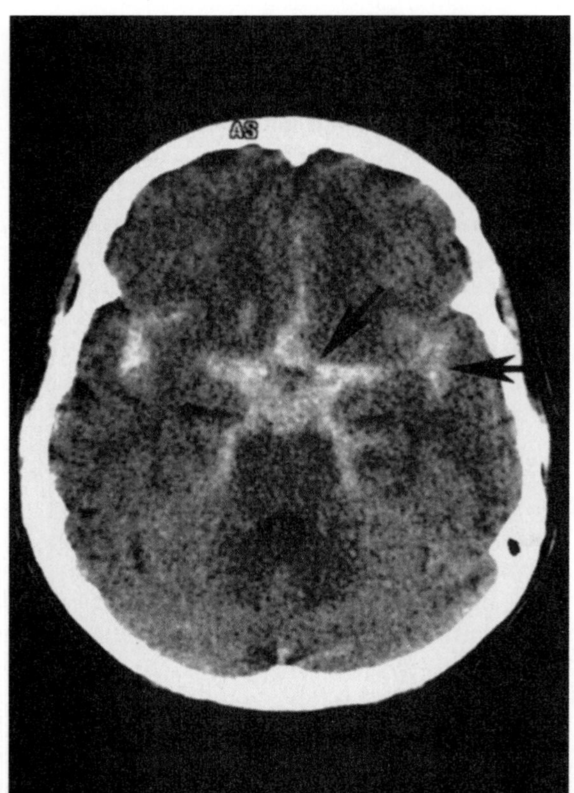

FIGURE 11–3 A nonenhanced computed tomography (CT) scan demonstrating a subarachnoid hemorrhage (SAH). Note the blood in the basal cisterns and the sylvian fissures.

revealing, an LP provides the proper diagnosis. Conventional interventional angiography is necessary to characterize the aneurysm.

c. **Therapy.** Treatment of aneurysmal SAH is aimed at **controlling complications,** which include rebleeding, vasospasm leading to delayed ischemic stroke, hyponatremia, acute or chronic hydrocephalus, intraparenchymal and intraventricular hematoma, and cardiac arrhythmias. Unfortunately, the mortality rate from aneurysmal rupture approaches 50%, although recent studies suggest an improved outcome. Interventional neuroradiologic techniques are playing a larger role in the management of aneurysms.
   (1) **Rebleeding** most frequently occurs in the first 48 hours after aneurysmal rupture. **Early intervention** to isolate the aneurysm should be performed when possible to eliminate the threat of rebleeding. Surgical "clipping" or endovascular therapy, which involves placing thrombogenic "coils" in the aneurysm, can be used to isolate the aneurysm.
   (2) The course of **vasospasm** can be followed with TCD and CTA studies.
      (a) The development of ischemic stroke from vasospasm is less likely when **nimodipine,** a calcium antagonist that may decrease small artery vasoconstriction or provide neuronal protection from ischemia, is administered.
      (b) Prophylaxis against symptomatic vasospasm also includes maintaining patients in a euvolemic state and avoiding hypotension.
      (c) If the aneurysm has been isolated from the circulatory system, symptomatic vasospasm may be treated with **hypervolemic therapy,** coupled with a moderate increase in blood pressure.
      (d) Refractory vasospasm may be amenable to angioplasty or selective intra-arterial papaverine or calcium antagonist infusion.
   (3) **Symptomatic hydrocephalus** can be treated with a ventricular drain, repeated LPs, or ventriculoperitoneal shunting, as dictated by clinical circumstances.

2. **Intraparenchymal hematoma**
   a. **Diagnostic considerations.** Chronic hypertension is often, but not invariably, associated with hemorrhage in the region of the putamen, thalamus, cerebellum, and pons.
      (1) An intraparenchymal hemorrhage that is not accompanied by a history of hypertension should prompt a search for an underlying cause of bleeding (e.g., coagulopathy, aneurysm, arteriovenous malformation, or tumor), particularly if the hemorrhage is not located in a region of the brain typically associated with hypertensive bleeding.
      (2) In elderly patients, lobar hematomas, especially if multiple, may be indicative of amyloid angiopathy. The APOE4 allele may be a risk factor for amyloid angiopathy and amyloid angiopathy-related hemorrhage.
      (3) Coagulopathies (especially when induced by thrombolytic therapy) and the use of drugs such as cocaine and sympathomimetics are associated with intraparenchymal hematoma.
   b. **Diagnosis**
      (1) **Clinical signs**
         (a) A **large putaminal hematoma** causes impaired consciousness, contralateral hemiparesis and sensory loss, and gaze preference to the side of the hemorrhage.
         (b) **Thalamic hemorrhage** can lead to impaired consciousness; contralateral motor and sensory loss; diminished vertical gaze; and small, poorly reactive pupils (i.e., Parinaud's syndrome).
         (c) Patients with **cerebellar hematomas** may present with impaired gait and stance and limb ataxia. If the hematoma is large, impaired consciousness, cranial nerve palsies (including eye movement abnormalities), and weakness can develop.
         (d) The classic signs of **pontine hematoma** include coma, pinpoint reactive pupils, impaired lateral ocular motility, and quadriplegia with decerebrate posturing. Small pontine hemorrhages cause more restricted pontine syndromes.

(2) **Diagnostic studies.** A CT scan is central to diagnosis. A coagulation profile and drug toxicology screen should be performed. Angiography may be appropriate in normotensive patients and in those with hemorrhage at atypical sites.

c. **Therapy**

(1) Taking measures to lower the elevated ICP associated with parenchymal hematoma can improve outcome.

(2) With cerebellar hematomas, surgical resection is a lifesaving measure. Surgical resection of hematomas at other sites is receiving increasing attention.

(3) A coagulopathy should be treated appropriately.

3. **Arteriovenous malformation.** Headaches, seizures, and intraparenchymal or, occasionally, SAHs may result. Therapeutic intervention may incorporate multiple modalities, including surgery, interventional radiology with embolization, and stereotactic radiosurgery.

IX SEIZURES

A seizure involves a **sudden abnormality of brain electrical activity.** Manifestations of a seizure can include impairment or loss of consciousness and sensory, motor, or behavioral abnormalities. The term **epilepsy** describes a syndrome characterized by recurrent seizures.

A Classification

Optimal management of seizure patients depends on proper classification of the seizure type. Seizures can be categorized as **generalized** or **partial.**

1. **Generalized seizures** are characterized by a sudden loss of consciousness.

a. **Generalized convulsive seizures** consist of tonic, clonic, or tonic–clonic (grand mal) motor activity. Generalized convulsions can result from a focal seizure disorder that has spread, involving the entire brain. **Postictal obtundation** and **confusion** commonly last minutes, and occasionally, hours. The EEG often shows generalized spikes or spikes and associated slow waves.

b. **Generalized nonconvulsive (absence) seizures** are characterized by a brief, sudden loss of consciousness and minor motor activity such as blinking, sporadic myoclonic jerks, or automatisms. Typically, the EEG demonstrates generalized spikes and associated slow waves.

2. **Simple partial (localization-related) seizures** are not accompanied by an impairment of consciousness. Generalized motor seizures may develop secondarily.

a. There may be isolated clonic or tonic activity of a limb or transient altered sensory perceptions.

b. The seizure activity may spread over one side of the body in a **jacksonian march** (e.g., the convulsive activity can start in the face, move to the ipsilateral arm and then to the leg, and may evolve into a generalized seizure).

c. The EEG may show a focal rhythmic discharge at the onset of a simple partial seizure, but occasionally, no ictal activity is detected. Interictally, focal spikes with associated slow waves are frequently present.

3. **Complex partial (localization-related) seizures** are often characterized by an **aura** followed by **impaired awareness.** The EEG often shows interictal spikes or spikes with associated slow waves in the temporal or frontotemporal areas and ictal focal rhythmic discharges. Generalized motor seizures may develop secondarily.

a. The **aura** may involve **hallucinations** (e.g., olfactory, visual, auditory, or gustatory) and complex **illusions** (e.g., of having experienced a new event or of never having experienced a commonplace event). However, patients frequently do not recall their aura.

b. Nausea or vomiting, focal sensory perceptions, and focal tonic or clonic activity may accompany a complex seizure.

c. After the aura, there may be an episode of impaired consciousness, lasting seconds to several minutes, during which time automatisms may be observed. Return to baseline cognitive abilities can take several minutes.

4. Status epilepticus is defined as an episode of repeated or ongoing seizure activity with impaired arousal lasting at least 30 minutes. Status epilepticus may involve both **convulsive** (generalized tonic–clonic activity) and **nonconvulsive** (absence or complex partial) seizures.
   a. Patients experiencing convulsive seizures are at risk for hypoxia, aspiration, acidosis, hypotension, hyperthermia, myoglobinuria, hypoglycemia, and multiple physical injuries.
   b. Patients experiencing nonconvulsive seizures can appear delirious. A fluctuating sensorium and subtle automatisms or myoclonic jerks are clues to the diagnosis, and the EEG is confirmatory.

B Etiology Table 11–7 outlines some of the many causes of seizures. Several seizure types have a defined genetic basis: autosomal dominant frontal lobe epilepsy (neuronal nicotinic acetylcholine receptor mutation) and autosomal dominant temporal lobe epilepsy with auditory features.

C Diagnosis

1. **Patient history** and **physical examination** can aid in the determination of whether a seizure or some other transient event was responsible for the patient's symptoms.
   a. A **family history** of **epilepsy** or a **history** of **febrile convulsions** is relevant.
   b. An **accurate description of the event by an observer** is helpful in defining the problem.
   c. **Urinary incontinence, back pain** (from a vertebral compression fracture), **myalgias,** and **oral lacerations** are clues to proper diagnosis.
   d. **Fever, fatigue, stress, alcohol withdrawal, medications,** and **menses** can provoke seizures.
2. **Differential diagnosis.** Other conditions that may produce sudden loss of consciousness are discussed in II A. Psychogenic seizures should be considered if patients exhibit nonstereotypic events, have an unexpected resistance to antiepileptic drugs, or have a psychiatric disorder.
3. **Diagnostic studies**
   a. The **EEG** is central to the evaluation of seizure patients. The best technique for fully characterizing a seizure disorder is continuous video EEG monitoring, but this is not usually used as an initial diagnostic test.
   b. An **MRI** scan is the most useful modality for detecting lesions that may cause seizures.
   c. **SPECT** and **positron emission tomography** (**PET**) can provide additional information to help localize a seizure focus.
   d. **Laboratory studies** are indicated to evaluate potential metabolic or toxic causes.

TABLE 11–7 Selected Causes of Seizures

Idiopathic	Infection
Genetic predisposition	Meningitis, abscess, and encephalitis
Mesial temporal sclerosis	Degenerative diseases
Metabolic abnormalities	Alzheimer's disease
Hyponatremia	Trauma
Hypo- or hyperglycemia	Eclampsia
Hypocalcemia	Drugs
Hypomagnesemia	Theophylline
Uremia	Lidocaine
Vascular disease and stroke	Cocaine
Infarction, especially cortical	Drug and substance withdrawal
Vascular malformation	Anticonvulsant medications
Vasculitis	Benzodiazepines
Inflammatory causes	Alcohol
Systemic lupus erythematosus (SLE)	Psychogenic causes
Neoplasia	
Metastatic and primary brain tumors	

D Therapy

1. **General considerations.** If a seizure is the suspected diagnosis, decisions about therapy depend on the underlying cause.
   a. Correction of hyponatremia, hypoglycemia, or drug intoxication may be all that is necessary.
   b. Patients with a neurologic condition known to be associated with recurrent seizures often require medication.
   c. Anticonvulsant therapy is often not initiated in patients with a single, unprovoked convulsion; a normal neurologic examination; and a normal brain imaging study and EEG unless they experience a second seizure.
2. **Medical therapy**
   a. **General principles.** An attempt is usually made to prevent subsequent seizures by using a **single agent,** to limit toxic effects. The drug should be administered in **progressive doses** until seizure control has been achieved or until drug toxicity occurs. Only if monotherapy fails should a second drug be added. If control is then obtained, the first agent might be carefully withdrawn.
   b. **Specific agents.** The choice of medication should be based on the seizure type, bearing in mind possible contraindications and side effects.
      (1) Typically, generalized convulsive, simple partial, and complex partial seizures are treated with carbamazepine, phenytoin, valproic acid, topiramate, levetiracetam, lamotrigine, or zonisamide.
      (2) Valproic acid or ethosuximide is used for generalized nonconvulsive spells (absence seizures).
      (3) Valproic acid is particularly effective for controlling myoclonic epilepsy of Janz (a disorder characterized by myoclonic seizures).
      (4) **Lamotrigine, gabapentin, tiagabine, oxcarbazepine,** and **topiramate** are adjunctive medications for the treatment of patients with refractory partial seizures.
3. **Surgical therapy.** Patients refractory to medical control of seizures may be candidates for surgery to control the epilepsy. **Temporal lobe resection, ablation** of a **cortical seizure focus,** and **corpus callosum sectioning** are able to reduce seizure frequency in some patients who meet specific criteria. **Vagus nerve stimulation** may help control seizures.
4. **Control of status epilepticus.** Generalized convulsive status epilepticus is a life-threatening condition; therefore, management of convulsive status epilepticus requires making certain that the airway is unobstructed and maintaining adequate oxygenation, blood pressure, and hydration. Definition of the underlying problem is essential.
   a. **Glucose** and **thiamine** should be administered after blood samples for glucose, electrolytes, renal function, anticonvulsant drug levels, and toxicology have been obtained.
   b. Often, **intravenous diazepam** or **lorazepam** is given to stop the convulsions. Lorazepam carries less of a risk of respiratory depression or arrest and remains effective for longer periods.
   c. Administration of a benzodiazepine is followed by administration of **phenytoin, fosphenytoin,** or **phenobarbital.**
   d. If convulsions continue after loading doses of phenytoin or fosphenytoin or phenobarbital have been administered, intravenous **midazolam, propofol,** or **pentobarbital** can be given in a carefully supervised setting, with continuous EEG monitoring, until the seizure discharges are eliminated from the EEG.
   e. Diminished cardiac output, bradycardia, and hypotension often limit the dose of intravenous anticonvulsants. **Fluid resuscitation** and **vasopressors** may be used.
5. **Psychosocial issues.** The following issues are important to consider when managing epilepsy.
   a. Patients may be depressed, have behavioral disturbances, and often require vocational support services. Frequently, community support services are available.

b. Reviews of the patient's driving status and work and play environment are necessary.
c. Family and friends need to be counseled as to how to manage a convulsion.
d. Women of childbearing age should be counseled about issues relating to pregnancy.

X MOVEMENT DISORDERS

A Parkinson's disease

1. **Pathogenesis**
   a. Parkinson's disease is characterized by a degeneration of cells in the substantia nigra, which causes a deficiency of dopamine (a neurotransmitter) in the CNS, leading to a series of changes in motor control pathways. The mechanism behind the degeneration of these cells is unknown, although hypotheses center about free radical damage and impaired mitochondrial oxidative function.
   b. Major insights into the genetics of Parkinson's disease are emerging. The *SNCA* gene codes for α-synuclein, the *PRKN* gene codes for parkin, and the *UCHL1* gene codes for a ubiquitin hydroxylase. Several other chromosome loci have been associated with Parkinson's disease.
   c. A common feature emerging from the genetics studies is that the pathophysiology of Parkinson's disease, as well as that of other neurodegenerative diseases, may involve abnormalities in pathways associated with ubiquitin-associated protein degradation.
2. **Diagnosis**
   a. **Clinical symptoms and signs**
      (1) Parkinson's disease patients often complain of "slowing up"; they have trouble dressing, arising from a seated position, climbing or descending stairs, writing, and turning over in bed.
      (2) On examination, **rigidity** and **akinesia** or **bradykinesia** are present and a **resting tremor** and **postural instability** are often evident. Signs are often asymmetrical early in the disease.
      (3) Cognitive impairment develops in over 50% of patients over time.
   b. **Differential diagnosis.** The diagnosis is a clinical determination, although, at times, testing to exclude other entities presenting as parkinsonism is indicated.
      (1) Sometimes **serial observations** are necessary to determine whether the parkinsonian state is the harbinger of another neurologic illness; this is of special concern in patients who do not have the **characteristic "pill-rolling"** or **resting tremor** of **Parkinson's disease** or fail to respond to levodopa therapy.
      (2) Conditions that may produce parkinsonian symptoms similar to those found in patients suffering from Parkinson's disease include NPH, multiple strokes, hypothyroidism, drug effects [e.g., neuroleptics (dopamine-blocking agents), metoclopramide, diltiazem, and reserpine], Wilson's disease, anoxic encephalopathy, and intoxication [e.g., by carbon monoxide, manganese, or n-methyl-4-phenyl-1,2,3,6-tetrahydropyridine (MPTP)].
      (3) Rare neurologic disorders that may have parkinsonian features are summarized in Table 11–8.
3. **Therapy.** Parkinson's disease is a progressive disease. Therefore, management protocols vary depending on the patient's symptoms and the extent of functional impairment.
   a. **Early therapy.** Several medications are available to treat Parkinson's disease.
      (1) **Carbidopa/levodopa combinations** are the mainstay of treatment for Parkinson's disease. This treatment should begin when the disease impairs the patient's functional status. A sustained release formulation of carbidopa/levodopa is available and provides a more uniform clinical response than conventional dosing.
         (a) **Levodopa** is converted to dopamine by the presynaptic neuron and therefore increases the amount of neurotransmitter available to the postsynaptic dopamine receptor.

TABLE 11–8 Key Features of Selected Conditions Causing Parkinsonism

Disorder	Distinguishing Clinical Characteristics
Progressive supranuclear palsy ("tauopathy")	Impaired vertical gaze; early axial rigidity with postural instability
Multiple systems atrophy (Shy-Drager syndrome)	Autonomic insufficiency; cerebellar dysfunction; upper and lower motor neuron dysfunction
Diffuse Lewy body disease ("Dementia with Lewy bodies")	Dementia early in illness, fluctuating cognition, visual hallucinations
Cortical-basal ganglionic degeneration ("tauopathy")	Asymmetric findings on examination of sensory loss and apraxia; unilateral rigidity; unilateral stimulus-sensitive myoclonus; dystonia
Frontotemporal lobar degeneration ("tauopathy")	Apathy, disinhibition, anomia, effortful speech
Huntington's disease	Parkinsonian features prominent in young patients; family history, choreoathetosis
Olivopontocerebellar atrophy*	Cerebellar dysfunction; autonomic dysfunction
Basal ganglia calcification	Calcification visible on computed tomography (CT) scan
Neuroacanthocytosis	Acanthocytes in wet peripheral blood smear

*May be the same as multiple systems atrophy.

(b) **Carbidopa** blocks systemic conversion of levodopa to dopamine, thereby decreasing the undesirable systemic effects of levodopa.

(2) **Dopamine agonists** are increasingly being used at initial therapy, especially in younger patients. They may have some neuroprotective benefits. Drugs include **pramipexole, ropinirole, pergolide, and bromocriptine.**

(3) **Anticholinergics,** which improve the cholinergic–dopaminergic balance in the basal ganglia, are particularly helpful in treating tremor. However, they may contribute to cognitive impairment.

(4) **Amantadine,** which increases the availability of dopamine to the postsynaptic neuron, can be effective early in the course of the disease or as an adjunctive therapy later in the disease course to help "smooth out" motor function.

b. **Advanced therapy.** In the later stages of the disease, therapy is directed at optimizing the patient's functional status and avoiding adverse effects of medication.

(1) **Dopamine agonists.** If the therapeutic response to carbidopa/levodopa therapy is inadequate, or if the patient cannot tolerate the medication, **pramipexole, ropinirole, pergolide, or bromocriptine** may be administered.

(a) These drugs are **direct postsynaptic dopamine-receptor agonists.**

(b) A combination of carbidopa/levodopa and a dopamine agonist seems to be particularly effective and is often well tolerated. Dopamine agonists help decrease motor fluctuations when used in conjunction with carbidopa/levodopa.

(2) **Management with disease progression.** Management of Parkinson's disease becomes increasingly difficult as the disease progresses. **"Wearing off"** effects, **dyskinesias,** and wide, random swings in patient mobility (**"on–off" phenomena**) develop. A sustained-release form of carbidopa/levodopa (alone or in combination with a dopamine agonist) can be used. **Catechol *O*-methyltransferase inhibitors,** which increase the synaptic availability of levodopa by blocking its degradation, also can be used to manage unstable patients.

c. **Ancillary therapy**

(1) Other therapeutic maneuvers include the **strategic reduction of medication** if patients are experiencing dyskinesia and **judicious use** of **psychotropic agents** to treat the various

untoward behavioral consequences of Parkinson's disease (e.g., insomnia, hallucinations, agitation).

(2) **Dietary manipulations** that **redistribute** or **limit protein** intake during the day may improve the efficacy of levodopa.

(3) **Physical therapy** and an **exercise program** help optimize mobility.

(4) **Pallidotomy** and **deep brain stimulation** offer new therapeutic options for refractory Parkinson's disease patients.

(5) The role of surgical implants of dopamine-containing cells for the treatment of Parkinson's disease remains experimental.

B Hyperkinetic disorders

1. **Tremor**
   a. **Benign essential tremor** is characterized by a posture-related 5–9-Hz oscillation of the hands and forearms that impairs performance of fine motor tasks.
      (1) This type of tremor is often **familial** and may be accompanied by **titubation (head tremor).**
      (2) Consumption of alcohol may temporarily suppress the tremor; stress, caffeine, or sleep deprivation may exacerbate the condition.
      (3) **β-Adrenergic blocking agents** and **primidone** are effective treatments.
   b. An **action (kinetic) tremor** is evident when patients move their arms; there may be a relatively mild accompanying postural and intention component. Treatment with **clonazepam** may be useful.
2. **Chorea** describes **rapid, "dance-like" distal limb** and **facial movements.** Causes include hyperthyroidism, drugs (e.g., birth control pills, levodopa), Sydenham's chorea, pregnancy, SLE, antiphospholipid syndrome, stroke, porphyria, Wilson's disease, Lyme disease, Huntington's disease, and neuroacanthocytosis.
3. **Athetosis** describes a **moderately rapid, principally distal, somewhat rotary "snake-like" movement in the distal extremities.** Causes include Wilson's disease, Huntington's disease, anoxic encephalopathy, trauma, birth control pills, and several rare hereditary disorders.
4. **Dystonia** describes **slow, writhing, sustained** and **involuntary contractions of the proximal limb, trunk,** and **neck musculature.** Dystonia is associated with Wilson's disease, Parkinson's disease, Huntington's disease, trauma, neuronal storage disorders, encephalitis, drugs (e.g., neuroleptics, levodopa), and other rare hereditary conditions.
   a. The TOR1A gene for autosomal dominant generalized torsion dystonia codes for torsin A, an ATP-binding and heat shock protein. Patients may respond to high doses of trihexyphenidyl.
   b. Some patients with autosomal dominant idiopathic dystonia are particularly responsive to carbidopa/levodopa therapy. This condition is associated with the DYT5 gene on chromosome 14 that codes for guanine triphosphate (GTP) cyclohydrolase I; a deficiency of this enzyme causes loss of dopamine synthesis.
   c. Focal dystonias such as writer's cramp, blepharospasm, spastic dysphonia, and torticollis can occur. Treatment with local botulinum toxin infiltration can be beneficial.
   d. Some patients with dystonia may exhibit chorea and athetosis.
5. **Hemiballismus** describes **wild, flinging, principally proximal movements** of the **arms** or **legs.** It is often caused by an infarct in the subthalamic nucleus. Haloperidol can decrease the involuntary movements.
6. **Blepharospasm** can occur in isolation or as part of a more widespread disorder such as Parkinson's disease, stroke, or Meige's syndrome (a syndrome distinct from that associated with ovarian cancer). Blepharospasm can be of such severity as to cause functional blindness.
   a. Many drugs have been tried in an attempt to control the problem with modest effect.
   b. Infiltration of botulinum toxin about the eyes can provide relief by decreasing neuromuscular transmissions.

7. **Neuroleptic-associated movement disorders** represent a spectrum of disorders related to the acute or chronic administration of neuroleptic medications (although for selected conditions, other drugs are implicated as well).
   a. **Acute dystonia** typically occurs shortly after the first few doses of a neuroleptic agent.
      (1) **Clinical signs** include uncontrollable face, neck, tongue, and eye muscle (oculogyric crisis) spasms.
      (2) **Therapy** consists of the administration of anticholinergics or diphenhydramine.
   b. **Parkinsonism** can develop with neuroleptic use. Therapy consists of decreasing the dose of the neuroleptic agent; changing to another neuroleptic drug; administering an anticholinergic agent; or using amantadine, a carbidopa/levodopa preparation, or an "atypical" neuroleptic such as clozapine, risperidone, or olanzapine.
   c. **Tardive dyskinesia** is an almost constant writhing movement of the tongue and oromandibular area, which may be accompanied by blepharospasm, respiratory grunts, choreoathetosis, and truncal hyperactivity. Ill-fitting dentures or an edentulous state can cause mouthing movements that are mistaken for tardive dyskinesia.
      (1) Tardive dyskinesia is usually an adverse side effect of neuroleptic agents; occasionally other drugs such as amphetamines, antihistamines, and carbamazepine are causally implicated.
      (2) If medication is implicated as the cause of the problem, the offending agent should be discontinued if possible. Clonazepam, reserpine, tetrabenazine, and other drugs have been used to treat tardive dyskinesia with variable success. Use of an "atypical" neuroleptic such as clozapine is another option.
   d. **Other neuroleptic-associated movement disorders** include tardive dystonia, akathisia (motor restlessness), and the rabbit syndrome (rhythmic lip movements).
   e. **Neuroleptic malignant syndrome (NMS)** is an idiosyncratic reaction to neuroleptic agents. It can also occur in Parkinson's disease patients after the abrupt discontinuation of antiparkinsonian medications. Dopamine receptor blockade is thought to be the cause of NMS.
      (1) **Clinical signs** include altered mentation, high fever, rigidity, autonomic instability, high creatine kinase (CK) levels, and myoglobinuria.
      (2) **Therapy** for this potentially lethal condition includes hydration, cooling blankets, antipyretics, dantrolene, and levodopa/carbidopa preparations or bromocriptine, although the use of antiparkinsonian drugs is controversial.

8. **Meige's syndrome (orofacial dystonia)** is an idiopathic condition that has features of dystonia and tardive dyskinesia, particularly blepharospasm.
   a. This diagnosis cannot be made if the patient has recently taken neuroleptic agents or other drugs implicated as a cause of tardive dyskinesia.
   b. No single medication is consistently effective in treating this condition; clonazepam is a reasonable first-line agent. Botulinum toxin infiltration can be used to treat the blepharospasm.

9. **Hemifacial spasm** describes lightning-quick spasms of muscles innervated by the facial nerve.
   a. The condition is most often caused by irritation of the facial nerve by a vascular "loop."
   b. Rarely, it occurs after facial nerve paralysis or is associated with tumors, MS, or other irritative processes.
   c. **Botulinum toxin infiltration, clonazepam,** and **carbamazepine** have been used to treat **hemifacial spasm;** microsurgical decompression may be successful.

10. **Tics** are brief involuntary movements, sounds, or sensations that occur within the context of normal neurologic function.
    a. **Types of tics**
       (1) **Simple motor tics** are isolated movements such as an eyeblink, shoulder shrug, or facial grimace. **Complex motor tics** include touching, smelling, and jumping.
       (2) **Simple phonic tics** include throat clearing, sniffling, and grunting. **Complex phonic tics** include the repetition of words and coprolalia.

(3) **Sensory tics** often accompany motor and phonic tics and are characterized by focal sensations of pressure, tickle, warmth, or cold.

b. Tourette's syndrome

(1) **Characteristics**

(a) Multiple motor and one or more phonic tics (that has been present at some time over the course of the illness)

(b) Tics that occur many times a day, nearly every day, for more than 1 year

(c) Tics that change over time in their anatomic location, number, frequency, complexity, type, and severity

(d) Onset of illness before age 21

(e) Absence of other conditions that can cause similar, but isolated, symptoms (e.g., neuroleptic drug effects, seizures, chorea)

(2) **Etiology.** Tourette's syndrome is thought to be inherited in a polygenic manner. Striatal dopamine receptor supersensitivity may be responsible for the clinical manifestations.

(3) **Associated behavioral disturbances. Obsessive–compulsive disorder** and **attention deficit hyperactivity disorder** may occur.

(4) **Therapy.** Treatment consists of education and counseling of the patient, family, and other appropriate parties. Clonidine, pimozide, or haloperidol can be used to manage disabling tics. Behavioral disturbances should respond to appropriate psychoactive medications.

XI DEMYELINATING DISEASES

A **Multiple sclerosis (MS)** is characterized by multiple foci of CNS demyelination. Patients either experience clinical remissions (often followed by relapses) or chronic, progressive symptoms.

1. **Pathophysiology.** Although the cause of MS remains unknown, a predominant theory contends that MS is an immunologic disorder associated with CNS immunoglobulin production and alteration of T and B lymphocytes. The **pathologic hallmark** of MS is inflammation associated with areas of **demyelination scattered about CNS white matter.** Recent findings have also documented **axonal disruption.**

2. **Diagnosis**

a. Clinical signs

(1) The diagnosis is most certain if neurologic problems occur over an extended length of time and involve several white matter pathways. MRI findings can be used as evidence of disease dissemination over time and anatomic space.

(2) Several patterns emerge that are suggestive of MS, including **optic neuritis** (a sign of which is the Marcus-Gunn pupil or afferent pupillary defect) and **internuclear ophthalmoplegia** or either of these conditions in association with corticospinal tract or cerebellar signs. Long-term follow-up indicates that 74% of women and 34% of men who present with isolated optic neuritis ultimately develop MS.

(3) Neurologic signs that can be localized to a single discrete area in the CNS such as the brain stem or craniocervical junction should suggest an alternate diagnosis such as a tumor or arteriovenous malformation.

b. Differential diagnosis. There is no specific diagnostic marker for MS; the physician needs to exclude other conditions that can masquerade as MS. Among these disorders are somatization disorder, SLE, brain stem or spinal vascular malformation, Sjögren's syndrome, Lyme disease, HIV infection, vitamin B_{12} deficiency, brain stem neoplasm, vasculitis, sarcoidosis, and adrenomyeloleukodystrophy.

c. Diagnostic studies

(1) **MRI** is an excellent technique for visualizing white matter lesions. Although its diagnostic specificity is poor, the contrast agent **gadolinium-DTPA** indicates areas of breakdown

of the blood-brain barrier. Serial MRI studies show white matter lesions that may come and go without clinical manifestations.

(2) **Examination of the CSF** can indicate a sterile inflammation with a mild protein elevation; modest, predominantly mononuclear pleocytosis; an elevated IgG index; oligoclonal bands; and increased myelin basic protein. Only occasionally do all of these abnormalities occur in a single patient.

(3) **Visual, brain stem–auditory,** and **somatosensory EPs** and **central motor conduction studies** can demonstrate clinically silent disruption of white matter tracts.

3. **Therapy.** There is no cure for MS.
   a. **Corticosteroid therapy** may hasten maximal recovery from an acute exacerbation. If optic neuritis is treated, high doses of intravenous corticosteroids are preferable to lower, oral doses.
   b. **Interferon-β** (IFN-β) therapy decreases the frequency of relapses, especially moderate and severe attacks. As judged by serial MRI studies, disease activity is lessened with IFN-β treatment.
   c. **Glatiramer acetate** also decreases the frequency of relapses, especially for patients with mild disease.
   d. Otherwise, treatment is directed at **symptoms.**
      (1) **Modafinil, amantadine,** and **pemoline** can improve **fatigue.**
      (2) **Baclofen, tizanidine,** and **diazepam** improve **spasticity.**
      (3) A **variety of agents** may help **urologic dysfunction,** depending on the specific problem.
   e. Patients with severe disease may respond to immunosuppressive therapy.

B Central pontine myelinolysis

1. **Etiology.** Demyelination of the basis pontis and other myelinated areas has been associated with the **excessively rapid correction** of **severe hyponatremia.** Central pontine myelinolysis has been seen in alcoholics, malnourished patients, and in association with diuretic use.
2. **Diagnosis.** Patients develop **impaired arousal, quadriparesis,** and **pseudobulbar signs. MRI** or **CT scan** confirms the diagnosis.
3. **Therapy.** Hyponatremia should be corrected **slowly,** and hypernatremia should be avoided.

XII MYELOPATHY AND OTHER SPINAL CORD DISORDERS

A Etiology

Selected causes of myelopathy are listed in Table 11–9.

TABLE 11–9 Selected Causes of Myelopathy

Vertebral column disorders	Multiple sclerosis
Trauma	Vascular disease
Cervical stenosis	Infarction
Disk protrusion	Vascular malformation
Odontoid subluxation	Metabolic diseases
Rheumatoid arthritis	Vitamin B_{12} deficiency (subacute combined degeneration)
Down syndrome	Vitamin E deficiency
Neoplasia	Adrenomyeloneuropathy
Epidural spinal cord compression	Radiation effects
Intradural extramedullary mass	Syringomyelia
Intramedullary mass	Spinocerebellar degeneration
Infection	
Spinal epidural abscess	
Human immunodeficiency virus (HIV)	
Human T-cell lymphotrophic virus type I (HTLV-I)	

B **Clinical signs** Disease affecting the spinal cord can present with principally **"long tract signs"** or a combination of long tract signs and **local radicular features.**

1. **Long tract motor signs** result from the disruption of descending corticospinal fibers, which causes **weakness, spasticity, and hyperreflexia.**
2. **Impaired sensation** results from disordered function of ascending spinothalamic and dorsal column pathways (Figure 11–4).
3. **Bowel, bladder, and erectile function may be compromised.**
4. **Local radicular symptoms and signs include radiating pain, weakness,** and **sensory loss** referable to one or several myotomes and dermatomes. These findings help define the rostral–caudal extent of a lesion (Figure 11–5).
5. The **Brown-Séquard syndrome** is caused by a lesion compromising the right or left hemispinal cord at a discrete level. There is caudal ipsilateral upper motor neuron weakness and loss of proprioception and vibratory sensibility as well as contralateral loss of pain and temperature sensation.

C **Selected conditions**

1. **Syringomyelia**
   a. **Definition.** Syringomyelia is a condition of unknown cause resulting in **cavitation of the spinal cord.** Syringomyelia can occur in isolation or in association with the **Arnold-Chiari malformation** (i.e., descent of the cerebellar tonsils into the cervical spinal canal).
   b. **Diagnosis**
      (1) **Signs of lower motor neuron dysfunction** develop on a segmental basis and are accompanied by **upper motor neuron signs** caudal to the cavity.
      (2) **Dermatomal loss of pain and temperature sensibility** results from local disruption of the spinothalamic tract by the cavity (syrinx). Impaired ascending dorsal column sensibility occasionally occurs caudal to the cavity.
      (3) **MRI** of the spine is the **optimal diagnostic test** (Figure 11–6).
   c. **Therapy. Surgery** is occasionally indicated to decompress the fluid-filled spinal cord cavity and to perform a biopsy of the wall to evaluate the possibility of a cavitary neoplasm. **Otherwise, treatment is supportive.**
2. **Transverse myelitis.** Inflammation of the spinal cord can cause an acute myelopathy.
   a. **Etiology.** Although many cases of segmental transverse inflammation are idiopathic, MS, SLE, and various infectious agents may cause transverse myelitis.

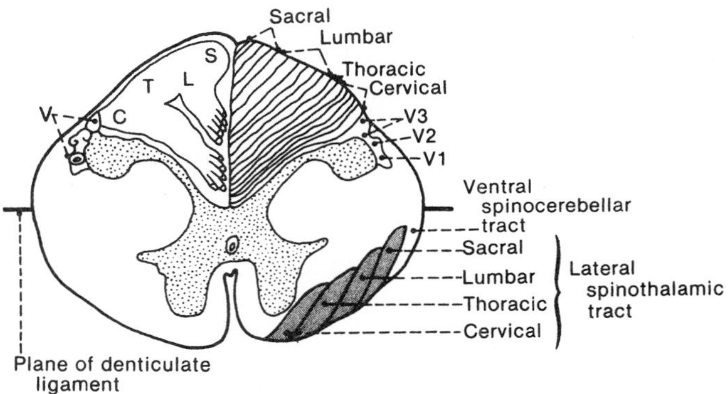

FIGURE 11–4 Cross section of the spinal cord at C1 that shows the lamination of ascending sensory axons by the level of entry in the dorsal columns (discriminative modalities) and ventrolateral columns (pain and temperature). V1, V2, and V3 refer to the first, second, and third sensory divisions of cranial nerve V, the trigeminal nerve. (Reprinted from NMS *Neuroanatomy*. Malvern, PA, Harwal Publishing, 1988, p 115.)

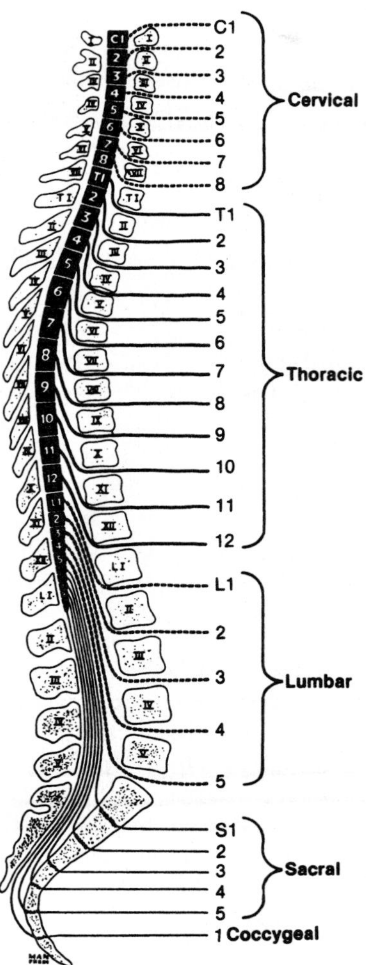

FIGURE 11–5 Topographic relationship among nerve roots, spinal cord segments, and the bodies and spinous processes of the vertebrae, which are indicated by *Roman numerals.* (Adapted from Haymaker W, Woodhall B: *Peripheral Nerve Injuries,* 2nd ed. Philadelphia, WB Saunders, 1953, p 32.)

b. **Diagnosis.** Patients may experience localized back or radicular pain, followed by prickling or burning sensations and progressive weakness in the legs. Bowel and bladder disturbances are usually present.

c. **Therapy. Corticosteroid treatment** is often advocated but is of unproven value.

3. **Anterior spinal artery occlusion**

a. **Etiology.** Blockage of a radicular artery to the spinal cord can cause an ischemic infarction.

(1) In many cases, the **artery of Adamkiewicz,** a branch of the aorta supplying the anterior two thirds of the lumbar spinal cord, is compromised.

(2) Thrombosis can be caused by aortic dissection, local atherosclerosis, vasculitis, and hyperviscosity.

b. **Diagnosis.** Patients present with flaccid, hyporeflexic paraplegia; impaired lower extremity pain and temperature sensation; and compromised bladder and bowel function. However, position and vibration senses are usually preserved.

c. **Therapy.** Treatment of the disease responsible for the spinal cord infarction.

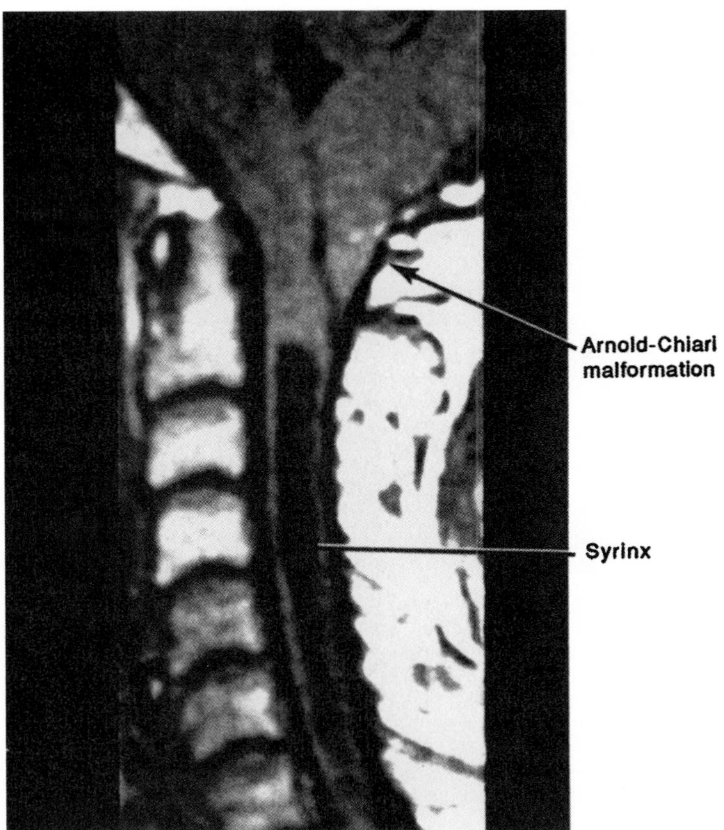

FIGURE 11–6 Nonenhanced T_1-weighted magnetic resonance imaging (MRI) scan demonstrating syringomyelia and an associated Arnold-Chiari malformation.

XIII NEUROPATHY

A Classification Neuropathies may be classified by:

1. **Course** (acute, subacute, or chronic)
2. **Type of symptoms and signs** (sensory, motor, autonomic, or any combination of the three)
3. **Presence of pain** (hyperesthesia or dysesthesia)
4. **Distribution** (generalized, focal, or multifocal)
5. **NCV/EMG features** (disruption of the axon, myelin sheath, or both)

B Etiology Selected causes of neuropathy are listed in Tables 11–10A and 11–10B.

C Therapy Control of the underlying disease process is critical.

1. If impaired sensation renders the patient prone to injury, protective measures should be taken.
2. Weakness (e.g., wrist or foot drops) calls for appropriate splinting and physical therapy.
3. Autonomic insufficiency is difficult to manage; orthostatic hypotension can be treated with agents that expand blood volume (e.g., fludrocortisone) and increase vascular tone (e.g., midodrine).
4. Tricyclic antidepressants, carbamazepine, phenytoin, and gabapentin, can help patients suffering from pain.

TABLE 11–10A Selected Types and Causes of Neuropathy

Neuropathy	Causes: Acute	Causes: Subacute or Chronic	
Sensory neuropathy		Diabetes mellitus Uremia Alcohol abuse Deficiencies Vitamins B_1, B_6, B_{12}, niacin HIV Hereditary neuropathies Drugs Vinca alkaloids Cisplatin Phenytoin 2′,3′-dideoxycytidine	Toxins Vitamin B_6 intoxication Sjögren's syndrome* Paraneoplastic (anti-Hu antibody)* Paraproteinemia Cryoglobulinemia Amyloidosis Leprosy
Motor neuropathy	Guillain-Barré syndrome Diabetes mellitus (proximal ischemic neuropathy) Critical illness polyneuropathy Porphyria	CIDP Lead intoxication Multifocal motor neuropathy Antibodies to GM_1 Charcot-Marie-Tooth disease	
Sensorimotor neuropathy		Diabetes mellitus Uremia Critical illness polyneuropathy Vasculitis Hypothyroidism Lyme disease Paraproteinemia† Cryoglobulinemia Paraneoplastic Drugs Toxins	CIDP/DADS† Charcot-Marie-Tooth disease Other hereditary neuropathies Metachromatic leukodystrophy Refsum disease Adrenomyeloneuropathy Lipoprotein deficiencies Sarcoidosis
Autonomic neuropathy	Guillain-Barré syndrome Porphyria	Diabetes mellitus Amyloidosis Familial dysautonomia	HIV Vincristine

HIV = human immunodeficiency virus; CIDP = chronic inflammatory demyelinating polyneuropathy; DADS = distal acquired demyelinating symmetric neuropathy.
*Also, sensory neuronopathy.
†Including myelin-associated glycoprotein (MAG) antibody and monoclonal gammopathy.

D Selected syndromes

1. **Compression neuropathies**
   a. **Pathophysiology**
      (1) Nerves can be damaged by repeated wear against firm surfaces, typically bone or fibrous tissue. Motor and sensory loss develop, referent to the affected nerve.
      (2) Common sites of compression leading to focal nerve dysfunction include the **median nerve** at the wrist (carpal tunnel), the **ulnar nerve** at the elbow, the **peroneal nerve** at the fibula head, and the **tibial nerve** at the ankle (tarsal tunnel).
   b. **Etiology.** The **carpal tunnel syndrome** can result from repetitive wrist movements, trauma, carpal tunnel stenosis, arthritides (rheumatoid arthritis and crystal-induced synovitis), dia-

TABLE 11–10B Selected Types and Causes of Neuropathy Classified by Other Features

Neuropathy	Causes
Dysesthetic neuropathy	Diabetes mellitus Alcohol abuse HIV 2′,3′-dideoxycytidine Vasculitis
Axonal neuropathy	Diabetes mellitus Uremia Drugs and toxins Critical illness polyneuropathy Vasculitis Paraproteinemia Cryoglobulinemia Vitamin B_{12} deficiency Hereditary neuropathies
Demyelinating neuropathy	Guillain-Barré syndrome CIDP Paraproteinemia* Hereditary neuropathies
Multifocal (mononeuritis multiplex) neuropathy	Diabetes mellitus Vasculitis Lyme disease Leprosy Sarcoidosis Hereditary liability to pressure palsy Malignant infiltrates

HIV = human immunodeficiency virus; CIDP = chronic inflammatory demyelinating polyneuropathy.
*Including myelin-associated glycoprotein (MAG) antibody and monoclonal gammopathy.

betes mellitus, myxedema, pregnancy, birth control pills, acromegaly, and infiltrative processes such as amyloidosis.

c. **Diagnosis.** An NCV study reveals a "conduction block" at the site of injury because of focal demyelination. If compression is severe, evidence of axonal injury may appear (e.g., muscle wasting, denervation on the EMG).

d. **Therapy. Treatment of underlying conditions** is important. Splinting often alleviates the condition, especially if aggravating maneuvers can be eliminated. Local corticosteroid injections may be beneficial. **Surgical decompression** of the nerve is necessary at times.

2. **Guillain-Barré syndrome**
   a. **Definition and etiology.** Guillain-Barré syndrome is a predominantly demyelinating motor polyneuropathy that usually occurs in otherwise healthy individuals. The illness can follow a nonspecific viral syndrome or be associated with HIV infection, *Campylobacter jejuni* infection, hepatitis, infectious mononucleosis, *Mycoplasma pneumoniae* infection, vaccination, surgery, lymphoma, or SLE.
   b. **Diagnosis**
      (1) **Clinical signs**
         (a) Classically, patients present with **foot** and **leg weakness** that ascends to involve other regions of the body; weakness can, however, begin in the arms or face. Progression of the disease should not extend beyond 4 weeks.
         (b) **Generalized paralysis** can develop gradually or relatively acutely, impeding respiratory function.

(c) Relatively minor sensory signs and symptoms occur; however, patients may complain of painful extremities.

(d) The **autonomic nervous system** is often involved. Involvement of the autonomic nervous system can lead to early mortality as a result of **cardiac arrhythmias** and **wide swings in blood pressure.**

(2) **Diagnostic studies**

(a) **Examination of the CSF** shows an elevated protein and less than 50 mononuclear cells/mm^3 (albuminocytologic dissociation).

(b) The motor NCV may be slowed.

(c) An abnormally small compound muscle action potential amplitude obtained with distal stimulation of a peripheral nerve (a measure of the integrity of the most distal parts of the axonal portion of the nerve) is associated with a poor prognosis.

c. **Therapy**

(1) **Plasmapheresis** can shorten the length of time that patients are dependent on a respirator and unable to ambulate. Criteria to initiate plasmapheresis include the inability to walk or rapid progression of the disease.

(2) **Intravenous immunoglobulin treatment** is also efficacious and is better tolerated than plasmapheresis.

3. **Diabetic neuropathy** (see also Chapter 9 IV A 7 d). Diabetes mellitus causes several neuropathic syndromes. The nerve injury may be secondary to chronic hypoxia (related to microvascular disease) that leads to axonal damage.

a. **Types**

(1) A predominantly sensory, distal, symmetric, small fiber polyneuropathy can be dysesthetic and involve pain and temperature modalities more than vibration and position senses.

(2) A predominantly sensory, distal, symmetric, large-fiber polyneuropathy may occur, affecting vibration and position modalities.

(3) A sensorimotor neuropathy can develop.

(4) An autonomic neuropathy or a mononeuropathy or mononeuritis multiplex can occur.

(5) Proximal diabetic neuropathy represents injury to large nerves that causes weakness and pain; it commonly involves the lumbosacral plexus.

b. **Therapy.** As a group, patients with better blood glucose control have a less severe polyneuropathy. However, in individual patients, symptoms usually do not respond to tighter blood glucose control.

4. **Chronic inflammatory demyelinating polyneuropathy (CIDP).** This condition, which can be idiopathic or associated with a monoclonal gammopathy, causes sensorimotor neuropathy. Antimyelin-associated glycoprotein antibodies may be detected or there may be an IgM monoclonal gammopathy. Several variants of CIDP have been defined based on characteristic clinical presentations, associated monoclonal proteins or antibodies, and response to therapy.

a. **Diagnosis.** NCV studies indicate slowing, and the CSF total protein is elevated.

b. **Therapy.** CIDP is responsive to corticosteroid therapy, plasmapheresis, and intravenous immunoglobulin administration, as well as several immunosuppressant drugs.

XIV DISORDERS OF THE NEUROMUSCULAR JUNCTION

A Myasthenia gravis

1. **Etiology.** Antibodies directed against the acetylcholine receptor on the muscle surface cause an increased rate of receptor destruction and lead to weakness.

2. **Diagnosis**

a. **Clinical signs.** Patients are often young women or older men. Complaints of double vision, difficulty swallowing and speaking, and limb weakness and fatigue are common. A thymoma is present in 10%–25% of patients.

b. **Diagnostic studies**
   (1) Administration of **intravenous edrophonium** (a cholinesterase inhibitor) usually produces a transient improvement in strength in patients suffering from myasthenia gravis. Patients with respiratory compromise or excessive oral secretions should not be given edrophonium because they may be unable to compensate for the increase in secretions that occurs after administration of this agent.
   (2) **Repetitive nerve stimulation studies** can demonstrate a decremental response of the motor unit action potential voltage.
   (3) **Acetylcholine receptor antibodies** can be detected in the blood of 80%–90% of patients.
   (4) A **thoracic CT** or **MRI scan** shows a thymoma, if present.

3. **Therapy**
   a. The mainstay of therapy is **administration** of a **cholinesterase inhibitor** (e.g., pyridostigmine).
   b. **Thymectomy** can often lead to improvement; the presence of a thymoma is a definite indication for surgery.
   c. **Corticosteroids, immunosuppressive agents, intravenous immunoglobulin,** or **plasmapheresis** are effective in patients with refractory disease.

B Eaton-Lambert myasthenic syndrome

1. **Pathophysiology.** This syndrome results when antibodies directed against the calcium channels on the presynaptic membrane of the neuromuscular junction interfere with the calcium-mediated release of acetylcholine vesicles in response to nerve stimulation. This syndrome is often associated with an underlying malignancy, especially small-cell carcinoma of the lung.

2. **Diagnosis**
   a. **Clinical signs.** Patients complain of weakness and fatigue, have diminished muscle stretch reflexes, and may have impaired autonomic function, leading to dry mouth and poor visual accommodation.
   b. **Diagnostic studies.** Repetitive nerve stimulation studies show an incremental response of the motor action potential voltage.

3. **Therapy.** Diaminopyridine, plasmapheresis, intravenous immunoglobulin, or immunosuppressive therapy may be helpful.

XV DISORDERS OF MUSCLE

A Muscular dystrophies

1. **Types of muscular dystrophies**
   a. **Duchenne muscular dystrophy** (**DMD**) is an X-linked recessive disorder caused by a defect in the dystrophin gene, which codes for a muscle membrane protein, dystrophin, that is not detectable in patients with DMD.
      (1) Although distal muscles are eventually affected as well, patients experience initial progressive proximal muscular weakness.
      (2) **Prednisone treatment** slows progression of weakness.
      (3) **Death** usually occurs in the third decade of life, often as a result of pneumonia.
   b. **Becker's muscular dystrophy** (**BMD**) is an X-linked recessive disorder of muscle caused by a defect in the dystrophin gene, which codes for a muscle protein, dystrophin, that is altered or present in reduced quantity in BMD. Patients with BMD have a **more benign course than those with DMD, with a 50%** survival rate beyond age 50.
   c. **Myotonic muscular dystrophy** is an autosomal dominant disorder localized to a gene, myotonin-protein kinase, located on chromosome 19. Patients with myotonic dystrophy have an increased number of CTG trinucleotide repeats in the kinase gene. The severity of the disease can increase in successive generations, and the CTG repeats increase proportionately (a phenomenon known as "anticipation").

(1) **Clinical signs** include a characteristic muscle myotonia (i.e., persistent muscle activity in response to contraction or percussion), distal weakness, cataracts, frontal balding, impaired intellect, hypersomnia, testicular atrophy, cardiomyopathy, mitral valve prolapse, and cardiac conduction defects.

(2) **Death** occurs in the fifth or sixth decade and typically is attributable to respiratory compromise or cardiac arrhythmia.

d. **Facioscapulohumeral muscular dystrophy** is an autosomal dominant disorder characterized by progressive weakness about the face, neck, upper torso, and proximal arms. The responsible gene is located on chromosome 4.

e. **Limb-girdle muscular dystrophy** is actually a group of autosomal dominant and recessive disorders characterized by progressive loss of motor strength of the trunk and proximal limbs.

(1) The disorder represents a group of conditions with different genotypic origins and similar phenotype.

(2) Some patients have a disorder of dystrophin. A mutation in the adhalin gene (which produces adhalin, a component of the muscle membrane dystrophin–glycoprotein complex) and other sarcolemmal protein genes can also cause the phenotypic appearance of limb-girdle muscular dystrophy.

2. **Diagnosis.** Patients typically have an **elevated serum CK level. EMG** demonstrates a "myopathic" pattern (i.e., brief, small amplitude muscle potentials). A **muscle biopsy** is often informative. **Genetic studies** are increasingly pursued.

B Acquired myopathy

1. **Etiology.** Muscle disease can be caused by inflammatory, toxic, or metabolic processes (Table 11–11).

2. **Diagnosis**

a. **Clinical signs.** A patient history and examination may provide clues to the diagnosis.

(1) Weakness is usually proximal and symmetric. Disease onset can be acute, subacute, or chronic.

(2) Swallowing and breathing can be compromised, and myoglobinuria may result from rapid muscle destruction, leading to renal insufficiency.

b. **Diagnostic studies.** The serum CK level may be elevated. The EMG reveals a "myopathic" pattern. A muscle biopsy is often informative.

TABLE 11–11 Selected Causes of Acquired Myopathy

Polymyositis
- Idiopathic
- Associated with other connective tissue diseases, infectious agents (including HIV), and drugs

Dermatomyositis
- Associated with malignancy

Inclusion body myositis

Electrolyte disorders
- Hypokalemia
- Hyperkalemia
- Hypercalcemia
- Hypomagnesemia
- Hypophosphatemia

Endocrine disorders
- Hypothyroidism
- Hyperthyroidism
- Cushing's disease and iatrogenic corticosteroid administration
- Addison's disease
- Acromegaly

Drugs (e.g., "statins" ϵ-aminocaproic acid, procainamide, zidovudine, phencyclidine, L-tryptophan)

HIV = human immunodeficiency virus.

3. **Selected syndromes**
   a. **Corticosteroid myopathy** is usually caused by chronic corticosteroid therapy and is associated with proximal muscle weakness and wasting. The serum CK level is normal, and the EMG is usually unremarkable.
   b. With **polymyositis,** the associated infiltration of lymphocytes destroys muscle fiber (see Chapter 10 IX D).
   c. **Inclusion body myositis** is an inflammatory myopathy characterized by a resistance to corticosteroid therapy and by distal and proximal weakness that may be asymmetric.
      (1) **Diagnosis.** Muscle biopsy demonstrates inflammation and inclusion bodies (including "rimmed vacuoles") that contain amyloid. Cytotoxic T (Tc) cells are active against a muscle antigen.
      (2) **Therapy.** There is **no accepted treatment.**
   d. **Polymyalgia rheumatica (PMR)** is not a myopathy but can masquerade as one.
      (1) **Clinical signs**
         (a) Patients often appear weak, but the major symptom is **painful (tender, aching,** and **stiff) muscles.**
         (b) Activities such as ascending stairs may be difficult to perform. On formal strength testing, patients may appear slightly weak, presumably because the pain prevents maximal effort. It has been found that if the pain can be relieved, strength is preserved.
         (c) **Temporal (giant cell) arteritis** is present in 15%–20% of patients.
      (2) **Diagnostic studies.** The erythrocyte sedimentation rate usually is significantly elevated but may be normal. The serum CK level is normal, and the EMG is unremarkable. Muscle histology is normal; biopsy is usually not performed.
      (3) **Therapy. NSAID or corticosteroid therapy** should bring about a rapid resolution of symptoms.

C **Nondystrophic myotonias (channelopathies)** are characterized by prolonged muscle relaxation after voluntary contraction or mechanical stimulation.

1. **Clinical signs.** Table 11–12 summarizes the clinical features of the nondystrophic myotonias.
2. **Therapy.** Treatment includes the use of quinine, procainamide, and phenytoin.

TABLE 11–12 Clinical Features of the Nondystrophic Myotonias

Feature	Sodium Channel Diseases		Chloride Channel Diseases: MYOTONIA CONGENITA	
	HYPERKALEMIC PERIODIC PARALYSIS	PARAMYOTONIA CONGENITA	THOMPSEN'S	BECKER'S
Periodic paralysis	Yes	Yes	No	Yes
Potassium-induced weakness	Yes	In some families	No	No
Cold-induced weakness	No	Yes	No	No
Paradoxical myotonia	Occasional	Yes	No	No
Progressive weakness	Variable	Variable	No	Rare
Systemic involvement	No	No	No	No
Genetic transmission/chromosome locus	AD/17	AD/17	AD/7	AR/7

Adapted from Ptacek LJ, Johnson KJ, Griggs RC: Genetics and physiology of the myotonic muscle disorders. *N Engl J Med* 1993;328(7):483.
AD = autosomal dominant; AR = Autosomal recessive.

D **Metabolic myopathies** include disorders of carbohydrate and lipid metabolism.

E **Myoglobinuria** can be caused by crush injuries, vascular occlusions, infection, toxins, drugs, metabolic myopathies, hyperthermia, and severe inflammation.

1. **Diagnosis** is aided by documenting an elevated serum CK level and urinary myoglobin. The latter can be suspected on the finding of dark (brownish) urine and a positive dipstick for blood along with a paradoxical absence of RBCs in the urine.
2. **Therapy** should be directed at the underlying cause. Patients must be kept vigorously hydrated to prevent kidney damage.

F **Acute quadriplegic myopathy** can develop as a complication of critical illness and the systemic inflammatory response syndrome. There is an association with the use of corticosteroids and nondepolarizing neuromuscular blocking agents. Treatment is supportive.

XVI INFECTION

A **Meningitis, encephalitis, and neurologic complaints associated with HIV infection** are discussed in Chapter 8.

B **Brain abscess**

1. **Etiology.** An abscess can occur after neurosurgery or penetrating head trauma, in association with otitis media or poor oral hygiene, in patients with a bacteremia, and in individuals with a pulmonary arteriovenous malformation or cardiac right-to-left shunt.
2. **Diagnosis**
   a. **Clinical signs.** Patients may present with headache, seizures, an altered sensorium, and focal neurologic symptoms and signs.
   b. **Diagnostic studies. CT** or **MRI scanning** can easily detect a brain abscess, although differentiation from a neoplastic lesion can be difficult.
3. **Therapy.** Empiric treatment should be directed against aerobic and microaerophilic gram-positive streptococci and anaerobes, including *Bacteroides fragilis.*
   a. **Antibiotic therapy** often includes penicillin, chloramphenicol, metronidazole, and cefotaxime or trimethoprim–sulfamethoxazole. The clinical setting can help define the most likely pathogen.
   b. Therapy is monitored by serial brain imaging techniques.
   c. Often, **surgical excision** of the abscess **can be avoided. Stereotactic biopsy and drainage of an abscess** occasionally is required.

C **A spinal epidural abscess** is usually caused by hematogenous seeding of an infective organism and is characterized by local pain and tenderness, fever, and neurologic signs and symptoms appropriate to the site of the infection.

1. **Diagnosis** can be aided by **spinal MRI** or **CT scans** and **myelography.**
2. **Surgical drainage** is indicated along with **antibiotic therapy.**

D **Neurosyphilis**

1. **Stages and clinical signs**
   a. **Asymptomatic disease.** CSF abnormalities may be the only sign of infection.
   b. **Acute syphilitic meningitis** usually develops within 2 years of primary infection. Headache, meningismus, hydrocephalus, and cranial nerve palsies can occur.
   c. **Cerebrovascular (meningovascular) syphilis** manifests months to years after primary infection. Affected patients present with ischemic strokes (often associated with headache) and behavioral abnormalities.

d. **General paresis** develops one to two decades after primary infection and is characterized by a progressive dementia.
e. **Tabes dorsalis** also manifests 10–20 years after primary infection with lightning pains, paresthesias, bladder dysfunction, gait instability, Argyll Robertson pupils (i.e., impaired pupillary light reaction with preserved pupillary constriction to accommodation, perhaps as a result of a midbrain tegmental lesion), areflexia (especially at the ankles), and loss of position and vibration sensibility.

2. **Diagnostic studies.** Patients with HIV infection are at particular risk for neurosyphilis.
   a. Almost all patients with neurosyphilis have a **reactive serum fluorescent treponemal antibody (FTA-ABS) test.** Patients with a nonreactive CSF FTA-ABS test do not have neurosyphilis.
   b. The **CSF VDRL** test is often reactive in neurosyphilis, but a nonreactive CSF VDRL test is found in 25% of patients with neurologic disease years removed from the primary infection.
   c. **Other CSF findings** include a predominantly mononuclear pleocytosis and an elevated protein and IgG index.
3. **Therapy.** Penicillin is the treatment of choice for neurosyphilis. Patients with concurrent HIV infection develop neurosyphilis earlier and may be more resistant to therapy than immunocompetent patients.

XVII PRIMARY CNS TUMORS

Although these tumors are relatively uncommon, they seem to be increasing in incidence.

A Astrocytic neoplasms

1. Astrocytomas are neoplasms with slight hypercellularity and pleomorphism. **Anaplastic astrocytomas** are characterized as having moderate cellularity and pleomorphism and some vascular proliferation.
   a. **Clinical signs.** Patients with astrocytomas and anaplastic astrocytomas typically present with focal hemispheric neurologic dysfunction, convulsions, or headache.
   b. **Therapy.** Anaplastic astrocytomas can be treated with **surgery** and **radiotherapy. Chemotherapy** may be helpful.
   c. **Prognosis.** Outcome is inversely related to the patient's age and the presence of tumor necrosis. The survival rate after 2 years is 38%–50%. Other predictors of outcome include the patient's functional status and the amount of residual tumor after initial surgery.
2. **Glioblastoma multiforme** has moderate-to-marked hypercellularity, pleomorphism, and necrosis; vascular proliferation may be present.
   a. **Clinical signs.** Clinical features are similar to those of less aggressive tumors. CT or MRI scans typically show an enhancing, irregular mass (Figure 11–7).
   b. **Therapy.** Treatment includes **corticosteroid therapy** (for edema reduction), **surgical debulking, radiation therapy,** and **chemotherapy,** both systemically or locally administered.
   c. **Prognosis.** The prognosis of glioblastoma multiforme is **poor,** with a survival rate of 10% after 24 months.

B Oligodendrogliomas

1. **Clinical signs.** Patients with these infiltrating tumors commonly present with headache and convulsions; focal neurologic deficits can develop.
2. **Therapy.** Anaplastic oligodendrogliomas seem to be responsive to **radiation therapy** and **chemotherapy. Surgery** is the mainstay of treatment.
3. **Prognosis.** The overall median length of survival is 53 months.

C Meningiomas are tumors that arise from the meninges and slowly enlarge, causing a mass effect that displaces normal structures. Angioblastic meningiomas are locally invasive.

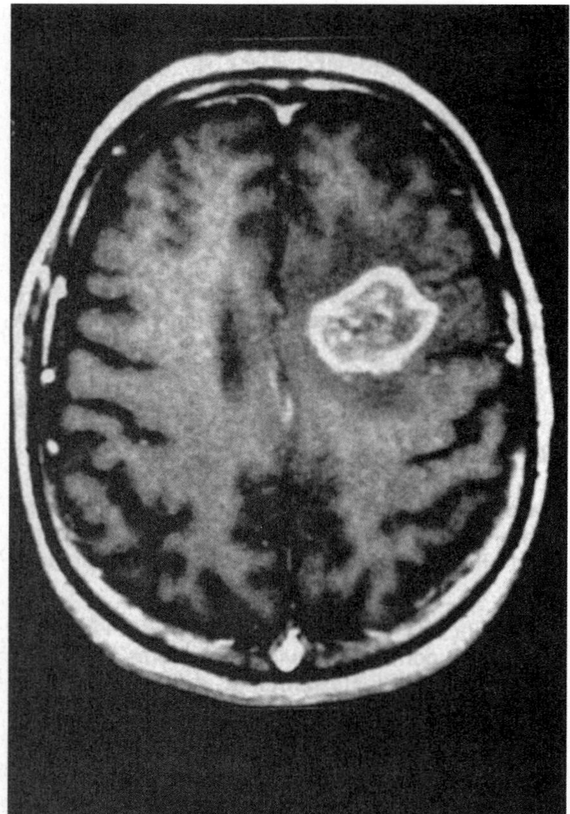

FIGURE 11–7 An enhanced T_1-weighted magnetic resonance imaging (MRI) scan demonstrating a glioblastoma multiforme.

1. **Clinical signs.** Headache, seizures, and focal neurologic signs can occur.
2. **Therapy.** Treatment is **surgical resection; radiation therapy** can be used for invasive tumors.
3. **Prognosis.** If the entire tumor can be surgically resected, the majority of patients do well. If the entire tumor cannot be removed, the patient may experience recurrence of symptoms.

D **Schwannomas** of the eighth cranial nerve (acoustic neuroma) typically arise from the vestibular component of the nerve. They can enlarge and displace structures about the cerebellopontine angle.

1. **Clinical signs.** Patients develop dizziness, hearing loss, and tinnitus. A diminished corneal reflex may be a sign of trigeminal nerve compromise by an enlarging mass.
2. **Diagnostic studies.** Diagnosis is best made with an enhanced MRI.
3. **Therapy.** Treatment options include **surgical resection or stereotactic radiation therapy.**
4. **Prognosis.** Small tumors can be surgically cured. If residual tumor remains, recurrent symptoms can develop, usually years later.

E **Primary CNS lymphoma** is increasing in incidence, especially in immunocompromised patients. Occasionally, primary CNS lymphoma presents as meningeal lymphomatosis.

1. **Diagnostic studies. Imaging studies** show one or more intensely enhancing lesions, typically in a periventricular distribution. The diagnosis can be established with stereotactic biopsy.
2. **Therapy.** Although initial treatment with corticosteroids can lead to a rapid decrease in the size of the mass, ultimate survival depends on radiation therapy and chemotherapy.

3. **Prognosis.** The development of multimodality treatment protocols has extended patient survival for years, especially in immunocompetent patients.

XVIII HEREDITARY DISORDERS

A Wilson's disease (hepatolenticular degeneration) This autosomal recessive disease is localized to an abnormality of the ATP7B gene on chromosome 13. It is associated with the accumulation of copper in the brain, liver, and other tissues because of a deficiency of the copper-binding protein ceruloplasmin.

1. **Clinical signs.** Presenting signs include hepatic disease, a Kayser-Fleischer ring in Descemet's membrane of the cornea, behavioral problems (including psychosis), movement disorders (e.g., incoordination, tremor, masked facies, dystonia, and athetosis), and hemolytic anemia.
2. **Diagnosis**
   a. Diagnosis is made by finding a low serum ceruloplasmin level, excessive 24-hour urine copper excretion, a Kayser-Fleischer ring on examination with a slit lamp, and increased levels of hepatic copper.
   b. MRI can reveal atrophy of the caudate and putamen with increased signal intensity on T_2-weighted images.
3. **Therapy.** Treatment consists of **copper chelation.**

B Neurofibromatosis (NF)

1. **Neurofibromatosis type 1 (NF 1, von Recklinghausen's disease)** is an autosomal dominant disorder. The responsible gene is located on chromosome 17, and the gene product is neurofibromin.
   a. Patients who meet two or more of the following criteria can be diagnosed as suffering from NF 1.
      (1) **Neurofibromas** (two or more, or one plexiform neurofibroma)
      (2) **Café-au-lait macules** (six or more measuring 1.5 cm in their greatest dimension)
      (3) **Freckling** in the **axillary or inguinal areas**
      (4) **Optic glioma**
      (5) Two or more **iris hamartomas (Lisch nodules)**
      (6) **Sphenoid dysplasia** or **thinning of the cortex of the long bones**
      (7) An **immediate relative** with NF 1
   b. **Complications** of NF 1 include astrocytic tumors, optic glioma, neurofibrosarcoma, compressive peripheral neuropathies, compressive myelopathy, pheochromocytoma, and scoliosis.
   c. **Therapy** is directed at the complications of the disease.
2. **Neurofibromatosis type 2 (NF 2)** is an autosomal dominant disorder localized to chromosome 22 and characterized by bilateral acoustic neurofibromas.

C von Hippel-Lindau disease This autosomal dominant disorder is localized to chromosome 3. **Cerebellar** and **retinal hemangioblastomas** are characteristic.

1. Hemangioblastomas also may be found throughout the CNS. The kidneys, pancreas, and liver can harbor hemangiomas. Pheochromocytomas may develop.
2. Polycythemia is associated with cerebellar hemangioblastoma.

D Osler-Weber-Rendu disease (hereditary hemorrhagic telangiectasia) This autosomal dominant disorder is associated with two genes (HHT 1 and 2). It is characterized by telangiectatic skin lesions, CNS vascular malformations, and pulmonary arteriovenous fistulae. Brain abscesses may occur, as may ischemic stroke, secondary to a paradoxical embolus via a pulmonary arteriovenous fistula.

E Tuberous sclerosis This autosomal dominant disorder is associated with two abnormal genes, TSC1 and TSC2.

1. **Criteria for diagnosis** include multiple facial angiofibromas, ungual fibromas, retinal hamartoma, cortical tubers, subependymal glial nodules (often calcified), and multiple renal angiomyolipomas.
2. **Some associated features** are hypomelanotic macules, a shagreen patch, multicystic kidneys, seizures, and mental retardation. Benign giant cell astrocytomas can develop, often near the foramen of Monro.

F Down syndrome (trisomy 21) This genetic disorder is characterized by mental retardation, epicanthal folds, Brushfield spots on the iris, a transverse palmar crease, and cardiac malformations. By age 50, most patients develop Alzheimer's disease. Myelopathy may develop because of atlantoaxial dislocation.

G Huntington's disease The gene that is responsible for this autosomal dominant disorder, which is localized to chromosome 4, has an excess of trinucleotide repeats and codes the protein huntingtin. Patients develop a progressive cognitive decline and choreoathetosis between 30 and 50 years of age. Depression frequently occurs. Atrophy of the caudate nucleus is characteristic.

H Cerebellar atrophies These conditions are associated with multisystem degenerative processes including abnormal oculomotor function, bulbar wasting and fasciculations, upper motor neuron signs, extrapyramidal dysfunction, cognitive decline, visual loss, and peripheral neuropathy.

1. **Etiology.** These diseases can be transmitted as autosomal dominant or recessive disorders, or they may be sporadic and presumably related to a new mutation.
2. **Types.** Approximately nine autosomal dominant spinocerebellar ataxias have been genetically identified. Most of these ataxias are characterized by an excess number of trinucleotide repeats and are identified as spinocerebellar atrophy type 1 (SCA-1), SCA-2, and so on.
   a. The phenotypic–genotypic correlations are often poor, making it difficult to accurately predict a patient's genotype from clinical evaluation alone.
   b. Molecular genetics will allow further genotypic classification of these disorders.
3. **Associated conditions.** Cerebellar atrophies have been associated phenotypically with deficiencies of glutamate dehydrogenase, pyruvate dehydrogenase complex, and hexosaminidase; vitamin E deficiency; mitochondrial disorders; and elevated very long–chain fatty acids.

I Peroxisome disorders The peroxisome is a cellular organelle that is involved with fatty acid oxidation.

1. **Adrenoleukodystrophy** is an X-linked disorder characterized by progressive intellectual decline, spasticity, and visual loss. **Adrenomyeloneuropathy,** also an X-linked disorder, is characterized by a progressive myelopathy and neuropathy.
   a. White matter changes are visible on CT and MRI scans in adrenoleukodystrophy.
   b. Both conditions result in excessive levels of very long–chain fatty acids in the blood, perhaps as a result of defective β-oxidation.
2. **Refsum disease** is an autosomal recessive disorder characterized by a sensorimotor neuropathy, retinal pigmentation, ataxia, anosmia, hearing loss, skin lesions, and elevated CSF protein.
   a. **Pathophysiology.** There is an excess of phytanic acid in the blood because of a defect in alpha-oxidation of this fatty acid.
   b. **Therapy.** Dietary control of phytanic acid intake and plasmapheresis can help control the neurologic problems.

J Mitochondrial disorders Mitochondrial DNA codes for components of the mitochondrial respiratory chain and oxidative phosphorylation enzymatic complexes. Disorders of mitochondrial DNA are transmitted by nonmendelian, maternal inheritance. The mitochondrial encephalopathies and myopathies have ragged red fibers in muscle. The ragged red fibers represent abundant abnormal mitochondria that are demonstrated by using a modified Gomori trichrome stain. Patients may have sensorineural hearing loss, short stature, or diabetes mellitus and often have elevated blood lactic acid levels.

1. **Kearns-Sayre syndrome** is characterized by progressive external ophthalmoplegia, pigmentary retinopathy, complete heart block, CSF protein levels greater than 100 mg/dL, ataxia, and myopathy. Deletions in the mitochondrial DNA are found.
2. **Myoclonic epilepsy with ragged red fibers (MERRF)** presents with myoclonus, epilepsy, and ataxia. There is a point mutation in the mitochondrial genome.
3. **Mitochondrial encephalomyopathy with lactic acidosis and stroke-like events (MELAS)** is characterized by intermittent vomiting and headaches, recurrent ischemic strokes, and seizures. Point mutations are present in the mitochondrial DNA.
4. **Leber's hereditary optic neuropathy** manifests as subacute bilateral central vision loss with retinal microangiopathy. It is caused by several point mutations in the mitochondrial genome.

XIX TOXIC AND METABOLIC DISORDERS

A Vitamin B_{12} deficiency

This vitamin deficiency results in combined systems degeneration.

1. **Pathophysiology.** Deprivation of vitamin B_{12} leads to demyelination and axonal degeneration, affecting the peripheral nerves, the spinal cord (where the posterior and lateral columns are demyelinated), and the cerebrum.
2. **Diagnosis**
   a. **Clinical signs.** Neurologic manifestations include cognitive impairment, diminished position and vibratory sensation, upper motor neuron signs with abnormal gait, and sensory peripheral neuropathy.
   b. **Diagnosis.** Patients typically have anemia, macrocytosis, and a low vitamin B_{12} level. However, neurologic disease can occur without anemia or macrocytosis. If the diagnosis remains suspect in a patient with a normal or marginally decreased serum vitamin B_{12} level, the finding of elevated serum methylmalonic acid and total homocysteine can confirm the presence of vitamin B_{12} deficiency.
3. **Therapy.** Treatment is administration of **cobalamin.**

B Acute intermittent porphyria

1. **Pathophysiology.** This autosomal dominant disorder is caused by a defect in the activity of uroporphyrinogen I synthetase, which leads to increased activity of Δ-aminolevulinic acid synthetase and elevated levels of Δ-aminolevulinic acid.
2. **Diagnosis.** Acute intermittent porphyria causes delirium, seizures, and autonomic, sensory, and motor neuropathies; a Guillain-Barré–like illness can develop. During an acute attack, the **Watson-Schwartz test** indicates elevated levels of urinary porphobilinogen.
3. **Therapy. Hematin administration** can decrease clinical manifestations. Precipitants such as barbiturates, phenytoin, starvation, and infection should be avoided in susceptible individuals.

C Complications of alcohol abuse

Alcohol may affect the nervous system by itself (i.e., alcohol intoxication, addiction, or withdrawal) or in tandem with a nutritional deficiency.

1. **Complications from intoxication, addiction, and withdrawal**
   a. **Acute alcohol intoxication** causes delirium and incoordination.
      (1) Severe intoxication can lead to metabolic coma with respiratory depression.
      (2) Alcoholic **"blackouts"** are characterized by the inability to form new memories in spite of preservation of consciousness.

b. **Alcohol withdrawal** causes early symptoms of tremulousness and hallucinosis. Delirium tremens is seen during late withdrawal from alcohol. Benzodiazepines may be used to treat alcohol withdrawal symptoms.

c. **Alcohol-related seizures ("rum fits")** are brief, generalized tonic–clonic convulsions that frequently occur in clusters.

(1) Classically, alcohol-related seizures were thought to occur primarily in the 48 hours after withdrawal from chronic alcohol intake. However, alcohol-related seizures also may be caused by chronic alcohol intoxication and represent a toxic effect of alcohol on the brain, not a withdrawal phenomenon.

(2) Typically, patients are alert shortly after the seizure. They do not have seizure discharges on an interictal EEG.

(3) **Therapy** should be directed at the underlying alcohol abuse. Anticonvulsant medications are not indicated for typical alcohol-related seizures.

d. Alcohol abuse is associated with **cerebral atrophy** and **cognitive impairments** and may **predispose patients to stroke.**

e. Alcoholic patients may develop a **myopathy** that is acute or chronic and predominantly affects the proximal muscles. **Rhabdomyolysis** can complicate the acute disorder.

2. **Complications related to nutritional deficiencies**

a. **Wernicke's encephalopathy** is seen in malnourished alcoholic patients who have a **thiamine deficiency.** Other conditions (e.g., hyperemesis, renal dialysis, malnutrition) are associated with thiamine deficiency and can lead to Wernicke's encephalopathy, even in patients who do not abuse alcohol.

(1) **Clinical signs.** Patients typically are delirious and have nystagmus, sixth cranial nerve palsies, and ataxia. Disorders of consciousness and hypothermia can occur.

(2) **Therapy.** Thiamine administration can resolve the acute illness.

b. **Korsakoff psychosis** is a chronic encephalopathy that is seen in alcoholic patients with a thiamine deficiency.

(1) **Clinical signs.** Features include retrograde and anterograde memory deficits, apathy, and impaired problem-solving abilities.

(2) **Therapy.** Patients may not improve with abstinence from alcohol or thiamine administration.

c. **Sensory neuropathy** is caused by alcohol and often leads to dysesthesia. Although this axonal (although some authors suggest demyelinative) neuropathy is probably related to concurrent malnutrition, alcohol itself may be toxic to nerves.

d. **Cerebellar degeneration** may occur in alcoholics. The anterior and superior vermis are particularly affected. Patients have difficulty with gait and stance; nystagmus and arm ataxia are not prominent.

D Drug abuse

1. Use of **cocaine** or **"crack"** can result in seizures, ischemic stroke, subarachnoid and intraparenchymal hemorrhage, and rhabdomyolysis. Hemorrhagic strokes may be associated with an underlying vascular lesion; definition of the vascular anatomy is usually indicated to search for an aneurysm or arteriovenous malformation.

2. Use of **heroin** can cause a metabolic coma; miosis is a characteristic finding in heroin users. Heroin has been associated with rhabdomyolysis, chronic myopathy, transverse myelitis, and peripheral neuropathies.

3. Ingestion of **phencyclidine (PCP)** can cause a wide range of neurologic disturbances ranging from acute psychosis to coma. Nystagmus, miosis, ataxia, myoclonus, dystonic posturing, generalized rigidity, dyskinesias, and seizures can occur.

4. Ingestion of **"ecstasy"** (an amphetamine analog) can cause delirium, hyperthermia, and rhabdomyolysis. This drug selectively damages serotoninergic neurons.

XX SLEEP DISORDERS

A **Narcolepsy** is characterized by hypersomnia with short latency periods for the onset of daytime sleep and the early development of rapid eye movement (REM) sleep. Patients awaken refreshed from sleep attacks.

1. **Etiology.** Narcolepsy is probably an autosomal dominant disorder with variable penetrance; it has been mapped to chromosome 6. The vast majority of patients have antigens for HLA-DR2 and HLA-DQB1.
2. **Clinical signs.** Features include **cataplexy** (i.e., transient episodes of diminished muscle tone), **sleep paralysis,** and **vivid dreams** at the beginning and end of sleep.
3. **Therapy.** Methylphenidate, pemoline, or modafinil can diminish the hypersomnia, and protriptyline or imipramine can decrease cataplexy.

B **Sleep apnea**, or hypoventilation during sleep, can be attributable to obstructive causes (e.g., obesity, a small oropharynx) or to nonobstructive (CNS) causes. Sleep apnea is commonly "mixed" and represents both CNS and obstructive problems.

1. **Clinical signs.** Patients have daytime hypersomnia and can develop nocturnal hypoxia, pulmonary hypertension, and cardiac arrhythmias.
2. **Therapy.** Treatment options include weight loss, continuous positive airway pressure (CPAP), uvulopalatopharyngoplasty (UPPP), tracheostomy, and several new, minimally invasive surgical techniques.

C **Periodic movements in sleep** involve flexor contractions in the legs. Patients can also experience sleep myoclonus and dystonia and restless legs syndrome while awake.

1. **Clinical signs.** Patients are momentarily aroused, and therefore nocturnal sleep quality is poor, leading to daytime hypersomnia.
2. **Therapy.** Treatment options include carbidopa/levodopa combinations, dopamine agonists, gabapentin, opiates, and clonazepam.

XXI TRAUMA

A **Brain injury**

1. A **concussion** is a momentary disruption of brain function after head injury that results in a brief loss of consciousness.
   a. **Clinical signs.** After awakening, patients complain of headache, impaired memory, poor concentration, blurred vision, tinnitus, dizziness, and nausea.
   b. **Duration of symptoms.** Symptoms can persist for days or weeks as the **postconcussion syndrome. Post-traumatic migraine** can develop but may be alleviated by using antimigraine agents.
2. **Severe head trauma** can cause brain contusion, epidural and subdural hematoma, penetrating brain injuries, SAH, and CSF leaks.
   a. **Clinical signs.** Progressive mental status changes leading to coma and focal neurologic signs can develop.
   b. **Diagnostic studies.** Emergent CT scanning can help delineate the extent of the problem.
   c. **Therapy.** Control of ICP and neurosurgical evaluation are indicated as appropriate.
3. A **subdural hematoma** can result from acute head trauma. Patients present with an altered sensorium and focal neurologic findings (e.g., hemiparesis). A subdural hematoma is also associated with minor trauma and can present with subtle subacute or chronic behavioral changes and mild focal deficits. At times, no history of trauma is elicited; this is especially true in elderly patients.
   a. **Diagnostic studies.** A CT scan is very helpful in documenting the presence of a subdural hematoma (Figure 11–8).

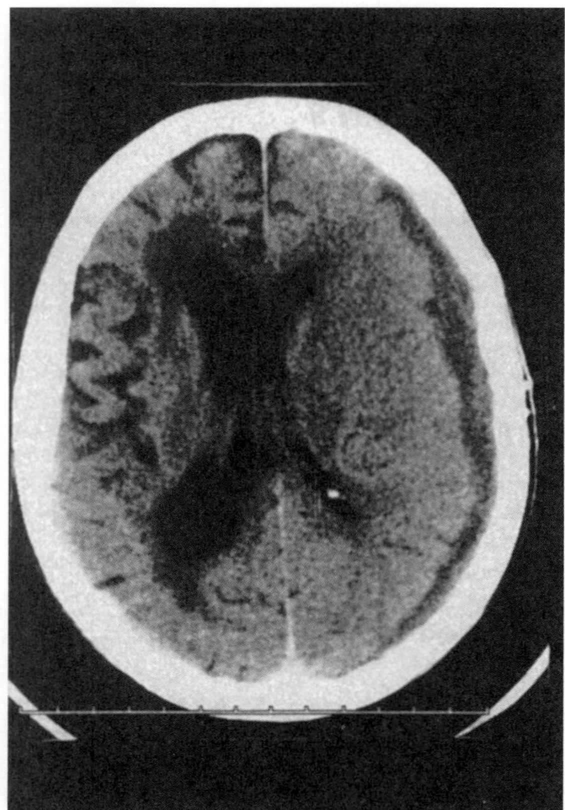

FIGURE 11–8 A nonenhanced computed tomography (CT) scan showing a chronic subdural hematoma. Note the mass effect on the lateral ventricle and the absence of sulci.

b. **Therapy.** Neurosurgical intervention is usually indicated for an acute subdural hematoma; a chronic subdural hematoma may not require surgery.

B **Spinal cord injury** can result in an acute paraparesis or quadriparesis. A central cord syndrome, which can follow a hyperextension injury to the cervical spinal cord, is characterized by lower motor neuron dysfunction affecting the cervical myotomes, mild sensory loss in the arms, and a myelopathy.

1. **Diagnostic studies.** Because the vertebral column may not be stable, patients should be immobilized while a radiographic assessment is made.
2. **Therapy.** High-dose methylprednisolone therapy given within 8 hours of injury can improve outcome.

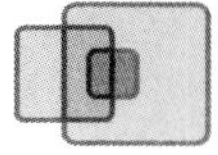

Study Questions

1. A 70-year-old man, a retired professor, complains of weakness and fatigue. Any physical activity is an effort, and he cannot find a comfortable position at rest. He has lost 5 pounds over the past month. Physical examination is normal. Which of the following diagnoses is most likely?

- A Depression
- B Hypokalemia
- C Temporal (giant cell) arteritis
- D Polymyalgia rheumatica (PMR)
- E Polymyositis

2. A 29-year-old woman suddenly develops a left hemiparesis. The patient experienced a deep venous thrombosis in her right leg 3 years ago. Which of the following conditions is the most likely cause of this patient's deficit?

- A Nonvalvular atrial fibrillation
- B Lupus anticoagulant
- C Mitral valve prolapse
- D Multiple sclerosis (MS)
- E Astrocytoma

3. An assembly-line worker complains of awakening at night with right-hand discomfort that resolves after several minutes. After 3 weeks of continuing symptoms, he seeks medical advice. Examination discloses mild weakness of thumb abduction and diminished pain sensibility on the palmar aspect of the thumb and index finger. Which of the following diagnoses is most likely?

- A Carpal tunnel syndrome
- B Cervical radiculopathy
- C Reflex sympathetic dystrophy
- D Tendinitis
- E Left middle cerebral artery ischemic attacks

4. A 32-year-old woman complains that she has had difficulty walking for the past week. Examination indicates leg weakness, and to a lesser extent, arm weakness and areflexia. The patient is unable to walk across the room. Which of the following medications would be the best treatment?

- A Corticosteroids
- B Penicillin
- C Phenytoin
- D Levodopa
- E Intravenous immunoglobulin (Ig)

5. A 73-year-old woman presents with a 6-month history of deteriorating gait and low back discomfort, which is exacerbated by walking. Examination is unremarkable except for hypoactive muscle stretch reflexes in the legs. Radiographs of the lumbosacral area show the expected degenerative changes associated with a woman of her age. Which of the following diagnoses is most likely?

- A Acute lumbar disk herniation
- B Lumbar stenosis
- C Myopathy
- D Normal pressure hydrocephalus (NPH)
- E Cervical stenosis

6. A 45-year-old right-handed man complains that he has had difficulty holding and using a writing instrument for the past year. He notes the development of right-hand and forearm spasms only when writing. Physical examination is unremarkable. Which of the following diagnoses is most likely?

A Parkinson's disease
B Focal dystonia
C Carpal tunnel syndrome
D Cervical radiculopathy
E Benign essential tremor

7. A previously healthy, 68-year-old woman develops auditory hallucinations. She cannot provide many details but believes her mother is speaking to her. She has difficulty cooperating during the interview and physical examination, which is unremarkable. Which of the following diagnoses is most likely?

A Complex partial seizures
B Adverse medication effect
C Alzheimer's disease
D Hyperthyroidism
E Peduncular hallucinosis

8. A 24-year-old construction worker with a 2-year history of low back pain complains of an acute onset of bilateral leg weakness and incontinence. Which of the following treatments would be the best management tactic?

A Administration of nonsteroidal anti-inflammatory drugs (NSAIDs)
B Emergency surgery
C Strict bed rest
D Lumbar traction
E Back exercises

9. A 32-year-old man presents with repetitive generalized motor convulsions that continue for 35 minutes until 2 mg of lorazepam are administered intravenously. The next course of action should be to administer which of the following?

A Phenytoin intravenously
B Carbamazepine orally
C Pentobarbital intravenously
D Ethosuximide orally
E Diazepam rectally

10. A 78-year-old woman complains of experiencing headaches and progressive confusion for the past month. She has a left hemianopia and cannot dress herself. A computed tomography (CT) scan demonstrates a large, irregularly enhancing mass in the right parietal lobe. There is no obvious systemic disease. Which of the following diagnoses is most likely?

A Brain abscess
B Glioblastoma multiforme
C Meningioma
D Metastasis
E Central nervous system (CNS) lymphoma

11. A 63-year-old woman develops intermittent dizziness. Examination shows a diminished right corneal reflex and mild hearing loss in the right ear. Which of the following diagnoses is most likely?

A Cerebellopontine angle tumor
B Benign paroxysmal positional vertigo (BPPV)
C Lateral medullary syndrome
D Meniere's disease
E Pontine infarction

12. A previously vigorous 80-year-old woman collapses when getting out of bed. Examination of her legs indicates bilateral weakness, loss of pain and temperature sensation, and areflexia. Her bladder is distended. The remainder of the examination is unremarkable. Which of the following diagnoses is most likely?

A Guillain-Barré syndrome
B Anterior cerebral artery occlusion
C Cauda equina syndrome
D Anterior spinal artery occlusion
E Thoracic spinal cord compression

13. A 70-year-old man reports that over the past 2 months, he has had progressive difficulty walking. Examination indicates distal (greater than proximal) weakness in the arms and legs and the absence of muscle stretch reflexes. Motor nerve conduction velocities (NCVs) are slowed. Which of the following diagnoses is most likely?

A Guillain-Barré syndrome
B Lead poisoning
C Chronic inflammatory demyelinating polyneuropathy (CIDP)
D Amyotrophic lateral sclerosis (ALS)
E Polymyositis

14. A 56-year-old man presents with a 2-year history of impotence and not feeling "right." Examination reveals masked facies, bradykinesia, rigidity, mild ataxia, and postural hypotension. The diagnosis is which of the following?

A Parkinson's disease
B Combined systems degeneration
C Multiple systems atrophy
D Spinocerebellar degeneration
E Vitamin E deficiency

15. A patient with a subarachnoid hemorrhage (SAH) caused by a right anterior communicating artery aneurysm undergoes successful surgery 2 days after the hemorrhage. Three days later, right arm weakness develops. Which of the following diagnoses is most likely?

A Hydrocephalus
B Meningitis
C Repeat hemorrhage
D Vasospasm
E Hyponatremia

16. A 17-year-old high school varsity diver develops a headache, dizziness, left-sided arm and leg clumsiness, and loss of pain and temperature sensation in the left facial and right body areas after a practice session. Which of the following diagnoses is most likely?

A Benign paroxysmal positional vertigo (BPPV)
B Multiple sclerosis (MS)
C Vertebral artery dissection

- D Astrocytoma
- E Labyrinthitis
- F Migraine with aura

17. A 26-year-old woman presents with recurrent throbbing headaches accompanied by nausea, emesis, photophobia, and sonophobia. She has been treating herself with acetaminophen and ice packs to her forehead. A reasonable therapeutic intervention might be to prescribe:

- A Baclofen
- B Amitriptyline
- C Indomethacin
- D Corticosteroids
- E Sumatriptan

18. A 76-year-old woman has been suffering from left temporal headaches for the prior 3 weeks. Over the prior 2 days she has had several brief episodes of cloudy vision in her left eye. On questioning, she notes a 5-pound weight loss over the past 2 weeks, which she attributes to discomfort when chewing. Therapy should be initiated with:

- A Baclofen
- B Amitriptyline
- C Indomethacin
- D Corticosteroids
- E Sumatriptan

19. A 57-year-old man has a 2-month history of severe, daily headaches that involve the right frontotemporoparietal area. The headaches typically last 60 to 90 minutes and occur once or twice daily. Over-the-counter medications have not provided relief. Chiropractic manipulation did not help. The patient is desperate for relief because he cannot work during the headache episodes. A reasonable treatment strategy is to initiate:

- A Baclofen
- B Amitriptyline
- C Indomethacin
- D Corticosteroids
- E Sumatriptan

20. A 53-year-old woman with the sudden onset of the worst headache of her life presents to the emergency department. She has a history of migraine but states that the current headache is not like her usual headaches. Results of her physical examination are unremarkable. The initial preferred diagnostic test is a:

- A Angiogram
- B CT scan
- C TCD
- D MRI
- E MR angiogram

21. A 78-year-old man with a history of type 1 (insulin-dependent) diabetes mellitus, hypertension, hypercholesterolemia, and remote smoking presents with the acute onset of aphasia. On examination, he has trouble expressing himself and has mild right facial and arm weakness. There is a left carotid bruit. The most definitive strategy for secondary stroke prevention will likely be:

- A Acute heparin administration followed by warfarin
- B Extracranial intracranial bypass surgery

C Warfarin and aspirin combined therapy
D Carotid endarterectomy
E Aspirin monotherapy

22. A 32-year-old woman who is 1 week postpartum presents with progressive headache and confusion. On examination she is afebrile with a blood pressure of 110/65 mm Hg. Papilledema is noted. The most likely diagnosis is:

A Pseudotumor cerebri
B Pituitary apoplexy
C Bacterial meningitis
D Sagittal sinus thrombosis
E Eclampsia

23. A 67-year-old woman with a history of hypertension, diabetes mellitus, and smoking presents to the emergency department at 8:30 AM with a mild expressive aphasia, right facial weakness, and mild right arm weakness. She had awakened at 7:00 AM and was speaking to her husband when her speech suddenly became difficult and weakness was noted. Her husband called 911, and she was transported to the hospital, where her blood pressure was 165/85 mm Hg. The preferred treatment is:

A Aspirin
B Heparin
C Warfain
D rt-PA
E Clopidogrel

24. A 62-year-old woman has a 2-month history of mild confusion. She occasionally has difficulty following a conversation. On the morning of presentation to the hospital, she developed 30 seconds of right face and arm twitching, followed by increased confusion. Examination shows difficulties in speech comprehension and a subtle right homonymous hemianopia. A brain CT scan shows a 2 × 3-cm ill-defined region of low density in the left parietal lobe. The most likely diagnosis is:

A Multiple sclerosis
B Stroke
C Astrocytoma
D Abscess
E Metastasis

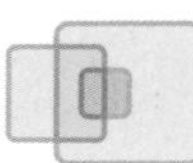

Answers and Explanations

1. The answer is D [IV B 5 a; XV B 3 d (1)–(2)]. Polymyalgia rheumatica (PMR) is characterized by muscle discomfort, and patients often present with vague complaints, as in this case. By definition, the results of the neuromuscular examination are normal.

Depression can cause fatigue and diminished activity, but discomfort is less frequently a complaint. A normal erythrocyte sedimentation rate, which is elevated in the presence of PMR, would support a diagnosis of depression. Hypokalemia can cause muscle weakness, but discomfort is not a typical feature. Temporal (giant cell) arteritis can occur with PMR, but this patient has no complaint of headache or symptoms referable to vision. Polymyositis can cause muscle discomfort, but there should be accompanying weakness. The serum creatine kinase (CK) level is often elevated.

2. The answer is B [VIII B 3 a 2, b, 7 b]. The lupus anticoagulant (an antiphospholipid antibody) is associated with peripheral venous thrombosis and ischemic (arterial) stroke. In patients with a history of deep venous thrombosis, the possibility of a paradoxical embolus causing a stroke (via a right-to-left cardiac shunt) should also be considered.

Nonvalvular atrial fibrillation is a common cause of stroke in the elderly, but there is no reason to suspect a rhythm disturbance in this patient. Mitral valve prolapse has been associated with cardiogenic emboli and stroke. However, a search for other causes of stroke should always be made, because mitral valve prolapse is a relatively common entity, and the association with stroke is weak. Multiple sclerosis (MS) and an astrocytoma can cause neurologic deficits in young patients; however, these conditions are not associated with deep venous thrombosis unless the patient is immobilized. These diagnoses should be considered in the evaluation of patients with hemiparesis, but the patient's history can often serve as a clue to guide diagnostic thinking.

3. The answer is A [XIII D 1 a–b]. People such as assembly-line workers or typists are particularly prone to carpal tunnel syndrome because their daily activities require repetitive wrist movements, which may, in time, compress the median nerve, causing neuropathy. Awakening at night with hand discomfort is a common complaint, and the findings on examination support the diagnosis.

A cervical radiculopathy can cause some of these findings. However, the history is more suggestive of carpal tunnel syndrome. Patients with a cervical radiculopathy often have a concurrent carpal tunnel syndrome and vice versa. The history and examination are not supportive of a diagnosis of tendinitis or reflex sympathetic dystrophy. Transient ischemic attacks (TIAs) rarely cause discomfort and are not associated with neurologic deficits after 24 hours have elapsed.

4. The answer is E [XIII D 2 b (1), c (2)]. The patient probably has Guillain-Barré syndrome, and administration of intravenous immunoglobulin has been found to hasten clinical improvement. Plasmapheresis is an alternate therapy.

Corticosteroids are not indicated for the treatment of Guillain-Barré syndrome but can be used to treat chronic inflammatory demyelinating polyneuropathy (CIDP). Patients with this illness can present with chronic progressive weakness, and, occasionally, subacute weakness, and it needs to be distinguished from the Guillain-Barré syndrome. Clues to a diagnosis of CIDP include early, marked slowing of nerve conduction velocities and disease progression beyond 4 weeks. Penicillin is used to treat Lyme disease, which can present with multiple radiculopathies and thereby cause difficulty ambulating. Examination of cerebral spinal fluid (CSF) typically reveals a pleocytosis. Phenytoin is used, on occasion, to treat painful polyneuropathies. There is no need for such treatment in this patient, because she has not complained of pain. Levodopa is inappropriate, because the patient has no stigmata of Parkinson's disease other than difficulty ambulating.

5. The answer is B [III B 4 a; VII A 2 b; XV B 2 a]. Lumbar stenosis is caused by degenerative changes in the lumbosacral spine, often in association with a congenitally small lumbosacral intraspinal space. The history is often that of vague low back discomfort associated with subtle findings on examination referable to impingement on motor and sensory roots. Diagnosis can be made by the characteristic finding of an "hourglass" appearance on magnetic resonance imaging (MRI) scans.

An acute disk herniation is characterized by low back discomfort and pain extending in a radicular fashion down one or both legs. Examination is often consistent with impingement on a single sensory or motor root. A myopathy can cause an impaired gait; low back discomfort because of weakness; and hypoactive muscle stretch reflexes, typically at the knees. However, this condition is much less common than lumbar stenosis and therefore is not the most likely diagnosis. Normal pressure hydrocephalus (NPH) causes an apractic gait (i.e., difficulty in walking in spite of an intact motor, sensory, and cerebellar examination), cognitive impairment, and urinary incontinence. The clinical picture is not consistent with this diagnosis. Cervical stenosis can cause a myelopathy and resultant gait problem. Because the patient does not exhibit signs of a myelopathy, this diagnosis is unlikely.

6. The answer is B [X A 2 a (1)–(2), B 1 a, 4 c; XIII D 1 a–b]. Writer's cramp is a focal dystonia of unknown cause. Patients develop symptoms of cramps or spasms with altered hand and arm posture when attempting the specific task of writing. Examination of the patient is otherwise normal.

Micrographia is a symptom of Parkinson's disease but is usually accompanied by signs of rigidity and bradykinesia, and often tremor. Carpal tunnel syndrome is caused by pressure on the median nerve as it enters the hand via the carpal tunnel. Median nerve dysfunction leads to hand weakness and loss of sensibility, which can affect writing. A cervical radiculopathy can lead to hand numbness and weakness and hyporeflexia. The exact distribution of findings depends on the nerve roots involved. A benign essential tremor is characterized by a distal upper extremity tremor during a task. There is no accompanying rigidity or bradykinesia. Handwriting in particular may suffer. Carpal tunnel syndrome, cervical radiculopathy, and benign essential tremor are all unlikely because the patient's examination shows no signs or symptoms other than difficulty with writing.

7. The answer is C [III B 3 d; IX A 3 a]. Alzheimer's disease is a cause of new-onset auditory hallucinations in the elderly. Typically, evidence of cognitive impairment is present, although on occasion, watchful waiting is necessary before other manifestations of Alzheimer's disease become apparent. Low doses of haloperidol can be quite helpful in treating auditory hallucinations associated with Alzheimer's disease.

Complex partial seizures can cause auditory hallucinations, but usually the patient reports simple sounds rather than words or complex sound patterns. Many medications can cause hallucinations, but this woman was "previously healthy"; therefore, it is unlikely that she was receiving medical therapy. Hyperthyroidism, especially apathetic hyperthyroidism, is a cause of delirium in the elderly. It is not particularly associated with auditory hallucinations. Peduncular hallucinations are primarily visual hallucinations due to rostral mesencephalic ischemia. This phenomenon is part of the top-of-the-basilar syndrome, which involves an ischemic insult to the territory of the rostral basilar artery.

8. The answer is B [VII A 2 a (2)–(3)]. The patient probably has an acute disk herniation causing a cauda equina syndrome, an indication for emergency surgery. Surgery should be considered as an elective intervention for those patients with sciatica, disabling neurologic deficits, and disk herniation (as demonstrated by appropriate imaging techniques) who fail to respond to 6 weeks of conservative management.

Nonsteroidal anti-inflammatory drugs (NSAIDs) can be helpful in the treatment of acute, and possibly chronic, low back pain; however, they are not indicated as primary therapy for patients with acute, severe neurologic disability. Strict bed rest is very helpful for the treatment of acute back pain, but this therapy is not appropriate for this patient. The intradisk pressure is lowest in the supine position. Bed rest for 2–7 days is usually suggested; prolonged bed rest results in deconditioning. Lumbar traction is probably not effective for the treatment of low back pain. Patients typically cannot exercise during the first few days of acute back pain. However, as the acute pain subsides, an exercise program may help prevent future problems.

9. The answer is A [IX D 2 b (1)–(2), 4 b, c]. Administration of intravenous lorazepam should be followed by the administration of phenytoin (or fosphenytoin) to control status epilepticus because the duration of action of lorazepam is limited. Therefore, unless there is a contraindication, the patient should receive a loading dose of phenytoin (or fosphenytoin) intravenously.

Carbamazepine is an effective anticonvulsant, but it cannot be given intravenously or intramuscularly. Therefore, a therapeutic level cannot be rapidly achieved given a drug half-life of 8–12 hours. Intravenous pentobarbital can be used to control repetitive seizures. However, because the patient is not currently convulsing, induction of barbiturate coma is not indicated. Ethosuximide is indicated for the treatment of absence seizures. Therefore, this is not an appropriate therapy for generalized motor convulsions. Rectal diazepam is used to abort seizures temporarily, especially in children.

10. The answer is B [XVI B 1, 2; XVII A 2, C, E 1]. A large, irregularly enhancing central nervous system (CNS) mass in an elderly patient without systemic cancer is highly suggestive of a glioblastoma multiforme. However, a biopsy is necessary before a definitive diagnosis can be made.

The patient has no predisposing condition for a brain abscess such as poor dentition or intravenous drug abuse. A meningioma can occur in the parietal area and distort the brain; however, a "convexity" meningioma is typically a homogeneously enhancing lesion. In the absence of systemic cancer, a brain metastasis is an unlikely cause of the patient's problem. However, without a biopsy, the diagnosis of metastatic disease cannot be excluded. CNS lymphoma typically manifests as a homogeneously enhancing mass lesion. Patients suffering from the human immunodeficiency virus (HIV) and other immunocompromised patients are prone to CNS lymphoma; in other populations, CNS lymphoma is rare.

11. The answer is A [VI B 2 b–c, e–f; XVII D 1–3]. A cerebellopontine angle tumor such as a schwannoma can cause intermittent dizziness. The tumor can arise from the eighth cranial nerve, thereby also affecting hearing, and can press on the trigeminal nerve, causing impairment of the corneal reflex.

Benign paroxysmal positional vertigo (BPPV) causes intermittent brief dizziness that is dependent on postural changes. Nystagmus is characteristic, but there are no other neurologic deficits. A lateral medullary syndrome usually causes constant dizziness that is exacerbated with movement. Although the corneal reflex can be depressed, hearing is normal. Meniere's disease causes intermittent dizziness and hearing loss, but the corneal reflex is not diminished. A pontine infarction does not cause intermittent symptoms; hearing loss is not expected as a result.

12. The answer is D [XII B 1–4; XII C 3 b; XIII D 2 b (1)]. Thrombosis of the caudal anterior spinal artery leads to a flaccid paraplegia, loss of pain and temperature sensation, and bowel and bladder dysfunction. The blood supply to the caudal spinal cord arises from the aorta via lumbar radicular arteries. The perfusion territory of the anterior spinal artery involves the anterior horn cells and the pain and temperature pathways.

In the Guillain-Barré syndrome, which rarely develops suddenly, loss of temperature and pain sensation can occur but rarely without a concurrent loss of position and vibration sense. Sensory loss is usually less severe than motor loss. Generalized areflexia is common. An anterior cerebral artery thrombosis, especially when bilateral, can cause leg weakness, but there is no sensory loss. Upper motor neuron signs are present in the leg. A cauda equina syndrome [VII A 2 (3) a] can cause a flaccid paraplegia, but all sensory modalities may be compromised because sensory nerve roots, which carry sensory fibers of all types, are involved in the disease process. Thoracic spinal cord compression is often associated with back pain and produces upper motor neuron dysfunction in the legs. In the acute condition, the bladder may be distended, but with time, its capacity is typically reduced.

13. The answer is C [V B 2 b (1); XIII D 2 b (1)–(2); Tables 11–10A and 11–10B]. Chronic inflammatory demyelinating polyneuropathy (CIDP) is characterized by progressive weakness that occurs over an extended time (e.g., ≥ 4 weeks), absent muscle stretch reflexes, and slowed motor nerve conduction velocities (NCVs).

Guillain-Barré syndrome should not cause progressive worsening of strength beyond 4 weeks. Typically, only some motor nerves demonstrate slowing, usually in a segmental, rather than a generalized, fashion. Lead poisoning can cause a motor neuropathy in children but only rarely in adults. Amyotrophic lateral sclerosis (ALS) causes progressive weakness, but motor NCVs are unremarkable and muscle stretch reflexes are often hyperactive. Polymyositis causes progressive proximal (greater than distal) weakness and is not associated with impaired motor NCVs. Muscle stretch reflexes are often preserved in proportion to the muscle strength.

14. The answer is C [V B 2 b (2) (j); X A 2 a (2); XIX A 2 a; Table 11–8]. The signs and symptoms are most consistent with multiple systems atrophy (Shy-Drager syndrome).

The early appearance of autonomic dysfunction (impotence and postural hypotension) and ataxia do not support the diagnosis of Parkinson's disease. Combined systems degeneration is due to vitamin B_{12} deficiency. Parkinsonian features are not a feature of the disease. Spinocerebellar degeneration is characterized by cerebellar dysfunction and an accompanying upper motor neuron syndrome. Extrapyramidal and autonomic dysfunction are not prominent features. Vitamin E deficiency can masquerade as spinocerebellar degeneration.

15. The answer is D [VIII C 1 c (2)]. Vasospasm can develop several days after an aneurysmal subarachnoid hemorrhage (SAH). Patients present with progressive weakness and alterations in consciousness. Early in the course, a computed tomography (CT) scan may not reveal an ischemic infarction.

Hydrocephalus can occur immediately after an SAH or weeks to months later. Symptoms are typically nonfocal and, if the hydrocephalus develops acutely, it is often accompanied by a depressed level of consciousness. Bacterial meningitis can develop after a craniotomy. Typically, there is fever and impaired arousal. Focal signs can develop but are rarely the presenting feature. Although a repeat hemorrhage can occur after clipping of an aneurysm if the aneurysm is not completely isolated from the circulation, it is unusual for this to happen and present with a focal deficit, as opposed to depressed consciousness. Hyponatremia, which can develop after SAH, can cause an altered sensorium and seizures but not unilateral weakness.

16. The answer is C [VI B 2 c, f; VIII B 4 c (1) (b)]. The patient has manifestations of a lateral medullary syndrome. In a young patient, who has subjected himself to strenuous neck movements, the most likely etiology is vertebral artery dissection.

Benign paroxysmal positional vertigo (BPPV) causes sudden episodes of dizziness, typically with changes in position. However, there are no associated neurologic symptoms or signs other than nystagmus. Multiple sclerosis (MS) can cause dizziness and clumsiness. However, the constellation of findings in this patient, which are referable to a single site within the brain and are of sudden onset, make the diagnosis of MS less likely. An astrocytoma can cause dizziness and unsteadiness. Often there is a headache. The onset is typically insidious, and the symptoms progressive. Labyrinthitis causes severe vertigo. Patients find it difficult to move about and prefer to remain still. Gait instability can occur because of the profound dizziness and no cerebellar deficits. There are no neurologic signs other than nystagmus. Migraine with aura is associated with headache and focal neurologic symptoms and signs. Unless patients have a history similar to that described, they should be evaluated for alternative diagnoses such as arterial dissection. Patients with migraine associated with focal neurologic deficits should be evaluated for alternate diagnoses before the problem is attributed to migraine with aura.

17. The answer is B [IV B 1 d (1)–(2) (a)]. Migraine headaches respond well to treatment with tricyclic antidepressants such as amitriptyline. This patient has been unresponsive to over-the-counter acetaminophen. Assuming she is having frequent headaches that are interfering with her lifestyle, it is reasonable to begin treatment with a prophylactic migraine medication.

Baclofen is not effective for migraine. Indomethacin is not commonly prescribed for migraine; though it may benefit an acute headache episode, it is not considered a prophylactic medication. Corticosteroids can be helpful in the treatment of a severe, acute migraine headache. However, corticosteroids are not commonly prescribed for migraine prophylaxis. Sumatriptan is an effective treatment for an acute migraine headache but it is not indicated as a prophylactic migraine therapy.

18. The answer is D [IV B 5 c]. This patient likely has giant cell (temporal) arteritis. The treatment of choice for giant cell arteritis is corticosteroids. An erythrocyte sedimentation rate and C-reactive protein assay should be obtained before beginning corticosteroid therapy, but waiting for a temporal artery biopsy should not delay initiation of therapy.

Neither baclofen, amitriptylene, indomethacin, or sumatriptan are indicated for giant cell arteritis.

19. The answer is C [IV B 8]. The patient's history is suggestive of paroxysmal hemicrania, an indomethacin-responsive disorder. In fact, a positive response to treatment with indomethacin can confirm a diagnosis of paroxysmal hemicrania.

Neither baclofen, amitriptylene, corticosteroids, or sumatriptan are considered beneficial for paroxysmal hemicrania.

20. The answer is B [VIII C 1 b; IV A 3 b]. The history is highly suggestive of subarachnoid hemorrhage (SAH). A brain computed tomography (CT) scan is the best test to screen for intracranial hemorrhage and should be emergently obtained to document subarachnoid blood. If the scan is normal and the history is suggestive of SAH, the woman should undergo a lumbar puncture (LP) to screen for blood before the physician concludes that she does not have a SAH.

Conventional angiography is necessary to evaluate patients with SAH to define the presence of an aneurysm and details of its anatomic configuration. Associated abnormalities such as vasospasm can also be assessed. However, an angiogram should not be the initial diagnostic test in a patient with a suspected SAH.

Transcranial Doppler (TCD) studies can detect cerebral artery vasospasm but not the presence of an aneurysm. Vasospasm typically develops a few days after SAH; therefore, it would not be expected to be apparent at the time of patient presentation.

Brain MRI is not as sensitive as brain CT for the detection of acute intracranial hemorrhage. Therefore, brain MRI is not considered the procedure of choice for the acute detection of SAH.

Although magnetic resonance (or computed tomography) angiography (MRA or CTA, respectively) can document the presence of an aneurysm, they are not as sensitive as conventional angiography. Neither MRA or CTA is adequate to determine the characteristics of the aneurysm fully and to direct therapy. Therefore, MRA or CTA are not the first test to be obtained in patients with a suspected SAH.

21. The answer is D [VIII B 4 c (1) (a), (3) (a)]. The patient has a non-disabling stroke. His risk factor profile and the presence of an ipsilateral bruit suggest that the most likely cause of his stroke is left internal carotid artery origin stenosis. The definitive intervention to prevent subsequent stroke is carotid endarterectomy.

Acute heparin administration and subsequent warfarin therapy have not been demonstrated to be effective for secondary stroke prevention in this setting. Likewise, there is no role for extracranial-intracranial bypass surgery to treat extracranial internal carotid artery origin stenosis. A combination of warfarin and aspirin has not been shown to be more effective than carotid endarterectomy for secondary stroke prevention for a patient such as this. Although aspirin is appropriate therapy for secondary stroke prevention for stroke due to arterial disease, treatment with aspirin should not preclude carotid endarterectomy in the appropriate setting. Aspirin should be administered after carotid endarterectomy to decrease the risk of postoperative stroke.

22. The answer is D [IV B 6]. The patient's presentation suggests sagittal sinus thrombosis. Although this condition is associated with the hypercoagulable state of pregnancy, further testing is indicated to evaluate the possibility of an underlying chronic hypercoagulable condition.

Pseudotumor cerebri (idiopathic intracranial hypertension) can present in association with pregnancy, and although it is characterized by headache and papilledema, confusion is not a part of pseudotumor cerebri.

Pituitary apoplexy can occur postpartum. It is characterized by headache and visual dysfunction. Papilledema and confusion are not common sequelae of pituitary apoplexy.

Although bacterial meningitis causes headache, confusion, and papilledema, patients are typically febrile.

Eclampsia can cause headache and confusion as well as papilledema. However, the patient's low blood pressure is evidence against this diagnosis. Also, there is no mention of proteinuria or seizures.

23. The answer is D [VIII B 1 c (1)]. The patient has had the acute onset of a neurologic deficit consistent with a stroke. She is presenting for medical care within 3 hours of symptom onset. No contraindications to IV thrombolytic therapy with rt-PA is mentioned. The patient should have an emergent brain CT scan and if no alternate diagnoses are suggested (tumor, subdural hematoma, etc.), IV rt-PA should be administered.

Aspirin is standard of care if the patient had presented more than 3 hours after symptom onset. There is little evidence that heparin or warfarin therapy are beneficial in this setting, and there is an increased incidence of bleeding with these anticoagulants. Clopidogrel is a therapeutic alternative for secondary stroke prevention, but its use should not take precedence over the administration of rt-PA.

If rt-PA is administered, aspirin administration should be delayed 24 hours. Also, if low-dose heparin is administered for deep venous thrombosis prophylaxis, its use should also be delayed for 24 hours before rt-PA use.

24. The answer is C [XVII A 1 a]. The patient presents with a 2-month history of progressive neurologic deficits. The CT scan shows an area of low density, and there is no mention of mass effect. The most likely diagnosis is an astrocytoma, which may not have much in the way of mass effect or enhancement on CT scan.

The progressive history is against a stroke. Multiple sclerosis rarely presents in this age group and would not be expected to cause a large area of decreased density on CT scan. An abscess or metastasis would have substantial mass effect and enhancement on CT scan.

chapter 12

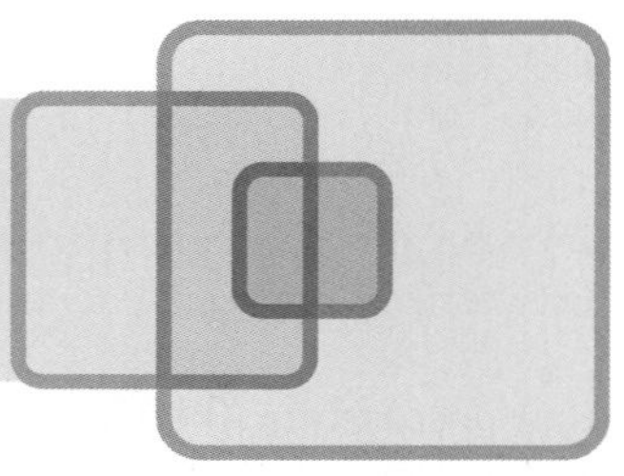

Dermatologic Disorders

STUART R. LESSIN

I STRUCTURE AND FUNCTION OF SKIN

A Structure The skin covers the subcutaneous fat (adipose or panniculus) and consists of two layers, the epidermis and dermis.

1. **Epidermis.** The epidermis is a stratified, squamous epithelium that is 0.1 mm thick. It produces keratin intermediate filaments and continually differentiates into the cornified (horny) layer that provides the barrier function to the skin. It renews itself every 28 days and gives rise to the following skin appendages: hair follicles, sebaceous glands, sweat glands, and nails.
   a. **Compartments** (Figure 12–1)
      (1) **Basal layer** or **stratum germinativum** is the layer of undifferentiated cells that contacts the basement membrane zone (BMZ).
      (2) **Spinous layer** or **stratum spinosum** is the layer in which keratin filament formation occurs.
      (3) **Granular layer** or **stratum granulosum** is the layer in which keratin filament pairing and assembly occurs.
      (4) **Cornified layer** or **stratum corneum,** the final differentiation product of the epidermis, is the barrier layer.
   b. **Cells**
      (1) **Keratinocytes** are the epithelial cells of the epidermis that undergo terminal differentiation.
      (2) **Melanocytes** are neural crest–derived cells that produce pigment (melanin). They are distributed along the basal cell layer and transfer pigment to basal keratinocytes to protect against ultraviolet (UV) irradiation.
      (3) **Langerhans cells** are bone marrow–derived, dendritic, antigen-presenting cells distributed within the epidermis that function in immune surveillance of the skin.
   c. **Epidermal proteins**
      (1) **Products of differentiation**
         (a) **Keratins** are intermediate filament proteins and are classified into two types based on molecular weight and charge. Type 1 keratins pair with type 2 keratins to form a tissue-specific keratin filament.
         (b) **Filaggrin** is a keratin-associated protein that forms a matrix for keratin filaments.
         (c) The **terminal cell envelope** encases keratin filaments. Together with **lipids,** the epidermal proteins provide the barrier function of the epidermis.
      (2) **Adhesion proteins** (Figure 12–2)
         (a) **Desmosomes** are multiprotein complexes that serve as points of attachment between keratinocytes. They contain intracellular and intercellular proteins (desmogleins, desmocollins, plakins).
         (b) **Hemidesmosomes** are multiprotein complexes that are located on the inferior side of basal layer keratinocytes and serve as points of attachment between keratinocytes and the BMZ. They contain intracellular and intercellular proteins (desmoplakin, collagen, plectin).

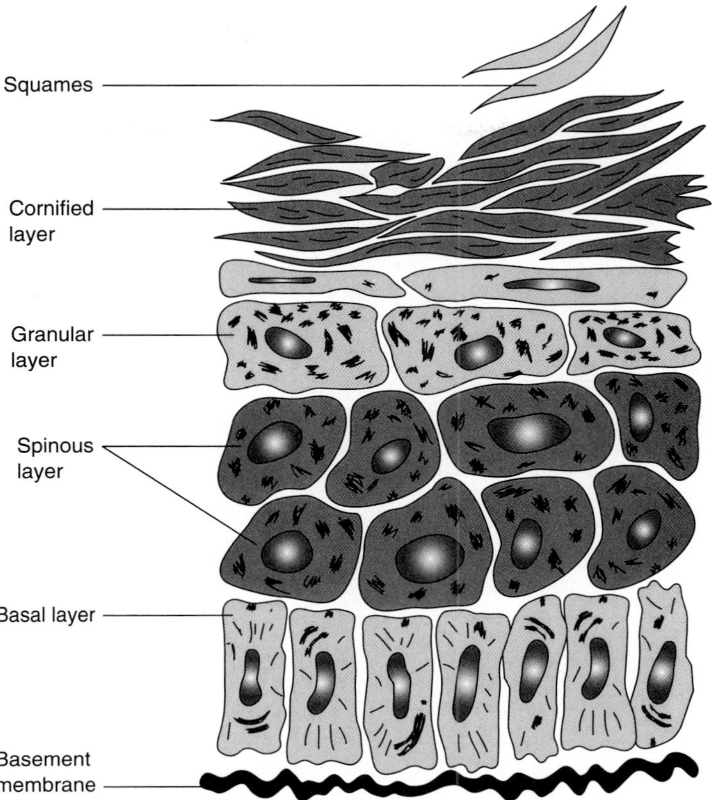

FIGURE 12–1 Compartments of the epidermis.

2. **Dermis.** The dermis is the layer beneath the epidermis that provides pliability and tensile strength. It is a matrix of fibrous and amorphous connective tissue that supports blood and lymphatic vessels, fibroblasts, skin appendages, and mast cells. It protects the body from mechanical injury, binds water, aids in thermal regulation, and contains receptors of sensory stimuli.
   a. **Compartments**
      (1) The **BMZ** is the **dermal–epidermal junction** (DEJ) that forms the interface between the epidermis and the dermis.
         (a) It consists of two layers: the **lamina lucida,** which lies directly beneath the basal layer, and the **lamina densa,** which lies directly beneath the lamina lucida.
         (b) It functions to anchor the epidermis to the dermis and provide resistance against external shearing forces.
         (c) It serves as a semipenetrable barrier and influences the polarity of basal cell growth and cytoskeleton organization.
      (2) The **papillary dermis** is the superficial portion of the dermis that lies directly below the BMZ.
      (3) The **reticular dermis** is the deeper portion of the dermis
   b. **Cells**
      (1) **Endothelial cells** are the cells that form cutaneous blood vessels and lymphatic channels.
      (2) **Fibroblasts** secrete macromolecules and the matrix components of the dermis.
      (3) **Mast cells** are bone marrow–derived cells that contain preformed inflammatory mediators (e.g., histamine, proteases) and participate in a variety of biologic responses, including urticaria and defense against parasites.

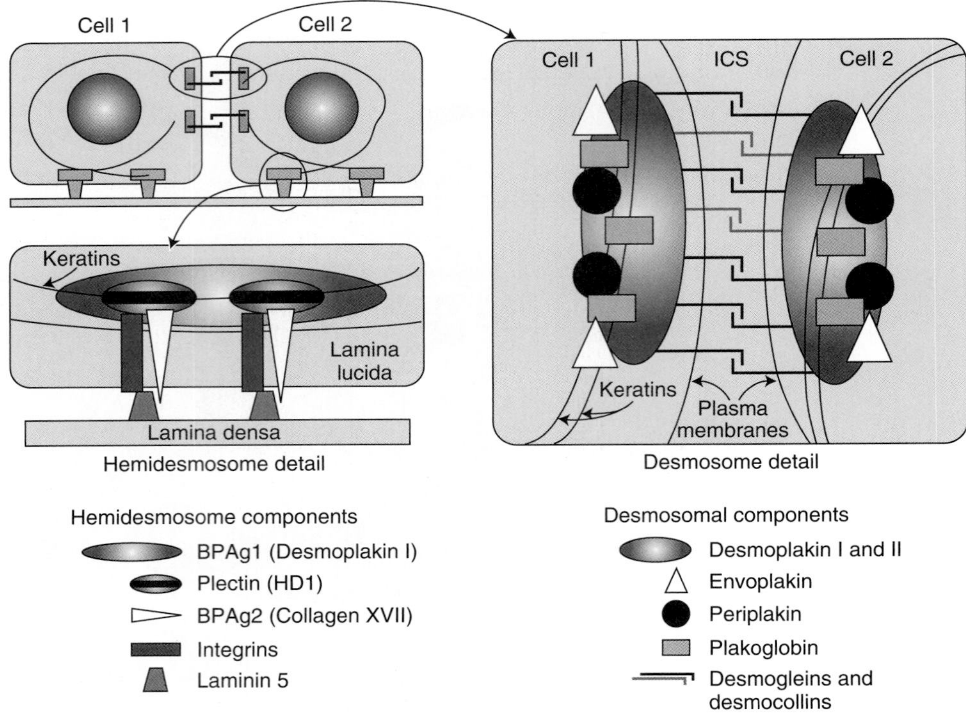

FIGURE 12–2 Adhesion molecules of the epidermis.

c. **Matrix**
   (1) **Collagen** is a macromolecule that gives tensile strength to the skin.
   (2) **Elastin** is a macromolecule that gives elasticity to the skin.
   (3) **Ground substance** forms the dermal matrix and consists of complex sugars (**mucopolysaccharides**) and proteins (**proteoglycans**).

d. **Nerves and nerve receptors.** These structures provide sensory input throughout the entire skin surface.

3. **Panniculus** (adipose). The panniculus is the subcutaneous fat layer that provides thermal insulation.
   a. **Hair follicles.** These epidermal appendages extend into the panniculus.
   b. **Sebaceous glands.** These glands empty into hair follicles, providing lubrication to the horny layer.
   c. **Sweat glands.** The glandular portion involved in sweat production extends into the panniculus, connecting to the skin surface through epithelium-lined ducts. These glands participate in thermoregulation and fluid and electrolyte balance.

B Functions

1. **Barrier.** The stratum corneum protects against water loss, entrance of microorganisms, and environmental toxins. The deeper layers of the skin protect from damage caused by UV irradiation, mechanical forces, and extreme environmental temperatures.
2. **Fluid and electrolyte balance.** Autonomic nerves innervate sweat glands that stimulate sweat production and assist in water and electrolyte regulation.
3. **Thermoregulation.** The skin serves as an outer shell that varies blood flow and sweat secretion to regulate heat exchange with the environment to maintain the body's core temperature.

4. **Vitamin D metabolism.** The skin is a major source of nondietary vitamin D. UV irradiation from sun exposure converts 7-dehydrocholesterol to vitamin D_3 (cholecalciferol), which is then hydroxylated in the liver and the kidney to form active vitamin D (1,25-dihydroxycholecalciferol).
5. **Sensory input.** A neural network provides sensory input for touch, pain, temperature, itch, and mechanical stimuli.
6. **Immune surveillance.** The skin is an important component of the immune system and participates in both innate and acquired immunity. Its resident immune cells (Langerhans cells); endogenous cytokines (interleukin-1 [IL-1], IL-3, IL-6); and growth factors [granulocyte colony stimulating factor (G-CSF), granulocyte-macrophage colony-stimulating factor (GM-CSF), macrophage colony-stimulating factor (M-CSF), tumor necrosis factor-α [TNF-α]) interact with circulating lymphocytes and macrophages. These immune factors participate in a wide range of physiologic and pathologic processes.

II DERMATOLOGIC DIAGNOSIS

A General considerations The foundation of dermatologic diagnosis relies on physical examination of the skin to first identify the morphology of the primary skin lesion(s). Based on morphology, a differential diagnosis is generated, and a final diagnosis is determined by using the dermatologic history and appropriate laboratory studies.

B Examination of the skin

1. **Inspection** of the skin defines morphology, color, distribution, and configuration.
   a. **Morphology.** Primary lesions of the skin are classified based on morphology (Table 12–1).
   b. **Distribution.** The location and extent of the primary eruption are important characteristics in defining the disease process.
      (1) Localized: involvement of limited areas of the skin
      (2) Diffuse: widespread involvement of the skin
      (3) Bilateral: symmetrical involvement
      (4) Dermatomal: involvement limited to skin over a dermatome (e.g., herpes zoster)
      (5) Acral: involvement of the skin of the distal extremities
   c. **Configuration** ***(Color Figures 12–1 through 12–4. See accompanying CD).*** Several features of primary lesions are important in defining the disease process.
      (1) Number (single versus multiple)
      (2) Spatial relationship (i.e., grouped)
      (3) Shape (i.e., annular, linear, serpiginous, polycyclic)
2. **Palpation** determines the texture, consistency, and depth of lesions, as well as the temperature, tenderness, and quality of erythema (i.e., blanchable).

C Dermatologic history

1. **History of the eruption.** The essential historical qualifiers for any cutaneous eruption include the following:
   a. Onset and progression
   b. Duration and course
   c. Symptoms
   d. Treatment and response
2. **Medical history.** A history of medical problems focused on cutaneous findings, including allergies, should be elicited.
3. **Medication history.** A detailed medication history is vital, especially when evaluating eruptions that may be triggered by medications. The medication history should include prescription and over-the-counter (OTC) medications, vitamins, eye drops, and herbal supplements.

TABLE 12–1 Terms Used in the Morphologic Description of Skin Lesions

Term	Description	Appearance
Macule	Flat lesion of variable size and shape that differs from surrounding skin because of its color	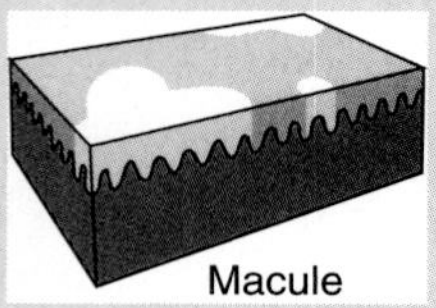 Macule
Papule	Small, solid, elevated lesion. Papules are generally smaller than 0.5 cm in diameter	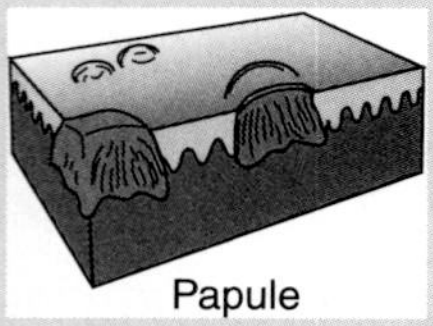 Papule
Plaque	Broad-based papule that occupies a relatively large surface area in comparison with its height above skin level	
Patch	Description of very large macules or a thin but large plaque	
Nodule	Palpable, firm, round to spheroid lesion with a depth of involvement greater than that of a papule	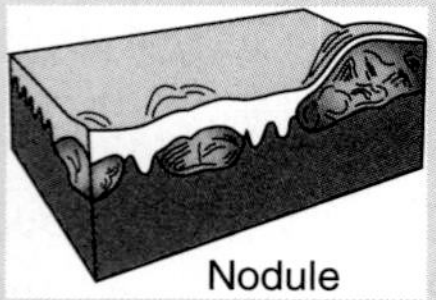 Nodule
Cyst	Epithelial-lined sac that contains liquid or semisolid material (fluid, cells, and cell products)	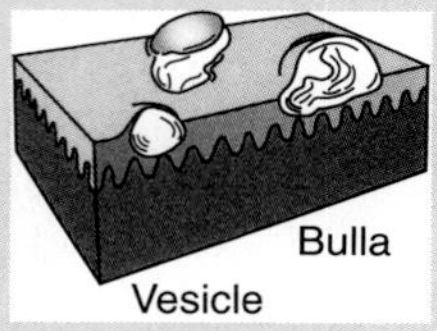 Bulla Vesicle
Vesicle	Fluid-filled, elevated lesion < 0.5 mm in diameter	
Bulla	Large vesicle (> 5 mm)	
Pustule	Raised lesion that contains purulent exudate (i.e., pus)	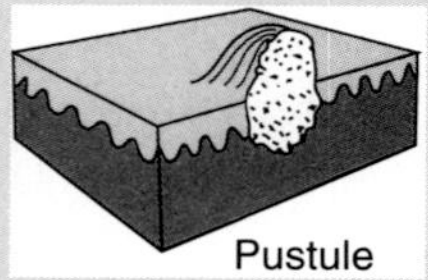 Pustule
Wheal	Flat-topped papule or plaque that is characteristically evanescent, disappearing within hours (i.e., hive)	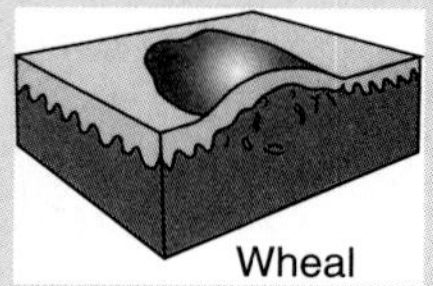 Wheal
Erosion	Circumscribed, superficial depression resulting from loss of all or portion of viable epidermis	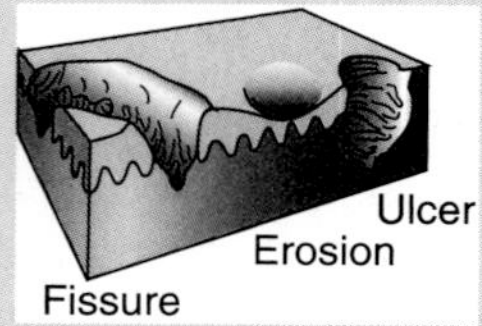 Ulcer Erosion Fissure
Ulcer	Deeper depression resulting from destruction of epidermis and at least upper (papillary) dermis	
Fissure	Linear crack in skin	
Furuncle	Deep necrotizing form of folliculitis with pus accumulation. Several furuncles may coalesce to form *carbuncle*	

(*continued*)

TABLE 12–1 Continued

Term	Description	Appearance
Abscess	Localized accumulation of purulent material so deep in dermis or subcutaneous tissue that pus is usually not visible on surface of skin	
Sinus	Tract leading from suppurative cavity to skin surface or between cystic or abscess cavities	
Atrophy	Epidermal atrophy: thinning of epidermis associated with decrease in number of epidermal cells Dermal atrophy: usually manifested as depression of skin; results from decrease in dermal connective tissue	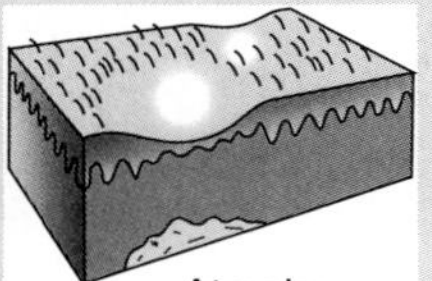 Atrophy
Sclerosis	Circumscribed or diffuse hardening or induration in skin	
Scaling	Abnormal shedding or accumulation of stratum corneum in perceptible flakes	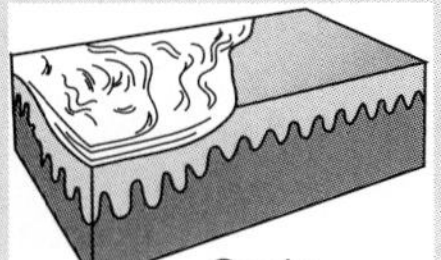 Scale
Papulosquamous	Eruptions consisting of scaling papules	
Crusts	Hardened deposits of dried serum, blood, or purulent exudate	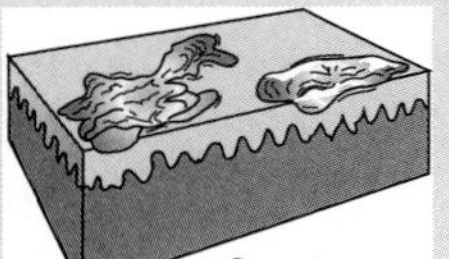 Crust
Excoriations	Superficial excavations of epidermis that may be linear or punctate and result from scratching	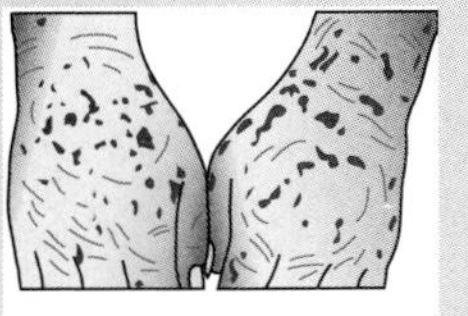 Excoriations
Lichenification	Thickening of the epidermis resulting from chronic scratching	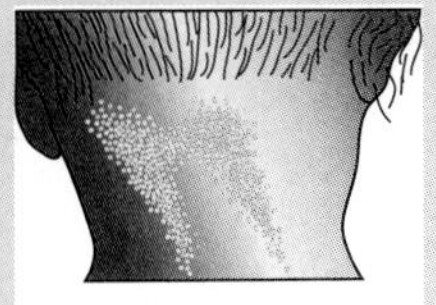 Lichenification
Poikiloderma	Combination of atrophy, telangiectasia, and pigmentary changes (hyperpigmentation and hypopigmentation)	

4. **Social history.** A detailed social history often provides diagnostic clues for cutaneous findings. The social history should focus on skin care (habits and products used), occupation, home environment, sexually transmitted diseases, and travel.
5. **Family history.** A family history is important in assessing skin disease predisposition and susceptibility, particularly for allergy, skin cancer, psoriasis, and rheumatic disease.

D Dermatology laboratory tests

1. **Direct microscopic examination.** Preparations of skin scrapings from scaling and blistering eruptions can provide important diagnostic information.
   a. **Potassium hydroxide (KOH) preparation.** KOH digests cellular material and facilitates the visualization of fungal hyphae, yeast forms, and scabies mites.
   b. **Tzanck smear.** Giemsa- or Wright-stained scrapings from herpetic vesicles reveal multinucleated giant cells.
   c. **Gram stain.** Gram-positive and gram-negative bacteria may be identified.
   d. **Darkfield microscopy.** Visualization of spirochetes (*Treponema pallidum*) from preparations of primary chancre and secondary lesions is diagnostic of syphilis.
2. **Skin cultures.** Bacterial, viral, and fungal cultures can be obtained from skin swabs or skin biopsies.
3. **Patch testing.** This method for identifying compounds responsible for contact dermatitis. Common and suspected compounds are placed on the skin under occlusion (i.e., patch) for 48–72 hours. Induction of cutaneous inflammation at specific patch sites identifies sensitizing agents.
4. **Phototesting and photopatch testing**
   a. **Phototesting** uses specialized light sources that deliver specific ranges and quantities of UV light to document photosensitivity in individuals with suspected photosensitivity.
   b. **Photopatch testing** combines patch testing and phototesting to identify photosensitizing compounds, which produce a photosensitivity reaction when exposed to UV light. Suspected photosensitizing compounds are patch tested with and without UV exposure.
5. **Skin biopsy** provides tissue for histopathologic evaluation.
   a. **Biopsy techniques**
      (1) **Punch biopsy** is a commonly used technique to obtain 2–6-mm cylindrical skin samples.
      (2) **Tangential (shave) biopsy** is a rapid technique used to obtain superficial skin samples.
      (3) **Incisional biopsy** is used to obtain large or deep (including panniculus) skin samples.
      (4) **Excisional biopsy** is used to obtain an entire lesion (e.g., suspicious pigmented lesion) for histologic review.
   b. **Examination of biopsy tissue**
      (1) **Light microscopy** is used to evaluate routine (hematoxylin and eosin) and special (e.g., periodic acid–Schiff) stains as well as immunohistochemical (monoclonal antibody) stains.
      (2) **Immunofluorescent microscopy** is used for identification of immunoreactants (e.g., autoimmune antibodies)
      (3) **Electron microscopy** is used for specialized studies that require visualizing subcellular structures.

III DERMATOLOGIC THERAPY

A General considerations Topical therapies are frequently used in treating dermatologic diseases and often provide alternatives to systemic therapies. The chief advantages of topical therapies may include higher efficacy and limited systemic toxicities, whereas the selection of topical therapies and systemic therapies for dermatologic diseases is guided by basic clinical management principles.

1. Therapeutic goals should be defined.
   a. Is therapy intended to cure or ameliorate (control) the disease?
   b. Is therapy intended to be short-term or long-term?
2. Therapy should maximize the benefit-to-risk ratio and minimize toxicity.
3. Patient compliance should be considered and promoted.
4. Cost-effectiveness should be evaluated as part of the therapeutic decision making.

B Topical Therapy

1. Two variables are involved in the selection of topical therapy. Both the medication and the vehicle to be used must be appropriate for the specific disorder being treated.
2. Generally, acute inflammation is treated with aqueous drying vehicles, and chronic inflammation is treated with more lubricating and moisturizing preparations (Figure 12–3).
3. Vehicle choice may be influenced by body site. For example, lotions, solutions, and sprays are more effective in hairy areas (e.g., scalp).
4. Water, oil, and particulate composition of a vehicle determine its characteristics.
   a. Creams are emulsions of oil, predominately in water.
   b. Ointments are emulsions of water, predominately in oil.
   c. Gels are semisolid emulsions of alcohol or acetone in an organic polymer (agar, gelatin).
   d. Lotions are powders in a water base.
   e. Solutions, sprays, and aerosols have a base of water, alcohol, or propylene glycol.
5. Topical corticosteroids are prescribed for a wide variety of inflammatory and pruritic conditions.
   a. Potency. Halogenated corticosteroids have the greatest potency. Potency of topical corticosteroids is measured by vasoconstrictive capacity and may be categorized as low, medium, or high (Table 12–2).
   b. Use
      (1) High-potency topical corticosteroids are used for the short-term treatment of acute and severe inflammatory eruptions. If prolonged topical steroid therapy is required, tapering to steroids of a lower potency is advised.
      (2) Mid-to-low potency topical steroids are used for treatment of mild to moderate inflammatory eruptions and for maintenance therapy or prolonged therapy.
      (3) Low-potency topical steroids are the only steroids to be prescribed for the face and intertriginous areas (skin folds of the axillae, inframammary region, abdominal panus, and groin) because of the increased risk of local side effects in these areas.
      (4) In general, prolonged use of topical steroids should be avoided. Tachyphylaxis and side effects are associated with prolonged topical steroid use.

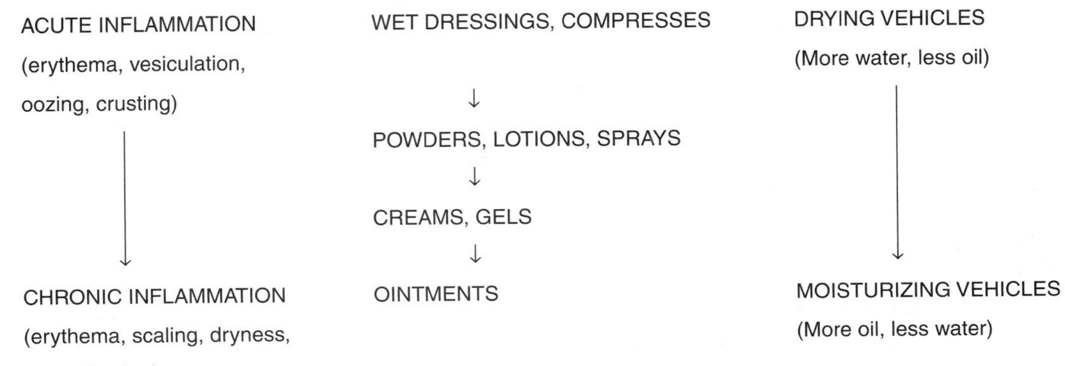

FIGURE 12–3 Vehicle suitability for topical skin therapy in terms of clinical setting.

TABLE 12–2 Potency of Topical Steroids

Compound	Concentration
Low potency	
Hydrocortisone acetate	0.5%,* 1%,*; 2.5%
Mid-potency	
Betamethasone benzoate	0.025%
Betamethasone valerate	0.1%
Clocortolone pivalate	0.1%
Desonide	0.05%
Flumethasone pivalate	0.03%
Fluocinolone acetonide	0.025%
Flurandrenolide	0.05%
Hydrocortisone butyrate	0.1%
Hydrocortisone valerate	0.2%
Triamcinolone acetonide	0.1%, 0.5%
High potency	
Amcinonide	0.1%
Betamethasone dipropionate	0.05%
Clobetasol propionate	0.05%
Desoximetasone	0.025%
Diflorasone diacetate	0.05%
Fluocinonide	0.05%
Halcinonide	0.1%
Halobetasol propionate	0.05%
Mometasone furoate	0.1%

*= available over-the-counter.

(5) Occlusion is an important adjuvant to topical therapy and increases absorption by increasing hydration and temperature. Materials such as plastic (Saran) wrap and gloves and shower caps can be used as occlusive dressings.

(6) Twice-daily application is generally recommended because of patient compliance. Individuals are more likely to treat their skin in the morning and evening when dressing and undressing. No compelling clinical data demonstrate an increase in efficacy with a frequency of application of more than twice-daily application.

c. Dispensing

(1) Prescribing the appropriate quantity of topical steroids is important for both compliance and safety. Table 12–3 presents guidelines for prescribing topical steroids.

(2) Most creams, ointments, and gels are commercially available in small (15 g, 30 g) or large (45 g, 60 g) tubes.

(3) Most solutions and lotions are commercially available in small (30 mL) or large (60 mL) bottles.

d. Complications of topical corticosteroids

(1) Local side effects occur with prolonged use, especially on intertriginous areas and on the face (Table 12–4).

(2) Systemic side effects may result from systemic absorption. Systemic absorption may result in hypothalamus-pituitary-adrenal (HPA) axis suppression. Risk factors for HPA axis suppression include impaired barrier function, increased surface area of treated skin, high potency, and prolonged use.

TABLE 12–3 Guidelines for Dispensing Topical Steroids

Area Treated	Amount for One Application (g)*	Amount for Twice-Daily Application for 7 Days (g)*
Face	1	15
Scalp	1	15
Hands	2	30
Arm	2	30
Feet	3	45
Leg	4	60
Anterior trunk	4	60
Posterior trunk	4	60
Entire body	30	425 (1 lb.)

*Amounts represent averages for creams in an adult population.

6. Topical antibiotics are useful agents for the treatment of secondary bacterial infection of superficial wounds; burns; and superficial, primary skin infections (e.g., impetigo). Agents include mupirocin cream or ointment, silver sulfadiazine cream, polymyxin B, and bacitracin ointment (nonprescription), and neomycin ointment (nonprescription).
7. Topical antifungals are prescribed for the treatment of superficial yeast (e.g., candidiasis) and fungal (e.g., dermatophyte) infections of the skin. Generally, the topical agent is available as a cream, but other formulations include powder, lacquer (for nails), spray, gel, solution, vaginal suppository, and oral troche. Topical antifungal agents are listed in Table 12–5.
8. Topical antiviral agents are available for the treatment of herpes simplex virus (HSV) infections of the face (fever blisters, cold sores) and human papilloma virus (HPV) infections (genital warts).
   a. HSV
      (1) Prescription drugs are purine analogs that are phosphorylated by viral thymidine kinase and inhibit viral DNA polymerase. Drugs include acyclovir 5% cream or ointment and penciclovir 1% cream.
      (2) A variety of nonprescription compounds are marketed for the treatment of cold sores, but only one has been approved by the Food and Drug Administration. Docosanol (10% cream) inhibits fusion between the human cell plasma membrane and the HSV envelope, thereby preventing viral entry into cells and subsequent viral replication.
   b. HPV. Imiquimod (5% cream) has been approved for the treatment of genital warts. It is an immune response modifier that induces cytokines, including interferon-α (IFN-α), at the treatment site.

C Systemic Therapy

1. **Systemic corticosteroids** are a mainstay of dermatologic therapy for severe inflammatory diseases of the skin that are not amenable to topical steroid therapy.

TABLE 12–4 Local Side Effects of Topical Steroids

Atrophy	Hypopigmentation
Candida superinfection	Rosacea-like eruption
Striae, stellate pseudoscars	Impaired wound healing
Miliaria	Acneiform eruption
Telangiectasia, purpura, erythema	Exacerbation of cutaneous infections, bacterial and dermatophyte infestations, scabies, or pediculosis
Periorofacial dermatitis	

TABLE 12–5 Topical Antifungal Agents

Agent	Formulation(s)	Rx/OTC
Polyene		
Nystatin*	C, O, OS, P, VT, T	Rx
Imidazoles		
Clotrimazole	C, L, S, T, VT	OTC
Econazole	C	Rx
Ketoconazole	C, Sh	C=Rx; Sh=OTC
Miconazole	C, L, S, P	OTC
Oxiconazole	C, L	Rx
Sulconazole	C, S	Rx
Allylamines and nonazole ergosterol synthesis inhibitors		
Amorolfine	NL	Rx
Butenafine HCl	C	Rx
Naftifine	C, O, P	Rx
Terbinafine	C, S	OTC
Other agents		
Ciclopirox olamine	C, L, NL, Sh	Rx
Haloprogin	C	Rx
Tolnaftate	C, S, P	OTC
Undecylenate	C, P, O, S	OTC

*Active against yeast (*Candida*) only.
C = cream; L = lotion; NL = nail lacquer; O = ointment; OS = oral suspension; P = powder; S = solution/spray; Sh = shampoo; T = troche; VT = vaginal tablet; Rx = prescription; OTC = over-the-counter (nonprescription)

a. **Prednisone** is the oral steroid of choice of the oral agents used for treatment of dermatologic diseases. Prednisone is metabolized in the liver to its active form, prednisolone, in a similar manner as cortisone is metabolized to hydrocortisone. Table 12–6 lists oral dose equivalents.
b. There are a variety of treatment regimens. For suppression of most inflammatory dermatoses in adults, an initial starting oral dose of 40–60 mg prednisone is commonly used. In most acute conditions, the prednisone is tapered over 10–20 days. If the course of therapy for suppression is too short, a flare and exacerbation may occur when prednisone is discontinued.
c. Long-term oral use requires tapering to an alternate-day dose, which decreases the frequency of most side effects except cataracts and osteoporosis. Table 12–7 lists the systemic side effects of corticosteroids.

TABLE 12–6 Oral Dose Equivalents for Corticosteroids

Drug	Dose (mg)
Cortisone	25
Hydrocortisone	20
Prednisone	5
Prednisolone	4
Methylprednisolone	4
Triamcinolone	4
Betamethasone	0.75
Dexamethasone	0.75

TABLE 12–7 Side Effects of Systemic Steroids

System Affected	Side Effect
Cardiovascular	Hypertension
Central nervous system	Mood alterations, psychosis, pseudotumor cerebri
Endocrine	Hypothalamus–pituitary–adrenal axis suppression
	Hirsutism, menstrual irregularities
	Truncal obesity, moon facies, buffalo hump
	Diabetes mellitus
Gastrointestinal	Peptic ulcer, pancreatitis
Hematologic	Lymphocytopenia, monocytopenia, neutrophilia
Immunologic	Opportunistic infections
Musculoskeletal	Osteoporosis, aseptic necrosis of femoral/humeral heads, myopathy
Ophthalmic	Glaucoma, cataracts (posterior subcapsular)
Renal	Sodium and fluid retention, hypokalemic alkalosis

2. Oral antihistamines are often used to treat pruritus associated with a wide range of skin diseases, particularly those that are mediated by type I histamine-mediated immune responses (e.g., urticaria).

a. Competitive antagonists for histamine H_1 receptors are commonly prescribed. These agents are metabolized in the liver. The shorter-acting agents last 3–6 hours, and the longer acting agents last 12–24 hours.

b. Complications of antihistamines include cholinergic side effects (e.g., glaucoma, constipation, xerostomia) and sedation. The longer-acting antihistamines produce less sedation.

c. In recalcitrant cases of pruritus, H_2 antagonists are added in combination with H_1 antihistamines. H_1 and H_2 receptor blockade also may be achieved with the use of doxepin, a tricyclic antidepressant with strong H_1 and H_2 antihistamine blocking effects. Both H_1 and H_2 antihistamines are available in prescription and nonprescription form (Table 12–8).

TABLE 12–8 Antihistamines Used in Dermatologic Treatments

Compound	Dosage (mg)	Rx/OTC
Short-acting H_1 antagonists		
Chlorpheniramine	4	OTC
Diphenhydramine	25, 50	OTC
Hydroxyzine	10, 25, 50, 100	Rx
Long-acting H_1 antagonists		
Cetirizine	5, 10	Rx
Desloratadine	10	Rx
Fexofenadine	60, 180	Rx
Loratadine	10	OTC
H_2 antagonists		
Cimetidine	200, 300, 400, 800	OTC
Famotidine	20, 40	OTC
Ranitidine	75, 150, 300	OTC
H_1/H_2 Antagonist		
Doxepin	10, 25	OTC

Rx = prescription; OTC = over-the-counter.

IV ACNE AND ROSACEA

A Acne vulgaris

1. **Definition.** Acne vulgaris is a common disorder of the **pilosebaceous unit** (hair follicle and sebaceous glands), located primarily on the face and trunk. It is manifested by follicular comedones with or without inflammatory papules, pustules, and nodules.

2. **Epidemiology.** Acne vulgaris affects 85%–100% of individuals to some degree during their lifetime.

3. **Etiology**
   a. The obstruction of sebaceous follicles is due to excessive sebum production by sebaceous glands in combination with excessive desquamation of the follicular epithelium.
   b. Inflammatory changes are linked to the presence of *Propionibacterium acnes,* a resident, lipophilic anaerobe. *P. acnes* proliferates in the microenvironment created by excess sebum and desquamated follicular cells. This bacterium produces chemotactic factors and proinflammatory mediators that contribute to inflammation.

4. **Pathophysiology**
   a. Acne begins in the prepubertal period, when increasing amounts of adrenal androgens (dehydroepiandrosterone sulfate [DHEAS]) stimulate sebaceous gland hyperplasia and increased sebum production.
   b. Abnormal follicular differentiation is coupled with this phenomenon, resulting in the development of the primary acne lesions, noninflammatory open and closed comedones ("blackheads" and "whiteheads," respectively).
   c. Dermal inflammation and follicular rupture lead to acne scarring.

5. **Clinical features** ***(Color Figure 12–5. See accompanying CD)***
   a. Sites of involvement include the **face** and **upper trunk.**
   b. **Noninflammatory (comedonal) acne** is dominated by open or closed comedones without inflammatory lesions.
   c. Mild **inflammatory acne** is characterized by inflammatory papules and comedones.
   d. Moderate inflammatory acne is characterized by comedones, inflammatory papules, and pustules.
   e. **Nodulocystic acne** is characterized by comedones, inflammatory papules/pustules, and inflammatory nodules (> 5 mm). **Scarring** is often evident.

6. **Diagnosis.** The diagnosis of acne vulgarus is clinical.

7. **Therapy.** Treatment is directed toward the pathogenic factors involved, including follicular dyskeratinization, excess sebum production, and *P. acnes.* The severity of the acne determines the type and level of therapy.
   a. **Topical therapy**
      (1) **Topical retinoids** are comedolytic and anti-inflammatory. The most commonly prescribed topical retinoids include adapalene, tazarotene, and tretinoin. They may be used alone or in combination with other treatments.
      (2) **Topical antibiotics** target *P. acnes.* Commonly prescribed topical antibiotics include erythromycin and clindamycin.
      (3) **Benzoyl peroxide** has antimicrobial properties against *P. acnes.* Benzoyl peroxide is the active ingredient in many OTC topical skin care products; it is available in a variety of formulations, including soaps, washes, lotions, creams, and gels. In addition, it is available by prescription. Benzoyl peroxide is often combined with topical antibiotics to improve efficacy and reduce antibiotic resistance.

b. Systemic therapy

(1) **Oral antibiotics.** Lipophilic antibiotics are most effective against *P. acnes.* Tetracycline, doxycycline, and minocycline are commonly prescribed for inflammatory acne. Trimethoprim, alone or in combination with sulfamethoxazole, as well as azithromycin, are also effective.

(2) **Isotretinoin.** This systemic retinoid is highly effective in treating severe and nodulocystic acne that is recalcitrant to oral antibiotic and topical therapies. It causes normalization of epidermal differentiation, depresses sebum production, is anti-inflammatory, and reduces levels of *P. acnes* in the skin. Isotretinoin is teratogenic, and pregnancy must be avoided. Informed consent with contraception counseling and baseline laboratory tests (including serum pregnancy test) are mandatory before the initiation of therapy.

(3) **Hormonal therapy.** This alternative to systemic antibiotics and isotretinoin in women with persistent acne involves treatment with estrogen or an antiandrogen. Oral contraceptives may be effective. Combination oral contraceptive pills (norgestimate–ethinyl estradiol) containing low levels of progestational compounds are preferred. Spironolactone, which reduces androgen production, may be used alone or in combination with an oral contraceptive.

B Rosacea

1. **Definition.** Rosacea is a disorder of the blood vessels and sebaceous glands of the face characterized by erythema, telangiectasia, flushing, and an inflammatory papulopustular eruption resembling acne.
2. **Epidemiology.** Rosacea is a common disorder that affects approximately 14 million adults in the United States. It is seen more frequently in fair-skinned individuals of European and Celtic descent.
3. **Etiology.** The precise etiology of rosacea is unknown. Clinical signs and symptoms result from the interaction of genetic susceptibility with environmental triggers (UV radiation, temperature changes) and dietary triggers (hot drinks, alcohol, spicy foods).
4. **Pathophysiology**
   a. Vascular lability results in intermittent facial flushing, leading to persistent redness and telangiectasias that affect the central face and occasionally the eyes.
   b. The pathogenesis of the sebaceous hyperplasia and the inflammatory papules and pustules is unclear. Mites of the genus *Demodex* (indigenous to human hair follicles) appear in greater numbers, but their etiologic role has not been established.
5. **Clinical features** (***Color Figure 12–6. See accompanying CD***)
   a. Flushing, erythema, and telangiectasia occur over the cheeks, forehead, and chin.
   b. Inflammatory papules and pustules involve the nose, forehead, and the cheeks, with an absence of comedones and scarring.
   c. Rhinophyma is a prominence of sebaceous glands of the nose that produces thickened skin and disfigurement in extreme cases.
   d. Ocular rosacea produces ocular signs that may include conjunctival injection, edema, chalazion, and episcleritis.
6. **Diagnosis.** The diagnosis is clinical. Overlapping features of acne vulgaris may sometimes be present, and it may be difficult of differentiate acne vulgaris and rosacea.
7. **Therapy.** Avoidance of environmental and dietary triggers is an important strategy to reduce signs and symptoms.
   a. **Topical antibiotics** (e.g., topical metronidazole) may be prescribed for mild disease.
   b. **Systemic antibiotics** (e.g., tetracycline, doxycycline, minocycline) are usually effective in treating acneiform lesions but have limited effectiveness in treating the facial erythema.

c. **Retinoids** (e.g., isotretinoin) are prescribed as a one-time course (similar to acne therapy) and may be an effective treatment for severe cases. Alternatively, long-term, low-dose isotretinoin can be used.

V AUTOIMMUNE BLISTERING DISEASES: PEMPHIGUS AND BULLOUS PEMPHIGOID

A General considerations

1. Autoimmune blistering diseases are characterized by blistering of the skin and mucous membranes associated with the deposition of autoantibodies.
2. Localization of autoantibodies to epitopes in the epidermis, BMZ, or dermis defines the specific clinical features, histopathology, and direct immunofluorescent staining pattern (Table 12–9).
3. Most autoimmune blistering diseases are idiopathic but may be associated with medications, such as pemphigus (see II B) and linear IgA dermatosis (see XII), pregnancy (herpes gestationis; see Table 12–9), autoimmune disease (bullous lupus erythematosus; see Table 12–9), or malignancy (paraneoplastic pemphigus; see XIII).
4. Two of the most commonly encountered forms of autoimmune blistering diseases are pemphigus and bullous pemphigoid.

B Pemphigus

1. **Epidemiology.** The incidence of pemphigus varies from 1 per 1,000,000 to 50 per 1,000,000 population depending on the type of pemphigus and ethnicity. Incidence is higher in Eastern European Jews and individuals of Mediterranean and Indian descent, suggesting some genetic

TABLE 12–9 Target Autoantibodies and Direct Immunofluorescence in Autoimmune Blistering Diseases

Autoimmune Blistering Disease	Ig Epitope	Direct Immunofluorescence (DIF) Findings
Pemphigus vulgaris	Desmoglein 1, 3	Intercellular IgG staining
Pemphigus foliaceus	Desmoglein 1	Intercellular IgG staining
Paraneoplastic pemphigus	Desmoglein 1, 3 Desmoplakin 1, 2 Envoplakin, periplakin, plectin	Intercellular IgG staining and linear BMZ C3 deposits
Bullous pemphigoid	Desmoplakin 1 Collagen XVII	IgG and linear C3 deposits along BMZ; on epidermal side of salt-split skin*
Cicatricial pemphigoid	Epiligrin Collagen XVII	IgG and linear C3 deposits along BMZ; on dermal side of salt-split skin
Herpes gestationis	Collagen XVII	IgG and linear C3 deposits along BMZ; on epidermal side of salt-split skin
Epidermolysis bullosa acquisita	Collagen VII	IgG and linear C3 deposits along BMZ; on dermal side of salt-split skin
Linear IgA dermatosis	Collagen VII Collagen XVII	Linear IgA deposit along BMZ and dermal side of salt-split skin
Bullous lupus erythematosus	Collagen VII	Linear IgA or granular IgG deposits along BMZ and dermal side of salt-split skin

BMZ = basement membrane zone.
*Salt-split skin = incubation of skin biopsy in 1 mol/L salt before performing the DIF results in cleavage through the lamina lucida of basement membrane.

predisposition. The onset of pemphigus is typically young to mid adulthood (< 35 years of age) and affects both sexes equally.

2. **Etiology.** Pemphigus is an immune-mediated disease associated with the production of IgG autoantibodies that target intraepidermal epitopes. The precise cause of autoantibody production is unknown. Certain drugs may trigger pemphigus in some individuals. Exacerbating drugs include penicillamine and angiotensin-converting enzyme inhibitors.
3. **Pathophysiology.** Pemphigus is mediated by IgG targeting of desmoglein, a transmembrane glycoprotein component of desmosomes. Desmosomes are responsible for intercellular adhesion of keratinocytes, and their binding by pemphigus autoantibodies results in separation of keratinocytes (acantholysis) and production of intraepidermal blisters.
   a. **Pemphigus vulgaris** develops from IgG targeting of desmoglein 3 (on keratinocytes of mucous membranes and skin) and desmoglein 1 (on keratinocytes of skin). Blistering results from splitting through the suprabasal portion of the epidermis.
   b. **Pemphigus foliaceus** develops from IgG targeting desmoglein 1, resulting in more superficial blistering within the subcorneal portion of the epidermis.
4. **Clinical features**
   a. **Pemphigus vulgaris** is characterized by dysphagia secondary to oral lesions (90% of cases) ***(Color Figure 12–7. See accompanying CD).*** Skin blisters are distributed predominately on the trunk and scalp. They are flaccid and break easily.
   b. **Pemphigus foliaceus** is characterized by more crusted or denuded lesions (due to the superficial nature of the blistering) with involvement of the face, scalp, and trunk. Oral involvement is rare.
5. **Diagnosis.** Inspection of the skin and identification of primary lesions provide a clinical diagnosis. **Skin biopsy** is required to confirm the clinical impression.
   a. **Histology** shows intraepidermal acantholysis at the suprabasal (pemphigus vulgaris) or subcorneal (pemphigus foliaceus) level.
   b. **Direct immunofluorescence** (**DIF**) of skin biopsy specimens shows IgG deposition throughout the intercellular spaces between keratinocytes.
   c. **Indirect immunofluorescence** (**IDIF**) detects circulating IgG autoantibodies in the patient's serum. Serum titer levels usually mirror disease activity.
6. **Therapy**
   a. **Systemic corticosteroids** are used to provide rapid control of the blistering process.
   b. **Immunosuppressants** are used in combination with corticosteroids and as steroid-sparing agents for long-term control and maintenance. These agents include azathioprine, mycophenolate mofetil, cyclophosphamide, methotrexate, cyclosporine, gold, intravenous immune globulin, and antibiotics.

C Bullous pemphigoid

1. **Epidemiology.** The exact incidence of bullous pemphigoid in the United States is unknown. The reported incidence in Europe is 6.6 cases per million annually. The average age at onset is 65 years.
2. **Etiology.** Bullous pemphigoid is an immune-mediated disease associated with the production of IgG autoantibodies that target basement membrane epitopes. The precise cause of autoantibody production is unknown. Bullous pemphigoid has been reported to be precipitated by phototherapy, radiation therapy, and exposure to certain medications. Drugs that exacerbate bullous pemphigoid include furosemide, nonsteroidal anti-inflammatory drugs (NSAIDs), captopril, penicillamine, and antibiotics.
3. **Pathophysiology.** The IgG autoantibodies of bullous pemphigoid target desmoplakin 1 (bullous pemphigoid antigen 1) and collagen XVII (bullous pemphigoid antigen 2), which are intracellular and transmembrane components, respectively, of hemidesmosomes. Hemidesmosomes are

responsible for the adhesion of basal keratinocytes with the basement membrane. The binding of antibodies at the basement membrane activates complement and attracts inflammatory cells to release proteases, leading to subepidermal blister formation.

4. **Clinical features**
   a. Tense bullae, with or without erythema, usually involve the trunk and flexural areas of the skin ***(Color Figure 12–8. See accompanying CD).***
   b. Mucosal involvement rarely occurs.
   c. Persistent urticarial lesions subsequently develop bullae.

5. **Diagnosis**
   a. **Clinical inspection** of the skin and identification of primary lesions yield a clinical diagnosis. Skin biopsy for histology and DIF is required to confirm the clinical impression.
      (1) **Histology** shows subepidermal split with an intact epidermis as the blister roof. Eosinophils often predominate in the dermal infiltrate.
      (2) **DIF** reveals linear IgG and C3 deposition along the DEJ. Bullous pemphigoid can be differentiated from other subepidermal autoimmune blistering diseases by incubating the skin biopsy sample in 1 mol/L salt before performing DIF. This process induces cleavage through the lamina lucida. DIF on salt-split skin shows IgG on the blister roof (epidermal side of split skin).
   b. **IDIF** can detect circulating IgG autoantibodies in the serum of most patients. However, titer levels do not correlate with disease activity.

6. **Therapy.** Mild cases may be controlled with antibiotics and topical steroids. Moderate and severe cases require systemic corticosteroids and steroid-sparing immunosuppressants, such as those used to treat pemphigus.

VI CUTANEOUS REACTION PATTERNS

Each dermatologic diagnosis included in this section represents a specific cutaneous reaction that can develop in response to multiple causes. The clinical diagnosis of each of these cutaneous reaction patterns requires a thorough investigation into the underlying cause that may vary from case to case.

A Erythema multiforme

1. **Epidemiology.** The true incidence of erythema multiforme in the United States is unknown.
   a. **Erythema multiforme minor** (less severe form) may account for up to 1% of dermatology office visits.
   b. **Erythema multiforme major** (more severe form) occurs at an incidence of 0.6 to 8.0 cases per million per year.

2. **Etiology.** Approximately 50% of cases are idiopathic; no underlying cause is identified.
   a. **Infection.** The most common causes of erythema multiforme are infectious (viral, bacterial, fungal). HSV is the most common infectious etiology, followed by *Mycoplasma pneumoniae*. Recurrent erythema multiforme (minor or major) can accompany recurrent HSV.
   b. **Drug reaction.** Another major cause is adverse drug reactions associated with malignancy, hormonal imbalances, collagen vascular diseases, and sarcoidosis.

3. **Pathophysiology.** Erythema multiforme is an acute hypersensitivity reaction to a variety of stimuli. It is a cytotoxic immunologic reaction resulting in epidermal keratinocyte necrosis associated with a dense lymphocytic infiltrate within the dermis. Immune complex deposition is nonspecific. Subepidermal bullae formation occurs in severe forms.

4. **Clinical features.** Based on severity of features and extent of mucous membrane involvement, erythema multiforme may be categorized into minor and major forms.
   a. **Erythema multiforme minor. Iris or target lesions** are erythematous macules or papules with concentric red borders and central purpura or vesicles ***(Color Figure 12–9. See accom-***

panying CD). Erythema multiforme tends to be symmetric and have an acral distribution with lesions involving the palms and soles. Lesions may involve extremities and face and coalesce and become generalized. Mild oral cavity blistering may be seen in up to 25% of cases. Resolution usually occurs within 2 weeks.

b. **Erythema multiforme major (Stevens-Johnson syndrome).** Skin findings are similar to erythema multiforme minor but are more severe. Mouth, lips, and bulbar conjunctivae are most commonly affected, with mucous membranes severely affected. Oral bullae break easily and create erosions that readily become secondarily infected, often causing pain and bloody, crusted lips.

5. **Diagnosis.** Clinical inspection of the skin and identification of primary skin lesions yields a clinical diagnosis. Skin biopsy confirms the clinical impression. Evaluation of the underlying cause should accompany a clinical diagnosis.

6. **Therapy.** Treatment of the underlying cause and withdrawal of any offending drugs is the first management step. Supportive care is initiated, as well as symptomatic relief of painful and secondarily infected mucocutaneous lesions. Systemic corticosteroids may be effective, but their use is controversial.

B Lichen planus

1. **Epidemiology.** The incidence is estimated at 1% of new patient office visits in the United States.
2. **Etiology.** The exact etiology of lichen planus is unknown. Most cases are idiopathic. A positive family history in a few cases suggests a genetic predisposition. Associated liver disease, including hepatitis C infection, chronic active hepatitis, and primary biliary cirrhosis, as well as autoimmune disorders such as ulcerative colitis, dermatomyositis, and myasthenia gravis, may occur. An adverse drug reaction (lichenoid drug reaction) may be the cause.
3. **Pathophysiology.** Lichen planus is a cell-mediated immunologic reaction targeting the epidermal keratinocytes. A dense lymphocytic infiltrate at the DEJ (lichenoid infiltrate) participates in the destruction of basal keratinocytes (basal vacuolization). Immunogenetic predisposition may play a role in the pathogenesis. Human leukocyte antigen DR1 (HLA-DR1) and HLA-DR10 is associated with idiopathic lichen planus, and HLA-B7 is associated with familial cases.
4. **Clinical features** ***(Color Figure 12–10. See accompanying CD).*** Most idiopathic cases are self-limiting, lasting 6 to 18 months. Other cases can be chronic and recurrent, particularly oral lichen planus.
   a. Polygonal papules are violaceous (purple), pruritic, and flat-topped (lichenoid), usually covered with fine scales. Lesions vary in size from 1 mm to more than 1 cm in diameter.
   b. The distribution of lesions typically involves flexor surfaces of the upper extremities (wrists), on the genitalia, and on the mucous membranes. Nails and scalp may be involved.
   c. Oral lesions involve the tongue and buccal mucosa and may be asymptomatic plaques displaying a white reticular pattern (Wickham striae). Erosive lesions are painful.
   d. Nail dystrophy with nail plate thinning and ridging may be seen in 10% of cases. Nail matrix involvement may lead to scarring of the nail bed (pterygium formation).
   e. Scalp involvement (lichen planopilaris) is seen more often in women and produces follicular inflammation, often resulting in scarring alopecia.
   f. Lesions resolve with residual postinflammatory hyperpigmentation.
5. **Diagnosis.** Clinical inspection of the skin and identification of primary skin lesions provides a clinical diagnosis. Skin biopsy confirms the clinical impression. Evaluation of the underlying cause and associated disorders should accompany a clinical diagnosis.
6. **Therapy.** Treatment of an identifiable underlying cause and **withdrawal of any offending drugs** is the first management step. **Antihistamines** and topical steroids are effective in mild, self-limiting cases. **Systemic corticosteroids** are used acutely to suppress more severe cases. Long-term control

of chronic cases may require **steroid-sparing immunosuppressants. Topical and systemic retinoids** as well as **topical and systemic cyclosporine** have been shown to be active in some cases.

C Urticaria Urticaria (hives) is a common cutaneous reaction pattern requiring investigation into its underlying etiology ***(Color Figure 12–11. See accompanying CD).*** It is covered in detail in Chapter 7, IV.

D Pyoderma gangrenosum

1. **Epidemiology.** The incidence of pyoderma gangrenosum in the United States is estimated at approximately 1 per 100,000 people each year.
2. **Etiology.** Pyoderma gangrenosum is an ulcerative skin disorder of unknown etiology. Several diseases are commonly associated with pyoderma gangrenosum (Table 12–10). No underlying disease association is present in 50% of cases.
3. **Pathophysiology.** The pathophysiology of pyoderma gangrenosum is poorly understood. It appears to be an immune-mediated reaction involving an intense and destructive neutrophilic infiltrate within the dermis. The dermal inflammatory reaction causes purulent ulceration. Immunocomplex deposition is nonspecific.
4. **Clinical features** ***(Color Figure 12–12. See accompanying CD).***
   - **a.** Initial presentation may be erythematous to violaceous painful nodules that quickly ulcerate.
   - **b.** Deep and purulent ulcers with highly inflammatory and tender borders develop.
   - **c.** Ulcer margins are typically undermined. Violaceous borders overhang the ulcer bed.
   - **d.** The lower extremities are typically affected. Variants may affect other areas.
   - **e.** **Pathergy,** the development of new lesions or aggravation of existing ones after trauma, may occur.
5. **Diagnosis.** Pyoderma gangrenosum is a clinicopathologic diagnosis of exclusion and is made after other causes of cutaneous ulcerations have been ruled out. There is no specific laboratory test, and the histopathology is only suggestive, not diagnostic. A **skin biopsy** with tissue sent for histology and cultures is required to establish a diagnosis. Appropriate laboratory studies, imaging studies, and diagnostic procedures (e.g., colonoscopy or bone marrow biopsy) should be ordered to identify any associated diseases (see Table 12–10).
6. **Differential diagnosis**
   - **a.** Bacterial infection (pseudomonas or anaerobic [clostridial] infections)
   - **b.** Atypical mycobacterial infection
   - **c.** Deep fungal infection (North American blastomycosis)
   - **d.** Amebiasis
   - **e.** Bromoderma and iododerma

TABLE 12–10 Diseases Associated with Pyoderma Gangrenosum
Inflammatory bowel disease: ulcerative colitis or Crohn's disease
Polyarthritis (usually symmetric; either seronegative or seropositive)
Hematologic diseases
Myeloid leukemias
IgA monoclonal gammopathy
Myelomas (IgA type, predominantly)
Hepatic diseases: hepatitis and primary biliary cirrhosis
Collagen vascular diseases: lupus erythematosus and Sjögren's syndrome

f. Rheumatoid vasculitis
g. Brown recluse spider bite
h. Wegener's granulomatosis

7. **Therapy.** Effective treatment of the associated underlying disease most often results in control of pyoderma gangrenosum.
   a. Local wound care and dressings are aimed at gentle cleansing of the ulcer base.
   b. **Surgical debridement** or surgical therapy (skin grafting) is contraindicated.
   c. Intralesional corticosteroid injections into new nodules or the borders of small ulcers may be effective as an early intervention.
   d. Systemic corticosteroids are often required to gain rapid control of the destructive skin changes. High doses of oral prednisone and intravenous pulsed methylprednisolone are effective. Other systemic therapies include cyclosporine, tacrolimus, mycophenolate mofetil, azathioprine, cyclophosphamide, chlorambucil, dapsone, thalidomide, and intravenous immune globulin.

E Erythema nodosum

1. **Epidemiology.** The incidence is unknown. Erythema nodosum occurs more frequently in young adults and in women.
2. **Etiology.** This immune-mediated reaction may occur in association with systemic disease (Table 12–11) or **adverse drug reaction,** or it may be **idiopathic.**
3. **Pathophysiology.** Erythema nodosum appears to be delayed-type hypersensitivity reaction targeting the subcutaneous fat (panniculus). A lymphohistiocytic infiltrate develops, resulting in nonsuppurative inflammatory nodules. No circulating immunocomplexes have been found.
4. **Clinical features** ***(Color Figure 12–13. See accompanying CD)***
   a. A prodrome of flu-like symptoms, including fever and arthralgia, may occur.
   b. Lesions begin as poorly defined red, tender nodules that are 2–6 cm in diameter.
   c. Lesions are typically distributed over the anterior lower leg but may appear on any surface.
   d. Individual lesions develop over 2 weeks, with gradual softening and a bruise-like appearance. The overlying skin usually desquamates. Leg pain and ankle swelling may persist for weeks.
   e. Thirty percent of idiopathic cases may last more than 6 months.
5. **Diagnosis.** Clinical inspection of the skin and identification of primary skin lesions provides a clinical diagnosis. An incisional skin biopsy with adequate sampling of the subcutaneous fat confirms the clinical impression and is reserved for diagnostically difficult cases. Evaluation of an underlying cause and associated disorders should accompany the clinical diagnosis.
6. **Therapy.** Treatment of an identifiable underlying cause and withdrawal of any offending drugs is the first management step. In idiopathic or self-limited cases, symptomatic relief with NSAIDs, compression dressings, and leg elevation is usually satisfactory. In persistent cases, systemic agents such as colchicine and liquid supersaturated potassium iodide have proven effective.

TABLE 12–11 Systemic Diseases Associated with Erythema Nodosum
Bacterial infections (streptococcal infections; most common bacterial cause)
Fungal infections (coccidioidomycosis; most common fungal infection)
Pregnancy
Sarcoidosis
Inflammatory bowel disease
Hodgkin's disease and lymphoma
Behçet disease

VII DERMATITIS

A General considerations The term *dermatitis* can be defined as inflammation of the skin. It is often used as a general term to describe skin findings, such as "rash"; however, it also is used in the diagnoses of specific cutaneous diseases. Three of the most prevalent dermatitides are described in this section.

B Atopic dermatitis

1. **Definitions**
   a. **Atopic dermatitis** (atopic eczema or eczema) refers to the chronic, relapsing cutaneous manifestations generated from pruritus and scratching, associated with an underlying allergic predisposition (atopy).
   b. **Atopy** is a hereditary predisposition toward developing hypersensitivity reactions, associated with elevated serum immunoglobulin E (IgE) levels, including asthma, allergic rhinitis, and atopic dermatitis.
2. **Epidemiology.** Atopic dermatitis affects as much as 12% of the US population.
3. **Etiology.** The precise etiology is unknown. There is a clear familial pattern of inheritance for atopic dermatitis and for all forms of atopy. Studies suggest an autosomal dominant inheritance pattern with variable penetrance. Genetic susceptibility interacts with various environmental and dietary triggers.
4. **Pathophysiology.**
   a. **Pruritus** (i.e., itchy skin) predominates and may be initiated by hypersensitivity to environmental, dietary, or endogenous triggers. Increased numbers of antigen-presenting cells are found in atopic skin. These antigen-presenting cells have increased numbers of high-affinity IgE receptors that bind IgE and may be involved in amplifying a cascade of inflammatory mediators (cytokines and chemokines) that propagate pruritus and inflammation.
   b. **Scratching,** a response to pruritus, propagates the cutaneous inflammatory process and leads to both acute and chronic skin changes. Exogenous triggers of atopic dermatitis include foods (milk, eggs, peanuts), dry skin from excessive bathing, contact with harsh skin care products (e.g., perfumes) or clothing (e.g., wool), and excessive or prolonged heat.
5. **Clinical features** ***(Color Figure 12–14. See accompanying CD)***
   a. Atopic dermatitis is primarily manifested in infancy and childhood. Approximately one third of the cases persist, to some degree, into adulthood.
   b. The disease has different **clinical stages,** which vary depending on severity.
      (1) The **acute stage** is associated with itchy and erythematous papules, vesicles with excoriated erosions, and serous exudate.
      (2) The **subacute stage** is associated with scaling and erythematous excoriated papules and plaques.
      (3) The **chronic stage** is associated with lichenification (thickening of the skin) with varying degrees of erythema, hyper- and hypopigmentation, and excoriated papules and nodules.
   c. The **flexor areas of the arms, legs, and neck** are primarily involved in children and adults. Severe cases may result in generalized erythroderma.
   d. Lesions often become secondarily infected with bacteria from scratching and are characterized by yellow crusting with impetigo.
   e. Hand and foot dermatitis may be the only manifestation of atopic dermatitis in adults with a history of atopy. Findings include erythema, scaling or peeling, and fissuring of the palms, soles, and fingers.
   f. Keratoconus is observed in severe cases. A cone-shaped cornea (requiring corneal transplant) may develop in the second or third decade of life.
6. **Diagnosis.** Atopic dermatitis is a clinical diagnosis. Serum IgE levels are usually elevated. A skin biopsy may be helpful in confirming the clinical diagnosis and ruling out other disorders.

7. Therapy

a. **Prevention** is effective in reducing acute exacerbations and complications.

(1) Exacerbating triggers should be identified and avoided.

(2) Good skin care maintenance should be practiced.

(a) Excessive bathing should be avoided. Short baths or showers in lukewarm water, with mild, moisturizing soaps are recommended.

(b) Use of moisturizers after bathing is recommended.

b. **Topical treatments**

(1) **Topical corticosteroids.** Medium- to high-potency topical steroids that can be tapered to low-potency topical corticosteroids are the best treatment for acute exacerbations.

(2) **Topical macrolide immunosuppressants.** Pimecrolimus ointment and tacrolimus ointment have been approved for the treatment of atopic dermatitis. These calcineurin inhibitors that are similar to cyclosporine are effective steroid-sparing therapies for the treatment of acute flares of atopic dermatitis.

(3) **Lubricants.** Moisturizing the skin with emollients should be used during treatment of acute flares as well as during maintenance therapy.

c. **Systemic treatments**

(1) **Systemic corticosteroids.** A short course of oral prednisone for treatment of acute and severe flares may be helpful in gaining rapid control.

(2) **Oral antibiotics.** Antibiotics are prescribed to treat secondary infections when present.

(3) **Antihistamines.** The pruritus of atopic dermatitis is not directly mediated by histamine, but H_1 and H_2 histamine blockade may be effective in recalcitrant cases. The sedative effects of antihistamines taken at bedtime may provide relief from scratching during sleep and thus reduce a perpetuating factor.

C Allergic contact dermatitis

1. Definitions

a. **Allergic contact dermatitis** is inflammation of the skin induced by a delayed-type hypersensitivity (allergy) reaction to a specific allergen that contacts the skin.

b. Irritant contact dermatitis is cutaneous inflammation induced by the direct contact and toxic effects of chemicals contacting the skin. Occupational dermatitis refers to allergic contact dermatitis or irritant contact dermatitis that occurs in the workplace.

2. Epidemiology. The incidence of both allergic and irritant contact dermatitis has been estimated to be 13.6 cases per 1000 population in the United States. Surveys indicate that contact dermatitis is one of the most frequent dermatologic diagnoses and represents between 5% and 9% of dermatology office visits. Occupational dermatitis represents up to 20% of all reported occupational diseases in the United States.

3. Etiology. Cutaneous contact with a specific allergen results in allergic contact dermatitis in susceptible individuals. Approximately 3000 chemical compounds have been documented as specific causes of allergic contact dermatitis. Table 12–12 lists some common chemicals.

4. Pathophysiology. Most compounds that induce allergic contact dermatitis are small molecules (haptens, <500 daltons) that bind to carrier proteins on epidermal antigen-presenting cells (Langerhans cells). Langerhans cells process antigenic molecules and present them on their surface within class II major histocompatability molecules. CD4+ T lymphocytes (helper T cells) interact with Langerhans cells and stimulate secretion of inflammatory mediators. Langerhans cells migrate from the epidermis to the regional draining lymph nodes and stimulate proliferation and activation of antigen-specific T cells. Expanded numbers of antigen-specific T cells circulate into the skin, recognize antigen at sites of contact, and amplify the inflammatory reaction. The initial sensitization may be acute or chronic. Usually, 10–14 days pass after an initial acute exposure to a strong contact allergen before an individual becomes sensitized. Some initial exposures may

TABLE 12–12 Common Allergens Frequently Inducing Allergic Contact Dermatitis

Allergen	Compounds Containing Allergen
Urushiol oil (*Rhus*)	Poison ivy, oak, sumac
Nickel sulfate	Gold jewelry
Cobalt dichloride	Cement, metal-plated objects, paints
Cinnamic alcohol	Fragrances
Balsam of Peru	Foods, cosmetics, fragrances, flavorings
Formaldehyde	Nail polish, cosmetics, plastics, glues
para-Phenylenediamine	Hair dyes, dyed textiles, and cosmetics
Mercaptobenzothiazole	Rubber products, adhesives
Thimerosal	Preservative in contact lens solutions and injectables
Neomycin	Topical antibiotics

not result in clinically apparent allergic contact dermatitis. Once an individual is sensitized to a chemical, allergic contact dermatitis develops within hours to several days of reexposure.

5. **Clinical features** *(Color Figure 12–15. See accompanying CD)*
   a. Acute disease is characterized by pruritic papules and vesicles on an erythematous base.
   b. Acute exposures result in cutaneous inflammation and pruritus lasting 2–3 weeks.
   c. The distribution tends to be asymmetrical and depends on the nature of the contact. Linear or geometric configurations often are present.
   d. Chronic allergic contact dermatitis, caused by chronic exposure to allergen, may produce lichenified, pruritic plaques.
   e. Occasionally, allergic contact dermatitis may generalize and produce a diffuse exfoliative erythroderma.
6. **Diagnosis.** The diagnosis is usually made on clinical grounds. **Skin biopsy** may support the clinical diagnosis in difficult cases. The initial site of dermatitis often provides the best clues regarding the potential cause of disease. **Patch testing** is required to confirm the diagnosis and identify the external chemicals to which the person is allergic.
7. **Therapy.** Prevention is the mainstay of therapy. Identification of the offending agent and avoidance reduces risk for chronic or recurrent dermatitis.
   a. **Topical treatments**
      (1) High-potency **topical corticosteroid** creams are effective when prescribed for 2-week courses.
      (2) **Drying agents,** such as calamine lotion or cool compresses (with saline or aluminum acetate solution), are helpful in soothing and drying acute, localized vesicular eruptions.
      (3) Individuals with widespread vesicular eruptions may obtain relief from cool oatmeal baths.
   b. **Systemic treatments**
      (1) **Corticosteroids.** Severe or diffuse disease often requires treatment with a 2–3-week course of oral prednisone. Short (5-day) courses of Solu-Medrol “dose packs” are inadequate. When discontinued, they usually result in flaring of symptoms.
      (2) Oral H_1 **antihistamines** often are helpful in diminishing pruritus.

D Seborrheic dermatitis

1. **Definition.** Seborrheic dermatitis (seborrhea) is a chronic and recurrent papulosquamous disorder with a distinctive distribution involving the scalp and central face, chest, axillae, and groin.
2. **Epidemiology.** Seborrheic dermatitis is a common disorder that affects as much as 5% of the population.

3. **Etiology**
   a. The precise etiology is unknown. An aberrant immune response to endogenous yeast forms (*Pityrosporum*) has been speculated.
   b. Triggers associated with flares include seasonal changes, trauma (e.g., scratching), emotional stress, and medications. Such medications, which may also induce seborrheic dermatitis, include psychotropic medications (e.g., chlorpromazine, haloperidol, lithium), benzodiazepines, cimetidine, ethionamide, gold, IFN-α, methyldopa, and psoralen. In addition, Parkinson's disease and acquired immunodeficiency syndrome (AIDS) are associated with flares.
4. **Pathophysiology.** Cutaneous inflammation may result from normal levels of *P. ovale*, releasing inflammatory free fatty acids. *P. ovale* is also able to activate the alternative complement pathway in affected individuals who have decreased humoral and cellular immune responses.
5. **Clinical features.** Seborrheic dermatitis affects adults but may be seen in infants (**cradle cap**).
   a. The scalp is usually involved in all cases. Disease may vary from mild, patchy scaling (dandruff) to widespread pruritic, erythematous, thick, adherent greasy scales.
   b. Disease usually moves from the scalp to the face, affecting the eyebrows and nasolabial folds (T-zone) ***(Color Figure 12–16. See accompanying CD).*** The chest, axillae, and groin also may be affected.
   c. A **seborrheic blepharitis** may occur, and rarely, a generalized exfoliative erythroderma may develop in severe cases.
6. **Diagnosis.** Seborrheic dermatitis is usually well recognized on clinical inspection and by history.
7. **Therapy.** Mild cases of scalp involvement (dandruff) respond to OTC shampoos that contain salicylic acid, tar, selenium, sulfur, zinc, or ketoconazole.
   a. **Topical corticosteroids** are effective for short-term treatment of acute flares.
   b. **Topical antifungals** are effective for prolonged treatment of the skin.

VIII PSORIASIS

A Definition Psoriasis is a chronic, relapsing skin disease that manifests as a papulosquamous eruption with variable clinical manifestations, but typically psoriasis occurs as inflammatory plaques with excessive white scaling in a predominately extensor distribution.

B Epidemiology Psoriasis affects approximately 2%–3% of the US population, or 6.4 million cases. Approximately 200,000 new cases occur annually. The median age at onset is 28 years.

C Etiology Psoriasis appears to be an autoimmune disease with a genetic predisposition. It is mostly likely inherited as a polygenic, autosomal dominant disease with variable penetrance. The precise target of the immune response is unknown. HLA-B13, HLA-B17, HLA-BW57, and HLA-CW6 are most frequently associated with psoriasis. As many as one third of patients report that one family member is affected. Psoriasis tends to flare during winter months and improve in the summer months as a function of sun (UV) exposure. Drugs that exacerbate psoriasis include β-adrenergic blockers, lithium, and angiotensin-converting enzyme inhibitors.

D Pathophysiology Psoriasis is an immune-mediated disease associated with a mixed inflammatory dermal infiltrate that initiates and maintains an increase in the proliferation rate of epidermal keratinocytes in affected areas. The increased keratinocyte turnover rate produces epidermal thickening (**acanthosis**) and disruption of normal epidermal differentiation, resulting in scaling. Disease onset and flares often follow upper respiratory infections (e.g., streptococcal pharyngitis), suggesting that superantigen activation of pathogenic T lymphocytes or molecular mimicry of cutaneous antigens plays a role in pathogenesis.

E Clinical features

1. **Plaque-type psoriasis** occurs as raised erythematous plaques covered with a white scale ***(Color Figure 12–17. See accompanying CD).*** Scratching the scale may lead to punctate bleeding (Auspitz sign).
2. The **distribution** of psoriatic lesions includes the **extensor surfaces** of the extremities (knees and elbows), scalp, and trunk (particularly the presacral area).
3. Psoriasis may affect the **nails** and cause pitting of the nail plates, yellow discoloration, and thickening and separation from the nail bed.
4. Lesions often develop at sites of cutaneous injury or trauma (Köbner phenomenon).
5. **Guttate (tear-shaped) psoriasis** is a clinical variant that develops rapidly, most often after a streptococcal upper respiratory infection. Multiple, small (< 1 cm) psoriatic lesions are distributed on the trunk and extremities.
6. **Pustular psoriasis** is a typically severe clinical variant that presents with sterile pustules appearing within plaques or diffusely.
7. **Erythrodermic psoriasis** is a severe clinical variant that presents as a generalized erythema with extensive scaling and exfoliation.
8. **Psoriatic arthritis** of varying severity affects approximately 10% of psoriatic patients (see Chapter 10 III B 3).

F Diagnosis

Psoriasis is usually well recognized on clinical inspection of the skin and usually distinguished from other papulosquamous eruptions. Skin biopsy confirms the clinical impression.

G Therapy

Treatment is tailored to the severity of psoriasis, which is usually estimated by the percentage of the body surface area involved. Topical therapies are used in mild cases, and phototherapy and systemic agents are used for moderate to severe cases.

1. **Topical agents** include keratolytic agents (salicylic acid), coal tar preparations, topical steroids, topical vitamin D_3 analogs (calcipotriene), and topical retinoids. **Phototherapy** with psoralen plus UV-A light or UV-B light is very effective in cases with generalized skin involvement.
2. **Systemic agents** include oral retinoids (acitretin), methotrexate (particularly for arthritis), cyclosporine, and biologic agents. Biologic agents include alefacept (a fusion protein that targets T-lymphocyte antigen molecule CD2), etanercept (a fusion protein that targets tumor necrosis factor), and efalizumab (an antibody that targets T-lymphocyte adhesion molecule CD11a). **Systemic corticosteroids should be avoided** because of severe rebound flares on withdrawal.

IX PITYRIASIS ROSEA

A Definition

Pityriasis rosea is a benign, self-limited **papulosquamous exanthem** with a distinctive distribution involving the **trunk.**

B Epidemiology

In children and young adults, the estimated incidence is 0.3%–3% of dermatology visits.

C Etiology

Pityriasis rosea appears to be an **infectious exanthem,** but no definitive etiologic agent has been identified. Case clusters among contacts have been reported. There appears to be a seasonal predilection to spring, autumn, and winter. The rate of recurrence is low (3%). Drug-induced pityriasis rosea associated with such agents as captopril, gold, and D-penicillamine has been described.

D Pathophysiology

An initial solitary lesion (**herald patch**) develops in 50%–90% of cases, followed by a secondary crop of lesions that appear over 2–21 days. Lesions spontaneously regress by 6 weeks.

E Clinical features *(Color Figure 12–18. See accompanying CD)*

1. The **herald patch** typically measures 1–3 cm in diameter and usually is located on the trunk or proximal extremities. The patch is oval or round and is erythematous with fine, peripheral (collarette) scaling.
2. The **secondary eruption** is similar in appearance but ranges in size from 0.5–1.0 cm. The lesion is symmetrical on the trunk and follows the lines of cleavage of the skin, producing a **"Christmas tree"** pattern on the back.
3. Lesions are usually asymptomatic but may be pruritic.

F Diagnosis

Pityriasis rosea is usually well recognized on clinical inspection of the skin and readily distinguished from other papulosquamous eruptions.

G Therapy

Pityriasis rosea is a self-limited disease, and no specific treatment is usually necessary. Topical steroids may be used to relieve pruritus. UV radiation therapy has been used to hasten the resolution of lesions.

X SKIN CANCERS

A Basal cell carcinoma

1. **Definition.** Basal cell carcinoma is a neoplastic growth of the basal cell layer of epidermis.
2. **Epidemiology.** Basal cell carcinoma is the most common type of cancer in the United States. Approximately 800,000 new cases occur each year.
3. **Etiology.** The multifactorial etiology includes genetic susceptibility and environmental exposure to UV light (sunlight).
4. **Pathophysiology**
   a. Neoplastic transformation of basal keratinocytes produces downward growth into underlying dermis and deeper tissues. Basal cell carcinoma is locally invasive without metastatic capacity. UV-induced mutations in the *ptch* gene pathway are detected in sporadic cases.
   b. **Basal cell nevus syndrome** (Gorlin syndrome) is a rare autosomal dominant syndrome with germline mutations in the *ptch* gene, resulting in increased basal cell carcinomas and developmental abnormalities of the skeletal system, genitourinary system, and central nervous system.
5. **Clinical features**
   a. A persistent skin lesion is usually in the 3–6-mm size range and on sun-exposed areas of the skin.
   b. Lesions are flesh colored to red, may be a plaque or a papule, and have a pearly or translucent quality *(Color Figure 12–19. See accompanying CD).*
   c. Some lesions may be brown to black (pigmented basal cell carcinoma) and often are associated with telangiectasias.
   d. The borders are rolled with central depressions, ulceration, or crusting (**rodent ulcer**).
   e. Lesions located on the central face (noses and eyes) and ears are at high risk for recurrence.
   f. Histologic variants include morpheaform basal cell carcinoma (scar-like quality and histologic fibrosis) and multicentric basal cell carcinoma (indistinct borders with histiologic skip areas) and are at high risk for recurrence.
   g. The risk of recurrence is high in immunosuppressed patients.
6. **Diagnosis.** The diagnosis is made by clinical inspection of skin and skin biopsy confirmation.
7. **Therapy**
   a. **Surgery.** The cure rate is 90%–99%, depending on the tumor site and surgical technique. Surgical techniques include technique excision, Mohs micrographic surgery, curettage with electrodesiccation, and cryosurgery.
   b. **Radiation therapy.** The cure rate is 93%–97%.

B Squamous cell carcinoma

1. **Definition.** Squamous cell carcinoma is a neoplastic growth of the suprabasal cell layer of epidermis.
2. **Epidemiology.** Squamous cell carcinoma is the second most common type of cancer in the United States. Approximately 400,000 new cases occur each year.
3. **Etiology.** The etiology is multifactorial and includes genetic susceptibility and environmental exposure to UV light (sunlight).
4. **Pathophysiology**
   a. Neoplastic transformation of suprabasal keratinocytes produces intraepidermal (in situ) foci leading to tumor invasion of underlying dermis and deeper tissues. UV-induced *p53* gene mutations are identified in precursor lesions (**actinic keratosis**), of which 0.1%–1.0% progress to squamous cell carcinoma in situ. Squamous cell carcinomas are locally invasive. Histopathology of lesions progresses from well differentiated to poorly differentiated. Metastatic progression to regional lymph nodes occurs in 1%–3% of cases.
   b. **Xeroderma pigmentosum** is an autosomal recessive syndrome with germ line mutations in one of the xeroderma pigmentosum nucleotide excision repair genes (*XPA* through *XPG*), resulting in photosensitivity and early onset and increased frequency of skin cancers, predominately squamous cell carcinoma.
5. **Clinical features** ***(Color Figure 12–20. See accompanying CD.)***
   a. Persistent lesions usually are detected on sun-exposed areas of the skin.
   b. The red, scaling plaques have variable degrees of firmness. Actinic keratoses are superficial without a palpable component.
   c. Large lesions (>1 cm) may be nodular with ulceration or secondary crusting.
   d. A subset of these carcinomas are considered high risk for metastasis. Risk factors for metastasis include location on the lower lip, histologic features such as poor differentiation, invasion more than 4 mm into the dermis, perineural invasion, occurrence in immunosuppressed patients, and development in burn sites.
6. **Diagnosis.** The diagnosis of squamous cell carcinoma is made by clinical inspection of skin and confirmed by skin biopsy.
7. **Therapy**
   a. **Surgery.** The cure rate is 90%–99% depending on the tumor site and surgical technique. Surgical techniques include excision, Mohs micrographic surgery, curettage with electrodesiccation, and cryosurgery.
   b. **Radiation therapy.** The cure rate is 93%–97%. Prophylactic postoperative radiation to regional lymph nodes is indicated in cases of perineural invasion.

C Melanoma

1. **Definition.** Melanoma is the neoplastic growth of melanocytes.
2. **Epidemiology**
   a. **Incidence.** Approximately 57,000 new cases of melanoma occur each year in the United States.
   b. **Risk factors**
      (1) **Genetic.** Ten percent of cases of melanoma are familial; at least one relative is affected. From 1% to 3% of cases of melanoma are hereditary; two or more first-degree relatives are affected with melanoma and have a germ line mutation in the *CDKN2A* gene.
      (2) **Previous melanoma.** Patients who have had one melanoma have a 5% probability of a second primary melanoma.
      (3) **Environmental.** The risk of melanoma increases with increased UV exposure, particularly with an increased number of severe sunburns in individuals younger than 20 years of age.

(4) **Pigmentation.** The following factors are associated with an increased risk of melanoma.
   (a) **Fair complexion** (readily sunburns and never tans, blue eyes, red or blonde hair)
   (b) **Increased number of melanocytic nevi (moles)** (>25)
   (c) Presence of **large melanocytic nevi** (>6 mm)
   (d) Presence of **atypical (dysplastic) nevi** (>5 mm with varying degrees of irregular clinical features [see X C 5]).

3. **Etiology.** The multifactorial etiology includes genetic susceptibility and environmental exposure to UV light (sunlight).
4. **Pathophysiology.** The initial stages of neoplastic transformation result in upward (pagetoid) growth of cytologically atypical melanocytes within epidermis (in situ). Tumor progression results in invasion of underlying dermis and deeper tissues. Regional lymph node metastasis usually precedes metastasis to distant sites, typically skin, lung, brain, and liver. In most cases, *BRAF* gene mutations are detected in early melanoma tumor progression.
5. **Clinical features.** The vast majority of cutaneous melanomas have unstable clinical features that change over time. Characteristic features may be remembered using the mnemonic "ABCD" ***(Color Figure 12–21. See accompanying CD).***
   a. **Asymmetry:** a deviation in the overall round to oval configuration
   b. **Border:** an irregular circumference of the lesion. The indistinct margins may blend in to the flesh-colored background.
   c. **Color:** nonuniformity of pigmentation with variations in color, including black, blue, and red hues
   d. **Diameter:** generally greater than 6 mm for detection
6. **Diagnosis.** The diagnosis of melanoma is made by clinical inspection of skin and confirmed by excisional biopsy.
7. **Prognosis.** The thickness of the melanoma (depth of invasion), measured in millimeters from the stratum corneum to the deepest penetration of the tumor, is thought to be the best predictor of the risk of metastatic disease (Table 12–13). Prognostic factors associated with increased risk for melanoma metastasis include the following:
   a. Primary tumor depth of invasion (>1 mm)
   b. Primary tumor ulceration
   c. Vascular or lymphatic invasion
   d. Age > 65 years
   e. Primary tumor located on trunk or head and neck
   f. Male sex
8. **Staging**
   a. Four clinical stages are defined for melanoma.
      (1) Stage I: skin involvement with a primary tumor < 2 mm in thickness
      (2) Stage II: skin involvement with a primary tumor > 2 mm in thickness

TABLE 12–13 Melanoma Prognosis and Survival

Thickness of Lesion	Risk Group	% Survival
0 mm (in situ)	Low	100
<1.00 mm	Low	98
1.00–2.00 mm	Intermediate	85
2.01–4.00 mm	High	69
>4.00 mm	Highest	33

(3) Stage III: any tumor with lymph node involvement (5-year survival = 30%)
(4) Stage IV: metastatic disease to distant skin and viscera (5-year survival < 4%).

b. **Sentinel lymph node mapping and biopsy** is a surgical staging procedure that identifies the most proximal lymph node draining the primary tumor. This technique is most often used in melanoma cases with primary tumors 1–3.99 mm in thickness and no evidence of lymphadenopathy or distant metastasis. The routine use of sentinel lymph node mapping and biopsy is not yet firmly established, although staging accuracy is well documented.

9. **Therapy**

a. **Surgery**

(1) **Primary excision.** Surgical excision of primary tumor with clear margins is primary therapy. Lesions less than 1 mm in depth can be safely excised with margins of 1 cm. Thicker lesions should be excised with wider margins (2–4 cm).

(2) **Nodal dissection.** Elective node dissection is controversial. Some investigators attribute a prophylactic benefit to node dissection for lesions 1.50–3.99 mm in depth. Lymphadenectomy is indicated for patients in whom adenopathy develops in the absence of metastatic disease.

b. **Chemotherapy** is of little benefit and does not confer a survival benefit in patients with metastatic disease. Drugs with documented activity include dacarbazine, cisplatin, and the nitrosoureas.

(1) **Dacarbazine** is considered the best single agent, with a 15% response rate. Neither tamoxifen nor IFN-α adds to the response seen with dacarbazine.

(2) The **combination of dacarbazine, carmustine, cisplatin, and tamoxifen** has been reported to have a 50% response rate. However, this rate has not been confirmed in randomized clinical trials.

c. **Biologic response modifiers** have modest antitumor activity in patients with metastatic disease.

(1) **IFN-α** has a 15%–20% response rate, primarily in soft tissue and lung metastases. Adjuvant IFN therapy may improve the disease-free and overall survival rates for stage III patients and those with nodal metastases that are resected.

(2) **High-dose IL-2** has elicited long-term complete responses in a small proportion of patients with metastatic melanoma. In phase II clinical trials, chemotherapy plus IL-2 and IFN-α had high response rates, but randomized phase III clinical trials have not confirmed these results.

(3) Other experimental procedures include **antitumor vaccines** and **monoclonal antibody therapy.** GM_2 ganglioside and peptide-containing vaccines derived from the gp100, **MART-1 and Melan-A, and MAGE-3** tumor regression antigens can induce protective T-cell immunity. In addition, when peptide vaccines are used alone or in conjunction with IL-2 therapy, they elicit objective responses in patients with metastatic disease.

10. **Prevention**

a. **Primary prevention** for melanoma involves sun avoidance. Recommendations include the following:

(1) Avoid mid-day sun (10:00 AM to 2:00 PM) and artificial tanning.
(2) Seek shade when possible.
(3) Use protective clothing (hats, long sleeves, sunglasses).
(4) Frequently apply sunscreen with a sun protection factor (SPF) of 30 or higher.

b. **Secondary prevention** for melanoma involves early detection and surveillance. Recommendations include the following:

(1) Perform regular, periodic skin self-examination.
(2) Have a skin examination and screening by a dermatologist (high-risk patients).
(3) Have a biopsy of clinically suspicious pigmented lesions.

D Cutaneous T-cell lymphoma

1. **Definition.** Cutaneous T-cell lymphoma (CTCL) constitutes a clonal proliferation of malignant T lymphocytes (T cells). CTCL begins as an indolent lymphoma involving the skin but may progress to involve lymph nodes, blood, and other visceral organs. CTCL has two clinical variants.
   a. **Mycosis fungoides** classically evolves slowly through progressive stages of cutaneous involvement from the patch and plaque stage (stages I–II), through the tumor or erythrodermic stage (stage III), with progression to extracutaneous involvement (stage IV).
   b. **Sézary syndrome,** the more rapidly progressing variant, presents as stage IV disease with diffuse skin involvement (erythroderma), lymphadenopathy, and leukocytosis characterized by the presence of lymphocytes with an atypical cerebriform nuclear morphology. These lymphocytes are referred to as Sézary cells.
2. **Epidemiology.** An estimated 1,000 new cases of CTCL occur each year in the United States.
3. **Etiology.** The etiology of CTCL is unknown. It appears to be an acquired disease with no known risk factors, case clustering, or genetic predisposition.
4. **Pathophysiology.** Infiltration of the skin is characterized by the presence of neoplastic T cells within the epidermis (epidermotropism) as single cells or in clusters (**Pautrier microabscess**). Immunophenotyping of the neoplastic T cells shows expression of CD4 (helper subset) antigen. The constellation of immunologic abnormalities associated with CTCL has been closely correlated to aberrant T_H2 cytokine expression and regulation.
5. **Clinical features**
   a. Early onset of lesions typically involve a **"bathing trunk" distribution,** including sun-protected areas: buttocks, hips, axillae, and women's breasts ***(Color Figure 12–22. See accompanying CD).***
   b. Lesions progress from patch, to plaque, and to tumors or erythroderma, and they involve an increasing percentage of the skin surface area.
      (1) **Patches** are red, scaling macules with variable size (1–15 cm), shapes (round, oval, crescent), and configurations (serpiginous, annular).
      (2) **Plaques** are red, variably infiltrated plaques that typically evolve from patches.
      (3) **Tumors** are reddish to violaceous nodules (1–15 cm) that often superficially ulcerate.
      (4) **Exfoliative erythroderma** is diffuse redness and exfoliative scaling often associated with hyperkeratosis of the palms and soles and lymphadenopathy.
6. **Diagnosis.** The diagnosis of CTCL is made by clinical inspection of skin and confirmed by skin biopsy.
7. **Therapy**
   a. **Skin-directed therapy.** These therapies are typically used in early stages with no evidence of extracutaneous involvement. They may be combined with systemic therapies in advanced stages.
      (1) Topical chemotherapy may be effective. Mechlorethamine (nitrogen mustard) or carmustine are mixed into a topical vehicle (water or ointment) and applied directly on the skin.
      (2) Topical retinoids are used. Bexarotene gel has been approved for topical use in CTCL.
      (3) Phototherapy is useful in CTCL.
      (4) Electron beam radiation therapy has been shown to be very effective in resolving CTCL.
   b. **Systemic therapies** are typically used in cases of evident extracutaneous involvement (blood, lymph nodes, or visceral organs).
      (1) Biologic response modifiers are often used as single agents or in combination.
         (a) IFN-α
         (b) Extracorporeal photopheresis
         (c) Retinoids (bexarotene)
         (d) IL-2 fusion toxin (denileukin diftitox)

(2) Drugs used in both single-agent and combination chemotherapy of T-cell non-Hodgkin lymphomas also are used to treat CTCL.

XI CUTANEOUS INFECTIONS AND INFESTATIONS

A **Bacterial skin infections** usually start in areas of trauma or impaired barrier function of the skin. *Staphylococcus aureus* and *Streptococcus pyogenes* are the predominant organisms that cause skin infection in healthy, nonimmunocompromised individuals.

1. **Clinical presentations**
   a. **Impetigo** is a superficial, intraepidermal, highly contagious vesiculopustular, often oozing eruption. Lesions have golden crusts ***(Color Figure 12–23. See accompanying CD).*** Frequency is highest in children.
   b. **Cellulitis** is an acute spreading infection of the dermis and subcutaneous tissue manifested by warmth, erythema, swelling, and tenderness. *S. pyogenes* infections are often associated with ascending lymphangitis ***(Color Figure 12–24. See accompanying CD.)***
   c. **Furuncle** is a deep necrotizing form of folliculitis that occurs as a warm, tender, erythematous, fluctuant, purulent nodule centered on a hair follicle. Several furuncles may coalesce, forming a carbuncle.
   d. **Abscess** is a localized accumulation of purulent material deep in the dermis or subcutaneous tissue. The pus is usually not visible on the surface of the skin.
2. **Therapy**
   a. **Impetigo.** Compresses to dry the area are necessary. Topical antibiotics (e.g., mupirocin) are used against ***Staphylococcus*** and ***Streptococcus.*** Systemic antibiotics also may be effective.
   b. **Cellulitis.** Systemic antibiotics are used against ***Staphylococcus*** and ***Streptococcus.***
   c. **Furuncles and abscesses.** Lesions should be drained, and systemic antibiotic therapy should be used.

B **Fungal skin infections**

1. **Clinical presentations**
   a. **Dermatophytoses.** Dermatophytes cause a superficial fungal infection of the dead keratin of skin, hair, and nails. *Epidermophyton, Microsporum,* and *Trichophyton* species infect humans. Infection is characterized by erythematous and scaling macules with active raised borders, often with central clearing (ringworm).
      (1) **Tinea capitis** is infection of scalp hair and produces alopecia.
      (2) **Tinea corporis** is infection of the trunk and extremities ***(Color Figure 12–25. See accompanying CD).***
      (3) **Tinea manuum** and **tinea pedis** are infections of the palms, soles, and interdigital webs. The resultant web space maceration often is the site of entry for secondary bacterial cellulitis.
      (4) **Tinea cruris** is infection of the groin.
      (5) **Tinea barbae** is infection of the beard area and neck. Males are typically affected.
      (6) **Tinea faciale** is infection of the face.
      (7) **Tinea unguium (onychomycosis)** is infection of the nail and produces thickened, yellow nails.
   b. **Candidiasis.** This superficial yeast infection (*Candida albicans*) affects moist intertriginous areas. Superficial pustules rapidly rupture, producing confluent erythematous, moist erosions with scaling borders, and satellite lesions on the periphery ***(Color Figure 12–26. See accompanying CD).***
   c. **Tinea versicolor.** Endogenous yeast forms (***Malassezia furfur***) cause numerous, well-marginated, finely scaly, oval-to-round pink, hypo- or hyperpigmented macules scattered over the trunk ***(Color Figure 12–27. See accompanying CD).***

2. **Diagnosis.** KOH preparations and fungal cultures of scales confirm the clinical diagnosis.
   a. **Dermatophytoses.** Long-branched hyphae are apparent on KOH examination.
   b. **Candidiasis.** Budding spores (pseudohyphae) are apparent on KOH examination.
   c. **Tinea versicolor.** Spores and short hyphae ("spaghetti and meatballs") are apparent on KOH examination.
3. **Therapy**
   a. **Dermatophytoses** are treated with topical antifungal agents. Tinea capitis requires oral griseofulvin. Onychomycosis responds best to oral agents (e.g., griseofulvin, itraconazole, terbinafine).
   b. **Candidiasis** is treated with topical antifungal creams. Care should be taken to keep areas of involvement dry. Rarely is systemic therapy needed.
   c. **Tinea versicolor** is treated with topical agents. It also responds to single doses of oral ketoconazole.

C Viral skin infections

1. **Clinical presentations**
   a. **Herpes simplex virus (HSV)** infections cause a prodrome of pain preceding the appearance of grouped vesicles on an erythematous base. Typically, HSV type 1 causes herpes labialis (cold sores, fever blisters), and HSV type 2 causes genital herpes. HSV infections tend to be recurrent and may be exacerbated by stress, the menstrual cycle, and immunosuppression ***(Color Figure 12–28. See accompanying CD).***
   b. **Herpes zoster** infections (shingles) cause a prodrome of pain radiating along a dermatome before an eruption of multiple erythematous vesicles, which have a dermatomal distribution. Herpes zoster infections, which are ultimately caused by **varicella-zoster virus (VZV),** represent the reactivation of latent varicella virus (chickenpox) from the dorsal ganglia of spinal and central nerves ***(Color Figure 12–29. See accompanying CD).***
   c. **Verruca vulgaris (warts)** are caused by **human papilloma virus** (HPV) infection of the epidermis. Fleshed-colored verrucous papules typically occur on the extremities ***(Color Figure 12–30. See accompanying CD).***
      (1) **Verruca plana (flat warts)** are 2–4-mm flat-topped flesh-colored papules that affect the face.
      (2) **Condyloma acuminata** are genital warts that tend to develop cauliflower-like macerated papules.
      (3) **Bowenoid papulosis** refers to genital warts that display histologic dysplasia and are associated with a risk of malignant transformation. Lesions tends to be recalcitrant and are most commonly induced by HPV type 16 infection.
2. **Diagnosis**
   a. **Tzanck smear** detects multinucleated giant cells of both HSV and VZV. DIF and culture of blisters identify HSV.
   b. **Skin biopsy** confirms the clinical impression of warts if needed and identifies lesions of bowenoid papulosis.
3. **Therapy**
   a. **HSV and herpes zoster. Topical antivirals** (acyclovir, penciclovir) are best used at the first clinical signs of herpes labialis infection. **Systemic antivirals** (acyclovir, valacyclovir, famciclovir) reduce viral shedding and time to heal.
   b. **Warts.** Therapy includes a variety of modalities such as **topical salicylic acid preparations, trichloroacetic acid, cryotherapy, laser therapy, curettage and electrodesiccation, and intralesional bleomycin or IFN-α.** Additional topical therapies for genital warts include **podophyllin** and **imiquimod.**

D Rickettsial diseases Rickettsiae are pleomorphic bacteria that are obligate intracellular parasites. Transmitted to humans by ticks and mites, they cause acute systemic infections that may be accompanied by a rash.

1. **Clinical presentations**
   a. **Rocky Mountain spotted fever.** Tick-borne ***Rickettsia rickettsii*** causes fever, myalgias, headache, and a petechial rash that typically begins around wrists and ankles or trunk. Involvement of the palms and soles may occur after the fifth day of symptoms.
   b. **Rickettsialpox.** Mouse mite–borne ***Rickettsia akari*** causes fever, headache, respiratory and abdominal symptoms, and an erythematous pustulonecrotic papule at the site of mite bites.
   c. **Epidemic typhus.** Body lice–borne ***Rickettsia prowazekii*** causes fever, chills, headache, malaise, and an erythematous macular and petechial rash involving the trunk.
2. **Diagnosis.** Serology confirms the diagnosis of rickettsial diseases. Skin biopsy specimens of petechial lesions show vasculitis.
3. **Therapy.** Rickettsial diseases are treated with antibiotic therapy and supportive therapy. Doxycycline is the drug of choice. Rickettsialpox is a self-limiting disease, and occasionally antibiotics may not be necessary.

E Infestations

1. **Clinical presentations**
   a. **Scabies.** This intensely pruritic and highly contagious infestation of the epidermis is caused by the ***Sarcoptes scabiei*** mite. The mite burrows into the skin. The resultant 1–3-mm burrows, papules, vesicles, and secondary excoriations are concentrated in the web spaces of the fingers, flexor aspects of the wrists, antecubital fossa, axilla, areola and nipples, umbilicus, buttocks, and feet ***(Color Figure 12–31. See accompanying CD).***
   b. **Pediculosis.** This infestation of the skin with **lice** (**ectoparasites**) is caused by ***Pediculus humanus capitis*** (**head louse**), ***Pediculus humanus corporis*** (**body louse**), and ***Pthirus pubis*** (**pubic louse**). Pediculosis spreads from person to person by close physical contact or through fomites (e.g., combs, clothes, hats, linens). All forms produce itching with 2–4-mm erythematous papules, excoriations, and often crusting. Lice and **nits** (**eggs attached to hairs**) are visible on clinical inspection ***(Color Figures 12–32A and B. See accompanying CD).***
2. **Diagnosis**
   a. **Scabies.** Diagnosis is confirmed with microscopic examination of skin scrapings from primary lesions showing scabies mites and eggs.
   b. **Pediculosis.** Diagnosis is confirmed with microscopic examination of nits and lice.
3. **Therapy**
   a. **Scabies.** Scabicides (e.g., **lindane, permethrin, crotamiton lotion or cream**) are prescribed for patients, household members, and close personal contacts. All bed linen and clothing should be washed in hot water. Symptomatic treatment may involve antihistamines.
   b. **Pediculosis.** Pediculicides (**permethrin, pyrethrin, lindane shampoo or lotion**) are applied topically and should be reapplied in 7 days. All contacts should be treated. Bed linen, clothing, and other materials (e.g., combs) should be washed in hot water.

XII CUTANEOUS DRUG REACTIONS

A Definition A cutaneous drug reaction is an adverse drug reaction involving the skin that results from exposure to a medication by ingestion, topical application, injection, instillation, insertion, or inhalation.

B Epidemiology As many as 5% of courses of drug therapy are complicated by adverse drug reactions. Approximately 30% of hospitalized medical patients develop at least one adverse drug reaction during the course of their hospitalization (3 million each year in the United States), and 2%–3% of these patients develop skin reactions (60,000–90,000 each year).

C **Etiology and pathophysiology** Various mechanisms are responsible for different types of adverse drug reactions.

1. **Overdose.** Usually the symptoms are an exaggeration of the pharmacologic action of the drug (e.g., hemorrhage resulting from overdosage of anticoagulants).
2. **Cumulation.** Cumulative effects may occur after prolonged administration of some drugs (e.g., argyria in patients using silver-containing nose drops).
3. **Pharmacologic side effects.** These are unwanted but known pharmacologic actions of drugs (e.g., alopecia in patients taking cytostatic drugs).
4. **Idiosyncrasy and intolerance**
   a. **Idiosyncrasy.** This qualitatively abnormal response is present only in certain people and is not dependent on immunologic mechanisms.
   b. **Intolerance.** An abnormally small dose of the drug produces the characteristic effects of the drug. Many of these reactions are a result of differences in enzymatic constitution (e.g., hemolytic anemia in patients with glucose-6-phosphate dehydrogenase deficiency who take primaquine).
5. **Ecological imbalance.** Reducing the flora of one species of microorganisms can result in overgrowth of another (e.g., anogenital moniliasis following use of broad-spectrum antibiotics).
6. **Exacerbation of existing latent or overt disease** (e.g., precipitation of porphyria by barbiturates)
7. **Jarisch-Herxheimer reaction.** This results from the administration of a drug highly effective in the treatment of an existing infection. The release of toxic substances caused by the destruction of the sensitive microorganisms causes exacerbations of existing lesions or the development of new ones (e.g., early syphilis treated with penicillin).
8. **Immunologic reactions**
   a. **IgE-dependent reactions.** IgE molecules fixed to sensitized mast cells or basophils are cross-linked by polyvalent drug–protein conjugates, causing release of biologically active materials (e.g., histamine, cytokines, chemokines).
   b. Immunocomplex-dependent drug reactions. Antigen–antibody complexes form 6 or more days after drug exposure ("serum sickness") and typically cause fever, arthritis, nephritis, neuritis, edema, and urticarial or papular rash.
   c. Cytotoxic drug reactions. Antigens or antigen–antibody complexes become attached to cell surfaces, which are damaged in the course of subsequent complement activation (e.g., hemolytic anemia induced by penicillin).
   d. Cell-mediated drug reactions. No circulating antibodies are found in this type of immune response (e.g., contact drug hypersensitivity).

D **Clinical features**

1. Cutaneous drug reactions vary in their presentation and include a wide array of primary lesions and skin findings (Table 12–14).
2. Some drugs are associated with an increased frequency of a particular cutaneous reaction. However, a drug may cause urticaria in one person, vasculitis in another, and erythema multiforme in another.
3. Some medications produce cutaneous reactions with greater frequency (Table 12–15).

E **Types of cutaneous drug reactions** The various cutaneous drug reactions are frequently associated with a prototype drug (Table 12–16).

TABLE 12–14 Skin Manifestations of Adverse Drug Reactions

Acne	Fixed eruption	Pruritus
Alopecia	Hirsutism	Purpura
Bulla	Hyperpigmentation	Pustule
Discoloration	Hypopigmentation	Striae
Eczema	Lichen planus	Telangiectasis
Epidermal necrolysis	Macule	Urticaria
Erythema multiforme	Nail dystrophy	Vasculitis
Erythema nodosum	Papule	Vesicle
Exfoliative dermatitis	Photosensitivity	

1. **Morbilliform eruption** *(Color Figure 12–33. See accompanying CD)*
   a. This measles-like eruption is the most common type of cutaneous drug reaction.
   b. The primary lesion is a minute, erythematous macule that often fades with pressure. Lesions form larger areas of confluence, causing widespread and symmetric erythema.
2. **Urticarial eruption**
   a. Urticaria is the second most common type of cutaneous drug reaction (see Chapter 7 IV).
   b. Drugs may cause urticaria by immunologic (IgE-dependent or immune complex-dependent) or nonimmunologic (direct histamine liberation) mechanisms.
3. **Lichenoid eruption.** Drugs may cause lichen planus-like eruptions (see VI C). Mucosal involvement is rare.
4. **Vasculitis** *(Color Figure 12–34. See accompanying CD)*
   a. Vasculitis occurs as palpable purpura as a result of blood vessel damage and extravasations of erythrocytes into the dermis.

TABLE 12–15 Drugs Frequently Associated with Cutaneous Reactions

Drug	Reaction Rate (per 1000)
Trimethoprim-sulfamethoxazole	59
Ampicillin	52
Semisynthetic penicillins	36
Corticotropin	28
Erythromycin	23
Sulfisoxazole	17
Penicillin G	16
Gentamicin sulfate	16
Practolol	16
Cephalosporins	13
Quinidine	12
Dipyrone	11
Mercurial diuretics	10
Nitrofurantoin	9
Heparin	8
Chloramphenicol	7
Trimethobenzamide	7
Phenazopyridine	7
Methenamine	6
Nitrazepam	6

TABLE 12–16 Cutaneous Drug Reactions and Frequently Associated Drugs

Drug Reaction	Associated Drug(s)
Morbilliform eruption	Prototype: ampicillin
Urticarial eruption	Prototype: penicillin
Lichenoid eruption	Prototype: gold
Vasculitis	Prototype: allopurinol Others: thiazides and sulfonamides
Erythema multiforme	Prototype: sulfonamides Others: barbiturates, hydantoins, thiazides
Exfoliative erythroderma	Prototype: diphenylhydantoin Others: sulfonamides, salicylates, antimalarials
Toxic epidermal necrolysis	Prototype: allopurinol Others: barbiturates, hydantoins, sulfonamides
Pigmentary alterations	Oral contraceptives (increased melanin production). Heavy metals (silver nitrate deposition) Amiodarone (deposition of lipofuscin)
Acneiform eruptions	Prototype: corticosteroids Others: lithium, diphenylhydantoin, oral contraceptives
Erythema nodosum	Prototype: oral contraceptives Others: sulfonamides, salicylates, bromides and iodides
Fixed drug eruption	Prototype: phenolphthalein (component of OTC laxatives) Others: barbiturates, sulfonamides, phenacetin
Lupus-like syndrome	Prototypes: hydralazine, procainamide
Photosensitivity eruptions	Prototype: thiazide diuretics Others: sulfonamides, sulfonylureas, phenothiazines
Drug-induced linear IgA dermatoses	Prototype: vancomycin Others: amiodarone, ampicillin, captopril

b. Patients often present with vasculitis in dependent areas (e.g., legs).
c. Allopurinol is the prototype causal drug. Thiazides and sulfonamides also may cause vasculitis.

5. **Erythema multiforme** (see V B). Sulfonamides are the prototype causal drugs. Barbiturates, hydantoins, and thiazides also may cause erythema multiforme.

6. **Exfoliative erythroderma.** ***(Color Figure 12–35. See accompanying CD)*** Exfoliative erythroderma occurs as a generalized erythema with exfoliative scaling. Mucous membranes are usually spared.

7. **Toxic epidermal necrolysis** (TEN) ***(Color Figure 12–36. See accompanying CD).*** TEN occurs as a fulminating, generalized sloughing of skin with complete necrosis of epidermis comparable to second-degree burn. Mucous membranes are severely affected.

8. **Pigmentary alterations.** These changes may occur in response to a medication through a variety of mechanisms.
   a. Increased melanin production often results in macular hyperpigmentation of the face termed **melasma** ***(Color Figure 12–37. See accompanying CD)*** and is often associated with oral contraceptives.
   b. Deposition of pigmented materials results from heavy metals (e.g., silver nitrate).
   c. Deposition of lipofuscin results from amiodarone.

9. **Acneiform eruption** ***(Color Figure 12–38. See accompanying CD).***
   a. Drug-induced acne has a rapid onset of acneiform lesions in a similar stage of development involving areas other than the face.
   b. Acneiform eruptions may occur at any age.

10. **Erythema nodosum** (see VI E).
11. **Fixed drug eruption** ***(Color Figure 12–39. See accompanying CD.)***
    a. A fixed drug eruption produces a demarcated oval or circular erythema that heals with residual hyperpigmentation. Lesions tend to be solitary but may be multiple.
    b. Reexposure to the offending drug causes lesions to develop in the same location.
12. **Lupus-like syndrome** ***(Color Figure 12–40. See accompanying CD).*** The cutaneous findings of drug-induced lupus are usually indistinguishable from systemic lupus erythematosus.
13. **Photosensitivity eruptions** ***(Color Figure 12–41. See accompanying CD).***
    a. Photosensitivity reactions require the presence of both light and the inciting drug.
    b. Specific wavelengths of light known as the "action spectrum" (285–425 nm) are required to initiate a photosensitive drug reaction.
    c. A **phototoxic reaction** (nonimmunologic) results from direct cellular injury when a drug is photoactivated by light.
    d. A **photoallergic reaction** (immune mediated) results when light interacts with a drug to produce an immunogenic intermediate or metabolite that stimulates an immune response.
14. **Drug-induced linear IgA dermatosis** (LAD) ***(Color Figure 12–42. See accompanying CD)***
    a. The heterogeneous pruritic lesions include tense bullae. There is a predominately extensor distribution with mucosal involvement in approximately 70% of cases.
    b. DIF of skin biopsy specimens shows linear deposits of IgA along the basement membrane that are identical to those found in idiopathic cases of LAD of adult and childhood.
    c. IgA autoantibodies target collagen XVII (BPAG 2) and type VII collagen.

F Diagnosis A cutaneous drug reaction should be suspected in any widespread rash of rapid onset.

1. It is critical to obtain a complete drug history.
    a. Ask specifically about tonics, laxatives, sedatives, tranquilizers, pain medications, vitamins, oral contraceptive pills, eye drops, inhalants, immunizations, and suppositories.
    b. In hospitalized patients, check the patient's chart for medication orders, including "prn" medications; "stat" orders; anesthetics; and diagnostic agents (e.g., contrast media, radioactive tracers).
2. Determine which drug is the most likely causal agent.
    a. Drugs started within 1 week before the appearance of the eruption are most likely causal.
    b. Drugs with a high frequency of cutaneous reactions are most likely causal.
    c. Drugs commonly causing the morphologic pattern present clinically should be suspected.
3. A skin biopsy may assist in making a diagnosis. Although there is no single histologic finding diagnostic of a drug eruption, other causes of the eruption may be ruled out.

G Therapy

1. The causal drug should be discontinued if possible. Some clinical situations prevent discontinuation of the causal drug.
2. Topical or systemic corticosteroids (for relatively severe eruptions) may produce symptomatic relief.
3. Antihistamines may help relieve associated pruritus.
4. Topical care consists of soothing baths or compresses and appropriate dressings. When present, secondary infections should be treated.

XIII SELECTED CUTANEOUS MANIFESTATIONS OF SYSTEMIC DISEASES

A General considerations The skin is often affected by systemic diseases. Cutaneous manifestations of systemic diseases may develop concurrently as a disease progresses or may be one of the early signs and symptoms leading to an initial diagnosis. Recognition of associated cutaneous manifestations aids in the diagnosis and management of many systemic diseases.

B Stasis dermatitis/lipodermatosclerosis

1. **Definitions**
   a. **Stasis dermatitis** is a common inflammatory skin disease that occurs on the lower extremities in individuals with chronic venous insufficiency. Stasis dermatitis is the earliest skin change associated with venous insufficiency and may lead to venous leg ulceration and fibrosis.
   b. **Lipodermatosclerosis** is the skin induration and hyperpigmentation of the legs that occurs in individuals with venous insufficiency. It involves a spectrum of acute inflammatory changes as well as chronic, fibrotic changes. Thus, the term *lipodermatosclerosis* is often preferred to *stasis dermatitis,* a misnomer in terms of the pathogenesis of the disease (see XIII B 4).
2. **Epidemiology.** The estimated prevalence of stasis dermatitis/lipodermatosclerosis is approximately 6%–7% in individuals older than 50 years of age.
3. **Etiology.** Venous insufficiency is the underlying cause of the cutaneous changes seen in stasis dermatitis/lipodermatosclerosis.
4. **Pathophysiology**
   a. Decreased competency of the one-way valvular system in the deep venous plexus of the legs results in backflow of blood from the deep venous system to the superficial venous system, producing venous hypertension. The link between venous hypertension and cutaneous changes is not precisely understood.
   b. Venous hypertension produces increased flow rates and high oxygen tension, contrary to early theories that hypothesized that an incompetent venous system lead to pooling of blood and reduced blood flow and oxygen tension in dermal capillaries. The pooling hypothesis led to the term *stasis dermatitis.*
   c. Increased venous hydrostatic pressure increases permeability of the dermal microcirculation and results in the formation of fibrin cuffs around dermal capillaries. However, fibrin cuffs have not been found to decrease oxygen diffusion significantly.
   d. Venous hypertension has been shown to result in leukocyte trapping in the microcirculation that may result in the increased release of inflammatory mediators and leukocyte sludging that contribute to tissue ischemia.
5. **Clinical features** ***(Color Figure 12–43. See accompanying CD)***
   a. Acute and chronic changes, including edema, varicosities, and diffuse red-brown discoloration representing dermal deposits of hemosiderin (from degraded, extravasated erythrocytes), may occur against a background of skin changes.
   b. Clinical changes occur bilaterally. The medial ankle is most frequently and severely involved.
   c. Early findings include erythematous scaling of a lower extremity.
   d. Exudative, weeping patches, and plaques may be associated with secondary infection.
   e. Ulceration may occur and generally tends to be medial with exudative bases. Healing results in scarring.
   f. Lichenification and hyperpigmentation may occur as a consequence of chronic scratching and rubbing. Induration, fibrosis, and scarring may result with constriction around the ankles, producing an inverted bowling pin appearance in the lower leg.
6. **Diagnosis.** Clinical inspection and venous Doppler studies establish the diagnosis of stasis dermatitis/lipodermatosclerosis in the setting of venous insufficiency. Skin biopsies are rarely indicated but rule out other diagnoses, especially when ulceration is present.
7. **Therapy**
   a. Topical therapy is directed at the relief of signs and symptoms. Treatments include compresses for weeping lesions, local wound care for ulcerations, and short-term use of mid-potency topical corticosteroids for reducing symptomatic inflammation and itching.

b. Obvious superficial infections (impetiginization) should be treated with topical mupirocin or a systemic antibiotic with activity against *Staphylococcus* and *Streptococcus* species.
c. Maintenance therapy requires use of moisturizers to prevent dryness and breakdown of the skin.
d. Compression stockings and elevation of legs at rest are important mainstays of maintenance and prevention. Arterial insufficiency is often present in patients with venous insufficiency; thus, assessing the patient's peripheral arterial circulation with a Doppler study is advised before recommending compression therapy.

C Cutaneous sarcoidosis

1. **Definition.** Sarcoidosis is characterized by noncaseating epithelioid granulomas that primarily affect the lungs. The lymphatic (especially pulmonary lymph nodes), ophthalmic, nervous, musculoskeletal, hepatic, cardiac, renal, and endocrine systems are also affected. In addition, the skin is often affected, and recognition and evaluation of these skin lesions often aids in establishing the diagnosis.
2. **Epidemiology.** The incidence of sarcoidosis is 1–40 per 100,000 population in the United States. It is more prevalent in African Americans than in Caucasians.
3. **Etiology.** The exact etiology of sarcoidosis has not been clearly defined. Immunogenetic susceptibility and environmental exposure influence disease expression. Etiologic agents may include infections, environmental agents, or autoantigens.
4. **Pathophysiology.** Impaired humoral and cellular responses have been documented in patients with sarcoidosis. Chronic antigen exposure may lead to a chronic T_H1 cytokine–driven response, which results in granuloma formation.
5. **Clinical features** ***(Color Figure 12–44. See accompanying CD)***
   a. Macular or papular sarcoidosis is the most common lesion in cutaneous sarcoidosis and is characterized by asymptomatic red-brown macules and papules often involving the face, periorbital, nasolabial folds, or extensor surfaces.
   b. **Lupus pernio** is the most distinctive of sarcoid skin lesions and is characterized by reddish to violaceous indurated plaques and nodules that usually affect the nostrils, cheeks, ears, and lips.
   c. Plaque sarcoidosis is characterized by round to oval, red-brown to violaceous infiltrated plaques, which are often distributed symmetrically and have an annular appearance. The center of the plaques may be atrophic or scaly.
   d. Subcutaneous nodular sarcoidosis (Darier-Roussy sarcoidosis) is characterized by nontender, firm, flesh-colored or violaceous 0.5–2-cm nodules that are commonly found on the extremities or on the trunk.
   e. Scars from previous trauma may become infiltrated and tender with a reddish or violaceous color.
   f. Erythema nodosum is a hypersensitivity reaction that may develop in the setting of sarcoidosis. It is often associated with hilar lymphadenopathy, anterior uveitis, or polyarthritis (Löfgren syndrome).
6. **Diagnosis.** Clinical inspection and skin biopsy demonstrating diagnostic noncaseating granulomas are the basis of diagnosis. Additional skin biopsy specimens should be sent for special stains and cultures to rule out infectious causes of granuloma formation, including mycobacterial and deep fungal infections.
7. **Therapy.** Treatment of underlying manifestations is paramount.
   a. Topical or intralesional corticosteroids (triamcinolone acetonide) may be used to treat cutaneous lesions.
   b. To avoid scarring, systemic immunosuppressants are used for recalcitrant lesions that do not respond to intralesional corticosteroids. Immunosuppressants for cutaneous sarcoidosis include methotrexate, azathioprine, and chlorambucil. Other reportedly useful therapeutic

agents include antimalarial drugs (hydroxychloroquine, chloroquine), cyclosporine, oral isotretinoin, allopurinol, and thalidomide.

D Paraneoplastic pemphigus

1. **Definition.** Paraneoplastic pemphigus is an autoimmune blistering disease characterized by severe mucosal involvement and association with an underlying malignancy.
2. **Epidemiology.** Paraneoplastic pemphigus is rare. Since its first description in 1990, only 60+ cases have been reported.
3. **Etiology**
   a. Development of autoantibodies associated with an underlying malignancy cross-react with epitopes in the skin and produce clinical blistering.
   b. The most common malignancy associated with paraneoplastic pemphigus is **non-Hodgkin's lymphoma.** Other associated malignancies include chronic lymphocytic leukemia, Castleman tumor, giant cell lymphoma (reticulum cell sarcoma), Waldenström macroglobulinemia, thymoma, poorly differentiated sarcoma, bronchogenic squamous cell carcinoma, and follicular dendritic cell sarcoma.
4. **Pathophysiology**
   a. An immune response to tumor antigens is thought to generate autoantibodies that recognize desmosome and hemidesmosome proteins in the skin and respiratory and gastrointestinal tracts.
   b. Autoantibodies target desmogleins 1 and 3, desmoplakins 1 and 2, envoplakin, periplakin, and HD1/plectin and an unidentified 170-kd protein.
5. **Clinical features**
   a. Painful oral mucosal erosions that usually present as mucositis with crusting are the dominant clinical feature.
   b. Mucosal membranes of the eyes, nose, pharynx, tonsils, and genitalia may be affected.
   c. Cutaneous eruption is typically polymorphous. Combinations of blisters, ulcerations, erythematous macules and papules, scaly plaques, urticarial plaques, diffuse erythroderma, and erosions have been reported.
6. **Diagnosis.** Skin biopsy and DIF confirm the diagnosis. Serum may be obtained for IDIF.
   a. Histopathologic changes include suprabasilar acantholysis, keratinocyte necrosis, and interface dermatitis.
   b. DIF shows immunoreactants, typically IgG and C3, within the epidermal intercellular spaces (as in pemphigus vulgaris) and at the epidermal basement membrane (as in bullous pemphigoid).
   c. IDIF detects circulating serum antibodies specific for stratified squamous or transitional epithelium.
   d. Once the diagnosis of paraneoplastic pemphigus is established, further evaluation for an underlying malignancy is warranted.
7. **Therapy.** Symptomatic relief and treatment of superinfection, if present, are necessary.
   a. Immunosuppressive agents used for pemphigus vulgaris and bullous pemphigoid should be tried [Sections V A and V B], but they are often ineffective.
   b. Treatment of underlying malignancy may not result in skin clearing.

E Dermatitis herpetiformis

1. **Definition.** Dermatitis herpetiformis is an autoimmune blistering skin disease associated with gluten-sensitive enteropathy (GSE).
2. **Epidemiology.** The estimated frequency of dermatitis herpetiformis in the United States is approximately 39 cases per 100,000 population.
3. **Etiology.** Deposits of IgA in the skin lead to pruritic blistering in patients with GSE.

4. **Pathophysiology**
   a. Pathogenesis is associated with the presence of GSE, an increased expression of HLA-A1, HLA-B8, HLA-DR3, and HLA-DQ2 haplotypes and granular deposition of IgA at the DEJ of the skin.
   b. Susceptible individuals, as determined by HLA haplotype, may develop a cell-mediated immune response resulting in T-cell activation in the small bowel mucosa exacerbated by a sensitivity to gluten, a protein present in barley, rye, and wheat but not in rice.
   c. Cutaneous inflammation is predominated by a dermal infiltrate of neutrophils with micro-abscesses formation and progression to subepidermal vesicle formation through the lamina lucida of the basement membrane zone. DIF shows a granular deposition of IgA.
5. **Clinical features**
   a. Skin lesions are extremely pruritic groups of erythematous vesicles, most frequently located on extensor surfaces.
   b. Lesions often are pustular or crusted from excoriation.
6. **Diagnosis.** Skin biopsy and DIF confirm the diagnosis.
7. **Therapy.** Diaminodiphenyl sulfone and sulfapyridine are the primary drugs used in treatment. Relief of symptoms may be seen within 24–48 hours of the start of therapy. Patients may choose to control the skin disease with a gluten-free diet.

F Calciphylaxis

1. **Definition.** Calciphylaxis is the phenomenon of vascular calcification and skin necrosis in end-stage renal disease (ESRD).
2. **Epidemiology.** Calciphylaxis is extremely rare in the general population, affecting 1%–4% of patients with ESRD.
3. **Etiology.** The precise etiology is uncertain, but hypercalcemia, hyperphosphatemia, elevated calcium-phosphate products, and secondary hyperparathyroidism associated with ESRD are contributing factors. In the absence of renal disease, there are case reports of occurrence of calciphylaxis in association with primary hyperparathyroidism, cirrhosis, and rheumatoid arthritis.
4. **Pathophysiology**
   a. The pathogenesis is poorly defined. Vascular calcification is a constant finding and may sensitize the vascular microenvironment to hypercoagulability or promote intimal hyperplasia and vascular occlusion.
   b. Alternatively, extensive endothelial calcification and intimal hyperplasia, which are known to compromise the luminal size of vessels in calciphylaxis, may result in vascular occlusion. These mechanisms remain hypothetical and have not yet been proven to lead to calciphylaxis.
5. **Clinical features**
   a. Early lesions of calciphylaxis develop suddenly and progress rapidly as nonspecific violaceous mottling or as erythematous papules, plaques, or nodules.
   b. Lesions progress with a stellate purpuric configuration with central necrosis and are extremely painful and tender.
   c. Lesions may be singular or numerous.
   d. Lesions may occur either distally on the lower legs or proximally in areas of body fat, such as the lower abdomen, thighs, and buttocks.
6. **Diagnosis.** The diagnosis is confirmed by incisional skin biopsy with adequate sampling of the subcutaneous tissue. Laboratory studies evaluating renal, endocrine, and coagulation status should be ordered.
7. **Therapy.** Local treatment involves wound care with debridement to avoid wound infection and sepsis. Hyperbaric oxygen therapy may be useful.

G Porphyria Cutanea Tarda

1. **Definition.** Porphyria cutanea tarda (PCT) is a photosensitive blistering disorder that results from a hereditary or acquired deficiency in the activity of the hepatic heme synthetic enzyme uroporphyrinogen decarboxylase (URO-D).
2. **Epidemiology.** The exact incidence of PCT in the United States is not known but is estimated to be approximately 3 per 100,000 people. PCT is the most common type of porphyria.
3. **Etiology.** Germ line mutations in the gene encoding URO-D are detected in individuals affected with familial forms of PCT. Clinical expression of both the familial and acquired forms often requires exposure to hepatotoxic agents or conditions including ethanol, estrogens, excess iron stores, hepatitis C virus, and human immunodeficiency virus (HIV).
4. **Pathophysiology.** Reduced hepatic URO-D activity results in overproduction of uroporphyrin (URO) and coproporphyrin (COPRO). Both URO and COPRO are water soluble and are excreted in elevated levels in the urine. In addition, they are photoactive molecules and absorb energy from visible light and produce a phototoxic reaction that results in increased mechanical fragility of the skin after sunlight exposure.
5. **Clinical features** (***Color Figure 12–44. See accompanying CD***).
   a. Fragility of sun-exposed skin after mechanical trauma is the most common finding. This leads to erosions and tense bullae on the dorsal aspects of the hands, forearms, and face.
   b. Healing of crusted erosions and blisters leaves scars, milia (tiny subepidermal keratinous cysts), and hyperpigmented and hypopigmented atrophic patches.
   c. Hypertrichosis and hyperpigmentation is often visible over the temporal and malar facial areas.
   d. Scleroderma-like changes may occur over the preauricular face, neck, chest and the back. These sclerodermoid plaques can develop dystrophic calcification.
   e. A urine sample is often grossly discolored with a tea- or wine-colored tint.
6. **Diagnosis**
   a. The diagnosis is confirmed by a history of photosensitivity, characteristic skin findings, a skin biopsy for histology and DIF (which is negative for immunoreactants), and elevated URO and COPRO levels in a 24-hour urine collection.
   b. Any underlying etiology or associated disorder should be evaluated with laboratory studies, including hematologic and iron profiles, liver function tests, and screening for hepatitis and HIV.
7. **Therapy**
   a. Exacerbating factors should be eliminated or minimized. Such measures include avoidance of sunlight, elimination of alcohol, and discontinuation of estrogen when possible.
   b. Therapeutic phlebotomy is often successful in reducing excess iron stores in tissue, which is followed by improvement of deregulated heme synthesis due to URO-D inhibition. One unit of whole blood is removed weekly every 2–3 weeks, as tolerated by the patient.
   c. When phlebotomy is contraindicated, low doses of chloroquine phosphate or hydroxychloroquine sulfate may be prescribed. These drugs displace hepatic iron stores. Large doses can cause severe hepatotoxicity.

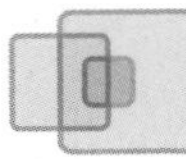

Study Questions

1. A middle-aged man who has recently begun taking captopril and hydrochlorothiazide for hypertension develops an itchy rash in sun-exposed areas. The most likely cutaneous diagnosis is

   A Urticaria
   B Erythema multiforme
   C Photosensitivity reaction
   D Erythema nodosum
   E Vasculitis

2. An adolescent girl presents with a 1-year history of acne that she has been treating with over-the-counter medications. Examination shows comedones and an occasional inflammatory papule on the face. She inquires about isotretinoin and would like to know whether it would be appropriate for her acne. You inform her that isotretinoin is indicated for the treatment of which of the following types of acne?

   A Comedonal acne
   B Mild inflammatory acne
   C Moderate inflammatory acne
   D Nodulocystic acne
   E Steroid acne

3. A young man presents with acute allergic contact dermatitis to poison ivy. Which of the following formulations is likely to be the most therapeutically effective?

   A Low-potency corticosteroid cream
   B High-potency corticosteroid cream
   C Mid- to high-potency corticosteroid solution
   D Mid- to high-potency corticosteroid ointment

4. A young woman develops an acute flare of plaque-type psoriasis on her trunk and extremities. Which of the following formulations is likely to be the most therapeutically effective?

   A Low-potency corticosteroid cream
   B High-potency corticosteroid cream
   C Mid- to high-potency corticosteroid solution
   D Mid- to high-potency corticosteroid ointment

5. A middle-aged man develops an acute flare of scalp psoriasis. Which of the following formulations is likely to be the most therapeutically effective?

   A Low-potency corticosteroid cream
   B High-potency corticosteroid cream
   C Mid- to high-potency corticosteroid solution
   D Mid- to high-potency corticosteroid ointment

6. A middle-aged woman develops an acute flare of seborrheic dermatitis affecting the nasolabial folds of her face. Which of the following formulations is likely to be the most therapeutically effective?

   A Low-potency corticosteroid cream
   B High-potency corticosteroid cream
   C Mid- to high-potency corticosteroid solution
   D Mid- to high-potency corticosteroid ointment

7. A 40-year-old woman develops painful ulcers in her mouth followed by a blistering eruption on the trunk. Examination shows erosions on the soft palate and pharynx as well as 0.5–1.5-cm crusted superficial erosions and flaccid bullae on the trunk. Skin biopsy reveals epidermal acantholysis and IgG intercellular staining. The most likely diagnosis is

- A Bullous pemphigoid
- B Pemphigus vulgaris
- C Paraneoplastic pemphigus
- D Erythema multiforme
- E Porphyria cutanea tarda

8. A 35-year-old woman with a history of Crohn's disease develops a painful nodule on her lower leg that soon ulcerates. Examination shows an extremely tender, deep, 8 × 10 cm ulceration with a purulent base and erythematous undermined borders. The most likely diagnosis is

- A Erythema nodosum
- B Stasis dermatitis
- C Pyoderma gangrenosum
- D Vasculitis
- E Calciphylaxis

9. A middle-aged man presents with a red rash on the abdomen. Examination shows a 5-cm erythematous scaling plaque with central clearing. A potassium hydroxide preparation from a scraping of the scales shows branched hyphae. The most accurate diagnosis is

- A Candidiasis
- B Tinea versicolor
- C Herpes simplex
- D Tinea capitis
- E Tinea corporis

10. An elderly woman with Parkinson's disease presents with a red scaling rash on the face that has waxed and waned for several months. Examination shows mild erythema with greasy scales predominately over the eyebrows and nasolabial folds with extension onto the malar surfaces of the face. The most likely diagnosis is

- A Psoriasis
- B Tinea versicolor
- C Lupus erythematosus
- D Seborrheic dermatitis
- E Allergic contact dermatitis

11. A 55-year-old man presents with a chronic rash over the buttocks and hips that has been unresponsive to topical steroids. It has recently started to itch. Examination shows 6–12-cm erythematous, scaling plaques in a "bathing trunk" distribution. Potassium hydroxide preparation is negative for evidence of a fungal infection. A skin biopsy indicates an atypical lymphocytic infiltrate with evidence of epidermotropism and Poutier microabscess formation. The mostly diagnosis is

- A Impetigo
- B Psoriasis
- C Cutaneous T-cell lymphoma (mycosis fungoides)
- D Tinea corporis
- E Atopic dermatitis

12. A 48-year-old woman with a fair complexion presents with a 4-mm pearly papule with a central crust located on the medial canthus of the right eye. A skin biopsy shows a well-circumscribed basal cell carcinoma. Which of the following clinical features makes the risk of recurrence of basal cell carcinoma high?

A Size of the lesion
B Fair complexion
C Histologic features
D Location of the lesion
E Gender

13. A 65-year-old man with a fair complexion presents with a 9-mm hyperkeratotic, erythematous plaque on the left jaw and no regional lymphadenopathy. A skin biopsy shows a poorly differentiated squamous cell carcinoma of skin with evidence of perineural invasion. Which of the following clinical features makes the risk of metastasis in squamous cell carcinoma high?

A Size of the lesion
B Fair complexion
C Histologic features
D Location of the lesion
E Gender

14. A middle-aged woman presents with an itchy eruption over her arms and trunk several days after gardening. Skin examination shows the changes seen in the figure ***(See Color Figure 12–46 on accompanying CD).*** The mostly likely diagnosis is

A Allergic contact dermatitis
B Herpes simplex infection
C Bullous pemphigoid
D Atopic dermatitis
E Vasculitis

15. An elderly man presents with a blistering eruption over the left thoracic back, flank, and chest. It developed shortly after he began to experience intense burning and pain in the affected areas. Examination shows grouped vesicles on an erythematous base in a dermatomal distribution over the left torso. A Tzanck smear from one of the vesicles shows the findings shown in the figure ***(See Color Figure 12–47 on accompanying CD).*** The mostly likely diagnosis is

A Scabies mite infestation
B Pemphigus vulgaris associated with acantholytic cells
C Herpes zoster associated with multinucleated giant cells
D Herpes simplex associated with multinucleated giant cells
E Impetigo associated with gram-positive cocci

16. A middle-aged woman complains of a severe sunburn 1 day after going to the beach and 2 days after initiating a course of oral sulfamethoxazole-trimethoprim for a bladder infection. Skin examination shows changes shown in the figure ***(see Color Figure 12–48 on accompanying CD).*** The mostly likely diagnosis is

A Lichen planus
B Atopic dermatitis
C Seborrheic dermatitis
D Psoriasis
E Photosensitivity reaction

17. A middle-aged woman notes an asymptomatic dark area on her trunk several weeks after taking over-the-counter laxatives for constipation. Skin examination shows the changes shown in the figure ***(see Color Figure 12–49 on accompanying CD).*** The mostly likely diagnosis is

- [A] Melasma
- [B] Melanocytic nevus (mole)
- [C] Fixed drug eruption
- [D] Melanoma
- [E] Psoriasis

18. A pregnant woman develops painful nodules on her legs. Skin examination shows the changes shown in the figure ***(see Color Figure 12–50 on accompanying CD).*** The mostly likely diagnosis is

- [A] Stasis dermatitis
- [B] Cellulitis
- [C] Vasculitis
- [D] Erythema nodosum
- [E] Erythema multiforme

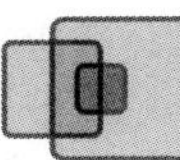

Answers and Explanations

1. The answer is C [XII E 13]. Hydrochlorothiazide is associated with a high frequency of photosensitivity. Captopril, an angiotensin-converting enzyme inhibitor, is associated with a high frequency of papulosquamous skin reactions. The clinical findings do not support the diagnoses of urticaria, erythema multiforme, erythema nodosum, or vasculitis.

2. The answer is D [IV A 7]. Isotretinoin is only indicated for the treatment of severe and recalcitrant nodulocystic acne. This agent should not be prescribed for milder forms of acne. Steroid acne responds to the discontinuation of systemic steroids and topical tretinoin.

3–6. The answers are: 3-B[III], **4-D**[III], **5-C**[III], **6-A**[III]. Both the potency and the vehicle of a topical corticosteroid must be appropriate for the specific clinical setting. High-potency topical steroids are used for the short-term treatment of acute and severe inflammatory eruptions. A cream has drying effects, and a high-potency steroid cream is well suited for treatment of a vesicular allergic contact dermatitis. An ointment has moisturizing effects, and a mid- to high-potency steroid ointment is highly effective for treating dry, scaly psoriatic plagues. Solutions and lotions are the vehicle of choice for the scalp; therefore, a mid- to high-potency steroid solution is effective for treating a flare of scalp psoriasis. Low-potency topical steroids are the only steroids used on the face. The drying effects of a cream are desirable for a greasy, scaling flare of seborrheic dermatitis in this location.

7. The answer is B [V B]. Pemphigus vulgaris typically affects middle-aged individuals and often presents dysphagia and oral involvement. Bullae are flaccid, and direct immunofluorescence shows IgG intercellular staining. Bullous pemphigoid rarely is characterized by oral involvement and tense bullae with linear IgG and C3 along the dermal–epidermal junction. Paraneoplastic pemphigus is characterized by severe oral involvement and heterogeneous skin lesions with histologic and direct immunofluorescent features of both pemphigus and pemphigoid. Erythema multiforme usually is characterized by target-like lesions on the palms and soles and distinct histopathology. Porphyria cutanea tarda is characterized by photosensitivity and tense bullae in a photo distribution and is associated with elevated urinary porphyrins.

8. The answer is C [VI D]. The clinical findings of a deep purulent and painful ulcer are typical of pyoderma gangrenosum, which often is associated with inflammatory bowel disease. Erythema nodosum is not an ulcerative process. Stasis dermatitis may be ulcerative but not to the extent of pyoderma gangrenosum. Palpable purpura is the hallmark of vasculitis (severe cases may result in ulceration). Calciphylaxis produces necrotic skin lesions.

9. The answer is E [XI B]. Dermatophyte infection of the body (tinea corporis) typically produces annular lesions that, on potassium hydroxide (KOH) preparation, show branched hyphae. Candidiasis produces pustules that form coalescent areas of erythema, typically in intertriginous areas, and KOH examination shows budding spores. Tinea versicolor produces confluent, scaling macules on the trunk, and KOH examination shows spores and nonbranched hyphae. Herpes simplex is a blistering eruption, and a Tzanck smear shows multinucleated giant cells. Tinea capitis is a dermatophyte infection that affects the scalp.

10. The answer is D [VII D]. Greasy scales along the T-zone of the face are typical of seborrheic dermatitis. Flares of seborrheic dermatitis are seen in patients with Parkinson's disease. Psoriasis and tinea versicolor rarely affect the face. Lupus erythematosus is characterized by a more prominent malar erythema and does not significantly involve the eyebrows and nasolabial fold. Allergic contact dermatitis is typically characterized by linear features to its configuration.

11. The answer is C [X D]. A papulosquamous eruption in a bathing trunk distribution can be seen with cutaneous T-cell lymphoma, tinea corporis, or possibly psoriasis. The skin biopsy shows diagnostic changes with atypical lymphocytes infiltrating the epidermis (epidermotropism) and forming clusters within the epidermis (Pautrier microabscess). Impetigo typically has golden crusts as a predominant feature. Atopic dermatitis predominantly affects flexor areas.

12. The answer is D [X, A]. The location of a basal cell carcinoma on the medial canthus of the eye determines where a lesion is at high risk for recurrence. The central face (eyes and nose) and ears are high-risk areas for recurrence of basal cell carcinoma. A fair complexion is associated with an increased incidence of basal cell carcinoma, both high- and low-risk lesions, and is not a clinical feature specific for high-risk basal cell carcinoma. Histologic features such as fibrosis (morpheaform basal cell carcinoma) and skip areas (multicentric basal cell carcinoma) are associated with high risk of recurrence for basal cell carcinoma. Gender is not a factor in determining the risk of basal cell carcinoma.

13. The answer is C [X, B]. Two histologic features of a squamous cell carcinoma that are associated with high risk for metastasis are poor differentiation and perineural invasion. Other factors such as location on the lower lip and size greater than 1 cm also contribute to metastasis. In this patient, the lesion is on the left jaw, and it is just less than 1 cm in size. Gender and complexion do not increase the risk for metastasis.

14. The answer is A [VII C]. The figure demonstrates erythematous macules and vesicles in a distinctive linear configuration. Such a configuration is typical of a contact dermatitis. Grouped vesicles, typical of herpes simplex infection, are not seen. Tense bullae, typical of bullous pemphigoid, is not present. Flexor involvement, typical of atopic dermatitis, is not seen. There is no evidence of palpable purpura, typical of vasculitis.

15. The answer is C [XI, C]. The figure demonstrates a Tzanck smear (stained with Giemsa stain) of scraping from blisters showing multinucleated giant cells. Multinucleated giant cells can be seen on Tzanck smears of herpes zoster and herpes simplex. The patient has a typical presentation of herpes zoster because of the clinical history of neuritic pain associated with blistering in a dermatomal distribution. Scabies can be visualized with scraping of web space burrows from patients with scabies. Acantholytic cells can be visualized when scraping blisters of pemphigus vulgaris. A Gram stain of impetigo reveals gram-positive cocci of *Staphylococcus* or *Streptococcus.*

16. The answer is E [XII E 13]. The figure demonstrates an erythematous maculopapular eruption with a sharp and discrete border, outlining the V of the neck, indicative of a photodistribution. The history indicates that the patient was started on sulfamethoxazole, which has a high frequency of photosensitive reactions. The distribution and clinical features seen in the figure are not typical of lichen planus, atopic dermatitis, seborrheic dermatitis, or psoriasis.

17. The answer is C [XII E 11]. The figure demonstrates a well-circumscribed, slate gray, hyperpigmented area typical of a fixed drug eruption. Phenolphthalein, a common ingredient of over-the-counter laxatives, is associated with a high frequency of fixed drug eruptions. Melasma is hyperpigmentation, typically on the face. The history and slate gray color is not typical of a melanocytic nevus. The lesion is well circumscribed with no features of asymmetry or pigment irregularity that can be seen in melanoma. Psoriasis does not produce pigmented lesions.

18. The answer is D [VI E]. The figure demonstrates inflammatory nodules on the lower extremity, which is typical of erythema nodosum. Pregnancy is associated with erythema nodosum. Stasis dermatitis is characterized by confluent changes about the ankles. Cellulitis typically affects one extremity with confluent erythema. Vasculitis is characterized by palpable purpura. Erythema multiforme is characterized by target lesions distributed peripherally.

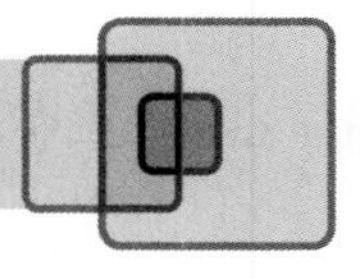

Case Studies in Clinical Decision-Making

CASE 1

Recurrent Sinopulmonary Infections in a Child

A 3-year-old boy is brought to your office for routine follow-up. It is noted that the child has another ear infection. On reviewing his chart, you note that the child has had many, many ear infections, several sinus infections, and three episodes of documented pneumonia. None of these infections has required hospitalizations. The child has always responded well to antibiotics.

QUESTIONS

- *What physical examination findings would make the practitioner question whether this child were immunologically normal?*
- *What is the normal number of infections for a child this age?*
- *What are other diseases that could be causing the recurrent infections?*

DISCUSSION

The child presented here has a common problem: recurrent sinopulmonary infections. The difference between a child who is having multiple infections versus immune deficiency is sometimes subtle. It is normal for a child of this age to have anywhere between 8 and 12 infections per year. Most of these would occur in the winter months.

If a child is presently in daycare, then that number of infections can rise to as many as 16. Also, it is sometimes very difficult to distinguish between a viral otitis media and a bacterial one; this can lead to an overuse of antibiotics.

The clinical signs that would indicate that the child may have an immune deficiency and not just a normal number of infections are the following: absence of lymphoid tissue for B cells that populate the lymphoid tissues. This is seen in X-linked agammaglobulinemia (XLA). Therefore, the child with XLA will have virtually no tonsillar or adenoidal tissue. When the examiner tries to palpate for lymph nodes, they will not be easily found. Also, children with this disease commonly have very severe ear infections, and the otoscopic examination will show scarred and deformed eardrums, which is very different from most children with recurrent ear infections. Pyogenic encapsulated bacteria such as *Streptococcus pneumonia, Haemophilus influenzae, Staphylococcus aureus,* and *Pseudomonas* species usually cause these infections. With all of these organisms, antibodies are important for opsonization and killing of the bacteria. Lastly, if the child had many episodes of pneumonia, they may have chronic scarring in the chest, but that is an unusual finding, which would not be identified by physical examination but rather by radiologic studies.

The differential diagnosis for this child includes anatomic abnormalities of the upper airway, gastroesophageal reflux, and potentially even atopy as the cause for recurrent otitis media and sinusitis. Allergic rhinitis would not commonly cause these symptoms to occur at a very young age. However, an anatomic abnormality or gastroesophageal reflux can cause this child to have ear and sinus infection from a very early age.

Other types of immune deficiencies also can cause recurrent infections. The most common would be a severe combined immune deficiency, but those children would almost always present before 1 year of life. Other immune deficiencies also can present at this age and would need to be evaluated (e.g., Wiskott-Aldrich and hyper IgE syndrome).

On careful examination, you note that the child has very scarred tympanic membranes. You also note that he has very small tonsils. You also review the chart carefully and note that this child has received antibiotics since the age of 1, almost on a monthly basis.

QUESTION

- *What immunologic and radiologic studies would be indicated?*

DISCUSSION

The serologic evaluation would center on the child's immunoglobulins. This could be done either in a stepwise fashion or as a comprehensive examination. The first step would involve measuring the quantitative IgG, IgM, IgA, and IgE. Other tests that could be done would involve functional antibodies to diphtheria and tetanus to evaluate the child's ability to mount an antibody response. A complete blood count with differential as well as an electrolyte panel and liver function tests also would be indicated. If the immunoglobulins were abnormal, then T-cell identification would be indicated to identify whether B cells are present. The radiologic studies that could be performed would include a chest x-ray, looking for scarring from previous pneumonias, a lateral neck film to evaluate adenoidal tissue, and possibly a barium swallow or milk scan to identify whether the child has any gastroesophageal reflux.

The laboratory values are available and indicate that the child does have x-linked agammaglobulinemia: IgG levels of 150 mg/dL (normal = 600–1500 mg/dL), antibody titers to diphtheria and tetanus were undetectable, T-cell indices were normal, and no B-cells were detected. In consultation with a pediatric immunologist, infusions of IV gamma globulins are started. The levels are measured, and a proper therapeutic value is obtained.

QUESTIONS

- *Should the child receive other medications beside the IV gamma-globulin?*
- *Does the child, now that he is receiving gamma-globulin, need immunizations?*

DISCUSSION

Many children with XLA will have chronic disease noted before their onset of therapy with IV gamma-globulin. Some of the patients will not need any other therapy beside the IV gamma-globulin. Many children will need chronic broad-spectrum antibiotics. These broad-spectrum antibiotics are routinely rotated to decrease the amount of resistance that is generated. The discontinuation of antibiotics usually triggers an immediate infection of the sinuses or ears.

Immunizations are not only unnecessary but in some cases contraindicated in this child. The child with XLA has no ability to generate an antibody response; therefore, no immunization will be helpful. In fact, immunizations with live viruses can be detrimental. A number of children with x-linked agammaglobulinemia who received live polio virus may have developed fulminate polio after the immunization. It was this population that was the impetus for the change from using a live polio virus to the killed vaccine that is currently in use.

The child is doing well, and the family is concerned about other issues they need to face. They are worried that even with the replacement therapy, his immune system is not normal.

QUESTIONS

- *Are there other infections and other manifestations that merit concern?*
- *Are these children susceptible to other infections?*

DISCUSSION

These children, before the advent of IV gamma-globulin, would commonly succumb to echovirus or Cocksackie virus infections. They would develop a chronic meningoencephalitis that would be insidious and have progressive neurologic symptoms. These infections would go on to be quite debilitating, if not fatal. These children less commonly are susceptible to a variety of other ailments, including protein-losing enteropathy, malabsorption, neutropenia, alopecia totalis, and amyloidosis. They also may have an autoimmune seronegative arthritis that is not related to an infection. The arthritis usually affects the large joints, causing hydrarthrosis and limited range of movement without joint pain or destruction.

These children handle most other infections quite well. They are not more susceptible to herpes infection or tuberculosis. When they do have these infections, they are no more serious than any normal patient and are self-limited. *Pneumocystis carinii* has been observed in a few patients with XLA, but those are usually extremely debilitated patients.

CASE 2

Oral Erosions and a Rash

A 29-year-old African-American man presents to the emergency department with the chief complaint of painful mouth erosions that have developed over 3 days. The initial symptom was a burning sensation of the left upper lip. Then tender sores developed on the gums and progressed to involve the entire mouth. Swallowing has become difficult because of increased secretions and pain. A rash has erupted on the patient's arms and legs within the past day.

Before the onset of symptoms, the patient was in good health. He has no ongoing or past medical problems. He takes no medications, vitamins, or herbal supplements. He has no known allergies and has no history of atopy. He works as a security officer and denies participating in any activities that pose a high risk for human immunodeficiency virus (HIV) infection. There is no family history of autoimmune disease or cancer. Review of systems is remarkable for a headache.

QUESTION

- *What is the differential diagnosis based on the history of oral erosions and a rash?*

DISCUSSION

The differential diagnosis of oral erosions includes infectious causes. Herpes simplex virus (HSV) infection produces localized blistering and secondary erosions that may affect the gingiva, buccal mucosa, and palate. Hand-foot-and-mouth disease (a coxsackievirus infection) produces blistering and erosions of the palate, buccal mucosa, gingiva, and tongue, as well as blisters on the hands and feet. Autoimmune blistering diseases such as pemphigus vulgaris and paraneoplastic pemphigus involve the oral mucosa and skin. An adverse reaction to a systemic medication can affect the mucous membranes. Erythema multiforme major and toxic epidermal necrolysis are the most severe forms of an adverse drug reaction. An allergic contact dermatitis to oral hygiene products (e.g., toothpaste, mouthwash) can produce inflammatory changes and erosions of the oral mucosa. Lichen planus is associated with erosive oral lesions. Systemic disorders such as inflammatory bowel disease, systemic lupus erythematosus, and Behçet's disease may involve the oral mucosa and cause erosive lesions.

The patient appears to be in mild distress and has a temperature of 99°F (37.2°C). Physical examination of the skin shows grouped erythematous vesicles and pustules on the left upper lip. The vermilion border is crusted with dried blood, and the anterior gingiva, buccal mucosa, and soft palate are bright red and eroded with serous exudate. The arms and legs show 0.5–1.0-cm erythematous round macules without scaling. The dorsum of the hands, palms, and soles have 1-cm erythematous target-like macules with a central violaceous hue. There is shotty submental and cervical lymphadenopathy.

QUESTION

- *What tests would you perform to narrow the differential diagnosis?*

DISCUSSION

A Tzanck smear should be taken from the grouped vesiculopustules of the left upper lip to identify the presence of HSV. The upper lip and oral mucosa should be swabbed, and bacterial and viral cultures should be obtained to confirm an infectious etiology. A skin biopsy from the buccal mucosa and one of the target-like lesions should be obtained, to confirm the diagnosis and rule out other causes of oral erosions, such as pemphigus vulgaris.

The Tzanck smear reveals multinucleated giant cells. Subsequent results demonstrate positive HSV type 1 cultures for the lip and skin biopsies of the buccal mucosa and hand characterized by histologic changes consistent with erythema multiforme.

QUESTIONS

- *What acute treatment should you provide?*
- *What are the long-term treatment issues?*

DISCUSSION

To reduce viral shedding and increase healing time, oral antiviral therapy should be initiated at appropriate doses for primary HSV infection. For oral pain relief, a topical anesthetic, such as viscous lidocaine, should be provided with instructions for the patient to swish and spit out up to four times a day. A short 10–14-day course of oral prednisone provides additional relief of acute inflammation of the erythema multiforme reaction.

The associated constitutional symptoms (headache and low-grade fever), lymphadenopathy, and no history of HSV indicate that the infection is primary and that the patient is at risk for recurrent episodes. The patient should be educated regarding the natural history of herpes labialis, its infectivity, and the signs and symptoms of recurrence. Because of the severe nature of the patient's reaction to his initiate eruption, he should be provided with a prescription for an oral antiviral agent with the instructions to initiate therapy at the first symptoms of recurrence. If the patient develops frequent eruptions such that the episodic antiviral therapy proves to be ineffective in suppressing erythema multiforme, then ongoing prophylactic doses of antiviral agents should be used for long-term suppression.

CASE 3

Polyarthritis

A 65-year-old woman presents to your office with a several-week history of pain and stiffness in her shoulders, hips, and hands, 2 weeks after visiting her grandchildren. Within a few weeks, she noted swelling in her hands and feet in addition to generalized stiffness lasting most of the morning. She did have a low-grade fever, but denied any chills, sweats, or weight loss. She had no associated headache, jaw claudication, or visual changes. She denied photosensitivity, oral ulcers, sicca symptoms, Raynaud's, serositis, history of miscarriages, or blood clots. She does have a family history of psoriasis.

QUESTIONS

- *What type of arthritis is this: inflammatory or noninflammatory?*
- *Does the pattern of joint involvement help in determining the type of arthritis?*
- *What are your initial concerns?*

DISCUSSION

The patient's history of morning stiffness lasting more than 1 hour suggests that inflammatory arthritis is the cause of her symptoms. At this juncture, the arthritis has been present only for a few weeks; thus, infectious etiologies must be considered. She does have a low-grade fever, but rarely does a bacterial arthritis present in a polyarticular fashion such as this, unless the patient is critically ill. Viral infections may present in this manner with a new-onset inflammatory arthritis. Of particular concern in this patient would be Parvovirus B19 infection, as she has been exposed to young children. Parvovirus B19 infection, or Fifth's disease, is endemic among school-aged children. Children typically present with a rash on their cheeks giving them a "slapped cheek" appearance in conjunction with a low-grade fever and mild constitutional symptoms. Adults infected with parvovirus B19 develop a flu-like illness and mild maculopapular rash on the extremities, with arthralgias and arthritis seen in approximately 20% of patients. The arthritis is symmetric and can be confused with rheumatoid arthritis (RA).

Young to middle-aged adult women are at highest risk for the arthropathy. Diagnostic testing soon after the onset of symptoms is helpful in making this diagnosis. A positive IgM antibody suggests active infection; a positive IgG antibody is consistent with prior exposure, but it is not helpful in the diagnosis given the high prevalence of seroconversion in the general population. Although the presence of fever raises the index of suspicion for an infectious process, many patients with noninfectious inflammatory arthritis can have low-grade fevers.

Other concerns in this patient given her age would include a paraneoplastic syndrome or polymyalgia rheumatica (PMR), especially in light of the proximal shoulder and pelvic girdle involvement. PMR may rarely have an associated inflammatory arthritis of the peripheral joints. Rheumatoid arthritis, systemic lupus erythematosus, scleroderma, and polymyositis all may present with an inflammatory symmetric polyarthritis. Psoriatic arthritis, although usually presenting in an asymmetric oligoarticular fashion, may present with a symmetric pattern of joint involvement, as can a crystalline arthritis such as gout (particularly in elderly women).

On examination, the patient is in obvious discomfort related to her joints. Her temperature is 38.0°C. She has a small, slightly raised erythematous scaly rash in her hairline and around her ears and in her umbilicus. No nail pits are present. There are no other mucocutaneous lesions. The temporal arteries have good pulsations and are nontender. There is no adenopathy. The cardiopulmonary and abdominal examinations are normal. The musculoskeletal examination is notable for limitation of motion of her shoulders secondary to pain and stiffness. She has obvious synovitis (synovial thickening with tenderness) of her bilateral wrists, metacarpophalangeal (MCPs), proximal interphalangeal (PIP) joints, ankles, and metatarsophalangeal joints (MTPJs). There are no "sausage digits" or evidence of an enthesopathy. She had mild warmth in both of her knees with moderate joint effusions. There was no sclerodactyly or muscle atrophy or weakness.

QUESTIONS

- *How do the findings on physical examination help you think about your differential diagnosis?*
- *What information should you seek from diagnostic tests at this time?*

DISCUSSION

The examination confirms the presence of a symmetric inflammatory polyarthritis. Thus, the differential includes RA, systemic lupus erythematosus (SLE), polymyalgia rheumatica, and less likely infectious, psoriatic and crystalline arthritis. The patient has the presence of a rash that has the appearance of psoriasis. Psoriatic arthritis develops in only 5% of patients with psoriasis. The risk of psoriatic arthritis increases with a family history of spondyloarthropathy or extensive nail pitting. There are five different patterns of psoriatic arthritis. See Chapter 10, Section IV B 3 d (2). It is possible that this patient has a pseudorheumatoid pattern of psoriatic arthritis. The differential diagnosis still includes viral illness such as parvovirus B19, rheumatoid arthritis, SLE, and malignancy. It is now unlikely based on the physical examination that the patient has scleroderma or an inflammatory myopathy. At this point, a complete blood count (CBC) and a comprehensive metabolic profile will help eliminate other systemic illnesses such as a viral hepatitis and malignancy. Systemic measures of inflammation such as an erythrocyte sedimentation rate (ESR) or C-reactive protein (CRP) are nonspecific indicators of inflammation and are not helpful in the diagnosis, but may be helpful in assessing response to treatment. Parvovirus serology should be evaluated, given her exposure to children. A rheumatoid factor (RF) and an antinuclear antibody (ANA) may be helpful in the diagnosis, given the symmetric presentation of her arthritis. It is important to keep in mind that 15% of patients with RA have a negative RF. A synovianalysis would be helpful in assessing the degree of synovial inflammation and to evaluate the presence of crystals.

The test results come back as follows: hemoglobin is 10.5 g/dL, the white blood cell (WBC) count is 8,300/µL, and the platelet count is 500,000/µL. The Westergren erythrocyte sedimentation rate is 78 mm/hr. A comprehensive metabolic profile is normal. The RF is positive at 349 IU/mL. The ANA is positive at 1:80 speckled. Parvovirus antibody IgG and IgM are negative. The x-rays of her hands and wrist show mild periarticular osteopenia around her MCPs. No erosions are seen. Synovial fluid analysis indicates 18,000 WBC with 80% polymorphonuclear cells (PMNs) and 20% lymphs. No crystals were seen.

QUESTIONS

- *What are the remaining diagnoses at this point?*
- *What additional diagnostic tests are appropriate to confirm the diagnosis?*
- *What therapeutic approach is most appropriate now?*

DISCUSSION

At this point, RA is the most likely diagnosis given the morning stiffness, symmetrical joint involvement, the presence of the serum RF, inflammatory synovial fluid, and the radiographic feature of periarticular osteopenia. There is no evidence of an associated malignancy, and PMR and psoriatic arthritis are less likely given the positive RF. Parvovirus has been excluded based on negative serologies, and viral hepatitis is unlikely with the normal transaminases. The patient must have arthritis for a period of 6 weeks to definitively diagnose RA, to ensure that other viral or self-limited entities are not contributing to the patient's arthritis. In the meantime, the patient is started on NSAID therapy and returns in 4 weeks.

On return 4 weeks later, the patient still has morning stiffness lasting most of the day. Her examination is notable for the presence of aggressive synovitis in her wrists, MCPs, PIPs, knee, ankle, and MTPJs. The results of the tests are reviewed with the patient, and therapeutic approach is outlined.

QUESTIONS

- *What therapies should be considered at this juncture?*
- *Should steroids be given?*

DISCUSSION

Now that it is clear that the arthritis has been present for 6 weeks, it is important that a disease-modifying antirheumatic drug (DMARD) be started immediately, as erosions occur early in the disease course. The gold standard in the treatment of RA is methotrexate. Before starting methotrexate, a baseline hepatitis screen and chest x-ray should be done. Additionally, it is becoming standard practice to obtain a test for tuberculosis [purified protein derivative (PPD)], because if the methotrexate is ineffective, an anti–tumor necrosis factor (TNF) agent may be considered. There have been documented cases of reactivation of tuberculosis while on anti-TNF therapy. While on the methotrexate, the patient must abstain from alcohol and have laboratory work every 6–8 weeks to monitor for toxicity. A short course of low-dose steroids may be helpful in controlling some of the symptoms while waiting for a DMARD to work, but a long-term course of steroids has no role in halting the progression of disease and is fraught with many potential side effects and long-term complications. The patient elects to start methotrexate therapy at 10 mg weekly, increasing the dose by 2.5 mg biweekly until a response recurs or 20 mg/week is reached. Folic acid 1 mg daily is prescribed to diminish the likelihood of stomatitis.

CASE 4

Severe Headache

A 62-year-old woman calls your office because of a severe headache that came on suddenly 1 hour ago. Her medical history is significant for headaches associated with menses, which ceased 12 years ago, and one or two throbbing headaches annually since menopause. She has hypertension controlled with an angiotensin-converting enzyme (ACE) inhibitor and beta-blocker, dyslipidemia treated with a statin, and she smokes one-half pack per day in spite of repeated urgings to stop smoking.

QUESTIONS

- *What are some possible causes of headache?*
- *What other questions would you like to ask this patient?*

DISCUSSION

The causes of headache are numerous. In a patient with headaches, it is useful to characterize each type of headache and develop a working hypothesis as to the cause of each headache. In this patient, there are potentially three types of headache: perimenstrual headaches, postmenopausal headaches, and the severe headache prompting her to seek medical assistance at this time.

Head pain is caused by disorders of the head or neck, including neurologic disorders. Problems as diverse as giant cell arteritis, acute glaucoma, sinusitis, dental abscess, temporomandibular joint dysfunction, trigeminal neuralgia, or cervical arthritis can cause head discomfort. Intracranial causes of headache include central nervous system (CNS) mass lesions such as primary or metastatic tumors, abscess, hydrocephalus, meningitis, superior sagittal sinus thrombosis, subarachnoid hemorrhage, and migraine.

One approach to the differential diagnosis of headache is to identify acute, life-threatening disorders such as meningitis and subarachnoid hemorrhage from chronic conditions such as migraine. Furthermore, it is helpful to target conditions that require specific, urgent intervention such as giant cell arteritis or acute glaucoma from more chronic disorders such as migraine or cervical arthritis.

Further history shows that the patient's perimenstrual headaches were characterized by holocephalic throbbing discomfort that started 1–2 days before menses and lasted 2–3 days. She graded the headache pain as 7/10. There was occasional nausea and photophobia. The patient found relief with nonsteroidal anti-inflammatory medications. Her postmenopausal headaches occurred every 3–4 months and again were holocephalic and throbbing, but only lasted a few hours or an entire day. The pain was 4–6/10 and was relieved with the same medications she had used for her perimenstrual headaches.

The patient denied visual symptoms including diplopia, jaw claudication, nasal drainage, dental pain, jaw "clicking," facial pain, or neck discomfort. She denied weakness or numbness in any limb and did not think she had a fever.

The patient did state that she had never had a headache like her current one, which was holocephalic and graded as 9–10/10. The pain was constant, and she had nausea and photophobia. She was gardening when the headache suddenly began and had momentarily collapsed to her knees. A dose of naproxen had not brought any relief.

QUESTIONS

- *What are your diagnostic considerations?*
- *What do you advise the patient to do?*

DISCUSSION

The patient's symptoms are not similar to her prior headache history, which are consistent with migraine. There are no symptoms to suggest local ocular, sinus, dental, or musculoskeletal sources of pain. Of concern is the sudden onset of severe, atypical head pain. It is not clear from the patient's history whether the collapse was due to brief weakness, loss of consciousness, or both. The collapse, accompanied by nausea, suggests a neurologic problem such as a stroke syndrome (vertebrobasilar disease, intracranial hemorrhage) or increased intracranial pressure [hydrocephalus, sagittal sinus thrombosis, subarachnoid hemorrhage (SAH)]. Her lack of focal neurologic symptoms is not supportive of vertebrobasilar disease or an intracerebral hematoma. The rapid onset of symptoms is not consistent with the presentation of sagittal sinus thrombosis.

Subarachnoid hemorrhage presents as "the worst headache of my life." The headache is typically of sudden onset, holocephalic, severe, and can be accompanied by nausea and brief loss of consciousness, probably reflecting a transient increase in intracranial pressure. Photophobia can occur, as can emesis. Typically there are no immediate focal neurologic symptoms or signs, although diplopia can reflect damage to the oculomotor nerve from the mass effect of a posterior communicating artery aneurysm. Smoking is a risk factor for SAH.

Because of your concern about SAH, you advise the patient to call 911 and have an ambulance transport her to the hospital. You contact the hospital to inform them about the patient's arrival and your diagnostic suspicion.

QUESTIONS

- *To which aspects of the physical examination should the ED physicians be particularly alert?*
- *What diagnostic tests are most essential to the patient's evaluation?*

DISCUSSION

Patients presenting with SAH frequently are quite hypertensive because of elevated catecholamine levels. Although patients with SAH can have a low-grade fever, elevated temperature should raise concern for an infective, rather than SAH-associated, meningitis. If a patient has impaired consciousness, there should be concern about airway protection, and intubation should be considered.

The ED physician should examine the head and neck for the causes of headache referred to previously. Although evidence of meningeal irritation, such as Kernig's and Brudzinski's signs, should be looked for in patients with a possible SAH, these signs are frequently absent early in the clinical course.

A critical determinant of outcome after SAH is the patient's level of consciousness on presentation, with progressively impaired arousal being associated with a worse prognosis. An oculomotor palsy in an alert patient is particularly suggestive of a posterior communicating artery aneurysm, and an abducens palsy suggests increased intracranial pressure (a "false localizing sign"). Alert or obtunded patients with SAH rarely have other focal neurologic signs such as a hemiparesis.

The "gold standard" for the diagnosis of SAH is the presence of subarachnoid blood on a brain computed tomography (CT) scan. If blood is present, there is no need to perform a lumbar puncture. A modest proportion of alert patients with SAH have an unremarkable CT scan; in these individuals, a lumbar puncture is indicated to document the presence of bleeding.

Clotting studies [platelet count, prothrombin time, and activated partial thrombin time (PT)] are appropriate to screen for a bleeding diathesis. A serum sodium should be obtained, because SAH patients are prone to disturbances in sodium concentrations. An electrocardiogram (ECG) may show findings such as peaked T-waves or arrhythmias, which may represent catecholamine-associated cardiac effects.

The patient's blood pressure was 185/95 mm Hg; she was afebrile. The patient had no neck rigidity and a normal head and neck examination. She was alert and cognitively intact. Her neurologic examination was normal.

A brain CT scan showed subarachnoid blood with mild dilation of the ventricles. Clotting studies, serum sodium concentration, and the ECG were normal.

QUESTIONS

- *What are the next management steps?*
- *At this time, to what complications should the patient's physicians be alert?*

DISCUSSION

Patients with SAH should be placed in an intensive care unit. There should be frequent neurologic evaluations. Extremes of blood pressure should be avoided. It is helpful to consider the relationship: cerebral perfusion pressure = mean arterial pressure – intracranial pressure. A cerebral perfusion pressure of 70–80 mm Hg is desirable. In an alert patient, who presumably does not have a critical elevation of intracranial pressure, a mean blood pressure of approximately 90–100 mm Hg can be targeted. Labetalol is a particularly effective antihypertensive agent in this setting because it does not cause an elevation in intracranial pressure.

Hydration with normal saline is appropriate so as to maintain a euvolemic state. Mild sedation and analgesia for headache should be considered, and agents to prevent straining at stool can be prescribed.

Nimodipine, a calcium channel antagonist, decreases the incidence of delayed ischemic deficits secondary to cerebral vasospasm. Unfortunately, it can cause excessive hypotension, which can exacerbate cerebral ischemia if not adequately treated.

Neurosurgical and radiologic consultation should be obtained, and urgent four-vessel angiography is necessary to document all aneurysms the patient may have.

Complications at this time include the development of hydrocephalus attributable to disruption of CSF flow patterns by subarachnoid (or intraventricular) blood, aneurysmal rebleeding, and hyponatremia. A decreased serum sodium level can be caused by overhydration, the syndrome of inappropriate secretion of antidiuretic hormone, and cerebral salt wasting. These complications can cause diminished consciousness, seizures, and, occasionally, focal neurologic signs.

The patient's blood pressure is successfully controlled with labetalol. Nimodipine is well tolerated. A cerebral angiogram indicates a single anterior communicating artery aneurysm measuring 10 mm in its largest diameter. The patient remains alert and cognitively intact. The patient, family, and physician team discuss treatment options to prevent rebleeding, including surgical "clipping" or endovascular "coiling" of the aneurysm. The patient decides on surgical intervention, which is performed on the second hospital day.

QUESTIONS

- *At this time, to what complications should the patient's physicians be alert?*
- *What management strategies should be pursued?*

DISCUSSION

An operative complication of anterior communicating artery aneurysm surgery is cognitive dysfunction because of injury to basal forebrain structures. After surgery, patients are still at risk for hydrocephalus and hyponatremia. With successful isolation of the aneurysm from the cerebral circulation, the risk of rebleeding should be nil. Of concern at this time is the development of delayed ischemic neurologic deficits because of cerebral vasospasm. This complication is thought to be attributable to the effects of subarachnoid blood on the intracranial arteries; there is vasoconstriction with associated histologic findings of intimal hyperplasia and smooth muscle proliferation. Patients can develop impaired consciousness and focal neurologic deficits.

Serial transcranial Doppler (TCD) studies can show increasing blood flow velocities, which can be a harbinger of subsequent clinically significant cerebral vasospasm. Medical management to prevent symptomatic vasospasm and symptomatic cerebral ischemia includes nimodipine and "triple H therapy": hemodilution, hypertension, and hypervolemia. Optimal oxygen transportation occurs at hematocrits in the 30–35 range. Elevation of the mean arterial blood pressure by 10%–20%, together with hypervolemia, can prevent or treat cerebral ischemia caused by vasospasm.

The patient is cognitively intact after surgery. Blood pressure and serum sodium levels are in an acceptable range. However, serial TCD studies show a progressive elevation of blood flow velocities in the middle and anterior cerebral arteries. Triple H therapy is begun. On the third postoperative day, the patient becomes obtunded, and a mild right hemiparesis develops in spite of

optimal medical management. A brain CT scan shows a left frontal ischemic infarction; there is no evidence of new hemorrhage.

QUESTIONS

- *What is the probable cause of the patient's new stroke?*
- *What management options might be considered?*

DISCUSSION

The patient has sustained an ischemic infarction caused by cerebral vasospasm. A cerebral angiogram should be obtained to define the extent of the vasospasm. Interventional neuroradiologic approaches to the treatment of medically refractory symptomatic vasospasm include angioplasty and intra-arterial infusion of papavarine.

The patient is taken to the angiography suite. Images demonstrate diffuse vasospasm, worse in the left middle cerebral artery. Angioplasty is performed and successfully dilates the left middle cerebral artery. Several papaverine infusions are directed at the distal branches of the anterior and middle cerebral arteries.

Over the next several days, the patient has a progressive decline in consciousness and develops a left hemiparesis. Repeat CT scans show multiple areas of ischemic infarction. A repeat angiogram shows severe diffuse vasospasm.

Two weeks after her SAH, the patient has lost all evidence of brain function and is declared brain dead.

COMMENT

In spite of many advances in neurologic intensive care, aneurysmal SAH remains a disease with a mortality rate approaching 50%. Patients are at risk for many complications, and even though they may appear quite intact on presentation, their clinical course can be perilous.

CASE 5

Deep Venous Thrombosis

A 28-year-old man consults his primary physician because of the sudden onset of shortness of breath and right pleuritic chest pain, having returned 3 days before the onset of symptoms from a business trip to Tokyo. He has been in excellent health all his life and takes no medications. His medical history is negative, with the exception of tonsillectomy at age 10 without bleeding complications and an appendectomy at age 18, which was followed 10 days later by an episode of right calf tenderness and swelling that resolved spontaneously without specific therapy. Family history indicated that his father died suddenly at age 35 of a "heart attack," and his sister died suddenly of unknown cause at age 25 postpartum. On physical examination, he is a physically fit–appearing man complaining of right-sided chest discomfort on deep inspiration and moderate distress with shortness of breath. Vital signs showed blood pressure (BP) = 110/60 mm Hg; pulse = 114 beats/min; respirations = 24 breaths/min; temperature = 37.5°C. Examination of the heart indicates a summation gallop at the apex with a prominent P2 at the base. Auscultation of the lungs discloses a pleural friction rub heard in the right axilla. Remainder of the physical examination is negative, with the exception of tenderness on palpation on the left calf, with pain elicited by dorsiflexion of the left foot. Subtle, but definite slight edema was present in the left ankle.

QUESTIONS

- *What is your differential diagnosis and the most likely explanation for his symptoms?*
- *What initial diagnostic studies should be carried out immediately to confirm the diagnosis?*

DISCUSSION

A chest x-ray was obtained, which showed no abnormality. An ECG showed sinus tachycardia with clockwise rotation and right axis deviation. An arterial blood sample was obtained, which showed the following results: $PaO_2 = 83$; $PaCO_2 = 31$; pH = 7.49, arterial oxygen saturation, 87%.

QUESTIONS

- *How do you interpret these finding?*
- *What diagnostic studies should be done next?*
- *Would you consider instituting any form of therapy based on the results at this point?*
- *Would you consider obtaining any further diagnostic studies before instituting therapy?*

DISCUSSION

The normal chest x-ray essentially excludes pneumonia or other pulmonary parenchymal pathology as the cause for the patient's symptoms. The ECG showed only nonspecific findings but is consistent with abnormalities observed in pulmonary embolic disease. The arterial blood gas studies show evidence of oxygen desaturation, mild respiratory alkalosis, and an abnormal A-a gradient that, in the absence of pulmonary parenchymal disease, strongly suggests a ventilation/perfusion abnormality such as is observed in acute pulmonary embolism (PE).

The correct diagnostic procedure is a ventilation/perfusion lung scan. Spiral CT scanning of the lung is also very good in the diagnosis of PE but has not replaced lung scanning as yet. However, before sending the patient to the radiology department, it would be appropriate to institute heparin therapy immediately based on a presumptive working diagnosis of PE, because the next embolus, if massive, might be fatal. However, before instituting heparin therapy, it would be desirable to obtain satisfactorily collected blood samples for preliminary investigation of a thrombophilic state, because the results from such a workup are difficult or impossible to interpret after anticoagulant therapy has been instituted. Even in the face of acute venous thromboembolic disease, some of the coagulation-based studies are not subject to definitive interpretation and therefore should also be repeated at a later date, when the patient is asymptomatic and not receiving anticoagulant therapy. At this point in the workup, venous blood samples can be obtained and properly stored for the following determinations pending the results of the V/Q scan:

Protein C
Protein S
Prothrombin 20210
Factor V Leiden
Lupus anticoagulant/anticardiolipin antibodies
Antithrombin III
Homocysteine

Of these studies, homocysteine, anticardiolipin antibodies, and genetic testing for prothrombin 20210 and Factor V Leiden will not be affected by the acute event or anticoagulant medicines.

In addition, a baseline prothrombin time and partial thromboplastin time (PTT) should be obtained before the institution of anticoagulant therapy. Finally, an assay for D-dimer will aid in diagnosis of an acute thrombosis.

The V/Q scan showed a large perfusion defect in the right middle lobe distribution with normal ventilation, a result consistent with a high probability for PE. If the V/Q scan were indeterminate or showed a low probability of PE, then a pulmonary angiogram should be done to rule in or rule out PE. Consideration also could be given to carrying out Doppler ultrasonography to investigate the possibility of deep vein thrombosis as the source of a PE, although, if the results of the V/Q scan definitively establish a diagnosis of PE, further investigation for deep vein thrombosis (DVT) is unnecessary. Assay for D-dimer was markedly elevated, 500 μg/dL (normal < 25), further confirming the presence of acute thrombosis.

QUESTION

- *Having established a diagnosis of pulmonary thromboembolism, what further therapy should be instituted?*

DISCUSSION

Concurrent administration of heparin therapy combined with an oral anticoagulant such as coumadin should be instituted. Heparin should be maintained for at least a 5-day period and warfarin for a variable time thereafter (see below).

QUESTIONS

- *What is the rationale for concurrent administration of heparin and oral anticoagulants?*
- *How are these two therapies monitored?*

DISCUSSION

The rationale for concurrent administration of heparin and oral anticoagulants is the following: heparin induces immediate anticoagulation by enhancing the activity of endogenous antithrombin III, whereas vitamin K antagonists such as coumadin (which inhibit the synthesis of factors VII, IX, and X, prothrombin, protein C, and protein S) require approximately 4–6 days to become fully effective based on the half-lives of the vitamin K–dependent protein. However, by decreasing the synthesis of protein C and protein S, coumadin actually can initially enhance the propensity to thromboembolism, resulting in "coumadin-induced skin necrosis" unless given simultaneously with heparin. Abrupt discontinuation of heparin therapy without coverage by oral anticoagulants can decrease the concentration of antithrombin III and is associated with a high relapse rate of thrombosis. Unfractionated heparin is monitored by the PTT, whereas warfarin therapy is monitored by the PT. Recently, the use of low-molecular-weight forms of heparin (LMWH) in place of standard heparin has increased. LMWH can be dosed on a weight basis with no need to monitor PTT, a big advantage.

QUESTIONS

- *Why is follow-up so important in the management of this patient?*
- *What should be the objective of follow-up management?*

DISCUSSION

This patient developed DVT and PE at a young age, has a suggestive prior personal history of thromboembolism, and has a strong family history suggestive of PE in the first-degree relatives. Therefore, he is a likely candidate for diagnosis of an inherited thrombophilia, such as deficiency of protein C, protein S, antithrombin III, the prothrombin 20210 polymorphism, or factor V Leiden. Studies to investigate these possibilities should be confirmed either using the aforementioned initially obtained specimens or after a 6-month to 12-month period of treatment with oral anticoagulants, followed by a 1–2-week period off oral anticoagulants to reestablish a normal level of these proteins. If deficiencies of one or more of these proteins are established, consideration should be given to long-term prophylaxis with oral anticoagulants.

The patient was treated with LMWH and did well. For completeness, a Doppler ultrasound was performed and was positive for DVT in the left leg. Initial hypercoagulable state workup indicated factor V Leiden heterozygous state by genetic testing. The epidemiology of this thrombotic event fits nicely into the current thinking, wherein "multiple hits" are responsible for most events. In this case, his genetic susceptibility (factor V Leiden) combined with unusual venous stasis (prolonged plane ride) to trigger a thromboembolic complication. Other triggering events include general anesthesia for >1 hour, immobilization by casting of the leg, and pregnancy and the postpartum state. This patient is currently on a long-term coumadin and is a candidate for indefinite anticoagulation because he has an underlying genetic hypercoagulable state and has experienced multiple thrombotic events.

CASE 6

Newly Discovered Renal Failure

A 62-year-old man visits his physician for a routine physical examination. He mentions that he has to get out of bed to urinate more frequently than he used to (two to three times each night) and that he has difficulty initiating and maintaining a urinary stream. In addition, he states that he has experienced mild shortness of breath on walking two to three flights of stairs and that his regular biweekly workouts at the gym have been much more difficult for him lately.

Physical examination shows moderate pallor, a blood pressure of 150/105 mm Hg, a pulse of 80 beats/min, and a respiratory rate of 18 respirations per minute. There is trace pedal edema. Examination of the chest and heart shows no abnormalities. Examination of the abdomen shows slight fullness in the lower abdomen but neither tenderness nor pain.

Laboratory work is obtained, including a complete blood count (CBC), electrolyte, glucose, calcium, and renal studies. The results of these studies are as follows: blood urea nitrogen (BUN), 88 mg/dL; creatinine, 6.4 mg/dL; sodium, 137 mEq/L; potassium, 5.9 mEq/L; chloride, 112 mEq/L; bicarbonate, 16 mEq/L; hemoglobin, 8.7 g/dL.

QUESTIONS

- *What is the first determination you should make with respect to this patient?*
- *What additional information might help you make this determination?*
- *What is the most likely cause of this patient's renal insufficiency? Does the patient's altered electrolyte and acid–base metabolism support this diagnosis?*

DISCUSSION

The determination of onset of renal failure is crucial to determine the proper therapeutic approach. Acute renal failure implies the potential for reversibility, and therefore every effort must be made to identify any ongoing injurious agents that adversely affect the kidney. In addition, acute support through some form of dialysis therapy may be required to sustain the patient until renal recovery can occur. Conversely, the presence of chronic renal failure suggests that the patient has sustained irreversible injury. The patient must then be treated in a way to prevent further loss of kidney function; chronic renal replacement therapy, either through dialysis support or through transplantation, may be necessary.

The determination of chronicity of renal failure can be difficult. In patients with acute renal failure, a clear precipitating event (e.g., exposure to nephrotoxic agents such as gentamicin, sepsis, shock) usually can be identified. The determination of the onset of chronic disease is more problematic. The time of initiation of subtle symptoms consistent with renal failure (e.g., pruritus) may be helpful in determining the onset of the disease. Renal ultrasound provides information about kidney size, which typically is reduced in chronic renal failure and normal in acute renal failure. Exceptions include diabetic nephropathy and amyloidosis, which may be associated with normal or enlarged kidneys, and polycystic kidney disease, which may be associated with extremely large kidneys despite coexistent renal failure. Chronic renal failure is typically associated with secondary hyperparathyroidism; subperiosteal resorption is typically seen radiographically. In addition, generalized bone demineralization, loss of bone mass at the acromial–clavicular joint, or mottling of the skull may be important findings. Anemia is typically seen in chronic renal failure because erythropoietin levels are reduced as kidney mass is reduced. However, anemia may develop rather rapidly, and occasionally, severe anemia is seen in both acute and chronic renal failure; it likely explains the dyspnea in this patient.

This patient most likely has acute renal insufficiency as a result of chronic obstructive uropathy. This conclusion stems from the history of difficulty voiding; the presence of bladder fullness on physical examination; and the findings of renal failure, hyperkalemia, and metabolic acidosis. Other common causes of acute renal failure in the ambulatory setting include toxic nephropathy from medication use and acute glomerulonephritis. In men, the most common cause of chronic obstructive nephropathy is prostatic hypertrophy, but bladder cancer or prostatic cancer is possible as well. The patient has hyperchloremic hypobicarbonatemia with associated hyperkalemia. This constellation of findings is common in patients with chronic renal insufficiency, particularly in association with obstructive uropathy. The hypobicarbonatemia suggests metabolic acidosis but also could be caused by chronic respiratory alkalosis.

The presence of renal insufficiency makes metabolic acidosis the most likely cause of the hypobicarbonatemia in this patient. The high chloride level reflects the fact that electrical neutrality must be maintained by body fluids, and as bicarbonate levels fall, preferential chloride reabsorption with sodium occurs in the renal tubules. Because the kidney is unable to generate new bicarbonate to restore the levels reduced by ingestion of dietary precursors of various mineral acids, bicarbonate levels fall. A reduced bicarbonate level is typical of all forms of renal failure.

The increase in serum potassium is an important indication of obstructive uropathy. Potassium is secreted in the distal nephron but requires adequate amounts of aldosterone as well as a normally responsive distal tubule potassium transport system for normal excretion. Chronic obstructive uropathy is associated with impairment of potassium excretion, occasionally secondary to reduced aldosterone levels but more typically due to a direct tubular abnormality. Correction of the underlying obstructive process leads to a normalization of potassium excretion and a return of serum potassium levels to the normal range.

Renal ultrasound is performed and confirms the diagnosis of obstructive uropathy. A Foley catheter is put in place.

QUESTION

- *What clinical problem should be anticipated after relief of obstruction?*

DISCUSSION

On relief of obstruction, it is typical for patients with obstructive uropathy to undergo a striking diuresis. The source of the diuresis is a combination of excretion of previously retained solutes and fluids as well as a mild residual tubular defect in sodium and water conservation. This massive diuresis typically remits once the patient's BUN and creatinine have leveled off.

Dialysis, either by hemodialysis or peritoneal dialysis, may be necessary in patients with renal insufficiency secondary to obstructive uropathy, but attempts should always be made to correct the obstructive uropathy before initiating hemodialysis. The decision to perform dialysis must be made on an individual basis and defies simple categorization. Hemodialysis is indicated in patients with pericarditis. Congestive heart failure (CHF) also may be an indication for dialysis therapy to achieve fluid removal. Institution of dialysis should not be made on the basis of the absolute BUN level alone, although most clinicians believe that the BUN should be maintained below 150 mg/dL.

CASE 7

Coma in a Diabetic Patient

A 20-year-old college student is rushed to the emergency department by ambulance after being found comatose by her roommate in her dormitory room. She is known to have type 1 (insulin-dependent) diabetes mellitus that has been well controlled by diet and insulin.

QUESTIONS

- *What are your immediate concerns about this patient?*
- *What are possible mechanisms of coma in a diabetic patient?*
- *What is at the top of your differential diagnosis?*

DISCUSSION

When the patient first arrives in the emergency department, an adequate airway should be ensured, vital signs should be measured to assess circulatory status, intravenous access should be established, and blood should be drawn for chemistries, arterial blood gas measurements, and a fingerstick glucose determination. Then additional information should be obtained from the patient's friend.

The causes of coma that are directly related to diabetes are diabetic ketoacidosis, hypoglycemia, and hyperosmolar nonketotic coma. The latter occurs mainly in elderly patients with type 2 (non–insulin-dependent) diabetes, so the first diagnostic impressions when this patient arrives in the emergency department are diabetic ketoacidosis and hypoglycemia.

Diabetic ketoacidosis occurs when there is a severe insulin deficiency, which causes an inability to utilize glucose and leads to hyperglycemia, ketosis, and acidosis. Hypoglycemia in a diabetic patient is usually the result of an imbalance between the factors that lower the blood glucose level, primarily administered insulin, oral hypoglycemic agents, and exercise, and the factors that raise the blood glucose level, namely food ingestion and hepatic output of glucose. Diabetic ketoacidosis and hypoglycemia should be ruled out before serious consideration is given to other causes of coma such as drug overdose, seizures, stroke, or meningitis.

The roommate recalls that the patient has been complaining of an "upset stomach" for 2 days, with some nausea, anorexia, mild diarrhea, and increasing abdominal pain. She seemed a bit groggy that morning and did not go to classes. Because she was unable to eat breakfast, she did not take her morning insulin dose. The roommate returned from class at 3:00 PM and found the patient lying in bed, breathing deeply and unresponsive to questions.

QUESTIONS

- *What risk factors does this patient have for the development of diabetic ketoacidosis?*
- *What is the significance of each of the patient's complaints?*

DISCUSSION

The apparently gradual onset over a period of hours, the preceding illness, and the omission of an insulin dose strongly suggest diabetic ketoacidosis rather than hypoglycemia as the most likely diagnosis. Illnesses such as upper respiratory infection or gastroenteritis may increase the need for insulin because of stress-related increases in catecholamines, cortisol, and glucagon; omitting insulin doses because of the illness makes matters worse. The gastrointestinal symptoms at the onset of illness suggest that gastroenteritis was the precipitating event, although the increasing abdominal pain could have been caused also by the developing ketoacidosis.

Why does abdominal pain sometimes occur in diabetic ketoacidosis? Gastric distention may be a factor, and it is known that ketosis from other causes such as starvation may lead to gastrointestinal symptoms such as anorexia, nausea, and vomiting. But the precise cause of abdominal pain in diabetic ketoacidosis is not known. The grogginess that the patient experienced earlier in the day suggests that the process leading to mental obtundation had already started. The symptoms of diabetic ketoacidosis are typically gradual in onset (over several hours), whereas the mental changes of hypoglycemia commonly have a relatively sudden onset, which is usually preceded by adrenergic symptoms such as sweating, tremor, and palpitations.

On examination, the patient is unresponsive, with dry skin and mucous membranes and rapid, deep respirations. Her blood pressure is 100/60 mm Hg supine, falling to 80/50 mm Hg when the head of the bed is raised. The neck veins are collapsed when the patient is lying supine. Her pulse rate is 110 beats/min, her respiratory rate is 24 breaths/min, and her temperature is 37.0°C. She winces when moderate pressure is applied to her abdomen. The deep tendon reflexes are hypoactive.

QUESTIONS

- *Do these physical findings aid in differentiating between diabetic ketoacidosis and hypoglycemia?*
- *What is the significance of the patient's respiratory pattern?*

DISCUSSION

These physical findings are highly suggestive of diabetic ketoacidosis. Insufficient insulin action makes glucose unavailable to the tissues, and the liver responds by producing ketones as an alternative fuel. The rising blood levels of glucose and ketones cause an osmotic diuresis, producing dehydration and intravascular volume depletion, with orthostatic hypotension. The osmotic diuresis leads to urinary losses of potassium and other electrolytes; hypokalemia causes muscle weakness and decreased reflexes. Abdominal pain and tenderness, perhaps caused by the ketosis, may be severe. The rapid, deep respirations, called Kussmaul's respirations, are caused by stimulation of the respiratory center by acidosis. This leads to respiratory alkalosis, which partially offsets the metabolic acidosis.

Blood glucose by fingerstick, determined soon after the patient's arrival in the emergency department, is found to be greater than 400 mg/dL. Urine dipstick testing is strongly positive for glucose and ketones. Treatment is started with an intravenous infusion of normal saline solution at a rate of 1000 mL/hr.

QUESTIONS

- *What is the rationale behind ordering these laboratory tests?*
- *What initial steps should be taken at this point to manage this patient's condition?*

DISCUSSION

The elevated blood and urine glucose levels and urine ketone levels confirm the diagnosis of diabetic ketoacidosis. The first priority in treatment is fluid replacement, which can be started while the initial laboratory results are awaited. An infusion of normal saline (1 L/hr for the first 2 hours) should be given if intravascular volume depletion is severe, as indicated by the orthostatic hypotension and decreased central venous pressure (decreased neck vein filling). Once the diagnosis of diabetic ketoacidosis is confirmed, insulin therapy should be started.

Intravenous infusion of regular insulin is started at a rate of 5 U/hr. Initial laboratory results include the following serum findings: glucose level of 520 mg/dL; sodium level of 132 mEq/L; potassium level of 3.3 mEq/L; and normal phosphate, calcium, and chloride levels. Blood urea nitrogen (BUN) and creatinine are slightly elevated, as is serum amylase. The white blood cell (WBC) count is 14,500/mm^3. Arterial blood gas analysis indicates a pH of 7.20, bicarbonate of 8 mEq/L, and a pattern consistent with high anion gap metabolic acidosis.

QUESTIONS

- *How do these laboratory values affect your differential diagnosis?*
- *What is the significance of the elevated amylase?*
- *What is the significance of the leukocytosis?*
- *What processes are included in your differential diagnosis for high anion gap acidosis?*

DISCUSSION

These laboratory findings are typical of moderately severe diabetic ketoacidosis. The metabolic acidosis is caused by the hepatic production of ketone bodies, which must be buffered by bicarbonate. Sodium tends to be low because of the osmotic effect of hyperglycemia, which increases extracellular water, thus diluting serum sodium. Potassium, although initially high because of movement out of cells, falls to low levels as urinary losses occur. Although serum phosphate may be normal initially, large urinary losses often lead to depletion of total body phosphate, which should be replaced. The BUN and creatinine tend to be slightly increased because of the effect of volume depletion on renal function.

Serum amylase often is increased, but this usually is attributed to transient leakage from the salivary glands as well as the pancreas and does not usually indicate pancreatitis.

Leukocytosis is common in diabetic ketoacidosis; if infection is not present, the increased WBC count may be attributed to dehydration and increased glucocorticoid activity, which occurs in response to stress and may cause leukocytosis.

The high anion gap is caused by the presence of an unmeasured anion, in this case ketone bodies. Other important causes of high anion gap acidosis include renal failure, alcoholic ketoacidosis, lactic acidosis, and toxic substances such as salicylates, ethylene glycol, and methanol.

After 6 hours of treatment, the patient is awake, breathing comfortably at a rate of 18 respirations per minute, and able to respond to questions. The serum glucose level is 210 mg/dL, the arterial blood pH is 7.34, and the serum bicarbonate level is 14 mEq/L. Urine ketones are now only weakly positive.

QUESTIONS

- *What other types of acute care might this patient require?*
- *What are some of the potential complications of diabetic ketoacidosis?*

DISCUSSION

Because insulin therapy is still needed to treat the resolving ketosis and acidosis, glucose should now be added to the intravenous fluids to prevent hypoglycemia. Potassium and phosphate should be replaced as indicated by blood values.

In spite of careful treatment, patients with diabetic ketoacidosis have a mortality rate of 5%–10%. Death may be caused by overwhelming infection, by irreversible shock, or by arterial thrombosis causing myocardial infarction (MI) or stroke. Cerebral edema occasionally occurs in young patients who appear to be responding well to treatment and may cause death. A more rapid decrease in glucose levels in blood than in the cerebrospinal fluid (CSF) causes fluid to enter the relatively hyperosmolar CSF compartment, leading to increased intracranial pressure (ICP) and cerebral edema.

CASE 8

Shortness of Breath in a Young Woman

A 38-year-old African-American woman comes to the emergency department with a chief complaint of shortness of breath on exertion that has progressively worsened in the past 6 months. Her symptoms have become so severe that she now has difficulty eating secondary to extreme dyspnea, and this has resulted in a 27-pound weight loss. She also notes a severe cough productive of white sputum but denies fevers, chills, or night sweats. Before the onset of symptoms (about 6 months ago), she was in good health.

QUESTIONS

- *What are your immediate concerns in this patient?*
- *How does the onset of symptoms help formulate a differential diagnosis?*
- *What are the most likely diagnostic considerations?*

DISCUSSION

On initial evaluation of this patient in the emergency department, care must be taken to ensure that she has an adequate airway. Her vital signs must also be assessed, with specific attention to respiratory rate, heart rate, and temperature. Supplemental oxygen should be provided to ensure an oxygen saturation of greater than 94%. Blood should be drawn for arterial blood gas analysis, complete blood count (CBC), and chemistries. A chest radiograph (posteroanterior and lateral views) and electrocardiogram (ECG) also should be ordered.

The causes of shortness of breath in this age group can include acute and chronic infections; cardiac malformations, including valvular dysfunction; anemia; and chronic lung disease, including interstitial lung disease. In general, cardiac causes are easy to exclude in two situations: (1) when the patient has no history of heart problems at birth (i.e., congenital) or in early childhood, and (2) when the cardiac examination is normal. In addition, anemia can be excluded when there is no history of continuing heavy menstrual blood loss or gastrointestinal hemorrhage.

The duration of this patient's symptoms makes an acute infection very unlikely and suggests a chronic infection or one of the interstitial lung diseases. However, the lack of a persistent fever, chills, or recurrent night sweats makes chronic infection less probable, although acquired immunodeficiency syndrome (AIDS)–related infections such as *Pneumocystis carinii* pneumonia (PCP) can present with a paucity of constitutional symptoms. Furthermore, this patient is at particular demographic risk for the development of sarcoidosis, a chronic granulomatous disorder of unknown cause that commonly affects young African-American women.

Other diagnostic considerations include pulmonary lymphangioleiomyomatosis, hypersensitivity pneumonitis, eosinophilic granuloma, idiopathic pulmonary fibrosis, and interstitial lung disease secondary to connective tissue disorders or vasculitis. Pulmonary lymphangioleiomyomatosis, a disorder characterized by proliferation of atypical smooth muscle cells, leads to parenchymal lung disease, pleural effusions, hemoptysis, and pneumothorax; however, it is exceedingly rare. Hypersensitivity pneumonitis also can occur in younger individuals after exposure to a variety of occupational and environmental triggers. Although it is usually self-limited, it can become chronic. Eosinophilic granuloma, a rare disorder, is characterized by abnormal proliferation of histiocytes, leading to infiltrative lung disease in the third and fourth decades of life. This condition, which occurs predominantly in smokers, is almost exclusively a disease of whites. Idiopathic pulmonary fibrosis often causes insidious, progressive respiratory impairment, but it is uncommon in patients younger than 40 years old. Pulmonary manifestations of vasculitis or connective tissue disorders, however, are most common in younger patients.

Until 3 months before the woman entered the hospital, she had to stop working because of severe exercise limitation. She has no history of occupational exposure to dusts or chemicals. A married woman, she has been in a monogamous relationship for many years. A test for human immunodeficiency virus (HIV) 3 months ago was negative. She is a Jehovah's Witness, denies use of tobacco or illicit drugs, and has lived in an urban neighborhood all her life. She denies skin rash, chest pain, or arthralgias but admits to seeing "spots before her eyes" and having occasional nausea and vomiting.

QUESTIONS

- *How does the patient's social and occupational history assist in narrowing the differential diagnosis?*
- *What is the significance of the patient's complaints?*

DISCUSSION

The social and family history contributes more to ruling out other causes of chronic lung disease than establishing a definitive diagnosis. Specifically, sarcoidosis is more common among nonsmokers, in contrast to eosinophilic granuloma, which is almost exclusively a disease of smokers. Furthermore, the patient's monogamous relationship, opposition to blood transfusion on religious grounds, and abstinence from intravenous drug use, as well as the negative HIV test, put her at a much lower risk for PCP infection, which usually occurs in patients with well-established HIV disease. The absence of a significant travel history also helps eliminate chronic fungal infection as a diagnostic possibility. Another pertinent negative factor is the lack of any significant environmental or occupational exposures, which makes hypersensitivity pneumonitis less likely. However, this condition cannot be excluded completely, because certain exposures are quite subtle or temporally remote; they can be missed without a rigorous exposure history.

A careful review of systems is critical to evaluate for disorders that can affect multiple organ systems. Ocular involvement can lead to photophobia, tearing, pain, and loss of vision. Gastrointestinal involvement can result in dysphagia, abdominal pain, jaundice, and nausea and vomiting. Infiltration of other organ systems can lead to skin rashes, syncope, irregular heart rhythm, chest pain, poor urine output, joint pain, and lymph node enlargement. Disorders that are particularly prone to manifest in multiple organ systems include the connective tissue disorders such as systemic lupus erythematosus (SLE) and scleroderma, as well as the vasculitides, including Wegener's granulomatosis. In addition, sarcoidosis may occur in almost any organ system of the body.

On examination, the woman is in mild distress secondary to dyspnea. Her pulse is 104 beats/min, her respiration rate is 28 breaths/min, her temperature is 35.8°C, and her blood pressure is 140/80 mm Hg. Her mucous membranes are dry. There is jugular venous distention with no significant adenopathy. She is not using accessory muscles of respiration, and lung examination shows coarse breath sounds bilaterally without wheezing, rales, dullness to percussion, or egophony. Cardiac examination indicates tachycardia, with a 2/6 systolic murmur at the left sternal border and an S_3 at the right sternal border. There is no hepatosplenomegaly. The extremities show 1+ pitting edema without clubbing, and there is no skin rash. Neurologic examination is unremarkable.

QUESTION

- *What is the significance of the findings on physical examination?*

DISCUSSION

Although many patients with interstitial lung disease present with clinically silent pulmonary involvement, some exhibit with advanced lung scarring and hypopexia. Physical findings, which are often absent early in the disease, become apparent only when advanced pulmonary hypertension and cor pulmonale have developed. These findings include the presence of a tricuspid regurgitation murmur, a right-sided S_3, a right ventricular or sternal heave, and congestion of the liver and lower extremities. In addition, patients with interstitial lung disease generally present with inspiratory rales, or crackles. However, these are less likely to be heard in patients with sarcoidosis or other granulomatous interstitial lung diseases. In addition, a careful search for any extrapulmonary manifestations should be undertaken.

The patient's initial laboratory findings include a pH of 7.44, a Pa_{CO_2} of 36.2 mm Hg, and a Pa_{O_2} of 52 mm Hg on room air. Blood urea nitrogen (BUN), creatinine, serum calcium, and serum albumin are normal. Chest radiographs (posteroanterior and lateral views) show bilateral reticulonodular interstitial infiltrates, with widening of the right paratracheal region, and fullness of both hila, suggestive of mediastinal lymphadenopathy. Minimal cardiomegaly is also noted. An ECG shows normal sinus rhythm with right atrial enlargement. Spirometry and lung volume analysis obtained shortly thereafter indicate a forced vital capacity (FVC) of 1.25 L (43% predicted), a forced expiratory volume in 1 second (FEV_1) of 1.02 L (43% predicted), and an FEV_1/FVC ratio of 82%. The total lung capacity (TLC) is 1.26 L (44%), and the diffusing capacity (DL_{CO}) is 7.3 mL/min/mm Hg (29% predicted).

QUESTIONS

- *What is the significance of the radiographic findings?*
- *How would you interpret the pulmonary function tests?*
- *What further tests should be performed to help make the diagnosis?*

DISCUSSION

The radiographic findings confirm the presence of interstitial lung disease; in fact, they are quite suggestive of pulmonary sarcoidosis. Intrathoracic lymphadenopathy, which occurs in 75%–90% of patients with sarcoidosis, is usually present in the bronchopulmonary, tracheobronchial, and paratracheal chains. This contrasts with lymphangioleiomyomatosis, hypersensitivity pneumonitis, connective tissue disorders, and vasculitis, in which intrathoracic lymphadenopathy is distinctly uncommon. The lung parenchyma also may be involved in sarcoidosis; affected patients usually demonstrate bilateral reticulonodular infiltrates, although a wide variety of other parenchymal abnormalities, including bullous changes, alveolar infiltrates, peripheral nodules, and fibrosis or "honeycombing," may be present.

The International Congress on Sarcoidosis has proposed the following radiographic classification of the disease: Stage 0, absence of abnormalities; stage 1, lymph node enlargement with parenchymal abnormalities; stage 2, lymph node enlargement and diffuse parenchymal disease; and stage 3, pulmonary fibrosis. The findings in this patient would be consistent with stage 2 disease.

The pulmonary function tests indicate a markedly reduced TLC, which is suggestive of severe restrictive lung disease with a significant impairment in the DL_{CO} and resting arterial hypoxemia. These findings correlate with the radiographic abnormalities just described and indicate an extensive parenchymal process. However, other diffuse interstitial processes can produce similar physiologic derangements, limiting the specificity of the test results. Of note, airflow obstruction resulting from granulomatous infiltration of the airways may be evident. However, the normal FEV_1/FVC ratio in this patient makes such obstruction unlikely.

Making a definitive diagnosis of sarcoidosis can be quite challenging. Tissue diagnosis, which is often pursued, may be falsely positive, especially if lymph node or liver biopsy is performed. When radiographic evidence of parenchymal disease is present, as in this patient, bronchoscopy with transbronchial biopsy is a preferred; the sensitivity of this method is 85%–90%. In certain patients, some noninvasive studies may be useful. These include the serum angiotensin-converting enzyme (ACE) level, percentage of lymphocytes in bronchoalveolar lavage (BAL) fluid, and gallium lung scanning.

The patient undergoes fiberoptic bronchoscopy and transbronchial lung biopsy. Review of the pathologic specimens indicates the presence of multiple noncaseating granulomas. Stains and cultures for acid-fast bacilli and fungi are negative. The serum ACE level is elevated at 111 U/L (range: 8–52). The echocardiogram is significant for a severely dilated right ventricle with preserved left ventricular function and an estimated pulmonary artery systolic pressure of 90 mm Hg. Moderate tricuspid regurgitation is present.

QUESTIONS

- *What is the significance of the pathologic findings and the elevated serum ACE level?*
- *How do you interpret the results of echocardiography?*
- *What treatment options are available?*

DISCUSSION

The presence of noncaseating granulomas in the correct clinical scenario is virtually pathognomonic for sarcoidosis. However, similar granulomas may occur in a wide variety of other diseases, including tuberculosis, fungal infection, malignancy, berylliosis, and foreign body reaction. Although the ACE level supports the diagnosis, it is relatively nonspecific and may be elevated in patients with tuberculosis, histoplasmosis, leprosy, and HIV infection. Nevertheless, the ACE level may be a useful marker of disease activity. It has been shown that a progressive decrease in the ACE level may reflect spontaneous remission of disease or response to therapy.

The results of echocardiography are consistent with the presence of severe pulmonary hypertension and cor pulmonale. These are expected sequelae of severe, diffuse parenchymal involvement and chronic hypoxemia. The presence of such extensive disease in vital organs such as the lungs and heart [and the eyes or central nervous system (CNS)] mandates the institution of definitive therapy. In patients with asymptomatic disease or involvement of nonvital organs, therapy may be withheld and patients closely followed. The rationale behind this approach is the observation that 30%–50% of cases spontaneously remit in a period of up to 3 years, with an additional 20%–30% of cases remaining relatively stable over the same period.

The most successful therapy for sarcoidosis has been the administration of systemic corticosteroids such as prednisone at a dosage of 20–60 mg by mouth daily. If patients respond, the treatment is continued at the lowest possible dose to maintain remission of disease for a period of several weeks or months before stopping. Occasionally, disease recurs with tapering of the steroid dose, and an upward adjustment is required. Unfortunately, the use of steroids can lead to multiple untoward effects, including the development of osteoporosis, cataracts, diabetes, hypertension, psychiatric disturbances, and immunosuppression. Although there has been much effort to develop alternative treatment regimens, including chloroquine and methotrexate, these have met with very limited success.

CASE 9

Syncope

A 64-year-old man is walking around a shopping mall with his wife when he suddenly loses consciousness and falls to the ground. An ambulance brings him to the emergency department. On arrival at the hospital, the man is awake and alert and complaining only of pain in his right elbow, which he apparently injured when he fell. He is placed on a cardiac monitor, and blood is drawn for laboratory work, which includes a complete blood count (CBC) and electrolyte, glucose, calcium, and cardiac enzyme studies.

QUESTIONS

- *What is the definition of syncope?*
- *What are some of the causes of a sudden loss of consciousness?*

DISCUSSION

Syncope is a sudden, temporary loss of consciousness caused by a lack of cerebral perfusion. The causes of sudden loss of consciousness can be divided into three major categories—cardiovascular, neurologic, and metabolic.

Cardiovascular syncope occurs when the cardiovascular system fails to maintain adequate blood pressure for cerebral perfusion. Inadequate stroke volume, inadequate heart rate, or inadequate total peripheral resistance all could be pathophysiologic causes of cardiovascular syncope. Impairment in stroke volume severe enough to cause syncope may be seen in ischemia and myocardial infarction (MI), dehydration or hemorrhage, or as a result of tachyarrhythmias, which impair ventricular filling. Mitral, aortic, or idiopathic hypertrophic subaortic stenosis, atrial myxoma, and pulmonary embolism also may cause syncope by obstructing cardiac inflow or outflow. Severe bradycardia (i.e., heart rate <40 beats/min) such as occurs in heart block and sick sinus syndrome may cause syncope. In some circumstances, cardiac output is adequate, but total peripheral resistance is reduced, leading to a decrease in blood pressure. Autonomic dysfunction or the use of vasodilators may reduce total peripheral resistance to the extent that syncope results. A common manifestation of syncope induced by reduced total peripheral resistance is the "vasovagal faint," which affects approximately 50% of the population at some point during the course of a lifetime.

Head trauma, stroke, or cerebrovascular disease may all cause loss of consciousness. Sudden increases in intracranial pressure (ICP) can compromise cerebral perfusion and cause a loss of consciousness, even in the setting of normal systemic blood pressure. A classic example is a colloid cyst of the third ventricle that acts as a ball valve and causes sudden obstructive hydrocephalus. Only rarely do disorders of the cerebrovascular system compromise perfusion to such an extent as to cause syncope. Therefore, syncope should not be viewed as a usual manifestation of a transient ischemic attack (TIA). Rarely, patients with compromise of distal basilar artery circulation (the top-of-the-basilar syndrome) experience a sudden loss of consciousness because of impaired perfusion of the ascending reticular activating system (RAS).

Another condition that is commonly considered in the differential diagnosis of syncope is seizure. However, seizures in adults rarely cause a loss of consciousness that is not associated with repetitive motor activity. It should be noted that some patients with syncope attributable to cardiac or circulatory failure have some generalized involuntary motor activity resulting from impaired cerebral perfusion, but this motor activity does not represent a primary convulsive event.

Finally, impaired delivery of essential nutrients to the brain (e.g., as a result of hypoglycemia or hypoxia) can cause a sudden loss of consciousness. However, metabolic disturbances usually worsen gradually and cause obtundation before loss of consciousness; therefore, the true definition of syncope is not generally met.

Additional history indicates that the fall was not preceded by an aura and that the patient remained continent during the episode. He awoke spontaneously and was not confused on awakening. The patient has had several previous episodes of light-headedness during exertion but says he never lost consciousness during those episodes. The patient does not recall anything unusual about the day before his syncopal episode, except that he experienced mild angina that was immediately relieved by a single sublingual nitroglycerin tablet.

QUESTIONS

- *What is significant about the onset and recovery of this syncopal episode?*
- *Based on the above limited history, what process do you most suspect as a cause of this patient's syncope?*

DISCUSSION

The abrupt onset of loss of consciousness is characteristic of a cardiac cause. There were no warning symptoms to suggest the aura of a seizure; no discrete neurologic symptoms characteristic of a TIA; and no diaphoresis, nausea, and wooziness such as would be associated with a vasovagal or hypoglycemic episode. That the patient remained continent during the event supports a cardiac or vasovagal cause, but this information is probably not very helpful in decision making; the continence of a patient during a seizure is more likely related to whether the patient's bladder is full at the time of the event. The lack of confusion on awakening argues against a seizure episode, although patients with atonic seizures can very rapidly regain normal cognition. Patients with a complex partial seizure do have a period of confusion often lasting several minutes. An important question to ask the patient's wife is whether her husband displayed any involuntary motor activity while unconscious. If he remained limp, this would argue strongly against the event being a seizure.

The patient's history of several prior episodes of light-headedness suggests an underlying abnormality of the cardiovascular system. In particular, this history in an older patient should direct attention to the heart. Two facts reinforce this impression: (1) the patient apparently has a history of angina, and (2) he has been taking nitroglycerin.

In summary, a cardiac cause of syncope is highly likely in this patient, because of the abrupt onset of the loss of consciousness and the history of angina. Because coronary disease should be particularly suspect in an individual of this patient's age, the possibility of an arrhythmia is particularly important to consider.

The patient's medical history is significant because of sporadic bouts of angina, for which he takes nitroglycerin. The angina has not recently increased in frequency or intensity. An exercise stress test performed 3 years ago was negative. The patient has had a heart murmur for many years but has been told that it is not significant. He takes no regular medications. His father died of a heart attack at age 60, and his mother had a mild stroke at 70 but did not die until 10 years later.

QUESTION

- *What is the significance of the patient's angina, stress test, family history, and heart murmur?*

DISCUSSION

The patient's angina suggests the possibility of coronary artery disease. Although the patient had a negative exercise stress test 3 years ago, this does not preclude the possibility of progression of atherosclerotic disease. It is entirely possible that mild coronary disease that was present then has now progressed to the point that it is causing symptoms. However, one must ask why the patient had a stress test. If he had it because of his chest pain, and his chest pain was not caused by ischemia 3 years ago (as suggested by the negative stress test), then his pain quite possibly may not be ischemic now.

The significance of the family history is hard to judge. Although a "heart attack" at age 60 in the patient's father does suggest premature coronary disease, many patients who are labeled as heart attack victims have not truly suffered an MI. The patient's mother's stroke at age 70 might represent atherosclerotic disease (at a relatively advanced age) or a hemorrhagic event. Certainly, the patient's history raises the possibility that atherosclerosis of the coronary or cerebral arterial circulation is causing the patient's symptoms. Although stroke or TIA due to large artery occlusive disease rarely is a cause of syncope, some patients with bilateral severe internal carotid artery stenosis can have syncopal events. The physician also should bear in mind the possibility of a top-of-the-basilar syndrome. The significance of the murmur is unclear from the history alone, but its existence suggests that underlying structural cardiac disease could be contributing to the patient's symptoms.

Although it is very likely that this patient has suffered syncope from a cardiovascular cause, the additional information does not help sway our clinical judgment one way or the other. It adds some "soft" features suggestive of coronary artery or valvular heart disease, which might in turn be responsible for a cardiac arrhythmia leading to syncope. However, this additional history is also entirely consistent with the absence of significant heart disease.

Physical examination shows a well-developed, well-nourished white man in no acute distress. His vital signs include a pulse of 88 beats/min, respirations of 14 breaths/min, blood pressure of 108/74 mm Hg, and a temperature of 37.2°C. The patient's skin is warm and dry, his pupils are equal and reactive to light and accommodation, and his lungs are clear. Cardiac examination indicates a normal S_1, a soft S_2, and an S_4. He has a harsh, late-peaking systolic ejection murmur that is loudest in the aortic area and radiates to both carotids, which demonstrate delayed upstroke and low volume. There are no carotid bruits and no jugular venous distention. Examination of the abdomen and extremities shows no abnormalities, with the exception of a bruise on the right elbow. Neurologic examination is completely within normal limits.

QUESTIONS

- *Which of these signs and symptoms are significant?*
- *How does this physical examination influence the differential diagnosis?*
- *What studies would you like to obtain?*

DISCUSSION

The patient's appearance does not suggest a systemic illness. Obtaining supine and upright blood pressure and pulse determinations is important in light of the patient's relatively low blood pressure. The patient does have a slightly high pulse, which suggests dehydration. That his skin is dry also raises the possibility of dehydration, as well as autonomic failure with resultant postural hypotension. His preserved pupillary accommodation attests to preservation of parasympathetic nervous function but leaves open the possibility of sympathetic nervous system failure. The harsh, late peaking, systolic ejection murmur, the delayed and reduced carotid upstrokes, and the soft S_2 are highly suggestive of aortic stenosis, an important cause of syncope. The lack of carotid bruits must be considered within the context of a loud precordial murmur that is already radiating into the neck; critical carotid stenoses can be missed because of masking sounds (as in this patient). Patients with preocclusive stenosis at the internal carotid artery origin may not have enough forceful perfusion to generate an audible bruit.

The information from the examination directs attention to the heart. Of particular concern is the possibility of structural heart disease as a cause of impaired aortic area outflow. Given the patient's history, consideration also should be given to the possibility of associated coronary artery disease and, less likely, carotid artery disease.

Usually the next studies that are ordered in patients suspected of having cardiac disease are the electrocardiogram (ECG) and the chest radiograph. However, in this case neither is likely to be very informative. The ECG may show evidence of left ventricular hypertrophy, but some patients with severe aortic stenosis fail to demonstrate this finding. Thus, a negative ECG should not dissuade one from the diagnosis. Typically, the chest radiograph in aortic stenosis shows a normal-sized heart, sometimes with a boot-shaped configuration indicative of concentric left ventricular hypertrophy. Again, this finding is not specific.

The most important study to be ordered at this time is an echocardiogram with Doppler evaluation of the aortic valve. The echocardiogram demonstrates the concentric left ventricular hypertrophy typical of aortic stenosis. Furthermore, it demonstrates severe restriction of the aortic valve leaflets. Both of these findings are consistent with the diagnosis but do not help quantify the severity of the disease. However, Doppler evaluation of the aortic valve can quantify the transvalvular aortic gradient precisely. In most cases the echo Doppler study is adequate to confirm the diagnosis and to arrive at a decision regarding surgery. Because this patient is in the coronary disease age group and because of the history of angina, cardiac catheterization to confirm the aortic valve gradient and to define the coronary anatomy with coronary arteriograms should also be performed.

An ECG shows left ventricular hypertrophy but no evidence of past or present ischemia. A chest radiograph is within normal limits, and a radiograph of the right elbow is also normal. Laboratory values are noncontributory. The patient is sent for an electroencephalogram (EEG) and for an echocardiogram with Doppler examination. The echocardiogram shows a calcified aortic value and left ventricular hypertrophy, both consistent with calcific aortic stenosis. The aortic valve gradient is 70 mm Hg. The patient is admitted to the hospital for a cardiac catheterization and probable aortic valve replacement, because only 50% of patients with aortic stenosis who have syncope achieve a 3-year survival if left untreated.

QUESTIONS

- *What are some of the causes of aortic stenosis?*
- *What is the pathophysiology underlying the physical signs and symptoms that characterize aortic stenosis?*

DISCUSSION

Causes of aortic stenosis include congenital, rheumatic, and calcific conditions. In this patient's age group, calcific aortic stenosis is of particular concern. There is no evidence of asymmetric septal hypertrophy, which is typical of subaortic stenosis, a primary cardiac muscle disease.

In aortic stenosis, the heart muscles force blood through a stenotic valve, which results in pressure overload on the left ventricle and subsequent concentric left ventricular hypertrophy. The clinical triad of angina, syncope, and heart failure are typical. The angina is the result of impaired blood flow limiting oxygen to the enlarged myocardium. The syncope can be caused by a decrease in the heart's ability to increase cardiac output across the stenotic valve. Syncope also can occur because of arrhythmias resulting from calcification within the cardiac conduction system. The patient's low systemic blood pressure is a consequence of his impaired cardiac output. The diminished S_2 is the result of impaired valve motion from the aortic disease. The S_4 is a result of decreased left ventricular compliance.

This patient illustrates that, with an appropriate history and physical examination, clues to the cause of a patient's syncope can be defined. Further evaluation can then be tailored to the patient. However, a cause for syncope is not readily evident in many patients. In these situations, a review of the patient's history may be informative. For example, did the syncope occur after a meal or during straining at defecation? In the patient with recurrent syncope, a Holter monitor to examine for arrhythmias, a stress test to try and induce the arrhythmia responsible for the syncope, autonomic testing to examine the integrity of postural reflexes, and an echocardiogram to search for underlying cardiac pathology are warranted. If arrhythmias are the suspected cause, electrophysiologic stimulation may provoke the causative arrhythmia. If occlusive cerebrovascular disease is suspected, a carotid duplex examination, magnetic resonance angiography (MRA), transcranial Doppler studies, or interventional angiography should be considered. If a neurologic etiology is suspected, an EEG to look for seizure activity and magnetic resonance imaging (MRI) to look for structural brain abnormalities are warranted.

CASE 10

Breast Lump

A 41-year-old white woman goes to her physician after discovering a lump in her left breast while doing a breast self-examination in the shower. She had thought in the past that she might have felt something in the same location, but now feels that the lump has gotten larger.

QUESTION

- *What additional historical information would you like to have from this patient?*

DISCUSSION

Eighty percent of women with breast lumps find the lump while performing a breast self-examination. As part of this patient's history, the physician should ask the patient about her risk factors for breast cancer. One should also ask the following questions: How long has the patient has been aware of the lump? What was its original size? When did it increase in size, and by how much? It also might help to know whether the mass changed in size in conjunction with the patient's menstrual period, because benign disease can regress after the menstrual cycle. If the mass is not clinically suspicious, it might be appropriate to reevaluate the patient after her next menstrual cycle when the flow ends—if the mass persists, intervention is necessary. Did the patient experience any discharge from the nipples? If so, was it bloody or clear? The presence of breast edema, discoloration, or pain is important to ascertain. Finally, the patient should be asked whether she has had any mammograms in the past.

Further history reveals that the patient first discovered the lump in the upper outer quadrant of her left breast about 4 months ago, but she did not seek medical attention because she has always had large, "lumpy" breasts. The patient's menstrual period does not seem to have affected the presence of the lump in any way. She has not experienced nipple discharge, breast edema or discoloration, or pain.

The patient has no previous medical or surgical history and takes no medications. One of her cousins died of breast cancer, but none of her other female relatives have had any cancer. Both of her parents are alive; her father has hypertension and coronary artery disease. The patient, who has experienced no symptoms of menopause, first began to menstruate at age 12 and has had regular periods lasting 4 days on a 30-day cycle. She has one 7-year-old daughter. She uses a diaphragm for birth control. Although the patient had a baseline mammogram at age 35, she has not had one since then, and she has not seen a gynecologist for over 1 year.

QUESTIONS

- *What risk factors does this patient have for developing breast cancer?*
- *What diseases might be included in your differential diagnosis at this point?*

DISCUSSION

The most important risk factors for breast cancer are family history (especially if the patient has a first-degree relative who developed premenopausal breast cancer), a history of fibrocystic disease, a history of previous breast biopsies, early onset of menarche, late onset of menopause, a first pregnancy after the age of 30, and, possibly, the use of high-dose estrogens by a postmenopausal patient. A patient's lack of risk factors for breast cancer should not dissuade the physician from performing the necessary procedures to rule out malignancy. Although most breast cancers are found in the upper outer quadrant, location should not change the physician's approach to excluding malignancy.

A young, premenopausal woman with a breast lump could have a benign mass such as a fibroadenoma or a cyst. Breast lumps are benign in 80% of cases, but malignancy must be ruled out. If the lump is indeed malignant, the patient has a higher chance of lymph node metastasis and micrometastatic disease as the tumor increases in size.

Physical examination shows a well-developed, thin, white woman who is slightly anxious but in no acute distress. The examination is normal except for the presence of a 2-cm mass in the upper, outer quadrant of the left breast. The mass appears firm and somewhat mobile. There is no obvious asymmetry between breasts, skin dimpling, or redness. No axillary nodes can be palpated, and there are no masses in the right breast.

QUESTION

- *What would you do next to evaluate this patient?*

DISCUSSION

All patients with a definable mass should have a mammogram; because this patient has not had a mammogram in 6 years, having one now would probably be especially worthwhile. A breast lump is visible on a mammogram alone in 20% of cases. However, mammograms are often difficult to interpret in premenopausal patients or postmenopausal patients taking estrogen, because estrogen causes dense, white, glandular tissue that may obscure white tumor masses of similar density. When a woman goes through menopause, the mammogram has a gray background, because the breast consists of mostly fibrofatty tissue. The gray serves as an ideal background for identification of new breast abnormalities, which appear whiter in contrast to the normal breast tissue. A negative mammogram does not necessarily imply that a patient's mass is not cancerous.

In addition to having a mammogram, this patient should be referred to a surgeon for needle aspiration to evaluate for the presence of fluid. If the mass disappears with aspiration of the fluid, then it is a benign cyst (assuming the cytology is negative). Less than 1% of patients in whom the mass totally disappears have malignant cells seen on cyst aspiration. If the mass is solid, the contents of the needle should be placed on a slide and submitted for cytology. Even if the cytology is benign, a malignant lesion still cannot be ruled out. If the mass persists after the patient's next menstrual period, an excisional biopsy should be performed to rule out cancer.

If an aspiration is not performed, ultrasound can determine whether the mass is solid or cystic. A cystic lesion seen on ultrasound examination should be the same size as the palpable mass. If there are no internal echoes within the cyst, then a solid lesion cannot be ruled out, and carcinoma is still a possibility.

Attempted fine-needle aspiration does not produce any fluid. A mammogram shows a well-defined 2.2-cm density in the left upper outer quadrant. No other densities or calcifications are noted.

The suspicious mammogram, coupled with the enlarging, palpable mass and the failure to aspirate fluid, lead the physician to recommend that the patient undergo a biopsy of the lesion. The patient is referred to a surgeon, who performs a biopsy with needle localization. The pathology report indicates an infiltrating adenocarcinoma.

QUESTIONS

- *How would you stage this patient's cancer?*
- *What would be your preferred mode of treatment?*
- *What is the patient's prognosis?*

DISCUSSION

This patient would be classified as having stage II disease, because the tumor measures between 2 and 5 cm in diameter and there are no fixed nodes or distant metastases. Most patients with stage I or II breast cancer can be offered the option of lumpectomy, axillary dissection, and radiation therapy to the breast (and node-bearing areas, if the nodes are positive). The cure rates associated with this mode of treatment are equivalent to those for a modified radical mastectomy, if the patient meets certain criteria. Because this particular patient does not have multicentric disease in the breast, more than one breast primary, or a tumor greater than 5 cm in diameter, she is an optimal candidate for radiation therapy.

Before the decision is made to perform a lumpectomy and axillary dissection, the patient should be seen by a radiation therapist. If the radiation therapist feels that the patient is not an optimal candidate, then a modified radical mastectomy is warranted. If the patient chooses to have a modified radical mastectomy, she has the option of undergoing breast reconstruction surgery at the time of the mastectomy or at some future time.

Adjuvant hormonal therapy, chemotherapy, and radiation therapy (i.e., radiation therapy for purposes other than breast conservation) also may play a role in treating patients with breast cancer.

Prognosis varies widely in breast cancer patients. Approximately 50% of patients with operable breast cancer develop recurrent disease unless they receive adjuvant chemotherapy or hormone therapy. Prognostic factors include the patient's axillary node status, the histopathology of the tumor, the patient's hormone receptor status, the S-phase fraction and DNA index, and oncogene expression.

CASE 11

Acute Low Back Pain

A 35-year-old man presents to the emergency department with a 2-day history of severe low back pain. The pain is worse when he sits up and better when he lies flat on his back. He claims to be well, although he recently experienced polyarthralgias, chills, and sweating. He reports that he was hospitalized for some form of hepatitis 2 years ago; he says it resolved uneventfully and he does not know what caused it. He denies alcohol or drug abuse.

QUESTIONS

- *What are your immediate concerns about this patient's low back pain?*
- *What are some of the mechanisms of low back pain?*
- *What additional information do you want to know about the pain?*

DISCUSSION

The history of chills and sweats makes one consider an infectious process more seriously than other possible causes of this low back pain. The man describes the pain as severe, which makes it more worrisome. The fact that the pain is worse when sitting upright and better with recumbency is not particularly helpful in suggesting a specific, potentially serious cause of this back complaint; most patients with discogenic and mechanical low back pain present in this manner.

Pain that is insidious in onset, associated with prolonged morning stiffness, relieved by exercise, and worsened by rest suggests underlying inflammatory back pain, typically the sacroiliitis of the spondyloarthropathies. In contrast, mechanical low back pain often is sudden in onset, worsened by exercise, and improved by rest. Pain that is ripping or tearing and perhaps associated with abdominal complaints is typical of an expanding abdominal aortic aneurysm. Pain associated with bladder or bowel incontinence and saddle anesthesia suggests a mid-line lumbar disk herniation with cauda equina compression; pain associated with leg sensory or motor complaints suggests lateral disk herniation and spinal nerve compression; and pain associated with gastrointestinal or genitourinary complaints suggests a need to investigate an intra-abdominal source as the cause. Constitutional complaints such as fever and chills make an infection more likely. Pain increasing with recumbency (the opposite of this patient's complaint) suggests a possible tumor; mid-line pain suggests either a tumor, an infection, or a compression fracture.

Ninety percent of low back pain is caused by self-limited biomechanical or strain problems, but it is important to look for features that make an acute medical condition more likely. There is important information still to be obtained about the nature of this patient's back pain.

On initial examination, the patient is writhing in discomfort and asking for intramuscular narcotics. His temperature is 38.3°C, and prominent needle tracks are observed on his hands and legs. Diffuse tenderness and guarding are noted on abdominal examination. Marked tenderness is noted over the entire low back paraspinal region, and prominent percussion tenderness is noted over several

lumbar and sacral vertebrae. The patient cooperates poorly with strength testing, but deep tendon reflexes and sensation are intact and anal wink and perianal sensations are normal. The patient complains of hamstring tenderness when either leg is raised in a straightened, extended position.

QUESTIONS

- *How do the findings on physical examination help you in thinking about your differential diagnosis?*
- *What conditions might cause referred back pain? Which should be ruled out?*
- *What information should you seek from laboratory tests and procedures at this time?*

DISCUSSION

Several findings on physical examination place self-limited musculoskeletal pain far down the differential diagnosis list. For one thing, it is known that the patient is likely abusing intravenous drugs, even though he denied this in the history. Narcotic drug-seeking behavior makes the physical examination more difficult to interpret, because exaggerated responses to physical examination maneuvers are common in drug-abusing patients. In addition, the patient has a fever and prominent findings on abdominal and back palpation as well as on spinal percussion. Intravenous drug abuse and fever make an infectious process (e.g., epidural abscess, paraspinal or perirectal collection, septic sacroiliitis) much more likely. No specific evidence for an aortic aneurysm exists on abdominal examination, and there is no neurologic evidence for cauda equina compression or discogenic nerve compression. No evidence has been presented for a potential referred source of pain such as a penetrating duodenal ulcer (gastrointestinal source) or a renal infection or stone (genitourinary source). There is no evidence of a spondyloarthropathy.

A complete blood count (CBC) might help with evaluation of an infectious process, particularly if leukocytosis is present. Amylase would be increased with pancreatitis and bowel emergencies (e.g., small bowel obstruction). The erythrocyte sedimentation rate is nonspecific, but significant elevation also might suggest an infection, particularly osteomyelitis. Urinalysis is important for discovering a potential genitourinary infection. Three sets of paired blood cultures should be obtained, because bacterial endocarditis can present with musculoskeletal complaints, and any bacterial process in the low back might be associated with bacteremia. Plain radiographs of the low back and sacroiliac joints quite likely might be normal, although patients with diskitis can have intervertebral narrowing and vertebral end-plate destruction; those with sacroiliitis can have sacroiliac joint erosions and sclerosis. A lumbar computed tomography (CT) scan would be of great help in evaluating bony detail for bone tumor or infection, and magnetic resonance imaging (MRI) would be best for evaluating soft tissue or intraspinal collections.

The test results come back as follows: hemoglobin is 11.3 g/dL, the white blood cell (WBC) count is 15,000/μL, and the platelet count is 500,000/μL. The Westergren erythrocyte sedimentation rate is 100 mm/hr. Chemistries indicate only an elevated alkaline phosphatase; amylase is normal. Urinalysis is negative. Chest radiograph, lumbar spine radiograph, and pelvic radiographs are unrevealing. MRI of the lumbar spine is scheduled for the following day.

One day later, the patient has required high doses of intramuscular narcotic for pain control but still complains of severe low back pain. He says that he is having difficulty walking to the bathroom because of leg weakness. His maximum temperature is 38.9°C. Physical examination indicates continuing poor cooperation with strength testing, but he appears to be severely weak (3/5 on muscle strength testing) in all lower extremity muscle groups. He also has decreased sensation to pinprick from the toes to the navel and prominent increased deep tendon reflexes in the lower extremities with four beats of clonus bilaterally.

QUESTIONS

- *What are the remaining most likely diagnoses at this point?*
- *What additional diagnostic tests are appropriate to confirm a diagnosis?*
- *What therapeutic approach is most appropriate now?*

DISCUSSION

The neurologic findings (leg weakness, abdominal sensory level, increased reflexes, and clonus) suggest spinal cord compression with features of an upper motor neuron lesion. When the history of intravenous drug abuse, fever, low back pain, and progressive neurologic deficit is added, the differential diagnosis narrows markedly. The patient's sensory level to about T12 suggests that the cord compression is occurring at this level, probably from an epidural abscess. Conditions such as transverse myelitis or an ischemic myelopathy at T12 cord level or a mid-line herniated thoracic disk are still possible, but these diagnoses are less likely to explain the fever or to be associated with intravenous drug abuse.

The best procedure for confirming a diagnosis would be an MRI scan. This test will best discriminate between an intrinsic cord lesion (e.g., transverse myelitis) and an extrinsic compression (e.g., due to an abscess or herniated disk). The test should be done emergently, because early surgical intervention is critical to preservation of lower extremity function.

The emergency MRI scan shows an epidural abscess at T12, and surgical débridement is carried out immediately. *Staphylococcus aureus* grows from one set of the blood cultures and the abscess.

QUESTION

- *What remaining treatment modalities should be used now?*

DISCUSSION

The patient should be treated for 4–6 weeks with antibiotics effective against *S. aureus,* initially intravenously. He should be carefully watched for features of bacterial endocarditis, despite the fact that only one blood culture was positive. Furthermore, the patient should receive intensive physical therapy once the acute pain subsides so that he can recover lower extremity strength and the ability to walk.

CASE 12

Gastrointestinal Bleeding

A 54-year-old white man presents to his general practitioner's office complaining of fatigue. He says that he tires easily and often feels light-headed and short of breath after climbing a single flight of steps or taking a short walk. He says that he is having difficulty at work because he is "just not himself."

QUESTIONS

- *What are some possible causes of generalized fatigue and weakness?*
- *What other questions would you like to ask this patient?*

DISCUSSION

Fatigue and weakness are common complaints that can be psychogenic or physical in origin. It is important to differentiate between these broad etiologic categories. Psychogenic causes consist of anxiety states and depression. Physical causes include infectious disease, metabolic disorders, blood dyscrasias, renal disease, liver disease, chronic pulmonary disease, chronic cardiovascular disease, neoplastic diseases, and neuromuscular disease. Specific examples of physical causes of fatigue include tuberculosis; diabetes mellitus; hypothyroidism; hyperparathyroidism; Addison's disease; anemia; lymphoma; leukemia; acute and chronic renal failure; acute and chronic hepatitis; cirrhosis; and common neoplastic diseases such as carcinoma of the lung, breast, colon, pancreas, prostate, ovary, or endometrium.

To narrow the diagnostic possibilities for this patient's fatigue and weakness, additional history should be obtained. The patient should be questioned about whether he has experienced weight loss, fever, chills, chest pain, paroxysmal nocturnal dyspnea, orthopnea, pedal edema, abdominal pain, changes in bowel habits, melena, hematochezia, polyuria, polydipsia, polyphagia, intolerance to heat or cold, or insomnia. A positive answer to these questions often, although not always, indicates a physical or organic cause of fatigue and weakness.

Further history indicates that the patient's symptoms started about 2 months ago and have steadily worsened. He claims he was in excellent health until this time; in fact, he has not had a routine physical examination in approximately 2 years because he has felt healthy. The patient takes no medications, except for the occasional use of acetaminophen or laxatives. He is an executive in a publishing company who smokes approximately half a pack of cigarettes per day and drinks a martini or two at lunch. He has no significant family history, except that an estranged older brother died after an abdominal operation for an unknown cause.

The patient denies chest pain or palpitations but has occasional shortness of breath and dyspnea on exertion, as described above. He has had no loss of appetite and even jokes that he can eat even on days when he is a bit "irregular." When asked about his constipation, he notes that he sometimes has difficulty passing his stool, but the stool is of normal consistency. He reports that his stools have seemed a bit darker lately, but he thought it might be due to laxatives he took for constipation; he has not noticed any bright red blood in the stool and denies hematemesis, nausea, vomiting, or diarrhea.

QUESTION

- *Which of these signs and symptoms concern you?*

DISCUSSION

This patient's history raises several points of concern. His symptoms began 2 months ago, meaning they are chronic complaints, and they have steadily worsened—an ominous sign. Acute complaints could be attributed to an acute viral or self-limited illness. That the patient was in excellent health until 2 months ago also indicates a change from a preexisting pattern. For example, a history of chronic abdominal pain and a change in bowel habits, if acutely present over 2–3 days or a week, could be compatible with an acute viral enteritis. Symptoms that have been present for a long time (2–3 years or more) suggest a chronic nonprogressive illness such as irritable bowel syndrome.

However, in a patient who was previously symptom-free and in excellent health, a 2-month history of symptoms that have steadily worsened would suggest a new and potentially serious change that could be compatible with inflammatory bowel disease, infectious states (e.g., giardiasis), or even malignant disease involving the gastrointestinal tract, particularly the colon.

The absence of medications would eliminate the possibility that a side effect of a drug (e.g., an antihypertensive agent) is responsible for the fatigue and shortness of breath. Smoking is clearly associated with numerous malignancies, including bronchogenic and pancreatic carcinoma, in addition to its known cardiovascular and pulmonary effects. The family history of an abdominal operation for an unknown cause raises the specter of possible colonic carcinoma, which has a two- to threefold increased incidence in first-degree relatives. Dyspnea on exertion could signify a cardiovascular cause but also could be associated with an anemic state. The "abnormally dark stools" might be indicative of melena, which would suggest that the upper gastrointestinal tract (above the ligament of Treitz) is the source of bleeding; dark red or mahogany-colored stools could indicate blood emanating from the right colon.

Physical examination shows a well-developed, overweight white man with a somewhat rapid respiratory rate (i.e., 20 respirations/min). Other vital signs show a pulse of 94 beats/min, a blood pressure of 110/60 mm Hg, and a normal temperature. The patient's skin is pale, as are his mucous membranes. His lungs are clear on auscultation, and his heart rhythm is regular, with a normal first and second heart sound (S_1 and S_2) and no third or fourth heart sound (S_3 or S_4). His abdomen is soft, without tenderness or obvious masses. His extremities show no cyanosis or edema; he has prolonged capillary refill. His rectal examination shows no palpable masses, but a dark, heme-positive stool is noted.

QUESTIONS

- *Based on this physical examination, what do you suspect is the cause of this man's fatigue?*
- *What are some of the causes of melena?*

- *What sorts of disorders produce hematochezia?*
- *How would you proceed in working up the heme-positive stool?*

DISCUSSION

Physical examination shows an individual whose skin and mucous membranes are pale and who has heme-positive stool. These signs suggest that the patient has gastrointestinal bleeding and is most likely anemic, possibly the reason he is feeling fatigued.

Melena is the passage of dark, tarry stools due to the presence of blood altered by intestinal juices. It is most commonly caused by upper gastrointestinal bleeding (e.g., duodenal ulcer disease, gastric ulcer disease, hemorrhagic gastritis, erosive esophagitis, esophageal varices or Mallory-Weiss tears, or vascular ectasia of the stomach). In an individual who is not acutely ill, peptic ulcer disease would be the most common cause; esophageal varices or a Mallory-Weiss tear of the distal esophagus would be unlikely.

Hematochezia is the passage of blood from the rectum, which varies in color from dark red or mahogany (from bleeding in the right colon) to bright red (as a result of bleeding from a more distal colonic source or the anal ring itself). Hematochezia may be caused by colonic diverticulosis and angiodysplasia, hemorrhoids, fissures, colon polyps, colon carcinoma, ulcerative colitis, infectious dysentery (especially *Shigella, Campylobacter,* and amebic colitis), and ischemic colitis. Unlike melena, hematochezia is often a sign of neoplastic lesions of the gastrointestinal tract; therefore, the patient should be evaluated for these disorders. Occasionally, an upper gastrointestinal source (e.g., brisk bleeding from a peptic ulcer) could lead to the passage of bright red blood from the rectum. Generally, this occurrence is seen in a patient who is otherwise hemodynamically unstable and would be identified by the finding of blood on the passage of a nasogastric tube into the stomach.

The initial workup for heme-positive stool depends on the patient's history and physical examination. If the history and examination are suggestive of an upper gastrointestinal source, initial evaluation should include an upper endoscopy. However, in most cases of occult gastrointestinal bleeding, a lower gastrointestinal evaluation would be indicated. Colonoscopy would be the appropriate initial evaluation. If this workup is unrevealing, an upper gastrointestinal source should be pursued, including evaluation of the small bowel. If no upper gastrointestinal source is identified, small bowel enteroclysis or small bowel enteroscopy would be indicated.

A nasogastric tube is inserted but does not reveal any evidence of blood. The physician has an anoscope in his office, but anoscopy does not show any obvious lesions. In-office hemoglobin and hematocrit tests give values of 9.4 g/dL and 36%, respectively. The physician decides to refer the patient immediately to a gastroenterologist for further workup of the gastrointestinal bleeding.

QUESTIONS

- *Why does the physician first look for evidence of upper gastrointestinal bleeding?*
- *What are the most common causes of lower gastrointestinal bleeding in this age group?*

DISCUSSION

The patient's history suggested a dark stool but, on the basis of the history, the physician could not determine whether the stool was black. Therefore, an upper gastrointestinal source was sought by the passage of a nasogastric tube. In approximately 75%–80% of cases, an upper gastrointestinal bleeding source can be identified by blood in the nasogastric tube. Occasionally, bleeding from a duodenal ulcer will be so slight it will cause a gastric aspirate to be negative for blood.

In individuals in this patient's age group, the two most common causes of lower gastrointestinal bleeding are diverticulosis and angiodysplasia. The differential diagnosis would also include those conditions known to cause hematochezia, as discussed earlier. A bleeding diathesis caused by a primary hematologic source such as leukemia, thrombocytopenia, hemophilia, or disseminated intravascular coagulation (DIC) should also be considered.

The gastroenterologist sees the patient immediately, and some laboratory tests are performed. A complete blood count (CBC) shows a white blood cell (WBC) count of 7.2/mm^3, a platelet count of 525,000/mm^3, and hemoglobin and hematocrit consistent with the previous values. Red blood cell (RBC) indices show a mean corpuscular volume (MCV) of 70 μm^3 and a mean corpuscular hemoglobin (MCH) of 25 pg. Serum iron and transferrin are decreased. Prothrombin time (PT) and partial thromboplastin (PTT) are normal, as are electrolyte, blood urea nitrogen (BUN), and creatinine levels.

QUESTIONS

- *What type of anemia do these values suggest?*
- *Which of the previously mentioned differential diagnoses can be ruled out by the laboratory values?*
- *What conditions are the highest on your differential?*
- *What are your immediate management plans?*

DISCUSSION

The laboratory findings suggest a microcytic, hypochromic anemia. The MCV of 70 mm^3 and the MCH of 25 pg are compatible with this diagnosis. An elevated platelet count is often seen in patients with chronic blood loss. The differential diagnosis of this type of anemia includes iron deficiency caused by poor intake or lack of absorption, or chronic blood loss. The usual source of chronic occult blood loss is from the gastrointestinal tract. Iron chelation therapy for lead intoxication also may cause this type of anemia. Congenital anemia such as thalassemia is also associated with hypochromic, microcytic anemia. Iron deficiency states are characterized by a low serum iron, a high total iron-binding capacity, and a low ferritin level.

The normal PT and PTT make a bleeding diathesis and a primary hematologic problem unlikely. Anemia of chronic renal insufficiency would be ruled out by the normal BUN and creatinine levels.

The most likely causes of this patient's problem are those involving chronic gastrointestinal blood loss (i.e., colonic polyp, colonic neoplasm, or angiodysplasia). Of particular concern is colonic neoplasm, in light of the patient's recent history of a change in bowel habits (constipation).

Immediate management goals include fluid replacement, correcting hypovolemia if present, monitoring serial hemoglobin and hematocrit values to be certain the patient does not have ongoing bleeding, arresting any active hemorrhage, and preventing recurrent hemorrhage.

The gastroenterologist arranges for a colonoscopy. During the colonoscopy, several polyps are noted in the descending portion of the colon. The polyps are 1–2 cm in size, and most are pedunculated. These lesions are removed by snare cautery and sent to pathology for evaluation.

QUESTIONS

- *What other procedures could have been used to investigate this problem?*
- *Why was colonoscopy useful in this case?*
- *What would have prevented colonoscopy from being a useful diagnostic tool?*

DISCUSSION

If bleeding were active and profuse, a technetium-labeled RBC scan, angiography, or both could locate a bleeding source, especially if the blood loss exceeded 0.2–1.0 mL/min. Otherwise, a high-quality air contrast barium enema and flexible sigmoidoscopy would have been an acceptable means of evaluating the colon. Colonoscopy is particularly useful, because it can be both diagnostic and therapeutic if a colonic polyp is discovered.

In this patient, colonoscopy was useful because there was no active bleeding to limit total examination of the colonic mucosa. However, if the bowel lumen had been coated with blood, a small polyp or arteriovenous malformation could have been missed. Also, if hemodynamic instability makes the patient a poor candidate for adequate sedation, a thorough evaluation of the colon may not be possible.

Pathology indicates villous adenomatous polyps with no foci of carcinoma. The patient is reassured, treated with iron supplements, and told to return in 1 year for a follow-up colonoscopy. If unremarkable, a repeat colonoscopy at 3–5 years would be indicated.

QUESTIONS

- *What factors about polyps increase the risk of adenocarcinoma?*
- *What would the treatment have been if foci of malignant cells had been found?*

DISCUSSION

Adenomatous and villous adenomatous polyps are considered precursors for adenocarcinoma. The risk of adenocarcinoma in patients with colonic polyps increases in proportion to the amount of villous tissue present in the polyp. Polyps that are sessile or greater than 2 cm in diameter also carry an increased risk for developing into carcinoma. Management of a malignant focus in a colonic polyp depends on the type of polyp. If a polyp is pedunculated on a long stalk and the carcinomatous cells have not invaded the stalk, the patient could be cured by simple colonoscopic polypectomy. However, if the carcinomatous cells have invaded the stalk, or if the polyp is sessile and the carcinomatous cells reach the margins of resection, the patient would require a segmental colonic resection. In either case, follow-up colonoscopy is indicated on a periodic basis in patients who have large or multiple colonic polyps, or if a malignancy is identified in any such lesions.

CASE 13

HIV Infection

A 37-year-old man, who was diagnosed with human immunodeficiency virus type 1 (HIV-1) infection 4 years ago, has experienced good overall health for 3 years despite a falling CD4 count. Although he was strongly encouraged to continue to take antiretroviral drugs, he stopped because of intolerable side effects. Fourteen months ago, he developed headaches and mild confusion at a time when his CD4 count was 94 cells/mm^3. Imaging studies and spinal fluid analysis confirmed the diagnosis of cryptococcal meningitis, and the patient responded well to antifungal therapy. He also consented to take antiretroviral drugs again.

QUESTIONS

- *What is the value of the CD4 count in monitoring patients who are infected with HIV-1?*
- *What are the major neurologic problems encountered in people with HIV-1 infection?*

DISCUSSION

When levels of circulating CD4 cells drop below certain thresholds, various interventions such as infection prophylaxis or antiretroviral therapy should be offered to the patient. [For example, when the CD4 count drops below 200 cells/mm^3, prophylaxis for *Pneumocystis carinii* pneumonia (PCP) should be initiated.] The CD4 count can be performed in many hospital and reference laboratories. The "viral load," as measured by quantitating the amount of viral nucleic acid in the blood, is primarily a measure of the rate of the disease's progression and of its response to drug therapy.

It is very common for patients infected by HIV-1 to experience a long period of clinical latency. Active viral replication occurs during all phases of the disease, but symptoms usually do not become apparent until there has been a substantial reduction in host immune function. Intervention with antiretroviral drugs can prevent, delay, or reverse this immune deterioration. Evaluation of clinical parameters (e.g., weight loss, decreasing functional capacity, development of one or more specific problems) and laboratory tests (e.g., enumeration of CD4 cells or quantitation of viral RNA) indicates the stage of HIV disease.

Several neurologic infections can complicate HIV-1 infection; the two most common conditions are cryptococcal meningitis and toxoplasmic encephalitis. Both of these infections occur relatively late in the course of HIV-1 infection, at a time when there are clinical or laboratory clues of strikingly diminished cellular immunity. Patients with cryptococcal infection commonly present with a chronic meningitis characterized by headache and diffuse, often mild, neurologic symptoms. Patients with toxoplasmosis more often present with focal neurologic findings or seizures. Dementia secondary to HIV-1 infection is also common late in the course of the disease. Less common neurologic complications include progressive multifocal leukoencephalopathy, central nervous system (CNS) lymphoma, neurosyphilis, *Listeria* meningitis, herpes simplex encephalitis, and cytomegalovirus (CMV) encephalitis.

The patient was able to return to work as a financial planner 14 months ago, and he seemed to be tolerating his medications. His drug regimen consisted of trimethoprim–sulfamethoxazole 3 days a week; isoniazid daily; fluconazole; and zidovudine, lamivudine, and lopinavir/ritonavir.

During this office visit, the patient says he is less peppy than usual after a bout of gastrointestinal illness consisting of watery diarrhea and crampy abdominal pain. He thinks he may have had some fevers over the past 2 weeks, but he has not taken his temperature.

QUESTIONS

- *What is the purpose of each of the medications the patient is currently taking?*
- *What is the differential diagnosis of watery diarrhea in advanced HIV infection?*
- *What diagnostic tests can be done to determine the cause of watery diarrhea?*
- *Of what significance is fever in individuals with advanced HIV infection?*

DISCUSSION

This patient is receiving a number of medications that are common to patients with HIV infection. Zidovudine, lamivudine, and lopinavir/ritonavir are four of the growing list of antiretroviral drugs available for direct suppression of HIV. Trimethoprim–sulfamethoxazole is used to prevent *P. carinii* infection, but it is also partly effective in preventing symptomatic toxoplasmosis and in reducing the number of bacterial infections. The fluconazole is given to prevent a recurrence of the patient's previously documented cryptococcal meningitis. Because the rate of symptomatic recurrence of cryptococcal meningitis is high, fluconazole should be given until the patient's immune function improves substantially. The isoniazid is used to prevent tuberculosis in a patient who has already been infected [i.e., one who tested positive using the purified protein derivative (PPD) test]. There is no accepted indication for monotherapy in patients with active tuberculosis.

Watery diarrhea is a common complication of HIV infection. Many cases are self-limited, and no specific etiology is determined. However, a wide variety of pathogens have been associated with this syndrome. The most common and perhaps the hardest to treat is *Cryptosporidium parvum.* Other protozoans that can cause diarrhea of this nature are *Giardia intestinalis,* microsporidia, and *Isospora belli.* Common bacterial agents of watery diarrhea include *Escherichia coli, Salmonella,* and *Campylobacter.* When a patient is undergoing or has recently completed a course of antibacterial therapy, diarrhea secondary to the toxin produced by *Clostridium difficile* should always be considered.

Diagnostic tests for watery diarrhea should be ordered when the diarrhea is persistent or extremely symptomatic. Usually, stool specimens are sent for microscopic assessment of protozoa (some laboratories call this test the ova and parasites test). The laboratory should be notified that cryptosporidia and other unusual protozoa are being sought. Stool cultures should also be sent. If a patient is currently undergoing or has just completed a course of antibacterial therapy, toxin tests for *C. difficile* should be ordered as well. If these noninvasive tests do not yield a result, further evaluation could entail endoscopic studies of the lower gastrointestinal tract or aspiration of the upper intestinal contents. A definitive diagnosis can be elusive if the first few stool tests are negative.

Fever is a very nonspecific problem in patients with advanced HIV infection. The development of new fever should prompt a careful history and physical evaluation. In addition to the large spectrum of infections that can produce a fever, a number of noninfectious processes such as malignancies and drug reactions should be considered. If the patient history, physical examination, chest radiographs, and routine laboratory tests do not suggest an organ-specific abnormality, disseminated infections such as

Mycobacterium avium-intracellulare (MAI), histoplasmosis, CMV, and HIV itself should be considered as causes of the fever.

On examination, the patient looks alert but pale. His temperature is 38°C, but otherwise, his vital signs are normal. The patient has lost 6 pounds since his last visit, 6 weeks earlier. Otherwise, there are no focal abnormalities. Laboratory testing shows a hemoglobin of 9.0 g/dL and a white blood cell (WBC) count of 3400 cells/mm^3 with a normal differential. The mean corpuscular volume (MCV) is 99 μm^3, and the serum vitamin B_{12} level is at the lower limit of normal. The patient's CD4 count is 32 cells/mm^3. Chemistries show mild elevation of aspartate aminotransferase (AST) and alanine aminotransferase (ALT).

QUESTIONS

- *What is the differential diagnosis of the macrocytic anemia?*
- *What is the significance of the weight loss?*
- *Why has this patient not responded to antiretroviral therapy?*

DISCUSSION

Macrocytic anemia is fairly common in patients with advanced HIV infection. Although nutritional deficiencies should be considered as potential causes of macrocytic anemia, the disorder is far more commonly associated with drug therapy—zidovudine or the antimetabolites of trimethoprim-sulfamethoxazole can cause macrocytic anemia. In many cases, the anemia is mild and only bears watching, but sometimes patients are given leucovorin (folinic acid) to combat the folate depletion brought on by zidovudine or trimethoprim-sulfamethoxazole. The serum levels of vitamin B_{12} can be depressed in patients with acquired immunodeficiency syndrome (AIDS), but there is rarely a response to injections of vitamin B_{12}.

Weight loss is a sign of active disease associated with HIV infection. In many patients, no obvious malabsorption, infection, or malignancy is present to account for weight loss, so efforts are directed at increasing the lean body weight. Nutritional supplements and hormonal manipulations are the most common interventions. Many infections are associated with weight loss, but in the absence of malabsorption or organ dysfunction, disseminated infections should be considered first.

The patient may not have responded to antiretroviral agents for several reasons. First, he may not have fully adhered to the treatment regimen; this noncompliance can result in both incomplete viral suppression or early emergence of resistant viral strains. Second, he may have been infected with a strain of HIV-1 that was already resistant to one or more of the antiretroviral drugs. Third, his initial viral load may have been so high that even perfect medication habits and a drug-susceptible viral strain will not have lowered his viral load sufficiently to allow for good immune reconstitution. Although a change in medications can help some of these patients, it is now clear that some individuals will not respond optimally to antiretroviral therapy despite all efforts. At this point, laboratory tests can help confirm which anti-retrovirals might be expected to work. Resistance tests (akin to bacterial tests for susceptibility or resistance) can be ordered. They are expensive and often difficult to interpret, but they can be extremely helpful in fashioning an effective treatment schedule. A review of medications with an emphasis on the importance of full adherence would be necessary with the next change of medications.

Blood cultures for mycobacteria are reported as positive 2 weeks later. The patient's fever has persisted, and he has lost 3 more pounds. He still has no localizing complaints. Repeat complete blood count (CBC) and chemistry tests show no change.

QUESTION

- *What is the most likely explanation for the positive blood cultures?*

DISCUSSION

Most likely, the positive blood cultures represent infection with *M. avium-intracellulare* rather than *Mycobacterium tuberculosis.* Disseminated tuberculosis without any organ involvement is rare, and it is even rarer to find positive blood cultures for *M. tuberculosis* at all (except in patients with overwhelming, possibly terminal, tuberculosis). In addition, it would be even more unusual (although not impossible) for cultures to be positive when the patient is on prophylactic isoniazid therapy.

M. avium-intracellulare is a commonly occurring late complication of HIV infection, which is not at all susceptible to isoniazid. MAI would most likely account for the weight loss seen in this patient. Patients with MAI infection have infiltration of many organs (with very little tissue reaction), with frequent high titers of mycobacteria in the blood and bone marrow. Many affected patients experience a partial or complete reversal of weight loss when the bacterial infection is brought under control.

The patient is started on therapy with three oral agents: ofloxacin, clarithromycin, and ethambutol. A gradual reduction in fever occurs, and he is able to return to work fulltime. His weight stabilizes, and he is comfortable except for intermittent nausea from the large number of pills that he takes daily. Laboratory tests show that his viral isolate is treatable with didanosine, emtricitabine, and tenofovir, which can be given in a once-a-day schedule.

QUESTION

- *What is the patient's prognosis?*
- *Could this infection have been prevented?*

DISCUSSION

MAI infection may be controlled but is essentially never cured in people with AIDS unless their immune dysfunction is reversed. Although MAI infection is rarely the direct cause of death in such individuals, mycobacteremia is a predictor of earlier mortality and increased morbidity. Treatment of mycobacteremia can benefit those people who tolerate the therapy and who are not moribund at its inception. Prevention of MAI infection is possible with the use of drugs in the macrolide and rifamycin classes. Rifamycins have significant interactions with many anti–HIV-1 medications and should be used cautiously. Macrolides such as azithromycin and clarithromycin can be used as prophylaxis in patients at risk (<75 CD4+ cells/mm^3). These provide significant though not complete protection from MAI infection. The simplification of his treatment might help him to maintain good adherence to treatment.

CASE 14

Dyspnea

A 58-year-old man calls an ambulance complaining that he "cannot get enough air" and that he is "suffocating." When the paramedics arrive, they find that the man is alert and oriented but that he cannot speak more than one or two words at a time because of shortness of breath. On the way to the emergency department, the paramedics insert an intravenous line and administer fluids. They also give the man oxygen at a rate of 15 L/min via mask.

QUESTIONS

- *How would you define dyspnea?*
- *What are your immediate concerns about this patient?*
- *What are some of the mechanisms that produce dyspnea?*

DISCUSSION

From his complaints and physical appearance, this man appears to be suffering from symptoms of dyspnea, a condition that is defined as any uncomfortable awareness of breathing. It involves both the perception of an abnormal sensation and a reaction to that perception. Dyspnea has many causes, most of which are cardiac or pulmonary in origin.

The overriding concern in a patient with dyspnea is to rule out the possibility of serious cardiac or pulmonary causes of the symptoms. Evaluation should begin with a check of vital signs, including blood pressure, pulse, respiratory rate, and temperature, to begin to narrow the list of potential major cardiac or pulmonary causes of dyspnea. Conditions that are associated with symptoms of dyspnea include pulmonary vascular disease [e.g., pulmonary embolism, pulmonary hypertension secondary to chronic obstructive pulmonary disease (COPD)], interstitial lung disease, asthma, neuromuscular disease, chest wall disease, and congestive heart failure (CHF) [including that caused by the various types of heart disease including valvular disease, hypertension, cardiomyopathy, and pulmonary edema]. Although chest pain would be a more common presenting symptom of myocardial infarction (MI) than dyspnea would be, MI should be considered and ruled out with cardiac enzyme studies and an electrocardiogram (ECG).

Another concern in this case (i.e., a new patient without a known cause of dyspnea) is the administration of oxygen at a high flow rate (i.e., 15 L/min), which may be the wrong approach if this man has obstructive pulmonary disease with carbon dioxide retention. Delivery of inspired oxygen at a high concentration can worsen carbon dioxide retention.

On arrival at the emergency department, the man is still short of breath and breathing at a rate of 28 respirations/min. His other vital signs show a pulse of 110 bpm, a blood pressure of 150/85 mm Hg, and a temperature of 38.1°C. Initial history reveals that 6 days ago, the patient developed an upper respiratory infection with rhinorrhea and a cough productive of thick yellow sputum. He has been short of breath for the past few days, but his symptoms worsened in the past several hours. He notes that he is more short of breath with minimal exertion and often begins to cough as a result of any effort. He denies chest pain or tightness.

The patient's past medical history is significant because of two previous hospital admissions for similar episodes. He also has a history of hypertension, for which he is supposed to take a mild diuretic once a day; however, he ran out of the drug and has not yet refilled his prescription. He uses an inhaler as needed but denies other medications or drug allergies. The patient says that he has smoked two packs of cigarettes per day for 30 years and that he drinks three to four beers per night. He is not married and recently lost his job in construction because he tires too easily.

QUESTIONS

- *How do these descriptions of the patient's symptoms help you in thinking about your differential diagnosis?*
- *How can you differentiate between cardiac and pulmonary causes of dyspnea?*

DISCUSSION

The subsequent history is more suggestive of an acute illness superimposed on an underlying chronic process (e.g., chronic lung disease with CHF or upper respiratory infection exacerbation) than of an acute process (e.g., acute MI, pulmonary embolism). The differential diagnosis at this point includes obstructive pulmonary disease, asthma, CHF, infection, and a tumor (a possibility in a patient with COPD and a history of cigarette smoking). The physician should also keep in mind the possibility of work-related exposures such as asbestos, asthma-sensitizers, and other occupational pulmonary toxins. Although the chronicity of symptoms points more toward a chronic than an acute process, the possibility of an acute MI should still be ruled out. Recurrent pulmonary embolism also is a possibility at this point, and ventilation-perfusion scanning with lower-extremity Doppler studies may be indicated.

Physical examination shows a well-developed, slightly overweight, white man in moderate respiratory distress with vital signs as noted above. His skin is moist without cyanosis, his neck shows mildly dilated jugular veins, his lungs reveal a prolonged expiratory phase with expiratory wheezes in all lung fields and poor respiratory effort, and examination of his heart reveals a prominent S_3 but no murmurs. Examination of his abdomen is unremarkable, revealing a slightly enlarged liver, and his extremities show 2+ peripheral edema.

QUESTIONS

- *What do these physical signs suggest?*
- *What disease process would be at the top of your differential diagnosis now?*
- *What laboratory tests or studies would you like to obtain?*

DISCUSSION

The expiratory wheezing and increased respiratory effort noted on physical examination of this patient suggest the presence of obstructive lung disease. Additionally, there is an S_3 gallop and peripheral edema. The S_3 and dilated jugular veins suggest left-sided heart failure, and the enlarged liver and peripheral edema suggest right-sided heart failure. The wheezes may be associated with either obstructive lung disease or CHF. At this point, it is essential to differentiate cardiac from pulmonary causes of this man's distress in order to plan an effective treatment. A chest radiograph along with an ECG, cardiac enzyme studies, and a complete blood count (CBC) with differential would help determine whether the patient has either or both underlying conditions.

The emergency department physician calls for the patient's old records, orders some laboratory tests (including arterial blood gas studies on oxygen, a CBC, a serum electrolyte panel, a cardiac enzyme analysis, a sputum culture, a "stat" ECG, and a portable radiograph). The ECG suggests some right axis deviation and sinus tachycardia but no ischemic changes. The results of the arterial blood gas studies are returned promptly and show a pH of 7.44, a PaO_2 of 81 mm Hg, a $PaCO_2$ of 50 mm Hg, and an O_2 saturation of 95% on 3 L FIO_2 by nasal cannula.

QUESTION

- *What sort of pattern do the arterial blood gas findings suggest?*

DISCUSSION

The arterial blood gas findings represent adequate oxygenation (normal PaO_2 = 80 mm Hg or above) with mild hypercarbia (normal $PaCO_2$ = 40 mm Hg) and a normal pH. The normal pH suggests a chronic process.

The patient's chest radiograph suggests a mild prominence of the pulmonary vascular markings. Otherwise, there are no radiographic changes.

QUESTION

- *Which diagnoses are less likely because of these radiographic results?*

DISCUSSION

The radiographic findings make the possibility of postobstructive pneumonitis, tumor, or pneumonia much less likely and are more compatible with a COPD exacerbation with some mild CHF. There is no mass to suggest a tumor and no infiltrates to suggest pneumonia.

Because the patient continues to have respiratory distress and is very uncomfortable without the oxygen, he is admitted to the hospital. His old records reveal that his previous admissions were for exacerbations of bronchitis. He is started on fluids, oxygen, diuretics, and a broad-spectrum antibiotic.

QUESTIONS

- *What are your goals for therapy for this patient?*
- *How can you prevent similar episodes from happening again?*

DISCUSSION

The goals for this patient are to control the exacerbation of his bronchitis with antibiotics and bronchodilators and to return him to baseline respiratory status. Peak flow measurements should be obtained before and after bronchodilators are administered, and the possibility of using corticosteroids along with the routine bronchodilator therapeutic regimen should be entertained. The possibility of underlying heart disease also should be addressed. An echocardiogram would be indicated at this time to determine if there is any cardiac functional abnormality. The most likely diagnosis here is chronic bronchitis exacerbated by an upper respiratory infection without pneumonia, with an underlying possibility of mild CHF. Future prophylaxis should include immunization against influenza as well as pneumococcal vaccine. In addition, the possibility of entering a pulmonary rehabilitation program should be discussed with the patient.

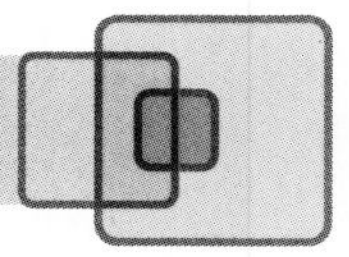

Comprehensive Examination

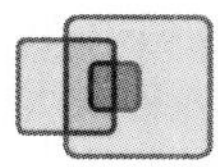

Questions

1. If present, which of the following features distinguishes upper tract (kidney) from lower tract (bladder) infection in women?

   A Fever > 38.5°C
   B Colony count > 10^5/mL
   C White blood cells (WBCs) in urinalysis
   D Burning on urination
   E Pubic tenderness

2. Which of the following is the most potent stimulus for the development of pulmonary hypertension in chronic obstructive pulmonary disease (COPD)?

   A Obliteration of the pulmonary vascular bed
   B Alveolar membrane damage
   C Left ventricular failure
   D Hypoxia
   E Acidosis

3. A 39-year-old woman comes to the emergency department complaining of cramps in her legs and numbness of her fingers. She had neck surgery 1 year earlier, but is not sure what was done. Chvostek's sign is positive: tapping on the facial nerve in front of the ear elicits a twitch of the upper lip. A positive sign suggests which of the following conditions?

   A Hypercalcemia
   B Hypocalcemia
   C Hyperkalemia
   D Acidosis
   E Hypophosphatemia

4. A 50-year-old woman complains of redness, swelling, and stiffness in the distal interphalangeal (DIP) joints of her hands but has no other joint complaints. Which of the following diagnoses is most likely?

   A Erosive osteoarthritis
   B Rheumatoid arthritis
   C Systemic lupus erythematosus (SLE)
   D Ankylosing spondylitis
   E Scleroderma

5. A patient with chronic renal failure caused by long-standing, severe hypertension is seen because of chest pain. The patient has received hemodialysis twice weekly for the last 2 years and has recently experienced episodes of hypotension at the beginning of treatment. The chest pain is located over the trapezius muscle. It is moderately reduced by assuming the upright position and exacerbated by deep breathing. Which of the following conditions is the most likely cause of this patient's chest pain?

   A Pericarditis
   B Coronary artery disease

C Diffuse esophageal spasm
D Pulmonary embolism
E Costochondritis

6. A 45-year-old man who has been in excellent health, except for mild obstructive lung disease as a result of smoking one pack of cigarettes per day (up until 3 years ago), is evaluated by his internist for weakness in the extremities. The internist refers the patient to a neurologist. The patient has a normal hematologic profile and chemistry panel. His neurologic examination is notable for 3+ strength in the legs, with mild sensory neuropathy in the hands accompanied by mild proprioception and vibratory loss. His physical examination otherwise is unremarkable. The patient has a normal chest radiograph. A computed tomography (CT) scan of the chest and abdomen reveals a 3.5 × 4-cm anterior mediastinal mass. Mediastinotomy is performed, and tissue is obtained, showing small-cell lung cancer (SCLC). An extensive metastatic workup shows no other evidence of disease outside of the mediastinum. Which of the following is the most appropriate therapy for this patient?

A Etoposide (VP-16-213), cisplatin, and concurrent radiation therapy to the chest
B VP-16-213, cisplatin, and bleomycin
C Cyclophosphamide, doxorubicin, vincristine, and prednisone
D Cyclophosphamide, doxorubicin, vincristine, and prednisone, followed by radiation to the chest if there is any residual abnormality in the anterior mediastinum
E Surgery followed by radiation therapy

7. A 30-year-old intravenous drug addict develops right-sided weakness and headache over a period of 2 days. Examination shows an afebrile, poorly nourished individual with a mild right hemiparesis. Which of the following is the most likely diagnosis?

A Bacterial endocarditis
B Human immunodeficiency virus (HIV) meningitis
C Brain abscess
D Cryptococcal meningitis
E Foreign body embolus

8. A previously normal 65-year-old African-American man presents with benign prostatic hypertrophy. A urinary infection is treated with trimethoprim-sulfamethoxazole. One week later, routine laboratory tests indicate new normocytic anemia, with hemoglobin 8.9 g/dL. Which of the following is the most likely diagnosis?

A Glucose-6-phosphate dehydrogenase (G6PD) hemolysis
B Occult blood loss from cecal carcinoma
C Occult blood loss from renal carcinoma
D Sickle cell trait
E Favism

9. A 45-year-old man with cirrhosis has had generalized abdominal pain for 24 hours without nausea or vomiting. His temperature is 38.3°C, and he has a distended abdomen with a clear fluid wave. There is diffuse tenderness on abdominal palpation. Paracentesis shows a clear fluid with 816 leukocytes/mm^3 (85% polymorphonuclear cells, 15% lymphocytes). Gram stain shows no bacteria. Which of the following diagnoses is most likely?

A Peptic ulcer disease
B Primary peritonitis
C Pancreatitis
D Cholecystitis
E Liver abscess

10. A 17-year-old boy arrives at the clinic complaining of swelling of his face and legs for the last several weeks. He has been in good health until the onset of this problem and has not seen a physician for the last 3 years, except for school examinations. He denies any medication use and any other medical problems.

On physical examination, the young man does not appear to be in any acute distress. His blood pressure is 110/80 mm Hg, his pulse is 60 beats/min, his respiratory rate is 15 breaths/min, and his temperature is 37°C. The only abnormalities relate to the marked peripheral edema, which is visible up to midthigh, and some facial puffiness. On laboratory examination, blood urea nitrogen (BUN) is 10 mg/dL, and creatinine is 1.1 mg/dL. The rest of the laboratory studies are normal. Urinalysis indicates 4+ protein and is negative for blood and glucose. Microscopic examination shows several hyaline casts but no other cellular elements. The urine protein is 16.4 g/24 hr. Which of the following diseases best explains this clinical disorder?

A Minimal change nephropathy
B Membranous glomerulonephritis
C Henoch-Schönlein purpura
D Acquired immunodeficiency syndrome (AIDS) nephropathy
E Systemic vasculitis

11. A 24-year-old woman complains of generalized weakness. Which of the following physical findings would be most suggestive of polymyositis as the cause of this weakness?

A Difficulty combing hair
B Difficulty unscrewing a lid from a jar
C Prominent tenderness in the weak muscles
D Difficulty with heel–toe walking
E Involvement of facial and skeletal muscles

12. A 65-year-old man reads in the newspaper that prostate-specific antigen (PSA) is a good screening test for cancer and asks his internist to have this drawn. The test reveals mildly elevated PSA levels of 10.4 ng/mL. Digital rectal examination indicates a normal-sized prostate, but ultrasound reveals a small hypoechoic area measuring 5×7 mm in the right lobe. Which of the following measures is the next appropriate step?

A Perform a bone scan
B Repeat assays for PSA in 3 months to check for further elevation
C Perform a transrectal biopsy of the abnormal area revealed by ultrasound
D Begin leuprolide depot therapy
E Perform a computed tomography (CT) scan of the retroperitoneum, pelvis, and prostate

13. Pulmonary crackles are frequently heard in patients with which one of the following conditions?

A Pneumothorax
B Pulmonary fibrosis
C Pleural effusion
D Lung cancer
E Cor pulmonale

14. Although most cases of acute viral hepatitis resolve spontaneously, complications may occur. Which of the following statements best describes the complications of hepatitis B virus (HBV) infection?

A The chronic carrier state is associated with an increased risk of hepatoma.
B Chronic persistent hepatitis usually leads to progressive deterioration of liver function and must be treated aggressively.

C Chronic active hepatitis can be diagnosed within 2–4 weeks of the acute infection with HBV.
D Chronic active hepatitis is characterized on liver biopsy by a periportal lymphocytic infiltrate without fibrosis or extraportal extension.
E Fulminant hepatitis is characterized by rapidly rising transaminase levels in an enlarging liver.

15. An 80-year-old woman with a history of congestive heart failure (CHF) develops angina pectoris. Her medications are adjusted to include furosemide, digoxin, nitroglycerin, and potassium supplements. Shortly thereafter, she develops intermittent frontal throbbing headaches. Which of the following should the physician do first?

A Perform a temporal artery biopsy
B Begin propranolol
C Begin sublingual ergotamine
D Obtain a brain computed tomography (CT) scan
E Discontinue nitroglycerin

16. A 55-year-old man who has smoked 30 cigarettes daily since he was 25 years of age is seen because of hemoptysis. He reports no symptoms except for a cough that produces 5–10 mL sputum each morning. Results found on physical examination and chest radiograph are normal. Which of the following is the most likely cause of this man's hemoptysis?

A Bronchogenic carcinoma
B Pulmonary tuberculosis
C Bronchiectasis
D α_1-Antitrypsin deficiency
E Chronic bronchitis

17. Which of the following statements regarding renovascular hypertension is correct?

A It is associated with an increased renin release.
B It does not respond to treatment with captopril.
C It is frequently seen in young men as a complication of fibromuscular disease.
D It is easy to control.
E It rarely produces severe hypertension.

18. A 45-year-old woman has a random serum glucose level of 180 mg/dL on routine examination. Which of the following studies should be performed next to evaluate this finding?

A Urine glucose
B Oral glucose tolerance test
C Fasting plasma glucose
D Repeat random plasma glucose
E Hemoglobin A_{1C} measurement

19. A 65-year-old patient presents with right knee pain, warmth, and swelling. Which of the following findings would be most useful for making a diagnosis of pseudogout in this patient?

A Enlarged proximal interphalangeal (PIP) and distal interphalangeal (DIP) joints
B Elevated serum uric acid level
C Negatively birefringent crystals in the knee fluid
D Meniscal calcium on a radiograph of the involved knee
E Inflammatory fluid on aspirate

20. A 25-year-old woman visits her family physician, complaining of nasal blockage and rhinorrhea. She is not pregnant and has not been taking medication recently, except for nasal decongestant spray, which she uses rarely to relieve her symptoms. She says a recent spell of humid weather has made the symptoms more severe. Anterior nasal speculum examination, skin tests, and cytologic nasal smear show no evidence of infection or of anatomic or immunologic abnormality. Which of the following diagnoses is most likely?

[A] Nasal decongestant spray abuse
[B] Allergic rhinitis
[C] Eosinophilic nonallergic rhinitis
[D] Vasomotor rhinitis
[E] Nasal polyposis

21. An 18-year-old man develops a persistent headache and fever and, after 5 days, has a focal seizure. A computed tomography (CT) scan of the head shows a ring-enhancing lesion in the right frontal lobe and an air–fluid level in the right frontal sinus. Neurosurgical aspiration of the lesion would be most likely to show which of the following?

[A] Small mononuclear cells suggestive of Burkitt's lymphoma
[B] *Toxoplasma gondii* cysts and tachyzoites (trophozoites)
[C] *Escherichia coli* and *Bacteroides fragilis*
[D] α-Hemolytic streptococcus and mixed anaerobes
[E] Budding yeast organisms with hyphal elements

22. A 20-year-old Asian woman presents with a new left lower extremity deep venous thrombosis. She has a history of mild thrombocytopenia and two miscarriages; she was treated for syphilis 2 years ago because of a positive rapid plasma reagin (RPR) test, even though antitreponemal antibody testing was negative. Which of the following conditions does her collective medical history most likely represent?

[A] Phospholipid antibody syndrome
[B] Systemic lupus erythematosus (SLE)
[C] Ro antibody syndrome
[D] Takayasu's arteritis
[E] Undifferentiated connective tissue disease (UCTD)

23. A 60-year-old gardener presents with a change in personality. The family states that several weeks ago he complained of a painful wrist, and 1 week ago he had transient facial asymmetry. Which of the following might be a particularly pertinent issue to consider?

[A] Toxin exposure
[B] Sexual habits
[C] Tick bite
[D] Mosquito bite
[E] Excessive vitamin consumption

24. A 40-year-old woman in good general health experiences sudden chest pain, fever, and shortness of breath. She is a heavy smoker and takes no medicines, except oral contraceptives. Tachypnea and a temperature of 38°C are found on physical examination. Chest auscultation, percussion, and radiographic findings are normal. Which of the following diagnoses is likely?

[A] Tracheobronchitis
[B] Atypical pneumonia
[C] Pulmonary embolus
[D] Bacterial pneumonia
[E] Lung cancer

25. A 25-year-old woman presents with fever and inflammatory arthritis affecting metacarpophalangeal (MCP) and proximal interphalangeal (PIP) joints. Which of the following features most strongly suggests systemic lupus erythematosus (SLE) rather than rheumatoid arthritis?

- A An active urinary sediment [red blood cells (RBCs), white blood cells (WBCs), cellular casts, no bacteria]
- B Inflammatory arthritis of the metacarpophalangeal (MCP) and proximal interphalangeal (PIP) joints
- C Pleural effusion on chest radiograph
- D Anemia
- E Abnormal liver function tests

26. A patient with lung carcinoma develops nausea, vomiting, and lethargy, and is found to have a serum calcium level of 13.4 mg/dL. Which of the following agents should be the first treatment step?

- A Intravenous pamidronate
- B Intravenous mithramycin
- C Intravenous glucocorticoids
- D Intravenous saline and furosemide
- E Subcutaneous calcitonin

27. A 27-year-old woman enters the emergency ward complaining of dyspnea and pleuritic chest pain. She also reports that over the past 4 days her right calf and thigh have become swollen and tender. Deep venous thrombosis, which may have led to pulmonary embolism, is suspected on the basis of the clinical presentation. Which of the following pieces of information in the patient history best supports this diagnosis?

- A History of smoking cigarettes
- B History of diabetes mellitus in the patient's family
- C History of lower extremity injury
- D History of hypertension
- E History of intravenous drug abuse

28. Which of the following procedures is the first test the physician should order to establish the diagnosis of deep venous thrombosis?

- A Cardiac catheterization
- B Contrast venography
- C Impedance plethysmography
- D Lung ventilation and perfusion scans
- E Computed tomography (CT) scan

29. The definitive diagnosis of pulmonary embolism is best made using which of the following?

- A Arterial blood gas analysis
- B Chest radiography
- C Electrocardiography (ECG)
- D Nuclear scanning of the lung
- E Pulmonary arteriography

30. A 42-year-old man with a history of seizure disorder experiences a grand mal seizure. His laboratory tests, taken shortly afterward, indicate the following: serum sodium = 140 mEq/L, serum potassium = 4.1 mEq/L, serum chloride = 97 mEq/L, plasma bicarbonate concentration [HCO_3^-] = 16 mEq/L, arterial pH = 7.15, and Pa_{CO_2} = 46 mm Hg. Which of the following best characterizes the acid–base disturbance?

A Respiratory acidosis
B Metabolic acidosis
C Metabolic acidosis plus respiratory acidosis
D Metabolic acidosis plus respiratory alkalosis

31. A 56-year-old woman has an elevated serum calcium level of 12.2 mg/dL. She has no history of any illness or treatment associated with hypercalcemia. Which of the following studies would be most helpful in making a diagnosis of primary hyperparathyroidism?

A Serum ionized calcium
B Serum phosphate
C Serum intact parathyroid hormone (PTH)
D Computed tomography (CT) of the neck
E 24-Hour urine calcium excretion

32. In a 23-year-old woman with a history of easy bruising and menorrhagia, coagulation laboratory studies indicate a normal prothrombin time (PT), a prolonged partial thromboplastin time (PTT), a normal platelet count, and a prolonged template bleeding time. Which of the following diagnoses is most likely?

A Hemophilia A
B Factor IX deficiency
C Factor VII deficiency
D Aspirin ingestion
E von Willebrand's disease (vWD)

33. A 23-year-old woman complains of generalized weakness and easy fatigability of 8 months' duration. She has no other symptoms. Her blood pressure is 126/86 mm Hg; otherwise, the physical examination is unremarkable. Laboratory studies show the following: serum sodium = 142 mEq/L, serum potassium = 2.2 mEq/L, serum chloride = 86 mEq/L, and plasma bicarbonate concentration [HCO_3^-] = 44 mEq/L. Which of the following conditions is the most likely cause of the patient's hypokalemic alkalosis?

A Primary aldosteronism
B Cushing's syndrome
C Chronic diarrhea
D Surreptitious vomiting
E Licorice abuse

34. A 27-year-old hospital employee has induration at the site of a purified protein derivative (PPD) test done as a part of routine screening. Which of the following features argues against chemoprophylaxis with isoniazid?

A Induration of 4-mm diameter
B Negative PPD skin test 1 year earlier
C Positive PPD skin test 1 year earlier
D Recent extensive exposure to a neighbor with active tuberculosis
E Prior hepatitis A virus (HAV) infection

35. A 66-year-old woman presents with a painless deterioration in walking. Examination shows a mildly spastic gait, poor position and vibration sense at the toes, 3+ muscle stretch reflexes at the knees, and absent ankle reflexes. Which of the following diagnoses is most likely?

A Multiple sclerosis (MS)
B Vitamin B_{12} deficiency

C Normal-pressure hydrocephalus (NPH)
D Human T-cell lymphotropic virus type I (HTLV-I) infection
E Adrenomyeloneuropathy

36. Which of the following statements best describes patients with obstructive sleep apnea?

A They have different clinical presentations than patients with other forms of sleep apnea.
B They respond well to respiratory stimulants.
C They respond well to nasal continual positive airway pressure (CPAP).
D They are not likely to fall asleep during the day.
E They are not likely to develop cor pulmonale.

37. A 30-year-old man develops pain and swelling in the right testicle. His physician orders an ultrasound, which shows a testicular mass measuring 2 × 2.5 cm. Inguinal exploration and orchiectomy are performed. The pathology indicates a pure seminoma. A computed tomography (CT) scan of the chest, abdomen, and pelvis shows two 3-cm retroperitoneal nodes that are enlarged. Blood counts, chemistries, and tumor markers are all within normal limits.

The oncologist and radiation therapist agree that the best therapeutic approach would involve which of the following?

A Surgical removal of all disease
B Radiation therapy to a total dose of 2500–3000 cGy to the ipsilateral iliac and retroperitoneal nodes
C Chemotherapy with three cycles of etoposide, cisplatin, and bleomycin, or four cycles of etoposide plus cisplatin
D Radiation therapy to a total dose of 2500–3000 cGy to the ipsilateral iliac and retroperitoneal nodes and mediastinum
E Observation

38. After definite therapy, for a stage II pure seminoma, testicular cancer a 40-year-old man is followed with monthly chest radiographs and computed tomography (CT) scans of his chest every 8–12 weeks. One year after completion of his radiation therapy, the patient's CT scan shows a 4-cm mediastinal mass. Tumor markers remain negative. The oncologist recommends which of the following?

A Mediastinal radiation
B Therapy with etoposide, cisplatin, and bleomycin
C Mediastinoscopy
D Needle biopsy of the mass, guided by CT
E Surgical resection

39. Which of the following juvenile rheumatoid arthritis patients is at greatest risk for developing chronic, erosive, disabling arthritis?

A A patient with oligoarthritis with axial spine involvement
B A patient with oligoarthritis without axial spine involvement
C A patient with systemic-onset juvenile rheumatoid arthritis
D A patient with polyarticular arthritis who is seropositive for rheumatoid factor
E A patient with polyarticular arthritis who is seronegative for rheumatoid factor

40. A 42-year-old woman has recently experienced fatigue, sleepiness, dry skin, constipation, and a 10-pound weight gain. Her thyroid is firm and twice the normal size. Which of the following laboratory tests is most likely to confirm the suspected diagnosis of hypothyroidism?

A Serum thyroxine (T_4)
B Serum triiodothyronine (T_3)

C T_3 resin uptake
D Serum thyroid-stimulating hormone (TSH)
E Antithyroid antibodies

41. A 71-year-old man presents with acute onset of gout. This problem has been recurrent for several years and has usually manifested itself as an acute monoarticular arthritis involving the first metatarsal proximal intertarsal joint. The patient also has a long history of chronic renal insufficiency, with serum creatinine values of 4–6 mg/dL over the past 5 years. In addition, he has long-standing hypertension, which has been treated with a variety of agents, including diuretics and α-adrenergic blocking agents.

On physical examination, his blood pressure is 170/105 mm Hg, his pulse is 72 beats/min, his respiratory rate is 15 breaths/min., and his temperature is 37°C. Examination further reveals moderate cardiomegaly with third heart sound (S_3) and fourth heart sound (S_4) gallops and a swollen, tender right first metatarsal joint. Laboratory studies indicate the following: blood urea nitrogen (BUN) = 63 mg/dL, creatinine = 5.1 mg/dL, serum sodium = 136 mEq/L, serum potassium = 5.9 mEq/L, serum chloride = 100 mEq/L, CO_2 = 19 mEq/L, and uric acid = 9.3 mg/dL. Which of the following is the most likely cause of this patient's condition?

A Chronic lead nephropathy
B Primary overproduction of uric acid
C Chronic interstitial nephritis related to analgesic abuse
D Hypertensive nephropathy
E Renovascular disease

42. A 28-year-old woman with a history of migraine develops a constant pressure-like headache associated with photophobia and a temperature of 39.1°C. A lumbar puncture (LP) demonstrates a cerebrospinal fluid (CSF) protein level of 62 mg/dL, a glucose level of 76 mg/dL, and 26 mononuclear cells/mm^3. Two days later, the patient is afebrile and has a headache only on arising. Which of the following is the most likely diagnosis for this patient at this time?

A Migraine
B Bacterial meningitis
C Aseptic meningitis
D Muscle contraction headache
E Post-LP headache

43. A 26-year-old woman is diagnosed with hypothalamic amenorrhea. Which of the following treatments would most likely restore normal ovulation and menstruation?

A Gonadotropin-releasing hormone (GnRH) injected every 24 hours
B GnRH injected every 4 hours
C GnRH injected every 90–120 minutes
D A long-acting GnRH analog injected every 24 hours
E A long-acting GnRH analog injected every 12 hours

44. A 17-year-old girl has a diffuse, red skin rash; a fever of 39.4°C; and mild, watery diarrhea. She had a sore throat recently, for which sulfamethoxazole was administered. She began her menses 3 days ago. Physical examination shows diffuse erythematous changes of the skin with early desquamation. The mouth and conjunctivae are red. Which of the following explains the entire process?

A *Salmonella* bacteremia
B Toxic shock syndrome (TSS)
C Tuberculosis
D Epstein-Barr virus mononucleosis
E Allergy to sulfamethoxazole

45. A 24-year-old woman complains that her hands turn white and then blue in the cold. Which of the following features is most suggestive of scleroderma as a cause of Raynaud's phenomenon in this patient?

- A Distal skin thickening extending proximally to the metacarpophalangeal (MCP) joints
- B Anticentromere antibody in serum
- C Antinuclear antibody (ANA) in serum
- D Distal capillary changes on evaluation of the nailbed
- E Esophageal spasm on manometry

46. A 73-year-old man attends a family dinner celebration and has a grand evening. As he leaves the restaurant, he collapses. Which of the following diagnoses is most likely?

- A Seizure
- B Cardiac arrhythmia
- C Carotid sinus hypersensitivity
- D Colloid cyst of the third ventricle
- E Postprandial syncope

47. A 36-year-old woman is evaluated for sore throat and cervical adenopathy. She has a temperature of 37°C, a pulse of 90 beats/min, and a blood pressure of 110/70 mm Hg. The right anterior cervical node measures 2.5 × 3 cm. No supraclavicular, axillary, epitrochlear, or inguinal adenopathy is palpable. The patient's abdominal examination is unremarkable. Over the next 6 months, the patient is reevaluated for recurrent upper respiratory tract infections. During this period, some regression of the cervical node occurred, but it seems to wax and wane in size in response to antibiotics. Because of her persistent adenopathy, the patient is referred to a surgeon, and a node biopsy is performed. Which of the following describes the histopathology corresponding to this patient's diagnosis?

- A Follicular small-cleaved cell lymphoma
- B Diffuse large cell lymphoma
- C Immunoblastic lymphoma
- D Burkitt's lymphoma
- E Normal lymph node

48. In human immunodeficiency virus (HIV) infection, diffuse lymphadenopathy in a person who is clinically well is usually a sign of which of the following?

- A Lymphoma
- B Kaposi's sarcoma
- C Tuberculosis
- D No specific infection or tumor
- E Syphilis

49. Which of the following pathophysiologic changes occur during a normal pregnancy?

- A Hyperuricemia
- B Proteinuria
- C Hypertension
- D A 40% increase in the glomerular filtration rate (GFR)
- E Metabolic alkalosis

50. A 35-year-old man with polyuria has a dehydration test. After fluid restriction, his maximum urine osmolality is 550 mOsm/kg and his plasma osmolality is 295 mOsm/kg. One hour after a subcutaneous injection of 5 U of aqueous vasopressin, his urine osmolality is 860 mOsm/kg. Which of the following diagnoses is likely?

A No disease
B Diabetes insipidus
C Partial diabetes insipidus
D Nephrogenic diabetes insipidus
E Diabetes mellitus

51. What percentage of patients with cystic fibrosis live to be 18 years of age or older?

A < 10%
B 10%–20%
C 20%–30%
D 30%–40%
E > 40%

52. A previously healthy 17-year-old girl has a total white blood cell (WBC) count of 500 cells/mm^3 (9% neutrophils, 91% lymphocytes) and a fever of 39.1°C. Piperacillin and amikacin therapy is initiated. Which of the following statements about this therapy is true?

A It is inappropriate because no antifungal therapy is included.
B It is appropriate because infection progresses quickly if untreated.
C It is inappropriate because no cultures are available to corroborate bacterial infection.
D It is appropriate because *Staphylococcus aureus* is the pathogen likely to be found.
E It is inappropriate because *Pseudomonas aeruginosa* is not likely to be inhibited.

53. The use of diuretics in the treatment of hypertension may be associated with side effects. These include which one of the following?

A Hypoglycemia
B Bronchospasm
C Prerenal azotemia
D Hemolytic anemia
E Hyperkalemia

54. A 42-year-old woman with menorrhagia from uterine fibroid tumors presents with anemia characterized by a hemoglobin level of 8.0 g/dL. The mean corpuscular volume (MCV) is 70 μm^3, and the blood smear indicates a uniform collection of both hypochromic and microcytic cells. Which of the following diagnoses is most likely?

A Pernicious anemia
B Sickle cell anemia
C Iron deficiency anemia
D Sideroblastic anemia
E Glucose-6-phosphate dehydrogenase (G6PD) deficiency

55. A 50-year-old patient with Down syndrome develops changes in personality, impaired memory, and difficulty with speech. Which of the following diagnoses is most likely?

A Hypothyroidism
B Multiple strokes
C Hydrocephalus
D Alzheimer's disease
E Creutzfeldt-Jakob disease
F Senile dementia of the Alzheimer type (SDAT)
G Dementia associated with prions

56. Which of the following is the most common nonalcoholic cause of acute pancreatitis in the United States?

A Thiazides
B Hypercalcemia
C Hyperlipidemia
D Gallstones
E Pancreas divisum

57. Eosinophilia is most likely to be found in which of the following settings?

A Pneumococcal pneumonia
B Diarrhea caused by *Giardia lamblia*
C Schistosomiasis
D Influenza
E Corticosteroid therapy

58. A 25-year old Peace Corps volunteer returns from his mission in Africa. He has noticed an enlarged lymph node in the left cervical region that is tender and seems to be enlarging at a fast rate. He has been experiencing some night sweats and has lost some weight. He spent most of his time in an HIV clinic while in Africa, working closely with patients. A needle biopsy of this mass reveals Burkitt's lymphoma. Which virus is associated with this type of lymphoma:

A HTLV-1
B HIV
C EBV
D Pox virus
E Adenovirus

59. A 62-year-old man has sudden onset of sharp right-sided chest pain. He has a long history of smoking (80 pack-years) and has used bronchodilators for 6 years. Six months earlier, he had a stroke, which resulted in dense left hemiplegia. He has a slight increase in cough with some reddish-yellow sputum, a temperature of 39.1°C, and diffuse rhonchi and wheezing without a noticeable increase in shortness of breath. The following test results were obtained:

Mycoplasma pneumoniae antibody: negative

Chest radiograph: patchy consolidation in right lower lobe

Noninvasive studies of leg veins: no evidence of clot

Sputum Gram stain: many polymorphonuclear cells, rare squamous cells, many short gram-negative rods, rare gram-positive cocci in chains, rare gram-negative cocci; culture results pending

Ventilation–perfusion scan: small, nonsegmental matched defects; larger defect in perfusion of right lower lobe

Which of the following drugs would be most reasonable?

A Heparin
B Penicillin
C Erythromycin
D Ceftriaxone
E Warfarin

60. While camping in late August, a 56-year-old man with a previous history of ischemic heart disease experiences sharp pain in the right forearm. Local erythema develops quickly, followed by diffuse urticaria and mild hoarseness. Within 20 minutes, the patient is brought to an emergency facility and found to be hypotensive, lethargic, and in moderate respiratory distress. Consultation with the patient's cardiologist indicates ongoing treatment with propranolol and an antihyperlipidemic agent. In light of this information, which of the following constitutes an appropriate immediate treatment measure?

A Intravenous pressors and hydrocortisone
B Nebulized β_2-adrenergic agonists
C Nebulized epinephrine
D Intravenous aminophylline
E Intravenous diphenhydramine

61. A 45-year-old white man enters the emergency department complaining of squeezing chest pain and nausea. The pain began approximately 1 hour before his arrival. On physical examination, his blood pressure is 110/70 mm Hg and his pulse is 72 beats/min and irregular. The patient is diaphoretic. Auscultation of the lungs indicates bibasilar rales. Cardiac examination is unremarkable. An electrocardiogram (ECG) indicates S-T segment elevation in leads V_1 through V_4, with S-T segment depression in leads 2, 3, and aVF. Which of the following diagnoses is the most likely?

A Inferior myocardial infarction (MI)
B Anterior MI
C Pulmonary embolism
D Peptic ulcer disease
E Pericarditis

62. A 45-year-old white man enters the emergency department complaining of squeezing chest pain and nausea. The pain began approximately 1 hour before his arrival. On physical examination, his blood pressure is 110/70 mm Hg and his pulse is 72 beats/min and irregular. The patient is diaphoretic. Auscultation of the lungs indicates bibasilar rales. Cardiac examination is unremarkable. An electrocardiogram (ECG) shows S-T segment elevation in leads V_1 through V_4, with S-T segment depression in leads 2, 3, and aVF. Which of the following is the most appropriate initial therapy for this patient?

A Close observation on a general ward
B Administration of thrombolytic therapy (provided there are no contraindications)
C Administration of atropine
D Intramuscular administration of morphine sulfate to relieve the patient's pain and anxiety
E Angiotensin-converting enzyme (ACE) inhibitor

63. A 44-year-old man calls the physician's office on Labor Day and complains of "the worst headache of his life." He is awake and oriented but does not want to leave the comfort, quiet, and darkness of his bedroom. The patient comes to the hospital and refuses to have a computed tomography (CT) scan. A difficult lumbar puncture (LP) yields a lightly blood-tinged sample with a red blood cell (RBC) count of 200,000/mm^3, a white blood cell (WBC) count of 5000/mm^3 (96% polymorphonuclear cells), a protein level of 104 mg/dL, and a glucose level of 20 mg/dL. Gram stain is negative for bacteria. Administration of which of the following is the most appropriate?

A ϵ-Aminocaproic acid
B Intravenous ceftriaxone
C Heparin
D Erythromycin
E Acyclovir

64. A 50-year-old man is admitted to the hospital with a temperature of 38.9°C and a tensely swollen right knee with markedly decreased range of motion. A 50-mL sample of purulent fluid, which has a white blood cell (WBC) count of 60,000/mm^3 (95% neutrophils) but contains no crystals or organisms, is removed from the patient's knee. Which of the following diagnoses is most likely?

A Bacterial infection
B Calcium pyrophosphate arthropathy
C Rheumatoid arthritis
D Gout
E Reactive (Reiter's) arthritis

65. A 44-year-old white woman presents to the emergency department complaining of acute shortness of breath on exertion. At 3:00 AM, she was awakened by the sudden onset of severe dyspnea. There was no associated chest pain; however, she did note a cough productive of pinkish sputum. The patient states that she has a history of both heart disease and emphysema.

On physical examination, she is dyspneic and in obvious distress. Her blood pressure is 200/110 mm Hg, pulse is 110 beats/min and regular, temperature is 37.8°C, and respiratory rate is 36 breaths/min. Her neck veins are not distended. Examination of the thorax indicates pulmonary rales up to the level of the scapulae and bilateral wheezes. The cardiac examination shows a summation gallop and no murmurs. There is no evidence of peripheral edema. An electrocardiogram (ECG) shows normal sinus rhythm and nonspecific S-T segment changes. A chest radiograph shows an enlarged heart and fluffy bilateral alveolar densities. Arterial blood gases drawn on room air show a Pa_{O_2} of 59 mm Hg, a Pa_{CO_2} of 25 mm Hg, and a pH of 7.45. Which of the following diagnoses is most likely?

A Emphysema exacerbated by pneumonia
B Pulmonary embolism
C Acute respiratory distress syndrome (ARDS)
D Acute cardiogenic pulmonary edema
E Hypertensive crisis

66. A 44-year-old white woman presents to the emergency department complaining of acute shortness of breath on exertion. At 3:00 AM, she was awakened by the sudden onset of severe dyspnea. There was no associated chest pain; however, she did note a cough productive of pinkish sputum. The patient states that she has a history of both heart disease and emphysema.

On physical examination, she is dyspneic and in obvious distress. Her blood pressure is 200/110 mm Hg, pulse is 110 beats/min and regular, temperature is 37.8°C, and respiratory rate is 36 breaths/min. Her neck veins are not distended. Examination of the thorax indicates pulmonary rales up to the level of the scapulae and bilateral wheezes. The cardiac examination shows a summation gallop and no murmurs. There is no evidence of peripheral edema. An electrocardiogram (ECG) shows normal sinus rhythm and nonspecific S-T segment changes. A chest radiograph shows an enlarged heart and fluffy bilateral alveolar densities. Arterial blood gases drawn on room air show a Pa_{O_2} of 59 mm Hg, a Pa_{CO_2} of 25 mm Hg, and a pH of 7.45. The most appropriate initial therapy for this patient is administration of which of the following?

A Oxygen
B Quinidine sulfate
C Digoxin
D Penicillin
E Heparin

67. A 73-year-old man presents to the emergency department because of the new onset of a left hemiparesis. He has no risk factors for stroke. A brain CT scan shows a right middle cerebral artery territory ischemic infarction. He is found to be anemic with occult blood in his stool; abnormal liver

function tests are documented. On further questioning, he admits to diminished appetite and a recent 15-pound weight loss; he denies fevers. The most likely diagnosis is:

A Gliobastoma multiforme
B Nonbacterial thrombotic endocarditis
C Metastatic tumor
D Bacterial endocarditis
E Lupus anticoagulant

68. A 56-year-old woman presents with a 4-month history of progressive difficulty walking. She denies pain, though she does note mild paresthesias in her feet. She has no bowel or bladder symptoms. On questioning, she thinks her hands may not be as strong as they should be. On examination, strength in her hands and distal legs is 4/5. There is mild sensory loss to all modalities to her knees. Muscle stretch reflexes are absent at the knees and ankles, and there is no Babinski response. The most likely diagnosis is:

A Vitamin B_{12} deficiency
B Cervical myelopathy
C Polymyositis
D Chronic inflammatory demyelinating polyneuropathy
E Guillain-Barré syndrome

69. An 82-year-old man has a chief complaint of painful feet for 6 months. The patient has a history of insulin-dependent diabetes mellitus, hypercholesterolemia, coronary artery disease, and mild congestive heart failure. On examination he has normal strength, diminished pain and temperature perception to his knees, and absent ankle reflexes. His discomfort is worsened during pain testing with a pin and when squeezing his foot. Plantar responses are flexor. The most likely diagnosis is:

A Chronic sensory polyneuropathy
B Vitamin B_{12} deficiency
C Lumbar stenosis
D Thoracic myelopathy
E Sciatica

70. A 37-year-old patient with AIDS presents with a 6-week history of progressive right-sided weakness and headache. MRI shows a left periventricular uniformly enhancing mass lesion. The most likely diagnosis is:

A Toxoplasmosis
B Abcess
C Astrocytoma
D Lymphoma
E Meningioma

71. A 43-year-old AIDS patient presents with a 2-week history of increasing confusion and headache. A CT scan with contrast indicates mild hydrocephalus. The initial results of a cerebrospinal fluid examination show a total protein of 122 mg/L, normal glucose, and 55 white blood cells per mm^3. The cells are 100% mononuclear. The most likely diagnosis is:

A Tuberculous meningitis
B HIV meningitis
C Cryptococcal meningitis
D Pneumococcal meningitis
E Syphilitic meningitis

Directions: *The response options for Items 72–75 are the same. You will be required to select one answer for each item in the set.*

A Cushing's disease caused by pituitary adrenocorticotropic hormone (ACTH) excess
B Cushing's syndrome attributable to an adrenal tumor
C Ectopic ACTH syndrome
D Adrenal insufficiency
E No adrenal disease

A patient is suspected of having Cushing's disease. For diagnostic purposes, dexamethasone is given in a low dose (2 mg daily) for 2 days and a high dose (8 mg daily) for 2 days. For each change in urinary 17-hydroxycorticoids and urinary free cortisol levels, select the diagnosis it indicates.

72. They fall distinctly with low-dose dexamethasone and high-dose dexamethasone.

73. They do not change with low-dose dexamethasone but fall distinctly with high-dose dexamethasone.

74. They do not fall with either low-dose or high-dose dexamethasone; the plasma ACTH level is elevated.

75. They do not fall with either low-dose or high-dose dexamethasone; the plasma ACTH level is low.

Directions: *The response options for Items 76–80 are the same. You will be required to select one answer for each item in the set.*

A Nitroblue tetrazolium (NBT) test
B Serum calcium level
C Platelet number and morphology
D Expression of CD18 on granulocytes
E Lymphocyte count

Match each of the immunodeficiency disorders listed below with the relevant assay.

76. Wiskott-Aldrich syndrome

77. Severe combined immunodeficiency (SCID)

78. Chronic granulomatous disease

79. DiGeorge syndrome

80. Leukocyte adhesion deficiency

81. A 25-year-old woman presents with progressive fatigue and difficulty breathing. Evaluation in the emergency department includes analysis of arterial blood gas: pH = 7.30, $Paco_2$ = 55 mm Hg, Pao_2 = 79 mm Hg, and calculated serum bicarbonate = 27 mEq/L. Which of the following conditions is typically associated with this acid–base abnormality?

A Normal pregnancy
B Cirrhosis
C Diuretic abuse

D Diabetic coma
E Myasthenia gravis

82. A 34-year-old woman was hospitalized for a 2-day history of progressive lethargy, muscle weakness, and shortness of breath. Her blood pressure was 105/78 mm Hg, and her pulse rate was 108 beats/min. Part of her evaluation included an analysis of arterial blood gas: pH = 7.60, $PaCO_2$ = 44 mm Hg, PaO_2 = 89 mm Hg, and calculated serum bicarbonate = 40 mEq/L. Which of the following conditions is typically associated with this acid–base abnormality?

A Hyporeninemic hypoaldosteronism
B Heroin overdose
C Diuretic abuse
D Impending shock
E Early gram-negative sepsis

83. A 44-year-old man is hospitalized for severe diarrhea. On physical examination, he has labored breathing without other significant findings. Laboratory studies (in mg/dL): Blood urea nitrogen = 60, serum creatinine = 1.2, and blood glucose = 126. The serum electrolytes (in mEq/L): Na^+ = 140, K^+ = 3.6, Cl^- = 114, and bicarbonate = 15. The arterial blood gas shows: pH = 7.29, $PaCO_2$ = 30 mm Hg, HCO_3^- = 14 mEq/L. Which of the following statements best describes the acid–base disturbance in this patient?

A No significant acid–base disturbance
B Mixed metabolic acidosis plus chronic respiratory acidosis
C Mixed metabolic acidosis plus chronic respiratory alkalosis
D Simple respiratory acidosis with appropriate renal compensation
E Simple metabolic acidosis with appropriate respiratory compensation

84. A 68-year-old man with hypertension is prescribed nifedipine (extended release) for better control of his blood pressure. Which one of the following statements best describes the mechanism of action of nifedipine as an antihypertensive agent?

A Inhibits sympathetic outflow from the central nervous system
B Reduces smooth muscle tone, producing vasodilatation
C Reduces renin secretion
D Directly dilates arteries and arterioles
E Antagonizes norepinephrine's stimulation of β-adrenergic receptors

85. A 78-year-old man has been in the hospital for 2 weeks because of a stroke. He is receiving intravenous fluids. His blood pressure in the supine position is 120/76 mm Hg, and his heart rate is 78 beats/min. The heart and lung examinations are normal, and there is no peripheral edema. His plasma and urine osmolality are 274 and 475 mOsm/Kg, respectively. Which of the following conditions is the most likely diagnosis?

A Syndrome of inappropriate antidiuretic hormone (SIADH)
B Extracellular fluid volume depletion
C Congestive heart failure
D Diabetes insipidus
E Compulsive water drinking

86. A 55-year-old man was found to have a serum Na^+ concentration of 160 mEq/L. His body weight is 78 kg. Assuming that the hypernatremia is due solely to electrolyte-free water loss, what would his total body water deficit be?

A 1 liter
B 3 liters

C 6 liters
D 9 liters
E 12 liters

87. A 32-year-old man with a 15-year history of type 1 diabetes mellitus is evaluated for end-organ complications. His medications are insulin and atenolol (50 mg/day). Pertinent findings are: blood pressure of 148/88 mm Hg, pulse 65 beats/min, serum creatinine of 1.7 mg/dL, moderate proliferative retinopathy, and a urinalysis showing +3 proteinuria. Optimal management of his disease should include which of the following?

A Dietary protein intake of at least 1 g/kg body weight per day
B Increase daily atenolol to 100 mg to reduce blood pressure to 135/80 mm Hg
C Treatment of hypertension and proteinuria with a thiazide diuretic and an angiotensin-converting enzyme inhibitor
D Target insulin therapy to achieve a hemoglobin A1c level of 8%
E Add glipizide to control hyperglycemia

88. A 70-year-old woman who was treated for a localized breast cancer about 10 years ago presents to an emergency room with the gradual onset of severe back pain. She recalls attempting to lift her grandson when the pain first appeared. The pain is described as a sharp, constant pain with a band-like distribution going around her lower thoracic vertebra. She has no other symptoms. Her neurologic examination is normal. The most serious potential diagnosis that must be immediately considered is:

A Osteoporotic fracture of spine
B Nerve root compression
C Bone metastasis with risk of cord compression
D Acute disc herniation
E Muscle spasm

89. A 75-year-old man has been diagnosed with localized prostate cancer. He is not a surgical candidate, and he is refusing radiation therapy. Prostate cancer would respond to:

A Androgen blockade
B Use of saw palmetto
C Tamoxifen
D Treatment with finasteride (Proscar)
E Radioimmunotherapy with Zevalin

90. A 46-year-old woman has been diagnosed with metastatic renal cell carcinoma metastatic to the lungs and several ribs. She is experiencing flank pain and occasional hematuria. The initial treatment at this point is:

A Chemotherapy
B Resection of primary tumor
C Radiation
D Resection of all metastatic lesions
E Supportive care

91. A 70-year-old man is about to undergo radiation therapy for a localized prostate cancer. This treatment is commonly associated with which side effect:

A Hematuria
B Osteopenia
C Infections
D Proctitis
E Disseminated intravascular coagulation

92. A 44-year-old man has undergone a chest x-ray evaluation secondary to persistence of shortness of breath. A large mediastinal mass is detected without evidence of other abnormalities. Routine laboratory evaluations indicate significant anemia. Biopsy of this mass is consistent with a thymoma. The anemia could be explained by which of the following:

- [A] DIC secondary to thymoma
- [B] Pure red blood cell aplasia
- [C] Bleeding within the thymoma
- [D] Bone marrow involvement by thymoma
- [E] Causes unrelated to the underlying disease

Directions: *The response options for Items 93–97 are the same. You will be required to select one answer for each item in the set.*

- [A] Ulcerative colitis
- [B] Laxative abuse
- [C] Pseudomembranous colitis
- [D] *Campylobacter* infection
- [E] Collagenous colitis

For each patient with diarrhea described below, select the most likely cause of the diarrhea.

93. A healthy 20-year-old man has an acute diarrheal disease characterized by bloody stool, crampy abdominal pain, and low-grade fever. His symptoms resolve spontaneously in 5 days and do not recur.

94. A healthy 20-year-old man has an acute onset of bloody diarrhea, crampy abdominal pain, and fever. His symptoms persist for several weeks, after which he consults a physician, who notes bleeding, friable mucosa on proctosigmoidoscopy.

95. A 30-year-old woman develops severe, watery diarrhea 2 weeks after undergoing antibiotic therapy for pelvic inflammatory disease (PID). Proctosigmoidoscopy shows plaque-like lesions covering the mucosa.

96. A 30-year-old woman complains of chronic watery diarrhea. Stool examination shows an osmolarity of 300 mEq/dL, a sodium concentration of 30 mEq/dL, and a potassium concentration of 45 mEq/dL. Shortly after she is hospitalized for evaluation and begun on a 48-hour fast, her diarrhea disappears.

97. A 56-year-old woman complains of intermittent nonbloody watery diarrhea over the past several years. All stool, radiographic, and endoscopic evaluations are normal, but the sedimentation rate is elevated slightly, and biopsy of the colon shows a prominent eosinophilic band in the subepithelial layer.

Directions: *The response options for Items 98–102 are the same. You will be required to select one answer for each item in the set.*

- [A] Folic acid deficiency
- [B] Vitamin B_{12} deficiency
- [C] Deficiency of either folic acid or vitamin B_{12}
- [D] No vitamin deficiency

For each condition described below, select the vitamin status with which it is most closely associated.

98. Pancytopenia with macrocytic anemia and megaloblastic marrow

99. Gastric carcinoma

100. An abnormal Schilling test

101. Neuropathy of the spinal cord

102. Alcoholism

Directions: *The response options for Items 103–106 are the same. You will be required to select one answer for each item in the set.*

A Hormone therapy
B Radical prostatectomy or radiation therapy
C Observation
D Chemotherapy
E Radical radiation therapy with boost doses to the prostate gland.

Match each of the following stages of prostatic carcinoma with its appropriate therapy.

103. Prostate nodule palpated on digital rectal examination

104. Prostate cancer that has spread beyond the capsule

105. Incidentally found prostate cancer

106. Metastatic prostate cancer

Directions: *The response options for Items 107–111 are the same. You will be required to select one answer for each item in the set.*

Items 107–111

	Pa_{O_2} (mm Hg)	O_2 Saturation (%)	Pa_{CO_2} (mm Hg)	$[HCO_3^-]$ (mEq/L)	pH
A	120	99	20	19	7.60
B	104	99	24	12	7.25
C	81	95	51	45	7.58
D	62	92	34	23	7.46
E	38	65	65	26.2	7.22

For each of the following clinical conditions, select the patient with the appropriate data.

107. Fulminant status asthmaticus

108. Long-standing pyloric obstruction

109. Hysterical hyperventilation

110. Diabetic ketoacidosis

111. Emphysematous chronic obstructive pulmonary disease (COPD)

Directions: *The response options for Items 112–114 are the same. You will be required to select one answer for each item in the set.*

- A IgG anti–insulin-receptor antibodies
- B IgE anti-insulin antibodies
- C IgG anti-insulin antibodies in circulating immune complexes
- D T-cell cytotoxicity
- E IgG anti-insulin antibodies

For each of the clinical scenarios described below, select the pathogenic mechanism with which it is likely to be associated.

112. After the initiation of insulin therapy, local erythema, swelling, and pruritus develop at multiple injection sites. Despite antihistamine therapy, subsequent injections of insulin lead to generalized urticaria and angioedema.

113. A gradually increasing insulin requirement is noted in a patient with a history of frequent local reaction and intermittent insulin therapy.

114. A 60-year-old diabetic woman requires increasing amounts of insulin. Arthralgias then develop, along with pigmented lesions of the axilla and groin.

Directions: *The response options for Items 115–119 are the same. You will be required to select one answer for each item in the set.*

- A Polycythemia vera
- B Anemia of chronic disease
- C Renal failure
- D Aplastic anemia
- E Secondary polycythemia of hepatoma

For each abnormality of erythropoietin described, match the correlating clinical condition.

115. High plasma erythropoietin titers; poor response to exogenous erythropoietin

116. Low-to-absent plasma erythropoietin

117. Diminished erythropoietin secretion; good response to exogenous erythropoietin

118. Near-normal to slightly elevated plasma erythropoietin; response to pharmacologic doses of exogenous erythropoietin

119. Extremely elevated plasma erythropoietin levels

Directions: *The response options for Items 120–124 are the same. You will be required to select one answer for each item in the set.*

- A Small-cell lung cancer (SCLC)
- B Testicular cancer
- C Breast cancer
- D Pancreatic cancer
- E Non-SCLC

Match each of the following syndromes with the appropriate tumor.

120. Eaton-Lambert syndrome

121. Syndrome of inappropriate antidiuretic hormone (SIADH)

122. Gynecomastia

123. Trousseau's syndrome [chronic disseminated intravascular coagulation (DIC) associated with malignancy]

124. Clubbing

Directions: *The response options for Items 125–127 are the same. You will be required to select one answer for each item in the set.*

- A Radiograph of sacroiliac joints
- B Joint fluid Gram stain and culture
- C Serum rheumatoid factor determination
- D Antibody titer to *Borrelia burgdorferi*
- E Erythrocyte sedimentation rate
- F Radiograph of lumbar spine
- G Paired blood cultures
- H Abdominal arteriogram

For each of the following case descriptions, select the most appropriate test to be used to arrive at a diagnosis.

125. A 28-year-old man complains of a 3-month history of morning low back pain, lasting 2 hours each day. He has also noticed a "sausage-like" swelling of his left second toe for 2 months, and has had pain in the bottoms of both heels when he walks. He reports that he had "pink eye" 1 year ago, around the time of an episode of bloody diarrhea that was treated by his family doctor with an antibiotic.

126. A 24-year-old woman has experienced extreme fatigue and polyarticular joint pain for 6 months. She has taken aspirin irregularly over that time with some relief, but she still complains of prolonged morning stiffness as well as bilateral pain and swelling in her wrists and metacarpophalangeal (MCP) and proximal interphalangeal (PIP) joints. She has no history of fever or other complaints. On physical examination, the only remarkable findings are swelling of the joints and mild limitation of motion of the involved joints because of pain.

127. During the summer, a 60-year-old man had a red, target-shaped rash on his leg. In September, he experiences fatigue, radicular left arm pain and numbness, and difficulty using his left hand for gripping. Two months later, he notices pain and swelling of the left wrist and right knee.

Directions: *The response options for Items 128–132 are the same. You will be required to select one answer for each item in the set.*

A Chronic lymphocytic leukemia (CLL)
B Chronic myelogenous leukemia (CML)
C Both CLL and CML
D Neither CLL nor CML

For each clinical situation, select the disease state with which it is most closely associated.

128. Elevated leukocyte alkaline phosphatase (LAP) level

129. Elevated lymphocyte count

130. Slow, steady disease progression

131. Termination in acute leukemia

132. Splenomegaly

Directions: *The response options for Items 133–138 are the same. You will be required to select one answer for each item in the set.*

A Pernicious anemia
B Dye and printing chemicals
C Asbestos
D Ulcerative colitis
E Epstein-Barr virus

Match each of the following tumors with the associated risk factor.

133. Burkitt's lymphoma

134. Bladder carcinoma

135. Gastric carcinoma

136. Colorectal carcinoma

137. Lung carcinoma

138. Nasopharyngeal cancer

Directions: *The response options for Items 139–141 are the same. You will be required to select one answer for each item in the set.*

A Acute urticaria
B Acute anaphylaxis
C Chronic cough
D Bronchospasm
E Interstitial nephritis
F Maculopapular eruption
G Photoallergic reaction

For each of the following patients, select the most likely clinical expression of an adverse drug reaction.

139. A 22-year-old man, who is in good health except for recurrent sinusitis, has elected to take 81 mg aspirin as antithrombosis therapy.

140. A 54-year-old woman with newly diagnosed hypertension has started enalapril at an appropriate dose.

141. A 34-year-old woman with human immunodeficiency virus (HIV) infection has started taking a prophylactic dose of sulfonamide three times each week.

142. A 28-year-old man with a family history of psoriasis has streptococcal pharyngitis. Shortly after the onset of the pharyngitis, he develops a rash consisting of 1–1.5-cm red scaling plaques distributed predominately on the trunk. Which of the following is the most common diagnosis of the rash?

A Plaque-type psoriasis
B Guttate psoriasis
C Pustular psoriasis
D Erythrodermic psoriasis
E Nail psoriasis

143. A young woman develops a persistent, red, itchy eruption on her finger under her engagement ring. Patch testing would most likely confirm the diagnosis of allergic contact dermatitis to

A Cobalt dichloride
B Balsam of Peru
C *Para*-phenylenediamine
D Mercaptobenzothiazole
E Nickel sulfate

144. A 65-year-old woman develops a blistering eruption over her abdomen and thighs. Examination shows 0.5–1.5-cm tense bullae, some of which have inflammatory bases. Skin biopsy shows a subepidermal blister and linear deposition of IgG and C3 along the dermal–epidermal junction. The most likely diagnosis is

A Bullous pemphigoid
B Pemphigus vulgaris
C Paraneoplastic pemphigus
D Erythema multiforme
E Porphyria cutanea tarda

145. A young man presents with an itchy rash on the arms and legs associated with a flare in his hay fever. Examination shows erythema; scaling, excoriated papules; and mild lichenification in the antecubital and popliteal fossae. The most likely diagnosis is

A Psoriasis
B Urticaria
C Atopic dermatitis
D Pityriasis rosea
E Lichen planus

146. A 55-year-old woman presents with tense bullae on the back of her hands that are exacerbated by sunlight. A skin biopsy shows a subepidermal blister, and direct immunofluorescence detects no immunoreactants. The most likely diagnosis is

A Porphyria cutanea tarda
B Pemphigus vulgaris
C Pemphigus foliaceus
D Bullous pemphigoid
E Paraneoplastic pemphigus

147. A 63-year-old man has a bleeding mole on his arm. A skin biopsy indicates a melanoma measuring 2.8 mm in depth with evidence of ulceration and vascular invasion. The only favorable prognostic factor is:

A Depth of primary tumor invasion > 1 mm
B Primary tumor ulceration
C Primary tumor vascular invasion
D Male sex
E Primary tumor located on an extremity

148. A young woman develops painful, red nodules on her shins 3 months after beginning to take oral contraceptive pills. The most likely cutaneous diagnosis is

A Erythema multiforme
B Erythema nodosum
C Lichen planus
D Pyoderma gangrenosum
E Urticaria
F Vasculitis

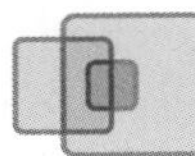

Answers and Explanations

1. **The answer is A** [Chapter 8 V F 3]. Fever is a variable feature in pyelonephritis and prostatitis but is never found with simple cystitis. Quantitative urine cultures do not distinguish between upper and lower tract infections. Although white blood cell (WBC) casts are formed in renal tubules and represent upper tract disease, WBCs are present in both upper and lower tract infections. Irritative voiding symptoms do not distinguish between upper and lower tract infections, and pubic tenderness can be seen in both upper and lower tract infections.

2. **The answer is D** [Chapter 2 VII C 1]. Pulmonary hypertension in patients with chronic obstructive pulmonary disease (COPD) is attributable primarily to the vasoconstrictive effect of hypoxia. This response may be increased by acidosis, which also has a direct, although less dramatic, vasoconstrictive effect on the pulmonary vasculature. Pulmonary vasoconstriction puts a strain on the right ventricle, leading to its eventual failure (cor pulmonale). Left ventricular failure occurs independently of right ventricular failure and usually is caused by atherosclerotic coronary artery disease. In patients with emphysema, a loss of the pulmonary capillary bed also may contribute to pulmonary hypertension.

3. **The answer is B** [Chapter 9 III B 3 a (1) (b)]. Chvostek's sign suggests hypocalcemia. A decrease in ionized calcium leads to increased neuromuscular irritability. In addition to Chvostek's sign, patients may have numbness and tingling of the extremities, twitching and cramps of the muscles, and muscular fatigue and weakness. Severe hypocalcemia, if untreated, can cause laryngeal spasm and seizures.

4. **The answer is A** [Chapter 10 V E 1]. Erosive osteoarthritis typically involves the distal interphalangeal (DIP) joints in middle-aged women. It is unlikely that such prominent distal joint symptoms would occur in a patient with rheumatoid arthritis or systemic lupus erythematosus (SLE) without more generalized joint complaints. No evidence suggests ankylosing spondylitis or scleroderma.

5. **The answer is A** [Chapter 6 Part I: III E 2]. The chest pain experienced by this patient is typical of pericarditis and inflammation of the pericardium, which are common complications in chronic renal failure patients on hemodialysis. These patients also may have inflammation in various serosal linings, including the peritoneum and pleura; the mechanism of this complication is unknown. Although coronary artery disease is common in dialysis patients, the characteristics of the pain in this individual suggest that this disease is not the diagnosis. Esophageal disease also is common in dialysis patients and should be specifically excluded as a possible cause. The apparent relationship to dialysis as well as the frequency of the symptoms both mitigate against pulmonary embolism as a cause of the chest pain. In addition, musculoskeletal pain due to various causes is typically seen in dialysis patients and may be attributable to the abnormalities of calcium and phosphorus metabolism, which lead to calcific deposits in various components of the musculoskeletal system.

6. **The answer is A** [Chapter 4 IV D 2–3, F 2 a (1) (a); Table 4–31]. Patients with small-cell lung cancer (SCLC) often present with paraneoplastic syndromes, including a variety that affect the central nervous system (CNS), the most common of which is Eaton-Lambert myasthenia. Other neuropathies, including sensory neuropathies, have been reported. SCLC can be cured if disease is limited to the chest. The most effective therapy is etoposide (VP-16-213) and cisplatin with concurrent radiation therapy. The role of surgery in SCLC is somewhat controversial, but it cannot replace combination chemotherapy.

7. **The answer is C** [Chapter 11 XVI B 1–2]. Intravenous drug addicts are prone to develop a bacteremia, which can in turn cause a brain abscess and progressive neurologic dysfunction. Patients with a brain abscess are typically afebrile unless there is an accompanying endocarditis or other endovascular source

of infection. Intravenous drug addicts are predisposed to develop bacterial endocarditis, and neurologic deficits can occur apoplectically because of a septic embolus to the brain. However, those patients are typically febrile. Human immunodeficiency virus (HIV) meningitis causes headache and evidence of meningeal irritation, but focal neurologic deficits typically do not occur at presentation. Cryptococcal meningitis typically presents with altered behavior and headache, and patients are afebrile. However, stroke-like events are rare. Finally, intravenous drug abuse can lead to a foreign body embolus but with apoplectic neurologic problems. An embolus can reach the brain via a right-to-left cardiac shunt or pulmonary arteriovenous malformation if the injection is venous. The embolus may enter the cerebral circulation directly if the injection is intracarotid.

8. The answer is A [Chapter 3 I C 2 b (2) (c) (i)]. Glucose-6-phosphate dehydrogenase (G6PD) deficiency is common in blacks, with a gene incidence of 10%. The gene is sex-linked, so hemolytic disease manifests mainly in males. The deficiency in African Americans is relatively mild, and only older red blood cells (RBCs) are critically enzyme deficient and liable for oxidant-induced hemolysis. Thus, hemolytic episodes are relatively mild (rarely is hemoglobin < 7.5 g/dL), well-tolerated, and quickly reversible. This presentation is very different from the Mediterranean variant, favism, in which the enzyme deficit is so severe that all RBCs are liable for hemolysis, and fatalities can result. Sulfa antibiotics are a classic precipitant. Occult blood loss causes chronic iron loss, and the resulting anemia would be expected to be microcytic. Sickle cell trait is asymptomatic hematologically, and an anemia would not be expected.

9. The answer is B [Chapter 8 V E 1 a]. The most likely diagnosis is primary peritonitis. Although it may be difficult to distinguish primary (spontaneous) peritonitis from rupture of a hollow viscus and peritoneal soiling, the presence of fever and the elevated white blood cell (WBC) count in the ascitic fluid suggest some kind of peritoneal infection. Pancreatitis is characterized by severe localized (midepigastric) pain, which radiates quickly to the back. Nausea and vomiting generally are not associated with acute pancreatitis. Abdominal pain in cholecystitis is in the right upper quadrant, and there is usually nausea and vomiting. Liver abscess tends to be a subacute illness without prominent peritoneal findings. In the presence of infected chronic ascites, peptic ulcer diseases is an unlikely possible cause.

10. The answer is A [Chapter 6 Part I: X B]. The most likely cause of this syndrome is minimal change nephropathy. This entity is the most common cause of nephrotic syndrome in children and adolescents. The disease has an excellent prognosis. Patients typically respond quite well to steroid therapy; although recurrent treatments are frequently necessary, complete remission eventually occurs in most patients. Renal biopsy is the only way to diagnose minimal change nephropathy definitively. Typically, no serologic abnormalities are associated with minimal change disease.

Poststreptococcal glomerulonephritis and Henoch-Schönlein purpura are associated with a nephritic picture—an active urinary sediment [red blood cells (RBCs) and casts] and heavy proteinuria. Acquired immunodeficiency syndrome (AIDS) nephropathy may present with a bland urinalysis and findings similar to those in minimal change nephropathy; however, associated renal insufficiency is much more common. The absence of systemic manifestations of human immunodeficiency virus (HIV) infection also makes this diagnosis highly unlikely in this patient. Finally, vasculitis rarely produces proteinuria as the sole renal manifestation. More frequently, vasculitis produces renal insufficiency, a glomerulonephritic picture, or both, along with systemic manifestations.

11. The answer is A [Chapter 10 IX E 1 d (1) (a)]. Difficulty combing hair and arising from a sitting position are cardinal symptoms of the proximal muscle weakness typical of polymyositis. Unscrewing a lid and heel–toe walking involve distal muscle strength, which would be more likely affected by a neuropathic problem. Tenderness in a muscle is a nonspecific finding that is not usually present in typical polymyositis; also, the avoidance of contracting a painful muscle could simulate weakness. Facial muscle involvement is not typical of polymyositis but is common in myasthenia gravis, in which involvement of eyelid and extraocular muscles is common.

12. The answer is C [Chapter 4 X C 4 a (3), b (1)]. Prostate-specific antigen (PSA) is a test that can be used to screen for prostate cancer. However, PSA levels can also be mildly elevated in benign prostatic hypertrophy. A transrectal ultrasound can identify small lesions not palpable on rectal examination. If patients have an elevated PSA and an ultrasound has confirmed an abnormal area, this area can be examined by transrectal biopsy under ultrasound guidance. Patients with prostate cancer generally undergo a metastatic workup, which includes a bone scan; chest radiograph; computed tomography (CT) scan of the retroperitoneum and pelvis; or magnetic resonance imaging (MRI) of the retroperitoneum and pelvis with special attention to the prostate, accompanied by laboratory studies. Metastatic prostate cancer can be treated with leuprolide, a luteinizing hormone–releasing hormone agonist that suppresses testicular testosterone production. Leuprolide therapy is equivalent to orchiectomy or estrogen therapy in the treatment of metastatic prostate cancer.

13. The answer is B [Chapter 2 XII D 2]. Crackles are produced by fluid in alveoli or by fibrotic airways. Therefore, they can be heard in patients with pulmonary fibrosis or congestive heart failure (CHF).

14. The answer is A [Chapter 5 IX A 1 f (1)–(3)]. The chronic carrier state for hepatitis B virus (HBV) is associated with an increased risk of hepatoma and is found in 0.2% of the population of the United States. Chronic active hepatitis cannot be diagnosed until at least 6 months after the acute infection with HBV. In chronic active hepatitis, the inflammation and fibrosis extend past the portal area and, thus, correlate with profuse deterioration of liver function, which may result in cirrhosis or liver failure. Fulminant hepatitis occurs in approximately 1%–2% of cases of HBV, hepatitis C (HCV), and non-A, non-B, non-C hepatitis. This rare complication usually is associated with falling transaminase levels as liver tissue is destroyed and the liver decreases in size.

15. The answer is E [Chapter 11 IV B 1 a (2), d (1) (a), 4 a–b]. Nitroglycerin can cause throbbing "vascular" headaches; therefore, the simplest management option is discontinuation of the nitroglycerin preparation and use of an alternate cardiac medication if possible. Temporal arteritis should always be considered as a possible cause of headache in patients older than 50 years of age. An elevated erythrocyte sedimentation rate; jaw claudication; arthralgias and myalgias; and a tender, indurated temporal artery make the diagnosis more likely. Propranolol is an effective antimigraine medication. However, before antimigraine medication is prescribed, potential precipitants of migraine should be eliminated. Ergotamine is an effective abortive therapy for migraine. However, because it is a vasoconstrictor, it should not be used in patients with angina pectoris. A brain computed tomography (CT) scan should be considered in the evaluation of an elderly patient with the new onset of headache. In this case, if the headache can be eliminated simply by stopping the nitroglycerin, a CT scan is unnecessary.

16. The answer is E [Chapter 2 II A 1 a, E 2 a (2); IV A 4 c]. By definition (i.e., cough and sputum production), this patient has chronic bronchitis. Normal results on chest radiograph do not absolutely rule out carcinoma but make it unlikely. The same is true for tuberculosis and bronchiectasis. A smoker in this age group would require bronchoscopy if the hemoptysis did not subside soon or if the clinical situation changed. α_1-Antitrypsin deficiency is a genetic factor that predisposes to emphysema. Unlike chronic bronchitis, emphysema is associated with little or no cough and expectoration.

17. The answer is A [Chapter 6 Part I: XIV C, Part III: II B 1]. Renovascular hypertension is associated with an increased renin release. Diminished renal blood flow stimulates the kidney to release increasing amounts of renin, which activate the renin–angiotensin–aldosterone axis, leading to hypertension. Because captopril prevents the conversion of angiotensin I to angiotensin II (a vasoconstrictor, this drug would be expected to be particularly effective in this disease). Young women, much more frequently than young men, develop fibromuscular obstruction of the renal arteries, leading to renovascular hypertension. Renovascular hypertension typically leads to very severe hypertension and is notoriously difficult to control. This difficulty in controlling blood pressure often raises the suspicion that renovascular hypertension is present.

18. The answer is C [Chapter 9 IV A 5, Table 9–10]. Although the oral glucose tolerance test (plasma glucose level 2 hours after 1 75-g glucose load) is more sensitive, the fasting plasma glucose is recommended as the primary test for the diagnosis of diabetes mellitus because of its greater convenience. A fasting plasma glucose level of 126 mg/dL or higher indicates a diagnosis of diabetes. Although a casual (random) glucose level greater than 200 mg/dL indicates diabetes in a patient with classic symptoms such as polyuria and polydipsia, it is not recommended for screening. Measurement of HbA_{1C} and, occasionally, urine glucose, may be useful in evaluating the glycemic control in patients with diabetes, but they are not sufficiently reliable or standardized to be very useful in the diagnosis of diabetes.

19. The answer is D [Chapter 10 IV B 5 b]. The finding of meniscal calcium on a radiograph of the involved knee is a diagnostic feature of calcium pyrophosphate dihydrate (CPPD) disease, which suggests that the knee inflammation is caused by pseudogout. Enlargement of proximal interphalangeal (PIP) and distal interphalangeal (DIP) joints suggests only osteoarthritis and not a specific cause. Serum urate elevation is associated with gout, not CPPD. The finding of positively birefringent crystals on red-compensated polarized light examination of synovial fluid is specific for a diagnosis of pseudogout. There are many causes of an inflammatory effusion other than CPPD.

20. The answer is D [Chapter 7 III E 2 a–h]. The woman's symptoms are likely caused by vasomotor rhinitis, which is a syndrome characterized by nasal blockage and rhinorrhea without evidence of immunologic or infectious nasal disease. Symptoms of vasomotor rhinitis often worsen after affected patients endure emotional stress or experience a change in body or environmental temperature, change in body position, or humid weather. Vasomotor rhinitis does not respond well to medication. Decongestant spray abuse is not indicated in the patient's history. The history and examination also rules out pregnancy and deviated septum, both of which are possible causes of rhinorrhea and nasal blockage. Allergic rhinitis, which is an IgE-mediated disorder, is characterized by a pale, boggy nasal mucosa, nasal eosinophilia, and positive skin tests. Although nasal blockage and rhinorrhea are symptoms of eosinophilic nonallergic rhinitis, this disorder is characterized by pronounced nasal eosinophilia, which would have been seen on the nasal smear. Nasal polyps are another symptom of eosinophilic nonallergic rhinitis. Symptoms related to nasal polyposis are not likely to be episodic.

21. The answer is D [Chapter 8 V A 3 a, b]. Neurosurgical aspiration of the lesion would most likely show α-hemolytic streptococcus and mixed anaerobes. Brain abscess may well occur in teenagers. Usually, frontal lobe disease is associated with sinusitis and reflects oral flora. *Escherichia coli* and *Bacteroides fragilis* are more commonly found in brain abscesses of otic origin. Primary brain lymphoma and toxoplasmosis are rarely seen in immunocompetent individuals. In people with severe acidosis, Zygomycetes can cause brain abscess, but these fungi have no yeast phase.

22. The answer is A [Chapter 10 VII F 1, 2 c, G 3 b]. This patient has several subtle manifestations of phospholipid antibody syndrome, which, taken together, make it a likely diagnosis. A positive rapid plasma reagin test (RPR) with negative treponemal test results probably reflects antibodies cross-reacting to the cardiolipin or phospholipid components of treponemal antigens. Thrombocytopenia is commonly seen in this situation, probably because of platelet–endothelial cell interactions and clotting induced by the antibodies. Miscarriages can be caused by clotting of small placental vessels. Deep venous thromboses or even major arterial clotting can be caused by the consequent hypercoagulability. No other evidence is presented for systemic lupus erythematosus (SLE), although phospholipid antibodies can be detected in approximately one third of patients. No features of the Ro antibody syndrome or undifferentiated connective tissue disease (UCTD) are described. Although Takayasu's arteritis classically occurs in young Asian women, no evidence is given for the large vessel arterial ischemia characteristic of this entity.

23. The answer is C [Chapter 8 VII F 3 b, c]. Lyme disease is transmitted by a tick bite. Neurologic complications include cranial neuropathy, radiculopathy, and encephalopathy. The patient's outdoor activities put him at risk for exposure to Lyme disease if he lives in an endemic area, and the suggestion of wrist arthritis is consistent with the systemic manifestations of Lyme disease. Toxin exposures can cause confusion but should not cause an arthritis or facial weakness. High-risk sexual behavior can predispose to human immunodeficiency virus (HIV) infection, which can cause a facial nerve palsy and encephalopathy. However, given this patient's history and presentation, Lyme disease is more likely. A mosquito bite can transmit viral encephalitis. However, there is no history of fever, and the wrist arthritis and facial weakness do not support a diagnosis of early viral encephalitis. Excessive vitamin consumption would not produce arthritis, carinal nerve neuropathy, and personality changes.

24. The answer is C [Chapter 2 VIII E 1, 2 a; Chapter 8 V C 3, 4]. The most likely diagnosis is a pulmonary embolus. Acute onset rules out atypical pneumonia and makes lung cancer very unlikely. Without evidence of productive cough, tracheobronchitis—also a subacute illness—is unlikely. Bacterial pneumonia is very unlikely in conjunction with a normal chest radiograph. Smoking and oral contraceptive use both predispose to deep venous thrombosis and pulmonary embolus.

25. The answer is A [Chapter 10 II G; VII G 1; Table 10–10]. An active urinary sediment suggests glomerulonephritis, a feature common in patients with systemic lupus erythematosus (SLE) but not in those with rheumatoid arthritis. Arthritis of the metacarpophalangeal (MCP) and proximal interphalangeal (PIP) joints, pleural effusions, and anemia could be seen in either disease. Abnormal liver function can be an atypical feature of SLE but would more commonly result from drug-related hepatic dysfunction [e.g., due to nonsteroidal anti-inflammatory drugs (NSAIDs)] in either disease.

26. The answer is D [Chapter 9 III A 6 a, b, d, 7 c (1), (3)]. Hypercalcemia caused by diseases other than hyperparathyroidism may be treated with intravenous saline and furosemide. Fluid replacement with intravenous saline, followed by forced diuresis with saline and intravenous furosemide, is a rapid and safe way to lower serum calcium and should be tried first. Pamidronate, mithramycin, or calcitonin may be added if additional lowering of the calcium level is needed. Glucocorticoids are effective in treating hypercalcemia caused by vitamin D excess, sarcoidosis, and some hematologic malignancies, but they do not lower calcium levels in most cases of hypercalcemia associated with solid tumors.

27–29. The answers are: 27—C [Chapter 1 VIII A 2 d, 3 a], **28—C** [Chapter 1 VIII A 4 a–b], **29—E** [Chapter 2 VIII E 6 a–c, 7, 8 a]. Lower extremity injury may lead to blood clot formation and the development of thrombophlebitis. Other factors that contribute to the development of deep venous thrombosis include the use of estrogen-containing compounds (e.g., oral contraceptives) and lower limb immobilization (e.g., during surgery or prolonged bed rest), which leads to venous stasis. Hypertension, diabetes mellitus, and intravenous drug abuse have no association with deep venous thrombosis. The dyspnea and pleuritic pain suggest that the suspected deep venous thrombosis has led to pulmonary embolism, which is most commonly caused by the migration of a thrombus from the veins in the lower extremities or pelvis to the pulmonary artery.

Lower extremity plethysmography is a noninvasive test that is useful for establishing a diagnosis of deep venous thrombosis. Contrast venography provides a definitive diagnosis in almost every case; however, this invasive test actually can cause thrombophlebitis in most cases. Cardiac catheterization, lung scanning, and computed tomography (CT) would be of no use in the diagnosis of deep venous thrombosis.

The most sensitive and specific test for pulmonary embolism is pulmonary arteriography. Nuclear scanning of the lung is another useful technique, but it is not as specific as arteriography. Although a normal scan virtually rules out pulmonary embolism, scanning results often fall into the intermediate probability range, making a definitive diagnosis impossible. In most cases of pulmonary embolism, the electrocardiogram (ECG) is normal. Acute right axis deviation noted on the ECG may lead to the erroneous diagnosis of anterior myocardial infarction (MI). Hypoxia, hypocapnia, and respiratory alkalosis are classic findings on arterial blood gas analysis but are not specific for pulmonary embolism. The chest radiograph may be normal, especially if infarction has not occurred.

30. The answer is C [Chapter 6 Part II: IV B–D]. The patient has significant acidemia (low arterial pH), which is associated with a low serum HCO_3^- concentration; thus, metabolic acidosis must be present. This condition is attributable to lactate accumulation, which is caused by seizure activity. Another clue is the elevated anion gap. In addition, the patient also has respiratory acidosis, as evidenced by the elevated $Paco_2$. Hypoventilation often accompanies grand mal seizure.

31. The answer is C [Chapter 9 III A 5 b]. An elevated level of serum intact parathyroid hormone (PTH), in the absence of renal failure or other cause of secondary hyperparathyroidism, is strong evidence for primary hyperparathyroidism. In hypercalcemia of other causes (e.g., with cancer, sarcoidosis, or excessive vitamin D intake), the PTH level is suppressed by the hypercalcemia and is low (or normal).

32. The answer is E [Chapter 3 V D 1 b]. Von Willebrand's disease (vWD) is a genetic defect with variable transmissions that results in the deficiency or derangement of the large antigenic portion of factor VIII (VIII^{ag}). This molecule is associated with both the intrinsic coagulation pathway and platelet–vessel wall interaction. Thus, in vWD, there is prolongation of both the partial thromboplastin time (PTT) [indicative of defects in the intrinsic coagulation cascade] and bleeding time (indicative of a defect in the platelet–VIII^{ag}–vessel wall interaction). The hemophilias, either factor VIII or factor IX varieties, affect males because of sex linkage of the genes. Isolated prolongations of PTT are characteristic. Other coagulation tests, including bleeding time, are normal. Factor VII is in the extrinsic arm of the coagulation cascade, and deficiency of this factor prolongs prothrombin time (PT) only. Aspirin, as well as many other nonsteroidal anti-inflammatory drugs (NSAIDs), inhibits platelet prostaglandin synthesis, which results in defective platelet function and prolongation of bleeding time. Results of other coagulation tests are normal.

33. The answer is D [Chapter 6 Part II: III B 2 a (1)]. Although hypokalemia can occur in each of these conditions, the hypokalemic alkalosis is most likely the result of surreptitious vomiting. Chronic diarrhea is characterized by acidosis rather than alkalosis. Although the remaining conditions are typically associated with alkalosis, surreptitious vomiting is the only condition associated with extracellular volume contraction and the absence of hypertension. The other conditions typically are associated with expansion of extracellular volume and hypertension, caused by increased mineralocorticoid activity.

34. The answer is A [Chapter 8 VII C 3]. Induration of 4-mm diameter at the site of a purified protein derivative (PPD) test would argue against chemoprophylaxis with isoniazid. All adults younger than 35 years with positive PPD test results should have isoniazid chemoprophylaxis unless they cannot tolerate isoniazid, have already received a full course, or are known to have been exposed to isoniazid-resistant tuberculosis. Usually, induration of at least 10 mm is required to call a test positive. A lesser degrees of induration may represent cross-reactions to other mycobacteria or fading skin test reactivity, and PPD testing may be repeated in a couple of weeks. Isoniazid can produce liver inflammation, but completely healed hepatitis is not a contraindication to isoniazid.

35. The answer is B [Chapter 11 III B 4 a; XI A; XIX A 2 a]. Vitamin B_{12} deficiency causes combined systems degeneration. Patients can present with a gait disturbance characterized by spasticity and diminished vibratory and position sense. A mild neuropathy may be present, causing depressed ankle reflexes. Because this is a treatable cause of abnormal gait, identification of vitamin B_{12} deficiency is important. Multiple sclerosis (MS) does not typically present in this age group. Absent ankle reflexes are not a common feature of MS; rather, hyperactive reflexes are consistent with the upper motor neuron findings commonly found.

Normal pressure hydrocephalus (NPH) is a cause of deteriorating gait. However, cognitive decline is often present and patients can have urinary incontinence. Impaired vibration and position sense and absent ankle reflexes are not typical of NPH. Human T-cell lymphotropic virus type I (HTLV-I) infection is a cause of myelopathy and should be suspected in patients who have had blood transfusions, abuse intravenous drugs, or have resided in endemic areas. It is not evident from the patient history that this patient has any risk factors for this infection. Adrenomyeloneuropathy is an X-linked recessive disorder related to adrenoleukodystrophy, typically presenting in young males. The disorder causes an accumulation of very-long-chain fatty acids because of an inability to catabolize these lipids. Female carriers may display a mild spastic paraparesis, but not the constellation of findings found in this patient.

36. **The answer is C** [Chapter 2 XV B–E]. Patients with obstructive apnea respond very well to nasal continual positive airway pressure (CPAP), which acts to splint the obstructed posterior pharynx. Patients with sleep apnea, whether central, obstructive, or mixed, are indistinguishable clinically; sleep studies are necessary to determine which type of apnea is present. Although some patients with obstructive apnea may respond to respiratory stimulants, others require more drastic measures. Patients with all forms of sleep apnea are sleepy during the day and, for reasons unknown, all are at risk for developing cor pulmonale.

37. **The answer is B** [Chapter 4 IX G 2]. Testicular cancer is the most common cancer in young adult males. The most common varieties are seminomas and nonseminomatous germ cell tumors, both of which are curable even in advanced stages. Seminomas are exquisitely sensitive to radiation therapy; therefore, patients with stage II disease (i.e., disease limited to the testicle and nodes below the diaphragm) may be treated with low doses of radiation. Because of bone marrow toxicity from mediastinal radiation therapy, prophylactic radiation to the mediastinum is no longer indicated. In this setting, enlarged retroperitoneal lymph nodes connote metastatic disease, and treatment is indicated.

38. **The answer is D** [Chapter 4 IV E 2–4]. Patients with a history of seminoma should be evaluated for recurrent disease. If disease recurs outside of the radiation field, patients should undergo diagnostic procedures to confirm the diagnosis, followed by combination chemotherapy with etoposide, cisplatin; bleomycin may be added in high-risk patients. The diagnosis may be made by needle biopsy under computed tomography (CT) guidance. If this does not provide the diagnosis, a mediastinotomy or mediastinoscopy may be required. Mediastinal radiation alone would not be sufficient to eliminate the recurrent disease. Occasionally, patients with germ cell tumors develop stable fibrosis in an area of previous tumor or develop teratomas that may undergo malignant degeneration. In some cases, future surgical exploration is required to exclude fibrosis or teratoma. However, fibrosis and teratomas occur uncommonly with apparently pure seminomas.

39. **The answer is D** [Chapter 10 XII E 2 c (1), H 2 a]. The subset of juvenile rheumatoid arthritis patients most likely to develop chronic, erosive, and severe arthritis is the polyarticular group that is seropositive for rheumatoid factor. This form of the disease is also most similar to adult rheumatoid arthritis and most likely to require a second-line agent.

40. **The answer is D** [Chapter 9 II A 5]. Serum thyroid-stimulating hormone (TSH) measurement is most likely to confirm a suspected diagnosis of hypothyroidism. In a mild case of primary hypothyroidism, TSH usually rises to abnormal levels before serum thyroxine (T_4) or serum triiodothyronine (T_3) have fallen below the normal range. T_3 resin uptake, which is not a highly accurate test of thyroid function, is used mainly to exclude abnormalities in thyroid hormone–binding proteins. A high titer of antithyroid antibodies would indicate the presence of chronic thyroiditis, the most common cause of hypothyroidism, but would not indicate whether hypothyroidism is present.

41. **The answer is A** [Chapter 6 Part I: XII B 2 b]. Chronic lead nephropathy is the most likely cause of this patient's condition. Lead nephropathy is associated with an impairment in uric acid excretion and typically is associated with the clinical syndrome of gout. Whereas gout and chronic renal failure from

other etiologies could coexist, the current evidence suggests that lead toxicity is responsible for the bulk of cases in which both diseases are concurrent. Analgesic abuse should not be associated with an increased incidence of gout, although the renal findings could be similar. Hypertensive nephropathy also may explain the findings, although it would not explain the occurrence of gout in this patient. Renovascular hypertension could be present in this patient but is typically associated with more severe hypertension when renal failure occurs. Furthermore, renovascular hypertension is not usually associated with gout. However, imaging of the renal vascular tree would be necessary to completely exclude this diagnosis.

42. The answer is E [Chapter 8 V A 1 a (1) (a)–(b); Chapter 11 IV C 2]. The patient most likely had a self-limited aseptic meningitis and developed a postural, post–lumbar puncture (LP) headache on arising. Associated symptoms can include nausea, blurred vision, tinnitus, and vomiting. Diminished cerebrospinal fluid (CSF) pressure may be the cause of an LP-associated headache. Treatment options include bed rest, analgesics, and a lumbar epidural blood patch that may, in part, plug a dural tear. Although the patient has a history of migraine, it is unusual for vascular headaches to occur only when standing. Bacterial meningitis is a rare complication of an LP. However, because the patient is afebrile and only has a headache when upright, this diagnosis is unlikely. Likewise, it is unlikely that the headache is caused by persistent aseptic meningitis. Patients can develop tender, tight cervical muscles after aseptic meningitis. This can be confused with persistent meningismus. However, it is more likely that this patient is suffering from a headache as a result of complications from the LP.

43. The answer is C [Chapter 9 VI B 1]. Normal hypothalamic secretion of gonadotropin-releasing hormone (GnRH) consists of pulsatile release every 90–120 minutes. If GnRh is injected by infusion pump in a way that mimics the normal pattern, luteinizing hormone (LH) and follicle-stimulating hormone (FSH) are secreted normally, and cyclic ovarian function may follow. Continuous, rather than pulsatile, blood levels of GnRH, which are produced by injection of long-acting analogs, have the opposite effect and suppress LH and FSH production.

44. The answer is B [Chapter 8 VII D 1 a, 2 b]. *Salmonella* bacteremia, toxic shock syndrome (TSS), tuberculosis, and Epstein-Barr mononucleosis can be accompanied by fever, but a diffuse desquamative rash should suggest TSS, severe drug reaction (e.g., Stevens-Johnson syndrome), Kawasaki disease, or scarlet fever. The skin rash associated with *Salmonella* is very subtle and evanescent (Rose spots). Tuberculosis is not characterized by diffuse skin and mucous membrane involvement or watery diarrhea. Although allergy to sulfamethoxazole can produce red skin and mucous membranes, it does not cause diarrhea.

45. The answer is A [Chapter 10 VIII F 1]. Skin thickening is a defining characteristic of scleroderma; if it is limited to distal areas, it may be a manifestation of the CREST variant of scleroderma (i.e., scleroderma that involves the coexistence of subcutaneous **C**alcinosis, **R**aynaud's phenomenon, **E**sophageal motility dysfunction, **S**clerodactyly, and **T**elangiectasia). Patients with Raynaud's phenomenon who are seropositive for antinuclear antibody (ANA) or anticentromere antibody or who exhibit digital capillary changes are at higher risk for developing scleroderma than a patient with Raynaud's phenomenon who does not have these features. Distal esophageal dysmotility, spasm, or stricture are possible features of scleroderma but are nonspecific.

46. The answer is E [Chapter 11 II A 3 a (2), b (2), d (1) (8)]. Postprandial syncope is a common cause of fainting in the elderly. Alcohol intake also can lead to syncope and often is a contributing factor. Postprandial syncope may occur when blood is shunted to the mesenteric bed, resulting in relative cerebral hypoperfusion. The patient shows no signs of convulsive activity; therefore, a seizure is unlikely. A cardiac arrhythmia and carotid sinus hypersensitivity can cause syncope and should always be considered in the elderly patient. However, the setting in which this patient fainted makes postprandial syncope a more likely cause. A colloid cyst of the third ventricle is a rare cause of sudden unconsciousness. The small cyst acts like a ball valve and obstructs flow through the foramen of Monro, causing acute hydrocephalus.

47. The answer is A [Chapter 4 XVI C 2, D 2]. Follicular small-cleaved cell lymphoma, previously called nodular poorly differentiated lymphocytic lymphoma, is one of the most common varieties of the indolent non-Hodgkin's lymphomas. Affected patients often present with stage III or IV disease. Even without treatment, patients may have waxing and waning of adenopathy, but over time, the disease progresses, and patients require chemotherapy. A small percentage of patients develop a more aggressive lymphoma, usually of the large cell or immunoblastic varieties.

48. The answer is D [Chapter 8 VIII G 1 b]. Diffuse lymphadenopathy in a human immunodeficiency virus (HIV)–infected person who is clinically well is usually a sign that there is no specific infection or tumor involved. Although all of the answers can be true, people with multiple enlarged lymph nodes, tuberculosis, or malignancy tend to be ill. Most often they also experience weight loss and fevers. Lymphoma is more likely to present with organ involvement in HIV-infected patients than in other patients. Kaposi's sarcoma may have lymphatic involvement, but generally this is found only in late-stage disease with extensive cutaneous and mucosal lesions. Moderate lymphadenopathy is a common finding in mid-stage HIV infection. Its exact cause is unknown, but the disappearance of long-standing lymphadenopathy may precede clinical deterioration. Syphilis may produce either local or diffuse adenopathy in patients with or without HIV infection. However, this adenopathy almost always accompanies some other feature of syphilis.

49. The answer is D [Chapter 6 Part I: XV A 1, 2]. The glomerular filtration rate (GFR) increases by approximately 40% in pregnancy. In fact, a fall in serum uric acid level typically occurs, as does a rise in uric acid clearance. Proteinuria normally is not seen in pregnancy, and the finding of increased urinary protein excretion suggests the presence of underlying renal disease or preeclampsia. The blood pressure typically falls in pregnancy; therefore, any degree of elevation represents important hypertension. Finally, respiratory alkalosis, not metabolic alkalosis, typically occurs, and this condition leads to a fall in serum bicarbonate level.

50. The answer is C [Chapter 9 I B 1 c; Table 9–2]. The patient probably has partial diabetes insipidus. The definite response by the patient to the injection of antidiuretic hormone (ADH) indicates that he did not produce maximally effective levels of ADH after fluid restriction and, therefore, he has either partial or complete diabetes insipidus. The ability to achieve normal or near-normal urine concentration, however, indicates that the ADH deficit is only partial. The response to ADH rules out nephrogenic diabetes insipidus. Diabetes mellitus, another cause of polyuria, is diagnosed by blood and urine glucose levels rather than studies of renal water handling.

51. The answer is E [Chapter 2 IV B 2 b]. More than 40% of patients with cystic fibrosis live to be 18 years of age or older. Until the 1960s, cystic fibrosis was purely a pediatric disease. At that time, the median age of cystic fibrosis patients shifted to the teens, primarily for two reasons: (1) availability of antibiotics that are more specific to the pathogenic bacteria, and (2) better understanding of the need for nutritional supplementation and exogenous pancreatic replacement. In 1998, the median age of patients with cystic fibrosis was over 32 years.

52. The answer is B [Chapter 8 II A 3 b; IV H]. Whereas recommendations about treatment regimens for patients with profound neutropenia always change, the general principle is that infection with enteric gram-negative rods and *Pseudomonas aeruginosa* is likely and quickly leads to a poor clinical outcome if left untreated. Piperacillin and amikacin may be good initial choices, depending on the antibiotic susceptibility of gram-negative rods in the community and the hospital. Antifungal therapy may be needed in a few days if there is no response to these antibiotics. Staphylococcal infections, common in patients with indwelling vascular catheters, are less likely to lead to cataclysmic deterioration.

53. The answer is C [Chapter 6 Part III: IV C 2 a (2)]. The use of diuretics in the treatment of hypertension may be associated with several side effects, including prerenal azotemia. Hypokalemia, hyperglycemia, hyperlipidemia, hyperuricemia, and hypercalcemia are also side effects of diuretic therapy. Bronchospasm is a side effect of β-blockade, and hemolytic anemia is a side effect of methyldopa, a centrally acting adrenergic antagonist. Both β-blockers and centrally acting adrenergic antagonists are alternative therapies for hypertension.

54. **The answer is C** [Chapter 3 I A 1]. The setting and history of this case are appropriate for a diagnosis of iron-deficiency anemia. The excessive menses represent a source of iron loss. The hypochromia and microcytosis indicated by the blood smear establish that there is no deficiency of vitamin B_{12}; therefore, pernicious anemia is unlikely. The blood smear also excludes sickle cell anemia. Although blood smears show a microcytic cell population in cases of sideroblastic anemia, it also shows a normal or slightly macrocytic population existing with the microcytic component. Glucose-6-phosphate dehydrogenase (G6PD) deficiency is unlikely because it presents as hemolysis, for which there is no evidence in this case.

55. **The answer is D** [Chapter 11 XVIII F]. Patients with Down syndrome are at high risk of developing Alzheimer's disease at approximately age 50 years. The pathology found is that of senile plaques and neurofibrillary tangles. Certainly hypothyroidism and hydrocephalus might occur in patients with Down syndrome, but the onset of dementia at age 50 is highly typical of developing Alzheimer's disease. Likewise, multiple strokes can lead to dementia, but stroke is not a usual cause of dementia in a 50-year-old Down syndrome patient. Creutzfeldt-Jakob disease, a rare disorder with no special propensity for Down syndrome patients, is associated with prions and causes dementia.

56. **The answer is D** [Chapter 5 VII A 1]. Like alcoholic pancreatitis, gallstone pancreatitis accounts for approximately 30%–40% of all cases of acute pancreatitis in the United States. Thiazide therapy, hypercalcemia, and pancreas divisum are less common causes of acute pancreatitis. Hyperlipidemia is an associated finding in 15% of cases, but it also may be causative.

57. **The answer is C** [Chapter 8 VII B 1, 2]. Of the choices, eosinophilia is most likely to be found in schistosomiasis. Eosinophilia is a characteristic finding in infections due to multicellular, tissue-invasive parasites such as *Schistosoma, Trichinella, Ascaris,* and *Strongyloides* species. Pinworm infestation is a purely luminal process, which does not elicit eosinophilia. Protozoal infections such as giardiasis and amebiasis rarely are associated with eosinophilia; the same is true of bacterial and viral infections such as influenza. Corticosteroids may be administered to individuals with underlying eosinophilia due to asthma or allergy to reduce the eosinophilia.

58. **The correct answer is C** [Chapter 4 XV B 2 a]. Classic Burkitt's lymphoma is clearly linked with this virus. Burkitt's lymphoma is a very aggressive type of non-Hodgkin's lymphoma, which could rapidly lead to death if left untreated. Patients with HIV infection could develop a non-Hodgkin's lymphoma, but this is not of the Burkitt type. Poxvirus does not lead to lymphoma in humans. HTLV-1 is associated with a T-cell lymphoma that is prevalent in Japan and the Caribbean islands.

59. **The answer is D** [Chapter 8 V C 4 c]. Although the studies do not completely exclude the possibility of a pulmonary embolus, bacterial pneumonia is likely. According to the Gram stain results, *Haemophilus influenzae* is the most likely causative organism, although pneumococcus is still possible. Ceftriaxone is effective against both. Bacterial resistance to penicillin and erythromycin make these suboptimal choices. In a less definite case of bacterial pneumonia, it might be prudent to offer azithromycin in combination with ceftriaxone to cover for the possibility of chlamydia and legionella. A broad-spectrum fluoroquinolone active against pneumococci would be an effective alternative in the face of allergy or the need for a completely oral course of therapy. Fluoroquinolones are effective in the treatment of community-acquired pneumonia, but there are two things to remember: ciprofloxacin has suboptimal effect on pneumococci, and this class of drug is very broad spectrum and might select for a highly resistant bacterial flora.

60. The answer is A [Chapter 7 V F 2 a–f]. A hypersensitivity reaction to an insect sting is likely to be the cause of the patient's symptoms. Immediately after such a sting, most individuals experience local discomfort. However, the progressive occurrence of diffuse pruritus or urticaria indicates a systemic hypersensitivity reaction, culminating in respiratory and cardiovascular embarrassment. Recent or concurrent use of β-antagonists such as propranolol reduces the efficacy of β-adrenergic agonists and predicts a more severe and protracted course of the anaphylactic reaction. In patients who have been taking β-blockers, measures not dependent on β-adrenergic receptor stimulation are preferred; thus, pressor agents and intravenous hydrocortisone are preferred over intravenous aminophylline, nebulized epinephrine, and nebulized β_2-adrenergic agonists. Intravenous glucagon also may be useful if anaphylaxis is only partially responsive to pressors and corticosteroids. Although diphenhydramine would be somewhat useful in the general treatment of anaphylaxis, it would not be appropriate acutely.

61. The answer is B [Chapter 1 III A 5 b (1), (2) (a)–(b)]. The patient is experiencing anterior myocardial infarction (MI). The S-T segment elevation in the anterior precordial leads indicates a current of myocardial injury. The S-T segment depression in the inferior leads is probably a reciprocal change reflecting the S-T segment elevation in the opposite (anterior) wall. Although pericarditis can mimic the clinical presentation of MI, the electrocardiogram (ECG) in pericarditis demonstrates diffuse S-T segment elevation without S-T segment depression.

62. The answer is B [Chapter 1 III A 5 b (4) (a) (i)–(ii), (5) (a)–(b)]. The most appropriate initial therapy for this patient would be the administration of thrombolytic therapy. Thrombolysis with streptokinase may allow for reperfusion of the myocardium, thus reducing infarct size and the chance of patient mortality. Reperfusion therapy is most effective within the first 4 hours after the beginning of the infarction. All patients with MI or suspected MI should be monitored in an intensive care unit, not a general ward. Administration of atropine would increase the heart rate, causing further increases in myocardial oxygen consumption and possibly worsening the MI. Pain relief is an important therapy in MI, but intramuscular injections should be avoided when treating this condition. By relieving pain, one relieves anxiety, which decreases oxygen consumption and may also decrease the incidence of arrhythmias.

63. The answer is B [Chapter 8 V A 1 a (1)]. Although all information is not in, the weight of the evidence suggests that this patient has bacterial meningitis, and IV ceftriaxone is the appropriate choice. The presence of blood can confuse the interpretation of lumbar puncture (LP) results. The number of white blood cells (WBCs) is more than expected for simple blood contamination. Although the clot stabilizer ϵ-aminocaproic acid may play a role in documented subarachnoid bleeds, the most urgent matter in this case is treatment of the possible bacterial meningitis. Oral or intravenous erythromycin plays no role in the treatment of meningitis. Heparin would be contraindicated until the diagnosis of subarachnoid bleed can be totally ruled out. Acyclovir is not appropriate; the clinical scenario and the cerebrospinal fluid (CSF) findings do not suggest herpes simplex meningitis. A severe headache and stiff neck seldom occurs with this form of meningitis, and CSF with a high WBC count is exceptionally rare.

64. The answer is A [Chapter 10 VI D, E]. Bacterial infection is the most likely diagnosis in any patient who presents with a fever and an inflammatory monoarthritis, unless crystals are seen under polarized light examination of the synovial fluid. The absence of crystals in this patient's joint fluid eliminates gout and pseudogout as diagnoses. A joint fluid white blood cell (WBC) count exceeding 50,000/mm^3 also makes the diagnosis of septic arthritis more likely.

65. The answer is D [Chapter 1 I D 1 e, 2 a–f, h]. The patient is suffering from acute cardiogenic pulmonary edema. The rapid onset of the symptoms, in addition to the pinkish sputum, the gallop rhythm, and the bilateral infiltrates on the chest radiograph, strongly suggest this diagnosis, particularly in a patient with antecedent heart disease. Although the possibility that a bilateral pneumonitis could be exacerbating the patient's emphysema cannot be ruled out, the acute onset and the absence of purulent sputum militate against this diagnosis. While her blood pressure is significantly elevated, this elevation is likely related to the stress of acute pulmonary edema and not hypertensive crisis, which has different clinical features.

66. The answer is A [Chapter 1 I F 2 b (1)]. Because the patient is dyspneic, hypoxic, and hypocarbic, administration of oxygen should be the first course of action. Although one must be cautious of administering oxygen to emphysemic patients, the fact that this patient is hypocarbic suggests that she will not retain carbon dioxide when a prudent amount of oxygen is administered. Because there is no evidence of an acute myocardial infarction (MI), her occasional extrasystoles do not require therapy with quinidine at this time. Although digoxin may be of some benefit in the long-range therapy of congestive heart failure (CHF), it has little immediate effect because it takes many hours to provide an adequate loading dose. Heparin has no known role in acute pulmonary edema. It would only be indicated if the pulmonary edema were secondary to an acute coronary syndrome, of which there is no evidence in this case.

67. The answer is B [Chapter 11 VIII B 3 a]. This patient most likely has a gastrointestinal malignancy, either stomach or colonic cancer metastatic to the liver. These mucinous carcinomas are associated with nonbacterial thrombotic endocarditis, which is a manifestation of systemic cancer-associated hypercoagulable state. Valvular vegetations can embolize to the cerebral circulation, causing an acute ischemic stroke.

A glioblastoma multiforme or metastatic tumor would appear as an enhancing lesion on brain CT scan with associated mass effect. This is not the pattern on the patient's CT scan. Bacterial endocarditis typically is associated with fever; this patient is afebrile. The lupus anticoagulant is associated with ischemic stroke as well as nonbacterial endocarditis. However, in this setting, with documented GI symptomatology, a cancer-associated hypercoagulable state is more likely than the lupus anticoagulant.

68. The answer is D [Chapter 11 XIII D 4]. Chronic inflammatory demyelinating polyneuropathy is a cause of progressive predominantly motor neuropathy leading to distal weakness with associated loss of reflexes. There can be sensory loss. Typically bowel and bladder control is retained, and there is a paucity of pain.

Vitamin B_{12} deficiency cause loss of lower extremity position and vibration perception. There can be mild leg weakness with evidence of an upper motor neuron lesion such as an extensor plantar response combined with hyporeflexia associated with a concurrent peripheral neuropathy. Cervical myelopathy causes lower extremity weakness with hyperreflexia. Sensory loss and bowel and bladder disordered function can be present. There is often neck discomfort. Upper extremity symptoms and signs can be present. Polymyositis causes predominantly proximal weakness without sensory changes. Myalgias can be present. By definition, the weakness associated with Guillain-Barré syndrome (acute inflammatory demyelinating polyneuropathy) does not progress beyond approximately 4 weeks. Therefore, the chronicity of this patient's progressive symptoms excludes this diagnosis.

69. The answer is A [Chapter 11 XIII D 3]. Diabetes is a common cause of painful feet. The small fiber chronic sensory polyneuropathy associated with diabetes is characterized by diminished pain and temperature sensibility. Patients have a heightened pain response during testing with a pin and may note increased discomfort with pressure on the skin surface. A small fiber polyneuropathy may be symptomatic early in the course of diabetes.

Vitamin B_{12} deficiency typically causes predominant loss of proprioception and vibration modalites. Painful feet are not characteristic of a vitamin B_{12}-associated polyneuropathy or myelopathy. Lumbar stenosis can cause loss of sensation in the feet, but typically the feet are not painful. Pin and temperature appreciation are not lost out of proportion to vibration and proprioception. A thoracic myelopathy can cause loss of sensory modalities in the lower extremities. There is frequently associated weakness and hyperreflexia, as well as leg spasticity. Pain in the feet can occur but is not characteristic. Sciatica can cause pain in a lower extremity, including the foot. However, sciatica is infrequently bilateral, and pain is not exacerbated with testing with a pin or with skin pressure. There can be associated weakness and diminished reflexes.

70. The correct answer is D [Chapter 11 XVII E; Chapter 8 VIII G 1 c 3]. CNS lymphoma is a complication of AIDS. It can present with focal neurologic deficits and is often in a periventricular location. CNS lymphoma is typically uniformly enhancing.

Toxoplasmosis is another AIDS complication. Typically there are multiple small enhancing lesions evident with brain MRI. There may be focal neurologic deficits, cognitive impairment, and seizures. An abscess can occur in any brain location, and typically the periphery of the lesion enhances. Similarly, an astrocytoma enhances about the periphery; it typically originates in hemispheral white matter locations, which may be periventricular. A meningioma often enhances uniformly, but a periventricular location would be most unusual.

71. The answer is D [Chapter 8 G 3 e]. Cryptococcal meningitis is a relatively common complication of AIDS. It causes headache and cognitive alterations; hydrocephalus can develop. The patient's CSF pattern is consistent with cryptococcal meningitis. A positive CSF India ink stain or cryptococcal antigen assay would help confirm the diagnosis pending culture results.

Tuberculous meningitis is often associated with a low CSF glucose level in relation to the blood glucose level. HIV-associated meningitis would not be expected to cause cognitive decline (as opposed to HIV-associated encephalopathy or AIDS-dementia complex) or hydrocephalus. Pneumococcal meningitis would not have a 2-week presentation; patients rapidly become ill. Syphilitic meningitis is not associated with hydrocephalus; patients can be cognitively impaired secondary to associated vascular compromise.

72–75. The answers are: 72—E, 73—A, 74—C, 75—B [Chapter 9 V B 3 d, e (1)]. Although basal cortisol levels may be increased by physical or emotional stress, even low doses of dexamethasone usually result in normal suppression in persons without adrenal disease.

The pituitary secretion of adrenocorticotropic hormone (ACTH) in Cushing's disease can be suppressed by dexamethasone or other glucocorticoids. However, larger-than-normal doses of dexamethasone are necessary for suppression.

The production of ACTH by oat cell carcinoma of the lung and other tumors is not suppressed by dexamethasone. Therefore, even high doses do not lower cortisol levels. The increased blood ACTH levels are helpful in distinguishing ectopic ACTH syndrome from adrenal tumors, in which ACTH (of pituitary origin) is suppressed.

Cortisol production by adrenal adenomas and carcinomas is autonomous; it is not under the control of pituitary ACTH. In fact, ACTH levels are suppressed by the increased circulating cortisol. Therefore, even high doses of dexamethasone do not lower cortisol levels by suppressing pituitary excretion of ACTH.

76–80. The answers are: 76—C [Table 7–7], **77—E** [Table 7–6], **78—A** [Table 7–5], **79—B** [Table 7–7], **80—D** [Table 7–5]. Wiskott-Aldrich syndrome is characterized clinically by susceptibility to infection during the first year of life, eczema, and purpura. The immunologic response deficiency is accompanied by a reduction in both the number and size of platelets.

Profound lymphopenia ($< 1500/mm^3$) is a cardinal feature of the severe combined immunodeficiency (SCID) disorders. This heterogeneous group of disorders usually develops in infancy; patients present with frequent bouts of otitis media, pneumonia, cutaneous infections, diarrhea, and sepsis. Opportunistic infections frequently lead to death before the age of 2 years.

The nitroblue tetrazolium (NBT) test is a simple screening procedure for chronic granulomatous disease; failure to reduce the nitroblue tetrazolium dye during phagocytosis constitutes a positive result. This disorder is characterized by an absence of the usual respiratory burst because of abnormal function of the reduced form of nicotinamide–adenine nucleotide phosphate (NADPH).

DiGeorge syndrome results from dysmorphogenesis of the third and fourth pharyngeal pouches, leading to aplasia or hypoplasia of the thymus and parathyroid glands. Neonatal tetany secondary to hypoparathyroid-induced hypocalcemia may be the first clinical manifestation; thus, assessing the serum calcium level is appropriate. Mandibular hypoplasia; hypertelorism; low-set, notched ears; and conotruncal heart lesions are common. The magnitude of the immune deficiency is variable, and patients with heart defects have the least favorable prognosis.

Delayed umbilical cord separation followed by persistent omphalitis suggests leukocyte adhesion deficiency. The diagnosis is confirmed by documenting deficient surface expression of CD18 membrane glycoprotein on granulocytes by flow cytometry. Affected children typically develop recurrent deep soft tissue or superficial cold abscesses.

81. The answer is E [Chapter 2 X A]. Myasthenia gravis and other myopathies may give rise to thoracic wall dysfunction and hypoventilation. The susequent retention of carbon dioxide leads to respiratory acidosis. Hypoxemia is often present. During normal pregnancy, progesterone stimulates the ventilatory center, producing a mild respiratory alkalosis. In liver diseases, a similar mild respiratory alkalosis is seen. Diabetic ketoacidosis is a form of metabolic acidosis associated with a wide anion gap that occurs secondary to ketone body formation in the insulin-deficient state.

82. The answer is C [Chapter 6 Part II: IV E 2 c]. Diuretic intake (e.g., thiazides, loop diuretics) cause urinary losses of Na^+ and Cl^-. The resulting volume depletion leads to augmented proximal reabsorption of sodium bicarbonate, causing metabolic alkalosis. The secondary hyperaldosteronism of volume depletion stimulates hydrogen ion secretion in the collecting duct, worsening the metabolic alkalosis. Kaluresis and hypokalemia are invariably present. Conditions associated with hyporeninemic hypoaldosteronism (e.g., diabetic nephropathy) give rise to hyperkalemia and metabolic asidosis (a condition often termed renal tubular acidosis type IV). Drugs that depress the central ventilatory center (e.g., heroin) induce hypoventilation, carbon dioxide retention, and respiratory acidosis. Conditions of tissue hypoperfusion, including severe decreases in cardiac output, lead to anaerobic glycolysis, increased lactate production, and decreased hepatic lactate metabolism. The result is lactic acidosis. Tachypnea and hyperpnea are early clinical signs of endotoxemia. The resulting decrease in $Paco_2$ leads to respiratory alkalosis. As septicemia proceeds to septic shock, lactic acidosis may supervene.

83. The answer is E [Chapter 6 Part II: IV D b 2]. The low bicarbonate concentration and the low arterial pH indicate the presence of metabolic acidosis, which in this case is attributable to the loss of alkali in the stools. The acid–base disturbance is a simple metabolic acidosis, because there is appropriate respiratory compensation. Winters' formula in this case is applicable:

$$\text{Expected } Paco_2 = (1.5 \times HCO_3) + 8 \pm 2 = (1.5 \times 14) + 8 \pm 2 = 29 \pm 2.$$

Note that the measured $Paco_2$ is 30, which is quite close to this value. This assessment effectively excludes the presence of other primary acid–base disorders such as respiratory acidosis or alkalosis. Note also that the anion gap is within the normal range, as is typically the case in diarrhea: $Na^+ - (Cl^- + HCO_3^-) = 140 - (115 + 14) = 11$.

84. The answer is B [Chapter 6 Part III: IV C (2) f]. Nifedipine, a calcium channel antagonist, modulates calcium release in smooth muscle, reducing smooth muscle tone and producing vasodilation. Drugs such as methyldopa or clonidine are centrally acting adrenergic antagonists that inhibit sympathetic outflow from the central nervous system (CNS) by stimulating central β-adrenoreceptors, which reduces peripheral resistance and blood pressure. The β-adrenergic blocking agents (e.g., metoprolol) are effective antihypertensive agents because they reduce cardiac output and blunt renin release. Vasodilator drugs such as minoxidil directly dilate arteries and arterioles. The β-adrenergic blocking agents (e.g., prazosin) reduce blood pressure by antagonizing norepinephrine's stimulation of β-adrenergic receptors.

85. The answer is A [Chapter 6 Part II: I B c; Chapter 9 I B 2]. Serum hypo-osmolarity associated with impaired renal water diluting capacity are hallmarks of the syndrome of inappropriate antidiuretic hormone (SIADH). This diagnosis is made after excluding conditions associated with renal hypoperfusion such as extracellular fluid volume depletion or congestive heart failure. The latter conditions also can give rise to serum hypotonicity and a relatively concentrated urine, but this patient has no clinical evidence for significant volume depletion or heart failure. Diabetes insipidus typically manifests by polyuria, dilute urine, and serum hyperosmolality if fluid intake is less than urine output. Compulsive water drinking also causes polyuria and a dilute urine, but the serum osmolality tends to be on the low side because of the large quantities of fluid intake.

86. The answer is C [Chapter 6 Part II: I C II]. In hypernatremic (hypertonic) states, water is lost from all body fluid compartments and not just from the plasma. This is because all cell membranes are freely permeable to water and all body fluid compartments have the same osmolality at equilibration. The routinely measured serum Na^+ concentration is equal to approximately half the plasma osmolality, and therefore can be considered as a good surrogate for the plasma osmolality (or for the osmolality of any body fluid compartment). With these considerations in mind, the electrolyte-free water loss can be readily calculated by the following formula:

$$(\text{serum Na}^+ \text{ concentration} \times \text{total body water})_{\text{current}} = (\text{serum Na}^+ \text{ concentration} \times \text{total body water})_{\text{normal}}$$

Assuming that total body water in adult males is equal to 0.6 × body weight and that the normal serum Na^+ concentration is 140 mEq/L, the current total body water is 140 × 0.6 × 78/160 = ~ 41 liters. The deficit in total body water comparing the current and the normal situations is therefore (0.6 × 78)–41, or approximately 6 liters.

87. The answer is C [Chapter 6 Part III; Chapter 9 IV 7 c (a)]. Strict control of hypertension is of paramount importance in the management of patients with diabetes mellitus, especially when albuminuria of any degree appears. The consensus recommendation for proteinuric patients is to reduce blood pressure close to 125/75 mm Hg, preferably with an agent that intercepts the renin-angiotensin axis (angiotensin-converting enzyme inhibitor or an angiotensin receptor blocker) with or without a diuretic. Multiple antihypertensive agents may be needed to achieve this target. It is desirable that dietary protein intake be restricted to 0.6 g/kg body weight per day and to target insulin therapy to achieve a hemoglobin A1c level of 7%. Oral hypoglycemic agents are ineffective and contraindicated in type I diabetes.

88. The correct answer is C [Chapter 4, V, 5, e]. Cord compression as a result of metastatic disease to the spine is a serious complication of breast cancer. Even though the patient's cancer was treated about 10 years ago, breast cancer can present itself in this fashion decades after initial treatment. If left untreated, cord compression can lead rapidly to permanent neurologic impairment. Therefore, if cord compression is suspected, it must be immediately ruled out by an MRI evaluation of the spine. The treatment consists of a combination of steroids and radiation treatment. Osteoporotic fractures and disk herniations usually have more localized pain distributions. Disk herniation is also often accompanied by neurologic deficits.

89. The correct answer is A [Chapter 4, Section IX C 6 b1]. Prostate cancer cells are responsive to testosterone withdrawal. Total androgen blockade can be accomplished by the administration of LH-RH antagonists and drugs that would block the biosynthetic pathway of testosterone production. Tamoxifen is an anti-estrogen agent that does not have a role in the treatment of prostate cancer. Both saw palmetto and Proscar are used for benign prostatic hypertrophy and do not have significant effects on prostate cancer cells, although new intriguing data suggest that Proscar might prevent prostate cancer in approximately 25% of the patients.

90. The correct answer is B [Chapter 4, Section IX A 7 1]. Renal cell carcinoma is the only malignancy in which even in the presence of metastatic disease, surgical resection of the primary tumor is commonly performed because it is associated with better outcomes. In rare cases, resection of the primary tumor is associated with the resolution of metastatic lesions. This is thought to be attributable to as yet undetermined immune processes. Moreover, this patient is experiencing occasional hematuria, which could further decline her quality of life, and resection of the tumor could resolve this issue. Chemotherapy and radiation do not play important roles in the treatment of this disease. Also, resection of multiple metastatic lesions is not feasible and does not change the overall poor outcome of the case.

91. **The correct answer is D** [Chapter 4 IX C 6 3]. Radiation proctitis is a difficult problem to manage. It significantly and adversely affects patient's quality of life. Fortunately, the incidence of this complication is low. Patients usually present with rectal pain and bloody diarrhea similar to a patient with Crohn's or ulcerative colitis. Treatment is directed toward the symptoms and usually involves the use of steroids. The other answers (hematuria, infection, or osteopenia) are not associated with external beam radiation. Myelosuppression, however, is associated with this treatment but it is not given as one of the choices.

92. **The correct answer is B** [Chapter 4, XVI, B, 1b]. Pure red blood cell aplasia is a classic paraneoplastic syndrome seen with thymomas. The exact cause is not known; however, it is thought to be related to the presence of autoantibodies that attack a component of red blood cell membrane and cause lysis of the cells. Treatment of the tumor usually leads to the resolution of the anemia. DIC can be a paraneoplastic syndrome with some other forms of malignancies such as acute promyelocytic leukemia but not thymomas. Bleeding into a mass is also rarely seen with thymomas. This disease does not have a tendency to metastasize to the bone marrow.

93–97. **The answers are: 93—D** [Chapter 5 IV D 4 f], **94—A** [Chapter 5 V D 2], **95—C** [Chapter 5 V I], **96—B** [Chapter 5 IV D 3 d], **97—E** [Chapter 5 V H]. *Campylobacter* infection is the most common cause of bacterial diarrhea. The diarrhea can be severe and bloody, and proctosigmoidoscopy during the acute phase can show ulcerated, friable mucosa. However, the disease is self-limited, and complete healing of the mucosa takes place.

Ulcerative colitis may manifest as an acute diarrheal illness that fails to resolve. Proctosigmoidoscopy shows diffuse friability, bleeding, and ulceration of the mucosa. Biopsy of the involved mucosa characteristically shows abscesses in the crypts of Lieberkühn.

Pseudomembranous colitis may arise as a complication of therapy with broad-spectrum antibiotics (e.g., clindamycin). Clindamycin suppresses most anaerobic bacteria of the colon but actually causes an overgrowth of the anaerobe *Clostridium difficile,* which produces an enterotoxin that is responsible for the development of pseudomembranous colitis. The characteristic lesion is a white plaque (pseudomembrane), which is seen in the sigmoid of 75%–90% of patients. The diagnosis can be established by measuring the toxin of *C. difficile* in the stool of patients in whom disease is confined to the right side of the colon.

Laxative abuse is an important cause of both secretory and osmotic diarrhea. Secretory diarrhea, which is diagnosed on the basis of the absence of an osmotic gap on stool electrolyte studies, may be caused by such laxatives as castor oil, bisacodyl, and phenolphthalein. Osmotic diarrhea, which is diagnosed on the basis of the presence of an osmotic gap, may be caused by such laxatives as milk of magnesia, lactulose, sorbitol, and magnesium-containing antacids. Because the only other causes of osmotic diarrhea are disaccharidase deficiency and maldigestion, the presence of an osmotic gap on stool electrolyte studies always should raise the suspicion of laxative abuse.

Collagenous colitis has been reported in middle-aged women who may have associated polyarthritis or thyroid disease. Detectable abnormalities may comprise only an elevated sedimentation rate (in approximately half of the patients) and a thickened colonic subepithelial collagen band (15–100 μm in diameter). Stool frequency is characteristic of a secretory diarrhea and may be attributable to incomplete absorption through the thickened band of collagen in the colonic submucosa.

98–102. The answers are: 98—C [Chapter 3 I B 3 a], **99—B** [Chapter 3 I B 3 a (1), 5 II B 1 6 (1)], **100—B** [Chapter 3 I B 3 c (3)], **101—B** [Chapter 3 I B 3 c (2)], **102—A** [Chapter 3 I B 3 a (2)]. Both folic acid and vitamin B_{12} deficiencies cause defective DNA synthesis and, thus, impaired cell maturation. Deficient DNA synthesis is the main characteristic of classic megaloblastic marrow (i.e., marrow cells with immature nuclei but mature cytoplasm) and macrocytic anemia. Because all marrow cell lines are affected, there is pancytopenia.

Vitamin B_{12} deficiency can result from absence of the gastric intrinsic factor needed to bind the vitamin and, thus, aid its absorption into the terminal ileum. This form of vitamin B_{12} deficiency, termed pernicious anemia, is associated with gastric atrophy, achlorhydria, and gastric carcinoma. The inability to absorb vitamin B_{12} into the ileum, which is corrected by administration of intrinsic factor, is identified by an abnormal Schilling test. Because of the role of vitamin B_{12} in myelin metabolism, deficiency causes neuropathy in the lateral and posterior columns of the spinal cord. Folic acid deficiency causes blood findings that are similar to those caused by vitamin B_{12} deficiency; however, folic acid deficiency is not associated with neuropathy. Usually, folic acid deficiency results from dietary deficiency because of poor intake (e.g., in the case of alcoholism).

103–106. The answers are: 103—B [Chapter 4 IX C 5 5 b, 6 a], **104—E** [Chapter 4 IX C 5 c], **105—C** [Chapter 4 IX C 5 a], **106—A** [Chapter 4 IX C 5 d, 6 b]. Stage T_2 tumors are the true, classic prostate nodules that are found on rectal examination. These tumors are confined to the gland and, therefore, theoretically can be cured with radical prostatectomy or radical radiation therapy (7000 cGy).

Stage T_3 tumors are cancers that are associated with metastasis to local structures (e.g., the seminal vesicles) but not to distant sites. These tumors cannot be treated surgically. However, radical radiation therapy with boost doses to the prostate gland has proved to be curative in some cases.

Stage T_{1A} prostatic tumors are low-morbidity lesions that usually are found in a routine examination for benign obstructive disease. Close follow-up may be adequate for stage T_{1A} tumors, which are well differentiated.

Stage M_2 tumors are cancers that have distant metastases, and, therefore, local measures do not suffice as therapy. Stage M_2 prostatic carcinoma requires systemic treatment such as hormone therapy.

107–111. The answers are: 107—E [Chapter 2 III E 3], **108—C** [Chapter 6 Part II: IV B, E], **109—A** [Chapter 6 Part II: IV C 1–2 a], **110—B** [Chapter 6 Part II: IV D 2 a (1), 4 b], **111—D** [Chapter 2 II E 2 a (1) (a)]. Patient E has status asthmaticus with respiratory failure. The patient has retained carbon dioxide from severe airway obstruction (as indicated by an arterial $Pa{CO_2}$ above the normal level of 40 mm Hg). The combination of abnormally high $Pa{CO_2}$ and abnormally low $Pa{O_2}$ (i.e., below the normal level of 80–100 mm Hg) in this patient indicates the presence of respiratory failure.

The blood gas data for patient C exemplify hydrochloric acid loss from pyloric outlet obstruction. The high arterial pH (i.e., above the normal value of 7.40), increased arterial $Pa{CO_2}$, and increased bicarbonate level (i.e., above the normal level of 24 mmol/L) indicate the presence of metabolic alkalosis with a compensatory respiratory acidosis.

A patient with hysterical hyperventilation has no obvious pulmonary disease and, therefore, should have no alveolar–arterial $Pa{O_2}$ gradient. This is the case with patient A. The excessive elimination of carbon dioxide by this patient results in pure respiratory alkalosis, which is characterized by below-normal arterial $Pa{CO_2}$ and bicarbonate levels and increased arterial pH.

Patient B does not have lung disease but, rather, shows a primary metabolic acidosis with a compensatory respiratory alkalosis. This condition is defined by a decrease in both arterial pH and arterial bicarbonate concentration and a lower than predicted arterial $Pa{CO_2}$ value (as determined using Winter's formula). This condition is seen in patients with diabetic ketoacidosis.

Patient D shows signs of the emphysematous type of chronic obstructive pulmonary disease (COPD). (The other classic type of COPD)—bronchitic COPD—is dominated by signs and symptoms of chronic bronchitis.) Pulmonary function testing in patients with emphysematous COPD reveals only mild hypoxia and hypocapnia, which are demonstrated in this patient by slight decreases in oxygen saturation and arterial $Pa{CO_2}$. In contrast, patients with bronchitic COPD demonstrate severe hypoxia and hypocapnia on pulmonary function testing.

112–114. The answers are: 112—B [Chapter 7 VII D 3 a (1)], **113—E** [Chapter 7 VII D 3 b (2)], **114—A** [Chapter 7 VII D 3 b (2)]. IgE-mediated hypersensitivity is implicated in local reactions at the site of insulin injections. Such reactions often subside in a few weeks. Improper injection techniques also may be responsible for local reactions to insulin.

High titers of circulating IgG antibodies to insulin may be associated with a rising insulin requirement (i.e., up to 200 U/day). An uncommon cause of insulin resistance, this phenomenon develops most frequently during the first year of therapy in patients with histories of local allergic reactions, intermittent insulin therapy, and administration of impure insulin preparations. Spontaneous remission is observed within 6 months in more than half of affected patients.

Elderly diabetic women are at risk of developing insulin resistance syndrome, a disorder characterized by an increasing insulin requirement, acanthosis nigricans, and lupus-like symptoms. Associated laboratory findings include IgG anti–insulin-receptor antibodies, elevated sedimentation rate, and antinuclear antibodies (ANAs). Spontaneous improvement is rare, and immunosuppressive therapy may be required.

115–119. The answers are: 115—D [Chapter 3 I C 1 a], **116—A** [Chapter 3 II C 2 b (2) (a)], **117—C** [Chapter 3 I C 1 c], **118—B** [Chapter 3 I A 2 a–b], **119—E** [Chapter 3 II C 2 b (1)]. Aplastic anemia patients have deficient stem cells and thus cannot respond to their own endogenously elevated erythropoietin or to exogenously administered erythropoietin.

Polycythemia vera is a neoplastic disease characterized by marrow synthesis of blood cells independent of erythropoietin and, therefore, lowered renal erythropoietin synthesis.

Renal failure patients lose renal erythropoietin synthetic ability along with renal function. Their erythropoiesis is intrinsically normal and responds well to exogenous erythropoietin.

In the anemia of chronic inflammatory disease, adaptive mechanisms result in marrow less responsive to either endogenous or exogenous erythropoietin. This is now known to be a result of the high plasma cytokine levels [e.g., interferon (IFN), tumor necrosis factor (TNF), interleukin-6 (IL-6)] present in inflammatory conditions. The marrow does respond to high doses of erythropoietin, and this maneuver has proved effective in acquired immunodeficiency syndrome (AIDS), rheumatoid arthritis, and Crohn's disease.

Secondary erythrocytosis syndromes associated with specific malignancies develop because of normal marrow responding to very high levels of tumor-synthesized erythropoietin analogs.

120–124. The answers are: 120—A [Table 4–31], **121—A** [Chapter 4 IV D 3 b], **122—B** [Chapter 4 XI D 4], **123—D** [Chapter 4 XVII B 2 a], **124—E** [Chapter 2 IV A 3]. Patients with small-cell lung cancer (SCLC) can present with Eaton-Lambert syndrome. These patients often have muscle weakness that improves with exercise. Skeletal muscles and the muscles of respiration may be affected.

Other neurologic paraneoplastic syndromes are also associated with SCLC. Many patients with SCLC have hyponatremia because of the syndrome of inappropriate antidiuretic hormone (SIADH). This improves with therapy.

Patients with nonseminomatous germ cell tumors and seminoma of the anaplastic variety can have elevations in human chorionic gonadotropin β-hCG). These tumors are associated with gynecomastia, which resolves as the tumor responds to therapy.

Trousseau's syndrome is chronic disseminated intravascular coagulation (DIC) associated with increased incidence of deep venous thrombosis in patients with malignancy. This occurs in patients with adenocarcinomas of the pancreas, stomach, and prostate, and occasionally with other tumor cell types of adenocarcinomatous histology.

Worsening clubbing is a common manifestation of non-SCLC.

125–127. The answers are: 125—A [Chapter 10 III B 1 d (2), e (4), 2 d, e (4) (b)], **126—C** [Chapter 10 II F], **127—D** [Chapter 8 VII F]. Radiographic evidence of sacroiliac and spinal involvement should be sought to confirm this patient's diagnosis. This patient's morning low back pain associated with prolonged stiffness sounds like the inflammatory symptoms associated with spondyloarthropathies. The "sausage toes" and heel pain are probably manifestations of the enthesopathic features of reactive arthritis (Reiter's syndrome), a diagnosis made more likely by the association with conjunctivitis. The onset after an episode of bloody diarrhea suggests that an infectious gastroenteritis triggered the reactive musculoskeletal findings.

This patient has had 6 months of a polyarticular inflammatory arthritis (prolonged morning stiffness and joint swelling suggest an inflammatory process), and the symmetrical involvement of wrists and the metacarpophalangeal (MCP) and proximal interphalangeal (PIP) joints is typical of rheumatoid arthritis. Certainly other diagnoses [e.g., systemic lupus erythematosus (SLE), sarcoidosis, psoriatic arthritis] must be considered, but the chronicity and character of the joint complaints are more typical of rheumatoid arthritis. Seropositivity for rheumatoid factor would help confirm the diagnosis; the erythrocyte sedimentation rate is likely to be elevated but nonspecific.

High levels of immunoglobulin M (IgM) antibody and increasing levels of IgG antibody to one or more *B. burgdorferi* antigens corroborate clinical suspicions of Lyme disease. The combination of a painful radiculitis and an oligoarthritis should support the likelihood of Lyme disease in an endemic area, even if no skin features are present and no tick bite was noted. Onset of these later features after the summer months is another piece of helpful evidence, because most cases start with a tick bite in the spring or summer.

128–132. The answers are: 128—D, 129—A, 130—A, 131—B, 132—C [Chapter 3 III A 2 b (1), B 3 a (3)]. Chronic lymphocytic leukemia (CLL) is a steadily progressive disease characterized by an accumulation of mature lymphocytes in the tissues and peripheral blood. Clinical manifestations of CLL vary with the extent of disease progression, which is broken down into stages (0 through 4). Examples include splenomegaly (a stage 2 CLL presentation) and anemia (a stage 3 CLL presentation). In time, CLL causes marrow failure and death.

Chronic myelogenous leukemia (CML) is characterized by excessive granulocytes and granulocyte precursors in the blood and tissues. These cells lack the normal leukocyte alkaline phosphatase (LAP) level. Splenomegaly is a common finding with CML. This disease, which often terminates in acute leukemia, is characterized by an accelerated progression.

133–138. The answers are: 133—E [Chapter 4 XVI B 2 a], **134—B** [Chapter 4 X B 2 a], **135—A** [Chapter 5 II B 1 b (1)], **136—D** [Chapter 4 VI A 2 d], **137—C** [Chapter 4 IV B 2], **138—E** [Chapter 4 XII B 6]. Studies have shown clustering of cases of non-Hodgkin's lymphomas, which suggests that infectious agents may play a causative role. In particular, Epstein-Barr virus has been implicated in the development of Burkitt's lymphoma, a disease commonly found in Africa.

Bladder carcinoma has been linked to tobacco as well as to certain chemical and biologic carcinogens. For example, there is a well-documented association between occupational exposure to dye and printing chemicals and the development of bladder tumors.

Several relationships have been noted in the etiology of gastric carcinoma. Up to 10% of patients with achlorhydria, atrophic gastritis, and pernicious anemia develop gastric cancer. An increased concentration of nitrosamine compounds in gastric juice has been suggested as an underlying factor in these relationships.

Colorectal carcinoma is a common malignancy in the United States, for which several precancerous lesions are known. Chronic ulcerative colitis of long duration has a documented and statistically significant association with the incidence of colorectal cancer.

In the United States, lung cancer is the primary cause of cancer-related deaths in men and is second only to breast cancer as the leading cause of cancer deaths in women. Cigarette smoking largely is implicated as a cause of lung cancer, but other etiologic factors such as exposure to industrial carcinogens have been noted. One of these factors, asbestos, classically has been linked to the more rare mesothelioma; however, asbestos exposure also has a clear and strong association with lung cancer.

Head and neck tumors are highly unusual in the Mormon population, which abstains from both alcohol and tobacco. This fact exemplifies the statistically based claims that the use of tobacco and alcohol is associated with an increased risk of head and neck cancers. Another noted risk factor is the Epstein-Barr virus, which has been linked to the unusual nasopharyngeal carcinoma that is unique to Asians.

139–141. The answers are: 139—D [Chapter 7 VII B 3 b, D 5], **140—C** [Chapter 7 VII E 4], **141—F** [Chapter 7 VII E 5]. Bronchospasm typically begins within 30 minutes after ingestion of aspirin and may be prolonged and severe. Individuals with preceding recurrent sinusitis may also have underlying chronic rhinitis and perhaps undiagnosed nasal polyposis. Aspirin-induced anaphylaxis does not occur in patients with underlying sinusitis or polyposis. The combination of asthma, nasal polyposis, and sinusitis is known as the aspirin triad.

Chronic cough has been reported in 5%—20% of patients taking angiotensin-converting enzyme (ACE) inhibitors. Symptoms may begin as early as 1 week or as late as 6 months after drug use. The cough is usually nonproductive and nocturnal. Angioedema also develops in 0.1%–0.2% of patients, and in certain clinical situations, ACE inhibitors are also known to exacerbate anaphylaxis.

A maculopapular eruption is seen in approximately 3% of all sulfonamide recipients and in more than 50% of those with human immunodeficiency virus (HIV) infection. The combination of trimethoprim-sulfamethoxazole is used for prophylaxis and treatment of *Pneumocystis carinii* infection in immunocompromised individuals. No in vitro or in vivo tests that reliably predict sensitivity are available, so an oral dose challenge and desensitization protocol is sometimes used in patients thought to be particularly vulnerable.

142. The answer is B [Chapter 12 VIII D, E]. All forms of psoriasis may flare after a streptococcal pharyngitis, but guttate psoriasis is the most frequently occurring type. Often, the first presentation of psoriasis in a young adult occurs in conjunction with streptococcal pharyngitis. Flares of psoriasis after streptococcal pharyngitis suggest involvement of superantigen activation of pathogenic T lymphocytes or molecular mimicry of cutaneous antigens in pathogenesis.

143. The answer is E [Chapter 12 VII C, Tables 12–13]. The clinical findings suggest that the patient has allergic contact dermatitis caused by her ring. Nickel sulfate, a component in gold jewelry, often causes allergic contact dermatitis in sensitized individuals. Cobalt dichloride is a common component in cement and often causes occupational dermatitis in cement workers. Balsam of Peru is a frequent additive in fragrances and flavorings. *Para*-phenylenediamine is a component of hair dyes. Mercaptobenzothiazole is a component of rubber products and adhesives.

144. The answer is A (Chapter 12 V C). Tense, subepidermal bullae with linear deposition of IgG and C3 along the dermal–epidermal junction defines bullous pemphigoid. Pemphigus vulgaris is characterized by flaccid blisters with intercellular IgG staining in the epidermis. Paraneoplastic pemphigus is characterized by severe oral involvement and heterogeneous skin lesions with histologic and direct immunofluorescent features of both pemphigus and pemphigoid. Erythema multiforme usually is characterized by target-like lesions on the palms and soles and distinct histopathology. Porphyria cutanea tarda is characterized by photosensitivity and tense bullae in a photo distribution and elevated urinary porphyrins.

145. The answer is C [Chapter 12 VII B]. Eczematous skin changes distributed over flexor areas are typical of atopic dermatitis, particularly with the history of flaring associated with allergic rhinitis (hayfever). Psoriasis tends to occur over extensor surfaces and flares during the winter months. Urticaria is characterized by evanescent itchy and inflammatory plaques. Pityriasis rosea is characterized by distinctive

"Christmas tree" distribution over the trunk. Lichen planus typically is characterized by flat-topped, violaceous, itchy plaques involving the wrists.

146. The answer is A [Chapter 12 V A, XIII G]. Clinical and histologic findings are consistent with porphyria cutanea tarda. The diagnosis is confirmed with the detection of elevated 24-hour urine levels of uroporphyrin and coproporphyrin. No immunoreactants are detected on direct immunofluorescence of skin biopsies. This finding is in contrast to autoimmune blistering diseases such as pemphigus vulgaris, pemphigus foliaceus, bullous pemphigoid, and paraneoplastic pemphigus.

147. The answer is E [Chapter 12 X C 2, 7, 8]. Melanomas located on the extremities have a better prognosis than melanomas located on the trunk. Other favorable prognostic factors that decrease the risk for the development of metastatic melanoma include primary tumor invasion depth < 1 mm, absence of ulceration, absence of vascular invasion, and female sex.

148. The answer is B [Chapter 12 VI E]. The clinical findings are consistent with erythema nodosum, which may be a reaction caused by hyperestrogen states, including oral contraceptive pills, estrogen replacement therapy, and pregnancy. Erythema multiforme is associated with target lesions on the hands and feet. Lichen planus is associated with a papulosquamous eruption. Pyoderma gangrenosum is associated with inflammatory and painful skin ulcers, typically on the lower extremities. Urticaria is associated with itchy evanescent plaques.

Index

Page numbers followed by an "f" denote figures; those followed by a "t" denote tables.